Aoife M

085 8149784

OXFORD HANDBOOK OF CLINICAL MEDICINE

Adequate urinary output = 0.5 mls/kg/hr

lady ~ 30mls
men ~ 40mls

Common haematology values *If outside this range, consult:*

Haemoglobin	men:	13–18g/dL	p318
	women:	11.5–16g/dL	p318
Mean cell volume, MCV		76–96fL	↓p320; ↑p326
Platelets		150–400 × 10^9/L	p358
White cells (total)		4–11 × 10^9/L	p324
neutrophils		40–75%	p324
lymphocytes		20–45%	p324
eosinophils		1–6%	p324

Blood gases

pH	7.35–7.45	p684
P_aO_2	>10.6kPa (75–100mmHg)	p684
P_aCO_2	4.7–6kPa (35–45mmHg)	p684
Base excess	±2mmol/L	p684

U&Es (urea and electrolytes) *If outside this range, consult:*

Sodium	135–145mmol/L	p686
Potassium	3.5–5mmol/L	p688
Creatinine	70–150μmol/L	p298–301
Urea	2.5–6.7mmol/L	p298–301
eGFR	>90	p683

LFTs (liver function tests)

Bilirubin	3–17μmol/L	p250, p258
Alanine aminotransferase, ALT	5–35iu/L	p250, p258
Aspartate transaminase, AST	5–35iu/L	p250, p258
Alkaline phosphatase, ALP	30–150iu/L (*non-pregnant adults*)	p250, p258
Albumin	35–50g/L	p700
Protein (total)	60–80g/L	p700

Cardiac enzymes

Troponin T	<0.1μg/L	p113
Creatine kinase	25–195iu/L	p113
Lactate dehydrogenase, LDH	70–250iu/L	p113

Lipids and other biochemical values

Cholesterol	<5mmol/L *desired*	p704
Triglycerides	0.5–1.9mmol/L	p704
Amylase	0–180 *Somorgyi* u/dL	p638
C-reactive protein, CRP	<10mg/L	p700
Calcium (total)	2.12–2.65mmol/L	p690
Glucose, fasting	3.5–5.5mmol/L	p198
Prostate specific antigen, PSA	0–4ng/mL	p538
T_4 (total thyroxine)	70–140mmol/L	p208
TSH	0.5–5.7mU/L	p208

For all other reference intervals, see p769–71

He moved N. 48

all the brightest gems N. 24

faster and faster towards the N.18

ever-growing bucket of lost hopes; N. 14
had there been just one more year

of peace the battalion would have made N. 12
a floating system of perpetual drainage.

A silent fall of immense snow came near oily N. 10
remains of the recently eaten supper on the table.

We drove on in our old sunless walnut. Presently N. 8
classical eggs ticked in the new afternoon shadows.

We were instructed by my cousin Jasper not to exercise by country N. 6
house visiting unless accompanied by thirteen geese or gangsters.

The modern American did not prevail over the pair of redundant bronze puppies. N. 5
The worn-out principle is a bad omen which I am never glad to ransom in August.

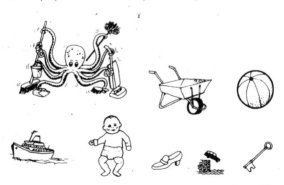

Reading tests. Hold this chart (well-illuminated) 30cm away, and record the smallest type read (eg N12 left eye, N6 right eye, spectacles worn) or object named accurately.

OXFORD HANDBOOK OF CLINICAL MEDICINE

EIGHTH EDITION

MURRAY LONGMORE
IAN B. WILKINSON
EDWARD H. DAVIDSON
ALEXANDER FOULKES
AHMAD R. MAFI

OXFORD
UNIVERSITY PRESS Great Clarendon Street, Oxford OX2 6DP

Oxford University Press is a department of the University of Oxford. It furthers the University's objective of excellence in research, scholarship, and education by publishing worldwide in: Oxford New York
Auckland Cape Town Dar es Salaam Hong Kong Karachi Kuala Lumpur Madrid Melbourne Mexico City Nairobi New Delhi Shanghai Taipei Toronto. *With offices in:* Argentina Austria Brazil Chile Czech Republic France Greece Guatemala Hungary Italy Japan Poland Portugal Singapore South Korea Switzerland Thailand Turkey Ukraine Vietnam

Oxford is a registered trade mark of Oxford University Press in the UK and in certain other countries

Published in the United States by Oxford University Press Inc., New York

First published 1985 (RA Hope & JM Longmore)
Second edition 1989
Third edition 1993
Fourth edition 1998
Fifth edition 2001 (JM Longmore & IB Wilkinson)
Sixth edition 2004
Seventh edition 2007
Eighth edition 2010

Translations:
Chinese
Czech
Estonian
French
German
Greek
Hungarian
Indonesian
Italian
Polish
Portuguese
Romanian
Russian
Spanish

British Library Cataloguing in Publication Data
Data available

Library of Congress Cataloging in Publication Data
Data available

Typeset by JML and MK (OUP); Printed in Italy by Rotolito Lombarda SpA.

ISBN 978-0-19-923217-8

Drugs

Except where otherwise stated, recommendations are for the **non-pregnant adult** who is **not breastfeeding** and who has reasonable **renal and hepatic function**. To avoid excessive doses in obese patients it may be best to calculate doses on the basis of ideal body weight (IBW): see p 621.

We have made every effort to check this text, but it is still possible that drug or other errors have been missed. OUP makes no representation, express or implied, that doses are correct. Readers are urged to check with the most up to date product information, codes of conduct, and safety regulations. The authors and the publishers do not accept responsibility or legal liability for any errors in the text, or for the misuse or misapplication of material in this work.

For updates/corrections, see www.oup.com/uk/ohcm8

Contents

We wrote this book not because we know so much, but because we know we remember so little...the problem is not simply the quantity of information, but the diversity of places from which it is dispensed. Trailing eagerly behind the surgeon, the student is admonished never to forget alcohol withdrawal as a cause of post-operative confusion. The scrap of paper on which this is written spends a month in the pocket before being lost for ever in the laundry. At different times, and in inconvenient places, a number of other causes may be presented to the student. Not only are these causes and aphorisms never brought together, but when, as a surgical house officer, the former student faces a confused patient, none is to hand.

We aim to encourage the doctor to enjoy his patients: in doing so we believe he will prosper in the practice of medicine. For a long time now, house officers have been encouraged to adopt monstrous proportions in order to straddle simultaneously the diverse pinnacles of clinical science and clinical experience. We hope that this book will make this endeavour a little easier by moving a cumulative memory burden from the mind into the pocket, and by removing some of the fears that are naturally felt when starting a career in medicine, thereby freely allowing the doctor's clinical acumen to grow by the slow accretion of many, many days and nights. From the preface to the 1st edition; RAH & JML 1985

Preface to the eighth edition

The world exists to end up in a book. So thought the French poet Mallarmé. This is not that book, but since it codifies more than half the sufferings of the world, it may partly assuage even that most hungry heart. Mallarmé banished all that was contingent and ephemeral from his work. Here we take a different approach, delighting in a thousand-and-one details of signs, symptoms, and doses. And where we have come across possibly universal truths, we have not shouted them from our roof-tops, but have hidden them like Easter eggs, between brackets and under footnotes, waiting for passing readers to fertilize them with their own thoughts. So will there be chicks inside these eggs? We hope so. Sometimes we see copies of this book strewn about lost wards, flaccid and as forlorn as an empty eggshell—all broken spines and torn type. Then we are happy to know that the chick has hatched. As we note elsewhere (p711), in order to be born we must first destroy our world. We hope you find pecking your way through these pages a liberating affair.

Our consultations are all theatrical stages, and the men and women whose exits and entrances we examine so closely are observing us more keenly than we ever know. They fly their symptoms as kites and spinnakers into the slipstreams of our wavering attention, for us to ignore or obsess about. As scientists, we rip these symptoms from their historical and social contexts and present them to each other as pure and simplified data to be held aloft, admired, and diagnosed. The invisible strings which attach these volatile symptoms to the real world seem irrelevant until one day we find that even though we have explained every symptom and cured every disease our patient's problem will not go away, and he remains stubbornly unimproved. If, for once, we ask "What must this person be feeling to have come up with this description of their condition?" we can reattach the string to the kite, and perhaps guide it safely home. "What does it feel like to have this symptom?" "Where are you in your understanding of the significance of this phenomenon?" Just the fact of our trying to address problems in different ways may be enough.

In most of what follows we fall into this trap of severing the kite from the earthly lives of our patients. But some readers will feel the cracks in our descriptions of diseases, through which their sighs and pangs are perpetually echoing. If we could listen more, we might come to *embody* our medical roles rather than play out caricatures of ourselves before an increasingly bemused audience. Let's at least try!

It is a great pleasure to have worked with Ahmad Mafi, Alexander Foulkes, and Edward Davidson to write this edition, which sees a full revision of the text, plus a complete rearrangement of ***signs and symptoms*** and the ***history and examination*** into a single chapter. We have every confidence that existing readers will appreciate their clarity and humanity, and that new readers will take for granted that learning medicine should be both logical and entertaining. **IBW & JML 2010**

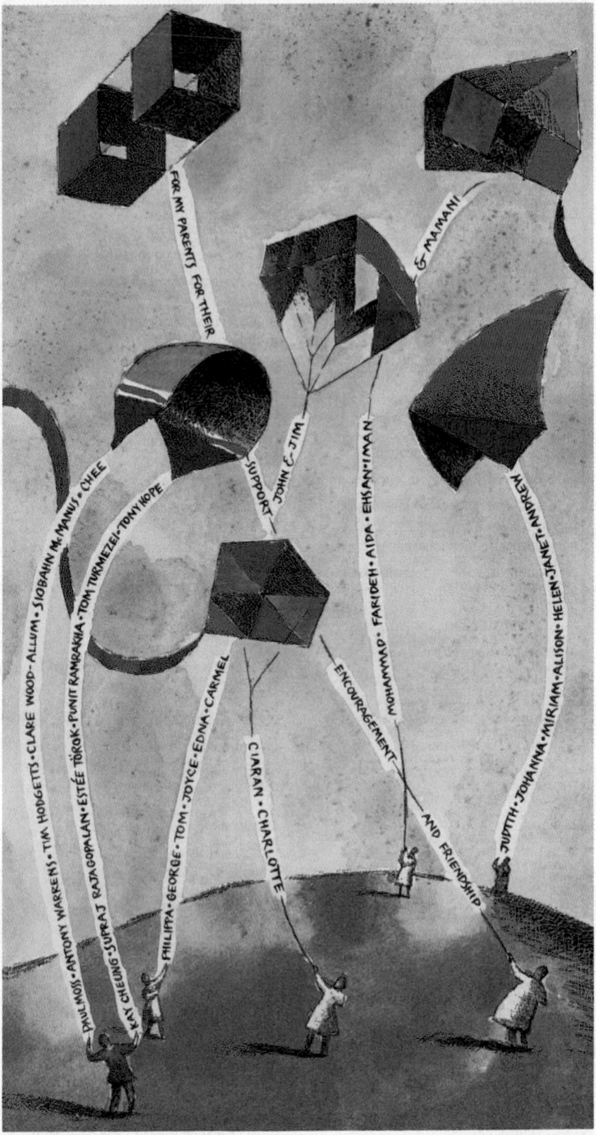
FOR MY PARENTS FOR THEIR
SUPPORT
ENCOURAGEMENT
AND FRIENDSHIP
G-MAMANI
JOHN & JIM
MOHAMMAD • FARIDEH • AIDA • EHSAN • IMAN
JUDITH • JOHANNA • MIRIAM • ALISON • HELEN • JANET • ANDREW
CIARAN • CHARLOTTE
PHILIPPA • GEORGE • TOM • JOYCE • EDNA • CARMEL
KAY CHEUNG • SUPRAJ RAJAGOPALAN • ESTÉE TÖRÖK • PUNIT RAMRAKHA • TOM TURMEZEI • TONY KOPE
PAUL MOSS • ANTONY WARRENS • TIM HODGETTS • CLARE WOOD-ALLUM • SIOBAHN McMANUS • CHEE

Symbols and abbreviations

- **►** this fact or idea is important.
- **►►** don't dawdle!—prompt action saves lives
- **💣** incendiary (controversial) topic
- **[ ]** non-BNF drug dose
- **🖫/★** reference available on our website www.oup.com/uk/ohcm8refs
- **♂:♀** male-to-female ratio. ♂:♀=2:1 means twice as common in males
- **@12** search Medline (pubmed.gov) with '12...' to get an abstract (omit '@')
- **∵** on account of
- **∴** therefore
- **~** approximately
- **-ve** negative (+ve is positive)
- **↑ ↓** increased or decreased (eg serum level)
- **↔** normal (eg serum level)
- **Δ** diagnosis
- **ΔΔ** differential diagnosis (list of possibilities)
- **A2** aortic component of the 2nd heart sound
- **A2A** angiotensin-2 receptor antagonist (p309; = AT-2, A2R, and AIIR)
- **Ab** antibody
- **ABC** airway, breathing, and circulation: basic life support (see inside back cover)
- **ABG** arterial blood gas: P_aO_2, P_aCO_2, pH, HCO_3
- **ABPA** allergic bronchopulmonary aspergillosis
- **ac** ante cibum (before food)
- **ACE(i)** angiotensin-converting enzyme inhibitor
- **ACTH** adrenocorticotrophic hormone
- **ADH** antidiuretic hormone
- **ad lib** as much/as often as wanted (ad libitum is Latin for at pleasure)
- **AF** atrial fibrillation
- **AFB** acid-fast bacillus
- **AFP** (or α-FP) alpha-fetoprotein
- **Ag** antigen
- **AIDS** acquired immunodeficiency syndrome
- **Alk phos** alkaline phosphatase (also ALP)
- **ALL** acute lymphoblastic leukaemia
- **AMA** antimitochondrial antibody
- **AMP** adenosine monophosphate
- **ANA** antinuclear antibody
- **ANCA** antineutrophil cytoplasmic antibody
- **APTT** activated partial thromboplastin time
- **AR** aortic regurgitation
- **ARA(B)** angiotensin receptor antagonist (p309; also AT-2, A2R, and AIIR)
- **ARDS** acute respiratory distress syndrome
- **ARF** acute renal failure
- **AS** aortic stenosis
- **ASD** atrial septal defect
- **ASO** antistreptolysin O (titre)
- **AST** aspartate transaminase
- **AT-2** angiotensin-2 receptor blocker (p309; also AT-2, A2R, and AIIR)
- **ATN** acute tubular necrosis
- **ATP** adenosine triphosphate
- **AV** atrioventricular
- **AVM** arteriovenous malformation(s)
- **AXR** abdominal X-ray (plain)
- **Ba** barium
- **BAL** bronchoalveolar lavage
- **bd** bis die (twice a day)
- **BKA** below-knee amputation
- **BMA** British Medical Association
- **BMJ** *British Medical Journal*
- **BNF** *British National Formulary*
- **BP** blood pressure
- **BPH** benign prostatic hyperplasia
- **bpm** beats per minute (eg pulse)
- **ca** cancer
- **CABG** coronary artery bypass graft
- **CAD** coronary heart disease
- **cAMP** cyclic adenosine monophosphate (AMP)
- **CAPD** continuous ambulatory peritoneal dialysis
- **CBD** common bile duct
- **CC** creatinine clearance (also CrCl)
- **CCF** congestive cardiac failure (ie left and right heart failure)
- **CCU** coronary care unit
- **CHB** complete heart block
- **CHD** coronary heart disease (related to ischaemia and atheroma)
- **CI** contraindications
- **CK** creatine (phospho)kinase (also CPK)
- **CLL** chronic lymphocytic leukaemia
- **CML** chronic myeloid leukaemia
- **CMV** cytomegalovirus
- **CNS** central nervous system
- **COC** combined oral contraceptive pill
- **COPD** chronic obstructive pulmonary disease
- **CPAP** continuous positive airways pressure
- **CPR** cardiopulmonary resuscitation
- **CRF** chronic renal failure
- **CRP** c-reactive protein
- **CSF** cerebrospinal fluid
- **CT** computer tomography
- **CVP** central venous pressure
- **CVS** cardiovascular system
- **CXR** chest x-ray
- **d** day(s); also expressed as /7; months are /12
- **DC** direct current
- **DIC** disseminated intravascular coagulation
- **DIP** distal interphalangeal
- **dL** decilitre
- **DoH** (or DH) Department of Health (UK)
- **DM** diabetes mellitus
- **DU** duodenal ulcer
- **D&V** diarrhoea and vomiting
- **DVT** deep venous thrombosis
- **DXT** deep radiotherapy
- **EBM** evidence-based medicine and its journal published by the BMA
- **EBV** Epstein-Barr virus
- **ECG** electrocardiogram
- **Echo** echocardiogram
- **EDTA** ethylene diamine tetraacetic acid (anti-coagulant coating eg in FBC bottles)
- **EEG** electroencephalogram
- **eGFR** estimated glomerular filtration rate (GFR; mL/min/1.73m^2—see p683
- **ELISA** enzyme-linked immunosorbent assay
- **EM** electron microscope
- **EMG** electromyogram
- **ENT** ear, nose, and throat
- **ERCP** endoscopic retrograde cholangiopancreatography; see also MRCP
- **ESR** erythrocyte sedimentation rate
- **ESRF** end-stage renal failure
- **EUA** examination under anaesthesia
- **FB** foreign body
- **FBC** full blood count
- **FDP** fibrin degradation products
- **FEV_1** forced expiratory volume in 1st sec
- **F_iO_2** partial pressure of O_2 in inspired air
- **FFP** fresh frozen plasma
- **FSH** follicle-stimulating hormone
- **FVC** forced vital capacity
- **g** gram
- **GA** general anaesthetic
- **GAT** *Sanford Guide to Antimicrobial Therapy*
- **GB** gall bladder
- **GC** gonococcus
- **GCS** Glasgow coma scale
- **GFR** glomerular filtration rate eGFR, p683
- **GGT** gamma glutamyl transpeptidase
- **GH** growth hormone
- **GI** gastrointestinal
- **GP** general practitioner
- **G6PD** glucose-6-phosphate dehydrogenase
- **GTN** glyceryl trinitrate
- **GTT** glucose tolerance test (OGTT: oral GTT)
- **GU(M)** genitourinary (medicine)
- **h** hour
- **HAV** hepatitis A virus
- **Hb** haemoglobin
- **HBsAg** hepatitis B surface antigen
- **HBV** hepatitis B virus
- **HCC** hepatocellular cancer
- **Hct** haematocrit
- **HCV** hepatitis C virus
- **HDV** hepatitis D virus
- **HDL** high-density lipoprotein, p704
- **HHT** hereditary haemorrhagic telangiectasia
- **HIDA** hepatic immunodiacetic acid
- **HIV** human immunodeficiency virus
- **HCM** hypertrophic obstructive cardiomyopathy
- **HONK** hyperosmolar nonketotic (diabetic coma)
- **HRT** hormone replacement therapy
- **HSV** herpes simplex virus
- **IBD** inflammatory bowel disease
- **IBW** ideal body weight, p446
- **ICD** implantable cardiac defibrillator
- **ICP** intracranial pressure
- **IDA** iron-deficiency anaemia
- **IDDM** insulin-dependent diabetes mellitus
- **IFN-α** alpha interferon
- **IE** infective endocarditis
- **Ig** immunoglobulin
- **IHD** ischaemic heart disease
- **IM** intramuscular
- **INR** international normalized ratio (prothrombin)

IP	interphalangeal
IPPV	intermittent positive pressure ventilation
ITP	idiopathic thrombocytopenic purpura
ITU	intensive therapy unit
iU/U	international unit
IVC	inferior vena cava
IV(I)	intravenous (infusion)
IVU	intravenous urography
JAMA	*Journal of the American Medical Assoc^n*
JVP	jugular venous pressure
K	potassium
KCCT	kaolin cephalin clotting time
kg	kilogram
KPa	kiloPascal
L	litre
LAD	left axis deviation on the ECG; also left anterior descending coronary artery
LBBB	left bundle branch block
LDH	lactate dehydrogenase
LDL	low-density lipoprotein, p704
LBW	lean body weight, p434
LFT	liver function tests
LH	luteinizing hormone
LIF	left iliac fossa
LKKS	liver, kidney (R), kidney (L), spleen
LMN	lower motor neuron
LOC	loss of consciousness
LP	lumbar puncture
LUQ	left upper quadrant
LV	left ventricle of the heart
LVF	left ventricular failure
LVH	left ventricular hypertrophy
μg	microgram
MAI	*Mycobacterium avium intracellulare*
MAOI	monoamine oxidase inhibitors
mane	morning (from Latin; the 'e' may be written 'é', but purists frown on this)
MC&S	microscopy, culture and sensitivity
MCP	metacarpo-phalangeal
MCV	mean cell volume
MDMA	3,4-methylenedioxymethamphetamine
ME	myalgic encephalomyelitis
MET	meta-analysis
mg	milligram
MI	myocardial infarction
min(s)	minute(s)
mL	millilitre
mmHg	millimetres of mercury
MND	motor neuron disease
MRCP	magnetic imaging cholangiopancreatography/member of Royal College of Physicians
MRI	magnetic resonance imaging
MRSA	methicillin-resistant *Staph aureus*
MS	multiple sclerosis (mitral stenosis)
MSU	midstream urine
NAD	nothing abnormal detected
NBM	nil by mouth
ND	notifiable disease
NEJM	*New England Journal of Medicine*
ng	nanogram
NG(T)	nasogastric (tube)
NHS	National Health Service (UK)
NICE	National Institute for Health and Clinical Excellence www.nice.org.uk
NIDDM	non-insulin-dependent diabetes mellitus
NMDA	N-methyl-D-aspartate
NNT	number needed to treat, for 1 extra satisfactory result (p671)
Nocte	at night
NR	normal range (=reference interval)
NSAID	non-steroidal anti-inflammatory drugs
N&V	nausea and/or vomiting
od	omni die (once daily)
OD	overdose
OGD	oesophagogastroduodenoscopy
OGS	oxogenic steroids
OGTT	oral glucose tolerance test
OHCS	*Oxford Handbook of Clinical Specialties 8*
om	omni mane (in the morning)
on	omni nocte (at night)
OPD	out-patients department
ORh−	blood group O, Rh negative
OT	occupational therapist
OTM	*Oxford Textbook of Medicine 5e* (OUP)
OTS	*Oxford Textbook of Surgery* (OUP)
P2	pulmonary component of 2nd heart sound
P_aCO_2	partial pressure of CO_2 in arterial blood
PAN	polyarteritis nodosa
P_aO_2	partial pressure of O_2 in arterial blood
PBC	primary biliary cirrhosis
PCP	*Pneumocystis carinii* (*jiroveci*) pneumonia
PCR	polymerase chain reaction (DNA diagnosis)
PCV	packed cell volume
PE	pulmonary embolism
PEEP	positive end-expiratory pressure
PEF(R)	peak expiratory flow (rate)
PERLA	pupils equal and reactive to light and accommodation
PET	positron emission tomography
PID	pelvic inflammatory disease
PIP	proximal interphalangeal (joint)
PMH	past medical history
PND	paroxysmal nocturnal dyspnoea
PO	per os (by mouth)
PPF	purified plasma fraction (albumin)
PPI	proton pump inhibitor, eg omeprazole^{etc}
PR	per rectum (by the rectum)
PRL	prolactin
PRN	pro re nata (Latin for as required)
PRV	polycythaemia rubra vera
PSA	prostate specific antigen
PTH	parathyroid hormone
PTT	prothrombin time
PUO	pyrexia of unknown origin
PV	per vaginam (by the vagina, eg pessary)
PVD	peripheral vascular disease
qds	quater die sumendus; take 4 times daily
qqh	quarta quaque hora: take every 4h
R	right
RA	rheumatoid arthritis
RAD	right axis deviation on the ECG
RBBB	right bundle branch block
RBC	red blood cell
RCT	randomized control trial
RFT	respiratory function tests
Rh	Rh; a contraction, not an abbreviation: derived from the rhesus monkey
RIF	right iliac fossa
RUQ	right upper quadrant
RV	right ventricle of heart
RVF	right ventricular failure
RVH	right ventricular hypertrophy
℞	recipe (treat with)
s/sec	second(s)
S1, S2	first and second heart sounds
SBE	subacute bacterial endocarditis (IE is any infective endocarditis)
SC	subcutaneous
SD	standard deviation
SE	side-effect(s)
SL	sublingual
SLE	systemic lupus erythematosus
SOB	short of breath
SOBE	short of breath on exercise
SPC	summary of product characteristics www.medicines.org.uk
SpO_2	peripheral oxygen saturation (%)
SR	slow-release (also MR, modified-release)
Stat	statim (immediately; as initial dose)
STD/I	sexually transmitted disease/infection
SVC	superior vena cava
SVT	supraventricular tachycardia
Sy(n)	syndrome
T°	temperature
T½	biological half-life
T3; T4	triiodothyronine; T4 is thyroxine
TB	tuberculosis
tds	ter die sumendus (take 3 times a day)
TFTs	thyroid function tests (eg TSH)
TIA	transient ischaemic attack
TIBC	total iron-binding capacity
tid	ter in die (Latin for 3 times a day)
TPR	temperature, pulse & respirations count
TRH	thyroid-releasing hormone
TSH	thyroid-stimulating hormone
U	units
UC	ulcerative colitis
U&E	urea and electrolytes and creatinine—in plasma, unless stated otherwise
UMN	upper motor neuron
URT(I)	upper respiratory tract (infection)
US(S)	ultrasound (scan)
UTI	urinary tract infection
VDRL	Venereal Diseases Research Laboratory
VE	ventricular extrasystole
VF	ventricular fibrillation
VMA	vanillyl mandelic acid (HMMA)
V/Q	ventilation/perfusion ratio
VSD	ventriculo-septal defect
VT	ventricular tachycardia
WBC	white blood cell
WCC	white blood cell count
wk(s)	week(s)
WR	Wassermann reaction (syphilis serology)
yr(s)	year(s)
ZN	Ziehl-Neelsen stain eg for mycobacteria

How to use this book

Through slow evolution, this book has accrued many features over the years that may help the reader. We hope that you will find some or all of the following useful.

Emergency, quick-ref lookup	Pages immediately inside covers.
Quick chapter lookups	Index on the back cover refers to and aligns with the coloured tabs on sides of the pages.
Disc symbol references	Reference materials used in writing the book. Details at **www.oup.com/uk/ohcm8refs**.
Star symbol references (☨)	Key reference materials. Also found on the web, but additionally reproduced at the end of the book.
Right-hand, vertical comments	At the side of some tables & topics: a cynic's interpolation
OHCS p321 etc.	Pages in the *Oxford Handbook of Clinical Specialties, 8th edition*: the essential companion volume to this book.
Comments, suggestions	*We thrive on your feedback*: please post comments to OUP or leave them at **www.oup.com/uk/ohcm8feedback** All are considered and many give rise to improvements.

Acknowledgements

Heartfelt thanks to our advisers on specific sections—each is acknowledged on the chapter's first page. For detailed work on the text we especially thank Dr Judith Collier, Mark Knowles, Jamie Hartmann-Boyce, and Dr Steve Emmett. We especially thank Rev. Gary Bevans for his kind permission to use the images on p225 and p566, from his beautiful Sistine Chapel sequences reproduced on the ceiling of the Church of the English Martyrs, Goring-by-Sea. IBW would like to acknowledge his clinical mentors Jim Holt and John Cockcroft. We thank the Department of Radiology at the Norfolk and Norwich University Hospital for their kind help in providing many images—as well as Professor P Scally and Dr J Harper both for images and for many thoughtful comments on the whole text. For further help we thank Dr F Rugg-Gunn, Dr D Werring, Dr J Burke, Dr Omid Zarghom, and Professor J McCormack.

Readers' comments These have formed a vital part of our endeavour to provide an accurate, comprehensive, and up-to-date text. We sincerely thank the many students, doctors and other health professionals who have found the time and the generosity to write to us on our Reader's Comments Cards, in editions past, or, in more recent times, via the web. These have now become so numerous for past editions that they cannot all be listed here. Here we would particularly like to thank Ali Almajed, Mark Lowenthal, Neil Long, and Dr Selby.

3rd-party web addresses We disclaim any responsibility for 3rd-party content.

Cosmological background to the 8th edition

In the beginning there was the Bed (*clinos*, in Greek): under the Bed there was Chaos comprising the Students and House Staff. At the head of the Bed was the Consultant, and at the foot was the Nurse. On the Bed lay the Patient, obediently lapping up the words of wisdom uttered by the Consultant and repeated by the Nurse—a theme with variations interspersed with laughter from the chorus under the Bed. Watching over this idyllic scene was the General Practitioner—the Infinity whence the Patient came, and to whom he will depart once the Operation has been completed.

This general cosmology held sway until one day in 1995 when the Patient got up off the Bed seemingly of his own Volition. And nothing was ever the same again. Because the Patient turned out, surprisingly, to be taller than everyone else, he was declared by the Paymaster to be the Infallible Judge of what constitutes Health. Ever since That Day, patients have been roaming the wards, seeping into libraries, going online, and congregating with the chorus under the Bed—and taking responsibility for their own Choices. And so the Era of Patient Centred Care came into being. And nobody knows what to make of it—but every so often when the laughter from under the Bed dies down, a little voice pipes up from where the Patient once lay, saying "Help me!" But nobody seems to be listening.

Prologue to clinical medicine: *Dag Hammarskjöld on teamwork*

Good doctors are good team players, because health care is complex, and nobody knows everything or how to relate to every patient and his or her unique needs. Because we are all fallible, we all see many examples of poor teams, where bad communication, power struggles, and personality clashes lead to poor outcomes. Stress, overwork, and resource restrictions contribute to this, but not inevitably. So it is worthwhile, at the outset of this journey through medicine, to commit oneself to being a good team member. 3 rules help: (1) All members are valuable; none is irreplaceable, and members are valued for who they are, not just for the resources they bring. (2) 'Innocence is no excuse'—ie you may not be 'to blame' for a group's malfunction but in the end each member is responsible for everything. (3) Every member needs encouragement. Just how important this is, is shown by this comment from a well-known statesman: "He was impossible. It wasn't that he didn't attend to his work. But his manner brought him into conflict with everybody ... When the crisis came, and the whole truth had to come out, he laid the blame on us: in his conduct there was nothing, absolutely nothing to reproach. His self-esteem was so strongly bound up, apparently, with the idea of his innocence, that one felt a brute as one demonstrated, step by step, the contradictions in his defence, and, bit by bit, stripped him naked before his own eyes. But justice to others demanded it. When the last rag of a lie had been taken from him, and we thought there was nothing more to be said, out it came with stifled sobs.

'But why did you never help me? You knew that I always felt you were against me. And fear and insecurity drove me further and further along the course for which you now condemn me. It's been so hard—everything. One day, I remember, I was so happy: one of you said that something I had produced was quite good—'

So, in the end, we were, in fact, to blame. We had not voiced our criticisms, but we had allowed them to stop us from giving him a single word of acknowledgement, and in this way had barred every road to improvement. It is always the stronger one who is to blame."

Markings; p47; Dag Hammarskjöld
Translated by WH Auden; Faber

Beyond the team

The team has moved on to more important tasks, leaving you detained in the crossfire from squinting eyes belonging to a patient with a stroke. No more to do. Unmendable, even by the best mender in the world. Move on? Health shattered—but what can I do? ***Health is soundness of body and mind.*** This definition works because it does not specify what the sound is, only that health cannot be considered in a vacuum (which implies no soundness at all). Your own health may be being eaten up by ceaseless demands delegated to you by the team. But here's a job that cannot be delegated or described or audited: making a relationship.

Let us accept that our happiness is encompassed by the quality of our relationships and move on from this to the idea that our health is defined by the health of our relationships, starting with our relationship with ourselves. We have all met children who have awful diseases but who don't yet know how to be ill. Their instinctive grasp of their own health is as yet uncracked, in their own bright eyes, as they have not yet been taught to be ill. We have met patients who are healthier after a stroke because a negative part of their personality has been ironed out by their lesion, and are leading richer lives despite being disabled. We have met diabetic patients who are healthier after getting their illness because they now teach fellow diabetics how to manage their illness and are forging satisfying networks of health-augmenting relationships. We have met patients who take their cancers for a walk on the greensward as if it was no more than an unruly pet. So, paradoxically, ***disease can be used as a vehicle to promote health.*** These people (not patients, now) have reached an accommodation with themselves that chalks up more health than was ever achieved in their angst-ridden but seemingly perfectly healthy adolescence. Note how creating this kind of health is not through teamwork or formulaic application of biopsychosocial models, but depends on flair, optimism, imagination, and a certain metaphysical dexterity—qualities which, we hope, will guide you through the forthcoming pages.

The Old Hippocratic oath ~425BC

I swear by Apollo the physician, and Aesculapius and Health and All-heal, and all the gods and goddesses, that, according to my ability and judgment, I will keep this oath and stipulation—to reckon him who taught me this Art equally dear to me as my parents, to share my substance with him, and relieve his necessities if required; to look upon his offspring in the same footing as my own brothers, and to teach them this Art, if they shall wish to learn it, without fee or stipulation, and that by percept, lecture, and every other mode of instruction, I will impart a knowledge of the Art to my own sons, and those of my teachers, and to disciples bound by a stipulation and oath according to the law of medicine, but to none other.

I will follow that system of regimen, which, according to my ability and judgment, I consider for the benefit of my patients, and abstain from whatever is deleterious and mischievous.

I will give no deadly medicine to anyone if asked, nor suggest any such counsel; and in like manner I will not give to a woman a pessary to produce abortion. With purity and with holiness I will pass my life and practise my Art.

I will not cut persons labouring under the stone, but will leave this work to be done by men who are practitioners of this work.

Into whatever houses I enter, I will go into them for the benefit of the sick, and will abstain from every voluntary act of mischief and corruption; and, further, from the seduction of females, or males, of freemen or slaves.

Whatever, in connection with my professional practice, I see or hear, in the life of men, which ought not to be spoken of abroad, I will not divulge, as reckoning that all such should be kept secret.

While I continue to keep this oath unviolated, may it be granted to me to enjoy life and practise this Art, respected by all men, in all times. Should I violate this Oath, may the reverse be my lot.

Addressed to gods we do not recognise, and entreating us to abhor operations for stones we never felt any compulsion to remove, we spent the first years of our training thinking that Hippocrates was merely quaint, until one day we took up work in a new hospital on the outskirts of small but quite well-known city in the middle of the country. There were carpets on the floor and all signs to the Labour Ward had been removed and replaced with ones to the 'Delivery Suite'. Everything was perfect and painless. There was even time for an introductory tour by the proud Administrator. As he droned on, our eyes roamed over the carpets, to the pictures on the walls, and settled on the ceiling—where there were undeniable squiggles of arterial blood. How had it got up there? And so soon after opening? Pain and calamity were seeping into that hospital even before the paint was dry. As our work unfolded, backs frequently to the wall, floored by vicious circumstances, and with ceilings caving in, Hippocrates seemed even further away, on his dark blue island of Cos, under his famous tree. No floors, no walls, and no ceilings. Then all became clear. What Hippocrates had at his back was no man-made wall but the bark of our living family tree, that most rooted of all our collective medical memories. Now, when our back is to the wall, we can sometimes hypnotize ourselves into feeling the rough contour of that supporting trunk; and now, when we look up, through the blood, we see sky.

A New Hippocratic oath ~2010AD

I promise that my medical knowledge will be used to benefit people's health. Patients are my first concern. I will listen to them, and provide the best care I can. I will be honest, respectful, and compassionate towards all.

I will do my best to help anyone in medical need, in emergencies. I will make every effort to ensure the rights of all patients are respected, including vulnerable groups who lack means of making their needs known.

I will exercise my professional judgment, uninfluenced by political or religious pressure, or the age, race, sexual orientation, social class, wealth, or celebrity of my patient. I will not put profit or my own career above my duty to my patient.

I recognize the special value of human life, but I also know that prolonging life is not the only aim of health care. If I agree to perform abortion, I agree it should take place only within an ethical and legal context.

I will not provide treatments that are pointless or harmful, or which an informed and competent patient refuses. I will help patients find the information and support they want to make decisions on their care.

I will be as truthful as I can, and respect patients' decisions, unless that puts others at risk of substantial harm. If I cannot agree with their requests, I will explain why.

If my patient has limited mental awareness, I will still encourage him or her to participate in decisions as much as they feel able. I will do my best to maintain confidentiality about all patients.

If there are overriding reasons preventing my keeping a patient's confidentiality I will explain them. I will recognize the limits of my knowledge and seek advice from colleagues as needed.

I will do my best to keep myself and my colleagues informed of new developments, and ensure that poor standards or bad practices are exposed to those who can improve them.

I will show respect for all those with whom I work and be ready to share my knowledge by teaching others what I know. I will use my training and professional standing to improve the community in which I work.

I will respect each of my roles, as expert, communicator, scholar, partner, manager, teacher, professional, and health advocate. I will promote fair use of health resources and try to influence positively those whose policies harm public health.

I recognise that I have responsibilities to humankind that transcend diktats and orders of States, and which no Legislature can countermand. I will oppose health policies that breach internationally accepted standards of human rights.

I will learn from my mistakes and seek help from colleagues to promote patient safety. While keeping within this framework, I will not be discouraged by failure, and will try to continue in a spirit of practical and rational optimism.

While I continue to keep this Oath unviolated,
may it be granted to me to enjoy life and the practice of the Art,
respected by all, in all times.

We take this oath not because we are doctors but because sooner or later we are all patients. Clause **1** is the central clause. It has a terrible beauty. For many, it is our family that is our main priority. Often we can strike an uneasy compromise with family life.
This page is dedicated to doctors for whom circumstances allow no such compromise: those who have *not* fled wars, or who have stayed at their posts during epidemics. Clause **3** is hareder to keep outside the UK NHS or similar free-access institution. ►It is better to create your own oath than use one off the peg, if it entails lying. The above is based on the BMA's *Revised Hippocratic Oath.*

Where should we keep this oath? Not in the dusty confines of a book, but in our limbic system (p436) where it has a every chance of influencing action, before our subverting cerebral cortex comes up with brilliant excuses as to why, in this case, the oath does not apply.

Decision and *intervention* are the essence of action: *reflection* and *conjecture* are the essence of thought: the essence of medicine is combining these realms in the service of others. We offer these ideals to stimulate both thought and action: like the stars, ideals are hard to reach, but they serve for navigation during the night. We choose Orion (**fig 1**) as our emblem for this navigation as he had miraculous sight (a gift from his immortal lover, Eos, to help him in his task of hunting down all dangerous things)—and, as his constellation is visible in the Northern *and* the Southern hemispheres (being at the celestial equator), he links our readers everywhere.

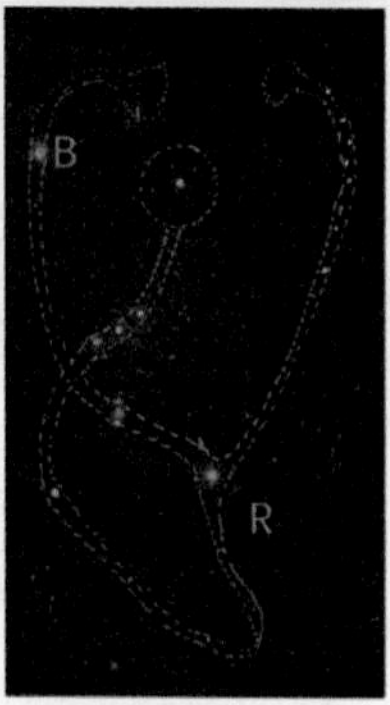

Fig 1. The constellation of Orion has 3 superb stars: *Bellatrix* (the stethoscope's bell), *Betelgeuse* (B) & *Rigel* (R). The 3 stars at the crossover (Orion's belt) are Alnitak, Alnilam, and Mintaka. ©JML & David Malin[2]

- ★Do not blame the sick for being sick.
- ★If the patient's wishes are known, comply with them.
- ★Work for your patients, not your consultant.
- ★Ward staff are usually right; respect their opinions.
- ★Treat the whole patient, not the disease, or the nurses.
- ★Admit people—not 'strokes', 'infarcts', or 'crumble'.
- ★Spend time with the bereaved; help them to shed tears.
- ★Give the patient (and yourself) time: time for questions, to reflect, to allow healing, and time to gain autonomy.
- ★Give patients the benefit of the doubt. Be optimistic. Optimistic patients who feel in charge live longer.[3]
- ★Use ward rounds to boost patients' morale, not your own.
- ★Be kind to yourself: you are not an inexhaustible resource.
- ★Question your conscience—however strongly it tells you to act.

Sleepwalking with our head in the clouds, we see neither the dozen stars above our head nor the tripwires at our feet, so we are frequently surprised to find ourselves falling head-over-heels in love with the idea that we are doing quite well. The great beauty of clinical medicine is that we are all levelled by our patients and their carers, whether we are students or professors, as this story shows. A man cut his hand and went round to his neighbour for help. This neighbour happened to be a doctor, but it was not the doctor but his 3-year-old daughter who opened the door. Seeing that he was hurt and bleeding, she took him in, pressed her handkerchief over his wound, and reclined him, feet up, in the best chair. She stroked his head and patted his hand, and told him about her marigolds, and then about her frogs, and, after some time, was starting to tell him about her father—when her father eventually appeared. He quickly turned the neighbour into a patient, and then into a bleeding biohazard, and then dispatched him to Casualty 'for suturing'. (The neighbour had no idea what this was.) He waited 3 hours in Casualty, had 2 desultory stitches, and an interview, with a medical student who suggested a tetanus vaccination (to which he developed an allergic reaction). He returned to his doctor next door a few days later, praising his young carer, but not the doctor (who had turned him into a patient), nor the hospital (who had turned him into an item on a conveyor belt), nor the student who turned him into a question mark (does a 50-year-old man with a full series of tetanus vaccinations need a booster at the time of injury?).

It was the 3-year-old who was his true nurse/physician and universal health worker, who took him in on his own terms, cared for him, and gave him time and dignity. Question her instinct for care as you will: point out that it could have led to harm; that it was not evidence-based; and that the hospital was just a victim of its own success. But remember that the story shows *there is*, as TS Eliot said, *at best, only a limited value in the knowledge derived from experience*, eg the knowledge encompassed in this book. The child had the innate understanding and the natural compassion that we all too easily lose amid the science, the knowledge, and our stainless-steel universe of organized health care.

The bedside manner and communication skills

On opening a window, to ventilate a stuffy consulting room, I got some candid feedback from the previous patient whose husband had asked how the consultation had gone "I suppose he got it right...pity about the bedside manner." I quickly shut the window! The point of this page is to slowly reopen the window, on the understanding that we have no special gifts in this area, just a rich catalogue of our errors to draw on. Doctors tends to write pompously about the bedside manner as if they were paragons, and patients may write with anger about it, without grasping the constraints (excuses?) which lead to our poor bedside manner. So let us start with *doctors who are patients*. You cannot get better than this doctor's report on her physician: "I felt he understood me: he asked all about how my illness interfered with my work and what I felt about it. He even seemed to remember parts of our previous consultation." It is simple to understand that words we use at the bedside are often misinterpreted: for example, 10% of patients say that jaundice means yellow vomit and remission is often taken to mean 'cure'. www.psycho-oncology.org When we analyse doctors who have become patients we realize there is an impasse in communication which no lexicon can remedy. Time itself flows differently for doctors and patients. "Just wait here and the radiographer will be with you right away" may presage a wait of 1 hour, which seems an age to the doctor-patient. "We will get the result soon" means weeks to doctors, and before lunch to patients.[4] If, when assessing risk, doctors who become patients tend to invert the meaning of "good" and "bad"—is there any hope that we can communicate well with our less rational patients?[5] Maybe these rules will help: • Give the most important details first • Check on retention and understanding • Be specific. "Drink 6 cups of water daily" is better than "Drink more fluids" • Give videos/written material with easy readability. Flesch's formula measures this: $F=206.835-(1.015 \times \text{ASL})-(84.6 \times \text{ASW})$ where ASL=average sentence length (number of words ÷ number of sentences) and ASW=average number of syllables/word. 100 is very easy; aim for >70. *F* for the 1st paragraph of this page is 71 but paragraph 2 is much more complex: *F*=39, as calculated by MS Word®'s automated Flesch score. It is sobering to display readability statistics for patient leaflets imported into Word®, and then fun to see if you can re-edit to get a score of >70. Language Therapy Departments are leading the way here.[6] ▶Don't assume everyone can read: naming the pictures but not the words on our test chart (see inside front cover) reveals this tactfully.

Ensure harmony between your view of what must be done and your patient's. We talk of *compliance* with our regimens, when what we should talk of is *concordance*, which recognizes the central role of patient participation in all good care plans.

Anxiety reduction or intensification Simple explanation of what you are going to do often defuses what can be a highly charged affair. With children, try more subtle techniques, such as examining the abdomen using the child's own hands, or examining his teddy bear first.

Pain reduction or intensification Compare: "I'm going to press your stomach. If it hurts, cry out" with "I'm going to touch your stomach. Let me know what you feel" and "I'll lay a hand on your stomach. Sing out if you feel anything." We can sound frightening, neutral, or joyful, and the patient will relax or tense up accordingly.

The tactful or clumsy invasion of personal space During ophthalmoscopy we must get much nearer to the patient than is acceptable in normal social intercourse. Both doctor and patient may end up holding their breath, which helps neither the patient keep his eyes perfectly still, nor the doctor to carry out a full examination. Simply explain "I need to get very close to your eyes for this." (Not "We need to get very close for this"—one of the authors was kissed repeatedly while conducting ophthalmoscopy by a patient with frontal lobe signs.)

In summary Our bedside manner must allow our patients to trust us, and enable the consultation to be a healing event in its own right. But it shouldn't be so delightful as to cause endless queues of eager, doctor-dependent patients. As another patient said to me: "All this babble...is it worth it? Your predecessor Dr W. would have cleared this waiting room in 1 hour, maximum, and then we could all go home."

Asking questions

We can all attend communications courses on how to make good use of focused and open-ended questions, ask fewer leading questions, and respond to patient cues. Does this influence what we do back at work? Randomized trials say "Yes!";[7] also, additional skills, not apparent at 3 months after courses, become evident, with 80% fewer interruptions, for example.[8] One reason for this acceleration of our skills is that good communication makes our work interesting, richer, and deeper. Tactful psychosocial probing is also evident.[9] But empathy may dry up over time[10] (one reason to refresh ourselves as often as possible).

Leading questions On seeing a bloodstained handkerchief you ask: "How long have you been coughing up blood?" "6 weeks, doctor", so you assume haemoptysis for 6 weeks. In fact, the stain could be due to a cut finger, or a nose bleed. On finding this out later (perhaps after expensive and unpleasant tests), you will be annoyed with your patient for misleading you, but he was trying to be polite by giving the sort of answer you were obviously expecting. Leading questions permit no opportunity to deny assumptions. "Is your chest pain sharp or dull?" is a common and commonly misleading question. It's as helpful as speaking to your patient in the wrong language.[11] Try "Tell me more about what you are feeling...what's it really like?" (p89).

Questions suggesting the answer "Was the vomit red, yellow, or black—like coffee grounds?"—the classic description of vomited blood. "Yes, like coffee grounds, doctor." The doctor's expectations and hurry to get the evidence into a pre-decided format have so tarnished the story as to make it useless.

Open questions The most open question is "How are you?" This suggests no particular answer, so the direction a patient chooses offers valuable information. Other examples are gentle imperatives such as "Tell me about the vomit" "It was dark" "How dark?" "Dark bits in it" "Like...?" "Like bits of soil in it." This information is gold, although it is not cast in the form of 'coffee grounds'.

Patient-centred questions "What do you think is wrong?" "Are there any other aspects of this we might explore?" "Are there any questions you want to ask?" (a closed question). Better still, try "What are the other things on your mind?[12] How does having this affect you? What is the worst thing? It makes you feel..." (The doctor is silent.) ►Unless you become patient-centred your patient may never be fully satisfied with you, or fully cooperative.

Casting your questions over the whole family This is most useful in revealing if symptoms are caused or perpetuated by psychological mechanisms. They probe the network of causes and enabling conditions which allow nebulous symptoms to flourish in family life. "Who else is important in your life? ... Are they worried about you? Who really understands you?" Until this sort of question is asked, illness may be refractory to treatment. Eg "Who is present when your headache starts? Who notices it first—you or your wife? Who worries about it most (or least)? What does your wife do when (or before) you get it?" Think to yourself: *Who* is his headache? We note with fascination research showing that in clusters of hard-to-diagnose symptoms, it is the spouse's view of them that is the best predictor of outcome: if the spouse is determined that symptoms must be physical, the outcome is worse than if the spouse allows that some symptoms may be psychological.

Echoes Try repeating the last words said as a route to new intimacies, otherwise inaccessible, as you fade into the distance, and the patient soliloquizes "...I've always been suspicious of my wife." "Wife ..." "My wife ... and her father together." "Together..." "I've never trusted them together." "Trusted them together..." "No, well, I've always felt I've known who my son's real father was... I can never trust those two together." Without any questions you may unearth the unexpected, important clue which throws a new light on the history.

►*If you only ask questions, you will only receive answers in reply.* If you interrogate a robin, he will fly away: treelike silence may bring him to your hand.

What is the mechanism? Finding narrative answers

Like toddlers, we should always be asking "*Why?*"—not just to find ultimate causes, nor to keep in step with our itineraries of veracity (although there is a place for this), but to enable us to find the simplest level for intervention. Some simple change early on in a chain of events may be sufficient to bring about a cure, but later on, such opportunities may not arise. For example, it is not enough for you to diagnose heart failure in your breathless patient. Ask: "*Why is there heart failure*?" If you do not, you will be satisfied with giving the patient an anti-failure drug—and any side-effects from this, such as uraemia or incontinence induced by diuretic-associated polyuria, will be attributed to an unavoidable consequence of necessary therapy.

If only you had asked "*What is the mechanism of the heart failure*?" you might have found a cause, eg anaemia coupled with ischaemic heart disease. You cannot cure the latter, but treating the anaemia may be all that is required to cure the patient's breathlessness. But do not stop there. Ask: "*What is the mechanism of the anaemia*?" You find a low MCV and a correspondingly low serum ferritin (p320)—and you might be tempted to say to yourself, I have the prime cause.

Wrong! Put aside the idea of prime causes, and go on asking "*What is the mechanism*?" Retaking the history (often the best 'investigation') shows a very poor diet. "*Why is the patient eating a poor diet*?" Is he ignorant or too poor to eat properly? You may find the patient's wife died a year ago, he is sinking into a depression, and cannot be bothered to eat. He would not care if he died tomorrow.

You come to realize that simply treating the patient's anaemia may not be of much help—so go on asking "*Why*?": "Why did you bother to go to the doctor if you aren't interested in getting better?" It turns out he only went to see you to please his daughter. He is unlikely to take your drugs unless you really get to the bottom of what he cares about. His daughter is what matters and, unless you include her, all your initiatives may fail. Talk to her, offer help for the depression, teach her about iron-rich foods and, with luck, your patient's breathlessness may gradually begin to disappear. Even if it does *not* start to disappear, you are learning to stand in your patient's shoes and you may discover what will enable him to accept help. And this dialogue may help you to be a kinder doctor, particularly if you are worn out by endless lists of technical tasks, which you must somehow fit into impossibly over-crowded days and nights. You never really know a man until you stand in his shoes and walk around in them. Harper Lee; *To Kill a Mockingbird*

Constructing imaginative narratives yielding new meanings Doctors are often thought of as being reductionist or mechanistic—but the above shows that asking "*Why?*" can enlarge the scope of our enquires into holistic realms. Another way to do this is to ask "***What does this symptom mean?***"—for this person, his family, and our world. A limp might mean a neuropathy, or falling behind with the mortgage, if you are a dancer; or it may represent a medically unexplained symptom which subtly alters family hierarchies both literally (on family walks) and metaphorically. Science is about clarity, objectivity, and theory in modelling reality. But there is another way of modelling the external world, which involves subjectivity, emotion, ambiguity, and arcane relationships between apparently unrelated phenomena. The medical humanities (p17) explore this—and have burgeoned recently[13]—leading to the existence of two camps: humanities and science. If while reading this you are getting impatient to get to the real nuts and bolts of technological medicine, you are in the latter camp. We are not suggesting that you leave it, only that you learn to operate out of both. If you do not, your professional life will be full of failures, which you may deny or remain in ignorance of. If you *do* straddle both camps, there will also be failures, but you will realize what these failures *mean*, and you will know how to *transform* them. This transformation happens through dialogue and reflection. We would achieve more if we did less: every hospital should have a department of reflection and it should be visited as often as the radiology department. In fact every hospital has many such departments, carved out of our own minds—it's just that their entrances are blocked by piles of events, tasks and happenings.

Compared with being born, death should be straightforward. As easy as falling off your blog or returning home. But nothing you can say to your patient can ever be relied upon to tame death's mystery. Luckily this is not required for a good death. But preparing people for death is more than control of terminal symptoms. It depends on understanding your own view of death. Something to be avoided at all costs?—or the yummiest chocolate in a rather uneven box? Tracking your own evolving views helps sensitize yourself to issues that confront your patient. Learn from your patients shamelessly. After all, rendering this service to you (and hence to others) may be your patient's last and only gift to humanity. A shared dialogue may be worth ten times its weight in morphine. Dying from pneumonia (the old man's friend) one patient said: "I want to do this right..."[14] This is a great starting point. Reflect on how to build on this universal (but rarely expressed) hope.

Death has got something of a bad press recently, but note that death is Nature's master stroke, albeit a cruel one, because it allows genotypes space to try on new phenotypes. The time comes in the life of any organ or person when it is better to start from scratch rather than carry on with the weight and muddle of endless accretions. Our bodies and minds are these perishable phenotypes—the froth, that always turns to scum, on the wave of our genes. These genes are not really *our* genes. It is we who belong to them for a few decades. It is one of Nature's great insults that she should prefer to put *all* her eggs in the basket of a defenceless, incompetent neonate rather than in the tried and tested custody of our own superb minds. But as our neurofibrils begin to tangle, and that neonate walks to a wisdom that eludes us, we are forced to give Nature credit for her daring idea. Of course, Nature, in her careless way, can get it wrong: people often die in the wrong order (one of our chief roles is to prevent this mis-ordering of deaths, not the phenomenon of death itself).

So we must admit that, on reflection, dying *is* a brilliant idea, and one that it is most unlikely we could ever have thought of ourselves.

The 4 causes of death **1** Homicide **2** Suicide **3** Misadventure **4** Natural causes.

Diagnosis Apnoea with no pulse or heart sounds, and fixed pupils. If on a ventilator, brain death may be diagnosed even if the heart is still beating, via the *UK brain death criteria* (USA criteria differ). Here, brain death is death of the brainstem, recognized by:

- Deep coma with absent respirations (hence on a ventilator).
- The absence of drug intoxication and hypothermia (<35°C).
- The absence of hypoglycaemia, acidosis, and U&E imbalance.

Tests: All brainstem reflexes should be absent.

- Unreactive pupils. Absent corneal response (no blink to a cotton-wool touch).
- No vestibulo-ocular reflexes, ie no eye movement occurs after or during slow injection of 20mL of ice-cold water into each external auditory meatus in turn. Visualize the ear-drum first to eliminate false-negative tests, eg due to wax.
- Stimulation in the cranial nerve distributions produces no motor response.
- No gag reflex or response to bronchial stimulation, and no respiratory effort on stopping the ventilator and allowing P_aCO_2 to rise to 6.7kPa.

Other considerations: Repeat tests after a suitable interval, eg 24h. Spinal reflexes are not relevant to diagnosing brain death; EEG is not required, nor is a neurologist. The doctor diagnosing brain death must be a consultant (or his deputy registered for >5yrs). The opinion of one other doctor (any) should also be sought.

Organ donation: The point of diagnosing brain death is partly that this allows organs (kidney, liver, cornea, heart, or lungs) to be donated and removed with as little hypoxic damage as possible. Don't avoid the topic with relatives. Many are glad to help.

After death Inform GP and the consultant. See the relatives. Sign death certificates promptly. If the cause is violence, injury, neglect, surgery, anaesthesia, alcohol, suicide, or poisoning, or is unknown, inform the Coroner/Procurator Fiscal.

The active management of death

When you might raise death with your patient, and you find yourself thinking it is better for him not to know, suspect that you mean: it is easier for me not to tell. ►Most patients are told less than they want.[15] Accepting death may involve passing through stages on a path. It helps to know where your patient is on this journey. At first there may be *shock* and *numbness*, then *denial* (which reduces anxiety), then *anger*, then *grief* and then, perhaps, *acceptance*.[16] Finally there may be intense longing for death as your patient moves beyond the reach of worldly cares. JS Bach *Ich habe genug*; Cantata 82

In the UK there are 12,000 deaths/week[17] and few hospice beds or palliative care experts, so the chances are that a death will be happening near you soon, and nobody will be in charge. The aim of this page is to give you courage to take charge: to find out about your patient's wishes, and comply with them. ►***Get help promptly from palliative care teams.*** Ensure you operate within the legal framework of the area you work in, and take into account GMC guidance[18] and current thinking expressed in the Liverpool care pathway/gold standards framework.[19] If a *living will/advance directive* is in existence, comply with it. The GMC is clear about this. Don't be mesmerized by legal or religious ambiguities: stick to your duty—promote your patient's autonomy. ►***At the end of life, autonomy trumps all else.***[1] Take strength from this clarity. No one we have talked to who is dying has said they want to be kept in limbo for weeks, drifting in and out consciousness, with inadequate doses of analgesia and swaddled in incontinence pads. Yet this can be the reality. So if this is happening on your ward in a patient who is dying, start by affirming that ***this must be wrong***. There must be a better way, eg ***the active management of death*** with leadership and authority (which you can help establish) used to enable patients' wishes to be acted on. Talk to the patient, the relatives, and staff. Get (and document[2]) consensus that the top priority is relief of suffering. If oral pain relief[3] keeps the patient happy and functioning, fine. But sometimes total sedation is needed to abolish symptoms, eg with regular (1-4hrly) injections,[4] or a syringe pump (p533).[5] Make sure your doses are adequate, not to cause death, but to leave no opportunity for pain and distress to re-emerge, if that is the patient's implied or stated wish.

If your doses are insufficient, you can get into a very undesirable circularity of coma, quasi-consciousness, distress and muddle, with each small dose increment achieving nothing but exhaustion in the relatives and limbo for your patient.[20] If the sedated patient shows any movement to physical stimulation, consciousness may be returning and dose increments may be needed.[6] Get help from the palliative care team, eg if you suspect opiate neurotoxicity (eg twitching) or hyperalgesia.

To comply with patients' wishes to be kept at peace, doses may well need to be at least doubled every 12h—or, if on a pump, increased by 50% ***every few hours***.[21] Active management needs geometric increments to avoid suffering. If you start with 10mg morphine/12h, and the need is for 200mg/12h, you are consigning your patient to weeks of misery if you use 5-10mg increments, but if you double doses every 12h, control will only take a few days *at most*. Your prescription ***must*** allow for this, and nursing staff must be brought in on decisions, with the rationale agreed at each handover. "This is what the patient wants" not "This is what the doctor says". Don't be frightened to use big or very big doses.[3,4,5] It's whatever the patient needs; this is very variable. Avoid transdermal drugs (dose escalation is slow and inefficient).[22]

1 Provided our humanity remains intact (NB: good palliative care will, in general, *enhance* humanity).
2 Establish & document that: ►The patient is dying and has initiated the request ►You have discussed doses with an experienced Dr ►Dose increases are proportionate and needed for symptom control.
3 Modified-release morphine sulfate 10-260mg/12h. Oxycodone is an alternative, eg Oxycontin®. In one study, the mean daily OxyContin® dose was ~80mg/d. 20% need at least 3 times as much.
4 For pain, morphine 2.5-100mg/1-4h SC. For larger doses use a pump or diamorphine (very soluble, so volumes can be *much* smaller). If the problem is distress or dyspnoea, midazolam 5mg/4h sc) + morphine rescue doses may be best. On demand doses are typically 25% of the background dose. If many rescue doses are needed, increase background analgesia by ≥50%. In one study, 91% needed 5-299mg of morphine/d), 7% needed 300-599mg/d, and 2% needed ≥600mg of morphine/d.
5 Morphine doses via a syringe driver range from 0.5 to 300mg/h. ***Example of dose escalation:*** if 10mg/h is not working, give a bolus of 10mg, and then increase the rate by ≥50% (15mg/h). If distress continues, re-bolus with 15mg, and ↑background to 22mg/h and so on until full comfort is achieved. It often helps to add midazolam 0.8-8mg/h; the buccal route works too: Epistatus®, p 836; 10mg/mL.
6 See Richmond Agitation-Sedation Scale. NB: validated protocols for dose escalation are lacking.

►Consult the *BNF* or *BNF for Children* or your local equivalent before giving any drug with which you are not thoroughly familiar; check interactions meticulously.

Before prescribing, ask if the patient is allergic to anything. The answer is often "yes"—but do not stop here. Characterize the reaction, or else you risk denying a possibly life-saving, and very safe, drug such as penicillin because of a mild reaction, eg nausea. Is the reaction a *true allergy* (anaphylaxis, p806, or a rash?), a *toxic effect* (eg ataxia is inevitable if given large doses of phenytoin), or a *predictable adverse reaction* (eg GI bleeding from aspirin), or an *idiosyncratic reaction*?

Remember *primum non nocere*: first do no harm. The more minor the illness, the more weight this carries. The more serious the illness, the more its antithesis comes into play: *nothing ventured, nothing gained*. ***Prescribing in renal failure*** and ***liver failure:*** p301 & p259. These **ten commandments** should be written on every tablet:

1 Explore alternatives to drugs—which often lead to doctor-dependency, paternalism, and medicalization of life. Drugs are also expensive: >£11 billion/yr[UK]; prices increase much faster than general inflation. There are 3 places to look:
- *The larder:* eg lemon and honey for sore throats, rather than penicillin.
- *The blackboard:* eg education about the self-inflicted causes of oesophagitis. Rather than giving expensive drugs, advise raising the head of the bed, and avoiding tight garments, too many big meals, smoking, and alcohol excess.
- *Lastly, look to yourself:* giving a piece of yourself, some real sympathy, is worth more than all the drugs in your pharmacopoeia to patients who are frightened, bereaved, or weary of life. One of us (JML) for many years looked after a lady who was paranoid: monthly visits comprised an injection and a hug, no doubt always chaperoned, until one day mental health nurses took over her care. She was seen by a different nurse each month. They didn't know about hugging, so after a while she stopped cooperating, and soon it fell to us to certify her death.

2 Are you prescribing for a minor illness because you want to solve all problems? Patients may be happy just to know the illness *is* minor. Knowing this may make it acceptable. Some people do not believe in drugs, and you must find this out.

3 Decide if the patient is responsible. If he now swallows *all* the quinine pills you have so attentively prescribed for his cramps, death will be swift.

4 Know of other ways your prescription may be misused. Perhaps the patient whose 'insomnia' you so kindly treated is even now selling it on the black market or grinding up your prescription prior to injecting himself, desperate for a fix. Will you be suspicious when he returns to say he has lost his drugs?

5 Address these questions when prescribing off the ward:
- How many daily doses are there? 1–2 is *much* better than 4. Good doctors spend much time harmonizing complex regimens. One reason for 'failure' of HIV drugs, for example, is that regimens are too complex. Drug companies know this, so keep abreast of new modified release (MR) preparations.
- The bottle/box: can the patient read the instructions—and can he open it?
- How will you know if the patient forgets to return (follow-up)?
- If the patient agrees, enlist the spouse's help in ensuring that he remembers to take the pills. Check, eg by counting the remaining pills at the next visit.

6 Discuss side effects and risk of allergy. We may downplay risk, but our drugs cause 1 million NHS admissions/yr (£1–2 billion/yr). Most drug deaths are avoidable.[23]

7 Use computerized decision support whenever you can. If the patient is on 7 drugs and has 5 complaints, the computer will help you find which of the drugs are possible culprits.[24] Computers also warn about drug interactions. Use them!

8 Agree with the patient on the risk : benefit ratio's favourability. Try to ensure there is true concordance (p3) between you and your patient.

9 Record how you will review the patient's need for each drug and progress towards agreed goals, eg pulse rate to mark degree of β-blockade.

10 List benefits of *this* drug to *this* patient for *all* drugs taken. Specify what each drug is for—and cooperate with national computer schemes (eg the 'NHS spine'), which aggregate drugs prescribed for your patient from *all* sources.

Surviving life on the wards

At the end of every day, with the going down of the sun (which we never see at the coalface of clinical medicine), we can momentarily cheer ourselves up by the thought that we are one day nearer to the end of life on earth—and our responsibility for the unending tide of illness that floods into our corridors and seeps into our wards and consulting rooms. Of course you may have many other quiet satisfactions, but if not, read on and wink with us as we hear some fool or visionary telling us that our aim should be to produce the greatest health and happiness for the greatest number.

When we hear this, we don't expect cheering from the tattered ranks of midnight on-call junior doctors: rather, our ears are detecting a decimated groan, because these men and women know that there is something at stake in on-call doctoring far more elemental than health or happiness: namely survival. Within the first weeks, however brightly your armour shone, it will now be smeared and splattered if not with blood, then with the fallout from very many decisions that were taken without sufficient care and attention. Not that you were lazy, but *force majeure* on the part of Nature and the exigencies of ward life have, we are suddenly stunned to realize, taught us to be second-rate: for to insist on being first-rate in all areas is to sign a death warrant for our patients, and for ourselves. Perfectionism cannot survive in our clinical world. To cope with this fact, or, to put it less depressingly, to flourish in this new world, don't keep re-polishing your armour (what are the 10 causes of atrial fibrillation—or are there 11?), rather furnish your mind—and nourish your body (regular food and drink make those midnight groans of yours less intrusive). Don't voluntarily deny yourself the restorative power of sleep. A good nap is the order of the day—and for the nights, sleep for as long as possible. Remember that sleep is our natural state, in which we were first created, and we only wake to feed our dreams.

We cannot prepare you for finding out that you are not at ease with the person you are becoming, and neither would we dream of imposing on our readers a recommended regimen of exercise, diet, and mental fitness. Finding out what can lead you through adversity is the art of living.

Junior doctors' first jobs are not just a phase to get through and to enjoy where possible (there are often *many* such possibilities); they are also the anvil on which we are beaten into a new and perhaps uncomfortable shape. Luckily not all of us are made of iron so there is a fair chance that one day we will spring back into something resembling our normal shape, and realize that it was our weaknesses, not our strengths, which served us best. The jobs of junior doctors encompass huge swings in energy, motivation, and mood, which can be precipitated by small events. If you are depressed for more than a day, speak to a sympathetic friend, partner, or counsellor. ►***When in doubt, communicate***. And use an integrative philosophy of medicine, as described in this next section, to reclaim yourself.

Integrative medicine: beyond biopsychosocial models

The biopsychosocial model is the medical teacher's Grand Theory of Everything. It's like a game of 'stones, scissors and paper': the patient presents with a physical symptom, and the clever doctor trumps you, who had taken the symptom at face value, by revealing the social background that allowed the symptom to flourish. If the problem is social (eg poor housing), the clever doctor reveals the hidden asthma that this is causing, and if the symptom is purely psychological, the doctor reveals and manages the social effects of this for the patient's family. It's a powerful game,[25] and much good comes from it.[26] But like all orthodoxy it needs challenging.[27] Let us consider Mr B, the builder, who comes to Casualty having nailed his testicle to a plank. Everybody gathers round, but the clever doctor is annoyed that nobody is listening to his biopsychosocial diagnosis. The nail is removed; the testicle is repaired, but Mr B does not go on his way rejoicing. A nurse, a better listener than our doctor, uses an individually tailored ***moral–symbolic–existential*** approach to reveal that the injury was self-inflicted. A ***spiritual–cultural–ritualistic*** model may be needed for his care.[28]

As the author of the biopsychosocial model knew, there is more to medicine than stones, scissors, and paper, or ***any*** triad that does not integrate a rethinking of the task of medicine with infrastructure of relationships and beliefs. George Engel 1977 [29] [30]

Quality, QALYs, and the interpretation of dreams

Resource allocation: who gets what Resource allocation is about cutting the health cake—whose size is *given*. What slice should go to transplants, new joints, and services for dementia? Cynics would say that this depends on how vociferous each group of patients (or doctors) is. Others try to find a rational way to allocate resources. Health economists (econocrats) have invented the QALY for this purpose. NB: focusing on how to cut the cake diverts attention from how large the cake should be (is it better to spend money on space exploration or incontinence pads?)

How much is a life worth? Some countries will spend $2–10 million to find a man on a life-raft; others will spend nothing ("he's just one more mouth to feed").[31,32] Totalitarian capitalist states (eg China) will take a different view to liberal democracies. In France, one life is worth a hundred cherry trees, if the blossom is fine.[33]

What is a QALY? 1 year of healthy life expectancy is worth 1 'quality adjusted life year'. 1 year of unhealthy life expectancy is worth <1 QALY (its value is lower the poorer health is).[34] If you are likely to live for 8yrs in perfect health on an old drug, you gain 8 QALYs; if a new drug would give you 16yrs but at a quality of life you rate at only 25% of the maximum, you would gain only 4 QALYs. The dream of a health economist is to buy most QALYs for his budget. Health assessment organizations (eg NICE) keep arbitrary figures in their head (~£30,000/QALY—not evidence-based—and some NHS trusts are paying more out of their own pockets).[35,36] If an intervention costs more than this, QALYs can be recalculated (on *very* dubious grounds)[37] after weighting for age and disease-seriousness[38] to give the politically correct answer.[1]

Cost per QALY In various studies, with undeclared assumptions, this was (£):

GP advice to stop smoking	220	Breast cancer screening	5780
Preventing stroke by BP treatment	940	Infliximab in Crohn's[39]	6700
Valve replaced (eg for aortic stenosis)	1140	Home dialysis	17,260
Hip replacement (♀ aged 60–69)[40]	1470	Abatacept (rheumatoid arthritis)	40,000
CABG for LAD stenosis (p111)	2090	Vaccination against rotavirus[41]	61,000
Kidney transplant	4710	Interferon in MS (p500)	834,000

QALYs *do* help in rationing, but problems include pricing and invidiousness in choosing between people; a *huge* snag is that if we accept that the quality of our life is the quality of our relationships (Anthony Robbins), and that this value is unquantifiable (1 wife is good, but 2 wives are not *exactly* twice as good),[2] then we can see why bodies such as NICE get excoriated over issues such as dementia drugs, when seemingly small improvements can cause disproportionate joy, as when a demented man becomes able to recall his wife's name.[42,43] Should the spouse put their own QALYs into the sum?

The inverse care law and distributive justice

> '*Availability of good medical care varies inversely with the need for it in the population served. This operates more completely where medical care is most exposed to market forces...the market distribution of medical care exaggerates maldistribution of resources.*'

There is much evidence in support of this famous thesis formulated by Tudor Hart,[44] and there is no doubt that if one wants to make a positive contribution to health, it is no good just discovering pathways, blocking receptors, and inventing drugs. The more this is done, the more urgent the need for distributive justice—that unyielding and perpetually problematic benchmark against which we are all judged.

If those who shout loudest get heard first, we need to know when to train our ears to be deaf, eg when deciding who to put on urgent operating lists.

1 Public pressure has manoeuvred NICE into the tricky position of granting extra value to prolonging the last months of life—so that the QALY test seems to be passed by new cancer drugs (only for rare diseases!—to save money). In doing so, NICE invalidates the whole calculation.

2 This is an example of a **non-parametric quantity**, ie a quantity where simple ordering *may* be valid, but not operations such as addition or multiplication. Most medical statistics are assumed to be parametric; this is often false, invalidating much research. statsoft.com/textbook/stnonpar.html

Psychiatry on medical and surgical wards

►Psychopathology is common in colleagues, patients, and relatives. ►Seek help for your own problems. Find a sympathetic GP and register with him or her. You are not the best person to plan your assessment, treatment, and referral.

Current mental state 'Move gently through her thoughts, as one might explore a new garden'. Ian McEwan 2001 *Atonement*; Vintage 150 What is in bloom now? Where do those paths lead? What is under that stone? *Focus on:* Appearance; behaviour (anxious? suspicious?); speech (rate; content); mood; beliefs; hallucinations; orientation; memory (current affairs recall, monarch's name); concentration. Note insight and degree of rapport. Non-verbal behaviour often gives more valid clues than words, *OHCS* p 82 & p324.

Depression This is common, and often ignored, at great cost to wellbeing. Thinking "I would be depressed in her shoes" may sap our will to help, and as biological features (early waking, ↓appetite, ↓weight, loss of interest in sex/hobbies) are common on all wards, we may not realize just how bad things have got. *The 2 'best questions' are:*[45] *"Have you been bothered by feeling down, depressed, or hopeless in the last month?"* If so, *"Have you been bothered by lack of interest or pleasure in doing things?"* If "yes", depression is likely. There may also be guilt and feelings of worthlessness. ►*Don't think it's not your job to treat depression.* It is as important as pain. Try to arrange activities to boost the patient's morale and confidence, and keep him in touch with his fellows. Share your thoughts with other team members: nurses, physio- and occupational therapists, as well as relatives, if the patient wishes. Among these, your patient may find a kindred spirit who can give insight and support. ►If in doubt, try an antidepressant, and see if it helps. For *selective serotonin reuptake inhibitors* (eg citalopram, 20mg/24h), see *OHCS* p340. Cognitive interventions are just as important as drugs (*OHCS* p370), so liaise with the patient's GP pre-discharge.

Alcohol/alcohol withdrawal is a common cause of problems on the ward (p282).

The violent patient Recognize early warning signs: visible distress, tachypnoea, clenched fists, shouting, chanting, restlessness, repetitive movements, pacing, gesticulations. Your own intuition may be helpful here. ► At the first hint of violence, get help. If alone, make sure you are nearer the door than the patient.

- Do not be alone with the patient; summon the police or porters if needed.
- Try calming and talking with the patient. Do not touch him. Use your body language to reassure (sitting back, open palms, attentive).
- Get his consent; if unforthcoming, emergency treatment can still be given to save life, or serious deterioration. Enlist the help of nurses who know the patient.
- Use minimum force to achieve his welfare (but this may entail 6 strong men).

Causes: Anger (long waiting times[46%], dissatisfaction with treatment[15%], disagreement with the physician[10%]),[46] *alcohol, drugs* (recreational; prescribed), *hypoglycaemia, delirium* (p488), *psychosis, psychopathy*. Do blood glucose, or give IV dextrose stat (p844). Before further tests, haloperidol may be needed: ~2mg IM (up to 10 or, rarely, 18mg stat; monitor pulse, T°, and BP every 15min–4h); maximum daily dose: 18mg.

If a rational adult refuses vital treatment, it may be as well to respect this decision, provided he is 'competent', ie he understands the consequences of his actions and what you are telling him, is able to retain this information, and form the belief that it is true. Competence is rarely all or nothing, so don't hesitate to get the opinion of others. Enlist the persuasive powers of someone the patient respects.

After a violent event: Attend to your own and others' wounds (get help as needed); report the event. Flashbacks, depression, insomnia, and need for time off are common.[47]

Mental Health Acts Familiarize yourself with local procedures and laws pertaining to your country before your period of duty starts (*OHCS* p402). In England, Common Law allows restraining a patient who is being violent on the ward.

►Only in the past 3 centuries has life expectancy risen much above 40 years. *An ageing population is a sign of successful social, health, and economic policies.*[48]

Healthy ageing is not a contradiction as health is not just 'complete mental and physical wellbeing (WHO) but also a process of adaptation, to changing environments, to growing up and ageing, to healing when damaged, to suffering, and death. Health embraces the future so includes anguish and the inner resources to live with it' (Illich, *OHCS* p470). ►Ageing reflects the cumulative effects of stressors (eg free radicals) and acquired mechanisms for dealing with them (as important as genetic effects).

Beware ageism! Old age is associated with disease but doesn't cause it *per se.*[49] Any deterioration is from treatable disease *until proved otherwise.*

1 Contrary to stereotype, most old people are fit.[50] 80% of those over 85yrs old do not live in institutions (95% if aged ~65yrs); 70% manage stairs and can bathe without help. Number of years in education and the number of comorbidities correlate inversely with difficulties in the activities of daily living.[51]
2 With any problem, find the cause; don't always be thinking: *this is simply ageing.* Look (within reason) for treatable disease, ↓fitness, and social factors.
3 Do not restrict treatment simply because of age. Old people vary. Age alone is a poor predictor of outcome and should not be used as a substitute for careful assessment of each patient's potential for benefit and risk.[52]

Characteristics of disease in old age There are differences of emphasis in the approach to old people compared with young people.[53]

1 ***Multiple pathology:*** Several disease processes may coincide: find out which impinge on each complaint (eg senile cataract + arthritis = falls).
2 ***Multiple causes:*** One problem may have several causes. Treating each alone may do little good; treating all may be of much benefit.[54]
3 ***Non-specific presentations:*** Some presentations are common in old people—eg the 'geriatric giants':[55] incontinence (p650);[56] immobility; instability (falls); and dementia/confusion (p488). Any disease may present with these. Also, typical signs and symptoms may be absent (myocardial infarction without chest pain; pneumonia, but no cough, fever, or sputum).
4 ***Rapid worsening if treatment is delayed:*** Complications are common.
5 ***More time is required for recovery:*** Points 4–6 reflect impairment in homeostatic mechanisms and loss of 'physiological reserve'.
6 ***Impaired metabolism and excretion of drugs:*** Doses may need lowering.
7 ***Rehabilitation is often needed*** to maximize independence; focus on balance & grip.
8 ***Social factors:*** These are central in aiding recovery and return to home.

Special points Assess all disabilities; get home details, eg stairs; access to toilet. Take a biopsychosocial approach[57] (look for and manage interactions between physical, psychological and social aspects of a person's life—relevant in any chronic disease).

- Drug concordance (p3): how many different tablets can he cope with? Probably not many more than 2. So which are the most important drugs? You may have to ignore other desirable remedies, or enlist the help of a friend, a spouse, or a pharmacist (who can batch morning, noon, and night doses in compartmentalized containers so complex regimens may be reduced to 'take the morning compartment when you get up, the noon compartment before lunch, etc').
- Social network (regular visitors; family and friends).
- Care details: what services are in operation?—meals delivered; community psychiatric or district nurse—who else is involved in the care?
- Speak to others (relatives; neighbours; carers; GP).
- Make a holistic *careplan.* Include nutrition. If food is dumped beside a blind man, and no one helps cut it up, he may starve. A passing doctor may arrange a CT 'for cachexia', when what he needs is food and cataract surgery.

On examination: Do BP lying and standing (postural drop >20/10mmHg ≈ falls). Rectal exam: impaction ≈ overflow incontinence. Detailed CNS exam may be needed if presentation is non-specific. This tires patients, so consider doing in batches.

Beyond the hospital: planning successful discharges (How to live and be frail in the community)

►*Start planning discharge from day 1.* A very common question on ward rounds is: "Will this patient get on OK at home?—we've got him as good as we can, but is discharge safe?" In answering this take into account:

- Does the patient live alone? Does any carer have support? Is he/she already exhausted by other duties (eg a handicapped toddler)?
- Is your patient in fact a carer for someone else even more frail?
- Most patients want to go home promptly. If not, find out why.
- Is the accommodation suitable? Stairs? Toilet on same floor?
- If toilet access is difficult, can he transfer from chair to commode?
- Can he open a tin, use the phone, plug in a kettle, cook soup?
- Is the family supportive—in theory or in practice?
- Are the neighbours friendly? "But I would not trouble them". Explore the validity of this sentiment by asking if they would want to know if they were reasonably fit, and a neighbour were in need.
- Are social services and community geriatric services well integrated? Or will the person who provides the lunch ignore the patient if she cannot gain access? Proper *case management programmes* with defined responsibilities, integrating social and geriatric services, really can help *and* save money (~20%).[58] Such integration is rare[59] but is possible in the UK thanks partly to the advent of Primary Care Trusts with overarching responsibilities for *both* medical *and* social care.

UK NHS national service framework (NSF) for older people

There are 8 standards of care http://bmj.com/cgi/content/full/326/7402/1300

1 *Rooting out age discrimination:* NHS services are to be provided regardless of age, on the basis of need alone. Social services will not use age in eligibility criteria or policies, to restrict access to available services.
2 *Person-centred care:* NHS services treat older people as individuals and enable them to make choices about their own care.
3 *Intermediate care:* Older people shall have access to intermediate care services at home or in designated care settings, to promote their independence by providing enhanced services from the NHS and councils to prevent unnecessary hospital admission. Rehabilitation services enable early discharge from hospital and prevent premature or unnecessary admission to long-term residential care.
4 *General hospital care:* Older people's care in hospital is delivered through appropriate specialist care and by hospital staff who have the right set of skills to meet their needs.
5 *Stroke:* People who are thought to have had a stroke must have access to diagnostic services, and be treated appropriately by a specialist stroke service, and subsequently, with their carers, participate in a multidisciplinary programme of secondary prevention and rehabilitation.
6 *Falls:* The NHS, working in partnership with councils, is required to take action to prevent falls and reduce fractures in older people and provide advice on fall prevention, through a specialist falls service.
7 *Mental health in older people* is to be promoted by access to integrated mental health services (from the NHS or councils) to ensure effective diagnosis, treatment, and support, for them and their carers.
8 *The promotion of health and active life in older age:* The health and wellbeing of older people are promoted through a coordinated programme of action led by the NHS with support from councils.

►NSFs attempt to improve services by central command and control: the least subtle and effective method.

On being busy: Corrigan's secret door

"I work much better in chaos." Francis Bacon [60] Chaos is not always an enemy: certainly there is no shortage of it in hospitals, consulting rooms, and other battle-grounds. Can we prepare ourselves to use chaos well? Being forewarned allows us to be forearmed, enabling us to adapt to being busy, or at least to wink at each other as we slide down the cascade of long hours→excessive paperwork→too few beds→effort-reward imbalance→compromised care from too few resources →trouble with superiors→difficult patients→too many deaths[61]→failure to reconcile personal and family life with professional roles.[62] Logistic regression shows our consequent problems are predicted by 5 stressors: **1** Lack of recognition of own contribution by others. **2** Too much responsibility. **3** Difficulties keeping up to date. **4** Making the right decision alone. **5** Effects of stress on personal/family life.[63]

We may think that it is modern medicine that makes us ever busier, but doctors have always been busy. Sir James Paget, for example, would regularly see over 60 patients each day, sometimes travelling many miles, on his horse, to their bedsides. Sir Dominic Corrigan was so busy 180 years ago that he had a secret door made in his consulting room to escape the ever-growing queue of eager patients.[64]

We are all familiar with the phenomenon of being hopelessly over-stretched, and of wanting Corrigan's secret door. Competing, urgent, and simultaneous demands make carrying out any task all but impossible: the junior doctor is trying to put up an intravenous infusion on a shocked patient when his 'bleep' sounds. On his way to the phone a patient is falling out of bed, being held in, apparently, only by his visibly lengthening catheter (which had taken the doctor an hour to insert). He knows he should stop to help but, instead, as he picks up the phone, he starts to tell Sister about "this man dangling from his catheter" (knowing in his heart that the worst will have already happened). But he is interrupted by a thud coming from the bed of the lady who has just had her varicose veins attended to: however, it is not her, but her visiting husband who has collapsed and is now having a seizure. In despair, he turns to the nurse and groans: "There must be some way out of here!" At times like this we all need Corrigan to take us by the shadow of our hand, and walk with us through a metaphorical secret door into a calm inner world. To enable this to happen, make things as easy as possible for yourself—as follows.

First, however lonely you feel, you are not usually alone. Do not pride yourself on not asking for help. If a decision is a hard one, share it with a colleague. Second, take any chance you get to sit down and rest. Have a cup of coffee with other members of staff, or with a friendly patient (patients are sources of renewal, not just devourers of your energies). Third, do not miss meals. If there is no time to go to the canteen, ensure that food is put aside for you to eat when you can: hard work and sleeplessness are twice as bad when you are hungry. Fourth, avoid making work for yourself. It is too easy for junior doctors, trapped in their image of excessive work and blackmailed by misplaced guilt, to remain on the wards reclerking patients, rewriting notes, or rechecking results at an hour when the priority should be caring for themselves. Fifth, when a bad part of the rota is looming, plan a good time for when you are off duty, to look forward to during the long nights.

However busy the 'on take', your period of duty will end. For you, as for Macbeth:

> **come what come may,**
> **time and the hour runs through the roughest day.**

Riding the wave In *Macbeth*, toil and trouble go hand in hand, but sometimes we work best when we are busy. This is recognized in the aphorism that *if you want a job done quickly, give it to a busy (wo)man.* Observe your colleagues and yourself during a busy day. Sometimes our energy achieves nothing but our own inundation. At other times, by jettisoning everything non-essential, we get airborne and accomplish marvellous feats. As with any sport, we have to break into a sweat before we can get into the zone, where every action meets its mark.

But note that what keeps us riding the wave of a busy day is not what we jettison but what we retain: humour, courtesy, a recognition of the work of others, and an ability to twinkle. A smile causes no delays, and reaches far beyond our lips.

Health and medical ethics

In our public medical personas, we often act as though morality consisted only in following society's conventions: we do this not so much out of laziness but because we recognize that it is better that the public think of doctors as old-fashioned or stupid, than that they should think us evil. But in the silences of our consultations, when it is we ourselves who are under the microscope, then, wriggle as we may, we cannot escape our destiny, which is to lead as often as to follow, in the sphere of ethics. To do this, we need to return to first principles, and not go with the flow of society's expectations. To give us courage in this enterprise, we can recall the aviator's and the seagull's law: it is only by *facing* the prevailing wind that we can become airborne, and achieve a new vantage point from which to survey our world.

Our analysis starts with our aim: to do good by making people healthy. *Good*[1] is the most general term of commendation, and entails four cardinal duties:

1 Not doing harm. We owe this duty to all people, not just our patients.[65]
2 Doing good by positive actions. We particularly owe this to our patients.
3 Promoting justice—ie distributing scarce resources fairly (p10) and respecting rights: legal rights, rights to confidentiality, rights to be informed, to be offered all the options, and to be told the truth.
4 Promoting autonomy. This is not universally recognized; in some cultures facing starvation, for example, it may be irrelevant, or even be considered subversive.

Health entails being sound in body and mind, and having powers of growth, development, healing, and regeneration. *How many people have you made healthy (or at least healthier) today?* And in achieving this, *how many cardinal duties have you ignored?* We cannot spend long on the wards or in our surgeries trying to 'make people healthy' before we have breached every cardinal duty—particularly (**3**) and (**4**). Does it matter? What is the point of having principles if they are regularly ignored? The point of having them is to provide a context for our negotiations with patients to form, where possible, a beneficial synthesis.

Synthesis When we must act in the face of two conflicting duties, ***one is not a duty***. How do we tell which one? Trying to find out involves getting to know our patient.

- Are the patient's wishes being complied with?
- What do your colleagues think? What do the relatives think? Have they his or her best interests at heart? Ask the patient's permission first.
- Is it desirable that the reason for an action be universalizable? (That is, if I say this person is too old for such-and-such an operation, am I happy to make this a general rule for everyone?—Kant's 'law'.)[2]
- If an investigative journalist were to sit on a sulcus of mine, having full knowledge of my thoughts and actions, would she be bored or would she be composing vitriol for tomorrow's newspapers? If so, can I answer her, point for point? Am I happy with my answers? Or are they merely tactical devices?
- What would a patient's representative think, eg the elected chairman of a patient's participation group (OHCS p496)? These opinions are valid and readily available (if a local group exists) and they can stop decision-making from being too medicalized.

Red flags on your wigwam For each patient use a check-list to avoid skating over ethical issues. If a red flag pertains, ethical aspects are likely to be very important.

- Wishes of the patient are unknown (find out if a living will is in existence).
- Issues regarding confidentiality/disclosure (eg HIV+ve but partner unaware).
- Goals of care: are these confused and contradictory in any way?
- Wants to discharge himself against advice? Is he fully informed and competent?
- Arguments among relatives as how best to proceed: have you listened to all sides?
- Money problems relating to cost of care or earnings lost through illness.[66]

1 Don't think of good and evil as forever opposite; good can come out of evil, and vice versa: this fundamental mix-up explains why we learn more from our dissolute patients than we do from saints.

2 There are problems with universalizability: only intuition can suggest how to resolve conflicts between competing universalizable principles. Also, there is a sense in which all ethical dilemmas are unique, so no moral rules are possible or required—so they *cannot* be universal (Sartre, Nietzsche).

"Unless both the doctor and the patient become a problem to each other, no solution is found." Jung's aphorism 67 is untrue for half our waking lives: for an anaesthetist there is no need for the patient to become a problem in order for the anaesthetic to work. But, as with all the best aphorisms, being untrue is the least of the problems they cause us. Great aphorisms signify because they unsettle. Our settled and smug satisfaction at finishing a period of duty without any problems is so often a sign of failure. We have kept the chaos at bay, whereas, if we were greater men or women, we would have embraced it. Half our waking professional lives we spend as if asleep, on automatic, following protocols or guidelines to some trite destination—or else we are dreaming of what we could do if we had more time, proper resources, and perhaps a different set of colleagues. But if we had Jung in our pockets he would be shaking us awake, derailing our guidelines, and saluting our attempts to risk genuine interactions with our patients, however much of a mess we make of it, and however much pain we cause and receive. (Pain, after all, is the inevitable companion to lives led authentically.)[1] To the unreflective doctor, and to all average minds, this interaction is anathema, to be avoided at all costs, because it leads us away from anaesthesia, to the unpredictable, and to destinations which are unknown.

After proposing that 'deep Thinking' can only be attained by someone capable of 'deep Feeling', Samuel Taylor Coleridge, in 1801, went on to calculate on the back of a jocular envelope that 'the Souls of 500 Sir Isaac Newtons would go to the making up of a Shakespeare or a Milton...Mind in his system is always passive...***and there is ground for suspicion that any system built on the passiveness of the mind must be a false system***'. 68 Newtonian models of the consultation in which the doctor remains unmoved are all tainted by this falsity. So when you find yourself being irritated, moved, or provoked by your patient, be half-glad, because these feelings welcome you to Shakespeare's and Coleridge's world where the imagination (p315) is the Prime Mover in the task of bringing about change in our patients.

So, every so often, be pleased with your difficult patients: those who question you, those who do not respond to your treatments, or who complain when these treatments *do* work. Often, it will seem that whatever you say is wrong, misunderstood, misquoted, and mangled by the mind you are confronting, perhaps because of fear, loneliness, or past experiences that you can only guess at. If this is happening, *shut up*—but don't *give up*. Stick with your patient. Listen to what he or she is saying and not saying. And when you have understood your patient a bit more, negotiate, cajole, and even argue—but don't bully or blackmail ("If you do not let your son have the operation he needs, I'll tell him just what sort of a mother you are ..."). When you find yourself turning to walk away from your patient, turn back and say "This is not going very well, is it? Can we start again?" Don't hesitate to call in your colleagues' help: not to win by force of numbers, but to see if a different approach might bear fruit. By this process, and by addressing the psychosomatic factors perpetuating your patient's illnesses, you and your patient may grow in stature. You may even end up with a truly satisfied patient. And a satisfied patient is worth a thousand protocols.

We all seek the reason for our own existence, and as we sit beside troubled, troubling, and troublesome patients we may dimly comprehend part of the reason, albeit in the background of our minds—even if, in the foreground, we are wondering why on earth this difficult patient has to exist, especially ***now*** when we are so busy and so stressed. The patient is likely to have their own unspoken metaphysical questions, for which you can be the midwife: "Why me?" "Why now?" Don't strangle these questions at birth: give them space to breathe, and who knows?

1 "Some say that the world is a vale of tears. I say it is a place of soul making"—John Keats, the first medical student to formulate these ideas about pain. They did not do him much good, as he died shortly after uttering them. But his ideas can do us good. Perhaps if each day we try at least once for authentic interactions with a patient, unencumbered by professionalism, research interests, defensive medicine, a wish to show off to our peers, or a wish to get though the day without fuss.

Medicine, art, and the humanities

If only we could live long enough to suffer from every disease, then we doctors, could be of real service to our patients. There would be no need for medical humanities, as we would understand angina from the inside, and the fire of zoster's pain would no longer mystify us. We could die a thousand deaths for our patients. But still death would be untamed, and our self-anecdotal knowledge of disease would be irrelevant to patients from foreign lands. All patients inhabit foreign lands, and even our own hearts are alien to us unless melted by narrative streams. It is only through the humanities that, prude or peasant, prince or prostitute, we can extend our horizons and universalize anecdotal experience, so that nothing human is foreign to us.

Doctor's and artist's methodologies overlap in that we both create new realities: artists do this by bewitchment and by suspending reality. Doctors do it by listening and suspending judgment. A patient one of us saw recently had been trapped in an abusive marriage for 52 years. She had tried telling one other person, who had not believed her. The relief of being believed and listened to shone through her tears, as we collaborated over plans to bring change to her life. It is good to aim to listen to our patients with as rapt attention as we display when reading a good book. While reading, there is no point in dissembling. We confront our subject with a steady eye because we believe, that, while reading to ourselves, we cannot be judged. Then, suddenly, when we are at our most open and defenceless, literature takes us by the throat—and that eye, which was so steady and confident a few minutes ago, is now perhaps misting over, or our heart is missing a beat, or our skin is covered in a goose-flesh more immediate than ever a Siberian winter produced. As the decades go by, not much in our mundane world sends shivers down our spines, but the power of art to do this ever grows, and sensitizes us to our patients' narratives, and shows us there are many valid routes to knowledge other than the strictly objective.

The reason for the ascendancy of art over science is simple. We scientists, when we are not adopting our listening role, are only interested in explaining reality. Artists are good at explaining reality too: but they also *create* it. Our most powerful impressions are produced in our minds not by simple sensations but by the association of ideas. It is a pre-eminent feature of the human mind that it revels in seeing something as, or through, something else: life refracted through experience, light refracted through jewels, or a walk through the woods transmuted into a Pastoral Symphony. Ours is a world of metaphor, fantasy, and deceit.

What has all this to do with the day-to-day practice of medicine? The answer lies in the word 'defenceless' above. When we read alone and for pleasure, our defences are down—and we hide nothing from the great characters of fiction. In our consulting rooms, and on the ward, we so often do our best to hide everything, beneath our avuncular bedside manner. So often, a professional detachment is all that is left after all those years inured to the foibles, fallacies, and frictions of our patients' tragic lives. It is at the point where art and medicine collide that doctors can re-attach themselves to the human race and re-feel those emotions that motivate or terrify our patients. We all have an Achilles heel: that part of our inner self which was not rendered invulnerable when we were dipped in the waters of our first disillusion. Art and literature may enable this Achilles heel to be the means of our survival as thinking and feeling human beings.

If it is true that all the great novels, songs, and drama defy any single interpretation it is all the more true for the patient sitting in front of us. If we are not getting very far it is because we are using light when we could be using shade—or harmony in place of disharmony, or we are only offering a monologue when what we should be risking is dialogue—and the forging of new meanings.

The American approach is to create Professors of Literature-in-Medicine and to conjure with concepts such as *the patient as text*, and most American medical schools do courses in literature in an attempt to inculcate ethical reasoning and speculation. Here, we simply intend to demonstrate, albeit imperfectly, in our writings and in our practice of medicine, that *every* contact with patients has an ethical and artistic dimension, as well as a technical one.

Contents

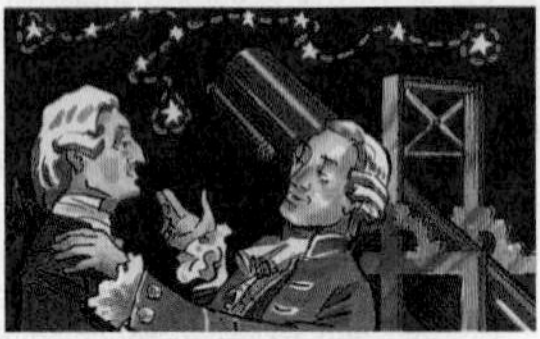

Fig 1. *Babbage* (looking at an astronomical image refracted through a prism): "I cannot see these lines you mention..."
Herschel: "An object is frequently not seen from not knowing how to see it, rather than from any deficit in the organ of vision. *I will instruct you how to see them...*".
...and so he did. Babbage was soon able to see the faint lines, the forerunners of the spectral lines which were to prove in 1861 that Betelgeuse, and subsequently every other known star is made of the elements we know on Earth (particularly sodium, calcium, magnesium, iron, chromium, nickel, barium, copper, and zinc). Herschel's great insight was that in seeing we do not simply register an image as in photography (a term he coined). The mind must be prepared for what we will see, otherwise it will remain obscure. This preparation is the purpose of this chapter. But who prepared the mind of the first observer of these spectral lines? Destiny, presumably. Many clinical signs have yet to be described. Keep looking. Sometimes a star is born (and whenever one is, it will be found to be made of familiar elements: precision, analogy, imagination, and curiosity).

Quote from Richard Holmes, 2008. *The Age of Wonder*, p440. Harper Press
(Babbage invented the first computer, and Herschel showed that our universe is an *evolving* structure).

Other relevant pages: acute abdomen (p608); lumps (p596-p606); hernias (p614-p616); varicose veins (p660); urine (p286); peripheral nerves (p456); dermatomes (p458). *In OHCS:* Vaginal examination (*OHCS* p242); abdominal examination in pregnancy (*OHCS* p40); the history and examination in children and neonates (*OHCS* p100-p102); examination of the eye (*OHCS* p412); visual acuity (*OHCS* p414); eye movements (*OHCS* p422); ear, nose, and throat examination (*OHCS* p536); skin examination (*OHCS* p584); examination of joints—see the contents page to *Orthopaedics and trauma* (*OHCS* p656).

A substantial number of images are taken from the **Oxford Handbook of Clinical Examination and Practical Skills (OHCEPS)**, *which gives an even more detailed account of this subject. Our thanks to Dr James Thomas and Dr Tanya Monaghan for their kind permission. We also thank Dr Owais Dar, who is our Specialist Reader for this chapter.*

Advice and experience

1 The way to learn physical signs is at the bedside, with guidance from an experienced colleague. This chapter is not a substitute for this process: it is simply an aide-mémoire both on the wards and when preparing for exams.

2 We ask questions to get information to help with differential diagnosis. But we also ask questions to find out about the lives our patients live so that we can respect them as individuals. The patient is likely to notice and reciprocate this respect, and it is this reciprocation that is the foundation of most of our therapeutic endeavours. Our challenge is to identify with as broad a range of humanity as possible, without getting exhausted by the scale of this enterprise. "Truth lies not only in what is said, but also in who says it, to whom, why, how, and under what circumstances". Vaclav Havel *Letters To Olga*.

3 Nobody set the puzzle that is the patient in front of you, so don't be surprised that some clues are ambiguous, and others are meaningless. Get good at recognizing patterns, but not so good that you create them when none are there. We all fall into this trap! Some signs will be your trusted friends for life; others such as the JVP will jilt you after your first date with them. We highlight the JVP here not because it is so important but because it teaches a lesson rarely alluded to: ***you can be a fine doctor without being able to elicit every sign.*** But because physical signs are fun, and bring out the Sherlock Holmes in us, and because the lay public haven't a clue about them, some insecure examiners insist that we should know them all—as our passport to the arcane inner sanctum of medicine. Don't go along with this! When baffled, don't bullshit: just say with quiet dignity: "Shall we move on?" or "Give me another clue."

The patient now waiting for you in cubicle 9...

The first news of your next patient will often be via a phone call: "There's an MI on the way in"—or "There's someone dementing in cubicle 9"—or "Can you take the overdose in resus?" On hearing such sanitized, dehumanized descriptions, our minds will start painting pictures, and the tone of these messages tends to colour these pictures. So when we arrive at the bedside, our mind is far from a *tabula rasa* or blank canvas on which the patient can paint his woes.

The mind always paints pictures, fills in gaps, and falls into traps. Perception is an active process, for, as Marcel Proust, that life-long all-knowing patient, observed[1]:

> *We never see the people who are dear to us save in the animated system, the perpetual motion of our incessant love for them, which before allowing the images that their faces present to reach us catches them in its vortex, flings them back upon the idea that we have always had of them, makes them adhere to it, coincide with it.*

So if you want to know your patient briefly contemplate him in the round before Proust's vortex whisks you off track. Divest yourself of those prejudices and expectations, which all good diagnosticians somehow ignore, and you will be all set for a gestalt recognition (p196) of incipient myxoedema (the cause of the dementia in cubicle 9—see p197), jaundice, anaemia, or, perhaps more important, the recognition that the person in front of you is frightened, failing, or dying.

Embracing the oral tradition

The written word has been with us only for a few thousand years. Even during this phase in history, epics, stories, methods, and teaching have still been passed on by word of mouth. It may be surprising, therefore, that we rely so much on the written word, given that so many important nuances can be missed.

In a working culture that has shifted from continuing care by multi-talented individuals towards an ever-changing team in a string of handovers, we might do well to uphold this oral tradition. So to keep the chain strong and care continuous, try to communicate face to face, at least when practical. At the least, to remain politic, we should continue to talk to each other.

1 *The Guermantes Way*, trans. CK Scott Moncrieff.

Taking (or receiving) histories is what most of us spend most of our professional life doing, and it is worth doing well. A good history is the biggest step towards correct diagnosis. History-taking, examination, and treatment begin the moment one reaches the bedside. (Divisions imposed by our page titles are somewhat misleading). Try to put the patient at ease: a good rapport may relieve distress. It often helps to shake hands. Introduce yourself and check whether patient is comfortable. Be conversational rather than interrogative in tone. General questions help break the ice and assess mental functions—sometimes important to establish early on.

Presenting complaint (PC) "What has been the trouble recently?" Record the patient's own words rather than eg 'dyspnoea'.

History of presenting complaint (HPC) When did it start? What was the first thing noticed? Progress since then. Ever had it before? '**SOCRATES**' questions: **s**ite; **o**nset (gradual, sudden); **c**haracter; **r**adiation; **a**ssociations (eg nausea, sweating); **t**iming of pain/duration; **e**xacerbating and alleviating factors; **s**everity (eg scale of 1-10, compared with childbirth/worst ever previous pain). ***Direct questioning*** (to narrow list of possible diagnoses) Specific questions about the differential diagnoses you have in mind (+risk factors, eg travel—p388) and a review of the relevant system.

Past medical history (PMH) Ever in hospital? Illnesses? Operations? Ask specifically about diabetes, asthma, bronchitis, TB, jaundice, rheumatic fever, high BP, heart disease, stroke, epilepsy, peptic ulcer disease, anaesthetic problems.

Drug history (DH) Any tablets, injections, 'off-the-shelf' or 'over-the-counter' drugs, herbal remedies, the Pill? Ask the features of allergies: may not have been one, or may have been a minor reaction of sensitization before full-blown anaphylaxis.

Social history (SH) Probe without prying. "Who else is there at home?" Job. Marital status. Spouse's job and health. Housing—any stairs at home? Who visits—relatives, neighbours, GP, nurse? Are there any dependents at home? Mobility—any walking aids needed? Who does the cooking and shopping? What can the patient not do because of the illness? The social history is all too often seen as a dispensable adjunct, eg while the patient is being rushed to theatre, but vital clues may be missed about the quality of life and it is too late to ask when the surgeon's hand is deep in the belly and she is wondering how radical a procedure to perform. It is worth cultivating the skill of asking a few searching questions of the admitting family doctor while you are conversing on the phone. If you are both busy, do not waste time on things you will shortly verify yourself but tap his knowledge of the patient and his 'significant others'. Remember: the GP is likely to be a specialist in his patients, whom he may have known for decades. He may even hold a 'living will' or advance directive to reveal your patient's wishes if he cannot speak for himself.

Alcohol, tobacco, recreational drugs How much? How long? When stopped? The CAGE questionnaire is useful as a screening test for alcoholism (p282). Quantify smoking in terms of **pack-years**: 20 cigarettes/day for 1 year equals 1 pack-year. Smoking is forbidden among Sikhs, so be tactful. We all like to present ourselves well, so be inclined to double stated quantities (Holt's 'law').

Family history (FH) Areas of the family history may need detailed questioning, eg to determine if there is a significant family history of heart disease you need to ask about the health of the patient's grandfathers and male siblings, smoking, tendency to hypertension, hyperlipidaemia, and claudication before they were 60 years old, as well as ascertaining the cause of death. Ask about TB, diabetes, and other relevant diseases. See BOX. ►**Be tactful when asking about a family history of malignancy.**

Functional enquiry (p22) helps uncover undeclared symptoms. Some of this may already have been incorporated into the history.

► Always enquire if your patient has any *ideas* of what the problem might be, if he/she has any particular *concerns* or *expectations*, and give him/her an opportunity to *ask you questions* or tell you *anything you may have missed*.

►Don't hesitate to retake the history after a few days: recollections change.

Drawing family trees to reveal dominantly inherited disease[1]

Advances in genetics are touching all branches of medicine. It is increasingly important for doctors to identify patients at high risk of genetic disease, and to make appropriate referrals. The key skill is drawing a family tree to help you structure a family history as follows:

1 Start with your patient. Draw a square for a male and a circle for a female. Add a small arrow (see below) to show that this person is the *propositus* (the person through whom the family tree is ascertained).

2 Add your patient's parents, brothers, and sisters. Record basic information only, eg age, and if alive and well (a&w). If dead, note age and cause of death, and pass an oblique stroke through that person's symbol.

3 Ask the key question "Has anybody else in your family had a similar problem as yourself?", eg heart attack/angina/stroke/cancer. Ask only about the family of diseases that relate to your patient's main problem. Do not record a potted medical history for each family member: time is too short.

4 Extend the family tree upwards to include grandparents. If you haven't revealed a problem by now, go no further—you are unlikely to miss important familial disease. If your patient is elderly it may be impossible to obtain good information about grandparents. If so, fill out the family tree with your patient's uncles and aunts on both the mother's and father's sides.

5 Shade those in the family tree affected by the disease. ● = an affected female; ■ = an affected male. This helps to show any genetic problem and, if there is one, will help demonstrate the pattern of inheritance.

6 If you have identified a familial susceptibility, or your patient has a recognized genetic disease, extend the family tree down to include children, to identify others who may be at risk, and who may benefit from screening. ►You must find out who is pregnant in the family, or may soon be, and arrange appropriate genetic counselling (*OHCS* p154).

The family tree below shows these ideas at work and indicates that there is evidence for genetic risk of colon cancer, meriting referral to a geneticist.

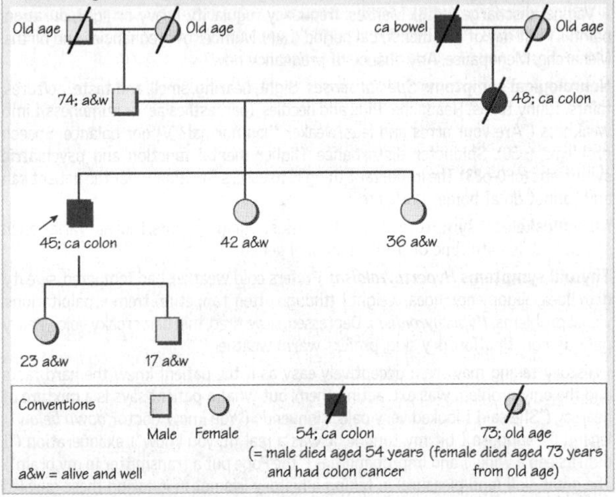

1 Use a different approach in paediatrics, and for autosomal or sex-linked disease. Ask if parents are related (consanguinity ↑risk of recessive diseases). This page owes much to Dr Helen Firth, whowe thank.

Just as skilled acrobats are happy to work without safety nets, so also older clinicians may operate without the functional enquiry. But to do this you must be experienced enough to understand all the nuances of the presenting complaint.

General questions may be the most significant, eg in TB, endocrine problems, or cancer: • Weight loss • Night sweats • Any lumps • Fatigue/malaise/lethargy • Sleeping pattern[1] • Appetite • Fevers • Itch or rash • Recent trauma[2]

Cardio-respiratory symptoms Chest pain (p88). Exertional dyspnoea (=breathlessness): quantify exercise tolerance and how it has changed, eg stairs climbed, or distance walked, before onset of breathlessness. Paroxysmal nocturnal dyspnoea (PND). Orthopnoea, ie breathlessness on lying flat (a symptom of left ventricular failure): quantify in terms of number of pillows the patient must sleep on to prevent dyspnoea. Oedema. Palpitations (awareness of heartbeats). Cough. Sputum. Haemoptysis (coughing up blood). Wheeze.

Gut symptoms Abdominal pain (constant or colicky, sharp or dull; site; radiation; duration; onset; severity; relationship to eating and bowel action; alleviating or exacerbating, or associated features). Other questions—think of symptoms throughout the GI tract, from mouth to anus:

- Swallowing (p240)
- Indigestion (p242)
- Nausea/vomiting (p240)
- Bowel habit (p246 & p248)
- Stool:
  - colour, consistency, blood, slime
  - difficulty flushing away (p280)
  - tenesmus or urgency

Tenesmus is the feeling of incomplete evacuation of the bowels (eg due to a tumour or irritable bowel syndrome). **Haematemesis** is vomiting blood. **Melaena** is altered (black) blood passed PR (p252), with a characteristic smell.

Genitourinary symptoms Incontinence (stress or urge, p650). Dysuria (painful micturition). Haematuria (bloody micturition). Nocturia (needing to micturate at night). Frequency (frequent micturition) or polyuria (the frequent passing of large volumes of urine). Hesitancy (difficulty starting micturition). Terminal dribbling.

Vaginal discharge (p418). Menses: frequency, regularity, heavy or light, duration, painful. First day of last menstrual period (LMP). Number of pregnancies and births. Menarche. Menopause. Any chance of pregnancy now?

Neurological symptoms *Special senses:* Sight, hearing, smell, and taste. Seizures, faints, 'funny turns'. Headache. 'Pins and needles' (paraesthesiae) or numbness. Limb weakness ("Are your arms and legs weaker than normal?"), poor balance. Speech problems (p80). Sphincter disturbance. Higher mental function and psychiatric symptoms (p80–p83). The important thing is to assess function: what the patient can and cannot do at home, work, etc.

Musculoskeletal symptoms Pain, stiffness, swelling of joints. Diurnal variation in symptoms (ie with time of day). Functional deficit.

Thyroid symptoms *Hyperthyroidism:* Prefers cold weather, bad tempered, sweaty, diarrhoea, oligomenorrhoea, weight↓ (though often ↑appetite), tremor, palpitations, visual problems. *Hypothyroidism:* Depressed, slow, tired, thin hair, croaky voice, heavy periods, constipation, dry skin, prefers warm weather.

►History-taking may seem deceptively easy, as if the patient knew the hard facts and the only problem was extracting them; but what a patient says is a mixture of hearsay ("She said I looked very pale"), innuendo ("You know, doctor, *down below*"), legend ("I suppose I bit my tongue; it was a real fit, you know"), exaggeration ("I didn't sleep a wink"), and improbabilities ("The Pope put a transmitter in my brain"). The great skill (and pleasure) in taking a history lies not in ignoring these garbled messages, but in making sense of them.

1 Too sleepy? Think of myxoedema or narcolepsy. Early waking? Think of depression. Being woken by pain is always a serious sign. ►For the significance of the other questions listed here, see Chapter 3.
2 Trauma is not just important because something may be broken, but because even if it seems trivial, it may provide the all-illuminating flash of insight which explains odd CNS features (eg post-traumatic subdural haemorrhage) or the vague prodromes of illnesses such as tetanus.

Presenting Mrs Dalloway, jargon, and confronting the whirlpool

We are forever presenting patients to our colleagues, almost never questioning the mechanisms and motivations that permeate these oral exchanges—and sometimes send them awry. By some ancient right we assume authority to retell the patient's story at the bedside, not in our own words but in highly stylized medical code: "Mrs Dalloway is a 51-year-old **Caucasian female**, a **known case of** menopausal dysphoria now presenting with intermittent delirium, **who complains of** paraesthesiae and weakness in her right **upper limb**… She **admits to drinking 21 units per week** and **other problems** are…" What is the purpose of this process of reverse alchemy by which we turn the gold of pure speech into the dross of medical jargon? The reason cannot be brevity, as if we are speaking in front of the patient, all that is in bold above could be omitted, or much curtailed. The next easy conclusion to confront is that we purposely use this jargon to confuse or deceive the patient. This is only sometimes the case. There must be deeper reasons for our medicalisms.

We get nearer to the truth when we realize that these medicalisms are used to sanitize and tame the raw data of our face-to-face encounters with patients—to make them bearable to us—so that however sordid or beautiful, however sad or profound, we can **think** about the patient rather than having to **feel** for him or her. This is quite right and proper—but only sometimes. We need the illusion that we are treading on well-marked-out territory when we are describing someone's pain—a problematic enterprise, not least because if the description is objective it is invalid (pain is, *par excellence*, subjective), and if it is subjective, it is partly incommunicable.

These medicalisms enrol us into a half-proud, half-guilty brotherhood. Proud because we hold the reins of life and death in our hands, and guilty because we are all dragged down by the unstated fear that our cures have never fully evolved from our ancient past of quackery and charlatanism. This is the reason why we are so pathologically loyal to each other and our jargon has the role of binding us into an unbeakable magic circle that ensures that what is unsayable remains unsaid.

The modulations of our voice, the stylized vocabulary, and the casual neglect of logic and narrative order ensure, in the above example, that we take on board so little of our patient that we remain upright, afloat, and (most dangerously) unfeeling, above the whirlpools of our patients' lives. So when you next hear yourself declaim in one breath that "Mrs D— is a 51-year-old Caucasian female with crushing central chest pain radiating down her left arm", take heed—what you may be communicating is that you have stopped thinking about this person—and pause for a moment. Look into your patient's eyes: confront the whirlpool...

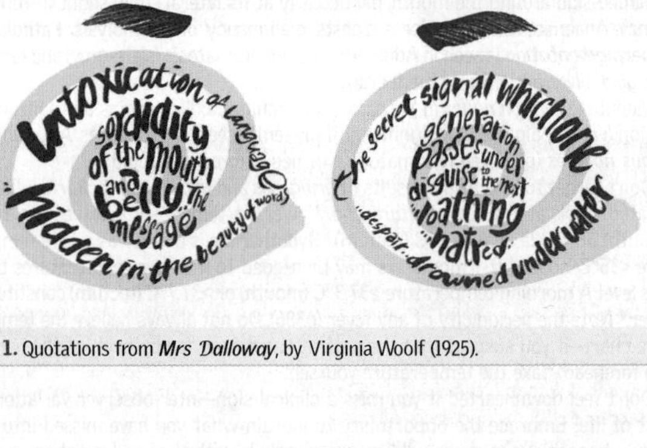

Fig 1. Quotations from *Mrs Dalloway*, by Virginia Woolf (1925).

The physical examination is not so much an extension of the history, but more of the first investigation, to confirm, exclude, define, or show the progress of the provisional diagnosis as revealed in the history. Even in the ED where the history may be brief, eg "trauma", the examination is to confirm a fracture, or to decide that a fracture is less likely, to define the blood loss, and to take baseline observations which may later reveal a subdural haematoma to be present. The examination sheds further light on the history. As you get better, your physical examination gets briefer. Establish your own routine—practice is the key.

Look at your patient as a whole to decide how sick he seems to be. Is he well or *in extremis*? Try to decide **why** you think so. Is he in pain? Does it make him lie still (eg peritonitis) or writhe about (eg colic)? What is the pattern of breathing: laboured; rapid; shallow; irregular; distressed? Is he obese or cachectic? Is his behaviour appropriate? Can you detect any unusual *smell* eg hepatic fetor (p258), cigarettes, alcohol? Also take a moment to look around the bed for other clues, eg inhalers, insulin administration kit, walking aids etc.

Specific diagnoses can often be made from ***the face and body habitus*** and these may be missed unless you stop and consider them: eg acromegaly, thyrotoxicosis, myxoedema, Cushing's syndrome, or hypopituitarism, see p196. Is there an abnormal distribution of body hair (eg bearded ♀, or hairless ♂) suggestive of endocrine disease? Is there anything about him to trigger thoughts about Paget's disease, Marfan's, myotonia, and Parkinson's syndrome? Look for rashes, eg the malar flush of mitral disease and the butterfly rash of SLE.

Assess the degree of ***hydration*** by examining the skin turgor, the axillae, and mucous membranes. Sunken orbits may also occur in dehydration. Check peripheral perfusion: eg press the nose/finger and time capillary return (CR)—it should be <2s in a well-hydrated individual. Record the temperature, and BP (lying and standing may suggest postural hypotension, a sign of shock).

Check for ***cyanosis*** (central and peripheral, p28). Is the patient *jaundiced*? Yellow skin is unreliable and may be produced by the lemon tinge of uraemia, pernicious anaemia, carotenaemia (in all these cases the sclerae are not yellow), or caecal carcinoma. The sign of jaundice is yellow sclerae seen in good daylight. ***Pallor*** is a nonspecific sign and may be racial, familial, or cosmetic. ***Anaemia*** is assessed from the palmar skin creases (when spread) and conjunctivae (**fig 1**, p319)—usually pale if Hb <8–9g/dL: you cannot conclude anything from **normal** conjunctival colour, but if they are pale, the patient is probably anaemic. Koilonychia and stomatitis (sore, dry, inflamed skin around the mouth, particularly at its lateral edge) suggest iron deficiency. Anaemia with jaundice suggests malignancy or haemolysis. Pathological ***hyperpigmentation*** is seen in Addison's, haemochromatosis (slate-grey) and ***amiodarone, gold, silver***, and ***minocycline*** therapy.

Palpate for ***lymph nodes*** in the neck (from behind), axillae, groins, and epitrochlear region (rarely palpable, but significant if present)—see p29 for causes. Any ***subcutaneous nodules*** (p597), eg rheumatoid, PAN, neurofibroma, sarcoid?

Don't forget to look at the results of ***urinalysis*** and ***urine output charts*** where indicated. Look at the ***temperature chart***. Average temperature values are 36.8°C (mouth), 36.4°C (axilla), 37.3°C (rectum).[1] **Hypothermia** is defined as a core temperature <35°C; special thermometers may be needed to measure temperatures below this level. A morning temperature ≥37.3°C (mouth) or >37.7°C (rectum) constitutes a **fever**.[2] Note the periodicity of any fever (p386). Do not always believe the temperature chart—if you suspect that the patient has a fever (eg by back-of-the-hand on the forehead), take the temperature yourself.

Don't feel downhearted if you miss a clinical sign—inter-observer variation is a fact of life! Embrace the opportunity to ingrain what you have missed into your own subconscious routine, building up your skills with time and practice.

1 The accuracy of different non-invasive methods for measuring T° is continually being assessed.
2 The nadir is at 6 AM, with a zenith at 6 PM; the mean amplitude of variability is 0.5°C.

Unexplained signs and symptoms: how to refer a patient for an opinion

►*When you don't know: ask.*

►*If you find yourself wondering if you should ask: ask.*

Frequently, the skills needed will lie beyond the team you are working on, so, during ward rounds, agree who should be asked for an opinion. You will be left with the job of making the arrangements. This can be a daunting task if you are very junior and have been asked to contact an intimidating registrar or consultant. Don't be intimidated: perhaps this may be an opportunity to learn something new. A few simple points can help the process go smoothly:

- Have the patient's notes, observations, and drug charts to hand.
- Be familiar with the history: you may be interrogated.
- Ask if it is a convenient time to talk.
- At the outset, state if you are just looking for advice or if you are asking if the patient could be seen. Make it clear exactly what the question is that you want addressed, "We wonder why Mr Smith's legs have become weak today...". This helps the listener to focus their thoughts while you describe the story and will save you wasting time if the switchboard has put you through to the wrong specialist.
- Give the patient's age and occupation to give a snapshot of the person.
- Run through a brief history including relevant past medical history. Do not present the case as if you are in finals—it will take ages to get to the point and the listener will get more and more irritated.
- If you would like the patient to be seen, give warning if they will be leaving the ward for a test at a particular time.
- It should not be necessary to write a long letter in the notes if you have given all the salient information available.
- The visiting doctor may be unfamiliar with your ward. When he or she arrives introduce yourself, get the notes and charts, and offer to introduce them to the patient. This will lead to all-round satisfaction and will make it easier to call the same doctor again.

Symptoms are features which patients report. **Physical signs** are elicited at the bedside. Together, they constitute the features of the condition in that patient. Their evolution over time, and interaction with the physical, psychological, and social spheres comprise the natural history of any disease. Throughout this chapter, we discuss symptoms in isolation and attempt to classify them into a 'system' or present them below as 'non-specific'. This is unnatural—but a good first step in learning how to diagnose. All doctors have to know about symptoms and their relief: this is what doctors are for. This chapter is disappointing in trying to explain *combinations* of symptoms and signs. It was this disappointment which was our stimulus to produce our electronic system, where over 20,000 signs, symptoms, and test results can be sifted in devious and diverse ways to help with difficult problems in differential diagnosis. See www.webmentorlibrary.com.

Itch

Itching (pruritus) is common and, if chronic, most unpleasant.

Local causes:	*Systemic:* (Do FBC, ESR, glucose, LFT, U&E, ferritin, TFT)	
Eczema, atopy, urticaria	Liver disease (bile salts eg PBC)	Old age; pregnancy
Scabies	Chronic renal failure	Drugs (eg morphine)
Lichen planus	Malignancy (eg lymphoma)	Diabetes mellitus
Dermatitis herpetiformis	Polycythaemia rubra vera	Thyroid disease
Spinal cord tumours (rare)[3]	Iron deficiency anaemia	HIV infection

Questions: Wheals (urticaria)? Worse at night? Others affected (scabies)? what provokes it? After a bath ≈ polycythaemia rubra vera (p360). Exposure, eg to animals (atopy?) or fibre glass (irritant eczema?) Look for ***local causes:*** Scabies burrows in finger webs, lice on hair shafts, knee and elbow blisters (dermatitis herpetiformis). ***Systemic:*** Splenomegaly, nodes, jaundice, flushed face or thyroid signs? ***Rx:*** Treat causes; try soothing bland emollients, eg E45®, ± emollient bath oils ± sedative antihistamines at night, eg chlorphenamine 4mg PO.

'Off-legs' - falls and walking difficulty

Common causes of admission in the elderly, and can lead to a spiral of loss of confidence and independence. Causes are often multifactorial: ***Intrinsic:*** typically osteo- or rheumatoid arthritis, but remember fractured neck of femur, CNS disease, vision↓, cognitive impairment, depression, postural hypotension, peripheral neuropathy, medication (eg antihypertensives, sedatives), pain eg arthritis, parkinsonism (eg drugs: prochlorperazine, neuroleptics, metoclopramide), muscle weakness, incontinence, UTI, pneumonia, anaemia, hypothyroidism, renal failure, hypothermia and alcohol. ***Environment:*** Poor lighting, uneven walking surface. Treatment includes addressing injuries, reducing risk factors, and reducing the risk of injury, eg treat osteoporosis (p696). A multidisciplinary multifactorial approach alongside occupational therapists and physiotherapists is likely to be beneficial.[4] See **gait disturbance,** p471.

If there is ataxia, the cause is not always alcohol: other chemicals may be involved (eg cannabis or prescribed sedatives). There may be a metastatic or non-metastatic manifestation of malignancy, or a cerebellar lesion.

►Bilateral weak legs may suggest a cord lesion: see p470. If there is associated urinary or faecal incontinence ± saddle anaesthesia or lower limb sensory loss, urgent imaging (MRI) and treatment for cord compression may well be needed.

Fatigue

So common that it is a variant of normality. Only 1 in 400 episodes of fatigue leads to visiting the doctor. ►Don't miss depression (p11). Even if depressed, still rule out common treatable causes—eg anaemia, hypothyroidism, diabetes. After history and examination: FBC, ESR, U&E, plasma glucose, TFT, ± CXR. Follow up to see what develops, and to address emotional problems.

Fevers, rigors, sweats

While some night sweating is common in anxiety, drenching sweats requiring changes of night-clothes are a more ominous symptom associated with infection (eg TB, brucellosis), lymphoproliferative disease, or mesothelioma. Patterns of fever may be relevant (see p386).

Rigors are uncontrolled paroxysms of shivering which occur as a patient's temperature rises rapidly. See p386.

Sweating excessively (hyperhidrosis) may be primary (eg hidradenitis suppurativa may be very distressing to the patient who may shun social encounters)—or be secondary to fever, pain or anxiety (cold & sweaty) or a systemic condition: the menopause, hyperthyroidism (warm & sweaty), acromegaly, malignancy, phaeochromocytoma, amyloidosis, or neuroleptic malignant syndrome (+hyperthermia). Or it may reflect gabapentin or opiate withdrawal, or a cholinergic or parasympathomimetic side effect (amitriptyline, bethanechol, distigmine, spider bites)—also hormonal drugs, eg levothyroxine, gonadorelin or somatostatin analogues, vasopressin, and ephedrine. Also amiodarone, ciprofloxacin, L-dopa, lisinopril, rivastigmine, ritonavir, pioglitazone, venlafaxine. At the bedside: Ask about all drugs, examine all over for nodes; any signs of hyperthyroidism? Any splenomegaly? Test the urine; do T°, ESR, TSH, FBC & blood culture. ℞: Antiperspirants (aluminium chloride 20%=Driclor®), sympathectomy, or iontophoresis may be tried.

Insomnia

This is trivial—until we ourselves have a few sleepless nights. Then sleep becomes the most desirable thing imaginable, and bestowing it the best thing we can do, like relieving pain. ►*No burden is heavier than perpetual consciousness.* Don't give drugs without looking for a cause.

- *Self-limiting:* Jet lag; stress; shift work; in hospital. We need less sleep as we age.
- *Psychic:* Depression; anxiety; mania; grief; psychomotor agitation/psychosis.
- *Organic:* Drugs (many; eg caffeine; mefloquine; nicotine withdrawal); nocturia; alcohol; pain (eg acid reflux—worse on lying down); itch; tinnitus; asthma; dystonias; obstructive sleep apnoea (p194); dementia. Rarities: restless leg syndrome (p712); encephalitis (eg West Nile virus) and encephalopathy (Whipple's; pellagra; HIV; prion diseases, eg CJD, p710, and fatal familial insomnia).

℞: **Sleep hygiene:** No daytime naps; don't turn in till you feel sleepy; regular bedtime routines. Keep a room for sleep; don't eat or work in it (not viable for much of the world). Less caffeine, nicotine, late exercise (but sexual activity may give excellent torpor) and alcohol (its abuse causes paradoxical pro-adrenergic tremor & insomnia).[5] Try monitoring quality with a sleep diary (unless already over-obsessive). There is no panacea for **non-restorative sleep**, but, as all *Sons and Lovers* know, "sleep is most perfect when it is shared with a beloved"[6]—hard in hospital. Music and relaxation may make sleep more restorative, and augment personal resources.[7]

Hypnotic drugs: give for a few nights only (addictive and cause daytime somnolence ± rebound insomnia on stopping). Warn about driving/machine use. Example: zopiclone 3.75–7.5mg. **Hypnosis** is a good alternative. *Obstructive sleep apnoea:* p194. *Parasomnias, sleep paralysis*, etc: *OHCS* p392. *Narcolepsy:* p714.

Cyanosis

Dusky blue skin (*peripheral*—of the fingers) or mucosae (*central*—of the tongue), representing ≥5g/dL of Hb in its reduced form, hence it occurs more readily in polycythaemia than anaemia. ***Causes:***

- ***Lung disease*** with inadequate oxygen transfer eg luminal obstruction, asthma, COPD, pneumonia, PE, pulmonary oedema—may be correctable by ↑ inspired O_2.
- ***Cyanotic congenital heart disease***, where there is admixture, eg transposition of the great arteries or right to left shunt (eg, VSD with Eisenmenger's syndrome; see p150)—cyanosis is *not* reversed by increasing inspired oxygen.
- ***Rare causes***: methaemoglobinaemia, a congenital or acquired red cell disorder.

►Acute cyanosis is a sign of impending emergency. Is there asthma, an inhaled foreign body, a pneumothorax (p763, **fig 1**) or pulmonary oedema? See p824.

Peripheral cyanosis will occur in causes of central cyanosis, but may also be induced by changes in the peripheral and cutaneous vascular systems in patients with normal oxygen saturations. It occurs in the cold, in hypovolaemia, and in arterial disease, and is therefore not a specific sign.

Pallor

May be racial or familial—or from anaemia, shock/faints, Stokes-Adams attack (p464, pale first, then flushing), hypothyroidism, hypopituitarism, and albinism. ►►If it's just one limb or digit, think of emboli. ***Anaemia*** is haemoglobin concentration below the normal range (p318). It may be assessed from the conjunctivae and skin creases. Koilonychia and stomatitis (p24) suggest iron deficiency. Anaemia with jaundice suggests haemolysis.

Skin discolouration

Generalized hyperpigmentation may be genetic (racial) or due to radiation; ↑ACTH (cross-reacts with melanin receptors, eg Addison's disease (p218), Nelson's syndrome (p32), ectopic ACTH in bronchial carcinoma); chronic renal failure (↑urea, p300); malabsorption; chloasma (seen in pregnancy or with the oral contraceptive pill); biliary cirrhosis; haemochromatosis ('bronzed diabetes'); carotenaemia; or drugs (eg chlorpromazine, busulfan, amiodarone, gold).

Obesity

(see *OHCS* p530)

This is defined by the World Health Organisation as a BMI of over 30kg/m^2. A higher waist to hip ratio, indicating central fat distribution, is commoner in ♂ and is associated with greater health risks, which include type 2 diabetes mellitus, IHD, dyslipidaemia, ↑BP, osteoarthritis of weight-bearing joints, and cancer (breast and bowel). The majority of cases are not due to specific metabolic disorders. Lifestyle change is key to treatment, to increase energy expenditure and reduce intake (p236). Medication ± surgery may be considered if the patient fulfils strict criteria. Conditions associated with obesity include: genetic (Prader-Willi syndrome, Lawrence-Moon syndrome), hypothyroidism, Cushing's syndrome and hypothalamic damage (eg tumour or trauma → damage to satiety regions).

Lymphadenopathy

Causes of lymphadenopathy are either reactive of infiltrative:

- **Reactive**
  - *Infective*
    - *Bacterial:* eg pyogenic, TB, brucella, syphilis.
    - *Viral:* EBV, HIV, CMV, infectious hepatitis.
    - *Others:* toxoplasmosis, trypanosomiasis.
  - ***Non-infective:*** sarcoidosis, amyloidosis, berylliosis, connective tissue disease (eg rheumatoid, SLE), dermatological (eczema, psoriasis), drugs (eg phenytoin).
- **Infiltrative**
  - *Benign histiocytosis—OHCS* p644, lipoidoses.
  - *Malignant*
    - *Haematological:* lymphoma or leukaemia: ALL, CLL, AML (p350).
    - *Metastatic carcinoma:* from breast, lung, bowel, prostate, kidney or head and neck cancers.

Oedema

(see p580)

Causes: ↑*Local venous pressure* eg DVT or right-heart failure ± ↓*intravascular oncotic pressure:* ↓plasma proteins, eg in cirrhosis, nephrotic syndrome, malnutrition, or protein-losing enteropathy: here water moves down the osmotic gradient into the interstitium to dilute the solutes there—Starling's principle. On standing, venous pressure at the ankle rises due to the height of blood from the heart (~100mmHg). This is short-lived if leg movement pumps blood through valved veins, but if venous pressure rises, or valves fail, capillary pressure rises and fluid is forced out causing oedema. ***Pitting oedema*** **(fig 1** & p580). ***Non-pitting oedema:*** (ie non-indentible) ≈ poor lymph drainage (lymphoedema), eg primary (Milroy's syndrome, p720) or secondary, due to radiotherapy, malignant infiltration, infection, filariasis. The mechanism is complex.[8]

Causes of eyelid oedema: Often contact dermatitis; angioedema; stings. If *proptosis* or T° ↑: cellulitis; cavernous sinus thrombosis; Graves' disease; EBV; sinusitis; Chagas' disease; anthrax; trichinella. If proteinuria: nephrosis; HSP (p716). Rarely: Wegener's disease; hypoalbuminaemia; SVC obstruction; dermatomyositis; SLE; sarcoid; amyloid; discoid lupus erythematosus; rosacea; cluster headache; sickle-cell disease; leukaemia; DIC.

Weight loss

This is a feature of chronic disease and depression; also of malnutrition, malignancy, chronic infections (eg TB, HIV/enteropathic AIDS), diabetes mellitus and hyperthyroidism (typically in the presence of increased appetite). Severe generalized muscle wasting is also seen as part of a number of degenerative neurological diseases and in cardiac failure (cardiac cachexia), although in the latter, right heart failure may not make weight loss a major complaint. Do not forget anorexia nervosa (*OHCS* p348) as an underlying cause of weight loss.

Focus on treatable causes, eg diabetes is easy to diagnose—TB can be very hard. For example, the CXR may look like cancer, so you may forget to send bronchoscopy samples for ZN stain and TB culture (to the detriment not just of the patient, but of the entire ward).

Cachexia

General muscle wasting from **famine,** or ↓**eating** (dementia; stroke; MND, p510; anorexia nervosa), **malabsorption** (enteropathic AIDS/slim disease/*Cryptosporidium*; Whipple's) or ↑**catabolism** (neoplasia; CCF; TB; chronic renal failure; leptin↑).[9]

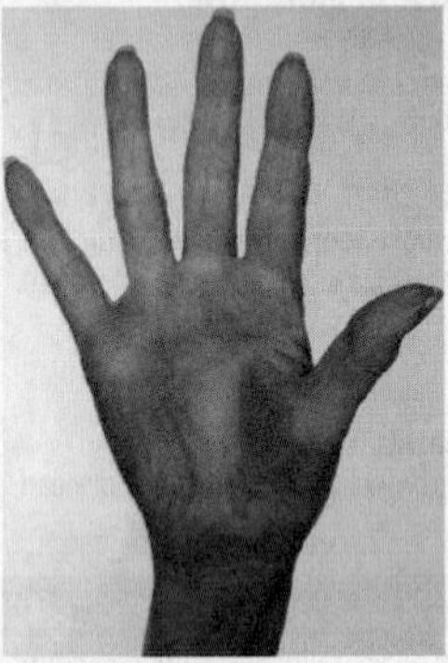

Fig 1. Palmar erythema.

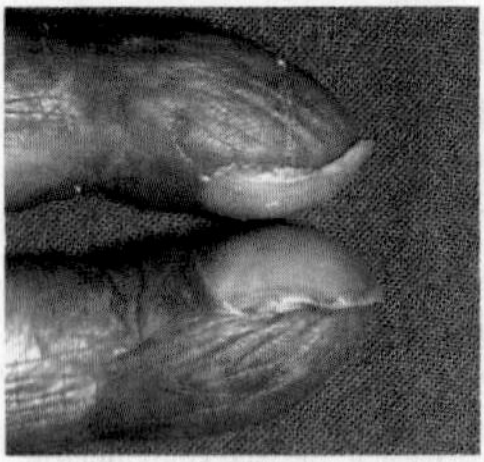

Fig 2. Finger clubbing.

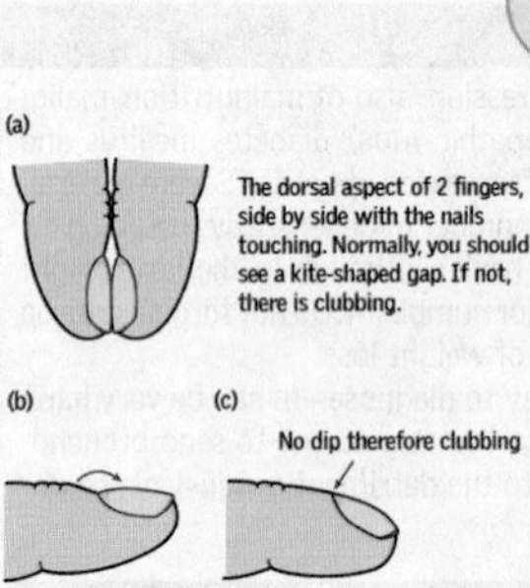

(a)
The dorsal aspect of 2 fingers, side by side with the nails touching. Normally, you should see a kite-shaped gap. If not, there is clubbing.
(b)
(c)
No dip therefore clubbing

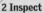

Fig 3. Testing for finger clubbing.

1 Introduction

Introduction, consent, position patient with hands resting on a pillow in patient's lap, expose arms (remove shirt). Enquire which hand, if any, is painful or tender.

2 Inspect

- *Skin:* palm and dorsum; erythema (fig 1), Dupytren's etc
- *Nails:* clubbing (see fig 2 & 3); pitting?
- *Muscle:* wasting?
- *Joints:* Heberden's , Bouchard's nodes
- *Bony deformities:* Boutonnière's, ulnar deviation, Z-deformity, swan neck, subluxation
- *Elbows:* rheumatoid nodules

3 Feel

- *Temperature:* of fingers and forearms, both sides
- *Tenderness:* palpate any abnormalities detected on inspection, palpate bones and joints systematically, and palpate anatomical snuff box (palpate areas where patient complains of tenderness last)

4 Move

- *Wrist:* test flexion: ask the patient to "put your hands together like this" **(fig 4)** and for extension: "and now like this" **(fig 5)**
- *Thumb:* with dorsum resting on pillow and palms facing the ceiling ask patient to "stick thumb out to the side (abduction), and don't let me push it back" (power), "now point thumb to ceiling" (abduction), "and don't let me push it back, and put thumb against palm" (adduction), "and don't let me pull it away, and finally touch your thumb to your little finger" (opposition), "and don't let me break the ring" (examiner must use little finger and thumb to attempt breaking the ring of examinee).
- *Fingers:* passively move each MCP and IP joint in turn assessing for limited range or crepitus, tell patient "spread your fingers" (abduction), "and don't let me push them together, now grip this piece of paper between your two fingers" (adduction), "and don't let me pull it away" (examiner must grip paper with same fingers as examinee), "now, squeeze my two fingers" (flexion and power grip).

5 Sensation

Detailed on p73

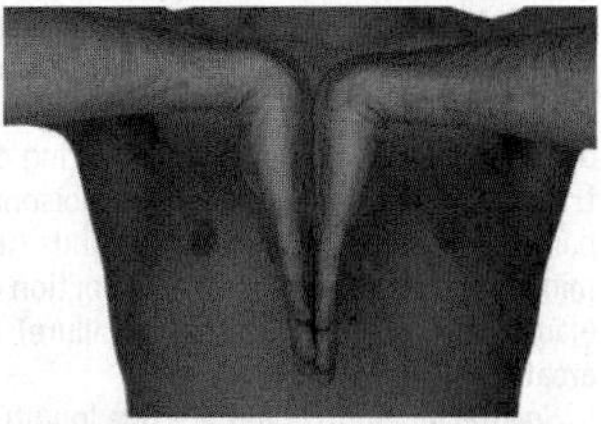

Fig 4. Wrist flexion tests: 'reverse-prayer position'.

6 Function

Ask patient to write name, fasten and unfasten a button, and pick up a coin from a flat surface

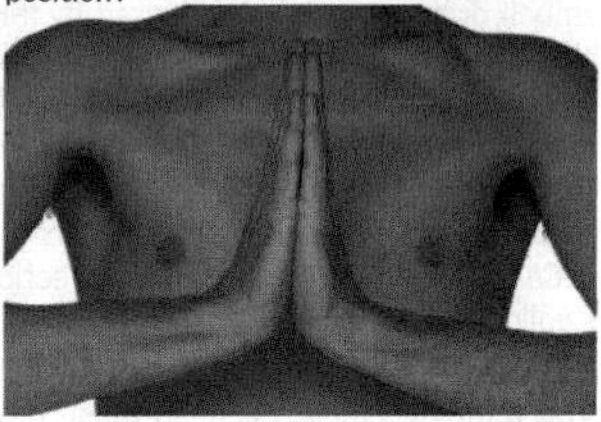

Fig 5. Wrist flexion tests: 'prayer position'.

7 Special tests

- *Tinel's sign:* percuss over distal skin crease of wrist—tingling? (carpal tunnel syndrome?)
- *Froment's sign:* "grasp paper between thumb and index finger"—?thumb flexes because can't adduct (ulnar nerve lesion).
- *Finkelstein's test:* get patient to flex thumb and ulnar deviate wrist—pain? (de Quervain's tenosynovitis?)
- *Phalen's test:* have patient make reverse prayer manoeuvre **(fig 4)** for 1 minute—tingling? (carpal tunnel syndrome?)

8 Complete examination

by examining neurological and vascular systems of the upper limb. Thank patient and wash hands.

A wealth of information can be gained from shaking hands and rapidly examining the hands of the patient. Is there a palsy or deformity—eg the patient may offer the other hand? Are they warm and well-perfused? Warm, sweaty hands signal hyperthyroidism while cold, moist hands may be due to anxiety. Are the rings tight with oedema? Lightly pinch the dorsum of the hand—persisting ridging of the skin means loss of tissue turgor (dehydration, or lack of connective tissue support from ageing). Are there any tar stains from tobacco use? Does the patient have difficulty releasing your hand after shaking it (dystrophia myotonica, p514)? Reluctance to let go is also a sign of loneliness. See also p540, p548 and p551)

Nails *Koilonychia* (spoon-shaped nails) suggests iron deficiency, fungal nail infection or Raynaud's. *Onycholysis* (nail destruction) is seen with hyperthyroidism, fungal infection, and psoriasis (**fig 2**, p553). *Beau's lines* (**fig 1**) are transverse furrows from temporary arrest of nail growth at times of ↑biological stress: malaria, typhus, rheumatic fever, Kawasaki disease, myocardial infarct, chemotherapy, Guillain-Barré & Raynaud's syndrome, trauma, high-altitude climbing, and deep sea diving.[11] As nails grow at ~0.1mm/d, the furrow's distance from the cuticle allows dating of the stress. *Mees' lines* are single white transverse bands seen in arsenic poisoning or renal failure. *Muehrcke's lines* are paired white parallel transverse bands (*without* furrowing)[12] seen eg in hypoalbuminaemia. *Terry's nails:* Proximal portion of nail is white/pink, nail tip is red/brown (causes: cirrhosis, chronic renal failure). *Pitting* is seen in psoriasis and alopecia areata.

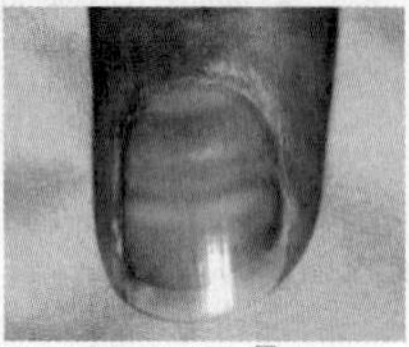

Fig 1. Beau's lines.[10]

Splinter haemorrhages are fine longitudinal haemorrhagic streaks (under nails), which in the febrile patient may suggest infective endocarditis. They may be microemboli, or be normal—being caused, by, for example, gardening. *Nail-fold infarcts* are characteristically seen in vasculitic disorders (OHCS, p 414).

Clubbing of the nails occurs with many disorders (p33). There is an exaggerated longitudinal curvature and loss of the angle between nail and nail fold (ie no dip). Also the nail feels 'boggy'. The cause is unknown but may be due to ↑blood flow through multiple arteriovenous shunts in the distal phalanges.

Chronic paronychia is a chronic infection of the nail-fold and presents as a painful swollen nail with intermittent discharge. Treatment: keep nails dry; antibiotics, eg *erythromycin* 250mg/6h PO and *nystatin* ointment.

The hands Changes occur in many diseases. *Palmar erythema* is associated with cirrhosis *et al* (see BOX 2). *Pallor* of the palmar creases suggests anaemia; *pigmentation* of the palmar creases (**fig 2**) is normal in Asians and blacks but is also seen in Addison's disease and Nelson's syndrome (↑ACTH after removal of the adrenal glands in Cushing's disease).[14] An odd rash on the knuckles (Gottron's papules) with dilated end-capillary loops at the nail fold suggests dermatomyositis (p554). *Dupuytren's contracture* (fibrosis and contracture of palmar fascia, p712) is seen in liver disease, trauma, epilepsy, and ageing.[15] Swollen proximal interphalangeal (PIP) joints with distal (DIP) joints spared suggest rheumatoid arthritis; swollen DIP joints suggest osteoarthritis, gout, or psoriasis. Look for *Heberden's* (DIP, **fig 3**) and *Bouchard's* (PIP) 'nodes'—osteophytes (bone over-growth at a joint) seen with osteoarthritis.

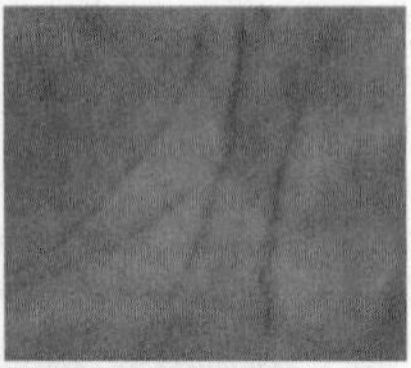

Fig 2. Hyperpigmented palmar creases.

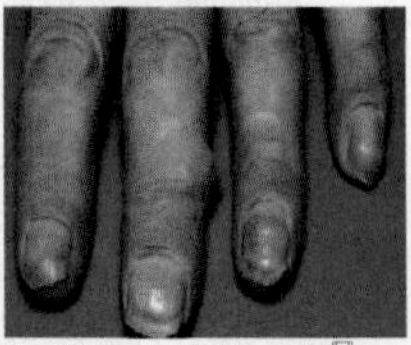

Fig 3. Heberden's node.[13]

Clubbing

Fingernails (± toenails) have ↑curvature in all directions and loss of the angle between nail and nail fold (**fig 2**, p30). The nail fold feels boggy. There are changes in local blood flow and ↑glucose metabolism,[16] but the exact mechanism is unclear. But as the causes (see below) are difficult to make sense of, and hence to remember, the platelet hypothesis is worth reflecting on (at least for some cases). Normal lung vascular beds retain platelet clumps and megakaryocytes, but if the lungs are: • Deranged, or there is • R-L shunting (hence cyanotic causes), or there are • AV malformations, or platelet clumps form on • damaged valves or • arterial grafts—then these clumps may impact in digital capillaries. Platelet-derived growth factor (±endothelial growth factor)[17] could explain all pathological changes in clubbing—and platelet clumps have been seen at necropsy in nail-bed capillaries of clubbed fingers.[18] Clubbing in liver disease is associated with multiple small pulmonary arteriovenous anastomoses (spider naevae are a related phenomenon) which could allow platelet clumps through. Also, chronic inflammatory conditions (such as Crohn's) are associated with ↑platelet production—and clubbing.

Hypertrophic osteoarthropathy entails clubbing, enlarged extremities, and symmetric painful periostitis (radius, fibula and, to a lesser degree, femur, humerus, metacarpals, and metatarsals). It may be primary (pachydermoperiostosis) or a nonmetastatic manifestation of lung cancer.

Causes

Thoracic:
- Bronchial lung ca (clubbing is twice as common in women); usually *not* small cell cancer)[19]
- Chronic lung suppuration
  - empyema, abscess
  - bronchiectasis
  - cystic fibrosis
- Fibrosing alveolitis
- Mesothelioma
- TB

GI:
- Inflammatory bowel disease (especially Crohn's)
- Cirrhosis
- GI lymphoma
- Malabsorption, eg coeliac

Rare:
Familial
- Thyroid acropachy (p564)
- Oesophageal cancer (rare)

Cardiovascular:
- Cyanotic congenital heart disease
- Endocarditis
- Atrial myxoma
- Aneurysms
- Infected grafts

Unilateral clubbing:
- (platelet hypothesis, above)
- Upper-limb artery aneurysm
- Brachial arteriovenous malformations

Palmar erythema

Causes: Pregnancy, hyperthyroidism, rheumatoid arthritis, polycythaemia, chronic liver disease—via ↓inactivation of vasoactive endotoxins by the liver. Also chemotherapy-induced palmar/plantar erythrodysaesthesia.[20]

History (see also p88) Ask about age, occupation, hobbies, sport, exercise and ethnic origin.

Presenting symptoms	**Direct questions**
Chest pain (see p88–9 and p796)	**S**ite? Central? **O**nset? (sudden? What was the patient doing?) **C**haracter? Ask patient to describe pain (crushing? heavy?) **R**adiation? Ask specifically if moves to arm, neck or jaw? **A**ssociations? Ask specifically about shortness of breath, nausea, sweating. **T**iming? duration? **E**xacerbating and alleviating factors? Worse with respiration or movement? (less likely to be angina), relieved by GTN? Worse on inspiration and better when sitting forwards (pericarditis)? **S**everity: out of 10? Also ask if patient is known to have angina or chest pain in the past; better/worse/same as usual pain; is it more frequent? Decreasing exercise tolerance? NB: 'heartburn' more likely if 'burning', onset after eating/drinking, or associated with dysphagia.
Palpitations (see BOX 1 & 2)	'Ever aware of your own heartbeat'? When & how did it start/stop? Duration? Onset sudden/gradual? Associated with blackout (how long)? Fast/slow? Regular/irregular? Ask patient to tap out the rhythm. Related to eating/drinking (especially coffee, tea, wine, or chocolate)?
Dyspnoea: (see BOX 3, p52; and p796)	Duration? At rest? On exertion? Determine exercise tolerance (And any other reason for limitation eg arthritis). NYHA classification (p131)? Worse when lying flat, how many pillows does the patient sleep with (**orthopnoea**)? Does the patient ever wake up in the night gasping for breath (**paroxysmal nocturnal dyspnoea**), and how often? Any ankle swelling?
Dizziness/ blackouts (see BOX and p464–467)	Did patient lose consciousness, and for how long (short duration suggests cardiac while longer duration suggests a neurological cause)? Any warning (**pre-syncope**)? What was patient doing at the time? Sudden/gradual? Associated symptoms? Any residual symptoms? How long did it take for patient to return to 'normal'? Any tongue biting (p 464–5), seizure, incontinence? Witnessed?
Claudication	SOCRATES? Specifically foot/calf/thigh/buttock? Quantify 'claudication distance', ie how long can patient walk before onset of pain? Rest pain?

(Screen for all above presenting symptoms before proceeding to past history.)

Past history Ask specifically about: angina, any previous heart attack or stroke, rheumatic fever, diabetes, hypertension, hypercholesterolaemia, previous tests/procedures (ECG, angiograms, angioplasty/stents, echocardiogram, cardiac scintigraphy, coronary artery bypass grafts (CABG)).

Drug history Particularly note aspirin/GTN/β-blocker/diuretic/ACE-i/digoxin/statin use

Ischaemic heart disease risk factors
• Smoking • Diabetes mellitus/BMI • Family history (1st degree relative <60yrs old with IHD) • Hypertension • Hyperlipidaemia • Renal disease • Deprivation

Family history Enquire specifically if any 1st degree relatives having cardiovascular events (especially if <60 years)

Social history Smoking, impact of symptoms on daily life

Palpitations

Palpitations represent to the patient the sensation of feeling his heart beat; to the doctor, the sensation of feeling his heart sink, as the symptom is notoriously elusive. Have the patient tap out the rate and rhythm of the palpitations. • Irregular fast palpitations are likely to be paroxysmal AF, or atrial flutter with variable block • Regular fast palpitations may reflect paroxysmal supraventricular tachycardia (SVT) or ventricular tachycardia (VT). • Dropped or missed beats related to rest, recumbency or eating are likely to be atrial or ventricular ectopics. • Regular pounding may be due to anxiety • Slow palpitations are likely to be due to drugs such as β-blockers, or bigeminus (**fig 1**, p122). Ask about associated chest pain, dyspnoea, and faints, suggesting haemodynamic compromise. Ask *when* it occurs: anxious people may be aware of their own heartbeat at night. Reassurance is vital and can often be therapeutic. If the diagnosis is not simply heightened awareness, do TSH and a 24h ECG. (Holter monitor, p102) Trans-telephonic event recording, if available, is better than 24h ECGs which miss some attacks.

Palpitations, Russian roulette, loose blood, and hypochondriasis

At night on my pillow the syncopated stagger
Of the pulse in my ear. Russian roulette:
Every heartbeat a fresh throw of the dice…
Hypochondria walked, holding my arm
Like a nurse, her fingers over my pulse…
The sudden lapping at my throat of loose blood.

Ted Hughes, *Birthday Letters*. Faber & Faber, by kind permission.

Dizziness

Dizziness is a loose term meaning: *vertigo* (p466), the illusion of rotation ± an unwilled need to cast oneself into any nearby abyss, ***or imbalance***, a difficulty in walking straight, from peripheral nerve, posterior column, cerebellar, or other central pathway failure ***or faintness***, ie 'light-headedness', seen in anaemia, ↓BP, postural hypotension, hypoglycaemia, carotid sinus hypersensitivity, and epilepsy. *'At the place where I stood, the hillside was cut away like a cliff, with the sea groaning at its foot, blue and pure. There was no more than a moment to suffer...how terrible was the dizziness of that thought! Twice I threw myself forward, and I do not know what power flung me back, still alive, on the grass which I kissed'* Gérard de Nerval 1837 (translated by Richard Holmes in *Footsteps*, 1996)

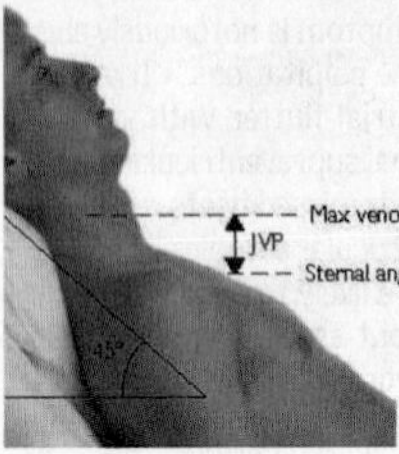

Fig 1. Measuring the JVP.

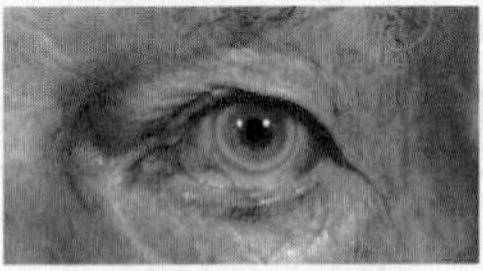

Fig 2. Corneal arcus.

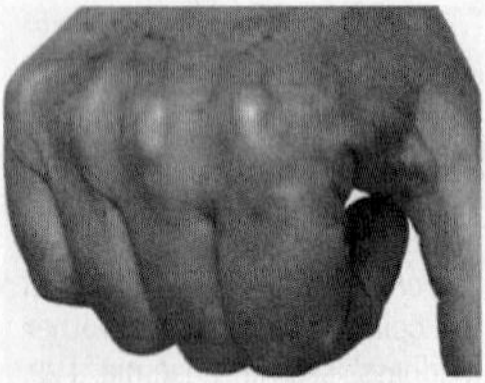

Fig 3. Tendon xanthomata.

Cardiovascular causes of clubbing
• Cyanotic congenital heart disease • Infective endocarditis • Atrial myxoma

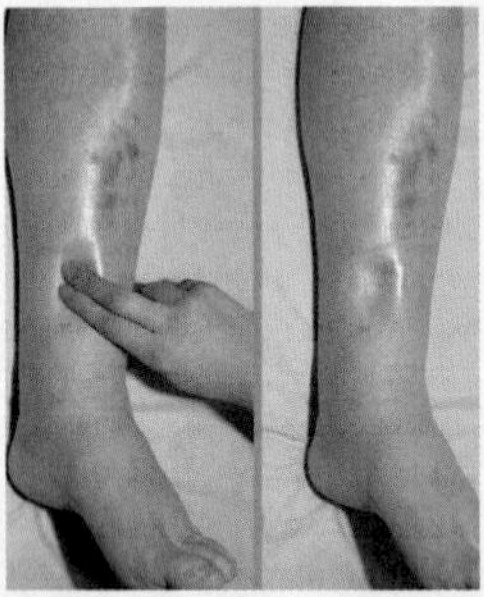

Fig 4. Pitting oedema, detected by applying firm pressure for a few seconds.

5 Face

- *Inspect:* jaundice, mitral flush, dental hygiene, xanthelasma, corneal arcus (**fig 2**), conjunctival pallor (warn patient before pulling down lower eyelid slightly; one side is sufficient), central cyanosis (ask patient to stick out tongue).

4 Blood pressure

3 Radial & brachial pulses

- *Radial:* (too far from heart to appreciate waveform) rate, rhythm; radial-radial delay (palpate pulse bilaterally simultaneously), radiofemoral delay (palpate ipsilateral pulses simultaneously), collapsing pulse (hold pulse with fingers of one hand, wrap the fingers of other hand around forearm, check "any pain in arm/shoulder?", lift arm up straight collapsing pulse, felt as 'waterhammer' pulsation in forearm).
- *Brachial:* (just medial to tendonous insertion of biceps). Waveform character.

2 Hands

- *Temperature*
- *Inspect:* clubbing (see MINIBOX), tobacco staining, cyanosis, tendon xanthomata (**fig 3**), signs of infective endocarditis: splinter haemorrhages, Janeway lesions, Osler's nodes.

1 General inspection

Introduction, consent, position patient sitting back at 45°, expose to waist and expose ankles (be considerate to ♀ patients, eg after general inspection use a towel to cover patient until palpating the chest (step 5). From foot of bed inspect for bedside clues ?Cyanosis (bluish tinge)/ pallor/malar flush/visible pulsations in the neck/appearance of breathlessness. Ask patient to sit forward; inspect for scars.
Whilst at the foot of the bed test for pitting oedema of the ankles (**fig 4**).

6 Neck
- *Carotid pulse:* (between larynx & sternomastoid) volume and character. Don't compress both carotids at once!
- *JVP:* ask patient to turn head away from you, press on liver and abdomen to aid identification (hepato- and abdominojugular reflux) (see **fig 1** and p40).

7 Palpating the praecordium
- '*Heaves*' & '*thrills*': place hand flat on chest to left then right of sternum (warn patient: "I'm going to examine your chest with my hands if that's OK"). **Heave:** sustained, thrusting usually felt at left sternal edge (= right ventricular enlargement). **Thrill:** palpable murmur felt as a vibration beneath your hand.
- *Apex beat (lowermost lateral pulsation):* **position:** displaced/undisplaced? Usually 5th intercostal space in mid-clavicular line; measure position in finger-breadths from mid-clavicular line, and by counting intercostal spaces (sternal notch lies at the level of 2nd intercostal space). **Character:** impalpable (?dextrocardia/COPD), tapping (palpable S_1)/double impulse/ sustained/strong. Count rate if pulse irregular (AF, p124); is there apical-radial pulse mismatch?

8 Auscultating the heart (see **fig 5**)
Feel for the pulse (felt at S_1, beginning of systole) at the same time as you listen, either at the apex or in the carotid artery.
Listen with bell and diaphragm at the apex (mitral area). Identify *1st & 2nd heart sounds*: are they normal? Listen for *added sounds* (p42) and *murmurs* (p44):
- At apex with bell, patient in left lateral position held in expiration ("Roll over onto your left side, now take in deep breath in and out...and hold it there" (*rumbling mid-diastolic murmur:* **mitral stenosis**?).
- At apex with diaphragm, patient held in expiration (*pansystolic murmur-* **mitral regurgitation**? If so listen for radiation in axilla).
- Lower left sternal edge (Tricuspid area) and pulmonary area (left of manubrium in the 2nd intercostal space): if suspect right-sided mumur, listen with patient's breath held in inspiration.
- Aortic area (right of manubrium in 2nd intercostal space; *ejection systolic murmur.* **aortic stenosis**? If so listen for radiation to the carotids).
- Sit the patient up and listen at the lower left sternal edge with patient held in expiration (*early diastolic murmur.* **aortic regurgitation**?)

9 Whilst patient is sitting forward...
- Palpate for *sacral oedema*
- *Lung bases:* auscultate for inspiratory crackles

10 Complete examination
Examine the abdomen, peripheral pulses, temperature chart, dip urine; examine retina by fundoscopy. Thank patient and wash hands.

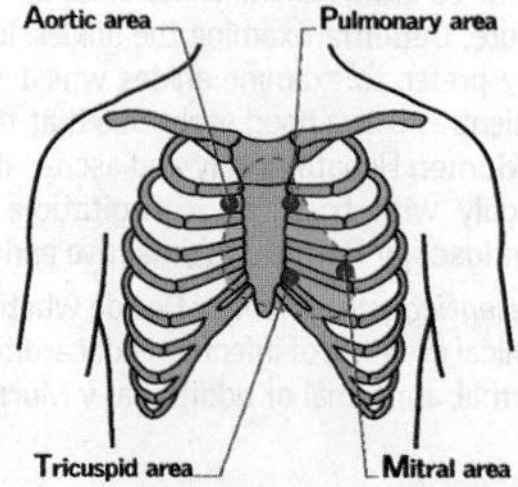

Fig 5. Auscultating the heart.
Figures 1-4 reproduced with permission from *Oxford Handbook of Clinical Examination and Practical Skills.*

1 General inspection Ill or well? In pain? Dyspnoeic? Are they pale, cold, and clammy? Can you hear the click of a prosthetic valve? Inspect for *scars*: median sternotomy (CABG; valve replacement; congenital heart disease). Inspect for any pacemakers.

2 Hands Finger clubbing occurs in congenital cyanotic heart disease and endocarditis. Splinter haemorrhages, Osler's nodes (tender nodules, eg in finger pulps) and Janeway lesions (red macules on palms, **fig 3**, p145) are signs of infective endocarditis. If found, examine the fundi for Roth's spots (retinal infarcts p386, **fig 1**). Are there nail fold infarcts (vasculitis, p558) or nailbed capillary pulsation (Quincke's sign in aortic regurgitation)? Is there arachnodactyly (Marfan's) or polydactyly (ASD)? Are there tendon xanthomata (**fig 3**, p36; hyperlipidaemia)?

3 Pulse See p42. Feel for *radio-femoral delay* (coarctation of the aorta) and *radio-radial delay* (eg from aortic arch aneurysm).

4 Blood pressure (see BOX) **Systolic BP** is the pressure at which the pulse is first heard as on cuff deflation; the **diastolic** is when the heart sounds disappear (Korotkov sound, K5) or become muffled (K4—use eg in the young, who often have no K5; state which you use). The *pulse pressure* is the difference between systolic and diastolic pressures. It is narrow in aortic stenosis and hypovolaemia, and wide in aortic regurgitation and septic shock. Defining hypertension is problematic: see p132. Examine the fundi for hypertensive changes (p133). **Shock** may occur if systolic <90mmHg (p804). *Postural hypotension* is defined as a drop in systolic >20mmHg or diastolic >10mmHg on standing (see BOX).

5 Face Is there corneal arcus (fig 2, p36) or xanthelasma (**fig 1**, p705, signifying dyslipidaemia, p704)? Is there a malar flush (mitral stenosis, low cardiac output)? Are there signs of Graves' disease, eg bulging eyes (exophthalmos) or goitre—p210)? Is the face dysmorphic, eg Down's syndrome, Marfan's syndrome (p720)—or Turner's, Noonan's, or William's syndromes (p143)?

6 Carotid pulse (p40) and **jugular venous pressure** (p41).

7 Praecordium Palpate the *apex beat*. Normal position: 5th intercostal space in the mid-clavicular line. Is it displaced laterally? Is it abnormal in nature: **heaving** (caused by outflow obstruction, eg aortic stenosis or systemic hypertension), **thrusting** (caused by volume overload, eg mitral or aortic incompetence), **tapping** (mitral stenosis, essentially a palpable 1st heart sound), **diffuse** (LV failure, dilated cardiomyopathy) or **double impulse** (H(O)CM, p146)? Is there dextrocardia? Feel for *left parasternal heave* (RV enlargement, eg in pulmonary stenosis, cor pulmonale, ASD) or *thrills* (transmitted murmurs).

8 Auscultating the heart Also auscultate for *bruits* over the carotids and elsewhere, particularly if there is inequality between pulses or absence of a pulse. Causes: atherosclerosis (elderly), vasculitis (young, p558).

9 and **10 Lungs** Examine the bases for creps & pleural effusions, indicative of cardiac failure. **Oedema** Examine the ankles, legs, sacrum, torso for pitting oedema. (You may prefer to examine ankles whilst standing at the foot of the bed inspecting patient as it is a good early clue that there may be further pathology to be found). **Abdomen** Hepatomegaly and ascites in right-sided heart failure; pulsatile hepatomegaly with tricuspid regurgitation; splenomegaly with infective endocarditis. **Fundoscopy** Roth spots (infective endocarditis) **Urine dipstick** Haematuria

Presenting your findings: Decide whether the patient has: **i** Signs of heart failure **ii** Clinical evidence of infective endocarditis **iii** Sinus/abnormal rhythm **iv** Heart sounds normal, abnormal or additional **v** Murmurs.

An unusual BP measurement

Don't interpret a BP value in isolation (p132). We cannot diagnose hypertension (or hypotension) on one BP reading, taken in isolation. Take into account pain, the 'white coat' effect, and equipment used.[21] Getting cuff size right is vital, as too small will give too high a reading, and too large will give a low reading. ►*Optimal cuff width is 40% of the arm circumference.* If you suspect a BP reading to be anomalous, check the equipment and review the observation chart for previous readings and other vital signs. Consider taking a manual reading with a different set yourself! Mercury sphygmomanometers are the type least likely to go wrong (and health risk is minimal).

Often a quiet chat will bring the BP down (yours and your patient's: keep your ears open, and the patient may reveal some new tangential but vital fact that the official history glossed over). Many things affect BP readings from background noise to how much you touch the patient. In general, professional touching (rather than social touching) *lowers* BP.[22] If BP ↑, eg ≥150/90, check both arms. If the systolic difference is >10mmHg, risk of MI and peripheral vascular disease is ↑;[23] [24] [25] reconfirm this: could he have a thoracic aortic aneurysm or coarctation (rare)? NB: right arm diastolic is normally 2.4–5mmHg higher than left.[26]

Postural hypotension

This is an important cause of falls and faints in the elderly. It is defined as a drop in systolic BP >20mmHg or diastolic >10mmHg after standing for 3min *vs* lying.[27] ***Causes:*** Hypovolaemia (early sign); drugs, eg nitrates, diuretics, antihypertensives; antipsychotics; Addison's (p218); hypopituitarism (↓ACTH), autonomic neuropathy (p509, DM, multisystem atrophy, p498), after a marathon run (peripheral resistance is low for some hours); idiopathic.

Treatment:

- Lie down if feeling faint.
- Stand slowly (with escape route: don't move away from the chair too soon!).
- Consider referral to a 'falls clinic', where special equipment is available for monitoring patient under various tilts.
- Manage autonomic neuropathy, p509.
- ↑Water & salt ingestion can help (eg 150mmol Na^+/d), but Na^+ has its problems.
- Physical measures: leg crossing, squatting, elastic abdominal binders/stockings (check dorsalis pedis pulse is present), and careful exercise may help.
- If post-prandial dizziness, eat little and often; ↓carbohydrate & alcohol intake.
- Head-up tilt of the bed at night ↑renin release, so ↓fluid loss and ↑standing BP.
- 1st-line drugs: fludrocortisone (retains fluid) 50µg/d; go up to 0.3mg/24h PO only if tolerated. Monitor weight; beware if CCF or ↓albumin: oedema worsens.[28] [29]
- 2nd-line: sympathomimetics, eg midodrine (not always available) or ephedrine;[30] pyridostigmine (eg if detrusor under-activity too);[31] erythropoietin. Some get a good response to half a Cafergot® suppository (caffeine 50mg + ergotamine 1mg).[32]

If these fail, turn things on their head and ask: *is this really supine hypertension?*

Xanthomata

Localized deposits of fat under the skin, occurring over joints (**fig 3**, p36), tendons, hands, and feet. They are a sign of dyslipidaemia (p704). ***Xanthelasma*** refers to xanthoma on the eyelid (p705, **fig 1**). ***Corneal arcus*** (**fig 2**, p36) is a crescentic-shaped opacity at the periphery of the cornea. Common in those over 60yrs, can be normal, but may represent hyperlipidaemia, especially in those under this age.

The internal jugular vein acts as a capricious manometer of right atrial pressure. Observe 2 features: the **height** (jugular venous pressure, JVP) and the **waveform** of the pulse. JVP observations are often difficult. Do not be downhearted if the skill seems to elude you. Keep on watching necks, and the patterns you see may slowly start to make sense—see BOX for the local venous anatomy. Relating the waveform to the arterial pulse (by concomitant palpation) will help to decipher patterns.

The height Observe the patient at 45°, with his head turned slightly to the left. Good lighting and correct positioning makes the examination a lot easier. Look for the right internal jugular vein as it passes just medial to the clavicular head of the sterno-cleidomastoid up behind the angle of the jaw to the ear lobes. The JVP is the vertical height of the pulse above the sternal angle (measured from the angle of Louis to the upper part of the JVP pulsation). It is raised if >4cm. Pressing on the abdomen normally produces a transient rise in the JVP. If the rise persists throughout a 15s compression, it is a **positive abdominojugular reflux sign.**[1] This is a sign of right ventricular failure, reflecting inability to eject the increased venous return.[33]

The waveform See BOX 1.

Abnormalities of the JVP

- ***Raised JVP with normal waveform:*** Fluid overload, right heart failure.
- ***Raised JVP with absent pulsation:*** SVC obstruction (p526).
- ***Large a wave:*** Pulmonary hypertension, pulmonary stenosis.
- ***Cannon a wave:*** When the right atrium contracts against a closed tricuspid valve, large 'cannon' a-waves result. *Causes:* complete heart block, single chamber ventricular pacing, ventricular arrhythmias/ectopics.
- ***Absent a wave:*** Atrial fibrillation.
- ***Large systolic v waves:*** Tricuspid regurgitation—look for earlobe movement.
- ***Constrictive pericarditis:*** High plateau of JVP (which rises on inspiration—Kussmaul's sign) with deep x and y descents.
- ***Absent JVP:*** When lying flat, the jugular vein should be filled. If there is reduced circulatory volume (eg dehydration, haemorrhage) the JVP may be absent.

Pulses

►Assess the radial pulse to determine rate and rhythm. **Character and volume** are best assessed at the brachial or carotid arteries. A **collapsing pulse** may also be felt at the radial artery when the patient's arm is elevated above his head. See BOX 2.

Rate Is the pulse fast (≥100bpm, p120) or slow (≤60bpm, p118)?

Rhythm An irregularly irregular pulse occurs in AF or multiple ectopics. A regularly irregular pulse occurs in 2° heart block and ventricular bigeminus.

Character and volume

- ***Bounding pulses*** are caused by CO_2 retention, liver failure, and sepsis.
- ***Small volume pulses*** occur in aortic stenosis, shock, and pericardial effusion.
- ***Collapsing ('waterhammer') pulses*** are caused by aortic incompetence, AV malformations, and a patent ductus arteriosus.
- ***Anacrotic (slow-rising) pulses*** occur in aortic stenosis.
- ***Bisferiens pulses*** occur in combined aortic stenosis and regurgitation.
- ***Pulsus alternans*** (alternating strong and weak beats) suggests LVF, cardiomyopathy, or aortic stenosis.
- ***Jerky pulses*** occur in H(O)CM.
- ***Pulsus paradoxus*** (systolic pressure weakens in inspiration by >10mmHg) occurs in severe asthma, pericardial constriction, or cardiac tamponade.

Peripheral pulses (See p34.) See p785 for arterial blood gas (ABG) sampling.

1 This sign was first described by W Pasteur in 1885, in the context of tricuspid incompetence. The term 'hepatojugular reflux' arose later, but was replaced by 'abdominojugular reflux' (not *reflex*!), as pressure over the middle of the abdomen, as well as over the liver, can be used to elicit the sign.

The jugular venous pressure wave

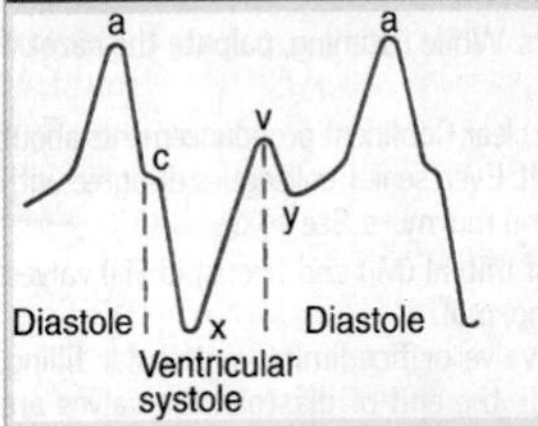

- a wave: atrial systole
- c wave: closure of tricuspid valve, not normally visible
- x descent: fall in atrial pressure during ventricular systole
- v wave: atrial filling against a closed tricuspid valve
- y descent: opening of tricuspid valve

The JVP drops as the x descent during ventricular systole because the right atrium is no longer contracting and the tricuspid valve is closed. This means that the pressure in the right atrium is dropping and this is reflected by the JVP.

The jugular venous system

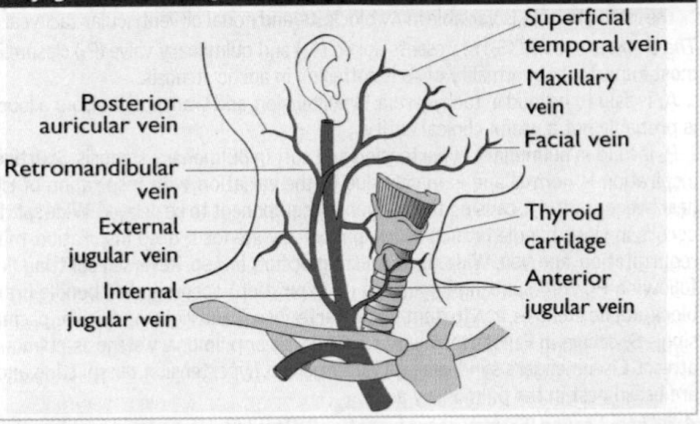

Is a pulse arterial or venous?

A venous pulse:
- Is not usually palpable.
- Is obliterated by finger pressure on the vessel.
- Rises transiently with pressure on abdomen (**abdominojugular reflux**) or on liver (**hepatojugular reflux**).
- Alters with posture and respiration.
- Usually has a double pulse for every arterial pulse.

Arterial pulse waveforms

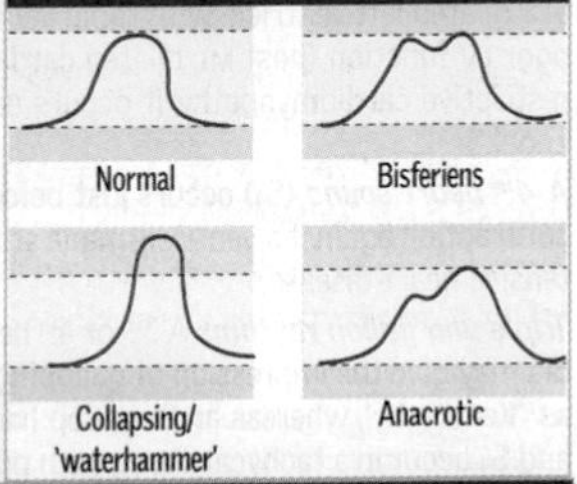

Inside the waterhammer

Before the age of video games, the waterhammer was a popular toy that consisted of a vacuum tube half-filled with water. On inversion, the whoosh of water produced an intriguing hammer-blow as it rushed from end to end. This is the alternative name for Corrigan's collapsing pulse—ie one in which the upstroke is abrupt and steep, whose peak is reached early and with abnormal force—before a rapid downstroke (as blood whooshes back into the left ventricle through an incompetent aortic valve).[34] Sometimes events conspire to put *us* in the waterhammer—rushing about in a vacuum tilted for the malicious pleasure of an unseen child. To let some air in, take a deep breath, and read all about Corrigan (p14).

Figs on this page after *Clinical Examination*, Macleod, Churchill & Aids to Undergraduate Medicine, J Burton, Churchill

►Listen systematically: sounds then murmurs. While listening, palpate the carotid artery: S_1 is synchronous with the upstroke.

Heart sounds The 1st and 2nd sounds are usually clear. Confident pronouncements about other sounds and soft murmurs may be difficult. Even senior colleagues disagree with one another about the more difficult sounds and murmurs. See BOX.

The 1st heart sound (S_1) represents closure of mitral (M_1) and tricuspid (T_1) valves. Splitting in inspiration may be heard and is normal.

In mitral stenosis, because the narrowed valve orifice limits ventricular filling, there is no gradual decrease in flow towards the end of diastole. The valves are therefore at their maximum excursion at the end of diastole, and so shut rapidly leading to a loud S_1 (the 'tapping' apex). S_1 is also loud if diastolic filling time is shortened, eg if the PR interval is short, and in tachycardia.

S_1 is soft if the diastolic filling time is prolonged, eg if the PR interval is long, or if the mitral valve leaflets fail to close properly (ie mitral incompetence).

The intensity of S_1 is variable in AV block, AF, and nodal or ventricular tachycardia.

The 2nd heart sound (S_2) represents aortic (A_2) and pulmonary valve (P_2) closure. The most important abnormality of A_2 is softening in aortic stenosis.

A_2 is said to be loud in tachycardia, hypertension, and transposition, but a loud A_2 is probably not a useful clinical entity.

P_2 is loud in pulmonary hypertension and soft in pulmonary stenosis. **Splitting** in inspiration is normal and is mainly due to the variation with respiration of right heart venous return, causing the pulmonary component to be delayed. **Wide splitting** occurs in right bundle branch block, pulmonary stenosis, deep inspiration, mitral regurgitation, and VSD. **Wide fixed splitting** occurs in ASD. **Reversed splitting** (ie A_2 following P_2, with splitting increasing on expiration) occurs in left bundle branch block, aortic stenosis, PDA (patent ductus arteriosus), and right ventricular pacing. A single S_2 occurs in Fallot's tetralogy, severe aortic or pulmonary stenosis, pulmonary atresia, Eisenmenger's syndrome (p150), large VSD, hypertension. **NB:** splitting and P_2 are heard best in the pulmonary area.

A 3rd heart sound (S_3) may occur just after S_2. It is low pitched and best heard with the bell of the stethoscope. S_3 is pathological over the age of 30yrs. A loud S_3 occurs in a dilated left ventricle with rapid ventricular filling (mitral regurgitation, VSD) or poor LV function (post MI, dilated cardiomyopathy). In constrictive pericarditis or restrictive cardiomyopathy it occurs early and is more high pitched ('pericardial knock').

A 4th heart sound (S_4) occurs just before S_1. Always abnormal, it represents atrial contraction against a ventricle made stiff by any cause, eg aortic stenosis or hypertensive heart disease.

Triple and gallop rhythms A 3rd or 4th heart sound occurring with a sinus tachycardia may give the impression of galloping hooves. An S_3 gallop has the same rhythm as '**Ken**-tucky', whereas an S_4 gallop has the same rhythm as 'Tenne-**ssee**'. When S_3 and S_4 occur in a tachycardia, eg with pulmonary embolism, they may summate and appear as a single sound, a summation gallop.

An ejection systolic click is heard early in systole with bicuspid aortic valves, and if BP↑. The right heart equivalent lesions may also cause clicks.

Mid-systolic clicks occur in mitral valve prolapse (p138).

An opening snap precedes the mid-diastolic murmur of mitral (and tricuspid) stenosis. It indicates a pliable (noncalcified) valve.

Prosthetic sounds are caused by nonbiological valves, on opening and closing: **rumbling sounds** ≈ ball and cage valves (eg Starr-Edwards); **single clicks** ≈ tilting disc valve (eg single disc: Bjork Shiley; bileaflet: St Jude—often quieter). Prosthetic mitral valve clicks occur in time with S_1, aortic valve clicks in time with S_2.

The cardiac cycle

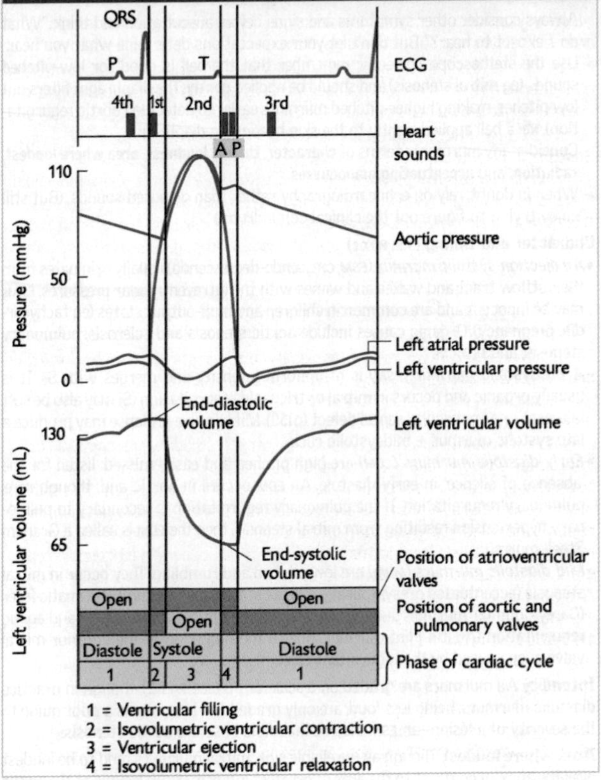
QRS
P
T
ECG
4th
1st
2nd
3rd
A
P
Heart sounds
110
50
0
Pressure (mmHg)
Aortic pressure
Left atrial pressure
Left ventricular pressure
End-diastolic volume
130
65
Left ventricular volume (mL)
Left ventricular volume
End-systolic volume
Open
Open
Open
Position of atrioventricular valves
Position of aortic and pulmonary valves
Diastole
Systole
Diastole
1
2
3
4
1
Phase of cardiac cycle
1 = Ventricular filling
2 = Isovolumetric ventricular contraction
3 = Ventricular ejection
4 = Isovolumetric ventricular relaxation

- ► Always consider other symptoms and signs before auscultation and think: "What do I expect to hear?" But don't let your expectations determine what you hear.
- ► Use the stethoscope correctly: remember that the bell is good for low-pitched sounds (eg mitral stenosis) and should be applied **gently**. The diaphragm filters out low pitches, making higher-pitched murmurs easier to detect (eg aortic regurgitation). NB: a bell applied tightly to the skin becomes a diaphragm.
- ► Consider any murmur in terms of **character, timing, loudness, area where loudest, radiation**, and **accentuating manoeuvres**.
- ► When in doubt, rely on echocardiography rather than disputed sounds. (But still enjoy trying to figure out the clinical conundrum!)

Character and timing (see BOX 1)

- *An ejection-systolic murmur* (ESM, crescendo-decrescendo) usually originates from the outflow tract and waxes and wanes with the intraventricular pressures. ESMs may be innocent and are common in children and high-output states (eg tachycardia, pregnancy). Organic causes include aortic stenosis and sclerosis, pulmonary stenosis, and H(O)CM.
- *A pansystolic murmur (PSM)* is of uniform intensity and merges with S_2. It is usually organic and occurs in mitral or tricuspid regurgitation (S_1 may also be soft in these), or a ventricular septal defect (p150). Mitral valve prolapse may produce a late systolic murmur ± midsystolic click.
- *Early diastolic murmurs (EDM)* are high pitched and easily missed: listen for the 'absence of silence' in early diastole. An EDM occurs in aortic and, though rare, pulmonary regurgitation. If the pulmonary regurgitation is secondary to pulmonary hypertension resulting from mitral stenosis, then the EDM is called a Graham Steell murmur.
- *Mid-diastolic murmurs (MDM)* are low pitched and rumbling. They occur in mitral stenosis (accentuated presystolically if heart still in sinus rhythm), rheumatic fever (Carey Coombs' murmur: due to thickening of the mitral valve leaflets), and aortic regurgitation (Austin Flint murmur: due to the fluttering of the anterior mitral valve cusp caused by the regurgitant stream).

Intensity All murmurs are graded on a scale of 1-6 (see TABLE), though in practice diastolic murmurs, being less loud, are only graded 1-4. Intensity is a poor guide to the severity of a lesion—an ESM may be inaudible in severe aortic stenosis.

Area where loudest Though an unreliable sign, mitral murmurs tend to be loudest over the apex, in contrast to the area of greatest intensity from lesions of the aortic (right 2nd intercostal space), pulmonary (left 2nd intercostal space) and tricuspid (lower left sternal edge) valves.

Radiation The ESM of aortic stenosis classically radiates to the carotids, in contrast to the PSM of mitral regurgitation, which radiates to the axilla.

Accentuating manoeuvres

- *Movements* that bring the relevant part of the heart closer to the stethoscope accentuate murmurs (eg leaning forward for aortic regurgitation, left lateral position for mitral stenosis).
- *Expiration* increases blood flow to the left side of the heart and therefore accentuates left-sided murmurs. *Inspiration* has the opposite effect.
- *Valsalva manoeuvre* (forced expiration against a closed glottis) decreases systemic venous return, accentuating mitral valve prolapse and H(O)CM, but softening mitral regurgitation and aortic stenosis. *Squatting* has exactly the opposite effect. *Exercise* accentuates the murmur of mitral stenosis.

Non-valvular murmurs *A pericardial friction rub* may be heard in pericarditis. It is a superficial scratching sound, not confined to systole or diastole. *Continuous murmurs* are present throughout the cardiac cycle and may occur with a patent ductus arteriosus, arteriovenous fistula, or ruptured sinus of Valsalva.

Typical waveforms of common heart murmurs

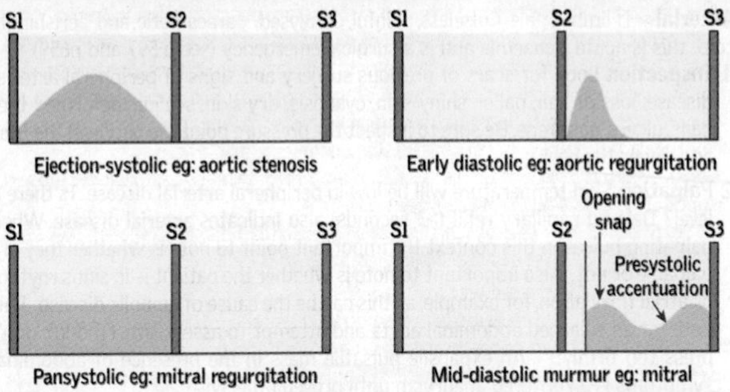

Grading intensity of heart murmurs

►The following grading is commonly used for murmurs—systolic murmurs from 1 to 6 and diastolic murmurs from 1 to 4, never being clinically >4/6.

Grade	Description
1/6	Very soft, only heard after listening for a while
2/6	Soft, but detectable immediately
3/6	Clearly audible, but no thrill palpable
4/6	Clearly audible, palpable thrill
5/6	Audible with stethoscope only partially touching chest
6/6	Can be heard without placing stethoscope on chest

Prosthetic valve murmurs

Prosthetic aortic valves All types produce a degree of outflow obstruction and thus have an ESM. Tilting single disc (eg Bjork Shiley) and bileaflet (eg St Jude) valves do not completely close and allow a regurgitant stream during diastole; hence they have a low-intensity diastolic murmur. The intensity of this murmur increases as the valve fails. Ball and cage valves (eg Starr-Edwards) and tissue valves **do** close completely in diastole and so any diastolic murmur implies valve failure.

Prosthetic mitral valves Ball and cage valves project into the left ventricle and can cause a low-intensity ESM as they interfere with the ejected stream. Tissue valves and bileaflet valves can have a low-intensity diastolic murmur. Consider any systolic murmur of loud intensity to be a sign of regurgitation and ∴ failure.

Arterial ▸▸ If limb is pale, pulseless, painful, paralysed, paraesthetic, and 'perishingly cold' this is acute ischaemia and is a surgical emergency (see p 597 and p659)

1 **Inspection** Look for scars of previous surgery and signs of peripheral arterial disease; loss of hair, pallor, shiny skin, cyanosis, dry skin, scaling, deformed toenails, ulcers, gangrene. Be sure to inspect the pressure points, ie between the toes and under the heel.

2 **Palpation** Skin temperature will be low in peripheral arterial disease. Is there a level? Delayed capillary refill (>3 seconds) also indicates arterial disease. When palpating pulses in this context the important point to note is whether they are palpable or not. Also important to note is whether the patient is in sinus rhythm or atrial fibrillation, for example, as this can be the cause of embolic disease. Palpate for an enlarged abdominal aorta and attempt to assess size. (Though don't press too firmly!) ▸▸An expansile pulsatile mass in the presence of abdominal symptoms is a ruptured aneurysm until proven otherwise.

3 **Auscultation** The presence of bruits suggests arterial disease.

4 **Special tests** ***Buerger's angle*** is that above the horizontal plane which leads to development of pallor (< 20° indicates severe ischaemia). ***Buerger's sign*** is the sequential change in colour from white to pink, upon return to the dependent position; if the limbs become flushed red (reactive hyperaemia) this is indicative of more severe disease.

5 Complete the examination by measuring the ABPI (p658), US doppler assessment for presence of pulses, and a neurological examination of the lower limbs.

Venous (see also p660)

1 **Inspection** Look for any varicosities and decide whether they are the long saphenous vein (medial), short saphenous vein (posterior, below the knee), or from the calf perforators (usually few varicosities but commonly show skin changes). Ulcers around the medial malleolus are more suggestive of venous disease, whereas those at the pressure points suggest arterial pathology. Brown haemosiderin deposits result from venous hypertension. There may also be atrophy and loss of skin elasticity (lipodermatosclerosis) in venous disease.

2 **Palpation** Warm varicose veins may indicate infection. Are they tender? Palpate the saphenofemoral junction (SFJ) for a saphena varix which displays a cough impulse. Similarly, incompetence at the saphenopopliteal junction (SPJ) may be felt as a cough impulse. If ulceration is present, it is prudent to palpate the arterial pulses to rule out arterial disease.

3 **Tap test** A transmitted percussion impulse from the lower limit of the varicose vein to the saphenofemoral junction demonstrates incompetence of superficial valves.

4 **Auscultation** Bruits over the varicosities means there is an arteriovenous malformation.

5 **Doppler** Test for the level of reflux. On squeezing the leg distal to placement of the probe you should only hear one 'whoosh' if the valves are competent at the level of probe placement.

6 **Tourniquet test** This is the more 'classical' test for the level of reflux. If the varicosities are controlled by the tourniquet then the level of incompetence is above the tourniquet. Note that all veins will refill eventually via the arterial system but rapid refill signifies superficial reflux. (Also ***Trendelenburg's test*** and ***Perthes' test***, p660)

7 Complete examination by examining the abdomen, pelvis in females and external genitalia in males (for masses).

Arterial

1 General inspection Introduction, consent, patient sitting back at 45°. Inspect skin (hair loss etc). Look between toes and lift up heels to inspect for ulcers.

2 Palpation
- *Temperature* bilaterally in thighs, legs, and feet
- *Capillary refill:* press/squeeze great toe until blanches, release, and measure time for colour to return
- *Peripheral pulses:* **Radial, brachial, carotid, femoral** (mid-inguinal point), **popliteal** (flex patient's knees slightly and press into centre of popliteal fossa; **fig 1**), **posterior tibial** (just posterior & inferior to medial malleolus) & **dorsalis pedis** (between bases of 1st & 2nd metatarsals); assess whether palpable bilaterally. Detect rate and rhythm. For brachial and carotid determine volume and character.
- *Abdominal aorta:* Palpate midline above umbilicus, position fingers either side of outermost palpable margins (**fig 2**).

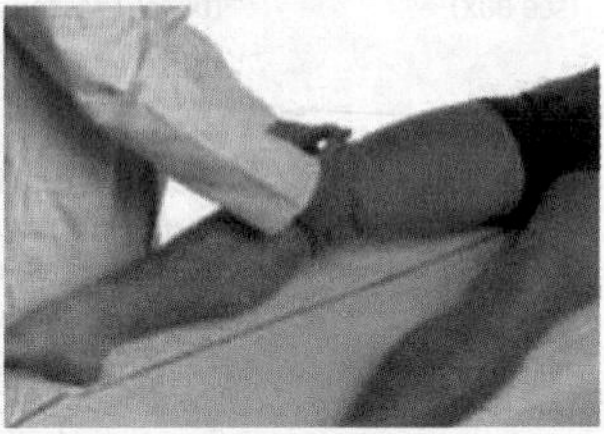

Fig 1. Peripheral pulses: popliteal.

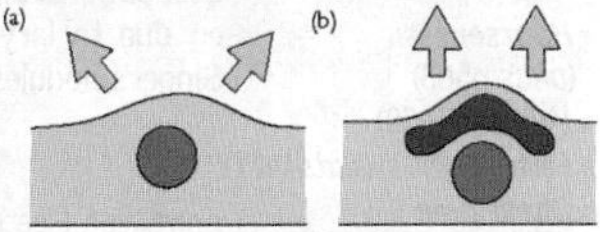

Fig 2. Pulses: Abdominal aorta
a) expansile (aneurysm?) b) transmitted.

Figures 1 and 2 reproduced with permission from *Oxford Handbook of Clinical Examination and Practical Skills*

3 Auscultation for carotid, femoral and aortic bruits

4 Special tests
Buerger's test: Lift both legs to 45° above the horizontal, supporting at heels. Allow a minute for legs to become pale. If they do, ask patient to sit up and swing around to lower legs to ground - observe colour change

5 Complete examination
Complete examination by using Doppler probe to detect pulses and measure ankle-brachial pressure index; conduct neurological examination of lower limbs.

Venous

1 Inspection Introduction, consent, patient sitting back at 45°. Inspect for varicosities & skin changes.

2 Palpation • *Temperature* of varicosities • Ask patient to cough while you *palpate for impulse at SFJ and SPJ.*

3 Tap test Percuss lower limit of varicosity & feel for impulse at SFJ.

4 Auscultation Listen for bruits over any varicosities.

5 Doppler Place probe over SFJ, squeeze calf & listen. Repeat with probe at SPJ.

6 Tourniquet test Elevate leg & massage veins to empty varicosities. Apply tourniquet to upper thigh. Ask patient to stand. If not controlled, repeat, placing tourniquet below knee.

7 Completion examinations of abdomen; rectum; pelvis (♀), genitals (♂).

History Age, race, occupation

Presenting symptoms	Direct questions
• ***Cough:*** (see BOX)	Duration? Character (eg brassy/barking/hollow)? Nocturnal (≈asthma, ask about other atopic symptoms, ie eczema, hayfever)? Exacerbating factors? Sputum (colour? How much?) Any blood/haemoptysis?
• ***Haemoptysis*** (see BOX)	Always think about TB (recent foreign travel?) and malignancy (weight loss?). Mixed with sputum? (Blood not mixed with sputum suggests pulmonary embolism, trauma, or bleeding into a lung cavity.), Melaena? (Occurs if enough coughed-up blood is swallowed).
• ***Dyspnoea:*** (see BOX) (p796)	Duration? Steps climbed/distance walked before onset? NYHA classification (p131)? Diurnal variation (≈asthma)? Focus on circumstances in which dyspnoea occurs (eg occupational allergen exposure).
• ***Hoarseness:*** (*OHCS* p568)	eg due to laryngitis, recurrent laryngeal nerve palsy, Singer's nodules, or laryngeal tumour.
• ***Wheeze*** (p50)	
• ***Fever/night sweats*** (p27)	
• ***Chest pain*** (p88 & p798)	SOCRATES (see p34)), usually 'pleuritic' if respiratory (ie worse on inspiration?)
• ***Stridor*** (see BOX)	

(Screen for all above presenting symptoms before proceeding to past history)

Past history Ask about: pneumonia/bronchitis; TB; atopy[1] (asthma/eczema/hay fever); previous CXR abnormalities; lung surgery; myopathy; neurological disorders.

Drug history Respiratory drugs (eg steroids, bronchodilators)? Any other drugs, especially with respiratory SE (eg ACE inhibitors, cytotoxics, β-blockers, amiodarone)?

Family history Atopy?[1] Emphysema? TB?

Social history Quantify smoking in 'pack-years' (20 cigarettes/day for 1 year = 1 pack-year). Occupational exposure (farming, mining, asbestos) has possible serious compensatory implications? Pets at home (eg birds)? Recent travel/TB contacts?

Stridor

Inspiratory sound due to partial obstruction of upper airways. Obstruction may be due to something within the lumen (eg foreign body, tumour, bilateral vocal cord palsy), within the wall (eg oedema from anaphylaxis, laryngospasm, tumour, croup, acute epiglottitis, amyloidosis), or extrinsic (eg goitre, oesophagus, lymphadenopathy, post-op stridor, after neck surgery). It's an emergency (↠p786) if gas exchange is compromised. **NB:** wheeze is an *expiratory* sound.

Characteristic coughs

Coughing is relatively nonspecific, resulting from irritation anywhere from the pharynx to the lungs. The character of a cough may, however, give clues as to the underlying cause:

- ***Loud, brassy coughing*** suggests pressure on the trachea, eg by a tumour.
- ***Hollow, 'bovine' coughing*** is associated with recurrent laryngeal nerve palsy.
- ***Barking coughs*** occur in croup.
- ***Chronic cough:*** Think of pertussis, TB, foreign body, asthma (eg nocturnal).
- ***Dry, chronic coughing*** may occur following acid irritation of the lungs in oesophageal reflux, and as a side effect of ACE inhibitors.

►Do not ignore a change in character of a chronic cough; it may signify a new problem, eg infection, malignancy.

1 Atopy implies predisposition to, or concurrence of, asthma, hay fever and eczema with production of specific IgE on exposure to common allergens (eg house dust mite, grass, cats).

Haemoptysis

Blood is *coughed up*, eg frothy, alkaline, and bright red, often in a context of known chest disease (*vomited* blood is acidic and dark).

Respiratory causes:

1 Infective	TB; bronchiectasis; bronchitis; pneumonia; lung abscess; COPD; fungi (eg aspergillosis); viruses (from pneumonitis, cryoglobulinaemia, eg with hepatitis viruses, HIV-associated pneumocystosis, or MAI, p411). Helminths: paragonimiasis (p445); hydatid (p444); schistosomiasis.[37]
2 Neoplastic	Primary or secondary.
3 Vascular	Lung infarction (PE); vasculitis (Wegener's; RA; SLE; Osler-Weber-Rendu); AV malformation; capillaritis.
4 Parenchymal	Diffuse interstitial fibrosis; sarcoidosis; haemosiderosis; Goodpasture's syndrome; cystic fibrosis.
5 Pulmonary hypertension	Pulmonary oedema; mitral stenosis; coarctation, idiopathic; Eisenmenger's syndrome (p150).
6 Coagulopathies	Any—eg thrombocytopenia, p338; DIC. (low platelets , p388).
7 Trauma/foreign body	eg post-intubation, or an eroding implanted defibrillator.
8 Pseudo-haemoptysis	Munchausen's (p720); aspirated haematemesis; red pigment (prodigiosin) from *Serratia marcescens* in sputum.[38]

Rare causes refuse to be classified neatly: vascular causes may have infective origins, eg hydatid cyst may count as a foreign body, *and* infection, *and* vascular if it fistulates with the aorta;[39] ditto for infected (mycotic) aneurysm rupture,[40] or TB aortitis. Infective causes entailing coagulopathy: dengue; leptospirosis.[41] Haemoptysis from *Pasteurella multocida* entails trauma (from cats) & infection.[42] Kaposi lung nodules are infectious & neoplastic.[43] In monthly haemoptysis, think of lung endometriosis.

℞ Haemoptysis may need treating in its own right, if massive (eg trauma, TB, hydatid cyst, cancer, AV malformation): call chest physician or surgeon (danger is drowning; lobe resection, endobronchial tamponade, or arterial embolization may be needed). Set up IVI, do CXR, blood gases, FBC, INR/APTT, crossmatch. If distressing, give *prompt* IV morphine, eg if inoperable malignancy.[44]

Dyspnoea

(see also p796)

Subjective sensation of shortness of breath, often exacerbated by exertion.

- *Lung*— airway and interstitial disease. May be hard to separate from cardiac causes; asthma may wake patient, and cause early morning dyspnoea & wheeze.
- *Cardiac*—eg ischaemic heart disease or left ventricular failure (LVF), mitral stenosis, of any cause. LVF is associated with ***orthopnoea*** (dyspnoea worse on lying; "How many pillows?") and *paroxysmal nocturnal dyspnoea* (PND; dyspnoea waking one up). Other features include ankle oedema, lung crepitations and ↑JVP.
- *Anatomical*—eg diseases of the chest wall, muscles, pleura. Ascites can cause breathlessness by splinting the diaphragm, restricting its movement.
- *Others* ►Any shocked patient may also be dyspnoeic (p804 & p609)—may be shock's presenting feature. Also anaemia or metabolic acidosis causing respiratory compensation, eg ketoacidosis, aspirin poisoning. Look for other clues—dyspnoea at rest *unassociated with exertion*, may be psychogenic: prolonged hyperventilation causes respiratory alkalosis. This causes a fall in ionized calcium leading to apparent hypocalcaemia. Features include peripheral and perioral paraesthesiae ± carpopedal spasm. Speed of onset helps diagnosis:

Acute	Subacute	Chronic
Foreign body	Asthma	COPD and chronic parenchymal diseases
Pneumothorax (p763, **fig 1**)	Parenchymal disease	Non-respiratory causes
Acute asthma	eg alveolitis	eg cardiac failure
Pulmonary embolus	pneumonia	anaemia
Acute pulmonary oedema	Effusion	

4 Neck
- *Trachea:* feel in sternal notch (deviated?), assess criocosternal distance in finger-breadths and feel for tracheal tug
- *Lymphadenopathy:* from behind with patient sat forward palpate lymph nodes of head and neck
- *JVP*

3 Face
- *Inspect:* for signs of Horner's, conjunctival pallor (warn patient before pulling down lower eyelid slightly- one side is sufficient), central cyanosis (ask patient to stick out tongue)

2 Hands
- *Inspect:* clubbing and tobacco staining
- *Asterixis:* ask patient to "hold arms out and cock your hands back like this" (see **fig 1**)
- *Pulse:* rate, rhythm, character
- *Temperature*
- *JVP*
- *Auscultation*

1 General inspection
Introduction, consent, position patient sitting back at 45°, expose to waist (be considerate to female patients, eg after general inspection use a towel to cover patient until palpating the chest (step 5). From foot of bed inspect for bedside clues? Cachectic/cyanosis (bluish tinge)/anaemia etc. Ask patient to sit forward; inspect for scars. Ask patient to take a deep breath in and out; any coughing/accessory muscle use/asymmetry etc?

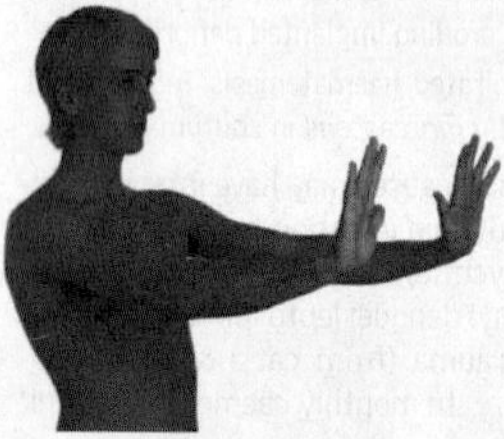

Fig 1. Asterixis. Looking for a flapping tremor: wrists are dorsiflexed and fingers spread.

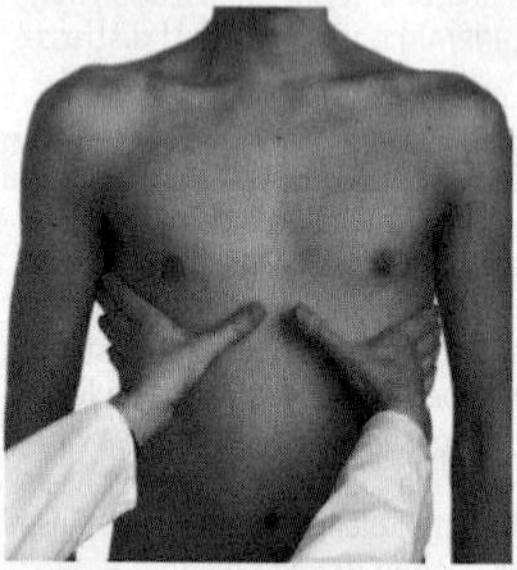

Fig 2. Placement of the hands for testing chest expansion: anchor with the fingers and leave the thumbs free-floating.

Respiratory causes of clubbing
• Lung carcinoma (usually not small cell) • Mesothelioma • Fibrosing alveolitis • Bronchiectasis • Cystic fibrosis • Empyema

5 Front of chest
(warn patient you are now going to examine their chest with your hands)

- *Apex beat*
- *Expansion:* Ask patient to "breathe all the way out", place hands as in **fig** 2, "now a deep breath in", and note distance thumbs to midline (same?); repeat with a hand on each lateral chest wall (symmetrical?), and in supramammary region with a hand flat either side of the midline (symmetrical?).
- *Tactile vocal fremitus:* Ask patient to repeat "99" each time they feel your hand while palpating the chest wall with the ulnar border of your hands over different respiratory segments (**fig 3**; test left and right of each before moving to next area).
- *Percussion:* Percuss (**fig 4**) over different respiratory segments, comparing right & left.
- *Auscultation:* Ask patient "can you take some deep breaths in and out through your mouth" (prompt with "keep going", or a demonstration if necessary!) and listen with diaphragm over different respiratory segments, comparing right and left.
- *Vocal resonance:* repeat auscultation asking patient to repeat "99" each time they feel the stethoscope. If marked $\uparrow$ resonance heard, repeat with asking patient to whisper "99"; if clearly heard this is termed 'whispering pectoriloquy'.

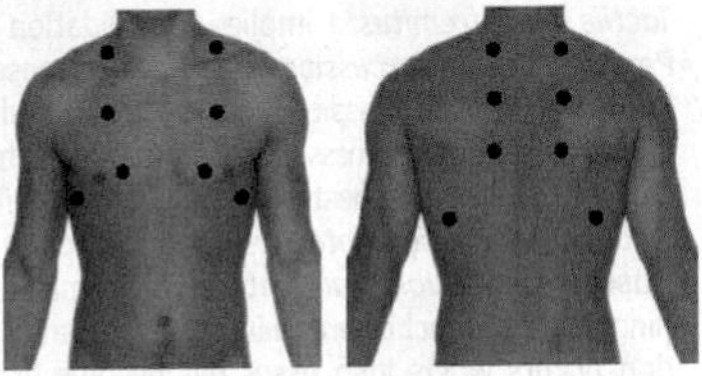

Fig 3. Areas of the chest to percuss. Test right versus left for each area, front and back.

6 Back of chest

- *Expansion*
- *Tactile vocal fremitus*
- *Percussion*
- *Auscultation*
- *Vocal resonance*

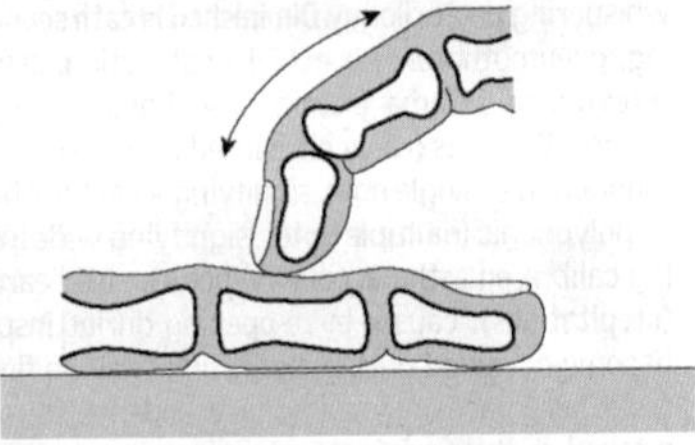

Fig 4. Percussing. Strike the firmly applied middle phalanx of the middle finger of the left hand, with the middle finger of the right hand.

Figures 1-4 reproduced with permission from *Oxford Handbook of Clinical Examination and Practical Skills*

7 Completion
Complete examination by examining sputum, temperature chart, O_2 saturation, and PEFR. Thank patient and wash hands.

Signs of respiratory distress
• Tachypnoea
• Nasal flaring
• Tracheal tug (pulling of thyroid cartilage towards sternal notch in inspiration)
• Use of accessory muscles (sternocleidomastoid, platysma, infrahyoid)
• Intercostal, subcostal and sternal recession
• Pulsus paradoxus (p40)

1 **General inspection** "Comfortable at rest" or unwell? Cachectic? **Respiratory distress**? (see MINIBOX; occurs if high negative intrapleural pressures needed to generate air entry). Stridor? **Respiratory rate, breathing pattern** (see BOX). Look for **chest wall & spine deformities** (see p55). Inspect for **scars** of past surgery, chest drains, or radiotherapy (skin thickening, tattoos demarcating irradiation field). **Chest wall movement**: symmetrical? (if not, pathology on restricted side). Paradoxical respiration? (abdomen sucked in with inspiration; seen in diaphragmatic paralysis, see p506).

2 **Hands** Clubbing, peripheral cyanosis, tar stains, fine tremor (β-agonist use), wasting of intrinsic muscles (T1 lesions, eg Pancoast's tumour, p722)? Tender wrists (hypertrophic pulmonary osteoarthropathy—cancer)? Temperature: warm (CO_2 retention)? Asterixis (CO_2 retention). Pulse: paradoxical (respiratory distress), bounding (CO_2 retention).

3 **Face** Ptosis & constricted pupil (Horner's syndrome, eg Pancoast's tumour, p722)? Bluish tongue and lips (central cyanosis, p28)? Conjunctival pallor (anaemia)?

4 **Neck** *Trachea* Central or displaced? (towards collapse or away from large pleural effusion/tension pneumothorax; slight deviation to right is normal). Cricosternal distance <3cm is hyperexpansion **Tracheal tug:** descent of trachea with inspiration (severe airflow limitation). *Lymphadenopathy:* TB/Ca? *JVP:* ↑ in cor pulmonale.

5 (& 6) Examining the chest:

- **Palpation** *Apex beat:* impalpable? (COPD/pleural effusion/dextrocardia?) *Expansion:* <5cm on deep inspiration is abnormal. ↓ expansion implies ipsilateral pathology. *Tactile vocal fremitus:* ↑ implies consolidation (< sensitive than vocal resonance).
- **Percussion** *Dull percussion note:* collapse, consolidation, fibrosis, pleural thickening, or pleural effusion (classically **'stony dull'**). **Cardiac dullness** usually detectable over the left side. Liver dullness usually extends up to 5th rib, right mid-clavicular line; below this, resonant chest is a sign of lung hyperexpansion (eg asthma, COPD). *Hyperresonant percussion note:* pneumothorax or hyperinflation (COPD).
- **Auscultation** *Quality and intensity:* Normal 'vesicular' breath sounds have a rustling quality. **Bronchial breathing:** hollow quality, gap between inspiration & expiration, occurs where lung tissue has become firm/solid, eg consolidation, localized fibrosis, above a pleural effusion, or next to a large pericardial effusion (Ewart's sign, p148). May be associated with increased tactile vocal fremitus, **vocal resonance**, and whispering pectoriloquy. **Diminished breath sounds:** pleural effusions, pleural thickening, pneumothorax, bronchial obstruction, asthma, or COPD. **Silent chest:** in life-threatening asthma (severe bronchospasm prevents adequate air entry. *Added sounds:* **Wheezes (rhonchi)**: caused by air expired through narrowed airways. May be monophonic (single note, signifying a partial obstruction of one airway, eg tumour) or polyphonic (multiple notes, signifying widespread narrowing of airways of differing calibre, eg asthma, COPD). Wheezes also heard in LVF ('cardiac asthma'). **Crackles (crepitations):** caused by re-opening, during inspiration, of small airways which have become occluded during expiration. May be fine and high pitched if coming from distal air spaces (eg pulmonary oedema, fibrosing alveolitis) or coarse and low pitched if they originate more proximally (eg bronchiectasis). Early inspiratory crackles suggest small airways disease (eg COPD), whereas late/pan-inspiratory crackles suggest disease confined to alveoli. Crackles disappearing on coughing are insignificant. **Pleural rubs:** caused by movement of visceral pleura over parietal pleura, when both surfaces roughened, eg by inflammatory exudate. Causes include adjacent pneumonia or pulmonary infarction. **Pneumothorax click:** produced by shallow left pneumothorax between layers of parietal pleura overlying heart, heard during cardiac systole

7 **Further examination** *Sputum* (see BOX), *temperature charts*, *O_2 sats*, PEFR.

Breathing patterns

Hyperventilation may be *fast* (tachypnoea, ie >20breaths/ min) or *deep* (hyperpnoea, ie tidal volume↑). Hyperpnoea is not unpleasant, unlike dyspnoea. It may cause respiratory alkalosis, hence paraesthesiae ± muscle spasm (Ca^{2+}↓). The main cause is anxiety: there is associated dizziness, chest tightness/pain, palpitations, and panic. Rare causes: response to metabolic acidosis; brainstem lesions.

- *Kussmaul respiration* is deep, sighing breaths in severe metabolic acidosis (it helps to blow off CO_2), eg diabetic or alcohol+fasting ketoacidosis,[45] renal failure.
- *Neurogenic hyperventilation* is produced by pontine lesions.
- The *hyperventilation syndrome* involves panic attacks associated with hyperventilation, palpitations, dizziness, faintness, tinnitus, alarming chest pain/tightness,[46] perioral and peripheral tingling (plasma Ca^{2+}↓). Treatment: relaxation techniques and breathing into a paper bag (↑ inspired CO_2 corrects the alkalosis).
- **NB:** the anxious patient in A&E with hyperventilation and a respiratory alkalosis may actually be presenting with an aspirin overdose (p856).

Cheyne–Stokes breathing Breaths get deeper and deeper, then shallower (±episodic apnoea) in cycles. *Causes:* Brainstem lesions or compression (stroke, ICP↑). If the cycle is long (eg 3min), the cause may be a long lung-to-brain circulation time (eg in chronic pulmonary oedema or ↓cardiac output). It is enhanced by opioids.

Sputum examination

Always inspect any sputum produced, however unpleasant this task may be. Send suspicious sputum for microscopy (Gram stain and auramine/ZN stain, if indicated), culture, and cytology.

- *Black carbon specks* in the sputum suggests smoking, the most common cause of increased sputum production.
- *Yellow/green sputum* suggests infection, eg bronchiectasis, pneumonia.
- *Pink frothy sputum* suggests pulmonary oedema.
- *Bloody sputum (haemoptysis)* may be due to malignancy, TB, infection, or trauma, and requires investigation for these causes. See p49.
- *Clear sputum* is probably saliva.

The respiratory segments supplied by the segmental bronchi

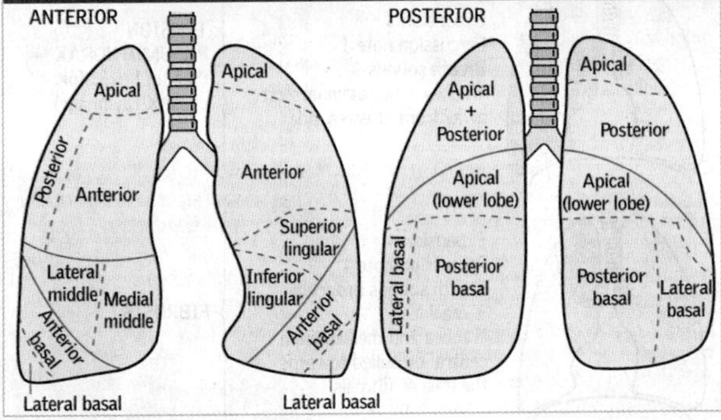

Physical signs on chest examination

Some physical signs

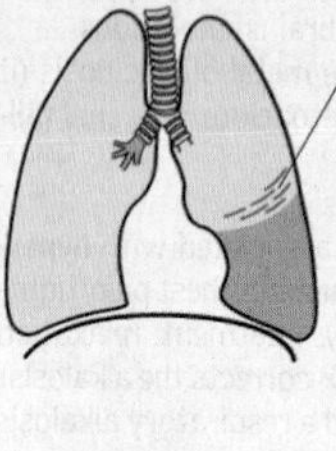

(There may be bronchial breathing at the top of an effusion)

Expansion: ↓
Percussion: ↓ (Stony dull)
Air entry: ↓
Vocal resonance: ↓
Trachea + mediastinum central (shift away from affected side only with massive effusions ≥1000mL)

} **PLEURAL EFFUSION**

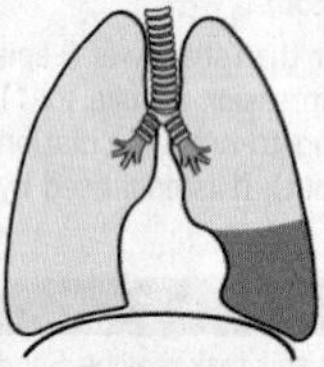

Expansion ↓
Percussion note ↓
Vocal resonance ↑
Bronchial breathing ± coarse crackles (with whispering pectoriloquy)
Trachea + mediastinum central

} **CONSOLIDATION**

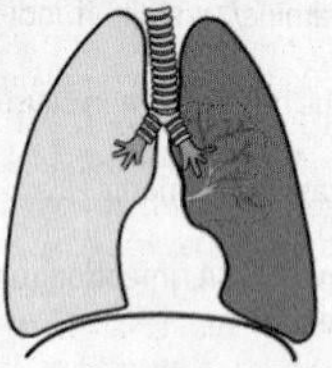

Expansion ↓
Percussion note ↑
Breath sounds ↓
Trachea + mediastinum shift towards the affected side

} **SPONTANEOUS PNEUMOTHORAX/ EXTENSIVE COLLAPSE (ΔΔ LOBECTOMY/ PNEUMONECTOMY)**

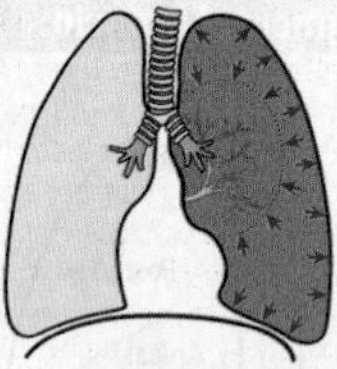

Expansion ↓
Percussion note ↑
Breath sounds ↓
Trachea + mediastinum shift away from affected side

} **TENSION PNEUMOTHORAX** (See fig 1 p763 for chest X-ray image)

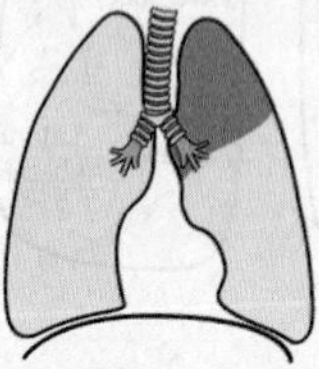

Expansion ↓
Percussion note ↓
Breath sounds bronchial ± crackles
Trachea and mediastinum central or pulled towards the area of fibrosis

} **FIBROSIS**

Chest deformities

- *Barrel chest:* AP diameter↑, tracheal descent and chest expansion↓, seen in chronic hyperinflation (eg asthma/COPD).
- *Pigeon chest (pectus carinatum):* See **fig 1**.
- *Funnel chest (pectus excavatum):* Developmental defect involving local sternum depression (lower end). See **fig 2**.
- *Kyphosis:* 'Humpback' from ↑ AP thoracic spine curvature.
- *Scoliosis:* Lateral curvature (*OHCS* p672); all of these may cause a restrictive ventilatory defect.

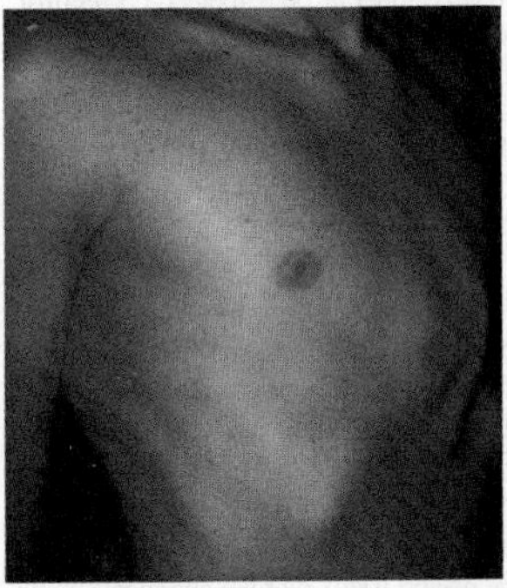

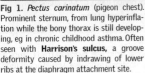

Fig 1. *Pectus carinatum* (pigeon chest). Prominent sternum, from lung hyperinflation while the bony thorax is still developing, eg in chronic childhood asthma. Often seen with **Harrison's sulcus,** a groove deformity caused by indrawing of lower ribs at the diaphragm attachment site.

Because these people hate exposing their chests they may become introverted, and never learn to swim. But it is wrong to let them sink without trace as merely a cosmetic problem. Be sympathetic, and remember Herr Minty, who inaugurated Graham Greene's theory of compensation: wherever a defect exists we must look for a compensating perfection to account for how the defect survives. In Minty's case, although "crooked and yellow and pigeon-chested he had his deep refuge, the inexhaustible ingenuity of his mind." *England Made Me*

Image courtesy of Prof Eric Fonkalsrud.[47]

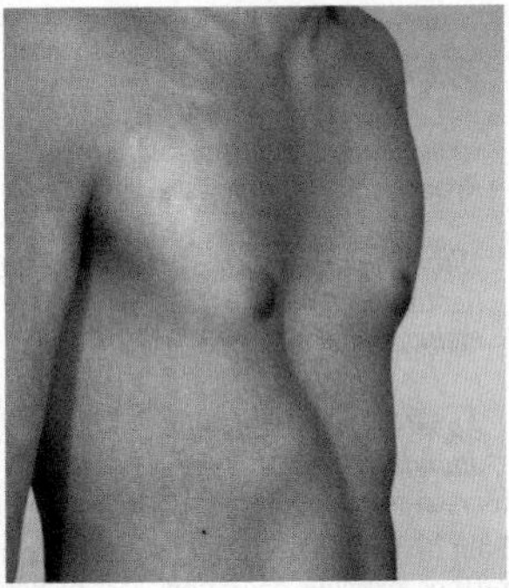

Fig 2. Pectus excavatum; the term for funnel or sunken chest. It is often asymptomatic, but may cause displacement of the heart to the left, and restricted ventilatory capacity ± mild air-trapping. Associations: scoliosis; Marfan's; Ehlers-Danlos syndrome. It is a common abnormality of the chest wall, often appearing during adolescent growth spurts. Exercise intolerance is the main symptom (from heart compression—do CXR/CT).[48] Psychological effects often exceed physical effects.[49] Indications for surgical correction: ≥2 of: a severe, symptomatic deformity; progression of deformity; paradoxical respiratory chest wall motion; pectus index >3.25 on CT; cardiac or lung compression; restrictive spirometry; cardiac pathology that might be from compression of the heart.[50]

Presenting symptoms	Direct questions
Abdominal pain (see BOX and p608)	'SOCRATES' (p34)
Distension (see BOX)	
Nausea, vomiting (see BOX)	Timing? Relation to meals? Amount? Content (liquid, solid, bile, blood) Frequency?
Haematemesis (p 252–4)	Fresh (bright red)/dark/'coffee grounds'? Consider neoplasia (weight loss, dysphagia, pain, melaena?), NSAIDs/Warfarin? Surgery? Smoking?
Dysphagia (p240)	Level? Onset? Intermittent? Progressive? Painful swallow (*odynophagia*)?
Indigestion/dyspepsia/reflux (p242)	Timing (relation to meals)?
Recent change in bowel habit	Consider neoplasia (weight loss, dysphagia, pain, melaena?)
Diarrhoea (p246), *constipation* (p248)	
Rectal bleeding (p631) or *melaena* (p252)	Pain on defecation? Mucus? Fresh/dark/black? Mixed with stool/ on surface/on paper/in the pan?
Appetite, weight change	Intentional? Quantify. Dysphagia? Pain?
Jaundice (p250).	Pruritus? Dark urine? Pale stools?

(Screen for all above presenting symptoms before proceeding to past history)

Past history Peptic ulcer disease, carcinoma, jaundice, hepatitis, blood transfusions, tattoos, previous operations, last menstrual period (LMP), dietary changes.

Drug history Especially steroids, the Pill, NSAIDs, antibiotics.

Family history Irritable bowel syndrome (IBS), inflammatory bowel disease (IBD), peptic ulcer disease, polyps, cancer, jaundice.

Social history Smoking, alcohol, recreational drug use, overseas travel, tropical illnesses, contact with jaundiced persons, occupational exposures, sexual orientation.

Vomiting

History is vital. Associated symptoms and past medical history often indicate cause. Examine for dehydration, distension, tenderness, abdominal mass, succussion splash (pyloric stenosis), or tinkling bowel sounds (intestinal obstruction).

Causes:

Gastrointestinal	CNS	Metabolic/endocrine
• Gastroenteritis	• Meningitis/encephalitis	• Uraemia
• Peptic ulceration	• Migraine	• Hypercalcaemia
• Pyloric stenosis	• ↑Intracranial pressure	• Hyponatraemia
• Intestinal obstruction	• Brainstem lesions	• Pregnancy
• Paralytic ileus	• Motion sickness	• Diabetic ketoacidosis
• Acute cholecystitis	• Ménière's disease	• Addison's disease
• Acute pancreatitis	• Labyrinthitis	
Alcohol and drugs:	**Psychiatric:**	**Others**[1]
• Antibiotics • Opiates	• Self-induced	• Myocardial infarction
• Cytotoxics	• Psychogenic	• Autonomic neuropathy
• Digoxin	• Bulimia nervosa	• Sepsis (UTI; meningitis)

[1] **How to remember the chief non-GI causes of vomiting?** Try **ABCDEFGHI**: **A**cute renal failure **A**ddison's disease; **B**rain (eg ↑ICP); **C**ardiac (myocardial infarct); **D**iabetic ketoacidosis; **E**ars (eg labyrinthitis, Ménière's disease); **F**oreign substances (alcohol; drugs, eg opiates); **G**ravidity (eg hyperemesis gravidarum) **H**ypercalcaemia/**H**yponatraemia; **I**nfection (eg UTI, meningitis).

Abdominal pain

Varies depending on the underlying cause. Examples: irritation of the mucosa (acute gastritis), smooth muscle spasm (acute enterocolitis), capsular stretching (liver congestion in CCF), peritoneal inflammation (acute appendicitis) and direct splanchnic nerve stimulation (retroperitoneal extension of tumour). The ***character*** (constant or colicky, sharp or dull), ***duration,*** and ***frequency*** depend on the mechanism of production. The ***location*** and ***distribution*** of referred pain depend on the anatomical site. ***Time of occurrence*** and ***aggravating*** or ***relieving factors*** such as meals, defecation, and sleep also have special significance related to the underlying disease process. The site of the pain may provide a clue:

- **Epigastric** Pancreatitis, gastritis/duodenitis, peptic ulcer, gall bladder disease, aortic aneurysm.
- **Left upper quadrant** Peptic ulcer, gastric or colonic (splenic flexure) cancer, splenic rupture, subphrenic or perinephric abscess, renal (colic, pyelonephritis).
- **Right upper quadrant** Cholecystitis, biliary colic, hepatitis, peptic ulcer, colonic cancer (hepatic flexure), renal (colic, pyelonephritis), subphrenic/perinephric abscess.
- **Loin** (lateral ⅓ of back between thorax and pelvis—merges with the flank, p567) Renal colic, pyelonephritis, renal tumour, perinephric abscess, pain referred from vertebral column. Causes of ***flank pain*** are similar (see index for fuller list).
- **Left iliac fossa** Diverticulitis, volvulus, colon cancer, pelvic abscess, inflammatory bowel disease, hip pathology, renal colic, urinary tract infection (UTI), cancer in undescended testis; zoster—wait for the rash! (p458). *Gynae:* Torsion of ovarian cyst, salpingitis, ectopic pregnancy. **Right iliac fossa pain** All causes of left iliac fossa pain plus appendicitis and Crohn's ileitis, but usually excluding diverticulitis.
- **Pelvic** *Urological:* UTI, retention, stones. *Gynae:* Menstruation, pregnancy, endometriosis (*OHCS* p288), salpingitis, endometritis (*OHCS* p274), ovarian cyst torsion.
- **Generalised** Gastroenteritis, irritable bowel syndrome, peritonitis, constipation.
- **Central** Mesenteric ischaemia, abdominal aneurysm, pancreatitis.
- ***Remember referred pain:*** Myocardial infarct → epigastrium; pleural pathology.

Abdominal distension (masses and the 'famous five' Fs)

Enid Blyton's Famous Five characters can generally solve any crime or diagnostic problem using 1950s methodologies steeped in endless school holidays, copious confection-laden midnight feasts, and lashings of homemade ginger beer.

Let's give them the problem of abdominal distension. The sweets and drinks used by the Famous Five actually contribute to the distension itself: fat, fluid, faeces, flatus, and fetus. If you think it far-fetched to implicate ginger beer in the genesis of fetuses, note that because it was homemade, like the fun, there was no limit to its intoxicating powers in those long-gone vintage summers.

Enid Blyton did her best to minimize the risks of unwanted pregnancies by gender reassignment (George) and by making one of her characters a dog (Timmy)—but accidents *must* have happened, even in the 1950s. The point is to think to ask "When was your last period?" *whenever* confronted by a distended abdomen.

Flatus will be resonant on percussion. Fluid will be dull, and can be from ascites (eg from malignancy or cirrhosis: look for shifting dullness), distended bladder (cannot get below it) or an aortic aneurysm (expansile). Masses can be pelvic (think of uterine fibroids or ovarian pathology) or tumours from colon, stomach, pancreas, liver, or kidney. Also see causes of ***ascites with portal hypertension*** (p606), ***hepatomegaly*** (p63), ***splenomegaly,*** and ***other abdominal masses*** (p606).

Faecal incontinence

This is common in the elderly. Do your best to help. Find out who does the washing: they may be severely stressed (Social Services may help with laundry). Causes: often multifactorial. Is it passive faecal soiling or urgency-related stool loss? The symptom may resolve if diarrhoea (p246) or constipation (p248) is treated (='overflow diarrhoea'—do PR to check for this, and anal tone, p633). ***GI causes:*** Rectal prolapse, tumour, sphincter laxity, severe piles, ↓storage capacity (inflammatory bowel disease, past surgery, irradiation). Others: see BOX. ***Tests:***[51] Anal sonography; barium defecography; anorectal manometry; puborectalis EMG; pelvic MRI.

Non-GI causes:

CNS	⏩spinal cord or cauda equina compression or trauma (S_2–S_4); myelitis/myeloradiculitis (treatable eg if infective—T°↑?; WCC↑?);[52] Parkinson's disease; stroke; MS; dementia.
Endocrine	Diabetes mellitus (autonomic neuropathy); hypothyroidism.
Pelvic floor lesions/ dysfunction	♀: prolapse; puborectalis or nerve root tears, or rectovaginal fistula at birth. Both sexes: weak pelvic floor muscles;[53] pelvic floor dyssynergia (paradoxical contraction of pelvic floor muscles with alternating constipation and incontinence—biofeedback helps).[54]
Drugs	Olanzapine and risperidone (due to reduced anal tone).[55]

►Do PR (overflow incontinence? Poor tone?). Refer to a specialist (esp. if rectal prolapse, anal sphincter injury, lumbar disc disease, or alarm symptoms for Ca. colon exist). Evacuation proctography and MRI may be needed.[56] ***Treat according to cause and to promote dignity:*** ►Never let your own embarrassment stop you from offering help. **Geography:** Ensure toilet is in easy reach. Plan trips away in the knowledge of toilet locations. **Behaviour:** Obey call-to-stool impulses (esp. after-meal, ie the gastro-colic reflex). **Knowledge:** Ensure access to latest continence aids and advice on use. **Pelvic floor rehabilitation:** for example can help faecal incontinence, squeeze pressure, and maximal tolerated volume.[57] Loperamide 2-4mg 45min before social engagements may prevent accidents outside home.[58] An anal cotton plug may help isolated internal sphincter weakness.[59] **Skin care. Support agencies.**[2007 NICE]

If all sensible measures fail, try a brake-and-accelerator approach: enemas to empty the rectum (twice weekly) and codeine phosphate, eg 15mg/12h on non-enema days to constipate. It's not a cure, but makes the incontinence manageable.

Flatulence

Normally, 400-1300mL of gas is expelled PR in 8-20 discrete (or indiscrete) episodes per day.[60] If this, with any eructation (belching) or distension, seems excessive to the patient, he may complain of flatulence. Eructation occurs in hiatus hernia—but most patients with 'flatulence' have no GI disease. Air swallowing (aerophagy) is the main cause of flatus; here N_2 is the chief gas. If flatus is mostly methane, H_2 and CO_2, then fermentation by bowel bacteria is the cause,[61] and reducing carbohydrate intake (eg less lactose and wheat) may help.[62] The more foetid the flatus, the more likely that malabsorption (eg coeliac) is to blame.[63]

Tenesmus

This is a sensation in the rectum of incomplete emptying *after* defecation. It's common in irritable bowel syndrome (p276), but can be caused by a tumour.

Regurgitation

Gastric and oesophageal contents are regurgitated effortlessly into the mouth—without contraction of abdominal muscles and diaphragm (so distinguishing it from true vomiting). It may be worse on lying flat, and can cause cough and nocturnal asthma. Regurgitation is rarely preceded by nausea, and when due to gastro-oesophageal reflux, it is often associated with heartburn. An oesophageal pouch may cause regurgitation. Very high GI obstructions (eg gastric volvulus, p613) cause non-productive retching rather than true regurgitation

Steatorrhoea

These are pale stools that are difficult to flush, and are caused by malabsorption of fat in the small intestine and hence greater fat content in the stool. ***Causes:*** ileal disease (eg Crohn's or ileal resection), pancreatic disease, and obstructive jaundice (due to ↓excretion of bile salts from the gall bladder).

Dyspepsia

Dyspepsia & indigestion (p240) are broad terms, used often to signify epigastric or retrosternal pain (or discomfort), which may be related to meals. Find out exactly what your patient is complaining of. 30% have no abnormality on endoscopy (p256).

Halitosis

Halitosis (fetor oris, oral malodour) results from gingivitis (Vincent's angina, p726), metabolic activity of bacteria in plaque, or sulfide-yielding food putrefaction eg in gingival pockets and tonsillar crypts.[64] Delusional halitosis is quite common.

Contributory factors: Smoking, drugs (disulfiram; isosorbide); lung disease, hang-overs (after one bad one, Lucky Jim thought "His mouth had been used as a latrine by some small creature of the night and then as its mausoleum...."). **℞:** Try to eliminate anaerobes: • Stand nearer the toothbrush • Dental floss • 0.2% aqueous chlorhexidine gluconate.[2007 Clinical evidence] • The very common halitosis arising from the tongue's dorsum is secondary to overpopulated volatile sulfur compound-producing bacteria. Locally retained bacteria metabolise sulfur-containing amino acids to yield volatile (∴ smelly) hydrogen sulfide and methylmercaptane, which perpetuate periodontal disease. At night and between meals conditions are optimal for odour production—so eating regularly may help. Treat by mechanical cleansing/scraping using tongue brushes or scrapes plus chemical solutions of essential oils, zinc chloride, and cetylpyridinium chloride.[65] Oral care products containing metal ions, especially Zn, inhibit odour formation, it is thought, because of affinity of the metal ion to sulfur. It is possible to measure the level of volatile sulfur-containing compounds in the air in the mouth directly by means of a portable sulfide monitor (a great way to plague your friends).

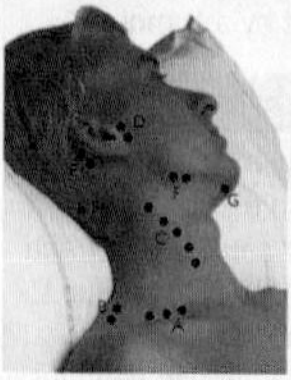

A= Supraclavicular
B= Posterior triangle
C= Jugular chain
D= Preauricular
E= Postauricular
F= Submandibular
G= Submental
H= Occipital

Fig 1. Cervical and supraclavicular nodes.

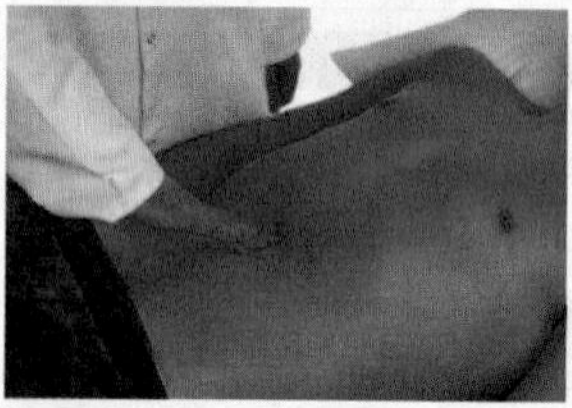

Fig 2. Palpation of the liver: align the lateral surface of the index finger with the costal margin and palpate from the right iliac fossa to ribs in a step-wise fashion.

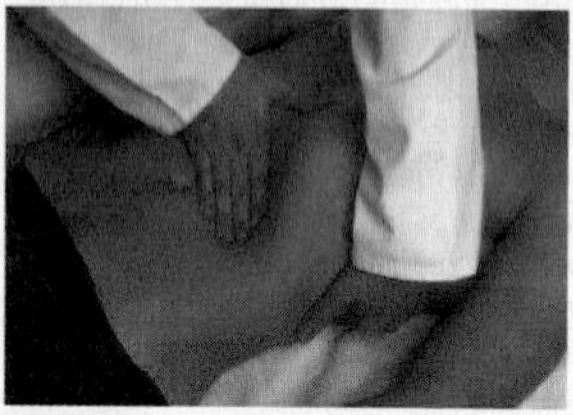

Fig 3. Palpation of the spleen: align the fingertips of your right hand with the left costal border and start palpating just below the umbilicus, working towards the left upper quadrant.

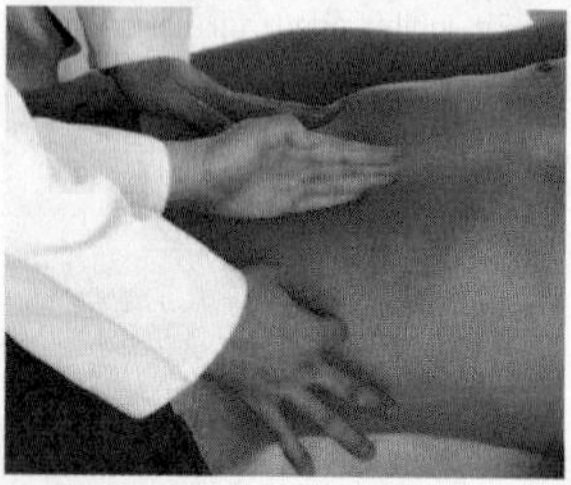

Fig 4. Testing for a fluid thrill. An assistant places a hand centrally on the abdomen preventing transmission of the impulse through the abdominal wall.

1 General inspection

Introduction, consent, position patient lying flat (with 1 pillow), expose ideally 'nipple to knee' (be considerate to patients, eg after general inspection use a towel to cover patient). Inspect general appearance (jaundice? pallor? body mass, state of hydration) for scars, stomas, signs of chronic liver disease,. Ask patients to "raise head off pillow" and "take deep breath", or cough, looking for abnormal contours/distension., and signs of pain.

2 Hands

- *Inspect:* clubbing, koilonychia, leuconychia, Muehrcke's lines, blue lunulae, palmar erythema, Dupuytren's contracture
- *Asterixis:* ask patient to "hold arms out and cock your hands back like this" (see **fig 1**, p50)
- *Pulse:* rate, rhythm, character (also check for an arteriovenous fistula)

3 Face

- *Inspect:* for jaundice, conjunctival pallor (warn patient before pulling down lower eyelid slightly; one side is sufficient), xanthelasma, Kayser-Fleischer rings, central cyanosis (ask patient to stick out tongue). Also inspect mouth for angular stomatitis, pigmentation, telangiectasia, ulcers, glossitis.

4 Neck

Examine cervical and supraclavicular lymph nodes (see **fig 1**).

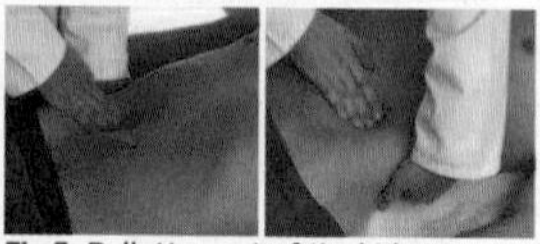

Fig 5. Ballottement of the kidneys.

5 Palpation
Squat by the side of the bed so that the patient's abdomen is at your eye level. Each of the 9 abdominal areas (p567) should be examined in turn with light and then deep palpation before focusing on specific organs Ask patient if there is any area of tenderness and remember to examine this part last. Watch the patient's face for signs of pain.

- *Light palpation:* if pain, determine whether worse when press or release (*'rebound tenderness'*). Any involuntary tension in muscles: general (*peritonitis*), local (*'guarding'*)? Consider special tests for appendicitis and cholecystitis (p610 & p636).
- *Deep palpation:* Should enable you to feel for any masses
- *Liver:* (see **fig 2**) Using the radial border of the index finger aligned with the costal margin start palpation from the RIF. Exert pressure and ask patient to take deep breath. If liver is not felt repeat the process with your hand 1-2cm more superior towards the ribs until the liver is felt.
- *Spleen:* (see **fig 3**) Start palpation just below the umbilicus in the mid-line and work towards the left costal margin asking the patient to take a deep breath in and feeling for the movement of the spleen under your fingers- much like palpating the liver.
- *Kidneys:* For each kidney: place one hand behind patient at the loin and move the kidney towards your other hand below the costal margin (see **fig 5**).
- *Aorta:* Palpate midline above umbilicus, Position fingers either side of outermost palpable margins; is it expansile? (**fig2**, p47).

↓

6 Percussion
Percuss 9 abdominal areas for 'percussion tenderness'.

- *Liver:* Percuss to map upper and lower border of liver.
- *Spleen:* Percuss from left costal margin towards mid-axillary line and lower left ribs for dullness of splenic enlargement.
- *Bladder:* Dullness to percussion in the suprapubic region may be helpful in identifying an enlarged bladder.
- *Ascites:* **Shifting dullness:** Percuss centrally to laterally until dull, keep your finger at dull spot and ask patient to lean onto opposite side. If the dullness was air-fluid level, fluid will now have moved by gravity and the previously dull area will be resonant. **Fluid thrill:** Assistant places hand centrally on abdomen (prevents transmission of impulse through abdominal wall) whilst you place hand on one side of the abdomen. Fluid thrill felt as a ripple when flicking the other side of the abdomen (**fig 4**).

↓

7 Auscultation

- *Bowel sounds:* Listen with the diaphragm just below the umbilicus
- *Bruits:* Listen over aorta and renal arteries (either side of midline above umbilicus).

↓

8 Completion
Complete examination by examining hernial orifices and external genitalia, performing a PR examination, and testing the urine. Thank patient and wash hands.

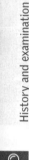

1 **Inspection** Does patient appear comfortable or in distress? Look for abnormal contours/distension. Tattoos? Cushingoid appearance may suggest steroid use post-transplant or IBD. Inspect (and smell) for signs of chronic liver disease:

- Hepatic fetor on breath (p258)
- Gynaecomastia
- Clubbing (rare)
- Purpura (purple stained skin, p338)
- Scratch marks
- Muscle wasting
- Spider naevi (**fig 1**, p261)
- Palmar erythema
- Jaundice
- Liver flap (coarse irregular tremor)
- Leuconychia (hypoalbuminaemia)

Inspect for signs of malignancy, anaemia, jaundice, Virchow's node. Note:

- Visible pulsation (aneurysm, p656)
- Peristalsis
- Scars
- Masses
- Striae (stretch marks, eg pregnancy)
- Distension
- Genitalia
- Herniae

If abdominal wall veins look dilated, assess **direction of flow**. In inferior vena caval (IVC) obstruction, flow below the umbilicus is up; in portal hypertension (*caput medusae*), flow radiates out from the umbilicus. *The cough test:* While looking at the face, ask the patient to cough. If this causes abdominal pain, flinching, or a protective movement of hands towards the abdomen, suspect peritonitis.

2 **Hands** Clubbing (see MINIBOX), *leuconychia* (whitening of the nails due to hypoalbuminaemia), *koilonychia* ('spooning' of the nails due to iron, B_{12}, or folate deficiency), *Muehrcke's lines* (transverse white lines due to hypoalbuminaemia), *blue lanulae* (bluish discoloration seen in Wilson's disease). *Palmar erythema* (chronic liver disease), *Dupuytren's contracture* (thickening and fibrous contraction of palmar fascia (see **fig 1**, p713; alcoholic liver disease). *Hepatic flap/asterixis* (hepatic encephalopathy), check pulse (and respiratory rate) (infection/sepsis?), palpate for arteriovenous fistulae in the forearm (access for haemodialysis in renal failure).

3 **Face** Assess for jaundice, anaemia, xanthelasma (PBC, chronic obstruction), *Kayser-Fleischer rings* (green-yellow ring at corneal margin seen in Wilson's disease). Inspect mouth for angular stomatitis (thiamine, B_{12} and iron deficiency), pigmentation (Peutz-Jeghers syndrome, p723, **fig 4**), telangiectasia (Osler-Weber-Rendu syndrome, p723, **fig 2**), ulcers (IBD), glossitis (iron, B_{12}, or folate deficiency).

4 **Cervical lymph nodes** Palpate for enlarged left supraclavicular lymph node (*Virchow's node/Troisier's sign*) (gastric carcinoma?).

5 **Palpation** Note any masses, tenderness, guarding (involuntary tensing of abdominal muscles- pain or fear of it), or rebound tenderness (greater pain on removing hand than on gently depressing abdomen—peritoneal inflammation); Rovsing's sign (appendicitis, p610);[66] Murphy's sign (cholecystitis, p636). *Palpating the liver:* Assess size (see BOX), regularity, smoothness, and tenderness. Pulsatile (tricuspid regurgitation)? *The scratch test* is an another way to find the lower liver edge (if it is below the costal margin): start with diaphragm of stethoscope at right costal margin. Gently scratch the abdominal wall, starting in the right lower quadrant, working towards the liver edge. A sharp increase in transmission of the scratch is heard when border of the liver is reached. *Palpating the spleen:* If suspect splenomegaly but cannot detect it, assess patient in the right lateral position with your left hand pulling forwards from behind the rib cage. *Palpating the kidneys:* see p46. Enlarged? Nodular? (MINIBOX) *Palpating the aorta:* Normally palpable transmitted pulsation in thin individuals.

6 **Percussion** Confirm the lower border and define the upper border of the liver and spleen (dull in the mid-axillary line in the 10th intercostal space). Percuss all regions of abdomen. If this induces pain, there may be peritoneal inflammation below (eg an inflamed appendix).[67] Some experts percuss first, before palpation, because even anxious patients do not expect this to hurt—so, if it does hurt, this is a very valuable sign. Percuss for the shifting dullness of ascites (p61 & p606). Ultrasound is a more reliable way of detecting ascites.

7 **Auscultation** Bowel sounds: absence implies ileus; they are enhanced and tinkling in bowel obstruction. Listen for bruits in the aorta, renal and femoral arteries.

8 **Further examination** Check for hernias (p614), perform a PR examination (p633).

Causes of hepatomegaly

(For hepatosplenomegaly, see p606)

- *Malignancy:* Metastatic or primary (usually craggy hepatomegaly).
- *Hepatic congestion:* Right heart failure—may be pulsatile in tricuspid incompetence, hepatic vein thrombosis (Budd-Chiari syndrome, p710).
- *Anatomical:* Riedel's lobe (normal variant).
- *Infection:* Infectious mononucleosis (glandular fever), hepatitis viruses, malaria, schistosomiasis, amoebic abscess, hydatid cyst.
- *Haematological:* Leukaemia, lymphoma, myeloproliferative disorders (eg myelofibrosis), sickle-cell disease, haemolytic anaemias.
- *Others:* Fatty liver, early cirrhosis, porphyria, amyloidosis, Gaucher's disease.

Splenomegaly

Abnormally large spleen. *Causes:* See p606. If massive, think of: chronic myeloid leukaemia, myelofibrosis, malaria (or leishmaniasis).

Features of spleen differentiating it from the kidney

- Cannot get above it (ribs overlie its top)
- Dull to percussion (kidney resonant because of overlying bowel)
- Moves more with inspiration (towards RIF)
- May have palpable notch on its medial side

GI causes of clubbing

- Inflammatory bowel disease (esp. Crohn's)
- Cirrhosis
- GI lymphoma
- Malabsorption, eg coeliac

Presenting symptoms	Direct questions
Dysuria (see BOX)	SOCRATES (p34). Fever? Sexual history. Urinary changes .
Loin/scrotal pain	Must rule out testicular torsion (p654).
Haematuria (p 285 and p649)	
Urethral/vaginal discharge (p418)	
Sex problems; painful intercourse/dyspareunia, (OHCS p310)	
Menses (OHCS p250)	Ask about menarche, menopause, length of periods, amount, pain? Intermenstrual loss? 1st day of last menstrual period (LMP)?

Detecting outflow obstruction (see BOX) eg prostatic hyperplasia; stricture; stone). Ask:

- On wanting to pass water, is there delay before you start? (**Hesitancy**)
- Does the flow stop and start? Do you go on dribbling when you think you've stopped, even after giving it a good shake? (**Terminal dribbling**)
- Is your stream getting weaker? Can you hit the wall OK? (**Poor stream**)
- Is your stream painful and slow/'drop-by-drop'? (**Strangury** eg from bladder stone)
- Do you feel the bladder is not empty after passing water?[i]
- Do you ever pass water when you do not want to? (**Incontinence**—p650)
- On feeling an urge to pass water, do you have to go at once? (**Urgency**)[i]
- Do you urinate often at night? (**Nocturia**)[i] In the day? (**Frequency**)[i] How often?

i = irritative (or 'filling') symptoms: they can be caused by, for example, UTI, as well as obstructions.

Past history Renal colic, urinary tract infection, diabetes; BP↑, gout, analgesic use (p306), previous operations.

Drug history Anticholinergics.

Family history Prostate carcinoma?

Social history Smoking, sexual orientation.

Dysuria

Be sure you mean the same as your patient and colleagues, as dysuria refers to both painful micturition ('**uralgia**'[68]) and difficult micturition (**voiding difficulty**, p65). Uralgia is typically from urethral, bladder or vaginal inflammation (UTI; bubble bath, spermicides, urethral syndrome, p292). If postmenopausal, look for a urethral caruncle—fleshy outgrowth of distal urethral mucosa, ≤1cm, typically originating from the posterior urethral lip. Also think of prostatitis, STI/urethritis (p418), vaginitis, and vulvitis, Rare causes: stones, urethral lesions (eg carcinoma, lymphoma,[69] papilloma),[70] appendix, or invasive placental pathologies.[71] [72]

Voiding difficulty is a sign of outflow obstruction, eg from an enlarged prostate, urethral stricture (traumatic, post-gonococcal, or vasculitic),[73] or urethral valves in boys.[74] Other features: straining to void, poor stream, retention, and incontinence. **Strangury** is urethral pain, referred from the bladder base, causing a constant distressing desire to urinate even if there is little urine to void. Causes: stones, catheters, cystitis, prostatitis, bladder neoplasia, bladder endometriosis,[75] schistosomiasis.[76]

Frequency

This is ↑frequency of micturition. Aim to differentiate ↑urine production (eg diabetes mellitus and insipidus, polydipsia, diuretics, alcohol, renal tubular disease, adrenal insufficiency) from frequent passage of small amounts of urine (eg in cystitis, urethritis, neurogenic bladder), or bladder compression or outflow obstruction (pregnancy, bladder tumour, enlarged prostate).

Oliguria/anuria

Oliguria means a urine output of <400mL/24h—a sign of shock (eg post-op, p578) or acute renal failure: causes: p298. **Anuria** means no urine output (▸▸p640; stones).

Polyuria

This is an increase in urine volume, eg >3L/24h. ***Causes:*** Over-enthusiastic IV fluid therapy; diabetes mellitus & insipidus (diabetes is Greek for fountain); ↑Ca^{2+}; psychogenic polydipsia/PIP syndrome (p232); polyuric phase of acute renal failure.

Irritative or obstructive bladder symptoms (see also p644)

Symptoms of prostate enlargement are miscalled 'prostatism'; it is better to talk about *irritative* or *obstructive* bladder symptoms as bladder neck obstruction or a stricture may be the cause. **1** ***Irritative bladder symptoms:*** Urgency, dysuria, frequency, nocturia[1] (the last two are also associated with causes of **polyuria**). **2** ***Obstructive symptoms*:** Reduced size and force of urinary stream, hesitancy and interruption of stream during voiding and terminal dribbling—the usual cause is enlargement of the prostate (prostatic hyperplasia), but other causes include a urethral stricture, tumour, urethral valves, or bladder neck contracture. The maximum flow rate of urine is normally ~18-30mL/s.

Terminal dribbling

Dribbling at the end of urination, often seen in conjunction with incontinence following incomplete urination, associated with prostatism.

Urinary changes

Cloudy urine suggests pus (UTI) but is often normal phosphate precipitation in an alkaline urine. ***Pneumaturia*** (bubbles in urine as it is passed) occurs with UTI due to gas-forming organisms or may signal an enterovesical (bowel-bladder) fistula from diverticulitis, Crohn's disease or neoplastic disease of the bowel. ***Nocturia*** occurs with 'irritative bladder', diabetes mellitus, UTI, and reversed diurnal rhythm (seen in renal and cardiac failure). ***Haematuria*** (RBC in urine) is due to neoplasia or glomerulonephritis (p294) until proven otherwise.

Voiding difficulty

This includes poor flow, straining to void, hesitancy, intermittent stream, incontinence (eg overflow), retention (acute or chronic), incomplete emptying (±UTI from residual urine). ►*Remember faecal impaction as a cause of retention with overflow.* ***Causes—CNS:*** Suprapontine (stroke); cord lesions (cord injury, multiple sclerosis); peripheral nerve (prolapsed disc, diabetic or other neuropathy); or reflex, due to pain (eg with herpes infections). ***Obstructive:*** Prostatic hyperplasia, early oedema after bladder neck repair, uterine prolapse, retroverted gravid uterus, fibroids, ovarian cysts, urethral foreign body, ectopic ureterocele, bladder polyp, or cancer. ***Bladder overdistension***—eg after epidural for childbirth. ***Detrusor weakness or myopathy*** causes incomplete emptying + dribbling overflow incontinence (do cystometry/electromyography;[77] causes include neurological disease and interstitial cystitis (*OHCM* p307); it may lead to a contracted bladder, eg requiring substitution enterocystoplasty).[78] ***Drugs:*** Epidural anaesthesia; tricyclics, anticholinergics.

1 In the elderly, nocturia (1-2/night) may be 'normal' because of: **i)** loss of ability to concentrate urine; **ii)** peripheral oedema fluid returns to the circulation at night; **iii)** circadian rhythms may be lost; **iv)** less sleep is needed and waking may be interpreted as a need to void (a conditioned Pavlovian response).

 (see p604-5)

Presenting symptoms	**Direct questions**
Breast lump	Previous lumps? Family history? Pain? Nipple discharge? Nipple inversion? Skin changes? Change in size related to menstrual cycle? Number of pregnancies? First/last/latest period? Drugs (eg HRT)? Consider metastatic disease (weight loss, breathlessness, back pain, abdominal mass?)
Breast pain (see BOX)	SOCRATES (p34). Bilateral/unilateral? Rule out cardiac chest pain (p88 & p796). History of trauma? Any mass? Related to menstrual cycle?
Nipple discharge (see BOX)	Amount? Nature (colour? consistency? any blood?)

(Screen for all above presenting symptoms before proceeding to past history)

Past history Any previous lumps and or malignancies. Previous mammograms, clinical examinations of the breast, USS, fine-needle aspirate (FNA)/core biopsies.

Drug history Ask specifically about HRT and the Pill.

Family history See p524

Social history Try and gain an impression of support network if suspect malignancy.

Breast pain

Is it premenstrual (*cyclical mastalgia, OHCS* p254)? Breast cancer (refer, eg for mammography if needed)? If non-malignant and non-cyclical, think of:

- Tietze's syndrome
- Angina
- Lung disease
- Oestrogens/HRT
- Bornholm disease[1]
- Gallstones
- Thoracic outlet syndrome

If none of the above, *wearing a firm bra* all day may help, as may NSAIDs.

Nipple discharge

Causes: Duct ectasia (green/brown/red, often multiple ducts and bilateral), intraductal papilloma/adenoma/carcinoma (bloody discharge, often single duct), lactation. *Management:* Diagnose the cause (mammogram, ultrasound, ductogram); then treat appropriately. Cessation of smoking reduces discharge from duct ectasia. Microdochectomy/total duct excision can be considered if other measures fail, though may give no improvement in symptoms.

1 Bornholm disease (Devil's grip) is due to Coxsackie B virus, causing chest and abdominal pain, which may be mistaken for cardiac pain or an acute surgical abdomen. It resolves within ~2 weeks.

The breast: examination

1 **Inspection** Assess size and shape of any masses as well as overlying surface. Which quadrant (see **fig 1**)? Note skin involvement; ulceration, dimpling (*peau d'orange*), and nipple inversion/discharge.
2 **Palpation of the breast** Confirm size, and shape of any lump. Is it fixed/tethered to skin or underlying structures (see BOX)? Is it fluctuant/compressible/hard Temperature? Tender? Mobile (more likely to be fibroadenoma)?
3 **Palpation of the axilla** Metastatic spread? Ipsilateral/bilateral? Matted? Fixed?
4 **Further examination** Examine abdomen for hepatomegaly, spine for tenderness, lungs (metastatic spread).

1 General inspection

►**Always have a chaperone present when examining the breast.**

Introduction, consent, position patient sitting at edge of bed with hands by her side, expose to waist. Inspect both breasts for obvious masses, contour anomalies, asymmetry, scars, ulceration, skin changes, eg *peau d'orange* (orange peel appearance resulting from oedema). Look for nipple inversion and nipple discharge. Ask her to "press hands hips" and then "hands on head" to accentuate any asymmetrical changes. Whilst patient has her hands raised inspect axillae for any masses as well as inspecting under the breasts.

2 Palpation of the breast

Position patient sitting back at 45° with hand behind head (ie right hand behind head when examining the right breast—see **fig 1**). Ask patient if she has any pain or discharge. Examine painful areas last and then ask her to express any discharge. Examine each breast with the 'normal' side first. Examine each quadrant in turn as well as the axillary tail of Spence (**fig 2**) or use a concentric spiral method (**fig 3**) using a flat hand to roll breast against underlying chest wall. Define any lumps/lumpy areas. If you discover a lump, to examine for fixity to the pectoral muscles ask the patient to push against your hand with her arm outstretched.

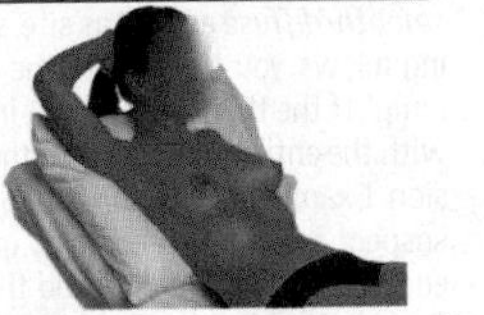

Fig 1. Correct patient position for breast examination

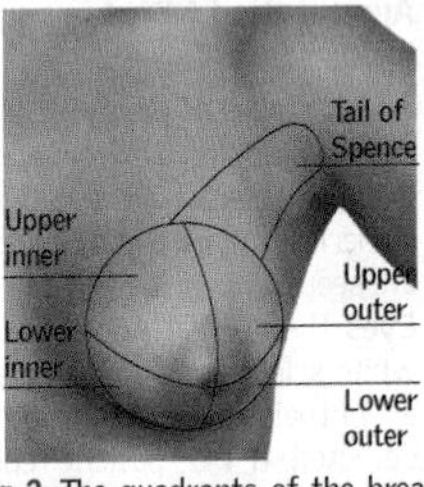

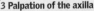

Fig 2. The quadrants of the breast with the axillary tail of Spence.

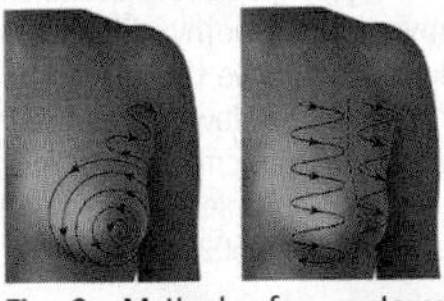

Fig 3. Methods for systematic breast palpation.

Figs 1-3 with permission from *OHCEPS*

3 Palpation of the axilla

Examine both axillae. When examining right axilla, hold the patient's right arm with your right hand and examine axilla with left hand. 5 sets of axillary nodes:

i) apical (palpate against glenohumeral joint)
ii) anterior (palpate against pectoralis major)
iii) central (palpate against lateral chest wall)
iv) posterior (palpate against latissimus dorsi)
v) medial (palpate against humerus)

4 Further examination

Complete examination by palpating down spine for tenderness, examining abdomen for hepatomegaly, and lungs for signs of metastases. Thank patient and wash hands.

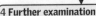

For symptoms of thyroid disease see p210 & p212. See also lumps in the neck, p600–2.

1 **Inspection** The key questions to ask oneself when presented with a lump in the neck are: Is this lump thyroid related or not? What is the patient's thyroid status? Inspect the neck; the normal thyroid is usually neither visible nor palpable. A midline swelling should raise your suspicion of thyroid pathology. Look for scars (eg collar incision from previous thyroid surgery). Examine the face for signs of hypothyroidism (puffiness, pallor, dry flaky skin, xanthelasma, corneal arcus, balding) as well as overall body habitus. Assess the patient's demeanour; do they appear anxious, nervous, agitated, fidgety (hyperthyroid)? Or slow and lethargic (hypothyroid)?

2 **Swallow test** Only goitres (p602), thyroglossal cysts (p600) and in some cases lymph nodes should move up on swallowing.

3 **Tongue protrusion test** A thyroglossal cyst will move up on tongue protrusion

4 **Palpation** (By this stage of the examination if the evidence is in favour of the lump not rising from the thyroid it is acceptable to examine the lump like any other (p596); assess site, size, shape, smoothness (consistency), surface (contour/edge/colour), and surroundings, as well as transilluminance, fixation/tethering, fluctuance/compressibility, temperature, tenderness and whether it is pulsatile). If a thyroid mass is suspected, standing behind the patient provides an opportunity to check for any proptosis (hyperthyroidism). Proceed to palpate each lobe attempting to decide whether any lump is *solitary or multiple, nodular or smooth/diffuse* as well as site, size etc. Repeating the swallow test whilst palpating allows you to confirm the early finding, but also attempt to 'get below the lump'. If the there is a distinct inferior border under which you can place you hand with the entire lump above it then the goitre is unlikely to have retrosternal extension. Examining for 'spread' to the lymph nodes is particularly important if you suspect a thyroid malignancy (p602). Complete palpation by assessing if the presence of the lump has caused the trachea to deviate from the midline.

5 **Percussion** A retrosternal goitre will produce a dull percussion note when the sternum is percussed.

6 **Auscultation** A bruit in a smooth thyroid goitre is suggestive of Graves' disease (p210)

The next stages of the exam are to examine the systemic signs of thyroid status.

7 **Hands** Clubbing ('thyroid acropachy') is seen in Graves' disease. Palmar erythema and a fine tremor are also signs of thyrotoxicosis. Assess temperature (warm peripheries if hyperthyroid) and the radial pulse; tachycardia and atrial fibrillation are seen in hyperthyroidism, while bradycardia is seen in hypothyroidism).

8 **Eyes** The 'normal' upper eyelid should always cover the upper eye such that the white sclera is not visible between the lid and the iris. In hyperthyroidism with exophthalmus there is proptosis as well as lid retraction and 'lid lag' may also be detected. If the patient reports double vision when eye movements are being tested this indicates ophthalmoplegia of hyperthyroidism.

9 Asking the patient to stand allows you to assess whether there is any proximal myopathy (hypothyroidism). Look for pretibial myxoedema (brown swelling of the lower leg above the lateral malleoli in Graves' disease). Finally, test the reflexes; these will be slow relaxing in hypothyroidism and brisk in hyperthyroidism

10 Thank the patient and consider whether the lump is a goitre, and if so whether it is single/multiple, diffuse/nodular, as well as the patient's thyroid status. Decide on a diagnosis (p602).

1 Inspection
Introduction, consent, position patient sitting on a chair (with space behind), adequately expose neck. Inspect from front and sides for any obvious goitres or swellings, scars, signs of hypo-/hyperthyroidism

↓

2 Swallow test
Standing in front of the patient ask them to "sip water...hold in your mouth ...and swallow" to see if any midline swelling moves up on swallowing

↓

3 Tongue protrusion test
Ask patient 'stick out your tongue'. Does the lump move up?

↓

If evidence favours lump not arising from thyroid, examine lump like any other p596

4 Palpation
Stand behind the patient.
- *Proptosis:* whilst standing behind the patient ask them to tilt their head back slightly; this will give you a better view to assess any proptosis than when assessing the other aspects of eye pathology from front on, as in **8**)
- *The thyroid gland:* Ask the patient "any pain?" Place middle 3 fingers of either hand along midline below chin and 'walk down' to thyroid. Assess any enlargement/ nodules
- *Swallow test:* repeat as before, now palpating; attempt to 'get under' the lump
- *Lymph nodes:* examine lymph nodes of head and neck (p60) Stand in front of the patient
- *Trachea:* palpate for tracheal deviation from the midline

↓

5 Percussion
Percuss the sternum for dullness of retrosternal extension of a goitre

↓

6 Auscultation
Listen over the goitre for a bruit

↓

7 Hands
- *Inspect:* for thyroid acropachy (clubbing) and palmar erythema
- *Temperature*
- *Pulse:* Rate and rhythm
- *Fine tremor:* ask patient to "hold hands out", place sheet of paper over out-stretched hands to help

↓

8 Eyes
- *Exophthalmos:* inspect for lid retraction and proptosis
- *Lid lag:* ask patient to "look down following finger" as you move your finger from a point above the eye to below.
- *Eye movements:* ask patient to follow your finger, keeping their head still, as you make an 'H' shape. Any double vision?

↓

9 Completion
Ask patient to stand up from the chair to asses for proximal myopathy, look for pretibial myxoedema, test ankle reflexes (ask patient to face away from you with knee resting on chair). Thank patient and wash hands.

History This should be taken from the patient and if possible from a close friend or relative as well for corroboration/discrepancies. The patient's memory, perception, or speech may be affected by the disorder making the history difficult to obtain. Note the progression of the symptoms and signs: gradual deterioration (eg tumour) *vs* intermittent exacerbations (eg multiple sclerosis) *vs* rapid onset (eg stroke). Ask about age, occupation and ethnic origin. Right- or left-hand dominant?

Presenting symptoms

- *Headache:* (p460 & p794) Different to usual headaches? Acute/chronic? Speed of onset? Single/recurrent? Unilateral/bilateral? Associated aura (migraine, p462)? Any meningism (p832)? Worse on waking (↑ICP)? Decreased conscious level? ►Take a 'worst-ever' headache very seriously. (See p763)
- *Weakness:* (p470) Speed of onset? Muscle groups affected? Sensory loss? Any sphincter disturbance? Loss of balance? Associated spinal/root pain?
- *Visual disturbance:* (*OHCS* p410) eg blurring, double vision (diplopia), photophobia, visual loss. Speed of onset? Any preceding symptoms? Pain in eye?
- *Special senses:* Hearing (p468), smell, taste.
- *Dizziness:* (p466) Illusion of surroundings moving (vertigo)? Hearing loss/tinnitus? Any loss of consciousness? Positional?
- *Speech disturbance:* (p80) Difficulty in expression, articulation, or comprehension (can be difficult to determine)? Sudden onset or gradual?
- *Dysphagia:* (p240) Solids and/or liquids? Intermittent or constant? Difficulty in coordination? Painful (odynophagia)?
- *Fits/faints/'funny turns'/involuntary movements:* (p464) Frequency? Duration? Mode of onset? Preceding aura? Loss of consciousness? Tongue biting? Incontinence? Any residual weakness/confusion? Family history?
- *Skin sensation disturbance:* eg numbness, 'pins & needles' (paraesthesiae), pain, odd sensations. Distribution? Speed of onset? Associated weakness?
- *Tremor:* (p71) Rapid or slow tremor? Present at rest? Worse on deliberate movement? Taking β-agonists? Any thyroid problems? Any family history?

Cognitive state If there is any doubt about the patient's cognition, an objective measure is a cognitive test—guessing has been shown to be inaccurate![79] The following 10 questions comprise the Abbreviated Mental Test Score (AMTS), a commonly used screening questionnaire for cognitive impairment:[80]

1. Tell patient an address to recall at the end (eg 42 West Street, Gateshead)
2. Age
3. Time (to nearest hour)
4. What year is it?
5. Recognize 2 people (eg doctor & nurse)
6. Date of birth
7. Dates of the Second World War
8. Name of present monarch
9. Name of hospital/institution
10. Count backwards from 20 to 1

A score of ≤*6* suggests poor cognition, acute (delirium), or chronic (dementia). AMTS correlates well with the more detailed Mini-Mental State Examination (MMSE™), though recent copyright means that its use has become more restricted.[81] **NB:** deaf, dysphasic, depressed, and uncooperative patients, as well as those who do not understand English, will also get low scores.[82] (TYM test: see p85).

Past medical history Ask about meningitis/encephalitis, head/spine trauma, seizures, previous operations, risk factors for vascular disease (p474, AF, hypertension, hyperlipidaemia, diabetes mellitus, smoking), and recent travel. Is there any chance that the patient is pregnant (eclampsia, *OHCS* p48)?

Drug history Any anticonvulsant/antipsychotic/antidepressant medication? Any psychotropic drugs (eg ecstasy)? Any medication with neurological side effects (eg *isoniazid* which can cause a peripheral neuropathy)?

Social and family history What can the patient do and not do, ie activities of daily living (ADLs)? What is the Barthel Index score?[83] Any neurological or psychiatric disease in the family? Any consanguinity?

Cramp

This is painful muscle spasm. Leg cramps are common at night or after exercise. Rarely, cramp signifies salt depletion, heat exhaustion,[84] muscle ischaemia (claudication DM), myopathy (McArdle, p718), dystonia (writer's cramp, p473), tetanus,[85] or rhabdomyolysis.[86] Forearm cramps suggest motor neurone disease. Night cramps may respond to passive exercise or quinine bisulfate 300mg at night PO.

Drugs causing cramp: Diuretics (? from $K^+\downarrow$), domperidone, salbutamol/terbutaline IVI, ACE-i; telmisartan, celicoxib, lacidipine, ergot alkaloids, levothyroxine

Paraesthesiae

'Pins & needles', numbness/tingling, which can hurt or 'burn' (dysaesthesia). **Causes:** ***Metabolic:*** $\downarrow Ca^{2+}$ (perioral); $P_aCO_2\uparrow$; myxoedema; neurotoxins (tick bite; sting). ***Vascular:*** ►►Limb emboli; Raynaud's; DVT; PAN;[87] plasma viscosity↑. ***Antibody-mediated:*** Paraneoplastic; SLE; ITP.[88] ***Infection:*** Lyme;[89] rabies. ***Drugs:*** ACE-i. ***Brain:*** Thalamic/parietal lesions. ***Cord:*** MS; myelitis/HIV; $B_{12}\downarrow$; ►►lumbar fracture;[90] cysticercosis.[91] ***Plexopathy/mononeuropathy:*** p506, cervical rib;[92] carpal tunnel; sciatica. ***Peripheral neuropathy*** (glove & stocking, p508, eg DM; CRF). If ***paroxysmal:*** Migraine;[93] epilepsy;[94] phaeochromocytoma.[95] If ***wandering:*** Strongyloides; loiasis.[96]

Tremor

Tremor is rhythmic oscillation of limbs, trunk, head, or tongue. 3 types:

1. ***Resting tremor***—worst at rest—eg from Parkinsonism (±bradykinesia and rigidity; tremor is more resistant to treatment than other symptoms). It is usually a slow tremor (frequency of 3–5Hz), typically 'pill-rolling' of the thumb over a finger.
2. ***Postural tremor***—worst if arms are outstretched. Typically *rapid* (8–12Hz). May be exaggerated physiological tremor (eg anxiety, hyperthyroidism, alcohol, drugs), due to brain damage (eg Wilson's disease, syphilis) or *benign essential tremor* (BET). This is often familial (autosomal dominant) tremor of arms and head presenting at any age. Cogwheeling may occur,[97] but there is no bradykinesia. It is suppressed by large-ish amounts of alcohol. Rarely progressive (unless onset is unilateral). Propranolol (40–80mg/8–12h PO) helps ⅓ of patients.
3. ***Intention tremor***—worst on movement, seen in cerebellar disease, with past-pointing and dysdiadochokinesis (see p503). No effective drug has been found.

Facial pain

CNS causes: migraine, trigeminal or glossopharyngeal neuralgia, (p461) or from any other pain-sensitive structure in the head or neck. ***Post-herpetic neuralgia:*** nasty burning-and-stabbing pain involves dermatomal areas affected by shingles (p400); it may affect cranial nerves V and VII in the face. It all too often becomes chronic and intractable (skin affected is exquisitely sensitive). Treatment is hard. Always give strong psychological support. Transcutaneous nerve stimulation, capsaicin ointment, and infiltrating local anaesthetic are tried. Amitriptyline eg 10–25mg/24h at night may help, as may carbamazepine (NNT≈4) and gabapentin (p508). **NB:** famciclovir or valaciclovir given in acute shingles may ↓ duration of neuralgia.[98]

Vascular and non-neurological causes:

Neck	Cervical disc pathology
Bone/sinuses	Sinusitis; neoplasia
Eye	Glaucoma; iritis; orbital cellulitis; eye strain; AVM
Temporomandibular joint	Arthritis or idiopathic dysfunction (common)
Teeth/gums	Caries; broken teeth; abscess; malocclusion
Ear	Otitis media; otitis externa
Vascular/vasculitis	Arteriovenous fistula;[99] aneurysm; or AVM at the cerebellopontine angle;[100] giant cell arteritis; SLE[101]

►The neurological system is usually the most daunting examination to learn, but the most satisfying once perfected. Learn at the bedside from a senior colleague, preferably a neurologist. Keep practising. Be aware that books present ideal situations: often one or more signs are equivocal or even contrary to expectation; don't be put off, consider the whole picture, including the history; try re-examining the patient.

Higher mental function Conscious level (Glasgow coma scale, p802), orientation in time, place, and person, memory (short- and long-term). See p70 for the AMTS and p85 for the *Test Your Memory* (TYM) test.

Speech Is there alteration in voice sound (**dysphonia** eg in laryngitis, recurrent laryngeal nerve palsy, MND, or vocal cord tumour)? **Dysphasia** & **dysarthria**: see p80?

Skull and spine Malformation. Signs of injury. Palpate scalp. If there is any question of spinal injury, **do not move the spine**: in-line immobilisation is required. Is there meningism (p832)? Auscultate for carotid/cranial bruits. Screening by listening for carotid bruits has a high specificity (91%) but a low sensitivity (56%), so if stenosis is suspected arrange a carotid ultrasound scan.[102]

Motor system Upper (below) or lower limb (p74) ►It is essential to discriminate whether weakness is upper (UMN) or lower (LMN) motor neuron (p451).

Sensation See dermatomes on p458. **Cranial nerves** See p76.

The neurological system: upper limb examination

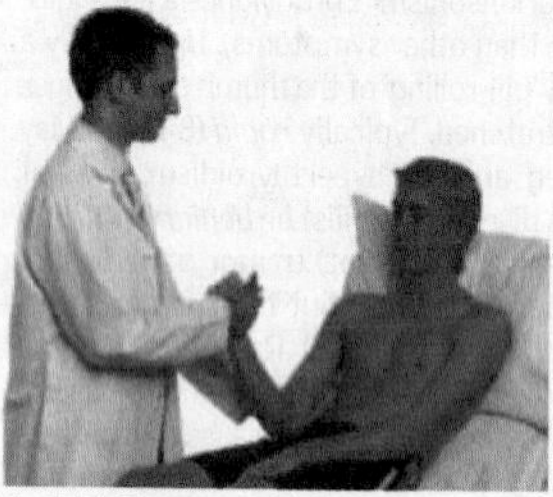

Fig 1. Testing upper limb tone.

2 Tone
Ask patient to 'relax/go floppy like a rag-doll'. Ask if patient has any pain in hands/arm/shoulder before passively flexing and extending limb while also pronating and supinating the forearm (fig 1). Any spasticity or rigidity?

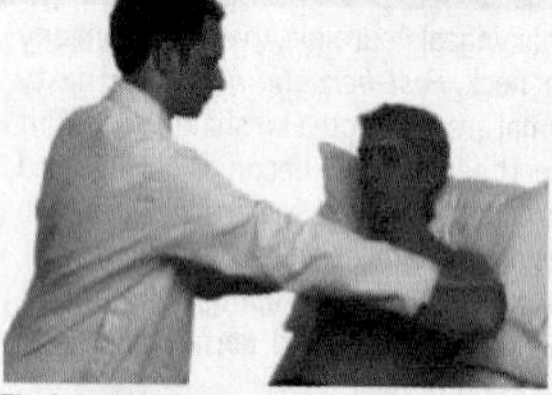

Fig 2. Testing upper-limb power: shoulders

1 General inspection
Introduction, consent, position patient sitting back at 45° with both upper limbs fully exposed. Inspect for abnormal posturing, asymmetry, abnormal movements (fasciculation/tremor/dystonia/athetosis), muscle wasting (especially small muscles of the hand)—symmetrical/asymmetrical? Local/general?

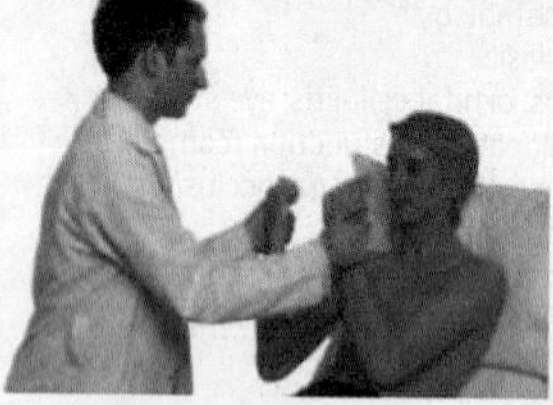

Fig 3. Testing upper-limb power: elbows

Figures 1-5 reproduced with permission from *Oxford Handbook of Clinical Examination and Practical Skills.*

3 Power Direct patient to adopt position and follow commands below while you as the examiner resist movements as appropriate to grade power (p451). Test each muscle group bilaterally before moving on to the next position. • Position as **fig 2**: "shrug shoulders and don't let me push down; push your arms out to the side against me; and try and pull them back in" • Position as **fig 3**: "hold arms up like this and pull me towards you ...and push me away" • Position as **fig 4**: "hold your hand out and don't let me push it down; now don't let me push it up" • Offer the patient two of your fingers and ask them to "squeeze my fingers" • Ask patient to "spread your fingers and stop me pushing them back together" then hand the patient a piece of paper to grip between two fingers. You as the examiner should grip the paper with your corresponding fingers whilst asking patient to "grip the paper and don't let me pull it away".

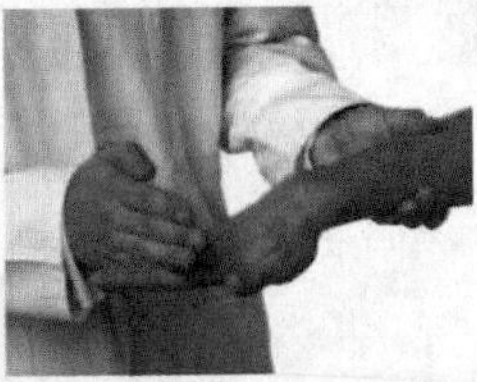

Fig 4. Testing upper-limb power: finger extension.

4 Reflexes For each reflex, test right, then left and compare. If absent attempt to elicit with 'reinforcement' by asking patient to clench their teeth on a count of 3 at which time you strike. Decide whether reflexes are absent/present (with reinforcement)/normal/brisk/exaggerated. • *Biceps*: (C5,6) • *Triceps*: (C7) • *Supinator*: (C6). See **fig 5**.

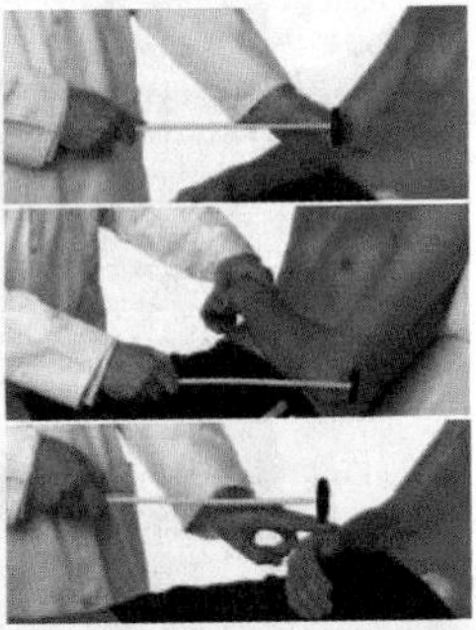

Fig 5. Testing tendon reflexes in biceps (top panel), triceps (middle panel) and supinator (bottom panel).

5 Coordination • *Finger-nose test*: Holding your finger in front of the patient instruct "touch my finger then your nose...as fast as you can". Look for intention tremor and 'past pointing'. • *Test for dysdiadokokinesis*: Ask patient to repeatedly pronate and supinate forearm, clapping the still hand each time. Test both limbs. You may have to demonstrate. Failure to perform rapidly alternating movements is dysdiadokokinesis. • *Test for pronator drift*: with patient's eyes closed and arms outstretched tap down on their up- facing palms look for a failure to maintain supination.

6 Sensation • *Light touch*: Tell patient "I'm going to touch you with this cotton wool". As you touch it to their sternum: "this is what it should feel like; say 'Yes' when you feel me touching you and tell me if it feels any different". Proceed to touch patient with cotton wool in all upper limb dermatomes (p458) comparing left and right. • *Pin prick*: Repeat as above using a neurological pin asking patient to tell you whether it feels sharp or dull. • *Temperature*: Repeat as above alternating hot and cold probes asking patient to say whether it feels hot or cold. • *Vibration*: Using a 128Hz tuning fork confirm with patient that they "can feel a buzzing" when you place the tuning fork on their sternum. Proceed to test at the most distal bony prominence and move proximally until patient confirms sensation. • *Joint position sense*: With the patient's eyes closed grasp distal phalanx of the index finger at the sides. Stabilise the rest of the finger. Move the joint up and tell patient "this is up", and down, saying "this is down". Flex and extend the joint, stopping at intervals to ask whether the finger tip is up or down.

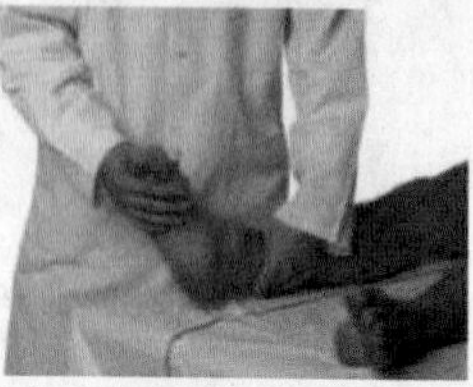

Fig 1. Ankle tone: testing for clonus.

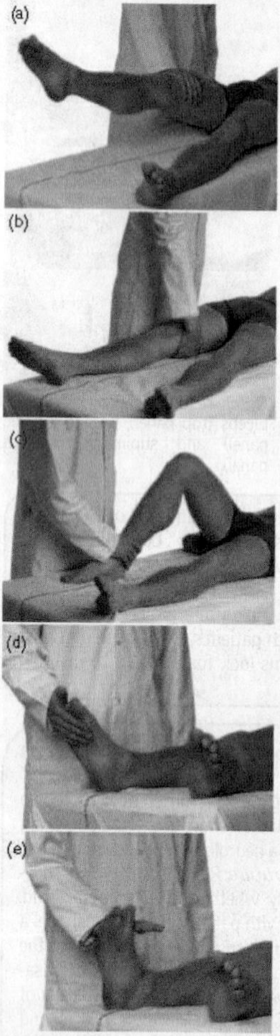

Fig 2. Testing lower limb power against resistance. See text for descriptions of tests.

1 General inspection

Introduction, consent, position patient sitting back at 45º with both lower limbs fully exposed. Inspect for abnormal posturing, muscle wasting, fasciculation (LMN lesion?), deformities of the foot (e.g pes cavus of *Friedreich's ataxia* or *Charcot-Marie-Tooth disease*). Is one leg smaller than the other (*old polio, infantile hemiplegia*)?

2 Tone

Ask patient to "relax/go floppy like a rag-doll". Ask if patient has any pain in feet/legs hips before passively flexing and extending limb while also internally and externally rotating. Hold the patient's knee and roll it from side to side. Put your hand behind the patient's knee and raise it quickly. The heel should lift slightly from the bed if tone is normal. Any spasticity/rigidity?

Clonus (**fig 1**) Plantar flex the foot then quickly dorsiflex and hold. More then 5 'beats' of plantar flexion is sustained clonus and considered abnormal. Hypertonia and clonus suggest an upper motor neuron lesion.

3 Power

Direct patient to adopt position and follow commands below while you as the examiner resist movements as appropriate to grade power (p451) Test each muscle group bilaterally before moving on to the next position. • Position as **fig 2a**: "keeping your leg straight, can you lift your leg off the bed, don't let me push it down" • Position as **fig 2b**: "and now using your leg, push my hand into the bed" • Position hands on outer thighs- "push your legs out to the sides" • Position hands on inner thighs- "and push your legs together" • Position as **fig 2c**: "bend your knee and bring your heel to your bottom, don't let me pull it away... and now kick out against me and push me away" • Position as **fig 2d**: "bend your foot down, pushing my hand away" • Position as **fig 2e**: "cock up your foot, point your toes at the ceiling, don't let me push your foot down".

4 Reflexes
For each reflex, test right, then left and compare. If absent attempt to elicit with 'reinforcement' by asking patient to clench their teeth on a count of 3, at which time you strike. Decide whether reflexes are absent/ present (with reinforcement)/ normal/ brisk/exaggerated
- *Knee:* (L3,4) See **fig 3**.
- *Ankle:* (L5,S1) See **fig 4**.
- ***Extensor plantar***: (L5, S1, S2) Stroke the patient's sole with an orange stick or similar as in **fig 5**. ***Babinski's sign*** is positive if there is dorsiflexion of the great toe (this is abnormal (upper motor neuron lesion) if patient age >6 months).

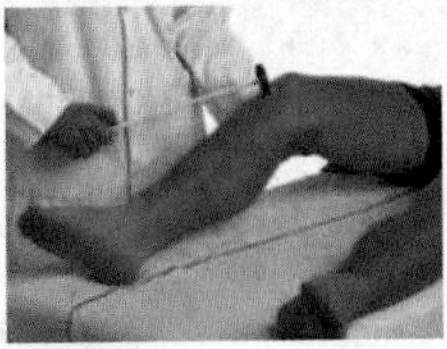

Fig 3. Testing knee reflexes

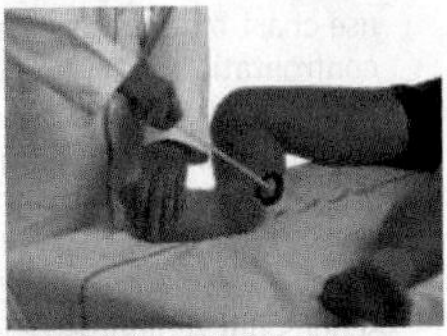

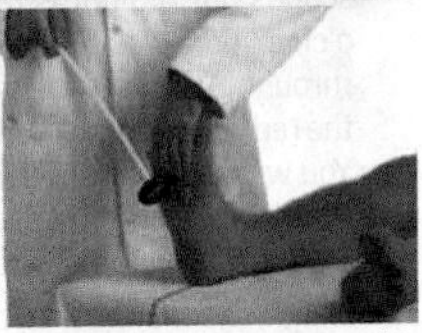

Fig 4. Methods for testing ankle reflexes.

Figs 1-4 with permission from *OHCEPS*

5 Coordination
Heel-shin test: using you finger on the patient's shin to demonstrate, instruct patient "put your heel just below your knee then run it smoothly down your shin, now up your shin, now down" etc. Repeat on other side.

6 Sensation
Light touch: Tell patient "I'm going to touch you with this cotton wool". As you touch it to their sternum: "this is what it should feel like; say 'Yes' when you feel me touching you and tell me if it feels any different". Proceed to touch patient with cotton wall in all lower limb dermatomes (p458) comparing left and right.
Pin prick: Repeat as above using a neurological pin asking patient to tell you whether it feels sharp or dull.
Temperature: Repeat as above alternating hot and cold probes asking patient to say whether it feels hot or cold.
Vibration: Using a 128Hz tuning fork, confirm with patient that they "can feel a buzzing" when you place the tuning fork on their sternum. Proceed to test at the most distal bony prominence, moving proximally until patient confirms sensation.
Joint position sense: With the patient's eyes closed grasp distal phalanx of the great toe at the sides. Stabilise the rest of the toe. Move the joint up and tell patient "this is up", and down. saying "this is down". Flex and extend the joint, stopping at intervals to ask whether the toe is up or down.

7 Gait (see also p471)
Ask patient to walk a few metres, turn and walk back to you. Note use of walking aids, symmetry, size of paces, arm swing. Ask patient to "walk heel-to-toe as if on a tightrope" to exaggerate any instability. Ask patient to walk on tiptoes, then on heels. Inability to walk on tiptoes indicates S_1 or gastrocnemius lesion. Inability to walk on heels indicates L4,5 lesion or foot drop.
Romberg's test: Ask patient to stand unaided with arms by their sides and close their eyes (be ready to support them). If they sway/lose balance the test is positive and indicates posterior column disease/ sensory ataxia.

Approach to examining the cranial nerves Where is the lesion? Think systematically. Is it in the brainstem (eg MS) or outside, pressing on the brainstem? Is it the neuromuscular junction (myasthenia) or the muscles (eg a dystrophy)? Cranial nerves may be affected singly or in groups. ►Face the patient (helps spot asymmetry). For causes of lesions, see BOX. For names of the nerves, see BOX, p83.

I *Smell:* Test ability of each nostril to distinguish familiar smells, eg peppermint.

II *Acuity:* test each eye separately, and its correctability with glasses or pin-hole; use chart on the pages inside the front covers. ***Visual fields:*** Compare during confrontation with your own fields or formally. Any losses/inattention? Sites of lesions: *OHCS* p428. ***Pupils:*** (p79) Size, shape, symmetry, reaction to light (direct and consensual), and accommodation if reaction to light is poor. ***Ophthalmoscopy:*** (*OHCS*, p412) Darken the room. Instil ***tropicamide*** 0.5%, 1 drop, if needed (►check for history of glaucoma beforehand). Select the focusing lens for the best view of the optic disc (pale? swollen?). This is found when the ophthalmoscope's dot of light is reflected from the cornea at 9 o'clock (right disc) or 3 o'clock (left disc). Follow vessels outwards to view each quadrant; rack back through the lenses to inspect lens and cornea. If the view is obscured, examine the red reflex, with your focus on the margin of the pupil, to look for a cataract. You will get a view of the fovea if you ask the patient to look at the ophthalmoscope's finest beam (after drops)—this is the sacred place: the **only** place with 6/6 vision. ►Pathology here merits prompt ophthalmic referral.

III^P, IV & VI Eye movements. ***IIIrd nerve palsy:*** Ptosis, large pupil, eye down and out. ***IVth nerve palsy:*** diplopia on looking down and in (often noticed on descending stairs)—head tilting compensates for this (ocular torticollis). ***VIth nerve palsy:*** Horizontal diplopia on looking out. ***Nystagmus*** is involuntary, often jerky, eye oscillations. Horizontal nystagmus is often due to a vestibular lesion (acute: nystagmus away from lesion; chronic: towards lesion), or cerebellar lesion (unilateral lesions cause nystagmus towards the affected side). If it is more in whichever eye is abducting, MS may be the cause (internuclear ophthalmoplegia, p78). If also deafness/tinnitus, suspect a peripheral cause (eg VIIIth nerve lesion, barotrauma, Ménière's, p466). If it varies with head position, suspect benign positional vertigo (p466). If it is up-and-down, ask a neurologist to explain what is going on—upbeat nystagmus classically occurs with lesions in the midbrain or at the base of the 4th ventricle, downbeat nystagmus in foramen magnum lesions. Nystagmus lasting ≤2 beats is normal, as is nystagmus at the extremes of gaze.

V ***Motor palsy:*** "Open your mouth": jaw deviates to side of lesion.
Sensory: Corneal reflex lost first; check all 3 divisions.

VII^P ***Facial nerve lesions*** cause droop and weakness. As the forehead has bilateral representation in the brain, only the lower two-thirds is affected in UMN lesions, but all of one side of the face in LMN lesions. Ask to "raise your eyebrows", "show me your teeth", "puff out your cheeks". Taste can be tested (though rarely done) with salt/sweet solutions.

VIII ***Hearing:*** p468. Ask to repeat a number whispered in an ear while you block the other. Perform Weber's and Rinne's tests (p468). ***Balance/vertigo:*** p466.

IX^P & X^P ***Gag reflex:*** Touch the back of the palate with a spatula to elicit a reflex contraction. The afferent arm of the reflex involves IX; the efferent arm involves X. X^th nerve lesions also cause the palate to be pulled to the normal side on saying "Ah".

XI ***Trapezii:*** "Shrug your shoulders" against resistance.
Sternocleidomastoid: "Turn your head to the left/right" against resistance.

XII ***Tongue movement:*** The tongue deviates to the side of the lesion.

P= Remember that these cranial nerves carry parasympathetic fibres. Sympathetic fibres originate from the thoracic chain and run with the arterial supply to distribute about the body (see also *OHCS*, fig 1, p629).

Causes of cranial nerve lesions

Any cranial nerve may be affected by diabetes mellitus; stroke; MS; tumours; sarcoidosis; vasculitis, p558, eg PAN (p558), SLE (p556); syphilis. Chronic meningitis (malignant, TB, or fungal) tends to pick off the lower cranial nerves one by one.

I Trauma; respiratory tract infection; frontal lobe tumour; meningitis.

II Field defects may start as small areas of visual loss (scotomas, eg in glaucoma). *Monocular blindness:* Lesions of one eye or optic nerve, eg MS, giant cell arteritis. *Bilateral blindness:* Methanol, tobacco amblyopia; neurosyphilis. **Field defects–*Bitemporal hemianopia:*** Optic chiasm compression, eg pituitary adenoma, craniopharyngioma, internal carotid artery aneurysm (**fig 1**, p452). *Homonymous hemianopia:* Affects half the visual field contralateral to the lesion in each eye. Lesions lie beyond the chiasm in the tracts, radiation, or occipital cortex, eg stroke, abscess, tumour.

Optic neuritis (pain on moving eye, loss of central vision, afferent pupillary defect, disc swelling from papillitis). **Causes:** Demyelination (eg MS); rarely sinusitis, syphilis, collagen vascular disorders.

Ischaemic papillopathy: Swelling of optic disc due to stenosis of the posterior ciliary artery (eg in giant cell arteritis).

Papilloedema (swollen discs, **fig 3**, p 562*):* **1** ↑ICP (tumour, abscess, encephalitis, hydrocephalus, idiopathic intracranial hypertension); **2** retro-orbital lesion (eg cavernous sinus thrombosis, p484).

Optic atrophy (pale optic discs and reduced acuity): MS; frontal tumours; Friedreich's ataxia; retinitis pigmentosa; syphilis; glaucoma; Leber's optic atrophy; optic nerve compression.[103]

III[c] *alone*[c]*:* Diabetes; giant cell arteritis; syphilis; posterior communicating artery aneurysm (+ surgery);[104] idiopathic; ↑ICP (if uncal herniation through the tentorium compresses the nerve). IIIrd nerve palsies without a dilated pupil are typically 'medical' (eg diabetes, BP↑). Early dilatation of a pupil implies a compressive lesion, from a 'surgical' cause (tumour, aneurysm) because the parasympathetic fibres run on the outer aspect of the nerve.

IV[c] *alone* Rare and usually due to trauma to the orbit.[105]

VI[c] *alone* MS, Wernicke's encephalopathy, false localizing sign in ↑ICP, pontine stroke (presents with fixed small pupils ± quadriparesis).[106]

V[c] *Sensory:* Trigeminal neuralgia (pain but no sensory loss, p461), herpes zoster, nasopharyngeal cancer, acoustic neuroma (p466). *Motor:* Rare.

VII *LMN:* Bell's palsy (p504), polio, otitis media, skull fracture, cerebello-pontine angle tumours, eg acoustic neuroma, malignant parotid tumours, herpes zoster (Ramsay Hunt syndrome p505, *OHCS* p652). *UMN:* (spares the forehead, because of its bilateral cortical representation)[107] Stroke, tumour.

VIII (p466 & p468) Noise, Paget's disease, Ménière's disease, herpes zoster, acoustic neuroma, brainstem CVA, drugs (eg aminoglycosides).

IX, X, XII Trauma, brainstem lesions, neck tumours.[108]

XI Rare. Polio, syringomyelia, tumour, stroke, bulbar palsy, trauma, TB.

Groups of cranial nerves VIII, then V, VI, IX and X: Cerebellopontine angle tumours, eg acoustic neuroma (p466; facial weakness is, surprisingly, not a prominent sign). V & VI (Gradenigo's syndrome): Lesion (eg a complication of otitis media) at the apex of the petrous temporal bone ('petroapicitis' on MRI).[109] **III, IV & VI:** Stroke, tumours, Wernicke's encephalopathy, aneurysms, MS.[110] **III, IV, V_a & VI:** Cavernous sinus thrombosis, superior orbital fissure lesions (Tolosa-Hunt syndrome, *OHCS* p654). **IX, X & XI:** Jugular foramen lesion. **ΔΔ***:* Myasthenia gravis, muscular dystrophy, myotonic dystrophy, mononeuritis multiplex (p506).

c= structures passing through the cavernous sinus; see BOX, p83.
NB: V_a is the only division of V to do so.

Internuclear ophthalmoplegia (INO) and its causes

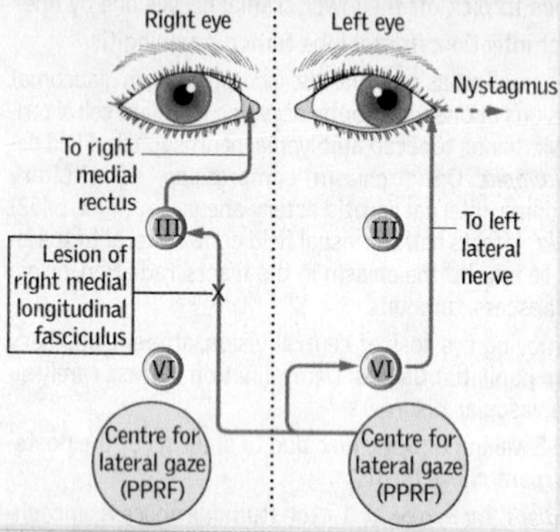

Fig 1. To produce synchronous eye movements, cranial nerves III, IV, and VI communicate through medial longitudinal fasciculus in midbrain. In INO, a lesion disrupts communication, causing weakness in adduction of ipsilateral eye with nystagmus of contralateral eye only when abducting. There may be incomplete or slow abduction of the ipsilateral eye during lateral gaze. Convergence is preserved. Causes: MS or vascular (more rarely: HIV; syphilis; Lyme disease; brainstem tumours; phenothiazine toxicity).[111]

Ptosis

Drooping of the upper eyelid. Best observed with patient sitting up, with head held by examiner. Oculomotor nerve (CN III) innervates main muscle concerned (levator palpebrae), but nerves from the cervical sympathetic chain innervate superior tarsal muscle, and a lesion of these nerves causes mild ptosis which can be overcome on looking up. ***Causes:*** **1** CN III lesions cause unilateral *complete* ptosis: look for other evidence of a CN III lesion: ophthalmoplegia with 'down and out' deviation of the eye, pupil dilated and unreactive to light or accommodation. If eye pain too, suspect infiltration (eg by lymphoma[112] or sarcoid).[113] If T°↑ or consciousness↓, suspect infection (any tick bites?) **2** Sympathetic paralysis usually causes unilateral *partial* ptosis. Look for other evidence of a sympathetic lesion, as in Horner's syndrome (p716): constricted pupil = *miosis*, lack of sweating on same side of the face (=*anhidrosis*). **3** Myopathy, eg dystrophia myotonica, myasthenia gravis (cause bilateral partial ptosis). **4** Congenital; usually partial & without other CNS signs.

Visual loss

►Get ophthalmic help. See *OHCS* p434–p455. Consider:
- Is the eye red? (*glaucoma, iritis* p562)
- Pain? *Giant cell arteritis*: severe temporal headache, jaw claudication, scalp tenderness, ↑ESR: ► urgent steroids (p558). *Optic neuritis*: eg in MS.
- Is the cornea cloudy: *corneal ulcer* (*OHCS* p432), *glaucoma* (*OHCS* p430)?
- Is there a contact lens problem (*infection*)?
- Any flashes/floaters? (*TIA, migraine, retinal detachment*?)
- Is there a visual field problem (*stroke, space-occupying lesion, glaucoma*)?
- Are there any focal CNS signs?
- Any valvular heart disease/carotid bruits (*emboli*)?; Hyperlipidaemia (p704)?
- Is there an afferent pupillary defect (p79)?
- Any past history of trauma, migraine, hypertension, cerebrovascular disease, MS, diabetes or connective tissue disease?
- Any distant signs: eg *HIV* (causes retinitis), *SLE, sarcoidosis, Behçet's disease*?

Sudden • Acute glaucoma • Retinal detachment • Vitreous haemorrhage (eg in diabetic proliferative retinopathy) • Optic neuritis (eg MS) • Temporal arteritis • Central retinal artery or vein occlusion • Migraine • CNS: TIA (amaurosis fugax), stroke, space occupying lesion • Drugs: quinine/methanol • Pituitary apoplexy.

Gradual • Optic atrophy • Chronic glaucoma • Cataracts • Macular degeneration • Tobacco amblyopia

Pupillary abnormalities

Key questions: • Equal, central, circular, dilated, or constricted? • React to light, directly and consensually? • Constrict normally on convergence/accommodation?
Irregular pupils: iritis, syphilis, globe rupture.
Dilated pupils: CN III lesions (►inc. ↑ICP, p840) & mydriatic drugs. *Always ask: is this pupil dilated, or is it the other which is constricted?*
Constricted pupils: old age, sympathetic nerve damage (Horner's, p716, & ptosis, p78), opiates, miotics (pilocarpine drops for glaucoma), & pontine damage.
Unequal pupils (anisocoria) may be due to unilateral lesion, eye-drops, eye surgery, syphilis, or Holmes-Adie pupil. Some inequality is normal.
Light reaction: Test: cover one eye and shine light into the other obliquely. Both pupils should constrict, one by direct, other by consensual light reflex (**fig 2**). Lesion site deduced by knowing pathway: from the retina the message passes up the IInd optic nerve (CNII) to the superior colliculus (midbrain) and thence to the CNIII nuclei bilaterally. The IIIrd cranial nerve causes pupillary constriction. If a light in one eye causes only contralateral constriction, the defect is 'efferent', as the afferent pathways from the retina being stimulated must be intact. Test for *relative afferent pupillary defect:* move torch quickly from pupil to pupil. If there has been incomplete damage to the afferent pathway, the affected pupil will paradoxically dilate when light is moved from the normal eye to the abnormal eye. This is because, in the face of reduced afferent input from the affected eye, the consensual pupillary relaxation response from the normal eye predominates. This is the ***Marcus Gunn sign***, and may occur after apparent complete recovery from the initial lesion.
Reaction to accommodation/convergence: If the patient first looks at a distant object and then at the examiner's finger held a few inches away, the eyes will converge and the pupils constrict. Afferent fibres in each optic nerve pass to the lateral geniculate bodies. Impulses then pass to the pre-tectal nucleus and then to the parasympathetic nuclei of the IIIrd cranial nerves, causing pupillary constriction.

- *Holmes–Adie (myotonic) pupil:* The affected pupil is normally moderately dilated and is poorly reactive to light, if at all. It is slowly reactive to accommodation; wait and watch carefully: it may eventually constrict more than a normal pupil. It is often associated with diminished or absent ankle and knee reflexes, in which case the Holmes-Adie syndrome is present. Usuall a benign incidental finding. Rare causes: Lyme disease, syphilis, parvovirus B19, HSV, autoimmunity. ♀:♂>1.
- *Argyll Robertson pupil:* This occurs in neurosyphilis. The pupil is constricted and unreactive to light, but reacts to accommodation (the prostitute's pupil accomodates, but does not react). Other possible causes: Lyme disease; HIV;[114] zoster; diabetes mellitus; sarcoidosis;[115] MS; paraneoplastic; B_{12}↓.[116] The iris may be patchily atrophied, irregular, and depigmented. The lesion site is not *always* near the Edinger-Westphal nucleus or even in the midbrain.[117] Pseudo-Argyll Robertson pupils occur in Parinaud's syndrome (p722).
- *Hutchinson pupil:* This is the sequence of events resulting from rapidly rising unilateral intracranial pressure (eg in intracerebral haemorrhage). The pupil on the side of the lesion first constricts then widely dilates. The other pupil then goes through the same sequence. ►See p840

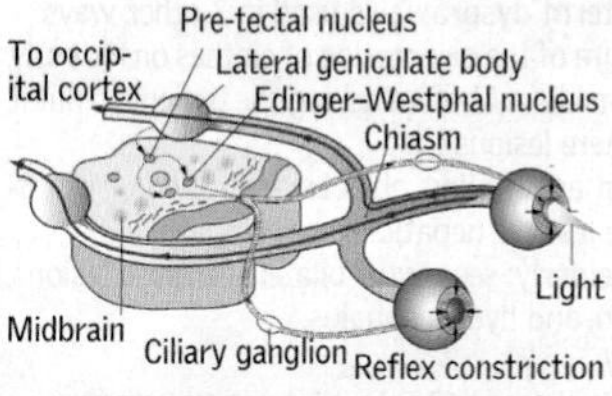

Fig 2. Light reflex. Action potentials go along optic nerve (red), traversing optic chiasm, passing synapses at pre-tectal nucleus, *en route* to Edinger-Westphal nuclei of CNIII. These send fibres to *both* irises' ciliary muscles (so *both* pupils constrict) via **ciliary ganglion** (also relays accommodation & corneal sensation, and gets sympathetic roots from C8–T2, carrying fibres to dilate pupil).

►Have mercy on those with dysphasia: they are suffocating because language is the oxygen of the mind.[1]

Dysphasia (Impairment of language caused by brain damage)

Assessment:

1 If speech is fluent, grammatical and meaningful, dysphasia is unlikely.
2 **Comprehension:** Can the patient follow one, two, and several step commands? (touch your ear, stand up then close the door).
3 **Repetition:** Can the patient repeat a sentence?
4 **Naming:** Can he name common and uncommon things (eg parts of a watch)?
5 **Reading and writing:** Normal? They are usually affected like speech in dysphasia. If normal, the patient is unlikely to be aphasic—is he mute?

Classification: • ***Broca's (expressive) anterior dysphasia:*** Non-fluent speech produced with effort and frustration with malformed words, eg 'spoot' for 'spoon' (or 'that thing'). Reading and writing are impaired but comprehension is relatively intact. Patients understand questions and attempt to convey meaningful answers. **Site of lesion:** infero-lateral dominant frontal lobe (see BOX 1 and **fig 1**).

- *Wernicke's (receptive) posterior dysphasia:* Empty, fluent speech, like talking ragtime with phonemic ('flush' for 'brush') and semantic ('comb' for 'brush') paraphasias/neologisms (may be mistaken for psychotic speech). He is oblivious of errors. Reading, writing, *and* comprehension are impaired (replies are inappropriate). **Site of lesion:** posterior superior dominant temporal lobe.
- *Conduction aphasia:* (Traffic between Broca's and Wernicke's area is interrupted.) Repetition is impaired; comprehension and fluency less so.
- *Nominal dysphasia:* Naming is affected in all dysphasias, but in nominal dysphasia, objects cannot be named but other aspects of speech are normal. This occurs with posterior dominant temporoparietal lesions.

►Mixed dysphasias are common. Discriminating features take time to emerge after an acute brain injury (**fig 1**). Consider speech therapy (of variable use).

Dysarthria Difficulty with articulation due to incoordination or weakness of the musculature of speech. Language is normal (see above).

- *Assessment:* Ask to repeat 'British constitution' or 'baby hippopotamus'.
- *Cerebellar disease:* Ataxia speech muscles cause slurring (as if drunk) and speech irregular in volume and scanning or staccato in quality. (see MINIBOX)
- *Extrapyramidal disease:* Soft, indistinct, and monotonous speech.
- *Pseudobulbar palsy:* (p511) Spastic dysarthria (**upper motor neuron**). Speech is slow, indistinct, nasal and effortful ('Donald Duck' or 'hot potato' voice from bilateral hemispheric lesions, MND (p510), or severe MS).
- *Bulbar palsy:* **Lower motor neuron** (eg facial nerve palsy, Guillain-Barré, MND, p510)—any associated palatal paralysis gives speech a nasal character.

Dysphonia Difficulty with speech volume due to weakness of respiratory muscles or vocal cords (myasthenia, p516; Guillain-Barré syndrome, p716). It may be precipitated in myasthenia by asking the patient to count to 100. Parkinson's gives a mixed picture of dysarthria and dysphonia.

Dyspraxia Poor performance of complex movements despite ability to do each individual component. Test by asking the patient to copy unfamiliar hand positions, or mime an object's use, eg a comb. The term 'dyspraxia' is used in 3 other ways:

- *Dressing dyspraxia:* The patient is unsure of the orientation of clothes on his body. Test by pulling one sleeve of a sweater inside out before asking the patient to put it back on (mostly nondominant hemisphere lesions).
- *Constructional dyspraxia:* Difficulty in assembling objects or drawing, eg a 5-pointed star (nondominant hemisphere lesions, hepatic encephalopathy).
- *Gait dyspraxia:* More common in the elderly; seen with bilateral frontal lesions, lesions in the posterior temporal region, and hydrocephalus.

1 *You cannot say, or guess, for you know only a heap of broken images ... connecting nothing with nothing.* TS Eliot, *The Wasteland*, 1922, Faber & Faber; ISBN 0571202705.

Problems with classifying dysphasias

The classical model of language comprehension occurring in Wernicke's area and language expression in Broca's area is too simple. Functional MRI studies show old ideas that processing of abstract words is confined to the left hemisphere, whereas concrete words are processed on the right are too simplistic.[1] It may be better to think of a mosaic of language centres in the brain with more or less specialized functions. There is evidence that tool-naming is handled differently and in a different area to fruit-naming.[118] There are also individual differences in the anatomy of these mosaics.[119] This is depressing for those who want a rigid classification of aphasia, but a source of hope to those who have had a stroke: recovery may be better than neuroimaging leads us to believe.[120] Where possible, be optimistic.

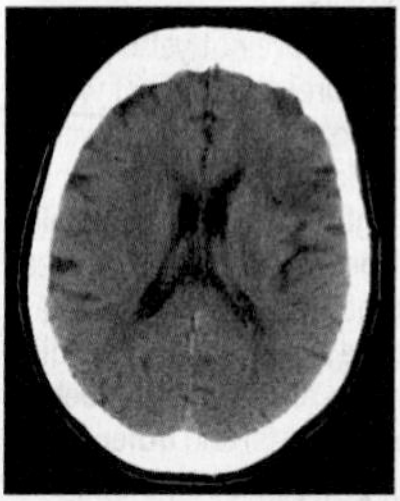

Fig 1. CT of the brain without IV contrast medium, showing a low attenuation area in the frontal lobe, corresponding to an area of acute infarction. This patient presented with a fractured right neck of femur: she had fallen onto her right side. After a few questions, it became clear that she was mostly only saying the word 'yes' in conversation. She was able to form a few phrases, but with difficulty and frustration at her errors. She intermittently understood 3-stage commands and repetition was reasonable, but she often misunderstood simple questions. On balance, she probably had an expressive dysphasia, but in the acute setting it was hard to tell. Courtesy of Norwich Radiology Department

Symptoms of movement disorders

Athetosis is due to a lesion in the putamen, causing slow sinuous writhing movements in the hands, which are present at rest. *Pseudoathetosis* refers to athetoid movements in patients with severe proprioceptive loss.

Chorea means *dance* (hence 'choreography')—a flow of jerky movements, flitting from one limb to another (each seemingly a fragment of a normal movement). Distinguish from athetosis/pseudoathetosis (above), and hemiballismus (p472). ***Causes:*** basal ganglia lesion (stroke, Huntington's, p716); streptococci (Sydenham's chorea; St Vitus' dance, p136); SLE (p556); Wilson's (p269); neonatal kernicterus; polycythaemia (p360), neuroacanthocytosis (genetic, with acanthocytes in peripheral blood with chorea, oro-facial dyskinesia, and axonal neuropathy), hyperthyroidism (p210), drugs (L-dopa, contraceptive steroids/HRT, chlorpromazine, cocaine's *crack dancing*). Early stages of chorea may be detected by feeling fluctuations in muscle tension while the patient grips your finger. ℞: Dopamine antagonists, eg tetrabenazine 12.5mg/12h (/24h if elderly) PO; increase, eg to 25mg/8h PO; max 200mg/d.

Hemiballismus is uncontrolled unilateral flailing movements of proximal limb joints caused by contralateral subthalamic lesions. See p472.

Cerebellar signs

- *Speech:* slurred/ataxic/staccato
- *Eye movements:* nystagmus
- *Tone and power:* hypotonia and reduced power
- *Coordination:* finger-to-nose test; test for dysdiadochokinesis, p503
- *Gait:* Broad based, fall to side of lesion. *Romberg test:* ask patient to stand with eyes closed. If he loses balance, test is positive and a sign of posterior column disease. Cerebellar disease is Romberg negative.

(Remember **DANISH**: **D**ysdiadochokinesis, **A**taxia, **N**ystagmus, **I**ntention tremor, **S**lurred speech, **H**ypotonia and reduced power)

1 While abstract words activate a sub-region of the left inferior frontal gyrus more strongly than concrete words, specific activity for concrete words can also be observed in the left basal temporal cortex.

Introduce yourself, ask a few factual questions (precise name, age, marital status, job, and who is at home). These will help your patient to relax.

Presenting problem Then ask for the main problems which have led to this consultation. Sit back and listen. Don't worry whether the information is in a convenient form or not—this is an opportunity for the patient to come out with his worries, ideas, and preoccupations unsullied by your expectations. After 3-5min it is often good to aim to have a list of all the problems (each sketched only briefly). Read them back to the patient and ask if there are any more. Then ask about:

History of presenting problem For each problem obtain details, both current state and history of onset, precipitating factors, and effects on life.

Check of major psychiatric symptoms Check those which have not yet been covered: **depression**—low mood, anhedonia (inability to feel pleasure), thoughts of worthlessness/hopelessness, sleep disturbance with early morning waking, loss of weight and appetite. Ask specifically about **suicidal thoughts and plans:** "Have you ever been so low that you thought of harming yourself?", "What thoughts have you had?" **Hallucinations** ("Have you ever heard voices when there hasn't been anyone there, or seen visions?"), and **delusions** ("Have you ever had any thoughts or beliefs which have struck you afterwards as bizarre?"); **anxiety** and **avoidance behaviour** (eg avoiding shopping because of anxiety or phobias); **obsessional thoughts** and **compulsive behaviour, eating** disorders, **alcohol** (see p283 for alcohol screening tests) and **other drugs**.

Present circumstances Housing, finance, work, marriage, friends.

Family history Ask about health, personality, and occupation of parents and siblings, and the **family's medical and psychiatric history.**

Background history Try to understand the context of the presenting problem.
- *Biography:* relationships with family and peers as a child; school and work record; sexual relationships and current relationships; and family. Previous ways of dealing with stress and whether there have been problems and symptoms similar to the presenting ones.
- *Premorbid personality:* mood, character, hobbies, attitudes, and beliefs.

Past medical and psychiatric history

Mental state examination This is the state **now**, at the time of interview.
- *Appearance:* Clothing, glasses, headwear? Unkempt/meticulous?
- *Observable behaviour:* Eg excessive slowness, signs of anxiety, gesture, gaze and mutual gaze, tears, laughter, pauses (while listening to voices?), attitude (eg withdrawn).
- *Mode of speech:* Include the rate of speech, eg retarded or gabbling (pressure of speech). Note its content. Flight of ideas? Knight's move? (See BOX 1)
- *Mood:* Note thoughts about harming self or others. Gauge your own responses to the patient. The laughter and grand ideas of manic patients are contagious, as to a lesser extent is the expression of thoughts from a depressed person.
- *Beliefs:* Eg about himself, his own body, about other people, and the future. Note abnormal beliefs (delusions), eg that thoughts are overheard, and abnormal ideas (eg persecutory, grandiose).
- *Unusual experiences or hallucinations:* Note modality, eg visual, auditory.
- *Orientation:* In time, place, and person. What is the date? What time of day is it? Where are you? What is your name?
- *Short-term memory:* Give a name and address and test recall after 5min. Make sure that he has got the address clear in his head before waiting the 5min.
- *Long-term memory:* Current affairs recall. Name of current political leaders (p 70 & p85). This tests many other CNS functions, not just memory.
- *Concentration:* Months of the year backwards.
- Note the degree of your *rapport* and the patient's *insight* into his current state.

Psychiatric symptoms

There are many different ways to think about psychiatric symptoms. One simple approach can be to consider negative and positive symptoms. *Negative symptoms* involve the absence of a behaviour, thought, feeling or sensation (eg lack of appetite, apathy, and blunted emotions in depression), whereas *positive symptoms* involve their presence when not normally expected (eg thought insertion, ie "Someone is putting thoughts into my head"). Understanding the difference between psychosis and neurosis is vital. *Psychosis* entails a thought disorder (eg thought insertion, thought broadcasting) ± delusions (abnormal beliefs which are held to despite all reasoning, and which run counter to the patient's cultural background) and abnormal perceptions (eg hallucinations). *Neurosis* entails insight—if there are intrusive ideas or odd experiential phenomena the person knows that they are false or illusory (and may be triggered by stress etc).

Interesting abnormalities of speech include *flight of ideas*, in which the speech races through themes, switching whimsically or through associations eg 'clang' association: "Yesterday I went down to the local shop. I didn't hop (*clang*), but I walked. Kangaroos hop, don't they? My friend Joey wasn't there, though...". *Knight's move* is an unexpected change in the direction of speech or conversation (akin to the lateral component of the move of the knight's piece in chess) and *neologism* is the formation of new words. They may be normal or indicate an organic brain condition or a psychosis.

Many psychiatric symptoms in isolation, to a lesser degree of severity, or even in a different culture, may well be considered part of 'normal' behaviour. For example, where would we be without language embracing brave new words? 121 As with so many aspects of medicine, in psychiatry there is a vast spectrum of behaviour, thought and perception, at least one extreme of which is considered to be 'abnormal'. It is in part our challenge to attempt to interpret these symptoms with relevance, insight and impartiality so that we may best benefit our patients and not form opinions that are set in stone. On acute medical wards psychiatric symptoms are usually due to stress, drug or alcohol withdrawal, U&E imbalance, or medication. When in doubt, ask a psychiatrist to help. **NB:** it is normal for the bereaved to hear the voice of the person who has died.

►Beware of simplistic formulations, eg *If you talk to God, you are praying. If God talks to you, you have schizophrenia* (Dr Thomas Szasz). It is not the auditory phenomenon that makes the diagnosis of psychosis: what matters is what the patient believes about the phenomenon, and whether they are associated with a thought disorder or a delusion.

The contents of the cavernous sinus and the cranial nerve names

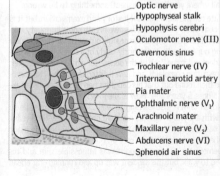

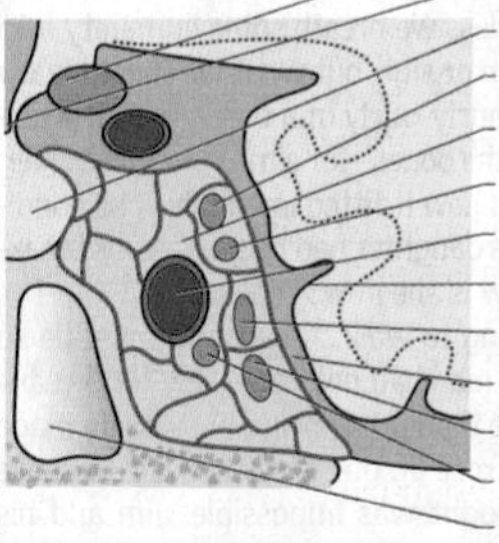

Cranial nerve names	
I	olfactory
II	optic
III	oculomotor
IV	trochlear
V	trigeminal
V_1	ophthalmic division
V_2	maxillary division
V_3	mandibular division
VI	abducens
VII	facial
VIII	vestibulocochlear
IX	glossopharyngeal
X	vagus
XI	accessory
XII	hypoglossal

1 Look at the patient. Healthy, unwell, or *in extremis*? This vital skill improves with practice. ►**Beware those who are sicker than they look**, eg cardiogenic shock; cord compression; nonaccidental injury.
2 Pulse, BP O_2 sats; T° (infrared tympanic[IRT] & liquid crystal[LC] devices avoid mercury).[1]
3 Examine nails, hands, conjunctivae (anaemia), and sclerae (jaundice). Consider: Paget's, acromegaly, endocrine disease (thyroid, pituitary, or adrenal hypo- or hyperfunction), body hair, abnormal pigmentation, skin.
4 Examine mouth and tongue (cyanosed; smooth; furred; beefy, eg rhomboid area denuded of papillae by *Candida*, after prolonged steroid inhaler use).
5 Examine the neck from behind: nodes, goitre.
6 Make sure the patient is at 45° to begin CVS examination in the neck: JVP; feel for character and volume of carotid pulse.
7 The praecordium. Look for abnormal pulsations. Feel the apex beat (character; position). Any parasternal heave or thrill? Auscultate (bell & diaphragm) apex in the left lateral position, then the other 3 areas (p39) and carotids. Sit the patient forward: listen during expiration.
8 Whilst sitting forward, look for sacral oedema.
9 Begin the respiratory examination with the patient at 90°. Observe (and count) respirations; note posterior chest wall movement. Assess expansion, then percuss and auscultate the chest with the bell.
10 Sit the patient back. Feel the trachea. Inspect again. Assess expansion of the anterior chest. Percuss and auscultate again.
11 Examine axillae & breasts, if indicated (+chaperone for *all* intimate examinations).
12 Lie flat (1 pillow) to inspect, palpate, percuss, and auscultate the abdomen.
13 Look at the legs: any swellings, perfusion, pulses, or oedema?
14 CNS exam: ***Cranial nerves:*** pupil responses; fundi; visual fields; visual acuity. Do corneal reflexes. "Open your mouth; stick your tongue out; screw up your eyes; show me your teeth; raise your eyebrows." ***Peripheral nerves:*** Look for wasting and fasciculation. Test tone in all limbs. "Hold your hands out with your palms towards the ceiling and fingers wide. Now shut your eyes." Watch for pronator drift. "Keep your eyes shut and touch your nose with each index finger." "Lift your leg straight in the air. Keep it there. Put your heel on the opposite knee (eyes shut) and run it up your own shin." You have now tested power, coordination, and joint position sense. Tuning fork on toes and index fingers to assess vibration sense.
15 Examine gait and speech. Any abnormalities of higher mental function to pursue?
16 Consider rectal and vaginal examination.
17 Examine the urine with dipstick and microscope if appropriate (p383).

►In general, go into detail where you find (or suspect) something to be wrong.

So now we have a template for the all-important history and examination, but it is no more than a tattered coat upon a stick 122 unless we breath some humanity into it. We start out nervous of missing some question or sign, but what we should really be nervous about is losing our humanity in the hurly-burly of a time-pressed interview. Here is how one student put some flesh on the bones—for a man in a wheelchair: she asked all about the presenting complaint, and how it fitted in with his CNS condition and life at home—and then found out that his daughter had had a nervous breakdown at the start of his illness, 5 years ago. "How is she now?" she asked "Fine—I've got two lovely grandchildren...Jim is just learning to walk..." "Oh...you must be so *busy*!" the student said with a joyful smile. This man had not been busy for 5 years, and was fed up with his passive dependency. The thought of being busy again made his face light up—and when the student left he rose up out of wheelchair to shake her by the hand, a movement we doctors thought was impossible. Jim and his grandfather were learning to walk, but this student was up and running—far ahead of her teachers.

1 IRT is better than forehead LC strips; LC is specific (100%) but not sensitive (39%).

The TYM (*Test Your Memory*) test

Please write your full name [2]

....

Today is ....day [1]

Today's date is the: [3]

...... of ...... (month) 20...

How old are you? .... years [1]

On what date were you born? [3]

........./......... (month) / 19....

Please copy the following sentence [2]

Good citizens always wear stout shoes

....

....

Please read the sentence again and try to remember it.

Who is the Prime Minister [2]

....

What year did the 1st world war start? [1]

....

Sums [4]

20 – 4 = ... 8 × 6 = ...

16 + 17 = ... 5 + 15 – 17 = ...

Please list 4 creatures beginning with 'S' (eg Shark) [4]

1. S................

2. S................

Why is a carrot like a potato? [2]

....

Why is a lion like a wolf? [2]

....

Remember:

Good citizens always wear stout shoes

Please name these items: [5]

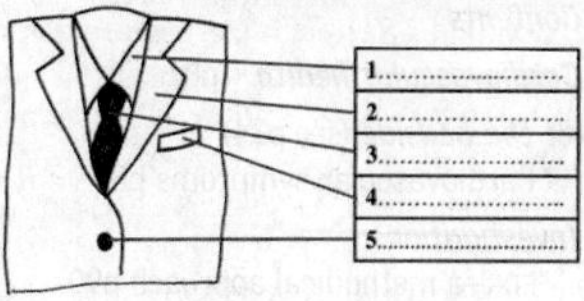

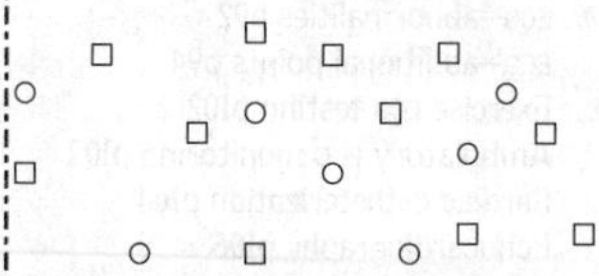

Please join the circles together to form a letter. [3]

Please draw in a clock face, put in the numbers 1 – 12, and put the hands at 9:20. [4]

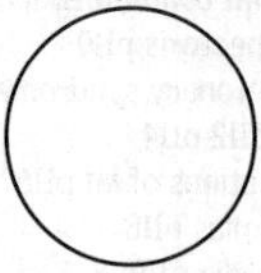

Without turning the page, please write down the sentence you copied earlier. [5]

....

....

For the TYM tester: help given? [5]

None⁵/trial⁴/minor³/moderate²/major¹

max 50

©Dr Jeremy Brown. BMJ 2009;338:b2030
www.bmj.com/cgi/data/bmj.b2030/dc1/1

(↑fold here)

In one preliminary study,[1] the controls' average score was 47/50. Those with Alzheimer's disease (AD) scored on average of 33/50. The TYM score correlates highly with other standard tests, but, uniquely, it is quick and can be self-administered. A score of <42/50 had a sensitivity of 93% and specificity of 86% for AD. TYM is more sensitive at detecting AD than the mini-mental exam (MMSE), detecting 93% of patients compared with 52% for MMSE. Negative & positive predictive values (p674) of TYM with a cut off of 42 were 99% & 42% (if prevalence of AD is 10%). If non-Alzheimer dementia, score was 39/50 (mean). This new test should not *make* any diagnosis—but it may suggest when further referral might help.

Use a **scoring sheet** for marking. www.elderguru.com/wp-content/uploads/2009/06/tym-test-score.pdf *Animals beginning with 'S':* 'Shark' and mythical creatures not allowed. *Carrot/potato:* Reasonable but less precise answer than "...vegetables..." eg "food", scores **1** point. 2 such statements score **2** eg "grows in ground...fierce" or "...food...4 legs..." scores **2** in total. *Jacket-naming:* Answers are collar, lapel, tie, pocket, button. **1** point each. Shirt is acceptable for item 1; jacket or blazer is OK for 2 or 4 (but not both). *Circles task:* **1** point if all circles joined even if not a letter W. *Clockface:* All numbers OK **1**; correct number position **1**; correct hands **1**. *Sentence:* **1** point for each word remembered up to a maximum of **5**.

[1] TYM for detection of Alzheimer's disease: cross sectional study. Brown J, Dawson K, Pengas G 2009 *BMJ* 338 1426.

Contents

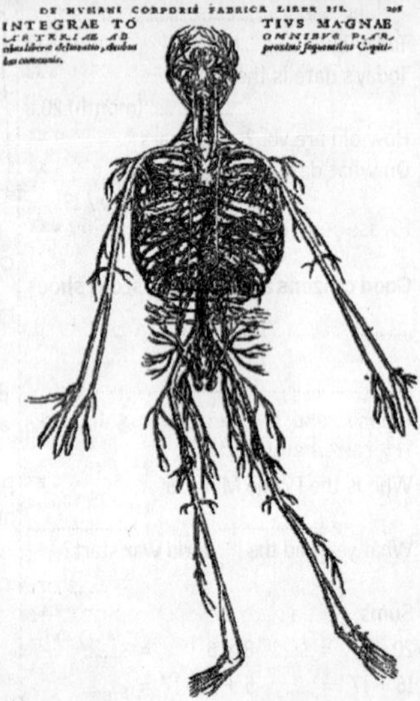

Fig 1. The vasculature, from Andreas Vesalius's, *De Humani Corporis Fabrica* (On the Fabric of the Human Body). The day after his finals he dissected a body with such vivid brilliance that he was at once made Professor of Surgery at Padua. By general acclamation, modern medicine began that day: December 6th, 1537.[1] Galen's infallibility was trumped by direct observation, experiment, and the painstaking accumulation of data.

Cardiovascular medicine has an unrivalled treasure house of such data, in the form of randomized trials. One of the chief pleasures of cardiovascular medicine lies in integrating these with clinical reasoning in a humane way. After a cardiac event, a protocol may 'mandate' statins, aspirin, β-blockers, ACE-i (p109), and a target BP and LDL cholesterol that makes your patient feel dreadful. What to do? Inform, negotiate, and compromise. Never reject your patient because of lack of compliance with your over-exacting regimens. Keep smiling, keep communicating, and keep up-to-date: the latest data may show that your patient was right all along.[2]

Other relevant pages: Emergencies: MI (p808); pulmonary oedema (p812); cardiac shock (p814); broad & narrow complex tachycardias (p816 & p818); *Cardiac arrest:* see inside back cover. CVS examination (p38); carotid bruit (p38); cyanosis (p28); dyspnoea (p49); haemoptysis (p49); oedema (p29); palpitations (p35); aneurysms (p600); dyslipidaemia (p704); risk factor analysis (p664); nuclear cardiology[et al] (p754).

We thank Dr James Rudd, our Specialist Reader for this chapter.

Cardiovascular health

Ischaemic heart disease (IHD) is the most common cause of death worldwide. Encouraging cardiovascular health is not *only* about preventing IHD: health entails the ability to *exercise*, and enjoying vigorous activity (within reason!) is one of the best ways of achieving health, not just because the heart likes it (BP↓, 'good' high-density lipoprotein, HDL↑)—it can prevent osteoporosis, improve glucose tolerance, and augment immune function (eg in cancer and if HIV+ve). People who improve *and maintain* their fitness live longer: ►*age-adjusted mortality from all causes is reduced by >40%*. Avoiding obesity helps too, but weight loss *per se* is only useful in reducing cardiovascular risk and the risk of developing diabetes when combined with regular exercise. Moderate alcohol drinking may also promote cardiovascular health.

Smoking is the chief risk factor for cardiovascular mortality. You *can* help people give up, and giving up *does* undo much of the harm of smoking. *Simple advice works*. Most smokers want to give up (unlike eaters of unhealthy diets who are mostly wedded to them by habit, and the pleasures of the palate). Just because smoking advice does *not always* work, do not stop giving it. Ask about smoking in consultations—especially those concerned with smoking-related diseases.

- Ensure advice is congruent with patient's beliefs about smoking.
- Getting patients to enumerate the advantages of giving up increases motivation.
- Invite the patient to choose a date (when there will be few stresses) on which he or she will become a non-smoker.
- Suggest throwing away all accessories (cigarettes, pipes, ash trays, lighters, matches) in advance; inform friends of the new change; practise saying 'no' to their offers of 'just one little cigarette'.
- ***Nicotine gum***, chewed intermittently to limit nicotine release: ≥ ten 2mg sticks may be needed/day. ***Transdermal nicotine patches*** may be easier. A dose increase at 1wk can help. Written advice offers no added benefit to advice from nurses. Always offer follow-up.
- ***Varenicline*** is an oral selective nicotine receptor partial agonist. Start 1 week before target stop date: initially 0.5mg/24h PO for 3 days, then 0.5mg/12h for 4 days, then 1mg/12h for 11 weeks (↓ to 0.5mg/12h if not tolerated). *SE:* appetite change; dry mouth; taste disturbance; headache; drowsiness; dizziness; sleep disorders; abnormal dreams; depression; suicidal thoughts; panic; dysarthria.
- ***Bupropion*** (=*amfebutamone*, p455) is said to ↑quit rate to 30% at 1yr *vs* 16% with patches and 15.6% for placebo (patches + bupropion: 35.5%):[3] consider if the above fails. *Dose:* 150mg/24h PO (while still smoking; quit within 2wks); dose may be twice daily from day 7; stop after 7-9wks. ***Warn of** SEs:* Seizures (risk <1 : 1000), insomnia, headache.
- Lipids and BP (p704 & p132) are the other major *modifiable* risk factors.

To calculate how risk factors interact, see **risk equation**, p664—and its caveats. NICE recommends a Framingham score with risk multiplied by 1.4 for south Asian men, but this doesn't cater for: • Asian diversity (eg multiply by 1.7 in Bangladeshi men) • Asian women • Deprivation effects • Double-counting problems if adjustment is made for ethnicity ***and*** family history. QRISK2 is better in UK patients.[4]

►Apply preventive measures such as healthy eating (p236) *early* in life to maximize impact, when there are most years to save, and before bad habits get ingrained.

For an example of implementation of cardiovascular health strategies, see the UK NHS national service framework: www.doh.gov.uk/nsf/coronary.htm

mitral stenosis
→ "tapping" apex beat
→ can feel
→ v. loud
+ v. quite end diastolic murmur

Chest pain ►Cardiac-sounding chest pain may have no serious cause, but always think *"Could this be a myocardial infarction (MI), dissecting aortic aneurysm, pericarditis, or pulmonary embolism?"*

Character: Constricting suggests angina, oesophageal spasm, or anxiety; a *sharp* pain may be from the pleura or pericardium. A prolonged (>½h), dull, central crushing pain or pressure suggests MI.

Radiation: To shoulder, either or both arms, or neck/jaw suggests cardiac ischaemia. The pain of aortic dissection is classically instantaneous, tearing, and interscapular, but may be retrosternal. Epigastric pain may be cardiac.

Precipitants: Pain associated with cold, exercise, palpitations, or emotion suggest cardiac pain or anxiety; if brought on by food, lying flat, hot drinks, or alcohol, consider oesophageal spasm/disease (but meals *can* cause angina).

Relieving factors: If pain is relieved *within minutes* by rest or glyceryl trinitrate (GTN), suspect angina (GTN relieves oesophageal spasm more slowly). If antacids help, suspect GI causes. Pericarditic pain improves on leaning forward.

Associations: Dyspnoea occurs with cardiac pain, pulmonary emboli, pleurisy, or anxiety. MI may cause nausea, vomiting, or sweating. Angina is caused by coronary artery disease—and also by aortic stenosis, hypertrophic cardiomyopathy (HCM), paroxysmal supraventricular tachycardia (SVT) and be exacerbated by anaemia. Chest pain with *tenderness* suggests self-limiting Tietze's syndrome.[1]

Pleuritic pain (ie exacerbated by inspiration) implies inflammation of the pleura from pulmonary infection, inflammation, or infarction. It causes us to 'catch our breath'. ΔΔ: Musculoskeletal pain;[1] fractured rib (pain on respiration, exacerbated by gentle pressure on the sternum); subdiaphragmatic pathology (eg gallstones).

Acutely ill patients: • Admit to hospital • Check pulse, BP in both arms, JVP, heart sounds; examine legs for DVT • Give O_2 by mask • IV line • Relieve pain (eg morphine 5–10mg IV slowly (2mg/min) + an antiemetic) • Cardiac monitor • 12-lead ECG • CXR • Arterial blood gas (ABG). *Famous traps:* Aortic dissection; zoster (p400); ruptured oesophagus; cardiac tamponade (shock with JVP↑); opiate addiction.

Dyspnoea may be from LVF, pulmonary embolism, any respiratory cause, or anxiety. *Severity:* ►►Emergency presentations: p796. Ask about shortness of breath at rest or on exertion, exercise tolerance, and in daily tasks. Is it episodic and triggered by lying flat (PND, p49)? *Associations:* Specific symptoms associated with heart failure are orthopnoea (ask about number of pillows used at night), paroxysmal nocturnal dyspnoea (waking up at night gasping for breath), and peripheral oedema. Pulmonary embolism is associated with acute onset of dyspnoea and pleuritic chest pain; ask about risk factors for DVT.

Palpitation(s) may be due to ectopics, AF, SVT and ventricular tachycardia (VT), thyrotoxicosis, anxiety, and rarely phaeochromocytoma. See p35. *History:* Ask about previous episodes, precipitating/relieving factors, duration of symptoms, associated chest pain, dyspnoea, or dizziness. *Did the patient check his pulse?*

Syncope may reflect cardiac or CNS events. Vasovagal 'faints' are common (pulse↓, pupils dilated). The history from an observer is invaluable in diagnosis. *Prodromal symptoms:* Chest pain, palpitations, or dyspnoea point to a cardiac cause, eg arrhythmia. Aura, headache, dysarthria, and limb weakness indicate CNS causes. *During the episode:* Was there a pulse? Limb jerking, tongue biting, or urinary incontinence? **NB:** hypoxia from lack of cerebral perfusion may cause seizures. *Recovery:* Was this rapid (arrhythmia) or prolonged, with drowsiness (seizure)?

1 25% of non-cardiac chest pain is **musculoskeletal**: look for pain on specific postures or activity. Aim to reproduce the pain by movement and, sometimes, palpation over the structure causing it. Focal injection of local anaesthetic helps diagnostically and is therapeutic. **Tietze's syndrome:** self-limiting costochondritis ± costosternal joint swelling. Causes: idiopathic; microtrauma; infection; psoriatic/rheumatoid arthritis. ℞: NSAIDs or steroid injections. Tenderness is also caused by: fibrositis, lymphoma, chondrosarcoma, myeloma, metastases, rib TB. Imaging: bone scintigraphy; CT.

How patients communicate ischaemic cardiac sensations

On emergency wards we are always hearing questions such as "Is your pain sharp or dull?", followed by an equivocal answer. The doctor goes on "Sharp like a knife—or dull and crushing?" The doctor is getting irritated because the patient must know the answer, but is not saying it. A true story paves the way to being less inquisitorial, and having a more creative understanding of the nature of symptoms. A patient came to one of us (JML) saying "Last night I dreamed I had a pain in my chest. Now I've woken up, and I'm not sure—have I got chest pain, doctor? What do you think?" How odd it is to find oneself examining a patient to exclude a symptom, not a disease. (It turned out that she *did* have serious chest pathology.) Odd, until one realizes that symptoms are often half-formed, and it is our role to give them a local habitation and a name. Dialogue can transform a symptom from 'airy nothingness' to a fact.[1] Patients often avoid using the word 'pain' to describe ischaemia: 'wind', 'tightening', 'pressure', 'burning', or 'a lump in the throat' (angina means to choke) may be used. He may say "'sharp" to communicate severity, and not character. So be as vague in your questioning as your patient is in his answers. "Tell me some more about what you are feeling (long pause)... as if someone was doing *what* to you?" "Sitting on me", or "like a hotness" might be the response (suggesting cardiac ischaemia). Do not ask "Does it go into your left arm". Try "Is there anything else about it?" (pause) ... "Does it go anywhere?" Note down your patient's exact words.

Note also non-verbal clues: the clenched fist placed over the sternum is a telling feature of cardiac pain (Levine-sign positive).

A good history, taking account of these features, is the best way to stratify patients likely to have cardiac pain. If the history is non-specific, and there are no risk factors for cardiovascular diseases, and ECG and plasma troponin T (p112) are normal (<0.2μg/L) 6-12h after the onset of pain, discharge will probably be OK.[5] When in doubt, get help. Features making cardiac pain unlikely:

- Stabbing, shooting pain
- Pain lasting <30s, however intense
- Well-localized, left sub-mammary pain ("In my heart, doctor")
- Pains of continually varying location
- Youth.

Do not feel that you must diagnose every pain. *Chest pain with no cause* is common, even after extensive tests. Do not reject these patients: explain your findings to them. Some have a 'chronic pain syndrome' which responds to a tricyclic, eg imipramine 50mg at night (this dose does not imply any depression). It is similar to post-herpetic neuralgia.

1 Dialogue-transformed symptoms explain one of the junior doctor's main vexations: when patients retell symptoms to a consultant in the light of day, they bear no resemblance to what you originally heard. But do not be vexed: your dialogue may have helped the patient far more than any ward round.

►First confirm the patient's name and age, and the ECG date. Then (see **fig 1**):

- *Rate:* At usual speed (25mm/s) each 'big square' is 0.2s; each 'small square' is 0.04s. To calculate the rate, divide 300 by the number of big squares per R-R interval (p91).
- *Rhythm:* If cycles are not clearly regular, use the 'card method': lay a card along ECG, marking positions of 3 successive R waves. Slide the card to and fro to check that all intervals are equal. If not, note if different rates are multiples of each other (ie varying block), or is it 100% irregular (atrial fibrillation (AF) or ventricular fibrillation, VF)? ***Sinus rhythm*** is characterized by a P wave (upright in II, III, & aVF; inverted in aVR) followed by a QRS complex. AF has no discernible P waves and QRS complexes are irregularly irregular. ***Atrial flutter*** (p125) has a 'sawtooth' baseline of atrial depolarization (~300/min) and regular QRS complexes. ***Nodal rhythm*** has a normal QRS complex but P waves are absent or occur just before or within QRS complexes. *Ventricular rhythm* has QRS complexes >0.12s with P waves following them (**ECG 6**).
- *Axis:* The mean frontal axis is the sum of all the ventricular forces during ventricular depolarization. The axis lies at 90° to the isoelectric complex (ie the one in which positive and negative deflections are equal). See BOX 2. *Normal axis* is between -30° and +90°. As a simple rule of thumb, if the complexes in leads I and II are both 'positive', the axis is normal. *Left axis deviation* (LAD) is -30° to -90°. Causes: left anterior hemiblock, inferior MI, VT from LV focus, Wolff-Parkinson-White (WPW) syndrome (some types). *Right axis deviation* (RAD) is +90° to +180°. Causes: RVH, PE, anterolateral MI, left posterior hemiblock (rare), WPW syndrome (some types). See BOX 3.
- ***P wave:*** Normally precedes each QRS complex. *Absent P wave:* AF, sinoatrial block, junctional (AV nodal) rhythm. Dissociation between P waves and QRS complexes indicates complete heart block. *P mitrale:* bifid P wave, indicates left atrial hypertrophy. *P pulmonale:* peaked P wave, indicates right atrial hypertrophy. Pseudo-P-pulmonale seen if $K^+\downarrow$.
- ***PR interval:*** Measure from start of P wave to start of QRS. *Normal range*: 0.12–0.2s (3–5 small squares). A *prolonged PR interval* implies delayed AV conduction (1st degree heart block). A *short PR interval* implies unusually fast AV conduction down an accessory pathway, eg WPW p120 (ECG p125).
- ***QRS complex:*** *Normal duration:* <0.12s. If ≥0.12s suggests ventricular conduction defects, eg a bundle branch block (p94 & p119). Large QRS complexes suggest *ventricular hypertrophy* (p94). *Normal Q wave* <0.04s wide and <2mm deep. They are often seen in leads V_5 and V_6, aVL and I, and reflect normal septal depolarization, which usually occurs from left to right. *Pathological Q waves* may occur within a few hours of an acute MI.
- ***QT interval:*** Measure from start of QRS to *end* of T wave. It varies with rate. Calculate *corrected QT interval* (QT^c) by dividing the measured QT interval by the square root of the cycle length, ie $QT^c = QT/\sqrt{RR}$. Normal QT^c: 0.38–0.42s. *Prolonged QT interval*: acute myocardial ischaemia, myocarditis, bradycardia (eg AV block), head injury, hypothermia, U&E imbalance ($K^+\downarrow$, $Ca^{2+}\downarrow$, $Mg^{2+}\downarrow$), congenital (Romano-Ward & Jervell-Lange-Nielson syndromes); sotalol, quinidine, antihistamines, macrolides (eg erythromycin), amiodarone, phenothiazines, tricyclics.
- ***ST segment:*** Usually isoelectric. Planar elevation (>1mm) or depression (>0.5mm) usually implies infarction (p113, **ECG 3,4**) or ischaemia (p103), respectively.
- ***T wave:*** Normally inverted in aVR, V_1 and occasionally V_2. Abnormal if inverted in I, II, and V_4–V_6. Peaked in hyperkalaemia (ECG 13, p689) and flattened in hypokalaemia.
- ***J wave*** see p861. Seen in hypothermia, subarachnoid haemorrhage and hypercalcaemia.

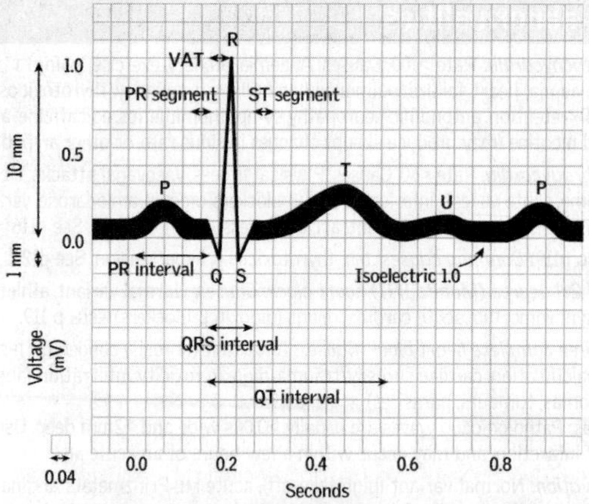

Fig 1. Schematic diagram of a normal ECG trace

Calculating the R–R interval

To calculate the rate, divide 300 by the number of big squares per R–R interval—if the UK standard ECG speed of 25mm/s is used (elsewhere, 50mm/s may be used: don't be confused!)

R–R duration (s)	Big squares	Rate (per min)
0.2	1	300
0.4	2	150
0.6	3	100
0.8	4	75
1.0	5	60
1.2	6	50
1.4	7	43

Determining the ECG axis

The axis lies at 90° to the isoelectric complex (the one in which positive and negative deflections are equal in size).

If the complexes in I and II are both predominantly positive, the axis is normal.

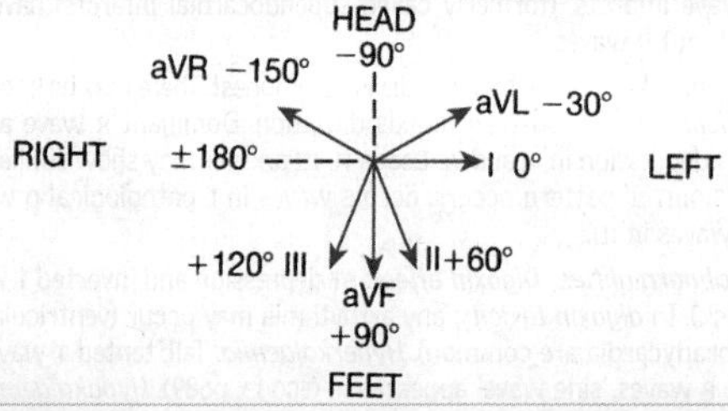

Causes of LAD (left axis deviation)	Causes of RAD (right axis deviation)
Left anterior hemiblock	RVH
Inferior MI	Pulmonary embolism
VT from LV focus	Anterolateral MI
WPW syndrome p120	WPW syndrome
	Left posterior hemiblock (rare)

Sinus tachycardia: Rate >100. Causes: Anaemia, anxiety, exercise, pain, ↑T°, sepsis, hypovolaemia, heart failure, pulmonary embolism, pregnancy, thyrotoxicosis, beri beri, CO_2 retention, autonomic neuropathy, sympathomimetics, eg caffeine, adrenaline, and nicotine (may produce abrupt changes in sinus rate, or other arrhythmia).

Sinus bradycardia: Rate <60. Causes: Physical fitness, vasovagal attacks, sick sinus syndrome, acute MI (esp. inferior), drugs (β-blockers, digoxin, amiodarone, verapamil), hypothyroidism, hypothermia, ↑intracranial pressure, cholestasis. See p116

AF: (ECG p119) *Common causes:* IHD, thyrotoxicosis, hypertension. See p124.

1st and 2nd degree (Mobitz I/II) heart block: Causes: Normal variant, athletes, sick sinus syndrome, IHD, acute carditis, drugs (digoxin, β-blockers). ECGs p 119.

3rd degree complete heart block: Causes: Idiopathic (fibrosis), congenital, IHD, aortic valve calcification, cardiac surgery/trauma, digoxin toxicity, infiltration (abscesses, granulomas, tumours, parasites). **ECG 5**, p 99.

Q waves: Pathological Q waves are usually >0.04s wide and >2mm deep. Usually as sign of infarction, and may occur within a few hours of an acute MI.

ST elevation: Normal variant (high take-off), acute MI, Prinzmetal's angina (p722), acute pericarditis (saddle-shaped), left ventricular aneurysm.

ST depression: Normal variant (upward sloping), digoxin (downward sloping), ischaemic (horizontal): angina, acute posterior MI.

T inversion: In V_1–V_3: normal (Blacks and children), right bundle branch block (RBBB), pulmonary embolism. In V_2–V_5: subendocardial MI, HCM, subarachnoid haemorrhage, lithium. In V_4–V_6 and aVL: ischaemia, LVH, associated with left bundle branch block (LBBB).

NB: ST and T wave changes are often non-specific, and must be interpreted in the light of the clinical context.

Myocardial infarction: (ECG p113)

- Within hours, the T wave may become peaked and ST segments may begin to rise.
- Within 24h, the T wave inverts, as ST segment elevation begins to resolve. ST elevation rarely persists, unless a left ventricular aneurysm develops. T wave inversion may or may not persist.
- Within a few days, pathological Q waves begin to form. Q waves usually persist, but may resolve in 10%.
- The leads affected reflect the site of the infarct: inferior (II, III, aVF), anteroseptal (V_{1-4}), anterolateral (V_{4-6}, I, aVL), posterior (tall R and ST↓ in V_{1-2}).

► 'Non-Q wave infarcts' (formerly called subendocardial infarcts) have ST and T changes without Q waves.

Pulmonary embolism: Sinus tachycardia is commonest. There may be RAD, RBBB (p91), *right ventricular strain pattern* (R-axis deviation. Dominant R wave and T wave inversion/ST depression in V_1 and V_2. Leads II, III and aVF may show similar changes). Rarely, the '$S_I Q_{III} T_{III}$' pattern occurs: deep S waves in I, pathological Q waves in III, inverted T waves in III.

Metabolic abnormalities: Digoxin effect: ST depression and inverted T wave in V_{5-6} (reversed tick). In *digoxin toxicity,* any arrhythmia may occur (ventricular ectopics and nodal bradycardia are common). *Hyperkalaemia:* Tall, tented T wave, widened QRS, absent P waves, 'sine wave' appearance (ECG 13, p689). *Hypokalaemia:* Small T waves, prominent U waves. *Hypercalcaemia:* Short QT interval. *Hypocalcaemia:* Long QT interval, small T waves.

Where to place the chest leads
V_1: right sternal edge, 4th intercostal space
V_2: left sternal edge, 4th intercostal space
V_3: half-way between V_2 and V_4
V_4: the patient's apex beat; all subsequent leads are in the same horizontal plane as V_4
V_5: anterior axillary line
V_6: mid-axillary line
(V_7: posterior axillary line)
(See fig 1.)
Finish 12-lead ECGs with a long rhythm strip in lead II.

Fig 1. Placement of chest leads.

Disorders of ventricular conduction
Bundle branch block (fig 5 p95, fig 1 & 3 p97) Delayed conduction is evidenced by prolongation of QRS >0.12s. Abnormal conduction patterns lasting <0.12s are incomplete blocks. The area that would have been reached by the blocked bundle depolarizes slowly and late. Taking V_1 as an example, right ventricular depolarization is normally +ve and left ventricular depolarization is normally –ve.

In RBBB, the following pattern is seen: QRS >0.12s, 'RSR' pattern in V_1, dominant R in V_1, inverted T waves in V_1–V_3 or V_4, deep wide S wave in V_6. Causes: normal variant (isolated RBBB), pulmonary embolism, cor pulmonale.

In LBBB, the following pattern is seen: QRS >0.12s, 'M' pattern in V_6, no septal Q waves, inverted T waves in I, aVL, V_5–V_6. Causes: IHD, hypertension, cardiomyopathy, idiopathic fibrosis. NB: if there is LBBB, no comment can be made on the ST segment or T wave.

Bifascicular block is the combination of RBBB and left anterior hemiblock, manifest as an axis deviation, eg LAD in the case of left anterior hemiblock.

Trifascicular block is the combination of bifascicular block and 1st degree heart block.

Ventricular hypertrophy There is no single marker of ventricular hypertrophy: electrical axis, voltage, and ST-wave changes should all be taken into consideration. Relying on a simple marker, such as voltage, may be unreliable as a thin chest wall may result in large voltage whereas a thick chest wall may mask it.

Suspect left ventricular hypertrophy (LVH) if the R wave in V_6 is >25mm or the sum of the S wave in V_1 and the R wave in V_6 is >35mm (see fig 4 p95).

Suspect right ventricular hypertrophy (RVH) if dominant R wave in V_1, T wave inversion in V_1–V_3 or V_4, deep S wave in V_6, RAD.

Other causes of dominant R wave in V_1: RBBB, posterior MI, some types of WPW syndrome (p120).

Causes of low voltage QRS complex: (QRS <5mm in all limb leads) hypothyroidism, chronic obstructive pulmonary disease (COPD), ↑haematocrit (intra-cardiac blood resistivity is related to haematocrit), changes in chest wall impedance (eg in renal failure, subcutaneous emphysema but not obesity), pulmonary embolism, bundle branch block, carcinoid heart disease, myocarditis, cardiac amyloid, adriamycin cardiotoxicity, and other heart muscle diseases, pericardial effusion, pericarditis.
See http://homepages.enterprise.net/djenkins/ecghome.html for masses of examples of ECGs

Where to place the chest leads

V1: right sternal edge, 4th intercostal space
V2: left sternal edge, 4th intercostal space
V3: half-way between V_2 and V_4
V4: the patient's apex beat (p64); all subsequent leads are in the same horizontal plane as V_4
V5: anterior axillary line
V6: mid-axillary line
(V_7: posterior axillary line)
(See **fig 1**).

Finish 12-lead ECGs with a long rhythm strip in lead II.

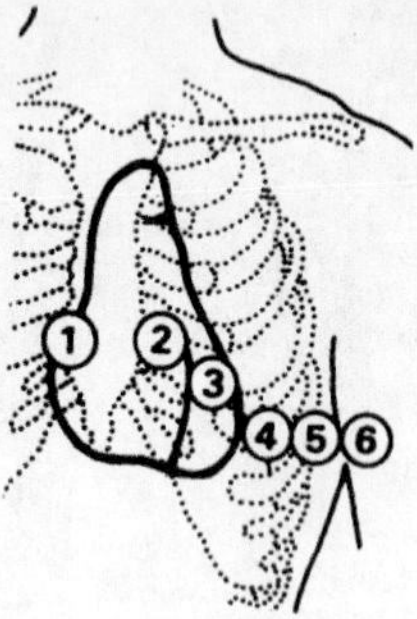

Fig 1. Placement of ECG leads.

Disorders of ventricular conduction

Bundle branch block (p95–p96, **ECGs 1 & 2**) Delayed conduction is evidenced by prolongation of QRS >0.12s. Abnormal conduction patterns lasting <0.12s are incomplete blocks. The area that would have been reached by the blocked bundle depolarizes slowly and late. Taking V_1 as an example, right ventricular depolarization is normally +ve and left ventricular depolarization is normally -ve.

In RBBB, the following pattern is seen: QRS >0.12s, 'RSR' pattern in V_1, dominant R in V_1, inverted T waves in V_1-V_3 or V_4, deep wide S wave in V_6. Causes: normal variant (isolated RBBB), pulmonary embolism, cor pulmonale.

In LBBB, the following pattern is seen: QRS >0.12s, 'M' pattern in V_5, no septal Q waves, inverted T waves in I, aVL, V_5-V_6. Causes: IHD, hypertension, cardiomyopathy, idiopathic fibrosis. ►**NB:** if there is LBBB, no comment can be made on the ST segment or T wave.

Bifascicular block is the combination of RBBB and left bundle hemiblock, manifest as an axis deviation, eg LAD in the case of left anterior hemiblock.

Trifascicular block is the combination of bifascicular block and 1st degree heart block.

Ventricular hypertrophy There is no single marker of ventricular hypertrophy: electrical axis, voltage, and ST wave changes should all be taken into consideration. Relying on a single marker such as voltage may be unreliable as a thin chest wall may result in large voltage whereas a thick chest wall may mask it.

Suspect *left ventricular hypertrophy* (LVH) if the R wave in V_6 >25mm or the sum of the S wave in V_1 and the R wave in V_6 is >35mm (**ECG 8** on p135).

Suspect *right ventricular hypertrophy* (RVH) if dominant R wave in V_1, T wave inversion in V_1-V_3 or V_4, deep S wave in V_6, RAD.

Other causes of *dominant R wave in* V_1: RBBB, posterior MI, some types of WPW syndrome (p120).

Causes of low voltage QRS complex: (QRS <5mm in all limb leads) Hypothyroidism, chronic obstructive pulmonary disease (COPD), ↑haematocrit (intra-cardiac blood resistivity is related to haematocrit), changes in chest wall impedance (eg in renal failure, subcutaneous emphysema but *not* obesity), pulmonary embolism, bundle branch block, carcinoid heart disease, myocarditis, cardiac amyloid, adriamycin cardiotoxicity, and other heart muscle diseases, pericardial effusion, pericarditis. 6

See http://homepages.enterprise.net/djenkins/ecghome.html for MRCP-ish examples of ECGs.

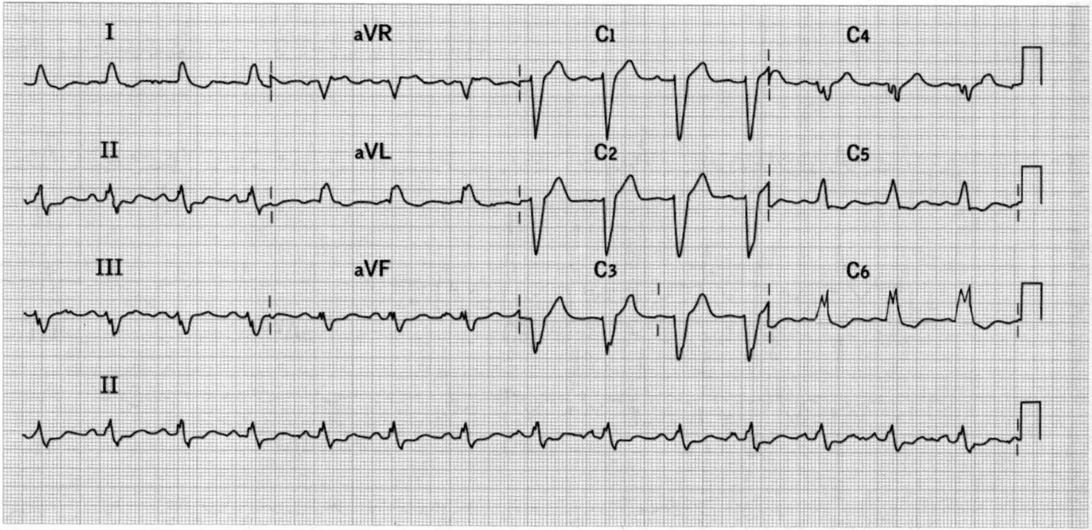

ECG 1—Left bundle branch block: note the W pattern in C1 (=V1) and the M pattern in C6 (=v6).

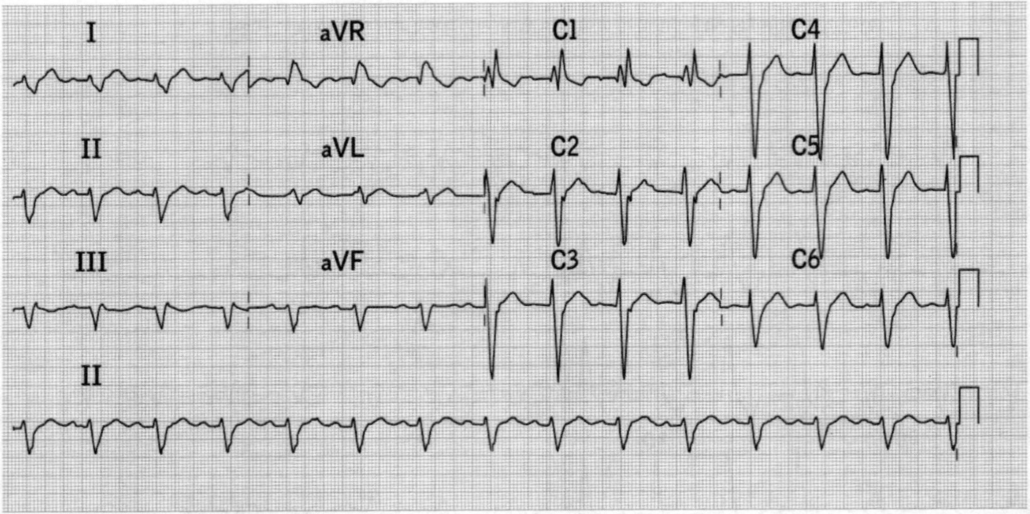

ECG 2—Right bundle branch block—M pattern in C1 and the W pattern in C5.

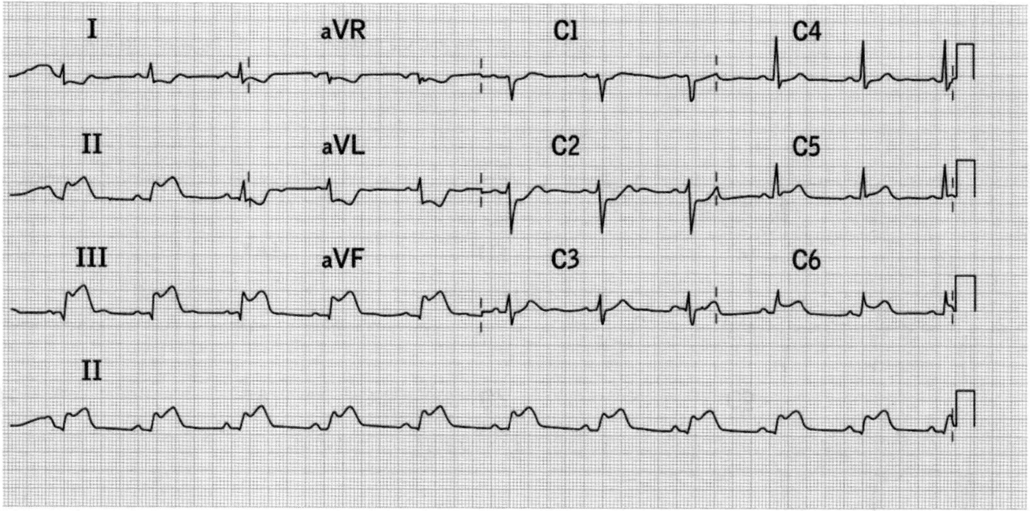

ECG 3—Acute infero-lateral myocardial infarction: marked ST elevation in the inferior leads (II, III, aVF), but also in C5 and C6, indicating lateral involvement as well. There is also 'reciprocal change' ie ST-segment depression in leads I and aVL. The latter is often seen with a large myocardial infarction.

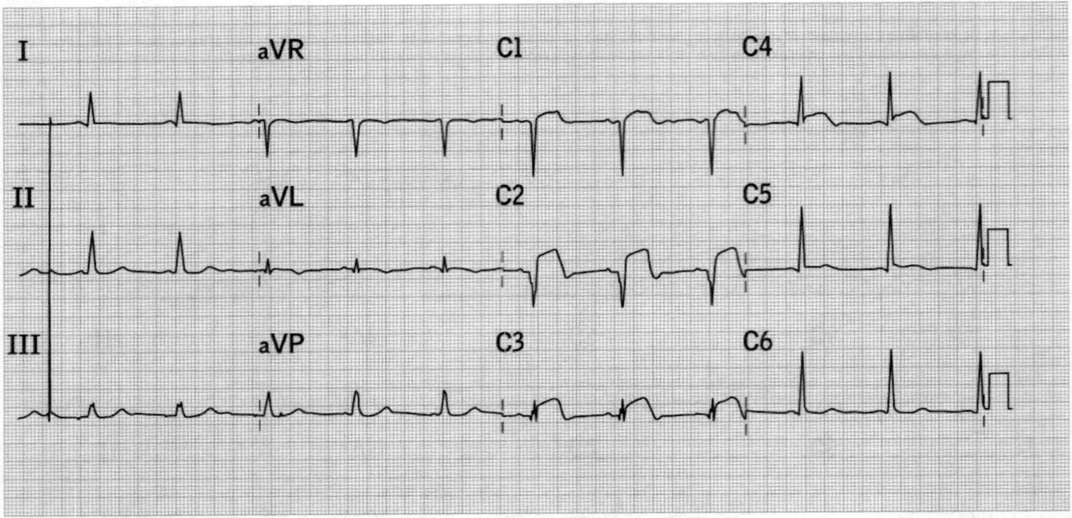

ECG 4—Acute anterior myocardial infarction—ST segment elevation and evolving Q waves in leads C1–C4.

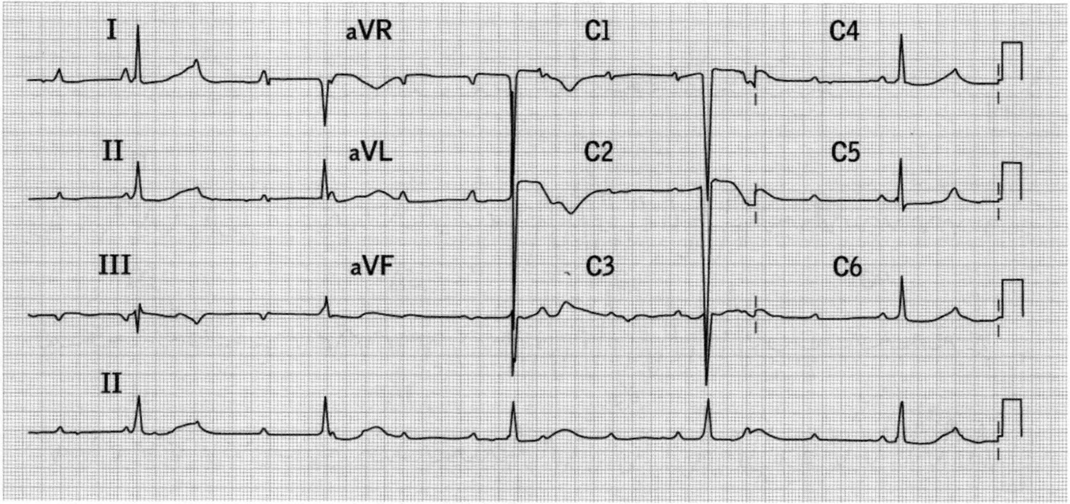

ECG 5—Complete heart block. Dissociation between the P waves and the QRS complexes. QRS complexes are relatively narrow, indicating that there is a ventricular rhythm originating from the conducting pathway.

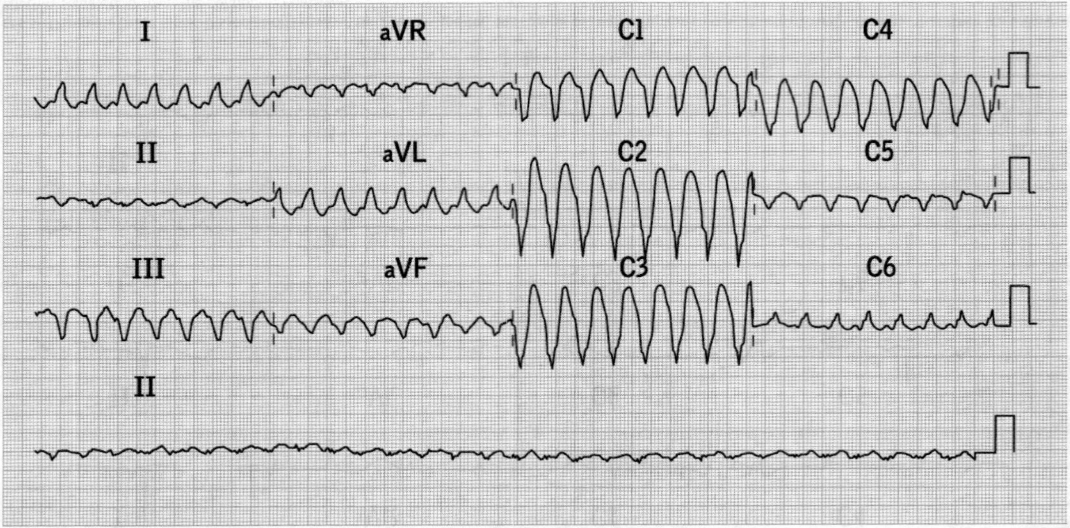

ECG 6—Ventricular tachycardia—regular broad complexes indicating a ventricular origin for the rhythm.

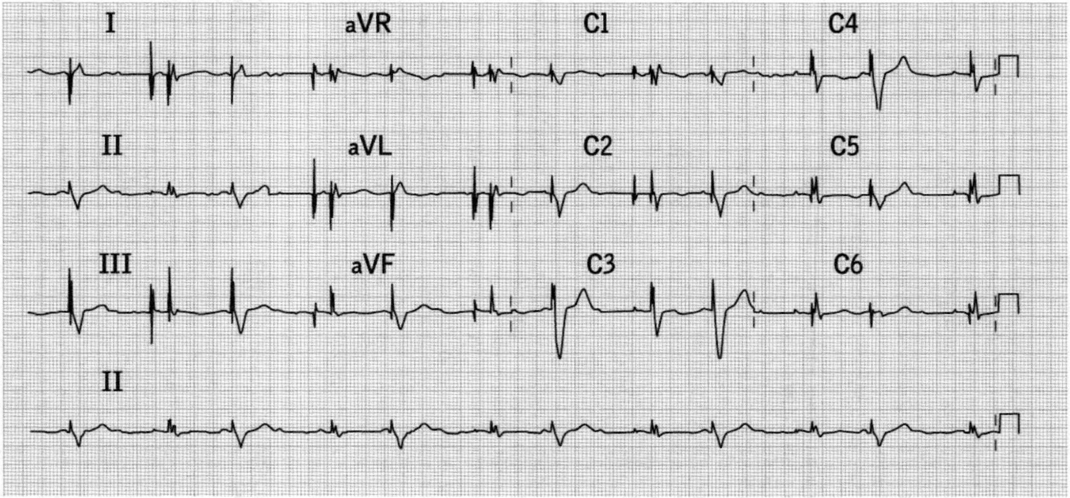

ECG 7—Dual chamber pacemaker. Pacing spikes occur before some of the P waves, and the QRS complexes.

Exercise ECG testing

The patient undergoes a graduated, treadmill exercise test, with continuous 12-lead ECG (**fig 1**) and blood pressure monitoring. There are numerous treadmill protocols; the 'Bruce protocol' is the most widely used.

Indications:

- To help confirm a suspected diagnosis of IHD.
- Assessment of cardiac function and exercise tolerance.
- Prognosis following MI. Was often done pre-discharge, but less so now.
- Evaluation of response to treatment (drugs, angioplasty, coronary artery bypass grafting, CABG).
- Assessment of exercise-induced arrhythmias.

Contraindications:

- Recent Q wave MI (<5 days ago) or unstable angina
- Severe AS
- Uncontrolled arrhythmia, hypertension, or heart failure
- Acute myocarditis or pericarditis
- Acute aortic dissection, acute pulmonary embolism

Be cautious about arranging tests that will be hard to perform or interpret:

- Complete heart block, LBBB
- Pacemaker patients, digoxin use
- Osteoarthritis, COPD, stroke, or other limitations to exercise.

Stop the test if:

- Chest pain, dyspnoea, cyanosis or pallor occurs.
- The patient feels faint, exhausted, or is in danger of falling.
- ST↑>1mm in leads without diagnostic Q waves (with or without chest pain).
- Atrial or ventricular arrhythmia (not just ectopics).
- Fall in blood pressure >10mmHg from baseline, failure of heart rate or blood pressure to rise with effort, SBP > 230mmHg and/or DBP >115mmHg.
- Development of AV block or LBBB.
- 90% maximal heart rate for age is achieved: [(220−age)±10].

Interpreting the test: A positive test only allows one to assess the *probability* that the patient has IHD. 75% with significant coronary artery disease have a positive test, but so do 5% of people with normal arteries (the false-positive rate is even higher in middle-aged women, eg 20%). The more positive the result, the higher the predictive accuracy. Down-sloping ST depression is much more significant than up-sloping, eg 1mm J-point depression with down-sloping ST segment is 99% predictive of 2-3 vessel disease.

Morbidity: 24 in 100,000. ***Mortality:*** 10 in 100,000.

Ambulatory ECG monitoring (eg Holter monitor)

Continuous ECG monitoring for 24h may be used to try and pick up paroxysmal arrhythmias. However, >70% of patients will not have symptoms during the period of monitoring. ~20% will have a normal ECG during symptoms and only up to 10% will have an arrhythmia coinciding with symptoms. Give these patients a recorder they can activate themselves during an episode. Recorders may be programmed to detect ST segment depression, either symptomatic (to prove angina), or to reveal 'silent' ischaemia (predictive of re-infarction or death soon after MI).

'Loop' recorders record only when activated by the patient—they cleverly save a small amount of ECG data *before* the event—useful if the arrhythmia causes loss of consciousness: the patient can press the button when they wake up. They are more expensive, but also more cost-effective than Holter monitors, as the pick-up rate of significant disease is higher. These may also be implanted just under the skin (eg Reveal Device), and are especially useful in patients with infrequent episodes.

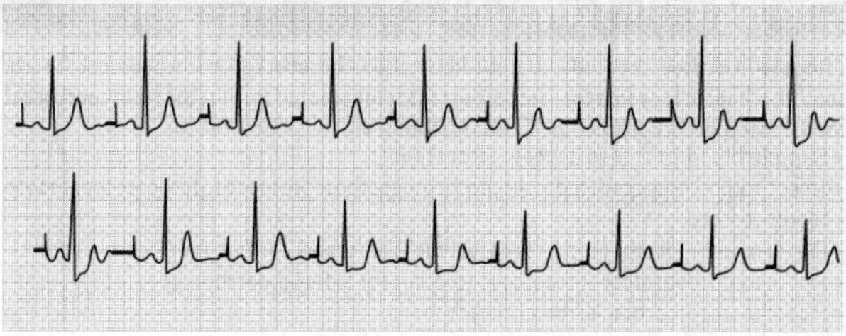

Each complex is taken from sample ECGs (lead C5) recorded at 1min intervals during exercise (top line) and recovery (bottom line). At maximum ST depression, the ST segment is almost horizontal. This is a positive exercise test.

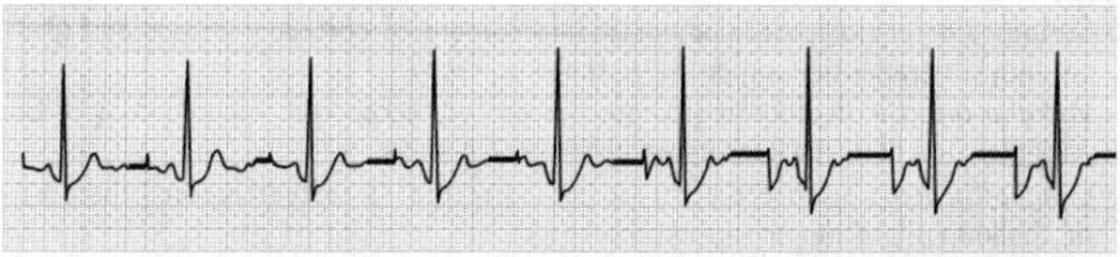

This is an exercise ECG in the same format. It is negative because although the J point is depressed, the ensuing ST segment is steeply up-sloping.

Fig 1. Exercise ECG testing. The J point is an isoelectric point between the T wave and the next P.

Exercise test or imaging for patients with ?angina

If the patient has an acute coronary syndrome, eg unstable angina, emergency admission is indicated. In those patients with undiagnosed chest pain which might be cardiac who do not require emergency admission, exercise ECG has been the next test to arrange after a resting ECG and routine blood (lipids and FBC etc). Alternatives are:

1 Tomography (CT) imaging for coronary artery calcium score.[1]
2 Myocardial perfusion scintigraphy (p754).
3 Dobutamine stress echocardiography.

1 The calcium score derived from CT images and is a summation of all calcified lesions in the coronary arteries. It reflects presence of plaques. The reported score is an individual's score, taking into account age and sex.

This involves the insertion of a catheter into the heart via the femoral (or radial/brachial) artery or vein. The catheter is manipulated within the heart and great vessels to measure pressures. Catheterization can also be used to:

- Sample blood to assess oxygen saturation.
- Inject radiopaque contrast medium to image the anatomy of the heart and flow in blood vessels.
- Perform angioplasty (± stenting), valvuloplasty, and cardiac biopsies. (see BOX 1)
- Perform intravascular ultrasound to quantify arterial narrowing.
- Perform intra-cardiac echocardiography.

During the procedure, ECG and arterial pressures are monitored continuously. In the UK, 70% of cardiac catheters are performed as day-case procedures (provided the patient can rest lying down for 4h). See BOX 2.

Indications:

- *Coronary artery disease:* diagnostic (assessment of coronary vessels and graft patency); therapeutic (angioplasty, stent insertion).
- *Valvular disease:* diagnostic (to assess severity); therapeutic valvuloplasty (if the patient is too ill or declines valve surgery). See BOX 3.
- *Congenital heart disease:* diagnostic (assessment of severity of lesions); therapeutic (balloon dilatation or septostomy).
- *Other:* cardiomyopathy; pericardial disease; endomyocardial biopsy.

Pre-procedure checks:

- Brief history/examination; **NB:** peripheral pulses, bruits, aneurysms.
- Investigations: FBC, U&E, LFT, clotting screen, CXR, ECG.
- Consent for angiogram (see BOX 4) ± angioplasty ± stent ± CABG. Explain reason for procedure and possible complications (below).
- IV access, ideally in the left hand.
- Patient should be nil by mouth (NBM) from 6h before the procedure.
- Patients should take all their morning drugs (and pre-medication if needed). Withhold oral hypoglycaemics.

Post-procedure checks:

- Pulse, blood pressure, arterial puncture site (for bruising or swelling? false aneurysm), peripheral pulses.
- Investigations: FBC and clotting (if suspected blood loss), ECG.

Complications:

- *Haemorrhage:* Apply firm pressure over puncture site. If you suspect a false aneurysm, ultrasound the swelling and consider surgical repair.
- *Contrast reaction:* This is usually mild with modern contrast agents.
- *Loss of peripheral pulse:* May be due to dissection, thrombosis, or arterial spasm. Occurs in <1% of brachial catheterizations. Rare with femoral catheterization.
- *Angina:* May occur during or after cardiac catheterization. Usually responds to sublingual GTN; if not give analgesia and IV nitrates.
- *Arrhythmias:* Usually transient. Manage along standard lines.
- *Pericardial tamponade:* Rare, but should be suspected if the patient becomes hypotensive and anuric.
- *Infection:* Post-catheter pyrexia is usually due to a contrast reaction. If it persists for >24h, take blood cultures before giving antibiotics.

Mortality: <1 in 1000 patients, in most centres.

Intra-cardiac electrophysiology This catheter technique can determine types and origins of arrhythmias, and locate (and ablate) aberrant pathways (eg causing atrial flutter or ventricular tachycardia). Arrhythmias may be induced, and the effectiveness of control by drugs assessed.

Coronary artery anatomy

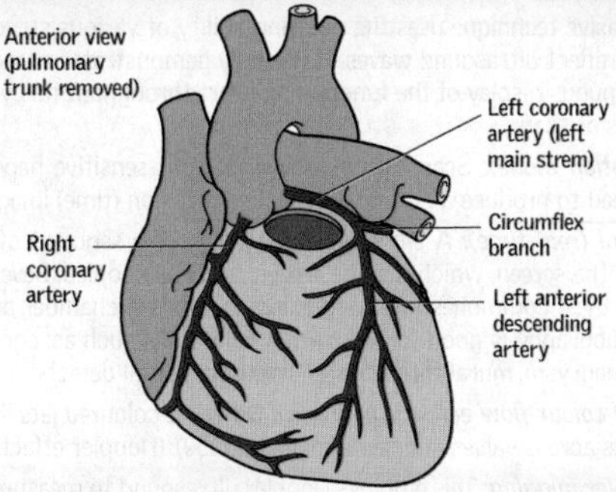

Normal values for intracardiac pressures and saturations

Location	Pressure (mmHg) Mean	Range	Saturation (%)
Inferior vena cava			76
Superior vena cava			70
Right atrium	4	0-8	74
Right ventricle			74
Systolic	25	15-30	
End-diastolic	4	0-8	
Pulmonary artery			74
Systolic	25	15-30	
Diastolic	10	5-15	
Mean	15	10-20	
Pulmonary artery	a	3-12	74
Wedge pressure	v	3-15	
Left ventricle			
Systolic	110	80-140	98
End-diastolic	8	≤12	
Aorta			
Systolic	110	80-140	98
Diastolic	70	60-90	
Mean	85	70-105	
Brachial			
Systolic	120	90-140	98
Diastolic	72	60-90	
Mean	83	70-105	

Gradients across stenotic valves

Valve	Normal gradient (mmHg)	Stenotic gradient (mmHg) Mild	Moderate	Severe
Aortic	0	<30	30-50	>50
Mitral	0	<5	5-15	>15
Prosthetic	5-10			

CT angiogram

CT angiogram permits contrast-enhanced imaging of coronary arteries during a single breath hold. It can diagnose significant (>50%) stenosis in CAD with an accuracy of 89%. Its negative predictive value is >99%, which makes it an effective non-invasive alternative to routine coronary angiography to rule out CAD. However, due to a high false-positive rate, especially in calcified vessels, its routine use is limited, but is expected to increase significantly in the future.[9 10]

This non-invasive technique uses the differing ability of various structures within the heart to reflect ultrasound waves. It not only demonstrates anatomy but provides a continuous display of the functioning heart throughout its cycle. There are various types of scan:

M-mode (motion mode): Scans are displayed on light-sensitive paper moving at constant speed to produce a permanent single dimension (time) image. See **fig 1**.

2-dimensional (real time): A 2-D, fan-shaped image of a segment of the heart is produced on the screen, which may be 'frozen' and hard-copied. Several views are possible and the 4 commonest are: long axis, short axis, 4-chamber, and subcostal. 2-D echocardiography is good for visualizing conditions such as: congenital heart disease, LV aneurysm, mural thrombus, LA myxoma, septal defects.

Doppler and colour-flow echocardiography: Different coloured jets illustrate flow and gradients across valves and septal defects (p150). (Doppler effect, p750)

Tissue Doppler imaging: This employs Doppler ultrasound to measure the velocity of myocardial segments over the cardiac cycle. It is particularly useful for assessing longitudinal motion—and hence long-axis ventricular function, which is a sensitive marker of systolic and diastolic heart failure.

Trans-oesophageal echocardiography (TOE) is more sensitive than transthoracic echocardiography (TTE) as the transducer is nearer to the heart. Indications: diagnosing aortic dissections; assessing prosthetic valves; finding cardiac source of emboli, and IE/SBE. Don't do if oesophageal disease or cervical spine instability.

Stress echocardiography is used to evaluate ventricular function, ejection fraction, myocardial thickening, and regional wall motion pre- and post-exercise. Dobutamine or dipyridamole may be used if the patient cannot exercise. Inexpensive and as sensitive/specific as a thallium scan (p754).

Uses of echocardiography

Quantification of global LV function: Heart failure may be due to systolic or diastolic ventricular impairment (or both). Echo helps by measuring end-diastolic volume. If this is large, systolic dysfunction is the likely cause. If small, diastolic. Pure forms of diastolic dysfunction are rare. Differentiation is important; as vasodilators are less useful in diastolic dysfunction as a high ventricular filling pressure is required.

Echo is also useful for detecting focal and global hypokinesia, LV aneurysm, mural thrombus, and LVH (echo is 5–10 times more sensitive than ECG in detecting this).

Estimating right heart haemodynamics: Doppler studies of pulmonary artery flow allow evaluation of RV function and pressures.

Valve disease: Measurement of pressure gradients and valve orifice areas in stenotic lesions. Detecting valvular regurgitation and estimating its significance is less accurate. Evaluating function of prosthetic valves is another role.

Congenital heart disease: Establishing the presence of lesions, and significance.

Endocarditis: Vegetations may not be seen if <2mm in size. TTE with colour Doppler is best for aortic regurgitation (AR). TOE is useful for visualizing mitral valve vegetations, leaflet perforation, or looking for an aortic root abscess.

Pericardial effusion is best diagnosed by echo. Fluid may first accumulate between the posterior pericardium and the left ventricle, then anterior to both ventricles and anterior and lateral to the right atrium. There may be paradoxical septal motion.

HCM (p146): Echo features include asymmetrical septal hypertrophy, small LV cavity, dilated left atrium, and systolic anterior motion of the mitral valve.

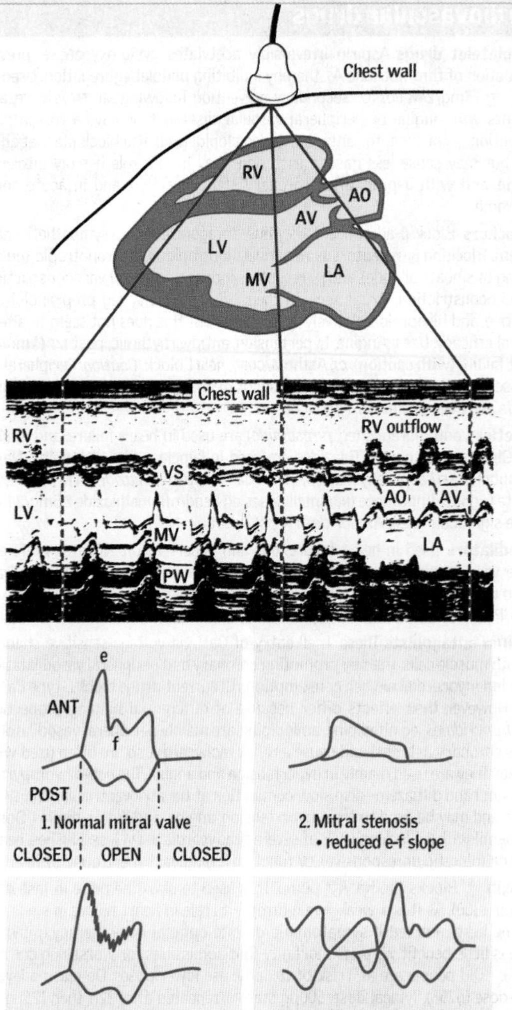

Fig 1. Normal M-mode echocardiogram (RV=right ventricle; LV=left ventricle; AO=aorta; AV=aortic valve; LA=left atrium; MV=mitral valve; PW=posterior wall of LV; IVS=interventricular septum). Adapted from R Hall *Med International* 17 774.

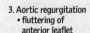

Antiplatelet drugs Aspirin irreversibly acetylates cyclo-oxygenase, preventing production of thromboxane A_2, thereby inhibiting platelet aggregation. Used in low dose (eg 75mg/24h PO) for secondary prevention following MI, TIA/stroke, and for patients with angina or peripheral vascular disease. May have a role in primary prevention.[11] ADP receptor antagonists (eg clopidogrel) also block platelet aggregation, but may cause less gastric irritation. They have a role if truly intolerant of aspirin, and with aspirin, after coronary stent insertion, and in acute coronary syndrome.

β-blockers Block β-adrenoceptors, thus antagonizing the sympathetic nervous system. Blocking β_1-receptors is negatively inotropic and chronotropic (pulse↓ by ↓firing of sinoatrial node), and β_2-receptors induce peripheral vasoconstriction and bronchoconstriction. Drugs vary in their β_1/β_2 selectivity (eg propranolol is non-selective, and bisoprolol relatively β_1 selective), but this does not seem to alter their clinical efficacy. *Uses:* Angina, hypertension, antidysrhythmic, post MI (↓mortality), heart failure (with caution). *CI:* Asthma/COPD, heart block. ***Caution:*** Peripheral vascular disease, heart failure/(but see carvedilol, p130). *SE:* Lethargy, erectile dysfunction, *joie de vivre*↓, nightmares, headache.

Diuretics Loop diuretics (eg *furosemide*) are used in heart failure, and inhibit the Na/2Cl/K co-transporter. Thiazides are used in hypertension and inhibit Na/Cl co-transporter. *SE: Loop:* dehydration, $\downarrow K^+$, $\downarrow Ca^{2+}$, ototoxic; *thiazides:* $\downarrow K^+$, $\uparrow Ca^{2+}$, $\downarrow Mg^{2+}$, ↑urate (±gout), impotence (**NB:** small doses, eg bendroflumethiazide 2.5mg/24h rarely cause significant SEs); *Amiloride:* $\uparrow K^+$, GI upset.

Vasodilators Used in heart failure, IHD, and hypertension. Nitrates preferentially dilate veins and the large arteries, ↓ filling pressure (pre-load), while hydralazine (often used with nitrates) primarily dilates the resistance vessels thus ↓ BP (after-load). Prazosin (an α-blocker) dilates arteries and veins.

Calcium antagonists These ↓cell entry of Ca^{2+} via voltage-sensitive channels on smooth muscle cells, thereby promoting coronary and peripheral vasodilatation and reducing myocardial oxygen consumption. All current drugs block L-type Ca^{2+} channels. However, their effects differ because of differential binding properties. The *dihydropyridines,* eg nifedipine, amlodipine, are mainly peripheral vasodilators (also dilate coronary arteries) and cause a reflex tachycardia, so are often used with a β-blocker. They are used mainly in hypertension and angina. The *non*-dihydropyridines—verapamil and diltiazem—also slow conduction at the atrioventricular and sinoatrial nodes and may be used to treat hypertension, angina, and dysrhythmias. Don't give verapamil with β-blockers (risk of severe bradycardia ± LVF). *SE:* Flushes, headache, oedema (diuretic unresponsive), LV function↓, gingival hypertrophy. *CI:* heart block.

Digoxin[12,13] Blocks the Na^+/K^+ pump. It is used to slow the pulse in fast AF (p124; aim for ≤100). As it is a weak +ve inotrope, its role in heart failure in sinus rhythm may be best reserved if symptomatic despite optimal ACE-i therapy (p109);[14] here there is little benefit *vis-à-vis* mortality (but admissions for worsening CCF are ↓by ~25%).[15] Old people are at ↑risk of toxicity: use lower doses. Do plasma levels >6h post-dose (p766). Typical dose: 500µg stat PO, repeated after 12h, then 125µg (if elderly) to 375µg/d PO (62.5µg/d is almost never enough). IV dose: 0.75-1mg in 0.9% NaCl over 2h. Toxicity risk↑ if: $K^+\downarrow$, $Mg^{2+}\downarrow$, or $Ca^{2+}\uparrow$. $t_{1/2} \approx 36$h. If on digoxin, use less energy in cardioversion (start at 5J). ►If on amiodarone, halve the dose of digoxin. *SE:* Any arrhythmia (supraventricular tachycardia with AV block is suggestive), nausea, appetite↓, yellow vision, confusion, gynaecomastia. In toxicity, stop digoxin; check K^+; treat arrhythmias; consider Digibind® by IVI (p854). *CI:* HCM; WPW syndrome (p120).

ACE-inhibitors p109; **Nitrates** p110; **Antihypertensives** p134.

Statins

(see also hyperlipidaemia, p704 and p705, fig 1)

Statins (eg simvastatin, p704) inhibit the enzyme HMG-COA reductase, which causes *de novo* synthesis of cholesterol in the liver. This increases LDL receptor expression by hepatocytes leading to ↓ circulating LDL cholesterol. More effective if given at night, but optimum dose, and target plasma cholesterol are unknown. SE: muscle aches, abdominal discomfort, ↑transaminases (eg ALT), ↑CK, myositis, rarely rhabdomyolysis (more common if used with fibrates). Besides lowering LDL cholesterol, statins may have other favourable or 'pleiotropic' effects:

- Anti-thrombotic and anti-inflammatory (CRP↓).
- Plaque stabilization; high doses *may* even reverse plaque growth but whether this leads to greater ↓morbidity/mortality is unclear.[16]
- Restoration of normal endothelial function.
- Reduction in cholesterol synthesis by within-vessel macrophages.
- Reduction of within-vessel macrophage proliferation and migration.

Statins are generally well tolerated. There are currently ~3 million people taking statins in England, which saves ~10,000 lives a year.

How to start ACE-inhibitors

Check that there are no contraindications/cautions:

- Renal failure (serum creatinine >200μmol/L; but not an absolute CI)
- Hyperkalaemia: K^+ >5.5mmol/L
- Hyponatraemia: caution if <130mmol/L (relates to a poorer prognosis)
- Hypovolaemia or hypotension (systolic BP <90mmHg)
- Aortic stenosis or LV outflow tract obstruction
- Pregnancy or lactation
- Severe COPD or cor pulmonale (not an absolute CI)
- Renal artery stenosis[1] (Suspect if arteriopathic, eg cerebrovascular disease, IHD, peripheral vascular disease. ACE-i ↓GFR and may precipitate acute renal failure)

Warn the patient about possible side effects:

- Dry cough (1:10)
- Hypotension, especially with 1st dose if CCF (so start at night)
- Taste disturbance
- Hyperkalaemia
- Renal impairment; this commonly co-exists with heart failure (atheroma is the reason for both, usually)—and is worsened by ACE-i (see below)
- Urticaria and angioneurotic oedema (<1:1,000)
- Rarely: proteinuria, leucopenia, fatigue

Starting ACE-inhibitors: ►Delay if intercurrent illness (esp. if dehydrated/D&V etc). Most patients can be safely started on ACE-i as outpatients. 1st-dose hypotension can be avoided by taking the 1st dose on going to bed. Use a long-acting ACE-i, eg **lisinopril** 10mg/d PO, 2.5mg/d in the elderly (or eGFR <30). Increase dose every 2wks until at target dose (equivalent of 30–40mg lisinopril a day if eGFR >30) or side effects supervene (↓BP, ↑creatinine). Review in ~1-2 wks; check U&E regularly. Patients on high doses of diuretics (>80mg furosemide a day) may need a reduction in their diuretic dose first. Before and after, check U&E . Expect a rise in creatinine (<20%; GFR↓ by <15%[17]) in ~ 2 wks after starting an ACE-i; a larger change may indicate underlying renal artery stenosis. Repeat U&E and ask a specialist's advice. Plasma K^+ may also rise. If >6mmol/L, ensure no NSAID is being taken, stop or reduce dose of K^+-sparing diuretics, and recheck U&E. The dose of loop diuretic may also need to be reduced (if there is no congestion). If ↑K^+ persists, ACE-i (or ARB) may need to be stopped.[18]

NB: the same cautions are needed when starting ARBs (eg candesartan). In patients with cardiac disease who are unable to tolerate ACE-i, an ARB can be used.

1 If renovascular disease precludes the use of ACE-i and furosemide is providing no answer, consider maximal vasodilatation with nitrates and hydralazine: seek expert advice.

Angina pectoris

This is due to myocardial ischaemia and presents as a central chest tightness or heaviness, which is brought on by exertion and relieved by rest. It may radiate to one or both arms, the neck, jaw or teeth. ***Other precipitants:*** Emotion, cold weather, and heavy meals. ***Associated symptoms:*** Dyspnoea, nausea, sweatiness, faintness.

Causes Mostly atheroma. Rarely: anaemia, AS; tachyarrhythmias; HCM; arteritis/small vessel disease (microvascular angina/cardiac syndrome X).

Types of angina *Stable angina:* induced by effort, relieved by rest. *Unstable (crescendo) angina:* angina of increasing frequency or severity; occurs on minimal exertion or at rest; associated with ↑↑risk of MI. *Decubitus angina:* precipitated by lying flat. *Variant (Prinzmetal's) angina* (see BOX 1): caused by coronary artery spasm (rare; may co-exist with fixed stenoses).

Tests ECG: usually normal, but may show ST depression; flat or inverted T waves; signs of past MI. If resting ECG normal, consider exercise ECG (p102), thallium scan (p754), cardiac CT or coronary angiography. Stress echo can detect changes in regional wall motion seen during ischaemia. Coronary Ca^{2+} score (measured by CT) is a strong predictor of CAD and is additive to the standard risk factors.[19] Exclude precipitating factors: anaemia, diabetes, hyperlipidaemia, thyrotoxicosis, temporal arteritis.

Management

Modify risk factors: stop smoking, encourage exercise, weight loss. Control hypertension, diabetes, etc., p87. If total cholesterol >4mmol/L give a statin—see p704.

Aspirin (75–150mg/24h) reduces mortality by 34%.

β-blockers: eg atenolol 50–100mg/24h PO, reduce symptoms unless contra-indicated (asthma, COPD, LVF, bradycardia, coronary artery spasm).

Nitrates: for symptoms, give GTN spray or sublingual tabs, up to every ½h. Prophylaxis: give regular oral nitrate, eg isosorbide mononitrate 20–40mg PO bd (have an 8h nitrate-free period to prevent tolerance) or slow-release nitrate (eg Imdur® 60mg/24h). Alternatives: adhesive nitrate skin patches or buccal pills. SE: headaches, BP↓.

Long-acting calcium antagonists: amlodipine 10mg/24h; diltiazem-MR 90–180mg/12h PO. They are particularly useful if there is a contraindication to ***β-blockers***.

K^+ channel activator, eg nicorandil 10–30mg/12h PO, if still not controlled.

Others: ivabradine inhibits the pacemaker ('funny') current in the SA node and thus reduces heart rate. Useful in those who cannot take a β-blocker, having similar efficacy. Trimetazidine inhibits fatty acid oxidation, leading the myocardium to use glucose, which is more efficient. Ranolazine inhibits the late Na^+ current.

►Unstable angina requires admission and urgent treatment: *emergencies*, p810.

Indications for referral Diagnostic uncertainty; new angina of sudden onset; recurrent angina if past MI or CABG (see BOX 2); angina uncontrolled by drugs; unstable angina. Some units routinely do exercise tolerance tests on those <70yrs old, but age alone is a poor way to stratify patients.

Percutaneous transluminal coronary angioplasty (PTCA) involves balloon dilatation of the stenotic vessel(s). *Indications:* poor response or intolerance to medical therapy; refractory angina in patients not suitable for CABG; previous CABG; post-thrombolysis in patients with severe stenoses, symptoms, or positive stress tests. Comparisons of PTCA *vs* drugs alone show that PTCA may control symptoms better but with more frequent early cardiac events (eg MI and need for CABG)[20] and little effect on mortality. However, early intervention may benefit high risk patients presenting with non-ST-segment elevation MI (p112).[21] Stenting reduces restenosis rates and the need for bailout CABG compared with angioplasty. *Complications:* Restenosis (20–30% within 6 months); emergency CABG (<3%); MI (<2%); death (<0.5%).

NICE recommends that >70% of angioplasties be accompanied by stenting. Antiplatelet agents, eg clopidogrel, reduce the risk of stent thrombosis, and IV glycoproteins IIb/IIIa-inhibitors (eg eptifibatide) reduce procedure-related ischaemic events.[22] Drug-coated stents reduce restenosis rates, but at the risk of increased late in-stent thrombosis. Long-term treatment with aspirin and clopidogrel may reduce this risk.

Prinzmetal angina

This is due to coronary artery spasm, which can occur even in normal coronary arteries. Pain usually occurs during rest (rather than during activity). ECG during pain shows ST segment elevation, which resolves as the pain subsides. Patients usually do not have the usual risk factors of atherosclerosis. ***Treatment:*** Calcium channel blockers ± long-acting nitrates. Aspirin can ***aggravate*** the ischaemic attacks in these patients. β-blockers (esp non-selective) should also be ***avoided*** as they can increase vasospasm. Prognosis is usually very good.

Coronary artery bypass graft (CABG)

CABG is performed in left main stem disease, multi-vessel disease; multiple severe stenoses; patients unsuitable for angioplasty; failed angioplasty; refractory angina.

Indications for CABG: to improve survival
- Left main stem disease
- Triple vessel disease involving proximal part of the left anterior descending

To relieve symptoms
- Angina unresponsive to drugs
- Unstable angina (sometimes)
- If angioplasty is unsuccessful

NB: when CABG and percutaneous coronary intervention (PCI, eg angioplasty) are both clinically valid options, NICE recommends that the availability of new stent technology should push the decision towards PCI. In practice, patients with single-vessel CAD and normal LV function usually undergo PCI, and those with triple-vessel disease and abnormal LV function more often undergo CABG.[23]

Compared with PCI, CABG results in longer recovery time and length of inpatient stay. Recent RCTs indicate that early procedural mortality rates and 5-year survival rates are similar after PCI and CABG. Compared with PCI, CABG probably provides more complete long-term relief of angina in patients, and less repeated revascularization. However, it is associated with ↑ risk of stroke.[24]

Procedure: Surgery is planned in the light of angiograms. Not all stenoses are bypassable. The heart is stopped and blood pumped artificially by a machine outside the body (cardiac bypass). Minimally invasive thoracotomies not requiring this are well-described,[25] but randomized trials are few. The patient's own saphenous vein or internal mammary artery is used as the graft. Several grafts may be placed. >50% of vein grafts close in 10yrs (low-dose aspirin helps prevent this). Internal mammary artery grafts last longer (but may cause chest-wall numbness).

On-pump or off-pump?

Off-pump CABG is associated with lower in-hospital mortality and complication rates than on-pump CABG (including short-term and probably long-term neurological complications), but long-term outcomes are comparable. Furthermore, on-pump CABG has been associated with less need for subsequent re-vascularization comparing with off-pump CABG.[26]

After CABG: If angina persists or recurs (from poor run-off from the graft, distal disease, new atheroma, or graft occlusion) restart anti-anginal drugs, and consider angioplasty. Mood, sex, and intellectual problems[27] are common early. Rehabilitation helps:
- Exercise: walk→cycle→swim→jog
- Drive at 1 month: no need to tell DVLA if non-HGV licences, p152
- Get back to work, eg at 3 months
- Attend to: smoking; BP; lipids
- Aspirin 75mg/24h PO forever; consider clopidogrel if aspirin CI

Definitions ACS includes unstable angina and evolving MI, which share a common underlying pathology—plaque rupture, thrombosis, and inflammation. However, ACS may rarely be due to emboli or coronary spasm in normal coronary arteries, or vasculitis (p558). Usually divided into *ACS with ST-segment elevation* or new onset LBBB—what most of us mean by acute MI; and *ACS without ST-segment elevation*—the ECG may show ST depression, T wave inversion, non-specific changes, or be normal (includes non-Q wave or subendocardial MI). The degree of irreversible myocyte death varies, and significant necrosis can occur without ST elevation.

Risk factors *Non-modifiable:* age, ♂ gender, family history of IHD (MI in first degree relative <55yrs). *Modifiable:* smoking, hypertension, DM, hyperlipidaemia, obesity, sedentary lifestyle. *Controversial* risk factors include: stress, type A personality, LVH, apoprotein A↑, fibrinogen↑, hyperinsulinaemia, homocysteine levels↑, ACE genotype, and cocaine use, and probably poor oral hygiene.

Incidence 5/1000 per annum (UK) for ST-segment elevation.

Diagnosis Acute MI is defined by several criteria.[28] The commonest is an↑ and then a ↓ in cardiac biomarkers (eg troponin) and either: symptoms of ischaemia, ECG changes of new ischaemia, development of pathological Q waves, or loss of myocardium on imaging.

Symptoms Acute central chest pain, lasting >20min, often associated with nausea, sweatiness, dyspnoea, palpitations. May present without chest pain ('silent' infarct) eg in elderly or diabetics. In such patients, presentations may include: syncope, pulmonary oedema, epigastric pain and vomiting, post-operative hypotension or oliguria, acute confusional state, stroke, diabetic hyperglycaemic states.

Signs Distress, anxiety, pallor, sweatiness, pulse↑ or ↓, BP↑ or ↓, 4th heart sound. There may be signs of heart failure (↑ JVP, 3rd heart sound, basal crepitations) or a pansystolic murmur (papillary muscle dysfunction/rupture, VSD). Low-grade fever may be present. Later, a pericardial friction rub or peripheral oedema may develop.

Tests *ECG* (see **fig 1**): Classically, hyperacute (tall) T waves, ST elevation or new LBBB occur within hrs of transmural infarction. T wave inversion and the development of pathological Q waves follow over hrs to days (p92). In other ACS: ST depression, T wave inversion, non-specific changes, or normal. ►*In 20% of MIs, the ECG may be normal initially. CXR:* Look for cardiomegaly, pulmonary oedema, or a widened mediastinum (aortic rupture). Don't routinely delay treatment whilst waiting for a CXR.

Blood: FBC, U&E, glucose, lipids.

Cardiac enzymes (see **fig 2**): ***Cardiac troponin*** levels (T and I) are the most sensitive and specific markers of myocardial necrosis. Serum levels ↑ within 3-12h from the onset of chest pain, peak at 24-48h, and ↓ to baseline over 5-14 days. If normal ≥6h after onset of pain, and ECG normal, risk of missing MI is tiny (0.3%).[29] Peak levels also help risk stratification.[30] ***Creatine kinase*** comprises 3 isoenzymes: CK-MM (found mainly in skeletal muscle; ↑after trauma (falls, seizures); prolonged exercise; myositis; AfroCaribbeans; hypothyroidism), CK-BB (predominantly in the brain); and CK-MB mainly in the heart. CK-MB levels ↑ within 3-12h of onset of chest pain, reach peak values within 24h, and return to baseline after 48-72h. Levels peak earlier if reperfusion occurs. Sensitivity is ~95%, with high specificity. ***Myoglobin*** levels rise within 1-4h from the onset of pain. They are highly sensitive but not specific.

Differential diagnosis (p88) Angina, pericarditis, myocarditis, aortic dissection (p656), pulmonary embolism, and oesophageal reflux/spasm.

Management See *emergencies*, p810. The management of ACS with and without ST-segment elevation varies. Likewise, if there is no ST elevation and symptoms settle without a rise in cardiac troponin, then no myocardial damage has occurred, the prognosis is good, and patients can be discharged. Therefore, the two key questions are: is there ST-segment elevation? Is there a rise in troponin?

Mortality 50% of deaths occur within 2h of onset of symptoms. Up to 7% die before discharge. Worse prognosis if: elderly, LV failure, and ST changes.[31]

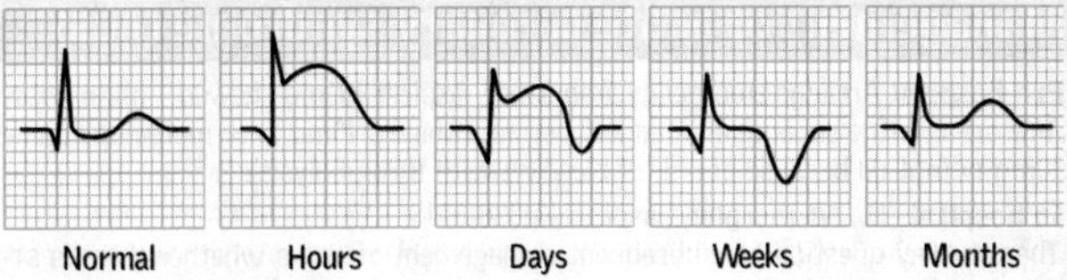

Fig 1. Sequential ECG changes following acute MI

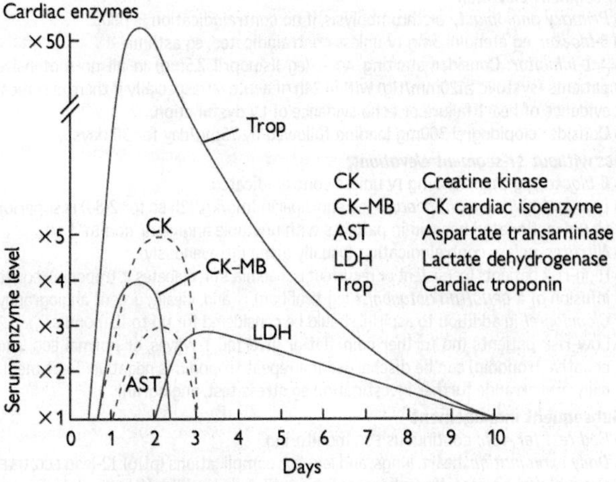

Fig 2. Enzyme changes following acute MI

Management of acute coronary syndrome (ACS)

Pre-hospital Arrange emergency ambulance. Aspirin 300mg chewed[32] (if no *absolute* CI) and GTN sublingual. Analgesia, eg morphine 5-10mg IV + metoclopramide 10mg IV (not IM because of risk of bleeding with thrombolysis).

In hospital—O_2, IVI, morphine, aspirin ▸▸p808-810

Then the key question for subsequent management of ACS is whether there is ST-segment elevation (includes new onset LBBB or a true posterior MI). See **fig 1**.

ST-segment elevation

- *Primary angioplasty* or thrombolysis, if no contraindication ▸▸ p808.
- *β-blocker*, eg atenolol 5mg IV unless contraindicated, eg asthma.
- *ACE-inhibitor*: Consider starting ACE-i (eg lisinopril 2.5mg) in all normotensive patients (systolic ≥120mm/Hg) within 24h of acute MI, especially if there is clinical evidence of heart failure or echo evidence of LV dysfunction.
- Consider clopidogrel 300mg loading followed by 75mg/day for 30 days[33].

ACS without ST-segment elevation[34]

- *β-blocker*, eg atenolol 5mg IV unless contraindicated.
- *Low molecular weight heparin* (eg enoxaparin 1mg/kg/12h SC for 2-8d) is superior to unfractionated heparin in patients with unstable angina or non-ST ↑ MI.
- *Nitrates*, unless contraindication (usually given intravenously).
- High-risk patients (persistent or recurrent ischaemia, ST↓, diabetes, ↑ troponin) require infusion of a *GPIIb/IIIa antagonist* (eg tirofiban),[35] and, ideally, urgent angiography. *Clopidogrel*, in addition to aspirin, should be considered for up to 12 months.[36]
- Low-risk patients (no further pain, flat or inverted T-waves, or normal ECG, **and** negative troponin) can be discharged if a repeat troponin is negative. Treat medically and arrange further investigation eg stress test, angiogram.

Subsequent management

- *Bed rest for 48h;* continuous ECG monitoring.
- *Daily examination:* heart, lungs, and legs for complications (p116); 12-lead ECG, U&E.
- *Prophylaxis against thromboembolism:* until fully mobile. If large anterior MI, consider warfarin for 3 months as prophylaxis against systemic embolism from LV mural thrombus.
- *Aspirin* (eg 75mg) ↓vascular events (MI, stroke, or vascular death) by 29%.
- Long-term β-blockade ↓mortality from all causes by ~25% in patients who have had a previous MI (eg metoprolol ~50mg/6h, enough to decrease the pulse to ≤60; continue for at least 1yr). If contraindicated, consider verapamil or diltiazem.
- *Continue* ACE-i in all patients. ACE-i in those with evidence of heart failure reduces 2yr mortality by 25-30%.
- *Start a statin* eg simvastatin 40mg.[37] Cholesterol reduction post-MI has been shown to be of benefit in patients with both elevated and normal cholesterol levels.
- *Address modifiable risk factors:* Discourage smoking (p87). Encourage exercise. Identify and treat diabetes mellitus, hypertension, and hyperlipidaemia.
- *Exercise ECG.* May be useful in risk stratification post-MI after 3-4wks, and in subjects without ST-segment elevation or a troponin rise.
- *General advice.* If uncomplicated, discharge after 5-7d. *Work:* He may return to work after 2 months. A few occupations should not be restarted post-MI: airline pilots; air traffic controllers; divers. Drivers of public service or heavy goods vehicles may be permitted to return to work if they meet certain criteria.[38] Patients undertaking heavy manual labour should be advised to seek a lighter job. *Diet:* A diet high in oily fish, fruit, vegetables, and fibre, and low in saturated fats should be encouraged. *Exercise:* Encourage regular daily exercise. *Sex:* Intercourse is best avoided for 1 month. *Travel:* Avoid air travel for 2 months.
- *Review at 5wks post-MI to review symptoms:* Angina? dyspnoea? palpitations? If angina recurs, treat conventionally, and consider coronary angiography.
- *Review at 3 months* Check fasting lipids.

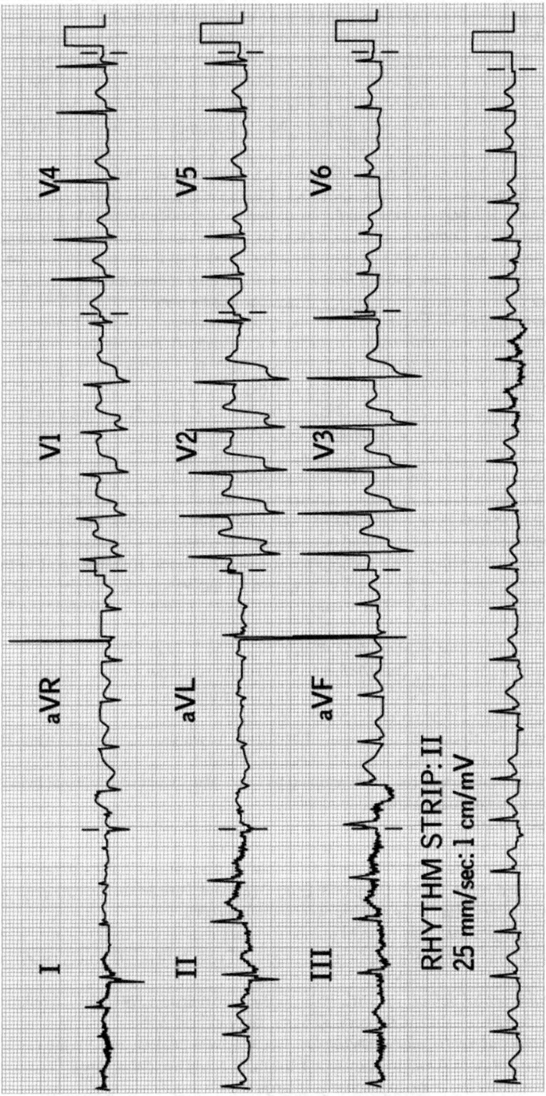

Fig 1. Acute postero-lateral MI.

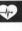

Cardiac arrest (inside backcover); ***cardiogenic shock*** (p814); LVF(p812).
Unstable angina: Manage along standard lines (p810) and refer to a cardiologist.
Bradycardias or heart block: *Sinus bradycardia:* treat with atropine 0.6-1.2mg IV. Consider temporary cardiac pacing if no response, or poorly tolerated by the patient. ↓BP which is not responsive to atropine in patients with inferior MI, may be due to RV infarction. *1st degree AV block:* Most commonly seen in inferior MI. Observe closely as approximately 40% develop higher degrees of AV block (in which case, calcium channel blockers and β-blockers should be stopped). *Wenckebach (Mobitz type I;* ECG, p119*) block:* Does not require pacing unless poorly tolerated. *Mobitz type II block:* Carries a high risk of developing sudden complete AV block; should be paced. *Complete AV block* (ECG, p90*):* usually resolves within a few days. Insert pacemaker (may not be necessary after inferior MI if narrow QRS and reasonably stable and pulse ≥40–50). *Bundle branch block:* MI complicated by trifascicular block or non-adjacent bifascicular disease should be paced.
Tachyarrhythmias: **NB:** K^+↓, hypoxia and acidosis all predispose to arrhythmias and should be corrected. *Sinus tachycardia* can ↑ myocardial O_2 demand. Pain and hypoxia are common causes (give O_2, analgesic). *SVT:* p120. *AF or flutter:* If compromised, DC cardioversion. Otherwise, control rate with digoxin (load with 0.5mg/12h PO for 2-3 doses; maintenance: 0.125–0.25mg/24h) ± β-blocker. In atrial flutter or intermittent AF, try amiodarone or sotalol (details p124). *Frequent PVCs* (premature ventricular contractions) are common after acute MI. They usually do not result in VF, and prophylactic antiarrhythmics are not recommended. *Non-sustained VT* (≥3 consecutive PVCs > 100 bpm and lasting <30s): if it happens at <48h after MI, antiarrhythmics are not recommended. However, if happens >48h, risk of sudden cardiac death is ↑ and electrophysiological studies should be considered. *Sustained VT* (≥3 consecutive PVCs > 100 bpm and lasting >30s): if compromised, give DC shock. If stable, treat with lidocaine or amiodarone. Recurrent VT may need pacing. *Ventricular fibrillation:* 80% occurs within 12h. If occur >48h, usually indicates pump failure or cardiogenic shock. ℞: DC shock.
Consider implantable cardiac defibrillator if ejection fraction <35% and VT.[39]
Right ventricular failure (RVF)/infarction: Presents with low cardiac output and JVP↑. Consider a Swan-Ganz catheter to measure right-sided pressures and guide fluid replacement. If BP remains low, give inotropes.
Pericarditis: Central chest pain, relieved by sitting forwards. ECG: saddle-shaped ST elevation. Treatment: NSAIDs. Echo to check for effusion.
DVT & PE: Patients are at risk of developing DVT & PE and should be prophylactically heparinized (enoxaparin) until fully mobile.
Systemic embolism: May arise from LV mural thrombus. After large anterior MIs, consider anticoagulation with warfarin for 3 months.
Cardiac tamponade: (p814) Presents with low cardiac output, pulsus paradoxus, JVP↑, muffled heart sounds. Diagnosis: Echo. Treatment: Pericardial aspiration (provides temporary relief ➡see p787 for technique), surgery.
Mitral regurgitation: May be mild (minor papillary muscle dysfunction) or severe (chordal or papillary muscle rupture or ischaemia). Presentation: Pulmonary oedema. Treat LVF (p812) and consider valve replacement.
Ventricular septal defect: Presents with pansystolic murmur, JVP↑, cardiac failure. Diagnosis: echo. Treatment: surgery. 50% mortality in first week.
Late malignant ventricular arrhythmias: Occur 1-3wks post-MI and are the cardiologist's nightmare. Avoid hypokalaemia, the most easily avoidable cause. Consider 24h ECG monitoring prior to discharge if large MI.
Dressler's syndrome: (p712) Recurrent pericarditis, pleural effusions, fever, anaemia and ESR↑ 1-3wks post-MI. Treatment: NSAIDs; steroids if severe.
Left ventricular aneurysm: This occurs late (4-6 weeks post-MI), and presents with LVF, angina, recurrent VT, or systemic embolism. ECG: persistent ST-segment elevation. Treatment: anticoagulate, consider excision.

Disturbances of cardiac rhythm or heart rate (arrhythmias) are:
- Common.
- Often benign (but may reflect underlying heart disease).
- Often intermittent, causing diagnostic difficulty.
- Occasionally severe, causing cardiac compromise.

Causes *Cardiac:* coronary artery disease, valvular (mitral) valve disease, cardiomyopathy, pericarditis, myocarditis, aberrant conduction pathways. *Non-cardiac:* caffeine, smoking, alcohol, pneumonia, drugs (β_2-agonists, digoxin, L-dopa, tricyclics, doxorubicin), metabolic imbalance (K^+, Ca^{2+}, Mg^{2+}, hypoxia, hypercapnia, metabolic acidosis, thyroid disease), & phaeochromocytoma.

Presentation With palpitation, chest pain, presyncope, syncope, hypotension, or pulmonary oedema. Some arrhythmias may be asymptomatic and incidental, eg AF.

History Take a detailed history of palpitations ([illegible]). Ask about precipitating factors, onset/offset, nature (fast or slow, regular or irregular), duration, associated symptoms (chest pain, dyspnoea, collapse). Review drug history. Ask about past medical history or family history of cardiac disease.

Tests FBC, U&E, glucose, Ca^{2+}, Mg^{2+}, TSH. ECG: look for signs of IHD, AF, short PR interval (WPW syndrome), long QT interval (metabolic imbalance, drugs, congenital), U waves (hypokalaemia). 24h ECG monitoring; several recordings may be needed. Echo: any structural heart disease, eg mitral stenosis, HCM? Provocation tests: exercise ECG, cardiac catheterization, electrophysiological studies may be needed.

Treatment If the ECG is normal during palpitations, reassure the patient. Otherwise treatment depends on the type of arrhythmia.

Bradycardia ([illegible]) If asymptomatic and rate >40bpm, no treatment is required. Look for a cause (drugs, sick sinus syndrome, hypothyroidism) and stop any drugs that may be contributing (β-blocker, digoxin). If rate <40bpm or patient is symptomatic, give atropine 0.6–1.2mg IV (up to maximum of 3mg). If no response, insert a temporary pacing wire ([illegible]). If necessary, start an isoprenaline infusion, or use external cardiac pacing.

Sick sinus syndrome Sinus node dysfunction causes bradycardia ± arrest, sinoatrial block or SVT alternating with bradycardia/asystole (tachy–brady syndrome). AF and thromboembolism may occur. Pace if symptomatic.

SVT ([illegible]) Narrow complex tachycardia (rate >100bpm, QRS width <120ms). Acute management: vagotonic manoeuvres, followed by adenosine if no result ([illegible]) or β-blocker/DC shock if compromised. Maintenance therapy: β-blocker or verapamil.

AF/flutter ([illegible]) May be treated [illegible] ventricular rate [illegible] digoxin [illegible] Alternatively [illegible] structural heart disease), DC shock if compromised ([illegible]).

VT ([illegible]) and other broad complex tachycardia (rate >100bpm, QRS width >120ms). Acute management: IV amiodarone or IV lidocaine. If no response or if compromised, DC shock. Give oral amiodarone loading dose 200mg/8h PO for 7d, then 200mg/12h for 7d followed by maintenance therapy (200mg/24h). SEs: corneal deposits, photosensitivity, hepatitis, pneumonitis, lung fibrosis, nightmares, INR↑ (warfarin potentiation), T4↑, T3↓. Monitor LFT and TFT.

Implanted permanent pacing may be used to override tachyarrhythmias, to treat bradycardia, or prophylactically if conduction disturbance ([illegible]). Implanted automatic defibrillators can save lives.

Disturbances of cardiac rhythm or arrhythmias are:

- Common
- Often benign (but may reflect underlying heart disease)
- Often intermittent, causing diagnostic difficulty
- Occasionally severe, causing cardiac compromise.

Causes *Cardiac:* MI, coronary artery disease, LV aneurysm, mitral valve disease, cardiomyopathy, pericarditis, myocarditis, aberrant conduction pathways. *Non-cardiac:* Caffeine, smoking, alcohol, pneumonia, drugs (β_2-agonists, digoxin, L-dopa, tricyclics, doxorubicin), metabolic imbalance (K^+, Ca^{2+}, Mg^{2+}, hypoxia, hypercapnia, metabolic acidosis, thyroid disease), & phaeochromocytoma.

Presentation is with palpitation, chest pain, presyncope/syncope, hypotension, or pulmonary oedema. Some arrhythmias may be asymptomatic and incidental, eg AF.

History Take a detailed history of palpitations (p35). Ask about precipitating factors, onset/offset, nature (fast or slow, regular or irregular) duration, associated symptoms (chest pain, dyspnoea, collapse). Review drug history. Ask about past medical history or family history of cardiac disease.

Tests FBC, U&E, glucose, Ca^{2+}, Mg^{2+}, TSH. ECG (see BOX): Look for signs of IHD, AF, short PR interval (WPW syndrome), long QT interval (metabolic imbalance, drugs, congenital), U waves (hypokalaemia). 24h ECG monitoring; several recordings may be needed. Echo: Any structural heart disease, eg mitral stenosis, HCM? Provocation tests: Exercise ECG, cardiac catheterization ± electrophysiological studies may be needed.

Treatment If the ECG is normal during palpitations, reassure the patient. Otherwise, treatment depends on the type of arrhythmia.

Bradycardia: (p119) If asymptomatic and rate >40bpm, no treatment is required. Look for a cause (drugs, sick sinus syndrome, hypothyroidism) and stop any drugs that may be contributing (β-blocker, digoxin). If rate <40bpm or patient is symptomatic, give atropine 0.6-1.2mg IV (up to maximum of 3mg). If no response, insert a temporary pacing wire (p814). If necessary, start an isoprenaline infusion or use external cardiac pacing.

Sick sinus syndrome: Sinus node dysfunction causes bradycardia ± arrest, sinoatrial block or SVT alternating with bradycardia/asystole (tachy-brady syndrome). AF and thromboembolism may occur. Pace if symptomatic.

SVT: (p120) Narrow complex tachycardia (rate >100bpm, QRS width <120ms). Acute management: vagotonic manoeuvres followed by IV adenosine or verapamil (if not on β-blocker); DC shock if compromised. Maintenance therapy: β-blockers or verapamil.

AF/flutter: (p124) May be incidental finding. Control ventricular rate with digoxin: loading dose (~500μg/12h×2-3) followed by maintenance dose (0.125-0.25μg/24h). Alternatives: verapamil, β-blocker, or amiodarone. Flecainide for pre-excited AF (caution if structural heart disease). DC shock if compromised (p806).

VT: (p122 and ECG 6) Broad complex tachycardia (rate >100bpm, QRS duration >120ms). Acute management: IV amiodarone or IV lidocaine, if no response or if compromised DC shock. Oral therapy: amiodarone loading dose (200mg/8h PO for 7d, then 200mg/12h for 7d) followed by maintenance therapy (200mg/24h). SE: Corneal deposits, photosensitivity, hepatitis, pneumonitis, lung fibrosis, nightmares, INR↑ (warfarin potentiation), T_4↑, T_3↓. Monitor LFT and TFT.

► Finally, permanent pacing may be used to overdrive tachyarrhythmias, to treat bradyarrhythmias, or prophylactically in conduction disturbances (p126). Implanted automatic defibrillators can save lives.

ECG diagnosis of bradycardias, AV block, and atrial fibrillation

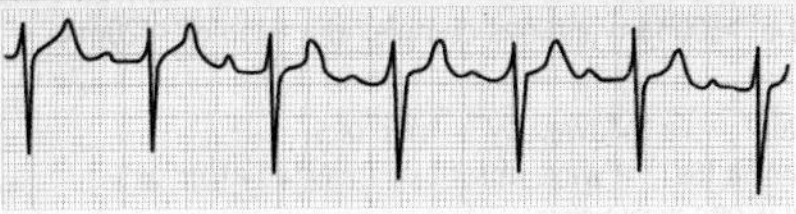

First degree AV block. P-R interval = 0.28s

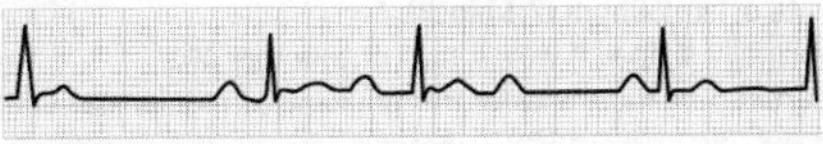

Mobitz type I (Wenckebach) AV block. With each succesive QRS, the P-R interval increases-until there is a non-conducted P wave.

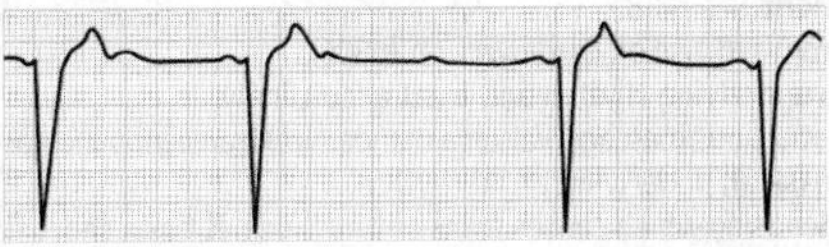

Mobitz type II AV block. Ration of AV conduction varies from 2:1 to 3:1

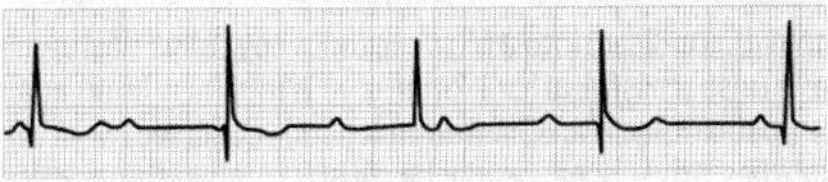

Complete AV block with narrow ventricular complex. There is no relation between atrial and the slower ventricular activity.

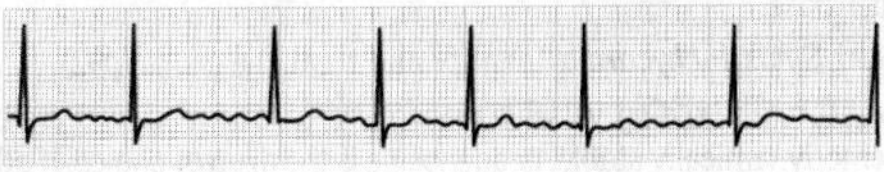

Atrial fibrillation

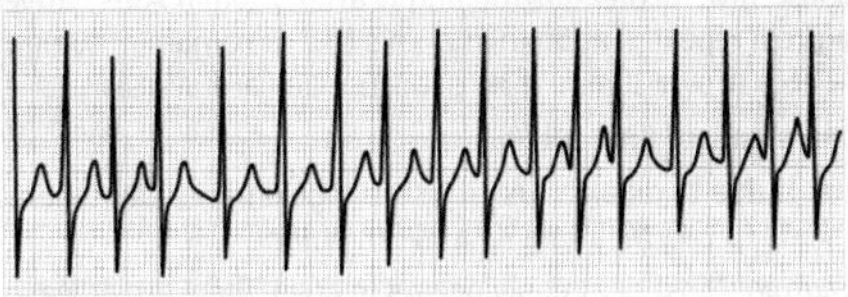

Atrial fibrillation with a rapid ventricular response. Diagnosis is based on the totally irregular ventricular rhythm.

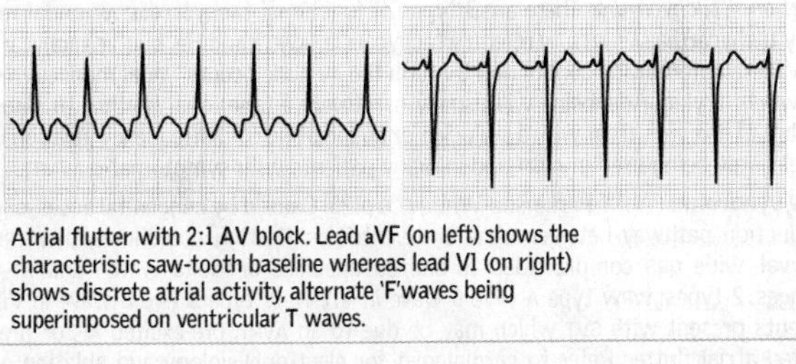

Atrial flutter with 2:1 AV block. Lead aVF (on left) shows the characteristic saw-tooth baseline whereas lead VI (on right) shows discrete atrial activity, alternate 'F'waves being superimposed on ventricular T waves.

Narrow complex tachycardia

Definition ECG shows rate of >100bpm and QRS complex duration of <120ms.

Differential diagnosis
- Sinus tachycardia: normal P wave followed by normal QRS.
- Supraventricular tachycardia (SVT): P wave absent or inverted after QRS.
- AF: absent P wave, irregular QRS complexes.
- Atrial flutter: atrial rate usually 300bpm giving 'flutter waves' or 'sawtooth' baseline (p119), ventricular rate often 150bpm (2:1 block).
- Atrial tachycardia: abnormally shaped P waves, may outnumber QRS.
- Multifocal atrial tachycardia: 3 or more P wave morphologies, irregular QRS complexes.
- Junctional tachycardia: rate 150–250bpm, P wave either buried in QRS complex or occurring after QRS complex.

Principles of management See p818.
- If the patient is compromised, use DC cardioversion (p806).
- Otherwise, identify the underlying rhythm and treat accordingly.
- Vagal manoeuvres (carotid sinus massage, Valsalva manoeuvre) transiently increase AV block, and may unmask an underlying atrial rhythm.
- If unsuccessful, give adenosine which causes transient AV block. It has a short t½ (10–15s) and works in 2 ways: by transiently slowing ventricles to show underlying atrial rhythm and by cardioverting a junctional tachycardia to sinus rhythm.

Adenosine dose: Give 6mg IV bolus (2sec) into a big vein; follow by saline flush, while recording a rhythm strip; if unsuccessful, after 1–2min, give 12mg, then 12mg again, unless on dipyridamole or post cardiac transplantation (change dose, see *BNF*). Warn of SE: transient chest tightness, dyspnoea, headache, flushing. CI: asthma, 2nd/3rd degree AV block, or sinoatrial disease (unless pacemaker). Drug interactions: potentiated by dipyridamole, antagonized by theophylline. Transplanted hearts are very sensitive; use a smaller dose.

Specific management *Sinus tachycardia* Identify and treat the cause (p92).

SVT: Vagal manoeuvres (breath-holding, valsalva manoeuvre, carotid massage) are 1st line treatments if haemodynamically stable. IV adenosine is the drug of choice. If adenosine fails, use verapamil 5mg IV over 2min, or over 3min if elderly (►not if already on β-blocker). If no response, give further dose of 5mg IV after 5–10min. Alternatives: atenolol 2.5mg IV at 1mg/min repeated at 5min intervals to a maximum of 10mg or sotalol 20–60mg (if eGFR >60) IV over 10min. If no good, use DC cardioversion.

AF/flutter: Manage along standard lines (p124).

Atrial tachycardia: Rare. If due to digoxin toxicity, stop digoxin; consider digoxin-specific antibody fragments (p854). Maintain K^+ at 4–5mmol/L.

Multifocal atrial tachycardia: Most commonly occurs in COPD. There are at least 3 morphologically distinct P waves with irregular P-P intervals. Correct hypoxia and hypercapnia. Consider verapamil or a β-blocker if rate remains >110bpm.

Junctional tachycardia: There are 3 types of junctional tachycardia: AV nodal re-entry tachycardia (AVNRT), AV re-entry tachycardia (AVRT), and His bundle tachycardia. Where anterograde conduction through the AV node occurs, vagal manoeuvres are worth trying. Adenosine will usually cardiovert a junctional rhythm to sinus rhythm. If it recurs, treat with a β-blocker or amiodarone. Radiofrequency ablation is increasingly being used in AVRT and in many patients with symptomatic AVNRT.[40]

WPW syndrome (Wolff-Parkinson-White ECG p125) Caused by congenital accessory conduction pathway between atria and ventricles. Resting ECG shows short PR interval, wide QRS complex (due to slurred upstroke or 'delta wave') and ST-T changes. 2 types: WPW type A (+ve δ wave in V_1), WPW type B (−ve δ wave in V_1). Patients present with SVT which may be due to an AVRT, pre-excited AF, or pre-excited atrial flutter. Refer to cardiologist for electrophysiology and ablation of accessory pathway.

Holiday heart syndrome 41 42

Binge drinking in a person *without* any clinical evidence of heart disease may result in acute cardiac rhythm and/or conduction disturbances, which is called holiday heart syndrome (note that recreational use of marijuana may have similar effects). The most common rhythm disorder is supraventricular tachyarrhythmia, and particularly AF (consider this diagnosis in patients without structural heart disease who present with new-onset AF).

The prognosis is excellent, especially in young patients without structural heart disease. As holiday heart syndrome resolves rapidly by abstinence from alcohol use, advise all patients against the excessive use of alcohol in future.

Broad complex tachycardia

ECG shows rate of >100 and QRS complexes >120ms (>3 small squares, p90). If no clear QRS complexes, it is VF or asystole, p766.

Principles of management
- Identify the underlying rhythm and treat accordingly.
- If in doubt, treat as ventricular tachycardia (VT)—the commonest cause.

Differential diagnosis
- VT; includes *torsade de pointes*, below, and BOX 2
- Supraventricular tachycardia (SVT) with aberrant conduction, eg AF, atrial flutter.

(**NB:** ventricular ectopics should not cause confusion when occurring singly; but if >3 together at rate of >120, this constitutes VT.)

Identification of the underlying rhythm may be difficult; seek expert help. Diagnosis is based on the history (IHD increases the likelihood of a ventricular arrhythmia), a 12-lead ECG, and the lack of response to IV adenosine (p120). ECG findings in favour of VT:
- Positive QRS concordance in chest leads
- Marked left axis deviation
- AV dissociation (occurs in 25%) or 2:1 or 3:1 AV block
- Fusion beats or capture beats (BOX 1).
- Also bear in mind the hard-to-remember QRS Brugada criteria (see BOX 3)

Concordance means QRS complexes are all +ve or -ve. *A fusion beat* is when an 'normal beat' fuses with a VT complex to create an unusual complex, and a *capture beat* is a normal QRS between abnormal beats (see BOX 1).

Management Connect to a cardiac monitor; have a defibrillator to hand.
- Give high-flow oxygen by face mask
- Obtain IV access and take blood for U&E, cardiac enzymes, Ca^{2+}, Mg^{2+}
- Obtain 12-lead ECG
- ABG (if evidence of pulmonary oedema, reduced conscious level, sepsis)

VT: Haemodynamically stable: correct low K^+ & hypomagnesaemia; monitor ECG. Then:
- Amiodarone 5mg/kg over 20-120min in 5% dextrose, repeat up to 1.2g in 24h. Unless a central line is used, phlebitis results, especially if concentration >2mg/mL.
- OR lidocaine 50mg over 2min repeated every 10min to 200mg max; see *BNF*.
- If this fails, or if cardiac arrest, use DC shock (p806 & inside back cover).
- After correction of VT, establish the cause from history/investigations.
- Maintenance antiarrhythmic therapy may be required. If VT occurs <24h after MI, give IV amiodarone or IVI lidocaine for 12-24h. If VT occurs >24h after MI, give IV lidocaine infusion and start oral antiarrhythmic, eg amiodarone.
- Prevention of recurrent VT: Surgical isolation of the arrhythmogenic area or implantation of tiny automatic defibrillators may help.

Ventricular fibrillation (VF): (ECG, see BOX 2) ►►Use asynchronized DC shock (p806): see also the *European Resuscitation Guidelines* (see inside back cover).

Ventricular extrasystoles (ectopics) are the commonest post-MI arrhythmia; they are also seen in health (≥10/h). Post-MI they suggest electrical instability, and the risk is VF if the 'R on T' pattern (ie no gap before the T wave) is seen (see **fig 1**). If frequent (>10/min), consider amiodarone IV as above. Otherwise, just observe patient.

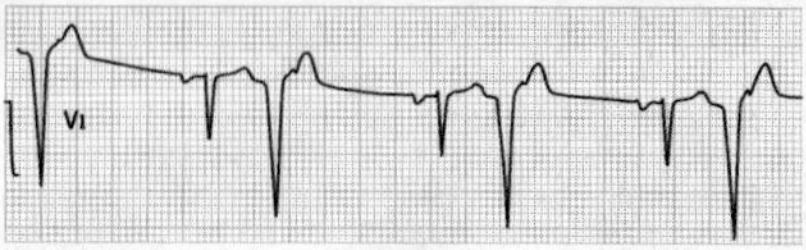

Fig 1. Ventricular extrasystoles may be intermittent, or have a fixed association with the preceding normal beat, ie 1:2 (bigeminy, as here) or 1:3 (trigeminy).[43]

Torsade de pointes: Looks like VF but is VT with varying axis (ECG, see BOX 2). It is due to ↑QT interval (a SE of antiarrhythmics, so consider stopping). ℞: Mg sulfate, 2g IV over 10 min ± overdrive pacing.

Fusion and capture beats

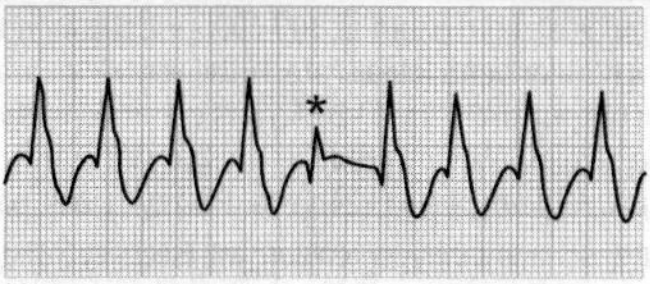

(a) A capture beat (*)

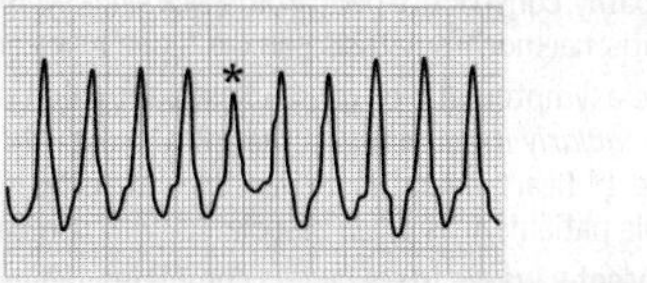

(b) A fusion beat (*)

Specimen rhythm strips

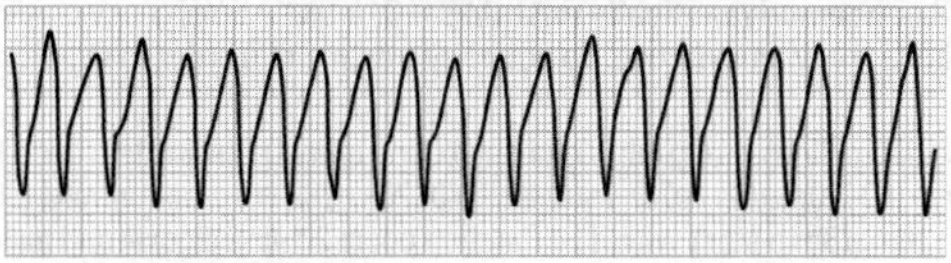

VT with a rate of 235/min.

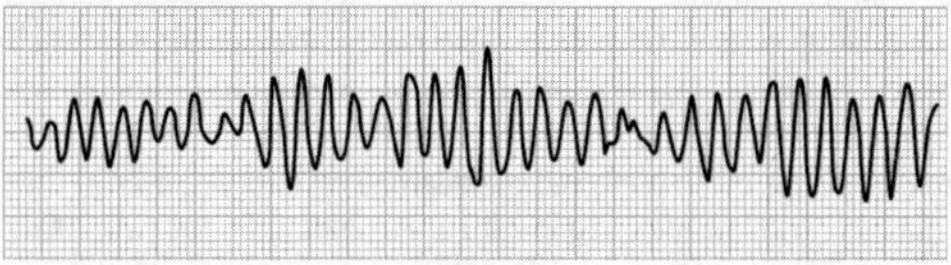

VF (p806).

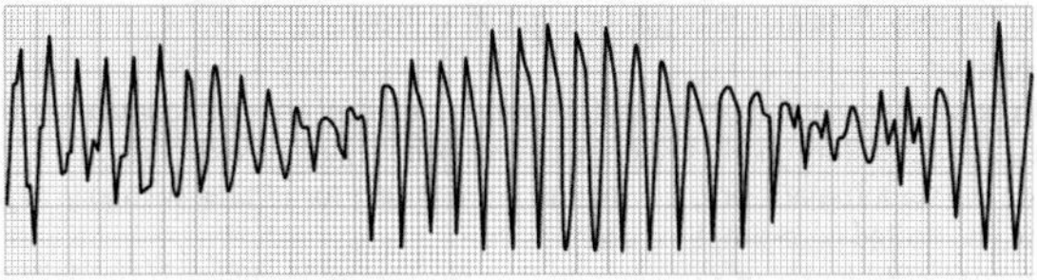

Torsade de pointes tachycardia.

The Brugada criteria may help differentiate SVT from VT... 44 45

Broad complexes + RBBB-like QRS

Lead V1:

- Monophasic R or QR or RS favours VT
- Triphasic RSR favours SVT

Lead V6

- R to S ratio <1 (R wave < S wave) favours VT
- QS or QR favours VT
- Monophasic R favours VT
- Triphasic favours SVT
- R to S ratio >1 (R wave > S wave) favours SVT

Broad complexes + LBBB-like QRS

Lead V1 or V2:

Any of these:

- R >30msec
- >60msec to nadir S
- Notched S favours VT

Lead V6

- Presence of any Q wave, QR or QS favours VT
- No Q wave in lead V6 favours SVT

Atrial fibrillation (AF) and flutter

ECG p119; NICE 2006

AF is a chaotic, irregular atrial rhythm at 300–600bpm; the AV node responds intermittently, hence an irregular ventricular rate. If the ventricles aren't primed reliably by the atria, cardiac output drops by 10–20%. AF is common in the elderly (≤9%). The main risk is embolic stroke. Warfarin reduces this to 1%/yr from 4%. So, *do an ECG on everyone with an irregular pulse* (±24h ECG if dizzy, faints, palpitations etc).

Causes Heart failure/ischaemia; hypertension; MI (seen in 22%);[47] PE; mitral valve disease; pneumonia; hyperthyroidism; caffeine; alcohol; post-op; K^+↓; Mg^{2+}↓.[48] ***Rare causes:*** Cardiomyopathy; constrictive pericarditis; sick sinus syndrome; lung ca.; atrial myxoma; endocarditis; haemochromatosis; sarcoid. 'Lone' AF means no cause found.

Symptoms May be asymptomatic or cause chest pain, palpitations, dyspnoea, or faintness. **Signs** *Irregularly irregular pulse*, the apical pulse rate is greater than the radial rate and the 1st heart sound is of variable intensity; signs of LVF (p812). ►Examine the whole patient: AF is *often* associated with non-cardiac disease.

Tests *ECG* shows absent P waves, irregular QRS complexes. *Blood tests:* U&E, cardiac enzymes, thyroid function tests. Consider echo to look for left atrial enlargement, mitral valve disease, poor LV function, and other structural abnormalities.

Acute AF (≤48h)

If **very ill** or **haemodynamically unstable:** ►►O_2 ►►U&E ►►Emergency cardioversion; if unavailable try IV amiodarone. Do not delay treatment in order to start anticoagulation.

Treat associated illnesses (eg MI, pneumonia). Control ventricular rate: a good 1st choice is **diltiazem** (60–120mg/8h PO) *or* **verapamil** (40–120mg/8h PO) *or* **metoprolol (**50mg/12h PO, or just 10mg/8h to start with if LV function poor). 2nd-line: **digoxin** and **amiodarone**. Start full anticoagulation with **LMWH**, to keep options open for cardioversion even if the 48h time limit is running out.[49] If the 48h period has elapsed, cardioversion without anticoagulation is OK if transoesophageal echo shows no intracardiac thrombus.

Cardioversion regimen: ►►O_2 ►►ITU/CCU ►►GA or IV sedation, monophasic ►►200J ►►360J ►►360J (biphasic; 200J). Relapses back into AF are common.

Drug cardioversion is often preferred: **amiodarone** IVI (5mg/kg over 1h then ~900mg over 24h via a central line max 1.2g in 24h) or PO (200mg/8h for 1wk, 200mg/12h for 1wk, 100–200mg/24h maintenance). Alternative (if stable and no known IHD or WPW): **flecainide** 2mg/kg IV over 10–30min, max 150mg (or 300mg PO stat); monitor ECG. Unfortunately, flecainide is a strong negative inotrope.

Chronic AF

Main goals in managing permanent AF are ***rate control*** and ***anticoagulation***. Rate control is at least as good as rhythm control,[50] but rhythm control may be appropriate if • symptomatic or CCF • younger • presenting for 1st time with lone AF • AF from a corrected precipitant (eg U&E↑↓).

Rate control β-blocker or rate-limiting Ca^{2+} blocker are 1st choice. If this fails, add **digoxin** (p108), then consider **amiodarone. Digoxin** as monotherapy in chronic AF is only OK in sedentary patients. ►*Don't give β-blockers with diltiazem or verapamil without expert advice (bradycardia risk).* Don't get fixated on a single figure to aim at: dialogue with patients tells what works best, and allows desired exercise levels, eg <90 at rest and on exertion 200–age (yrs) if ambulatory.

Rhythm control If cardioversion is chosen, do echo 1st; pre-treat for ≥4wks with **sotalol** or **amiodarone** if there is ↑risk of cardioversion failure (past failure, or past recurrence). Pharmacological cardioversion: **flecainide** is 1st choice if no structural heart disease (IV **amiodarone** if structural heart disease). AV node ablation, maze procedure, pacing, and pulmonary vein ablation are options to ask about.[51]

Anticoagulation see BOX 1.

In paroxysmal AF 'pill in the pocket' (eg sotalol or flecainide PRN) may be tried if: infrequent AF, BP >100mmHg systolic, no past LV dysfunction. Anticoagulate (BOX 1).

Anticoagulation and AF

Acute AF: Use *heparin* until a full risk assessment for emboli (see below) is made—eg AF started <48h ago and elective cardioversion is being planned (if >48h, ensure ≥3wks of therapeutic anticoagulation before elective cardioversion; NB trans-oesophageal-guided cardioversion is also an option here). Use *warfarin* (target INR: 2.5; range 2-3) if risk of emboli **high** (past ischaemic stroke, TIA or emboli; ≥75yrs with BP↑, DM; coronary or peripheral arterial disease; evidence of valve disease or ↓LV function/CCF—only do echo if unsure).[52] Use ***no anti-coagulation*** if *stable* sinus rhythm has been restored **and** no risk factors for emboli, **and** AF recurrence unlikely (ie no failed cardioversions, no structural heart disease, no previous recurrences, no sustained AF for >1yr).

Chronic AF: Anticoagulate with *warfarin* aim for an INR of 2-3.[53] Less good alternative is *aspirin* ~300mg/d PO—eg if warfarin contraindicated or at very low risk of emboli (<65yrs, and no hypertension, diabetes, LV dysfunction, ↑LA size, rheumatic valve disease, MI, or past TIA). *CI to warfarin in AF:*[54] Bleeding diathesis; platelets $<50\times10^9$/L; BP>160/90 (consistently); compliance issues around dosing or INR monitoring; patient choice, after risks discussed. Factors such as age ≥75–80yrs old, frequent falls, on NSAIDs, past intracranial bleeds, Hb↓, and polypharmacy are CI according to some authorities,[55] but are less evidence-based. Risk of major bleeds is ~13/100-person-yrs if ≥80yrs old (4 if <80yrs).[56] [57] ►Discuss with patient: *let him decide*. The CHADS score quantifies risk of stroke and may help in decision making.[58] ***Dabigatran:*** This is a direct thrombin inhibitor which doesn't need regular lab monitoring and dose adjustment. Despite its expense, it may be an alternative to warfarin (eg if warfarin is declined or has SE/CI, or monitoring INR is intrusive). In one trial, 110mg/12h PO it was as good as warfarin in preventing stroke and emboli in AF, and it caused fewer bleeding problems.[59] CI: severe renal/liver impairment; active bleeding; lesion at risk of bleeding; ↓clotting factors. Warn to report signs of bleeding. Interactions: heparin, clopidogrel, NSAIDs, GPiib/GPiia antagonists, p-glycoprotein inhibitors (verapamil, amiodarone, clarithromycin) etc. ↓Dose if eGFR <50 (avoid if <30).

Note on atrial flutter

See p119 for ECGs.

ECG: continuous atrial depolarization (eg ~300/min, but very variable) produces a sawtooth baseline ± 2:1 AV block (as if SVT at, eg 150bpm). **Carotid sinus massage** and IV **adenosine** transiently block the AV node and may unmask flutter waves.

Treatment Cardioversion may be indicated (anticoagulate before, see p124). Anti-AF drugs may not work—but consider amiodarone to restore sinus rhythm, and amiodarone or sotalol to maintain it. Aim to control rate as opposite; if the IV route is needed, a β-blocker is preferred (eg p819). Cavotricuspid isthmus ablation (this 'flutter isthmus' is low in the right atrium) may be tried.[60]

Wolff-Parkinson-White (WPW) syndrome

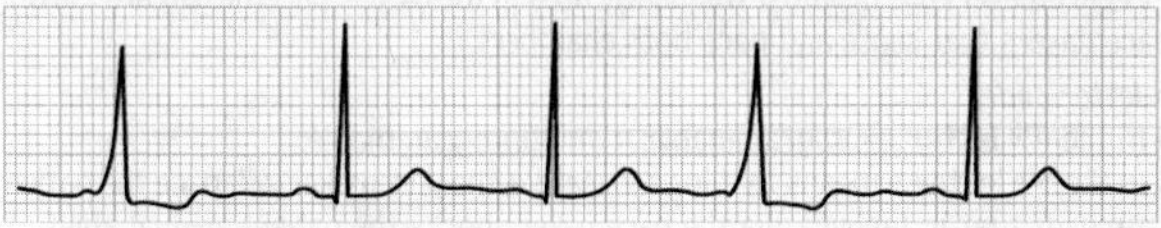

ECG of WPW syndrome (p120) in 1st & 4th beats; compared with the other beats, it can be seen how the delta wave both broadens the ventricular complex and shortens the PR interval. ►If WPW is the underlying cause of AF, avoid AV node blockers such as diltiazem, verapamil and digoxin—but flecainide may be used.

Pacemakers

Pacemakers supply electrical initiation to myocardial contraction. The pacemaker lies subcutaneously where it may be programmed through the skin as necessary. Pacemakers usually last 5-10yrs, but usually only the box needs replacing.

Indications for temporary cardiac pacing

- Symptomatic bradycardia, unresponsive to atropine.
- After acute *anterior* MI, prophylactic pacing is required in:
  - Complete AV block
  - Mobitz type I AV block (Wenckebach)
  - Mobitz type II AV block
  - Non-adjacent bifascicular or trifascicular block (p94).
- After *inferior* MI, pacing may not be needed in complete AV block if reasonably stable, rate is >40-50, and QRS complexes are narrow.
- Suppression of drug-resistant tachyarrhythmias, eg SVT, VT.
- Special situations: During general anaesthesia; during cardiac surgery; during electrophysiological studies; drug overdose (eg digoxin, β-blockers, verapamil).

►See p814 for further details and insertion technique.

Indications for a permanent pacemaker

- Complete AV block (Stokes-Adams attacks, asymptomatic, congenital)
- Mobitz type II AV block (p119)
- Persistent AV block after anterior MI
- Symptomatic bradycardias (eg sick sinus syndrome, p118)
- Drug-resistant tachyarrhythmias

Some say persistent bifascicular block after MI requires a permanent system: this remains controversial.

Pre-operative assessment: FBC, clotting screen, hepatitis B status. Insert IV cannula. Consent for procedure under local anaesthetic. Consider pre-medication. Give antibiotic cover (eg flucloxacillin 500mg IM and benzylpenicillin 600mg IM) 20min before, and 1 and 6h after.

Post-op management: Prior to discharge, check wound for bleeding or haematoma; check position on CXR; check pacemaker function. During 1st week, inspect for wound haematoma or dehiscence. Count apical rate (p37): if this is ≥6 bpm below the rate quoted for the pacemaker, suspect malfunction. Other problems: lead fracture; pacemaker interference (eg from patient's muscles). Driving rules: p152.

3-letter codes These enable pacemaker identification:

- the **1st letter** indicates the chamber paced (A=atria, V=ventricles, D=dual chamber);
- the **2nd letter** identifies the chamber sensed (A=atria, V=ventricles, D=dual chamber, O=none),
- the **3rd letter** indicates the pacemaker response (T=triggered, I=inhibited, D=dual, R=reverse).

VVI pacemakers are the most frequently used in the UK. **DDD** pacemakers are the only pacemakers that sense and pace both chambers.

5-letter codes

- In the **4th letter**, P=programmable; M=multiprogrammable.
- In the **5th letter**, P means that in tachycardia, the pacemaker will pace the patient. S means that in tachycardia the pacemaker shocks the patient. D=dual ability to pace and shock. O=neither of these.

ECG of paced rhythm: (**ECG 7** p101, and **fig 1** for rhythm strip) If the system is on 'demand' of 60bpm, a pacing spike will be seen only if the intrinsic heart rate is <60bpm. If it is cutting in at a higher rate, its sensing mode is malfunctioning. If it is failing to cut in at slower rates, its pacing mode is malfunctioning, ie the lead may be dislodged, the pacing threshold is too high, or the lead (or insulation) is faulty. If you see spikes but no capture (ie no systole), suspect dislodgement.

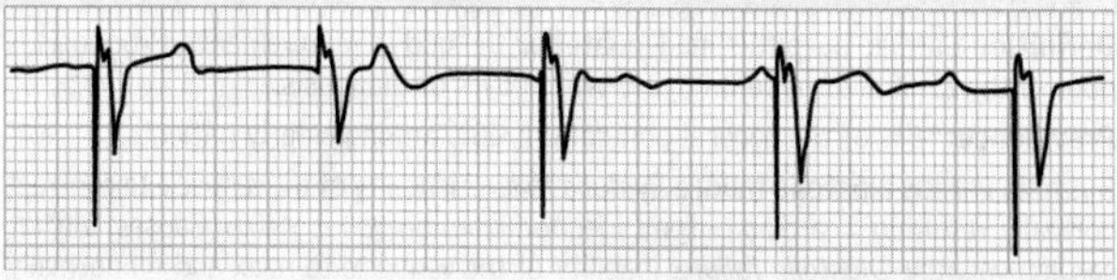

Fig 1. ECG of paced rhythm.

Some confusing pacemaker terms

Fusion beat: Union of native depolarization and pacemaker impulse.
Pseudofusion: The pacemaker impulse occurs just after cardiac depolarization, so it is ineffective, but it distorts the QRS morphology.
Pseudopseudofusion beat: If a DVI pacemaker gives an atrial spike within a native QRS complex, the atrial output is non-contributory.
Pacemaker syndrome: In single-chamber pacing, retrograde conduction to the atria, which then contract during ventricular systole. This leads to retrograde flow in pulmonary veins, and ↓cardiac output, dyspnoea, palpitations, malaise, and even syncope.
Pacemaker tachycardia: In dual-chamber pacing, a short-circuit loop goes between the electrodes, causing an artificial WPW-like syndrome. Solution: Single-chamber pacing. For ECG images, see www.monroecc.edu./depts/pstc/backup/paracar6.htm

Definition Cardiac output is inadequate for the body's requirements. Prognosis is poor with ~25-50% of patients dying within 5yrs of diagnosis.

Prevalence: 1-3% of the general population; ~10% among elderly patients.[65]

Systolic versus diastolic failure *Systolic failure:* inability of the ventricle to contract normally, resulting ↓cardiac output. Ejection fraction (EF) is <40%. Causes: IHD, MI, cardiomyopathy. *Diastolic failure:* inability of the ventricle to relax and fill normally, causing ↑ filling pressures. EF is >50%. Causes: constrictive pericarditis, tamponade, restrictive cardiomyopathy, hypertension. NB: systolic and diastolic failure usually coexist.

Left-sided versus right-sided failure *Left ventricular failure* (LVF) and *right ventricular failure* (RVF) may occur independently, or together as *congestive cardiac failure* (CCF). *Left ventricular failure:* Symptoms: Dyspnoea, poor exercise tolerance, fatigue, orthopnoea, paroxysmal nocturnal dyspnoea (PND), nocturnal cough (±pink frothy sputum), wheeze (cardiac 'asthma'), nocturia, cold peripheries, weight loss, muscle wasting. *Right ventricular failure:* Causes: LVF, pulmonary stenosis, lung disease. Symptoms: Peripheral oedema (up to thighs, sacrum, abdominal wall), ascites, nausea, anorexia, facial engorgement, pulsation in neck and face (tricuspid regurgitation), epistaxis.

Acute versus chronic heart failure ***Acute heart failure*** is often used exclusively to mean new onset acute or decompensation of chronic heart failure characterised by pulmonary and/or peripheral oedema with or without signs of peripheral hypoperfusion. ***Chronic heart failure*** develops or progresses slowly. Venous congestion is common but arterial pressure is well maintained until very late.

Low-output versus high-output failure *Low-output heart failure:* cardiac output is ↓and fails to ↑normally with exertion. ***Causes: Pump failure:*** Systolic and/or diastolic HF (see above), ↓ heart rate (eg β-blockers, heart block, post MI), negatively inotropic drugs (eg most antiarrhythmic agents). ***Excessive preload:*** eg mitral regurgitation or fluid overload (eg NSAID causing fluid retention). Fluid overload may cause LVF in a normal heart if renal excretion is impaired or big volumes are involved (eg IVI running too fast). More common if there is simultaneous compromise of cardiac function, and in the elderly. ***Chronic excessive afterload:*** eg aortic stenosis, hypertension.
High-output heart failure: This is rare. Here, output is normal or increased in the face of ↑↑needs. Failure occurs when cardiac output fails to meet these needs. It will occur with a normal heart, but even earlier if there is heart disease. ***Causes:*** anaemia, pregnancy, hyperthyroidism, Paget's disease, arteriovenous malformation, beri beri.
Consequences: Initially features of RVF; later LVF becomes evident.

Signs For diagnosis to be made there should be symptoms of HF *and* objective evidence of cardiac dysfunction (at rest). Diagnosis can be made using *Framingham* criteria (see BOX).[66] Other signs: exhaustion, cool peripheries, cyanosis, ↓BP, narrow pulse pressure, pulsus alternans, displaced apex (LV dilatation), RV heave (pulmonary hypertension), murmurs of mitral or aortic valve disease, wheeze (cardiac asthma).

Investigations According to NICE,[67] if ECG and B-type natriuretic peptide (BNP; p131), are normal, heart failure is unlikely, and an alternative diagnosis should be considered; if either is abnormal, then echocardiography (p106) is required.

Blood tests: FBC; U&E; BNP; ***CXR:*** Cardiomegaly (cardiothoracic ratio >50%), prominent upper lobe veins (upper lobe diversion), peribronchial cuffing, diffuse interstitial or alveolar shadowing, classical perihilar 'bat's wing' shadowing, fluid in the fissures, pleural effusions, septal (formerly called 'Kerley B') lines (variously attributed to interstitial oedema[68] and engorged peripheral lymphatics[69]). ***ECG*** may indicate cause (look for evidence of ischaemia, MI, or ventricular hypertrophy). It is rare to get a completely normal ECG in chronic heart failure. ***Echocardiography*** is the key investigation.[70] It may indicate the cause (MI, valvular heart disease) and can confirm the presence or absence of LV dysfunction. ***Endomyocardial biopsy*** is rarely needed.

Prognosis If admission is needed, 5yr mortality≈75%. Don't be dogmatic: in one study, 54% of those dying in the next 72h had been expected to live for >6months.[71]

Framingham criteria for congestive cardiac failure (CCF)

Diagnosis of CCF requires the simultaneous presence of at least 2 major criteria or 1 major criterion in conjunction with 2 minor criteria.

Major criteria:

- Paroxysmal nocturnal dyspnoea
- Neck vein distention
- Crepitations
- Acute pulmonary oedema
- S_3 gallop
- Hepatojugular reflux
- Cardiomegaly (cardiothoracic ratio >50% on chest radiography)
- Increased central venous pressure (>16cmH_2O at right atrium)
- Weight loss >4.5kg in 5 days in response to treatment

Minor criteria:

- Bilateral ankle oedema
- Nocturnal cough
- Dyspnoea on ordinary exertion
- Hepatomegaly
- Tachycardia (heart rate >120/min.)
- Pleural effusion
- Decrease in vital capacity by ⅓ from maximum recorded

The CXR in left ventricular failure

(see also fig 2 p737)

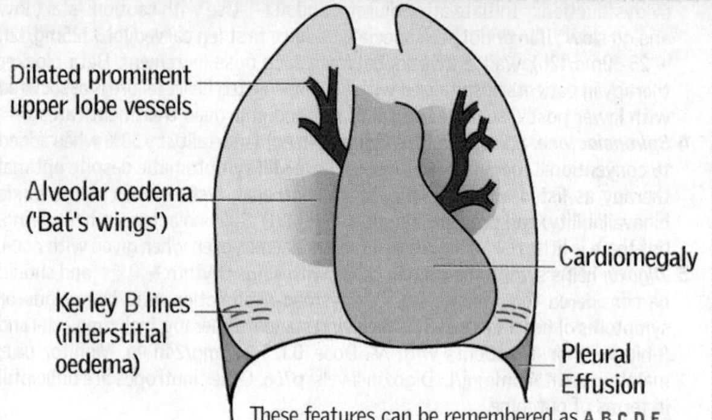

These features can be remembered as **A B C D E.**

Acute heart failure ▸▸This is a medical emergency (p812).

Chronic heart failure ▸Stop smoking. Eat less salt. Optimize weight & nutrition.
- Treat the cause (eg if dysrhythmias; valve disease).
- Treat exacerbating factors (anaemia, thyroid disease, infection, ↑BP).
- Avoid exacerbating factors, eg NSAIDs (fluid retention) and verapamil (-ve inotrope).
- Drugs: the following are used:

1 *Diuretics:* Diuretics can reduce the risk of death and worsening heart failure.[73] Give loop diuretics to relieve symptoms eg **furosemide** 40mg/24h PO or **bumetanide** 1-2mg/24h PO. Increase dose as necessary. SE: K^+↓, renal impairment. Monitor U&E and add K^+ sparing diuretic (eg **spironolactone**) if K^+ <3.2mmol/L, predisposition to arrhythmias, concurrent digoxin therapy (↓K^+ increases risk of digoxin toxicity), or pre-existing K^+-losing conditions. If refractory oedema, consider adding a thiazide, eg **metolazone** 5-20mg/24h PO.

2 *ACE-i:* Consider in all those with left ventricular systolic dysfunction; improves symptoms and prolongs life (see p108). If cough is a problem, an *angiotensin receptor blocker* (ARB) may be substituted (eg **candesartan** 4mg/d; max 32mg PO). These are occasionally used in combination by specialists; SE ↑K^+.

3 *β-blockers* (eg **carvedilol**) decrease mortality in heart failure.[74] These benefits appear to be additional to those of ACE-i in patients with heart failure due to LV dysfunction.[75] Initiate after diuretic and ACE-i. Use with caution: 'start low and go slow'; if in doubt seek specialist advice first (eg carvedilol 3.125mg/12h → 25-50mg/12h); wait ≥ 2weeks between each dose increment. Beta-blocker therapy in patients hospitalized with decompensated heart failure is associated with lower post-discharge mortality risk and improved treatment rates.[76]

4 *Spironolactone:* Spironolactone (25mg/24h PO) ↓mortality by 30% when added to conventional therapy.[77 RALES trial] Use in those still symptomatic despite optimal therapy as listed above. It improves endothelial dysfunction (↑nitric oxide bioavailability) and prevents remodelling (p131). Spironolactone is K^+-sparing, but there is little risk of significant hyperkalaemia, even when given with ACE-i.

5 *Digoxin* helps symptoms even in those with sinus rhythm;[78 RADIENCE trials] and should be considered for patients with LV systolic dysfunction who have signs or symptoms of heart failure while receiving standard therapy, including ACE-i and β-blockers, or in patients with AF. Dose: 0.125-0.25mg/24h PO. Monitor U&E; maintain K^+ at 4-5mmol/L. Digoxin levels: p766. Other inotropes are unhelpful in terms of outcome.

6 *Vasodilators:* The combination of **hydralazine** (SE: drug-induced lupus) and **isosorbide dinitrate** should be used if intolerant of ACE-i and ARBs as it reduces mortality. It also reduces mortality when added to standard therapy (including ACE-i) in Black patients with heart failure.[79]

Intractable heart failure Reassess the cause. Are they taking the drugs?—at maximum dose? Switching furosemide to **bumetanide** (one 5mg tab≈200mg furosemide) might help: absorption may be better.[80]. Consider admitting for:
- Strict bed rest ± Na^+ & fluid restriction (≤1.5L/24h PO).[81] [82]
- Metolazone (as above) and IV furosemide (p812).
- Opiates and IV nitrates may relieve symptoms (p812).
- Weigh daily. Do frequent U&E (beware K^+↓).
- DVT prophylaxis: heparin + TED stockings (p580).

In extremis, try IV inotropes (p814; it may be difficult to wean patients off them). Consider a heart transplant. **NB:** reports of the Jarvik thumb-sized titanium axial-flow impeller pump seem promising.[83] It is implanted in to the LV. A graft takes the blood to the descending aorta—making surgery hazardous.

Palliative care Treat/prevent comorbidities (eg flu vaccination). Good nutrition (allow alcohol!).[84] Involve GP: continuity of care and discussion of prognosis is much appreciated.[85] Dyspnoea, pain (from liver capsule stretching), nausea, constipation, and ↓mood all need tackling.[86] Opiates help pain and dyspnoea. O_2 may help.[87]

New York classification of heart failure: summary

I Heart disease present, but no undue dyspnoea from ordinary activity.
II Comfortable at rest; dyspnoea on ordinary activities.
III Less than ordinary activity causes dyspnoea, which is limiting.
IV Dyspnoea present at rest; all activity causes discomfort.

Natriuretic peptides

Secretory granules have long been known to exist in the atria, and if homogenized atrial tissue is injected into rats, their urine volume (and Na^+ excretion) rises. This is evidence of endocrine action via the effects of atrial natriuretic peptide (ANP). BNP is a similar hormone originally identified from pig brain (hence the B), but most BNP is secreted from ventricular myocardium. Plasma BNP is closely related to LV pressure. In MI and LV dysfunction, these hormones can be released in large quantities. Secretion is also increased by tachycardia, glucocorticoids, and thyroid hormones. Vasoactive peptides (endothelin-1, angiotensin II) also influence secretion. ANP and BNP both increase GFR and decrease renal Na^+ resorption; they also decrease preload by relaxing smooth muscle. ANP partly blocks secretion of renin and aldosterone.

BNP as a biomarker of heart failure[88 89 90] As plasma BNP reflects myocyte stretch; BNP is used to diagnose heart failure. ↑BNP distinguishes heart failure from other causes of dyspnoea more accurately than LV ejection fraction, ANP, and N-terminal ANP (sensitivity: >90%; specificity: 80–90%). BNP is highest in decompensated heart failure, intermediate in left ventricular dysfunction but no acute heart failure exacerbation, and lowest if no heart failure or LV dysfunction.

What BNP threshold for diagnosing heart failure? If BNP >100ng/L, this 'diagnoses' heart failure better than other clinical variables or clinical judgement (history, examination, and CXR). BNP can be used to 'rule out' heart failure if <50ng/L—negative predictive value (PV) 96%, ie the chance of BNP being <50ng/L given that heart failure is absent in 96%, see p672.

In those with heart failure, BNP is higher in systolic dysfunction than in isolated diastolic dysfunction (eg hypertrophic or dilated cardiomyopathy), and is highest in those with systolic *and* diastolic dysfunction. BNP also increases in proportion to right ventricular dysfunction, eg in primary pulmonary hypertension, cor pulmonale, PE, and congenital heart disease, but rises are less than in left ventricular disorders.

Prognosis in heart failure: The higher the BNP, the higher the cardiovascular and all-cause mortality (independent of age, NYHA class, previous MI and LV ejection fraction). ↑BNP in heart failure is also associated with sudden death. Serial testing may be important: persistently ↑ BNP despite vigorous anti-failure treatment predicts adverse outcomes. In one study, those with heart failure randomized to get N-terminal BNP-guided (rather than symptom-guided) therapy had ↓adverse events.

Prognosis in angina and MI: BNP has some prognostic value here (adverse left ventricular remodelling; LV dysfunction; death post-MI).[91]

Cautions with BNP: A BNP >50ng/L does not exclude other co-existing diseases such as pneumonia. Also, assays vary, so liaise with your lab.

Hypertension

Hypertension is a major risk factor for stroke and MI. It is usually asymptomatic, and regular screening (eg 3-yrly) is a *vital* primary care task. It causes ~50% of all vascular deaths (8×10^6/yr). Most preventable deaths are in areas without universal screening.[92]

Defining hypertension Blood pressure has a skewed normal distribution (p765) within the population, and risk is continuously related to blood pressure, so it is impossible to define 'hypertension'.[93] We choose to select a value above which risk is significantly increased, and the benefit of treatment is clear cut, see below. Assess BP over a period of time (don't rely on a single reading). The 'observation' period depends on the BP and the presence of other risk factors or end-organ damage.

Whom to treat All with BP ≥160/100mmHg (sustained; p133). For those ≥140/90, the decision depends on the risk of coronary events, presence of diabetes or end-organ damage; see BOX 4. The recent HYVET study showed that there is even substantial benefit in treating the over-80s.[94]

Systolic (SBP) or diastolic (DBP) pressure? For many years diastolic pressure was considered to be more important than systolic pressure. However, evidence from the Framingham and the MrFIT studies indicates that systolic pressure is the more important determinant of cardiovascular risk in the over-50s.

Isolated systolic hypertension (ISH): The most common form of hypertension in the UK—affects >50% of the over-60s, and results from stiffening of the large arteries (arteriosclerosis). It is not benign: doubles risk of MI, triples risk of CVA. Treatment reduces this excess risk, and is as, if not more, effective than treating moderate hypertension in middle-aged patients.

'***Malignant' hypertension:*** This refers to severe hypertension (eg systolic >200, diastolic>130mmHg) + bilateral retinal haemorrhages and exudates; papilloedema may or may not be present. Symptoms are common, eg headache ± visual disturbance. Alone it requires urgent treatment. It may also precipitate acute renal failure, heart failure, or encephalopathy, which are hypertensive emergencies. Untreated, 90% die in 1yr; treated, 70% survive 5yrs. Pathological hallmark is fibrinoid necrosis. It is more common in younger patients and in Blacks. Look hard for any underlying cause.

Essential hypertension (primary, cause unknown). ~95% of cases.

Secondary hypertension ~5% of cases. Causes include:

- ***Renal disease:*** The most common secondary cause. 75% are from *intrinsic renal disease:* glomerulonephritis, polyarteritis nodosa (PAN), systemic sclerosis, chronic pyelonephritis, or polycystic kidneys. 25% are due to *renovascular disease,* most frequently atheromatous (elderly ♂ cigarette smokers, eg with peripheral vascular disease) or rarely fibromuscular dysplasia (young ♀).
- ***Endocrine disease:*** Cushing's (p216) and Conn's syndromes (p220), phaeochromocytoma (p220), acromegaly, hyperparathyroidism.
- ***Others:*** Coarctation, pregnancy (*OHCS* p48), steroids, MAOI, 'the Pill'.

Signs & symptoms Usually asymptomatic (except malignant hypertension, above). Headache is no more common than in the general population. Always examine the CVS system fully and check for retinopathy. Are there features of an underlying cause (phaeochromocytoma, p220 etc.), signs of renal disease, radio-femoral delay, or weak femoral pulses (coarctation), renal bruits, palpable kidneys, or Cushing's syndrome? Look for end-organ damage: LVH, retinopathy and proteinuria—indicates severity and duration of hypertension and associated with a poorer prognosis.

Tests *To help quantify overall risk:* Fasting glucose; cholesterol. *To look for end-organ damage:* ECG (any LV hypertrophy? past MI?); urine analysis (protein, blood). *To 'exclude' secondary causes:* U&E (eg K^+↓ in Conn's); Ca^{2+} (↑ in hyperparathyroidism). *Special tests:* Renal ultrasound/arteriography (renal artery stenosis); 24h urinary VMA×3 (p220); urinary free cortisol (p217); renin; aldosterone.

Echocardiography and 24h ambulatory BP monitoring may help sometimes, eg in 'white coat' or borderline hypertension. Ambulatory readings are always lower; add on 12/7mmHg to 'convert' to clinic pressures for decision-making.

Defining hypertension

Category	Systolic	Diastolic
Optimal BP	<120 mmHg	<75 mmHg
Normal BP	120-129 mmHg	75-84 mmHg
High normal BP	130-139 mmHg	85-89 mmHg
Mild hypertension	140-159 mmHg	90-99 mmHg
Moderate hypertension	160-179 mmHg	100-109 mmHg
Severe hypertension	≥180 mmHg	≥110 mmHg

Grading hypertensive retinopathy

I Tortuous arteries with thick shiny walls (silver or copper wiring, p544, fig 1)
II A-V nipping (narrowing where arteries cross veins, p544, fig 2)
III Flame haemorrhages and cotton wool spots
IV Papilloedema, p544, fig 3.

Measuring blood pressure: mercury sphygmomanometers

- Use the correct size cuff. The cuff width should be >40% of the arm circumference. The bladder should be centred over the brachial artery, and the cuff applied snugly. Support the arm in a horizontal position at mid-sternal level.
- Inflate the cuff while palpating the brachial artery, until the pulse disappears. This provides an estimate of systolic pressure.
- Inflate the cuff until 30mmHg above systolic pressure, then place stethoscope over the brachial artery. Deflate the cuff at 2mmHg /second.
- *Systolic pressure:* appearance of sustained repetitive tapping sounds (Korotkoff I).
- *Diastolic pressure:* usually the disappearance of sounds (Korotkoff V). However, in some individuals (eg pregnant women) sounds are present until the zero point. In this case, the muffling of sounds, Korotkoff IV, should be used. State which is used for a given reading. For children, see *OHCS* p156.
- For advice on using automated sphygmomanometers, and a list of validated devices see http://www.bhsoc.org/how_to_measure_blood_pressure.stm.

Recommendations on preventing coronary heart disease[1]

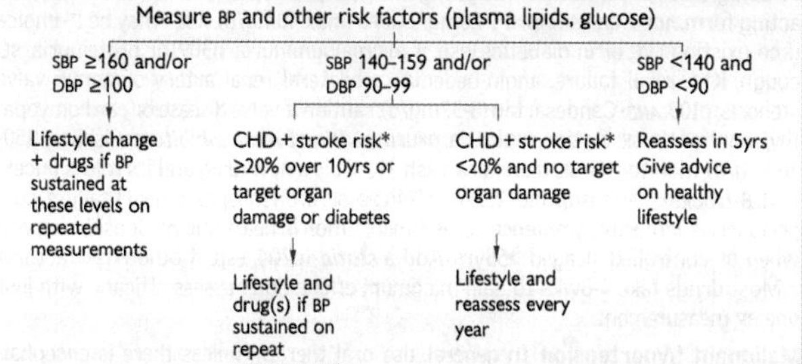
Measure BP and other risk factors (plasma lipids, glucose)
SBP ≥160 and/or DBP ≥100
SBP 140–159 and/or DBP 90–99
SBP <140 and DBP <90
Lifestyle change + drugs if BP sustained at these levels on repeated measurements
CHD + stroke risk* ≥20% over 10yrs or target organ damage or diabetes
CHD + stroke risk* <20% and no target organ damage
Reassess in 5yrs Give advice on healthy lifestyle
Lifestyle and drug(s) if BP sustained on repeat measurements
Lifestyle and reassess every year

All values are mmHg; SBP=systolic; DBP=diastolic.

Target pressure is <140/90mmHg, but in diabetes mellitus, aim for <130/80mmHg, and <125/75 if proteinuria.

*To quantify this, see **www.bhsoc.org. NB:** most sources older than 2004 just tabulate CHD risk, not CHD + stroke. The new CHD + stroke threshold of 20% ≈ 15% for CHD alone.[1] Examples of target (end-organ) damage: • LVH • PMH of MI or angina • PMH of stroke/TIA • Peripheral vascular disease • Renal failure.

1 Data from various sources. See British Cardiac Society & British Hyperlipidaemia Association & British Hypertension Society (BHS) & British Diabetic Association *Heart* 2005 **91** (1); see also USA Joint National Committee regimen (JNC 7) 2003 *JAMA* **289** 2560-72; BHS-IV *2004 Guidelines, BMJ* 2004 **328** 634.

Look for and treat underlying causes (eg renal disease, alcohol↑: see p132). Drug therapy reduces the risk of cardiovascular disease and death. Almost any adult over 50 would benefit from the antihypertensives below, *whatever their starting BP*.[97] Treatment is especially important if: BP is persistently ≥160/100mmHg **or** cardiovascular risk ↑ (10yr risk of vascular disease ≥20%) **or** existing vascular disease **or** target organ damage (eg brain, kidney, heart, retina) with BP >140/90mmHg. Essential hypertension is not 'curable' and long-term treatment is needed.

Treatment goal <140/85mmHg (<130/80 in diabetes). Reduce blood pressure *slowly*; rapid reduction can be fatal, especially in the context of an acute stroke.

Lifestyle changes ↓Concomitant risk factors: stop smoking; low-fat diet. Reduce alcohol and salt intake; increase exercise; reduce weight if obese.

Drugs The ALLHAT study suggests that adequate BP reduction is more important than the specific drug used.[98] However, β-blockers seem to be less effective than a comparator drug at reducing major cardiovascular events, particularly stroke. β-blockers and thiazides may increase the risk of new onset diabetes, Ca^{2+} channel blockers appear neutral, and ACE-i or ARB may reduce the risk.[99]

Monotherapy If ≥55yrs, and in Black patients of any age, 1st choice is a Ca^{2+} channel blocker or thiazide. If <55, 1st choice is ACE-i (or ARB if ACE-i intolerant, eg cough). β-blockers are not 1st-line for hypertension, but consider in younger people, particularly: if intolerance or contraindication to ACE-i/ARB (angiotensin receptor blockers) exists, or she is a women of child-bearing potential, or there is ↑sympathetic drive.

Combination therapy ACE-i + a Ca^{2+}-channel blocker or diuretic is logical, and has been commonly done in trials. There is little evidence on using 3 drugs so the recommendation is based on the most straightforward option:[100] try ACE-i, Ca^{2+}-channel blocker and thiazide. If BP still uncontrolled on adequate doses of 3 drugs, add a 4th (consider: higher-dose thiazide, or another diuretic, eg spironolactone (monitor U&E), or β-blockers, or selective α-blockers) and get help. If only on a β-blocker and a 2nd drug is needed, add a Ca^{2+} blocker, not a thiazide to ↓ risk of developing diabetes.

Dose examples ***Thiazides:*** eg chlortalidone 25–50mg/24h PO *mane*. SEs: K^+↓, Na^+↓, postural hypotension, impotence. CI: gout. ***Ca^{2+} channel blockers:*** eg nifedipine MR, 30–60mg/24h PO. SE: flushes, fatigue, gum hyperplasia, ankle oedema; avoid short acting form. ***ACE-i:*** eg lisinopril 5–20mg/24h PO (max 40mg/d). ACE-i may be 1st choice if co-existing LVF, or in diabetics (esp. if microalbuminuria, p309) or proteinuria. SE: cough, K^+↑, renal failure, angio-oedema. CI bilateral renal artery or aortic valve stenosis; p109. ***ARB:*** Candesartan (8–32mg/d); caution if valve disease or cardiomyopathy; monitor K^+. SE: vertigo, urticaria, pruritus. ***Direct renin inhibitors*** aliskiren (150–300mg/d); monitor K^+. SE: diarrhoea, rash ↑K^+. It is a new drug and its role is uncertain. ***β-blockers:*** eg bisoprolol 2.5–5mg/24h PO. SE: bronchospasm, heart failure, cold peripheries, lethargy, impotence. CI: asthma; caution in heart failure. Consider ***aspirin*** when BP controlled, if aged >55yrs. Add a ***statin*** (p704, esp. if other risk factors).

►Most drugs take 4–8wks to gain maximum effect: don't assess efficacy with just one BP measurement.

Malignant hypertension In general, use oral therapy, unless there is encephalopathy or CCF. The aim is for a controlled reduction in blood pressure over days, not hours. Avoid sudden drops in BP as cerebral autoregulation is poor (so stroke risk↑). Bed rest; there is no ideal hypotensive, but atenolol or long-acting Ca^{2+} blockers may be used PO.

Encephalopathy (headache, focal CNS signs, seizures, coma): aim to reduce BP to ~110mmHg diastolic over 4h. Admit to monitored area. Insert intra-arterial line for pressure monitoring. Furosemide 40–80mg IV; then either IV labetalol (eg 50mg IV over 1min, repeated every 5min, max 200mg) or sodium nitroprusside infusion (0.5μg/kg/min IVI titrated up to 8μg/kg/min, eg 50mg in 1L dextrose 5%; expect to give 100–200mL/h for a few hours only, to avoid cyanide risk).

►Never use sublingual nifedipine to reduce BP (∵ big drop in BP and stroke risk).[101]

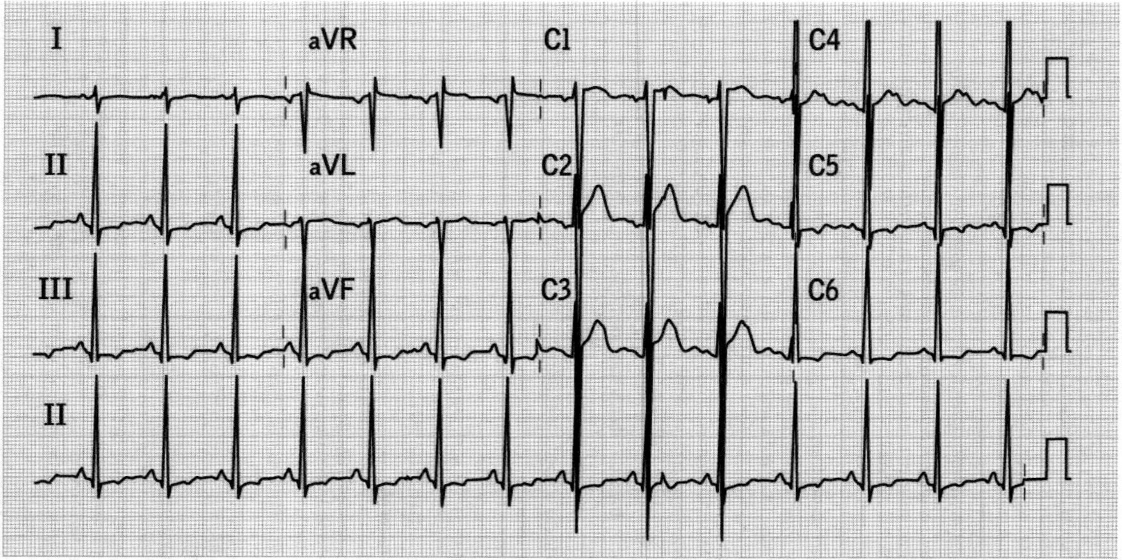

ECG 8—Left ventricular hypertrophy—this is from a patient with malignant hypertension—note the sum of the S-wave in C2 and R-wave in C6 is greater than 35mm.

Rheumatic fever

This systemic infection is still common in developing countries but increasingly rare in the West. Peak incidence: 5-15yrs. Tends to recur unless prevented. Pharyngeal infection with Lancefield group A β-haemolytic streptococci triggers rheumatic fever 2-4wks later, in the susceptible 2% of the population. An antibody to the carbohydrate cell wall of the streptococcus cross-reacts with valve tissue (antigenic mimicry) and may cause permanent damage to the heart valves.

Diagnosis Use the *revised Jones criteria* (may be over-rigorous). There must be evidence of recent strep infection plus 2 major criteria, or 1 major + 2 minor.

Evidence of group A β-haemolytic streptococcal infection:
- Positive throat culture (but this is usually negative by the time symptoms of rheumatic fever appear)
- Rapid streptococcal antigen test
- Elevated or rising streptococcal antibody titre (eg ASO or DNase B titre)
- Recent scarlet fever

Major criteria:
- *Carditis:* Tachycardia, murmurs (mitral or aortic regurgitation, Carey Coombs' murmur, p44), pericardial rub, CCF, cardiomegaly, conduction defects (45–70%). An apical systolic murmur may be the only sign.[102]
- *Arthritis:* A migratory, 'flitting' polyarthritis; usually affects larger joints (75%).
- *Subcutaneous nodules:* Small, mobile painless nodules on extensor surfaces of joints and spine (2-20%).
- *Erythema marginatum:* (**fig 1**) Geographical-type rash with red, raised edges and clear centre; occurs mainly on trunk, thighs, arms in 2-10% (p564).
- *Sydenham's chorea* (St Vitus' dance): Occurs late in 10%. Unilateral or bilateral involuntary semi-purposeful movements. May be preceded by emotional lability and uncharacteristic behaviour.[103]

Minor criteria:
- Fever
- Raised ESR or CRP
- Arthralgia (but not if arthritis is one of the major criteria)
- Prolonged PR interval (but not if carditis is major criterion)
- Previous rheumatic fever

Management
- Bed rest until CRP normal for 2wks (may be 3 months).
- Benzylpenicillin 0.6-1.2g IM or penicillin V 250-500mg 2-3 times daily PO for 10 days (if allergic to penicillin, give erythromycin or azithromycin for 10 days).[104]
- Analgesia for carditis/arthritis: aspirin 100mg/kg/d PO in divided doses (max 8g/d) for 2d, then 70mg/kg/d for 6wks. Monitor salicylate level. Toxicity causes tinnitus, hyperventilation, and metabolic acidosis. Alternative: NSAIDs (p548). If moderate-to-severe carditis is present (cardiomegaly, CCF, or 3rd-degree heart block), add oral prednisolone to salicylate therapy. In case of heart failure, treat appropriately (p130)
- Immobilize joints in severe arthritis.
- Haloperidol (0.5mg/8h PO) or diazepam for the chorea.

Prognosis 60% with carditis develop chronic rheumatic heart disease. This correlates with the severity of the carditis.[105] Acute attacks last an average of 3 months. Recurrence may be precipitated by further streptococcal infections, pregnancy, or use of the Pill. Cardiac sequelae affect mitral (70%), aortic (40%), tricuspid (10%), and pulmonary (2%) valves. Incompetent lesions develop during the attack, stenoses years later.

Secondary prophylaxis Penicillin V 250mg/12h PO. Alternatives: sulfadiazine 1g daily (0.5g if <30kg) or erythromycin 250mg twice daily (if penicillin allergic). ***Duration:*** If carditis+persistent valvular disease, continue at least until age of 40 (sometimes lifelong). If carditis but no valvular disease, continue for 10 yrs. If there is no carditis, 5 yrs prophylaxis (until age of 21) is sufficient.[106]

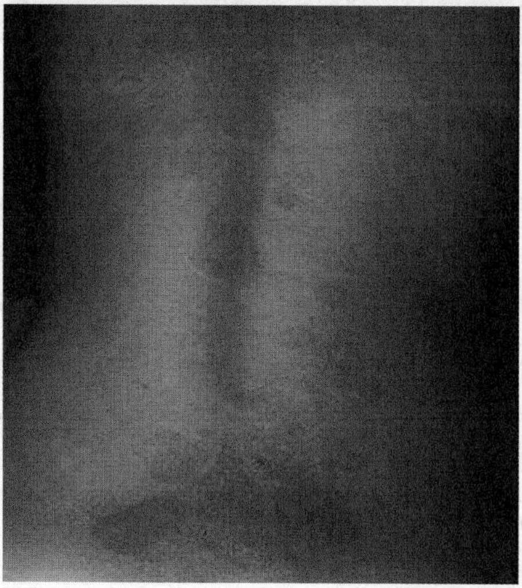

Fig 1. Erythema marginatum.

Image courtesy of Dr Maria Angelica Binotto.

Mitral stenosis *Causes:* Rheumatic; congenital, mucopolysaccharidoses, endocardial fibroelastosis, malignant carcinoid (p278; rare), prosthetic valve.

Presentation: Normal mitral valve orifice area is ~4-6cm². Symptoms usually begin when the orifice becomes <2 cm²: dyspnoea; fatigue; palpitations; chest pain; systemic emboli; haemoptysis; chronic bronchitis-like picture ± complications (below).

Signs: Malar flush on cheeks (due to ↓ cardiac output); low-volume pulse; AF common; tapping, non-displaced, apex beat (palpable S_1). On auscultation: loud S_1; opening snap (pliable valve); rumbling mid-diastolic murmur (heard best in expiration, with patient on left side). Graham Steell murmur (p44) may occur. *Severity:* The more severe the stenosis, the longer the diastolic murmur, and the closer the opening snap is to S_2.

Tests: *ECG:* AF; P-mitrale if in sinus rhythm; RVH; progressive RAD. *CXR:* left atrial enlargement (double shadow in right cardiac silhouette); pulmonary oedema; mitral valve calcification. *Echocardiography* is diagnostic. Significant stenosis exists if the valve orifice is <1cm²/m² body surface area. Indications for *cardiac catheterization:* previous valvotomy; signs of other valve disease; angina; severe pulmonary hypertension; calcified mitral valve.

Management: If in AF, *rate control* (p124) *is crucial*; anticoagulate with warfarin (p345). Diuretics ↓preload and pulmonary venous congestion. If this fails to control symptoms, balloon valvuloplasty (if pliable, non-calcified valve), open mitral valvotomy or valve replacement. SBE/IE prophylaxis for GI/GU infected procedures (p144). Oral penicillin as prophylaxis against recurrent rheumatic fever (p136).

Complications: Pulmonary hypertension; emboli, pressure from large LA on local structures, eg hoarseness (recurrent laryngeal nerve), dysphagia (oesophagus), bronchial obstruction; infective endocarditis (rare).

Mitral regurgitation *Causes:* Functional (LV dilatation); annular calcification (elderly); rheumatic fever, infective endocarditis, mitral valve prolapse, ruptured chordae tendinae; papillary muscle dysfunction/rupture; connective tissue disorders (Ehlers-Danlos, Marfan's); cardiomyopathy; congenital (may be associated with other defects, eg ASD, AV canal); appetite suppressants (eg fenfluramine, phentermine).

Symptoms: Dyspnoea; fatigue; palpitations; infective endocarditis. *Signs:* AF; displaced, hyperdynamic apex; RV heave; soft S_1; split S_2; loud P_2 (pulmonary hypertension) pansystolic murmur at apex radiating to axilla. *Severity:* The more severe, the larger the left ventricle.

Tests: *ECG:* AF ± P-mitrale if in sinus rhythm (may mean left atrial size↑); LVH. *CXR:* big LA & LV; mitral valve calcification; pulmonary oedema.

Echocardiogram to assess LV function and aetiology (trans-oesophageal to assess severity and suitability for repair rather than replacement). *Doppler echo* to assess size and site of regurgitant jet. *Cardiac catheterization* to confirm diagnosis, exclude other valve disease, assess coronary artery disease.

Management: Control rate if fast AF. Anticoagulate if: AF; history of embolism; prosthetic valve; additional mitral stenosis. Diuretics improve symptoms. Surgery for deteriorating symptoms; aim to repair or replace the valve before LV irreversibly impaired. Antibiotics to prevent endocarditis.

Mitral valve prolapse is the most common valvular abnormality (prevalence: ~5%). Occurs alone or with: ASD, patent ductus arteriosus, cardiomyopathy, Turner's syndrome, Marfan's syndrome, osteogenesis imperfecta, pseudoxanthoma elasticum, WPW (p120). *Symptoms:* Asymptomatic—or atypical chest pain and palpitations. Some patients have symptoms of autonomic dysfunction (anxiety, panic attack, syncope). *Signs:* Mid-systolic click and/or a late systolic murmur. *Complications:* Mitral regurgitation, cerebral emboli, arrhythmias, sudden death. *Tests:* *Echocardiography* is diagnostic. *ECG* may show inferior T wave inversion. *℞:* β-blockers may help palpitations and chest pain. In case of severe mitral regurgitation, surgery is needed.

Aortic stenosis (AS) *Causes:* Senile calcification is the commonest. Others: congenital (bicuspid valve, William's syndrome—p642), rheumatic heart disease.

Presentation: Think of AS in any elderly person with chest pain, exertional dyspnoea or syncope. The classic triad includes angina, syncope, and heart failure (usually after age 60). Also: dyspnoea; dizziness; faints; systemic emboli if infective endocarditis; sudden death. *Signs:* Slow-rising pulse with narrow pulse pressure (feel for diminution and delayed carotid upstroke—*parvus et tardus*); heaving, non-displaced apex beat; LV heave; aortic thrill; ejection systolic murmur (heard at the base, left sternal edge and the aortic area, radiates to the carotids). S_1 is usually normal. As stenosis worsens, A_2 is increasingly delayed, giving first a single S_2 and then reversed splitting. But this sign is rare. More common is a quiet A_2. In severe AS, A_2 may be inaudible (calcified valve). There may be an ejection click (pliable valve) or an S_4 (said to occur more often with bicuspid valves, but not in all populations).

Tests: ECG: P-mitrale, LVH with strain pattern; LAD (left anterior hemiblock), poor R wave progression; LBBB or complete AV block (calcified ring). CXR: LVH; calcified aortic valve (fig 1, p143); post-stenotic dilatation of ascending aorta. Echo: diagnostic (p110). Doppler echo can estimate the gradient across valves: severe stenosis if peak gradient ≥50mmHg and valve area <0.5cm². If the peak jet velocity is >4m/s (or is increasing by 0.3m/s per yr) risk of complications is increased. Cardiac catheter can assess valve gradient, LV function, coronary artery disease; but risks emboli.

Differential diagnosis: Hypertrophic cardiomyopathy (HCM, p146).

Management: If symptomatic, prognosis is poor without surgery: 2–3yr survival if angina/syncope; 1–2yr if cardiac failure. If moderate-to-severe and treated medically, mortality can be as high as 50% at 2yrs, therefore prompt valve replacement (p142) is usually recommended. In asymptomatic patients with severe AS and a deteriorating ECG, valve replacement is also recommended. If the patient is not medically fit for surgery, percutaneous valvuloplasty/replacement may be attempted.

Aortic sclerosis is senile degeneration of the valve. There is an ejection systolic murmur, no carotid radiation, and normal pulse (character and volume) and S_2.

Aortic regurgitation (AR) *Acute:* Infective endocarditis, ascending aortic dissection, chest trauma. *Chronic:* Congenital, connective tissue disorders (Marfan's syndrome, Ehlers–Danlos), rheumatic fever, Takayasu arteritis, rheumatoid arthritis, SLE, pseudoxanthoma elasticum, appetite suppressants (eg fenfluramine, phentermine), seronegative arthritides (ankylosing spondylitis, Reiter's syndrome, psoriatic arthropathy), hypertension, osteogenesis imperfecta, syphilitic aortitis.

Symptoms: Exertional dyspnoea, orthopnoea, and paroxysmal nocturnal dyspnoea. Also: palpitations, angina, syncope, CCF. *Signs:* Collapsing (water-hammer) pulse (p37); wide pulse pressure; displaced, hyperdynamic apex beat; high-pitched early diastolic murmur (best heard in expiration, with patient sitting forward). Eponymous signs: Corrigan's sign: carotid pulsation; de Musset's sign: head nodding with each heart beat; Quincke's sign: capillary pulsations in nail beds; Duroziez's sign: in the groin, a finger compressing the femoral artery 2cm proximal to the stethoscope gives a systolic murmur; if 2cm distal, gives a diastolic murmur as blood flows backwards; Traube's sign: 'pistol shot' sound over femoral arteries; an Austin Flint murmur (p44) denotes severe AR.

Tests: ECG: LVH. CXR: cardiomegaly; dilated ascending aorta; pulmonary oedema. *Echocardiography* is diagnostic. Cardiac catheterization to assess: severity of lesion; anatomy of aortic root; LV function; coronary artery disease; other valve disease.

Management: The goal of medical therapy is to reduce systolic hypertension; ACE-i are helpful. Echo every 6–12 months to monitor. Indications for surgery include: increasing symptoms; enlarging heart on CXR/echo; ECG deterioration (T wave inversion in lateral leads); or infective endocarditis refractory to medical therapy. Aim to replace the valve before significant LV dysfunction occurs. Predictors of poor post-operative survival: ejection fraction <50%, NYHA class III or IV (p130), duration of CCF >12 months.

Aortic stenosis (AS) *Causes:* Senile calcification is the commonest.[107] Others: congenital (bicuspid valve, William's syndrome, p143), rheumatic heart disease.

Presentation: Think of AS in any elderly who presents with chest pain or exertional dyspnoea. The classic triad includes angina, syncope, and heart failure (usually after age 60). Also: dyspnoea; dizziness; faints; systemic emboli if infective endocarditis; sudden death. *Signs:* Slow rising pulse with narrow pulse pressure (feel for diminished and delayed carotid upstroke—*parvus et tardus*); heaving, non-displaced apex beat; LV heave; aortic thrill; ejection systolic murmur (heard at the base, left sternal edge and the aortic area, radiates to the carotids). S_1 is usually normal. As stenosis worsens, A_2 is increasingly delayed, giving first a single S_2 and then reversed splitting. But this sign is rare. More common is a quiet A_2. In severe AS, A_2 may be inaudible (calcified valve). There may be an ejection click (pliable valve) or an S_4 (said to occur more often with bicuspid valves, but not in all populations).[108]

Tests: *ECG:* P-mitrale, LVH with strain pattern; LAD (left anterior hemiblock); poor R wave progression; LBBB or complete AV block (calcified ring). *CXR:* LVH; calcified aortic valve (see **fig 1**); post-stenotic dilatation of ascending aorta. *Echo:* diagnostic (p106). *Doppler echo* can estimate the gradient across valves: severe stenosis if gradient ≥50mmHg and valve area <0.5cm². If the aortic jet velocity is >4m/s (or is increasing by >0.3m/s per yr) risk of complications is increased.[109] *Cardiac catheter* can assess: valve gradient; LV function; coronary artery disease; but risks emboli.

Differential diagnosis: Hypertrophic cardiomyopathy (HCM, p146).

Management: If symptomatic, prognosis is poor without surgery: 2-3yr survival if angina/syncope; 1-2yr if cardiac failure. If moderate-to-severe and treated medically, mortality can be as high as 50% at 2 yrs, therefore prompt valve replacement (p142) is usually recommended. In asymptomatic patients with severe AS and a deteriorating ECG, valve replacement is also recommended. If the patient is not medically fit for surgery, percutaneous valvuloplasty/replacement may be attempted.

Aortic sclerosis is senile degeneration of the valve. There is an ejection systolic murmur, no carotid radiation, and normal pulse (character and volume) and S_2.

Aortic regurgitation (AR) *Acute:* Infective endocarditis, ascending aortic dissection, chest trauma. *Chronic:* Congenital, connective tissue disorders (Marfan's syndrome, Ehlers-Danlos), rheumatic fever, Takayasu arteritis, rheumatoid arthritis, SLE; pseudoxanthoma elasticum, appetite suppressants (eg fenfluramine, phentermine), seronegative arthritides (ankylosing spondylitis, Reiter's syndrome, psoriatic arthropathy), hypertension, osteogenesis imperfecta, syphilitic aortitis.

Symptoms: Exertional dyspnoea, orthopnoea, and paroxysmal nocturnal dyspnoea. Also: palpitations, angina, syncope, CCF. *Signs:* Collapsing (water-hammer) pulse (p40); wide pulse pressure; displaced, hyperdynamic apex beat; high pitched early diastolic murmur (heard best in expiration, with patient sitting forward). Eponyms: **Corrigan's sign:** carotid pulsation; **de Musset's sign:** head nodding with each hear beat; **Quincke's sign:** capillary pulsations in nail beds; **Duroziez's sign:** in the groin, a finger compressing the femoral artery 2cm *proximal* to the stethoscope gives a systolic murmur; if 2cm *distal*, it gives a diastolic murmur as blood flows backwards; **Traube's sign:** 'pistol shot' sound: over femoral arteries; an **Austin Flint** murmur (p44) denotes *severe* AR.

Tests: *ECG:* LVH. *CXR:* cardiomegaly; dilated ascending aorta; pulmonary oedema. *Echocardiography* is diagnostic. *Cardiac catheterization* to assess: severity of lesion; anatomy of aortic root; LV function; coronary artery disease; other valve disease.

Management: The main goal of medical therapy is to reduce systolic hypertension. ACE-i are helpful. Echo every 6-12 months to monitor. Indications for surgery: increasing symptoms; enlarging heart on CXR/echo; ECG deterioration (T wave inversion in lateral leads); IE refractory to medical therapy. Aim to replace the valve before significant LV dysfunction occurs. Predictors of poor post-operative survival: ejection fraction <50%, NYHA class III or IV (p131), duration of CCF >12 months.

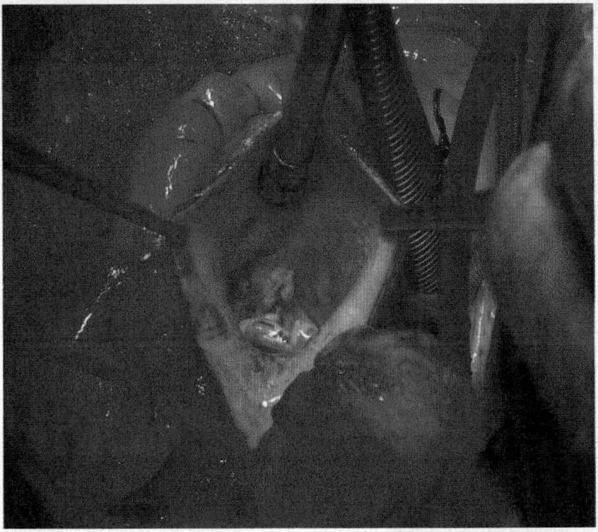

Fig 1. Severely calcified aortic valve.

Reproduced with permission from Hamid Reza Taghipour.

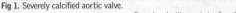

Right heart valve disease

Tricuspid regurgitation *Causes:* Functional (RV dilatation; eg due to pulmonary hypertension induced by LV failure); rheumatic fever; infective endocarditis (IV drug abuser[1]); carcinoid syndrome; congenital (eg ASD, AV canal, Ebstein's anomaly, ie downward displacement of the tricuspid valve—see *OHCS* p642), drugs (eg ergot-derived dopamine agonists, p498, fenfluramine). ***Symptoms:*** Fatigue; hepatic pain on exertion; ascites; oedema and also dyspnoea and orthopnoea if the cause is LV dysfunction. ***Signs:*** Giant *v* waves and prominent *y* descent in JVP (p41); RV heave; pansystolic murmur, heard best at lower sternal edge in inspiration; pulsatile hepatomegaly; jaundice; ascites. ***Management:*** Treat underlying cause. Drugs: diuretics, digoxin, ACE-inhibitors. Valve replacement (~10% 30d mortality). Tricuspid regurgitation resulting from myocardial dysfunction or dilatation has a mortality of up to 50% at 5 yrs.

Tricuspid stenosis *Cause:* Main cause is rheumatic fever, which almost always occurs with mitral or aortic valve disease. Also: congenital, infective endocarditis. ***Symptoms:*** Fatigue, ascites, oedema. ***Signs:*** Giant *a* wave and slow *y* descent in JVP (p41); opening snap, early diastolic murmur heard at the left sternal edge in inspiration. AF can also occur. ***Diagnosis:*** Echo. ***Treatment:*** Diuretics; surgical repair.

Pulmonary stenosis *Causes:* Usually congenital (Turner's syndrome, Noonan's syndrome, William's syndrome, Fallot's tetralogy, rubella). Acquired causes: rheumatic fever, carcinoid syndrome. ***Symptoms:*** Dyspnoea; fatigue; oedema; ascites. ***Signs:*** Dysmorphic facies (congenital causes); prominent *a* wave in JVP; RV heave. In mild stenosis, there is an ejection click, ejection systolic murmur (which radiates to the left shoulder); widely split S_2. In severe stenosis, the murmur becomes longer and obscures A_2. P_2 becomes softer and may be inaudible. ***Tests:*** ECG: RAD, P-pulmonale, RVH, RBBB. ECHO/TOE (p106). *CXR:* prominent main, right, or left pulmonary arteries caused by post-stenotic dilatation. Cardiac catheterization is diagnostic. ***Treatment:*** Pulmonary valvuloplasty or valvotomy.

Pulmonary regurgitation is caused by any cause of pulmonary hypertension (p194). A decrescendo murmur is heard in early diastole at the left sternal edge (the Graham Steell murmur if associated with mitral stenosis and pulmonary hypertension).

Cardiac surgery

Valvuloplasty can be used in mitral or pulmonary stenosis (pliable, non-calcified valve, no regurgitation). A balloon catheter is inserted across the valve and inflated.

Valvotomy Closed valvotomy is rarely performed now. Open valvotomy is performed under cardiopulmonary bypass through a median sternotomy.

Valve replacements *Mechanical valves* may be of the ball-cage (Starr-Edwards), tilting disc (Bjork-Shiley), or double tilting disc (St Jude) type. These valves are very durable but the risk of thromboembolism is high; patients require lifelong anticoagulation. *Xenografts* are made from porcine valves or pericardium. These valves are less durable and may require replacement at 8–10yrs. Anticoagulation is not required unless there is AF. *Homografts* are cadaveric valves. They are particularly useful in young patients and in the replacement of infected valves. *Complications of prosthetic valves:* systemic embolism, infective endocarditis, haemolysis, structural valve failure, arrhythmias.

CABG See p104.

Cardiac transplantation Consider this when cardiac disease is *severely* curtailing quality of life, and survival is not expected beyond 6–12 months. Refer to a specialist centre.

1 This list is easier to remember once we recall that it is the tricuspid valve which is the valve most vulnerable to events arriving by vein, eg pathogens from IV drug abusers reach the tricuspid valve first; likewise for drugs and toxins from distal carcinoid tumours.

The heart in various, mostly rare, systemic diseases

This list reminds us to look at the heart *and* the whole patient, not just in exams (where those with odd syndromes congregate), but always.

Acromegaly: (p230) BP↑; LVH; hypertrophic cardiomyopathy; high output cardiac failure; coronary artery disease.

Amyloidosis: (p364) Restrictive cardiomyopathy. Bright myocardium on echo.

Ankylosing spondylitis: Conduction defects; AV block; AR.

Behçet's disease: (p708) Aortic regurgitation; arterial ± venous thrombi.

Cushing's syndrome: (p216) Hypertension.

Down's syndrome: (*OHCS* p152) ASD; VSD; mitral regurgitation.

Ehlers–Danlos syndrome: (*OHCS* p642) Mitral valve prolapse + hyperelastic skin ± aneurysms and GI bleeds. Joints are loose and hypermobile; mutations exist, eg in genes for procollagen (COL3A1); there are 6 types.

Friedreich's ataxia: (p712) Hypertrophic cardiomyopathy, dilatation over time.

Haemochromatosis: (p262) AF; cardiomyopathy.

Holt–Oram syndrome: ASD or VSD with upper limb defects. [110]

Human immunodeficiency virus: (p408) Myocarditis; dilated cardiomyopathy; effusion; ventricular arrhythmias; SBE/IE; non-infective thrombotic (marantic) endocarditis; RVF (pulmonary hypertension); metastatic Kaposi's sarcoma.

Hypothyroidism: (p212) Sinus bradycardia; low pulse pressure; pericardial effusion; coronary artery disease; low voltage ECG.

Kawasaki disease: (*OHCS* p646) Coronary arteritis similar to PAN; commoner than *rheumatic fever* (p136) as a cause of acquired heart disease.

Klinefelter's syndrome: ♂ (*OHCS* p646) ASD. Psychopathy; learning difficulties; libido↓; gynaecomastia; sparse facial hair and small firm testes. XXY.

Marfan's syndrome: (p720) Mitral valve prolapse; AR; aortic dissection. Look for long fingers and a high-arched palate.

Noonan's syndrome: (*OHCS* p650) ASD; pulmonary stenosis ± low-set ears.

PAN: (p558) Small and medium vessel vasculitis + angina; MI; arrhythmias; CCF; pericarditis and conduction defects.

Rheumatoid arthritis: Conduction defects; pericarditis; LV dysfunction; aortic regurgitation; coronary arteritis. Look for arthritis signs, p548.

Sarcoidosis: (p186) Infiltrating granulomas may cause complete AV block; ventricular or supraventricular tachycardia; myocarditis; CCF; restrictive cardiomyopathy. ECG may show Q waves.

Syphilis: (p431) Myocarditis; ascending aortic aneurysm.

Systemic lupus erythematosus: (p556) Pericarditis/effusion; myocarditis; Libman-Sacks endocarditis; mitral valve prolapse; coronary arteritis.

Systemic sclerosis: (p554) Pericarditis; pericardial effusion; myocardial fibrosis; myocardial ischaemia; conduction defects; cardiomyopathy.

Thyrotoxicosis: (p210) Pulse↑; AF ± emboli; wide pulse pressure; hyperdynamic apex; loud heart sounds; ejection systolic murmur; pleuropericardial rub; angina; high-output cardiac failure.

Turner's syndrome: ♀ Coarctation of aorta. Look for webbed neck. XO.

William's syndrome: Supravalvular aortic stenosis (visuospatial IQ↓).

Infective endocarditis (IE)

►Fever + new murmur = endocarditis until proven otherwise. *Any* fever lasting >1wk in those known to be at risk[1] must prompt blood cultures.[111] Classification: 50% of all endocarditis occurs on *normal valves*. It follows an ***acute course***, and presents with acute heart failure ± emboli. Chief cause:[112] *S. aureus*. Risk factors: dermatitis; IV injections; renal failure; organ transplantation; DM; post-op wounds. Entry is usually via the skin. Mortality: 5–50% (related to age and embolic events). Endocarditis on *abnormal valves* tends to run a ***subacute course***. Risk factors: aortic or mitral valve disease; tricuspid valves in IV drug users; coarctation; patent ductus arteriosus; VSD; prosthetic valves. Endocarditis on prosthetic valves may be 'early' (during surgery, poor prognosis) or 'late' (haematogenous).

Causes *Bacteraemia:* This is occurring all the time, eg when we chew (not just when we have dentistry or medical interventions—which is why routine prophylaxis for such procedures does not make sense).[113] *Strep viridans* is common cause (>35%). Others: enterococci; *Staph aureus/epidermidis*; diphtheroids; microaerophilic streps. Rarely: **HACEK** Gram –ve bacteria (*Haemophilus-Actinobacillus-Cardiobacterium-Eikenella-Kingella*); *Coxiella burnetii*; *Chlamydia*. *Fungi: Candida; Aspergillus; Histoplasma*. *Other causes:* SLE (Libman-Sacks endocarditis); malignancy.

Signs *Septic signs:* Fever, rigors, night sweats, malaise, weight loss, anaemia, splenomegaly, and clubbing (**fig 1**). *Cardiac lesions:* Any new murmur, or a changing pre-existing murmur, should raise the suspicion of endocarditis. Vegetations may cause valve destruction and severe regurgitation, or valve obstruction. An aortic root abscess causes prolongation of the PR interval, and may lead to complete AV block. LVF is a common cause of death. ***Immune complex deposition:*** Vasculitis (p558) may affect any vessel. Microscopic haematuria is common; glomerulonephritis and acute renal failure may occur. Roth spots (boat-shaped retinal haemorrhage with pale centre; p386 **fig 1**); splinter haemorrhages (**fig 2**); Osler's nodes (painful pulp infarcts in fingers or toes) and Janeway lesions (**fig 3**; painless palmar or plantar macules) are pathognomonic. ***Embolic phenomena:*** Emboli may cause abscesses in the relevant organ, eg brain, heart, kidney, spleen, gut (or lung if right-sided IE).

Diagnosis Use the *Duke* criteria (BOX 1).[114] *Blood cultures:* Do 3 sets at different times from different sites at peak of fever. 85–90% are diagnosed from the 1st 2 sets; 10% are culture-negative. *Blood tests:* Normochromic, normocytic anaemia, neutrophilia, high ESR/CRP. Also check U&E, Mg^{2+}, LFT. *Urinalysis* for microscopic haematuria. *CXR* (cardiomegaly). *ECG* (long PR interval) at regular intervals. *Echocardiogram* TTE (p106) may show vegetations, but only if >2mm. TOE (p106) is more sensitive, and better for visualizing mitral lesions and possible development of aortic root abscess.

℞: Liaise early with microbiologist and cardiologists. Antibiotics: see BOX 2. *Consider surgery if:* heart failure, valvular obstruction; repeated emboli; fungal endocarditis; persistent bacteraemia; myocardial abscess; unstable infected prosthetic valve.[115]

Mortality 30% with staphs; 14% if bowel organisms; 6% if sensitive streptococci.

Prevention Antibiotic prophylaxis solely to prevent IE is not recommended because:

- There is no proven association between having an interventional procedure (dental or non-dental) and the development of IE.
- The clinical effectiveness of antibiotic prophylaxis is not proven.
- Antibiotic prophylaxis against IE for dental procedures may lead to ↑deaths through fatal anaphylaxis compared with a strategy of no antibiotic prophylaxis.

Recommendations: Give clear information about prevention, including:

- The benefits and risks of antibiotic prophylaxis.
- The importance of maintaining good oral health.
- Symptoms that may indicate IE and when to seek expert advice.
- The risks of invasive procedures, including non-medical procedures such as body piercing or tattooing.[116]

1 Past IE or rheumatic fever; IV drug abuser; damaged or replaced valve; structural congenital heart disease (but not simple ASD or fully repaired VSD or patent ductus); hypertrophic cardiomyopathy.

Duke criteria for infective endocarditis

Major criteria:

- Positive blood culture:
  - typical organism in 2 separate cultures or
  - persistently +ve blood cultures, eg 3, >12h apart (or majority if ≥4)
- Endocardium involved:
  - positive echocardiogram (vegetation, abscess, dehiscence of prosthetic valve) *or*
  - new valvular regurgitation (change in murmur not sufficient).

Minor criteria:

- Predisposition (cardiac lesion; IV drug abuse)
- Fever >38°C
- Vascular/immunological signs
- Positive blood culture that does not meet major criteria
- Positive echocardiogram that does not meet major criteria.

How to diagnose: Definite infective endocarditis: 2 major **or** 1 major and 3 minor **or** all 5 minor criteria (if no major criterion is met).

Antibiotic therapy for infective endocarditis

Consult a microbiologist early. The following are guidelines only:

Empirical therapy: **benzylpenicillin**[1] 1.2g/4h IV + **gentamicin**, eg 1mg/kg/8h IV for 4wks. Do gentamicin levels (p767; in IE/SBE, the *BNF* recommends a serum peak of 3–5mg/L & a pre-dose trough of <1mg/L; see p767). If acute, add **flucloxacillin** 2g/6h IV to cover staphylococci.

Enterococci: **amoxicillin**[1] 1g/6h IV + **gentamicin** as above.

Streptococci[1]: **benzylpenicillin**[1] 1.2g/4h IV for 2–4wks; then **amoxicillin** 1g/8h PO for 2wks. Monitor minimum inhibitory concentration (MIC). Add **gentamicin**.

Staphylococci: **flucloxacillin**[2] 2g/6h IV + **gentamicin** as above IV. Treat for 6–8wks; stop gentamicin after 1wk. If prosthetic valve or MRSA suspected, substitute flucloxacillin with **vancomycin** plus **rifampicin**.

Coxiella: **doxycycline** 100mg/12h PO indefinitely + **co-trimoxazole**, **rifampicin**, or **ciprofloxacin**.

Fungi: **flucytosine** 50mg/kg/6h IVI over 30min followed by **fluconazole** 50mg/24h PO (higher doses may be needed). **Amphotericin** (p168) if flucytosine resistance or *Aspergillus*. **Miconazole** if renal function is poor.

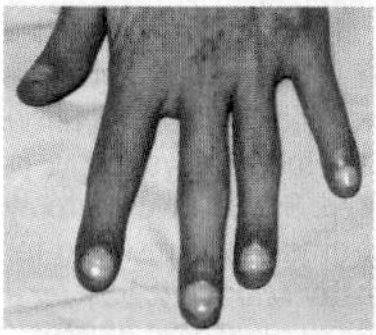

Fig 1. Clubbing with endocarditis.

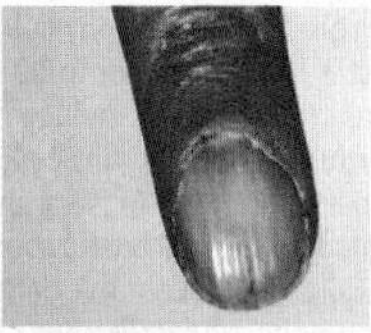

Fig 2. Splinter haemorrhages are normally seen under the fingernails or toenails. They are usually red-brown in colour.

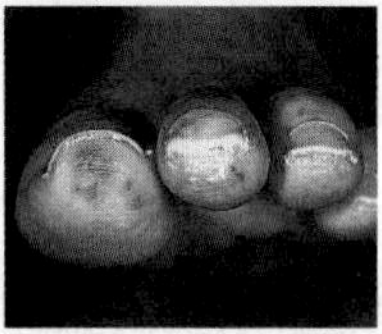

Fig 3. Janeway's lesions are non-tender erythematous, haemorrhagic, or pustular lesions, often on the palms or soles.

1 If *Strep bovis* is cultured, do colonoscopy, as a colon neoplasm is the likely portal of entry.
2 For penicillin allergy, use **vancomycin** 1g/12h IV.

Acute myocarditis This is inflammation of myocardium. ***Causes:*** Idiopathic (~50%), viral (flu, hepatitis, mumps, rubeola, Coxsackie, polio, HIV); bacterial (Clostridia, diphtheria, TB, meningococcus, mycoplasma, brucellosis, psittacosis); spirochaetes (leptospirosis, syphilis, Lyme); protozoa (Chagas' p426); drugs(cyclophosphamide, herceptin, penicillin, chloramphenicol, sulfonamides, methyldopa, spironolactone, phenytoin, carbamazepine); toxins; vasculitis, p558. ***Signs & symptoms:*** Fatigue, dyspnoea, chest pain, fever, palpitations, tachycardia, soft S_1, S_4 gallop (p42). ***Tests:*** ECG: ST elevation or depression, T wave inversion, atrial arrhythmias, transient AV block. In proper clinical setting (and absence of MI) +ve troponin I or T confirms the diagnosis. Negative antimyosin scintigraphy also excludes active myocarditis. ***℞:*** Supportive. Treat the underlying cause. Patients may recover or get intractable heart failure (p130).

Dilated cardiomyopathy A dilated, flabby heart of unknown cause. Associations: alcohol, ↑BP, haemochromatosis, viral infection, autoimmune, peri- or postpartum, thyrotoxicosis, congenital (x-linked). ***Prevalence:*** 0.2%. ***Presentation:*** Fatigue, dyspnoea, pulmonary oedema, RVF, emboli, AF, VT. ***Signs:*** ↑Pulse, ↓BP, ↑JVP, displaced, diffuse apex, S_3 gallop, mitral or tricuspid regurgitation (MR/TR), pleural effusion, oedema, jaundice, hepatomegaly, ascites. ***Tests:*** *Blood:* plasma BNP is sensitive and specific in diagnosing heart failure. ↓Na^+ indicates a poor prognosis. *CXR:* cardiomegaly, pulmonary oedema. *ECG:* tachycardia, non-specific T wave changes, poor R wave progression. *Echo:* globally dilated hypokinetic heart and low ejection fraction. Look for MR, TR, LV mural thrombus. ***℞:*** Bed rest, diuretics, digoxin, ACE-i, anticoagulation, biventricular pacing, ICDs, cardiac transplantation. ***Mortality:*** Variable, eg 40% in 2yrs.

Hypertrophic cardiomyopathy *HCM≈LV* outflow tract (LVOT) obstruction from asymmetric septal hypertrophy. HCM is the leading cause of sudden cardiac death in the young. ***Prevalence:*** 0.2%. Autosomal dominant inheritance, but 50% are sporadic. 70% have mutations in genes encoding β-myosin, α-tropomyosin, and troponin T. May present at any age. Ask about family history of sudden death. ***Symptoms & signs:*** Sudden death may be the first manifestation of HCM in many patients (VF is amenable to implantable defibrillators), angina, dyspnoea, palpitation, syncope, CCF. Jerky pulse; *a* wave in JVP; double-apex beat; systolic thrill at lower left sternal edge; harsh ejection systolic murmur. ***Tests:*** *ECG:* LVH; progressive T wave inversion; deep Q waves (inferior + lateral leads); AF; WPW syndrome (p120); ventricular ectopics; VT. *Echo:* asymmetrical septal hypertrophy; small LV cavity with hypercontractile posterior wall; midsystolic closure of aortic valve; systolic anterior movement of mitral valve. *Cardiac catheterization* may provoke VT. It helps assess: severity of gradient; coronary artery disease or mitral regurgitation. Electrophysiological studies may be needed (eg if WPW, p120). Exercise test ± Holter monitor (p102) to risk stratify. ***℞:*** β-blockers or verapamil for symptoms (the aim is reducing ventricular contractility). Amiodarone (p124) for arrhythmias (AF, VT). Anticoagulate for paroxysmal AF or systemic emboli. Dual-chamber pacing (p126) is rarely used. Septal myomectomy (surgical, or chemical, with alcohol, to ↓LV outflow tract gradient) is reserved for those with severe symptoms. Consider implantable defibrillator. ***Mortality:*** 5.9%/yr if <14yrs; 2.5%/yr if >14yrs. *Poor prognostic factors:* age <14yrs or syncope at presentation; family history of HCM/sudden death.

Restrictive cardiomyopathy ***Causes:*** Idiopathic, amyloidosis; haemochromatosis; sarcoidosis; scleroderma; Löffler's eosinophilic endocarditis, endomyocardial fibrosis. ***Presentation*** is like constrictive pericarditis (p148). Features of RVF predominate: ↑JVP, with prominent *x* and *y* descents; hepatomegaly; oedema; ascites. ***Diagnosis:*** Cardiac catheterization. ***℞:*** Treat the cause.

Cardiac myxoma (fig 1) Rare benign cardiac tumour. Prevalence ≤5/10,000, ♀:♂≈2:1. Usually sporadic, but may be familial (Carney complex: cardiac and cutaneous myxomas, skin pigmentation, endocrinopathy, etc, p215). It may mimic infective endocarditis (fever, weight loss, clubbing, ↑ESR), or mitral stenosis (left atrial obstruction, systemic emboli, AF). A 'tumour plop' may be heard, and signs may vary according to posture. ***Tests:*** Echo. ***℞:*** Excision.

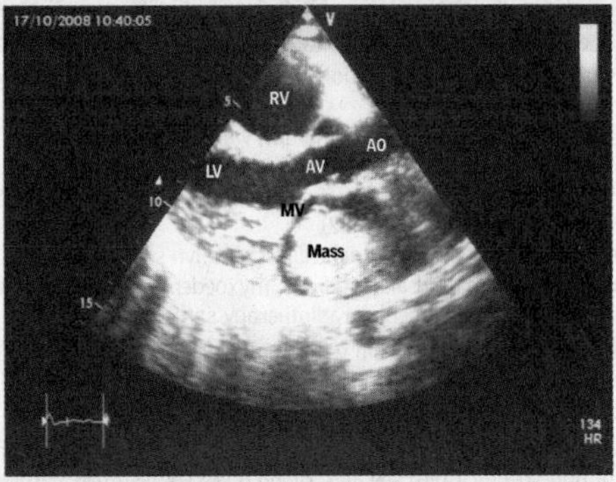

Fig 1a. Echocardiogram of a 35yr old patient who presented with severe exertional dyspnoea and several episodes of syncope. Look at the large mass (cardiac myxoma) in left atrium. **Abbreviations:** RV: right ventricle; LV: left ventricle; AV: aortic valve; AO: Aorta; MV: mitral valve.

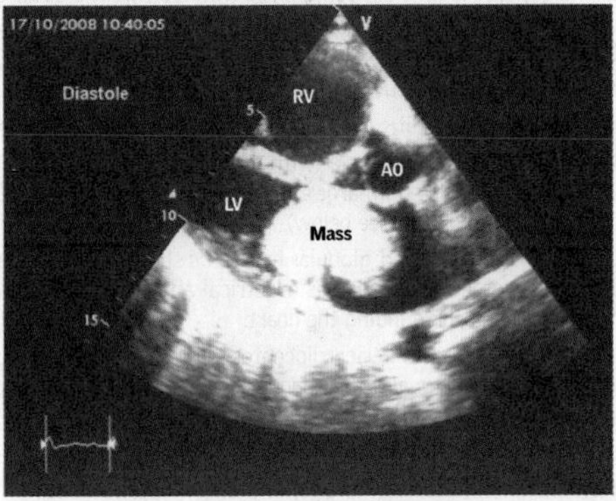

Fig 1b. Echocardiogram of the same patient during diastole. Notice how the large mass of myxoma protrudes into the left ventricle during diastole, and obstructs the mitral valve almost completely. **Abbreviations:** RV: right ventricle; LV: left ventricle; AO: Aorta.

Acute pericarditis This is inflammation of the pericardium. It may be idiopathic or secondary to:
- Viruses (Coxsackie, flu, Epstein-Barr, mumps, varicella, HIV)
- Bacteria (pneumonia, rheumatic fever, TB, staphs, streps, MAI in HIV, p410)
- Fungi
- Myocardial infarction, Dressler's (p712)
- Drugs: procainamide, hydralazine, penicillin, cromolyn sodium, isoniazid.
- Others: uraemia, rheumatoid arthritis, SLE, myxoedema, trauma, surgery, malignancy (and anti-neoplastic agents), radiotherapy, sarcoidosis.

Clinical features: Central chest pain worse on inspiration or lying flat ± relief by sitting forward. A pericardial friction rub (p44) may be heard. Look for evidence of a pericardial effusion or cardiac tamponade (see below). Fever may occur.

Tests: *ECG* classically shows concave (saddle-shaped) ST segment elevation, but may be normal or non-specific (10%); see **fig 1**. *Blood tests:* FBC, ESR, U&E, cardiac enzymes (*NB: troponin may be raised*), viral serology, blood cultures, and, if indicated, autoantibodies (p555), fungal precipitins, thyroid function tests. Cardiomegaly on *CXR* may indicate a pericardial effusion. *Echo* (if suspected pericardial effusion).

Treatment: Analgesia, eg ibuprofen 400mg/8h PO with food. Treat the cause. Consider colchicine before steroids/immunosuppressants if relapse or continuing symptoms occur. 15–40% *do* recur.[117] Steroids may increase the risk of recurrence.

Pericardial effusion Accumulation of fluid in the pericardial sac.

Causes: Any cause of pericarditis (see above).

Clinical features: Dyspnoea, raised JVP (with prominent x descent, p40), bronchial breathing at left base (Ewart's sign: large effusion compressing left lower lobe). Look for signs of cardiac tamponade (see below).

Diagnosis: *CXR* shows an enlarged, globular heart. *ECG* shows low-voltage QRS complexes and alternating QRS morphologies (electrical alternans). *Echocardiography* shows an echo-free zone surrounding the heart.

Management: Treat the cause. Pericardiocentesis may be *diagnostic* (suspected bacterial pericarditis) or *therapeutic* (cardiac tamponade). See p809. Send pericardial fluid for culture, ZN stain/TB culture, and cytology.

Constrictive pericarditis The heart is encased in a rigid pericardium.

Causes: Often unknown (UK); elsewhere TB, or after *any* pericarditis.

Clinical features: These are mainly of right heart failure with ↑JVP (with prominent x and y descents, p41); Kussmaul's sign (JVP rising paradoxically with inspiration); soft, diffuse apex beat; quiet heart sounds; S_3; diastolic pericardial knock, hepatosplenomegaly, ascites, and oedema.

Tests: CXR: small heart ± pericardial calcification (if none, CT/MRI helps distinguish from other cardiomyopathies). *Echo*; cardiac catheterization.

Management: Surgical excision.

Cardiac tamponade Accumulation of pericardial fluid raises intra-pericardial pressure, hence poor ventricular filling and fall in cardiac output.

Causes: Any pericarditis (above); aortic dissection; haemodialysis; warfarin; trans-septal puncture at cardiac catheterization; post cardiac biopsy.

Signs: Pulse↑, BP↓, pulsus paradoxus, JVP↑, Kussmaul's sign, muffled S_1 & S_2.

Diagnosis: *Beck's triad:* falling BP; rising JVP; small, quiet heart. *CXR:* big globular heart (if >250mL fluid). *ECG:* low voltage QRS ± electrical alternans. *Echo* is diagnostic: echo-free zone (>2cm, or >1cm if acute) around the heart ± diastolic collapse of right atrium and right ventricle.

Management: Seek expert help. The pericardial effusion needs urgent drainage (p809). Send fluid for culture, ZN stain/TB culture and cytology.

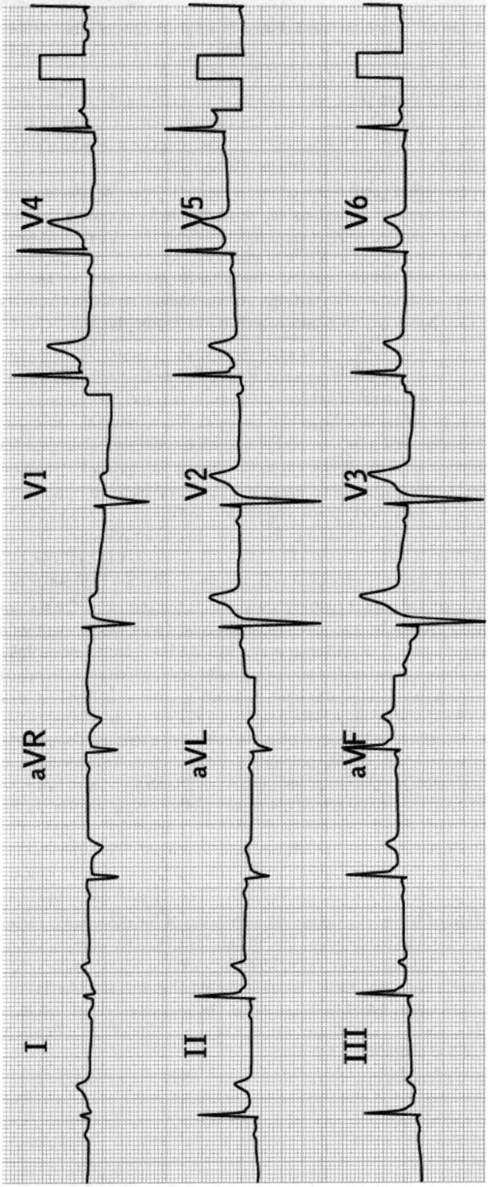

Fig 1. Pericarditis.

The spectrum of congenital heart disease in adults is considerably different from that in infants and children; adults are unlikely to have complex lesions. The commonest lesions, in descending order of frequency, are:

Bicuspid aortic valve These work well at birth and go undetected. Many eventually develop aortic stenosis (needing valve replacement) ± aortic regurgitation predisposing to IE/SBE ± aortic dilatation/dissection. Intense exercise may accelerate complications, so do yearly echocardiograms on affected athletes.[118]

Atrial septal defect (ASD) A hole connects the atria. *Ostium secundum* defects (high in the septum) are commonest; *ostium primum* defects (opposing the endocardial cushions) are associated with AV valve anomalies. Primum ASDs present early. Secundum ASDs are often asymptomatic until adulthood, as the L→R shunt depends on compliance of the right and left ventricles. The latter decreases with age (esp. if BP↑), so augmenting L→R shunting (hence dyspnoea/heart failure, eg at age 40–60). There may be pulmonary hypertension, cyanosis, arrhythmia, haemoptysis, and chest pain.

Signs: AF; ↑JVP; wide, fixed split S_2; pulmonary ejection systolic murmur. Pulmonary hypertension may cause pulmonary or tricuspid regurgitation. ↑ freq of migraine.

Complications: • Reversal of left to right shunt, ie Eisenmenger's complex: initial L→R shunt leads to pulmonary hypertension, hence shunt reversal, causing cyanosis (±heart failure & chest infections). • Paradoxical emboli (vein→artery via ASD; rare).

Tests: ECG: RBBB with LAD and prolonged PR interval (primum defect) or RAD (secundum defect). CXR: small aortic knuckle, pulmonary plethora, progressive atrial enlargement. Echocardiography is diagnostic. Cardiac catheterization shows step up in O_2 saturation in the right atrium. *Treatment:* In children closure is recommended before age 10yrs. In adults, if symptomatic, or if pulmonary to systemic blood flow ratios of ≥1.5:1. Transcatheter closure is now more common than surgical.

Ventricular septal defect (VSD) A hole connects the ventricles. *Causes:* congenital (prevalence 2:1000 births); acquired (post-MI). *Symptoms:* May present with severe heart failure in infancy, or remain asymptomatic and be detected incidentally in later life. *Signs:* These depend on size and site: smaller holes, which are haemodynamically less significant, give louder murmurs. Classically, a harsh pansystolic murmur is heard at the left sternal edge, with a systolic thrill, ± left parasternal heave. Larger holes are associated with signs of pulmonary hypertension. *Complications:* AR, infundibular stenosis, IE/SBE, pulmonary hypertension, Eisenmenger's complex (above). *Tests:* ECG: normal (small VSD), LAD + LVH (moderate VSD) or LVH + RVH (large VSD). CXR: normal heart size ± mild pulmonary plethora (small VSD) or cardiomegaly, large pulmonary arteries and marked pulmonary plethora (large VSD). Cardiac catheter: step up in O_2 saturation in right ventricle. *Treatment:* This is medical, at first, as many close spontaneously. Indications for surgical closure: failed medical therapy, symptomatic VSD, shunt >3 : 1, SBE/IE. Endovascular closure is also possible [119].

Coarctation of the aorta Congenital narrowing of the descending aorta; usually occurs just distal to the origin of the left subclavian artery. More common in boys. *Associations:* Bicuspid aortic valve; Turner's syndrome. *Signs:* Radio-femoral delay (femoral pulse later than radial); weak femoral pulse; BP↑; scapular bruit; systolic murmur (best heard over the left scapula). *Complications:* Heart failure; infective endocarditis. *Tests:* CT or MRI-aortogram, CXR shows rib notching. *Treatment:* Surgery, or balloon dilatation ± stenting.

Pulmonary stenosis may occur alone or with other lesions (p142).

Fallot's tetralogy: what the non-specialist needs to know

Tetralogy of Fallot (TOF) is the most common cyanotic congenital heart disorder (prevalence: 3-6 per 10,000), and it is also the most common cyanotic heart defect that survives to adulthood, accounting for 10% of all congenital defects.[120] It is believed to be due to abnormalities in separation of the truncus arteriosus into the aorta and pulmonary arteries that occur in early gestation (**fig 1**).

The 4 features typical of TOF include:

1 Ventricular septal defect (VSD)
2 Pulmonary stenosis
3 Right ventricular hypertrophy
4 The aorta overriding the VSD

Occasionally, a few children also have an atrial septal defect, which makes up the pentad of Fallot.[121]

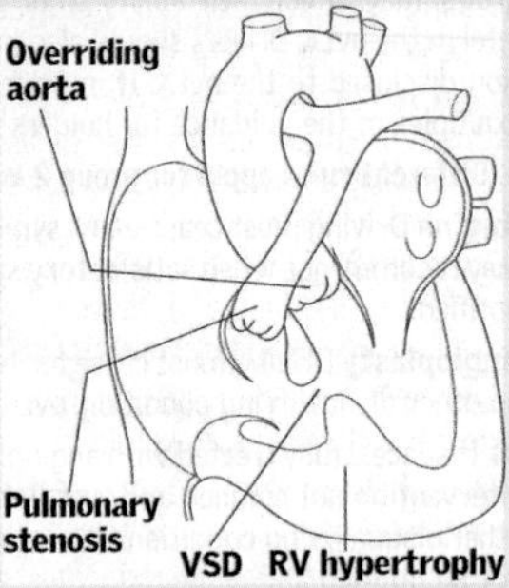

Fig 1. Tetralogy of Fallot.
Adapted with permission from *Cardiothoracic Surgery*. © OUP 2006.

Presentation: Severity of illness depends greatly on the degree of pulmonary stenosis. Infants may be acyanotic at birth, with a pulmonary stenosis murmur as the only initial finding. Gradually (especially after closure of ductus arteriosus) they become cyanotic due to decreasing flow of blood to the lungs as well as right-to-left shunt across the VSD. During a hypoxic spell, the child becomes restless and agitated, and may cry inconsolably. Toddlers may squat, which is typical of TOF, as it increases peripheral vascular resistance and decreases the degree of right to left shunt.[122] Also: difficulty in feeding, failure to thrive, clubbing. Adult patients are often asymptomatic. In the unoperated adult patient, cyanosis is common, although extreme cyanosis or squatting is uncommon. In repaired patients, late symptoms include exertional dyspnoea, palpitations, RV failure, syncope, and even sudden death.[123] ***ECG*** shows RV hypertrophy with a right bundle-branch block.

CXR may be normal, or show the hallmark of TOF, which is the classic boot-shaped heart (**fig 2**). *Echocardiography* can show the anatomy as well as the degree of stenosis. Cardiac *CT* and *cardiac MRI* can give valuable information for planning the surgery.[124]

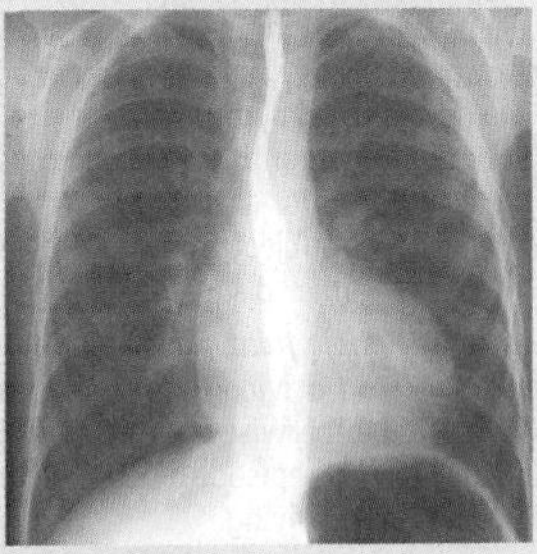

Fig 2. Boot-shaped heart.
Courtesy of Dr Edward Singleton.

Management: Give O_2. Place the child in knee-chest position. Morphine can sedate the child as well as relaxing the pulmonary outflow. Long-term β-blockers may be needed. Give endocarditis prophylaxis. Without surgery, mortality rate is ~95% by age 20. Surgery is usually done before 1yr of age, with closure of the VSD and correction of the pulmonary stenosis. 20-yr survival is ~90-95% after repair.

UK licences are inscribed "You are required by law to inform Drivers Medical Branch, DVLA, Swansea SA99 1AT at once if you have any disability (physical or medical), which is, or may become likely to affect your fitness as a driver, unless you do not expect it to last more than 3 months". It is the responsibility of drivers to inform the DVLA, and that of their doctors to advise patients that medical conditions (and drugs) may affect their ability to drive and for which conditions patients should inform the DVLA. Drivers should also inform their insurance company of any condition disclosed to the DVLA. If in doubt, ask your defence union. The following are examples of the guidance for holders of standard licences.

Different rules apply for group 2 vehicle licence-holders (eg lorries, buses).

Angina Driving must cease when symptoms occur at rest or with emotion. Driving may recommence when satisfactory symptom control is achieved. DVLA need not be notified.

Angioplasty Driving must cease for 1wk, and may recommence thereafter provided no other disqualifying condition. DVLA need not be notified.

MI If successfully treated with angioplasty cease driving for 1 week provided urgent intervention not planned and LVEF (left ventricular ejection fraction) >40%, and no other disqualifying condition. Otherwise, driving must cease for 1 month. DVLA need not be notified.

Dysrhythmias *Sinoatrial including AF/flutter:* Driving must cease if the dysrhythmia has caused or is likely to cause incapacity. Driving may recommence 4 weeks after successful control provided there is no other disqualifying condition.

Significant atrioventricular conduction defects: Driving may be permitted when underlying cause has been identified and controlled for >4wks. DVLA need not be notified unless there are distracting/disabling symptoms.

Pacemaker implant Stop driving for 1wk.

Implanted cardioverter/defibrillator The licence is subject to annual review. Driving may occur when these criteria can be met:

- The 1st device has been implanted for at least 6 months.
- The device has not administered therapy (shock and/or symptomatic antitachycardia pacing) within the last 6 months (except during testing).
- Any previous therapy has not been accompanied by *incapacity* (whether caused by the device or arrhythmia).
- A period of 1 month off driving must occur following any revision of the device (generator and/or electrode) or alteration of antiarrhythmics.
- The device is subject to regular review with interrogation.
- There is no other disqualifying condition.

Syncope *Simple faint:* no restriction. *Unexplained syncope* with low risk of recurrence 4wks off driving, high risk of recurrence 4wks off driving if cause identified and treated; otherwise 6 months off. See driving and epilepsy (BOX). Patients who have had a single episode of loss of consciousness (no cause found) still need to have at least 1yr off driving.

Hypertension Driving may continue unless treatment causes unacceptable side effects. DVLA need not be notified.

1 See www.dvla.gov.uk/medical/ataglance.aspx

Other conditions: UK DVLA[1] state they must be informed if:

- An epileptic event. A person who has suffered an epileptic attack while awake must not drive for 1yr from the date of the attack. A person who has suffered an attack while asleep must also refrain from driving for 1yr from the date of the attack, unless they have had an attack while asleep >3yrs ago and have not had any awake attacks since that asleep attack. In any event, they should not drive if they are likely to cause danger to the public or themselves.
- Patients with TIA or stroke should not drive for at least 1 month. There is no need to inform the DVLA unless there is residual neurological defect after 1 month, eg visual field defect. If TIAs have been recurrent and frequent, a 3-month period free of attacks may be required.
- Sudden attacks or disabling giddiness, fainting, or blackouts. Multiple sclerosis, Parkinson's (any 'freezing' or on-off effects), motor neuron diseases are relevant here.
- Severe mental handicap. Those with dementia should only drive if the condition is mild (do not rely on armchair judgements: on-the-road trials are better). Encourage relatives to contact DVLA if a dementing relative should not be driving. GPs may desire to breach confidentiality (the GMC approves) and inform DVLA of demented or psychotic patients (tel. 01792 783686). Many elderly drivers (~1 in 3) who die in accidents are found to have Alzheimer's.
- A pacemaker, defibrillator, or anti-ventricular tachycardia device fitted.
- Diabetes controlled by insulin or tablets.
- Angina while driving.
- Parkinson's disease.
- Any other chronic neurological condition.
- A serious problem with memory.
- A major or minor stroke with deficit continuing for >1 month.
- Any type of brain surgery, brain tumour. Severe head injury involving inpatient treatment at hospital.
- Any severe psychiatric illness or mental disorder.
- Continuing/permanent difficulty in the use of arms or legs which affects ability to control a vehicle.
- Dependence on or misuse of alcohol, illicit drugs, or chemical substances in the past 3yrs (do not include drink/driving offences).
- Any visual disability which affects *both* eyes (do not declare short/long sight or colour blindness).

Vision (new drivers) should be 6/9 on Snellen's scale in the better eye and 6/12 on the Snellen scale in the other eye and (wearing glasses or contact lenses if needed) and 3/60 in each eye without glasses or contact lenses.

1 DVLA is the UK Driving and Vehicle Licensing Authority.

Contents

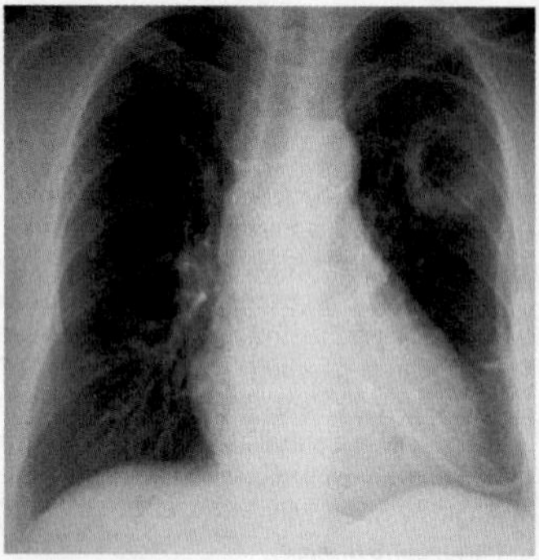

Fig 1. Smoke ring sign: cavitating lung carcinoma (OTM)

Relevant pages in other sections:

Symptoms and signs: The respiratory history & examination (p48–p54); chest deformities (p55); chest pain (p88); clubbing (p33); cough (p48); cyanosis (p28); dyspnoea (p49); haemoptysis (p49); sputum (p53); stridor (p48).

Radiology: CXR (p736); chest CT (p744); V/Q scan (p753).

Procedures: Aspirating pleural effusions (p778); pleural biopsy (p778); chest drains (p780); pneumothorax aspiration (p781); arterial blood gas sampling (p785).

▸▸*Emergencies:* Asthma (p820); COPD (p822); tension pneumothorax (p824); pneumonia (p826); pulmonary embolism (p828).

Others: Sickle-cell acute chest (p335); acid-base balance (p684); tuberculosis (p398).

We thank Dr Phillippa Lawson, who is our Specialist Reader for this chapter.

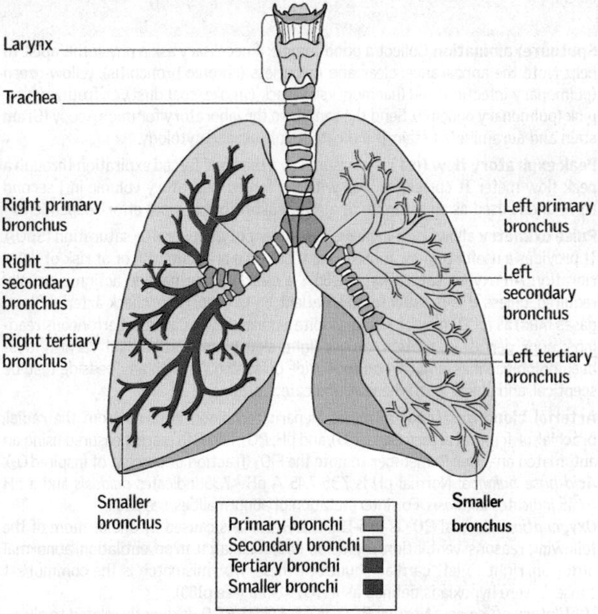

Fig 2. Lung anatomy. The left lung has two lobes and the right has 3 lobes.

Sputum examination Collect a good sample; if necessary ask a physiotherapist to help. Note the appearance: clear and colourless (chronic bronchitis), yellow-green (pulmonary infection), red (haemoptysis), black (smoke, coal dust), or frothy white-pink (pulmonary oedema). Send the sample to the laboratory for microscopy (Gram stain and auramine/ZN stain, if indicated), culture, and cytology.

Peak expiratory flow (PEF) is measured by a maximal forced expiration through a peak flow meter. It correlates well with the forced expiratory volume in 1 second (FEV_1) and is used as an estimate of airway calibre, but is more effort-dependent.

Pulse oximetry allows non-invasive assessment of peripheral O_2 saturation (SpO_2). It provides a useful tool for monitoring those who are acutely ill or at risk of deterioration. An oxygen saturation of ≤80% is clearly abnormal and action is usually required, unless this is usual for the patient, eg in COPD. Here, check arterial blood gases (ABG) as P_aCO_2 may be rising despite a normal P_aO_2. Causes of erroneous readings: poor perfusion, motion, excess light, skin pigmentation, nail varnish, dyshaemoglobinaemias, and carbon monoxide poisoning. As with any bedside test, be sceptical, and check ABG, whenever indicated (p181).

Arterial blood gas (ABG) analysis Heparinized blood is taken from the radial, brachial, or femoral artery (see p785), and pH, P_aO_2, and P_aCO_2 are measured using an automated analyser. Remember to note the FiO_2 (fraction or percent of inspired O_2).
Acid–base balance: Normal pH is 7.35–7.45. A pH <7.35 indicates *acidosis* and a pH >7.45 indicates *alkalosis*. For interpretation of abnormalities, see p684.
Oxygenation: Normal P_aO_2 is 10.5–13.5kPa. Hypoxia is caused by one or more of the following reasons: ventilation/perfusion (V/Q) mismatch, hypoventilation, abnormal diffusion, right to left cardiac shunts. Of these, V/Q mismatch is the commonest cause. Severe hypoxia is defined as a P_aO_2 <8kPa (see p180).
Ventilatory efficiency: Normal P_aCO_2 is 4.5–6.0kPa. P_aCO_2 is directly related to alveolar ventilation. A P_aCO_2 <4.5kPa indicates *hyperventilation* and a P_aCO_2 >6.0kPa indicates *hypoventilation*.
Type 1 respiratory failure: is defined as P_aO_2 <8kPa and P_aCO_2 <6.0kPa.
Type 2 respiratory failure: is defined as P_aO_2 <8kPa and P_aCO_2 >6.0kPa.

Alveolar–arterial O_2 concentration gradient may be calculated from the FiO_2, P_aO_2, and P_aCO_2: see BOX 1.
Aa normal range breathing air: 0.2–1.5kPa aged 25yrs; ↑ to 1.5–3.0 at 75yrs.
A high Aa indicates a problem with O_2 transfer, whereas a normal Aa gradient in the context of hypoxia suggests hypoventilation.

Spirometry measures functional lung volumes. Forced expiratory volume in 1s (FEV_1) and forced vital capacity (FVC) are measured from a full forced expiration into spirometer (Vitalograph®); exhalation continues until no more breath can be exhaled. FEV_1 is less effort-dependent than PEF. The FEV_1/FVC ratio gives a good estimate of the severity of airflow obstruction; normal ratio is 75–80%. See BOX 2.
Obstructive defect (eg asthma, COPD) FEV_1 is reduced more than the FVC and the FEV_1/FVC ratio is <75%.
Restrictive defect (eg lung fibrosis) FVC is ↓ and the FEV_1/FVC ratio is ↔ or ↑. Other causes: sarcoidosis; pneumoconiosis, interstitial pneumonias; connective tissue diseases; pleural effusion; obesity; kyphoscoliosis; neuromuscular problems.

(Aa)PO_2: the Alveolar-arterial (Aa) oxygen gradient

This is the difference in the O_2 partial pressures between the alveolar and arterial sides. In type II respiratory failure it helps tell if hypoventilation is from lung disease or poor respiratory effort. (Aa)$PO_2 = P_AO_2 - P_aO_2$. P_AO_2, the partial pressure of oxygen in the alveoli depends on **R**, the respiratory quotient (≈0.8, nearer to 1 if eating all carbohydrates); barometric pressure ($P_B \approx$ 101kPa at sea level), and P_{H_2O}, the water saturation of airway gas ($P_{H_2O} \approx$ 6.2kPa as inspired air is usually fully saturated by the time it gets to the carina). P_AO_2 also depends on F_iO_2, the fractional concentration of O_2 in inspired air (eg F_iO_2 is 0.5 if breathing 50% O_2, and 0.21 if breathing room air). So...

$$P_AO_2 = (P_B - P_{H_2O}) \times F_iO_2 - (P_aCO_2/R)$$
$$= (101 - 6.2) \times F_iO_2 - (P_aCO_2/0.8) \text{ (at sea level)}$$
$$= (94.8 \times F_iO_2) - (P_aCO_2 \div 0.8)$$

See A Williams *BMJ* 1998 **317** 1213

If breathing air and a P_aCO_2 of 8kPa, the $P_AO_2 = 94.8 \times 0.21 - (1.25 \times 8) = 10$kPa.

Examples of spirograms

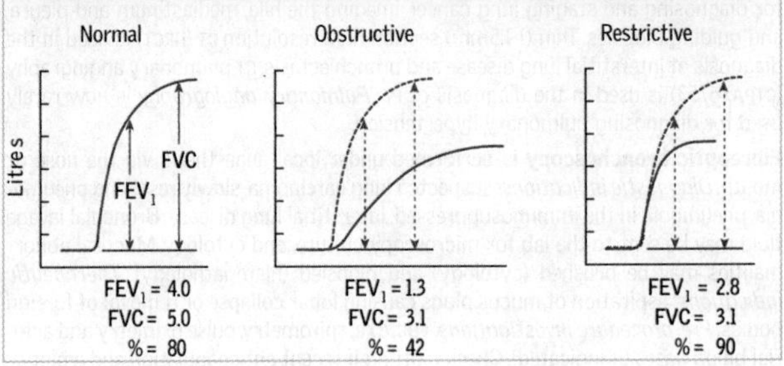

Lung function tests PEF, FEV_1, FVC (see p156). ***Total lung capacity*** (TLC) and ***residual volume*** (RV) are useful in distinguishing obstructive and restrictive diseases. TLC and RV are increased in obstructive airways disease and reduced in restrictive lung diseases and musculoskeletal abnormalities. The ***gas transfer*** coefficient (KCO) represents the carbon monoxide diffusing capacity (DLCO) corrected for alveolar volume. It is calculated by measuring carbon monoxide uptake from a single inspiration in a standard time (usually 10s) and lung volume by helium dilution. Low in emphysema and interstitial lung disease, high in alveolar haemorrhage.[3] ***Flow volume loop*** measures flow at various lung volumes. Characteristic patterns are seen with intra-thoracic airways obstruction (asthma, emphysema) and extra-thoracic airways obstruction (tracheal stenosis).

Radiology ***Chest x-ray*** see p736. ***Ultrasound*** is used in the diagnosis and to guide drainage of pleural effusions (particularly loculated effusions) and empyema. ***Radionuclide scans*** *Ventilation/perfusion (V/Q, p752) scans* are used to diagnose pulmonary embolism (PE) (unmatched perfusion defects are seen). *Bone scans* are used to diagnose bone metastases. ***Computed tomography*** (CT, p744) of the thorax is used for diagnosing and staging lung cancer, imaging the hila, mediastinum and pleura, and guiding biopsies. Thin (1-1.5mm) section high resolution CT (HRCT) is used in the diagnosis of interstitial lung disease and bronchiectasis. CT pulmonary angiography (CTPA, p753) is used in the diagnosis of PE. ***Pulmonary angiography*** is now rarely used for diagnosing pulmonary hypertension.

Fibreoptic bronchoscopy is performed under local anaesthetic via the nose or mouth. *Diagnostic indications:* suspected lung carcinoma, slowly resolving pneumonia, pneumonia in the immunosuppressed, interstitial lung disease. Bronchial lavage fluid may be sent to the lab for microscopy, culture, and cytology. Mucosal abnormalities may be brushed (cytology) and biopsied (histopathology). *Therapeutic indications:* aspiration of mucus plugs causing lobar collapse or removal of foreign bodies. *Pre-procedure investigations:* FBC, CXR, spirometry, pulse oximetry and arterial blood gases (if indicated). Check clotting if recent anticoagulation and a biopsy may be performed. *Complications:* respiratory depression, bleeding, pneumothorax (**fig 1**, p763). *Diagnostic sensitivity* for cancer in smokers: 53% (may be improved in the future to 95% by additional gene profiling of cell samples).[4] [5]

Bronchoalveolar lavage (BAL) is performed at the time of bronchoscopy by instilling and aspirating a known volume of warmed, buffered 0.9% saline into the distal airway. *Diagnostic indications:* suspected malignancy, pneumonia in the immunosuppressed (especially HIV), suspected TB (if sputum negative), interstitial lung diseases (eg sarcoidosis, extrinsic allergic alveolitis, histiocytosis X). *Therapeutic indications:* Alveolar proteinosis.[1] *Complications:* hypoxia (give supplemental O_2), transient fever, transient CXR shadow, infection (rare).

Lung biopsy may be performed in several ways. ***Percutaneous needle biopsy*** is performed under radiological guidance and is useful for peripheral lung and pleural lesions. ***Transbronchial biopsy*** performed at bronchoscopy may help in diagnosing diffuse lung diseases, eg sarcoidosis. If these are unsuccessful, an ***open lung biopsy*** may be performed under general anaesthetic.

Surgical procedures are performed under general anaesthetic. ***Rigid bronchoscopy*** provides a wide lumen, enables larger mucosal biopsies, controlling bleeding, and removal of foreign bodies. ***Mediastinoscopy*** and ***mediastinotomy*** enable examination and biopsy of the mediastinal lymph nodes/lesions. ***Thoracoscopy*** allows examination and biopsy of pleural lesions, drainage of pleural effusions, and talc pleurodesis.

1 **Pulmonary alveolar proteinosis** causes cough, dyspnoea, and restrictive spirometry. It is caused by accumulation of surfactant-derived acidophilic phospholipid/protein compounds which fill alveoli and distal bronchioles. Diagnosis may require lung biopsy. Cause: primary genetic or antibody problem, or secondary to inflammation caused by inhaling silica, aluminium or titanium.

Lung volumes: physiological and pathological[6]

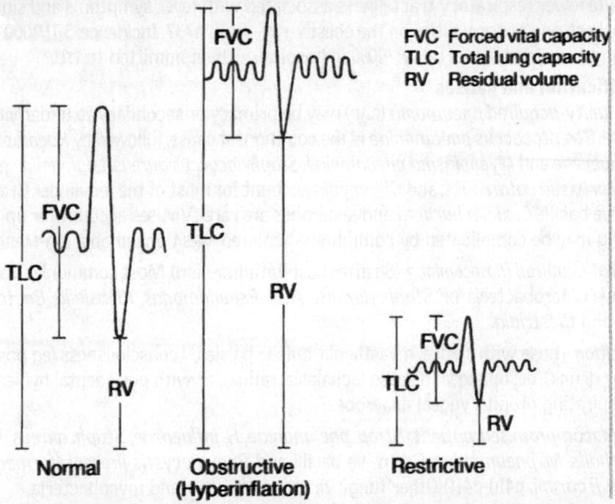

Flow volume loops[7]

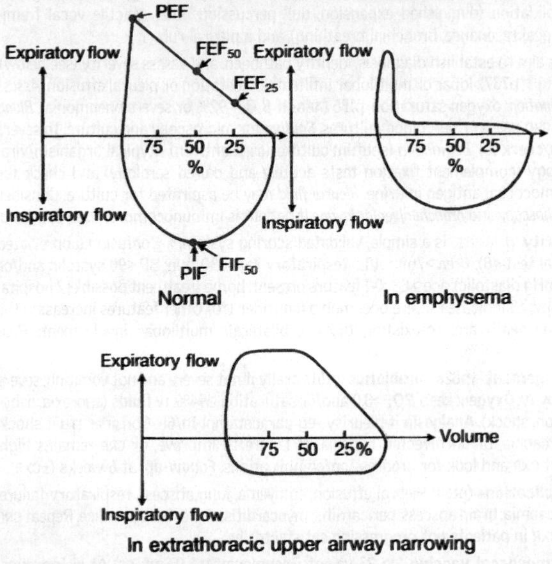

PEF=peak expiratory flow; FEF50=forced expiratory flow at 50% TLC; FEF25=forced expiratory flow at 25% TLC; PIF=peak inspiratory flow; FIF50=forced inspiratory flow at 50% TLC.

An acute lower respiratory tract illness associated with fever, symptoms and signs in the chest, and abnormalities on the chest x-ray—**fig 1**, p737. Incidence: 5-11/1000 (↑ in young and elderly). Mortality: ~10% in hospital, ~30% if admitted to ITU.

Classification and causes

Community-acquired pneumonia (CAP) may be primary or secondary to underlying disease. *Streptococcus pneumoniae* is the commonest cause, followed by *Haemophilus influenzae* and *Mycoplasma pneumoniae. Staphylococcus aureus, Legionella* species, *Moraxella catarrhalis*, and *Chlamydia* account for most of the remainder. Gram negative bacilli, *Coxiella burnetii* and anaerobes are rarer. Viruses account for up to 15%. Flu may be complicated by community-acquired MRSA pneumonia (CA-MRSA)

Hospital-acquired (nosocomial; >48h after hospital admission). Most commonly Gram negative enterobacteria or *Staph. aureus*. Also *Pseudomonas, Klebsiella, Bacteroides*, and *Clostridia*.

Aspiration Those with stroke, myasthenia, bulbar palsies, ↓consciousness (eg post-ictal or drunk), oesophageal disease (achalasia, reflux), or with poor dental hygiene, risk aspirating oropharyngeal anaerobes.

Immunocompromised patient: Strep. pneumoniae, H. influenzae, Staph. aureus, M. catarrhalis, M. pneumoniae, Gram -ve bacilli and *Pneumocystis jiroveci (formerly named P. carinii*, p410–p411). Other fungi, viruses (CMV, HSV), and mycobacteria.

Clinical features *Symptoms:* Fever, rigors, malaise, anorexia, dyspnoea, cough, purulent sputum, haemoptysis, and pleuritic pain. *Signs:* Fever, cyanosis, confusion (may be the only sign in the elderly), tachypnoea, tachycardia, hypotension, signs of consolidation (diminished expansion, dull percussion note, ↑tactile vocal fremitus/vocal resonance, bronchial breathing), and a pleural rub.

Tests aim to establish diagnosis, identify pathogen, and assess severity (see below). *CXR* (**fig 1**, p737): lobar or multilobar infiltrates, cavitation or pleural effusion. *Assess oxygenation:* oxygen saturation, p156 (ABGs if S_aO_2 <92% or severe pneumonia). *Blood tests:* FBC, U&E, LFT, CRP, blood cultures. *Sputum* for microscopy and culture. In severe cases, check for *Legionella* (sputum culture, urine antigen), atypical organism/viral serology (complement fixation tests acutely and paired serology) and check for pneumococcal antigen in urine. *Pleural fluid* may be aspirated for culture. Consider *bronchoscopy* and *bronchoalveolar lavage* if patient is immunocompromized or on ITU.

Severity 'CURB-65' is a simple, validated scoring system: **C**onfusion (abbreviated mental test ≤8); **U**rea >7mmol/L; **R**espiratory rate ≥30/min; **B**P <90 systolic and/or 60mmHg diastolic); age ≥**65**. 0–1 feature present: home treatment possible; 2 hospital therapy; ≥3 indicates severe pneumonia (consider ITU). Other features increasing the risk of death are: co-existing disease; bilateral/ multilobar involvement; P_aO_2 <8kPa/S_aO_2 <92%.

Management ▸▸p826. **Antibiotics** (p161): orally if not severe and not vomiting; severe give by IV. **Oxygen:** keep P_aO_2 >8.0 and/or saturation ≥94%. **IV fluids** (anorexia, dehydration, shock). **Analgesia** if pleurisy—eg paracetamol 1g/6h. Consider ITU if shock, hypercapnia, or uncorrected hypoxia. If failure to improve, or CRP remains high, repeat CXR and look for progression/complications. **Follow-up:** at 6 weeks (±CXR).

Complications (p164) Pleural effusion, empyema, lung abscess, respiratory failure, septicaemia, brain abscess, pericarditis, myocarditis, cholestatic jaundice. Repeat CRP and CXR in patients not progressing satisfactorily.

Pneumococcal vaccine (eg 23-valent Pneumovax II®, 0.5mL SC) At-risk groups: • ≥65yrs old • Chronic heart, liver (eg cirrhosis), renal (eg renal failure, nephrosis*, post-transplant*) or lung conditions • Diabetes mellitus • Immunosuppression, eg spleen function↓ (eg splenectomy, asplenia*, sickle cell* or coeliac disease), AIDS, or on chemotherapy or prednisolone >20mg/d). CI: pregnancy, lactation, T°↑. If at ↑risk of fatal pneumococcal infection (* above), re-vaccinate after 6yrs. Children: *OHCS* p151.

Empirical treatment of pneumonia

Clinical setting	Organisms	Antibiotic (further dosage details: p378 & p379)
Community-acquired		
Mild not previously Rx	*Streptococcus pneumoniae* *Haemophilus influenzae*	Oral amoxicillin 500mg-1g/8h or clarithromycin 500mg/12h or doxy-cycline 200mg loading then 100mg/12h
Moderate	*Streptococcus pneumoniae* *Haemophilus influenzae* *Mycoplasma pneumoniae*	Oral amoxicillin 500mg-1g/8h + clarithromycin 500mg/12h or doxy-cycline 200mg loading then 100mg/12h. If IV required: amoxicillin 500mg/8h + clarithromycin 500mg/12h
Severe	As above	Co-amoxiclav 1.2g/8h IV or cephalosporin IV (eg cefuroxime 1.5g/8h IV) AND clarithromycin 500mg/12h IV. Add flucloxacillin if staph suspected; vancomycin (or teicoplanin) if MRSA suspected. Treat for 10d (14-21d if staph, legionella, or Gram –ve enteric bacteria suspected).
Atypical	*Legionella pneumophilia*	Consider adding rifampicin; treat for 14-21d. See p162.
	Chlamydophila species	Tetracycline
	Pneumocystis jiroveci	High-dose co-trimoxazole (p410-p411)
Hospital-acquired		
	Gram negative bacilli Pseudomonas Anaerobes	Aminoglycoside IV + antipseudomonal penicillin IV or 3rd gen. cephalosporin IV (p379)
Aspiration		
	Streptococcus pneumoniae Anaerobes	Cefuroxime 1.5g/8h IV + metronidazole 500mg/8h IV
Neutropenic patients		
	Gram positive cocci Gram negative bacilli	Aminoglycoside IV + antipseudomonal penicillin IV or 3rd gen. cephalosporin IV
	Fungi (p168)	Consider antifungals after 48h

3rd gen=3rd generation, eg cefotaxime, p379; gentamicin is an example of an aminoglycoside (p381). Ticarcillin is an example of an antipseudomonal penicillin.

For antibiotic doses, see p378 & p380. TB: ►see p398.

Pneumococcal pneumonia is the commonest bacterial pneumonia. It affects all ages, but is commoner in the elderly, alcoholics, post-splenectomy, immuno-suppressed, and patients with chronic heart failure or pre-existing lung disease. Clinical features: fever, pleurisy, herpes labialis. CXR shows lobar consolidation. Treatment: amoxicillin, benzylpenicillin, or cephalosporin.

Staphylococcal pneumonia may complicate influenza infection or occur in the young, elderly, intravenous drug users, or patients with underlying disease, eg leukaemia, lymphoma, cystic fibrosis, (CF). It causes a bilateral cavitating bronchopneumonia. Treatment: flucloxacillin. MRSA: contact lab; consider vancomycin.

Klebsiella pneumonia is rare. Occurs in elderly, diabetics and alcoholics. Causes a cavitating pneumonia, particularly of the upper lobes, often drug resistant. Treatment: cefotaxime or imipenem.

Pseudomonas is a common pathogen in bronchiectasis and CF. It also causes hospital-acquired infections, particularly on ITU or after surgery. Treatment: anti-pseudomonal penicillin, ceftazidime, meropenem, or ciprofloxacin + aminoglycoside.

Mycoplasma pneumoniae occurs in epidemics about every 4yrs. It presents insidiously with flu-like symptoms (headache, myalgia, arthralgia) followed by a dry cough. CXR: reticular-nodular shadowing or patchy consolidation often of 1 lower lobe, and worse than signs suggest. Diagnosis: mycoplasma serology. Cold agglutinins may cause an autoimmune haemolytic anaemia. Complications: skin rash (erythema multiforme, **fig 3**, p546), Stevens-Johnson syndrome, meningoencephalitis or myelitis; Guillain-Barré syndrome. Treatment: clarithromycin or tetracycline or a fluroquinolone (such as ciprofloxacin or norfloxacin).

Legionella pneumophilia colonizes water tanks kept at <60°C (eg hotel air-conditioning and hot water systems) causing outbreaks of Legionnaire's disease. 'Flu-like symptoms (fever, malaise, myalgia) precede a dry cough and dyspnoea. Extra-pulmonary features include anorexia, D&V, hepatitis, renal failure, confusion, and coma. CXR shows bi-basal consolidation. Blood tests may show lymphopenia, hyponatraemia, and deranged LFTs. Urinalysis may show haematuria. Diagnosis: *Legionella* serology/urine antigen. Treatment: clarithromycin (p380) ± rifampicin (300–600mg/12h PO) or a fluoroquinolone for 2-3wks. 10% mortality.

Chlamydophila pneumoniae is the commonest chlamydial infection.[14] Person-to-person spread occurs causing a biphasic illness: pharyngitis, hoarseness, otitis, followed by pneumonia. Diagnosis: *Chlamydophila* serology (non-specific).[15] Treatment: tetracycline or clarithromycin.

Chlamydiophila psittaci causes psittacosis, an ornithosis acquired from infected birds (typically parrots). Symptoms include headache, fever, dry cough, lethargy, arthralgia, anorexia, and D&V. Extra-pulmonary features are legion but rare, eg meningo-encephalitis, infective endocarditis, hepatitis, nephritis, rash, splenomegaly. CXR shows patchy consolidation. Diagnosis: *Chlamydophila* serology. Treatment: tetracycline or clarithromycin.

Viral pneumonia The commonest cause is influenza (p402 and BOX). Other viruses that can affect the lung are: measles, CMV, and varicella zoster.

Pneumocystis pneumonia (PCP) causes pneumonia in the immunosuppressed (eg HIV). The organism responsible was previously called *Pneumocystis carinii*, and now called *Pneumocystis jiroveci*.[16] It presents with a dry cough, exertional dyspnoea, fever, bilateral crepitations. CXR may be normal or show bilateral perihilar interstitial shadowing. Diagnosis: visualization of the organism in induced sputum, bronchoalveolar lavage, or in a lung biopsy specimen. Drugs: high-dose co-trimoxazole (p410–p411), or pentamidine by slow IVI for 2-3 weeks (p411). Steroids are beneficial if severe hypoxaemia. Prophylaxis is indicated if the CD4 count is $<200\times10^6$/L or after the 1st attack.[17]

Avian influenza

Avian-to-human transmission of the H5N1 strain of influenza A causes serious infection in humans with a ≥50% mortality, often from a rapidly progressive pneumonia. Human-to-human transmission is reported but is unusual. Oseltamivir (Tamiflu®) can reduce morbidity from influenza A by 1-2 days (see p402; note that oseltamivir-resistant H5N1 has been reported).[18] A vaccine is under development, but the most likely cause of a pandemic of flu is a new mutant developing between human and avian influenza virus (genetic reassortment, p403) which may require a different vaccine.

►Suspect avian flu if undiagnosed fever and dyspnoea/pneumonia rapidly progresses to acute respiratory distress syndrome, especially if there is lymphopenia or thrombocytopenia.[19] There may also be a history of close contact with poultry. **NB:** D&V, abdominal pain, pleuritic pain, and bleeding from the nose and gums are reported to be an early feature in some patients.[20]

Diagnosis: Viral culture ± reverse transcriptase-PCR with H5 & N1 specific primers.[21]

Management: ►Get help. Contain the outbreak (use your pandemic preparedness plan[1], p403, in the UK, via your consultant in communicable disease control, CCDC). Ventilatory support + O_2 and antivirals may be needed. Nebulizers & high-air flow O_2 masks are implicated in nosocomial spread (only use with meticulous precautions).[22]

Precautions for close contacts:
Use appropriate hand hygiene, do not share utensils, avoid face-to-face contact with suspected or proven cases, wear high-efficiency masks and eye protection.

Start empirical antiviral treatment and do diagnostic testing if fever (T° >38°C) and cough, shortness of breath, diarrhoea, or other systemic symptoms develop.

In case of close contact or sharing a defined setting (household, extended family, hospital or other residential institution, or military service) with a patient with proven or suspected avian influenza A (H5N1) infection, monitor body temperature twice daily, check for symptoms for 7d after the last exposure, and start post-exposure prophylaxis with **oseltamivir**: 75mg once daily for 7-10d.[23]

SARS[24]

Severe acute respiratory syndrome (SARS) is caused by SARS-CoV virus—a coronavirus. Major features are persistent fever >38°C, chills, rigors, myalgia, dry cough, headache, diarrhoea, and dyspnoea—with an abnormal CXR and WCC↓. Respiratory failure is the big complication; >50% need supplemental O_2; ~20% progress to acute respiratory distress syndrome requiring invasive ventilation.[25]

Mortality is 1-50%, depending on age. Close contact with an index case, or travel to an area with known cases should raise suspicion. The mechanism of transmission of SARS-CoV is only by close contact with other patients.

Management is supportive. No drugs have convincing efficacy (experts may advise on antivirals). Rapid diagnosis, early isolation, and good infection control measures are vital. Communicate with your consultant in infectious diseases.[26]

[1] Therapeutic or prophylactic antivirals are said to be the most effective single intervention followed by vaccine and basic public health measures. But oseltamivir resistance and unavailability of a suitable vaccine during the early stages of a pandemic make non-drug interventions all the more important.

Respiratory failure (See p180.) Type 1 respiratory failure (P_aO_2 <8kPa) is relatively common. Treatment is with high-flow (60%) oxygen. *Transfer the patient to ITU if hypoxia does not improve with O_2 therapy or P_aCO_2 rises to >6kPa.* Be careful with O_2 in COPD patients; check ABGs frequently, and consider elective ventilation if rising P_aCO_2 or worsening acidosis. Aim to keep SaO_2 at 90–94%.

Hypotension may be due to a combination of dehydration and vasodilatation due to sepsis. If systolic BP is <90mmHg, give an intravenous fluid challenge of 250mL colloid/crystalloid over 15min. If BP does not rise, insert a central line and give intravenous fluids to maintain the systolic BP >90mmHg. If systolic BP remains <90mmHg despite fluid therapy, request ITU assessment for inotropic support (adrenaline, noradrenaline).

Atrial fibrillation (p124) is quite common, particularly in the elderly. It usually resolves with treatment of the pneumonia. Digoxin or β-blocker may be required to slow the ventricular response rate in the short term.

Pleural effusion Inflammation of the pleura by adjacent pneumonia may cause fluid exudation into the pleural space. If this accumulates in the pleural space faster than it is reabsorbed, a pleural effusion develops (**fig 2**, p737). If this is small it may be of no consequence. If it becomes large and symptomatic, or infected (empyema), drainage is required (p184 & p780).

Empyema is pus in the pleural space. It should be suspected if a patient with a resolving pneumonia develops a recurrent fever. Clinical features and the CXR indicate a pleural effusion. The aspirated pleural fluid is typically yellow and turbid with a pH <7.2, glucose↓, and LDH↑. The empyema should be drained using a chest drain, preferably inserted under radiological guidance. Adhesions and loculation can make this difficult.

Lung abscess is a cavitating area of localized, suppurative infection within the lung (see **fig 1**).

Causes: • Inadequately treated pneumonia • Aspiration (eg alcoholism, oesophageal obstruction, bulbar palsy) • Bronchial obstruction (tumour, foreign body) • Pulmonary infarction • Septic emboli (septicaemia, right heart endocarditis, IV drug use) • Subphrenic or hepatic abscess.

Clinical features: Swinging fever; cough; purulent, foul-smelling sputum; pleuritic chest pain; haemoptysis; malaise; weight loss. Look for: finger clubbing; anaemia; crepitations. Empyema develops in 20–30%.

Tests: Blood: FBC (anaemia, neutrophilia), ESR, CRP, blood cultures. *Sputum* microscopy, culture, and cytology. *CXR:* walled cavity, often with a fluid level. Consider CT scan to exclude obstruction, and bronchoscopy to obtain diagnostic specimens.

Treatment: Antibiotics as indicated by sensitivities; continue until healed (4–6 wks). Postural drainage. Repeated aspiration, antibiotic instillation, or surgical excision may be required.

Septicaemia may occur as a result of bacterial spread from the lung parenchyma into the bloodstream. This may cause metastatic infection, eg infective endocarditis, meningitis. Treatment with IV antibiotic according to sensitivities.

Pericarditis and myocarditis may also complicate pneumonia.

Jaundice This is usually cholestatic, and may be due to sepsis or secondary to antibiotic therapy (particularly flucloxacillin and co-amoxiclav).

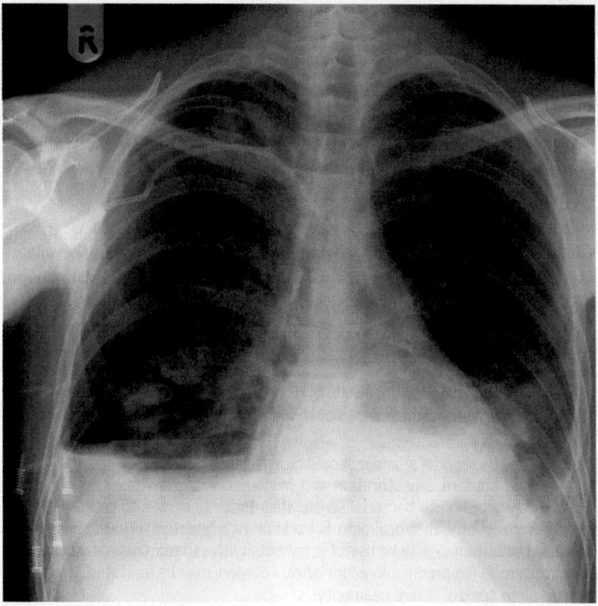

Fig 1. PA chest radiograph showing multiple rounded ring lesions of differing sizes in the right lower zone, at the right apex and in the left lower zone. The lesions are largest in the right lower zone, where they can be seen to contain air-fluid levels, typical appearance of infection in a pneumatocele (=air cyst) or cavitating lesion. A moderate right-sided hydropneumothorax can also be seen, suggesting that one of these lesions may have ruptured into the pleural cavity. The patient also has a right subclavian central venous catheter for the administration of antibiotics. The diagnosis in this case was that of multiple pulmonary abscesses in a patient who was an intravenous drug user.

Image courtesy of Derby Hospitals NHS Foundation Trust Radiology Department

Bronchiectasis

Pathology Chronic infection of the bronchi and bronchioles leading to permanent dilatation of these airways. Main organisms: *H. influenzae; Strep. pneumoniae; Staph. aureus; Pseudomonas aeruginosa.*

Causes *Congenital:* cystic fibrosis (CF); Young's syndrome; primary ciliary dyskinesia; Kartagener's syndrome (*OHCS* p646). *Post-infection:* measles; pertussis; bronchiolitis; pneumonia; TB; HIV. *Other:* Bronchial obstruction (tumour, foreign body); allergic bronchopulmonary aspergillosis (ABPA, p168); hypogammaglobulinaemia; rheumatoid arthritis; ulcerative colitis; idiopathic.

Clinical features *Symptoms:* persistent cough; copious purulent sputum; intermittent haemoptysis. *Signs:* finger clubbing; coarse inspiratory crepitations; wheeze (asthma, COPD, ABPA). *Complications:* pneumonia, pleural effusion; pneumothorax; haemoptysis; cerebral abscess; amyloidosis.

Tests *Sputum* culture. *CXR:* cystic shadows, thickened bronchial walls (tramline and ring shadows); see **fig 1**. *HRCT chest:* (p158) to assess extent and distribution of disease. *Spirometry* often shows an obstructive pattern; reversibility should be assessed. *Bronchoscopy* to locate site of haemoptysis or exclude obstruction. *Other tests:* serum immunoglobulins; CF sweat test; *Aspergillus* precipitins or skin-prick test.

Management • *Postural drainage* should be performed twice daily. Chest physiotherapy may aid sputum expectoration and mucous drainage. • *Antibiotics* should be prescribed according to bacterial sensitivities. Patients known to culture *Pseudomonas* will require either oral ciprofloxacin or IV antibiotics. • *Bronchodilators* (eg nebulized salbutamol) may be useful in patients with asthma, COPD, CF, ABPA (p168). • *Corticosteroids* (eg prednisolone) for ABPA. • *Surgery* may be indicated in localized disease or to control severe haemoptysis.

Cystic fibrosis (CF)

See *OHCS* (Paediatrics, p162)

One of the commonest life-threatening autosomal recessive conditions (1 : 2000 live births) affecting Caucasians. Caused by mutations in the CF transmembrane conductance regulator (CFTR) gene on chromosome 7 (>800 mutations have now been identified). This is a Cl^- channel, and the defect leads to a combination of defective chloride secretion and increased sodium absorption across airway epithelium. The changes in the composition of airway surface liquid predispose the lung to chronic pulmonary infections and bronchiectasis.

Clinical features *Neonate:* Failure to thrive; meconium ileus; rectal prolapse.

Children and young adults: *Respiratory:* cough; wheeze; recurrent infections; bronchiectasis; pneumothorax; haemoptysis; respiratory failure; cor pulmonale. *Gastrointestinal:* pancreatic insufficiency (diabetes mellitus, steatorrhoea); distal intestinal obstruction syndrome (meconium ileus equivalent); gallstones; cirrhosis. *Other:* male infertility; osteoporosis; arthritis; vasculitis (p558); nasal polyps; sinusitis; and hypertrophic pulmonary osteoarthropathy (HPOA). *Signs:* cyanosis; finger clubbing; bilateral coarse crackles.

Diagnosis *Sweat test:* sweat sodium and chloride >60mmol/L; chloride usually > sodium. *Genetics:* screening for known common CF mutations should be considered. *Faecal elastase* is a simple and useful screening test for exocrine pancreatic dysfunction.

Tests *Blood:* FBC, U&E, LFT; clotting; vitamin A, D, E levels; annual glucose tolerance test (p198). *Bacteriology:* cough swab, sputum culture. *Radiology: CXR;* hyperinflation; bronchiectasis. *Abdominal ultrasound:* fatty liver; cirrhosis; chronic pancreatitis; *Spirometry:* obstructive defect. *Aspergillus serology/skin test* (20% develop ABPA, p168). *Biochemistry:* faecal fat analysis.

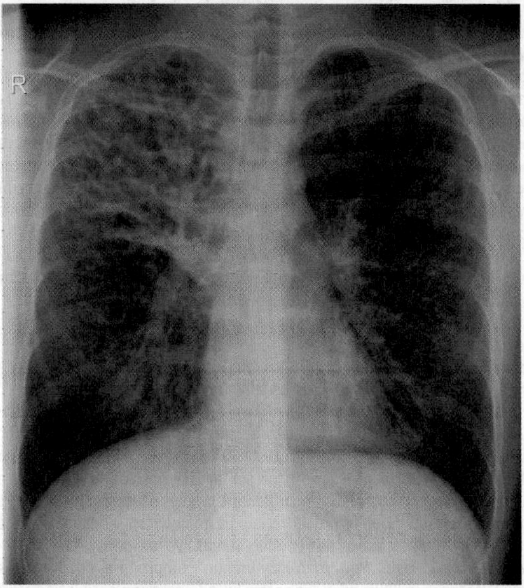

Fig 1. PA chest radiograph showing marked abnormal dilatation of the airways throughout the right upper lobe, along with similar changes to a lesser degree throughout the rest of the lung (most notably in the periphery of the left upper zone). Appearances are that of bronchiectasis, which in this case was congenital. The fine background reticular pattern in the lungs suggests that there may also be some interstitial lung disease present.

Image courtesy of Nottingham University Hospitals NHS Trust Radiology Department

Management of cystic fibrosis

Patients with cystic fibrosis are best managed by a multidisciplinary team, eg physician, GP, physiotherapist, specialist nurse, and dietician with attention to psychosocial as well as physical well-being. Gene therapy (transfer of CFTR gene using liposome or adenovirus vectors) is not yet possible.

Chest: Physiotherapy regularly (postural drainage, active cycle breathing techniques or forced expiratory techniques). Antibiotics are given for acute infective exacerbations and prophylactically (PO or nebulized). Mucolytics may be useful (eg DNase, ie Dornase alfa, 2.5mg daily nebulized, *OHCS* p163). Bronchodilators.

Gastrointestinal: Pancreatic enzyme replacement; fat soluble vitamin supplements (A, D, E, K); ursodeoxycholic acid for impaired liver function; cirrhosis may require liver transplantation.

Other: Treatment of CF-related diabetes; screening for and treatment of osteoporosis; treatment of arthritis, sinusitis, and vasculitis; fertility and genetic counselling.

Advanced lung disease: Oxygen, diuretics (cor pulmonale); non-invasive ventilation; lung or heart/lung transplantation.

Prognosis: Median survival is now over 30yrs.

Aspergillus This group of fungi affects the lung in 5 ways:

1 *Asthma:* Type I hypersensitivity (atopic) reaction to fungal spores, p172.

2 *Allergic bronchopulmonary aspergillosis (ABPA):* This results from a type I and III hypersensitivity reaction to *Aspergillus fumigatus*. Early on, the allergic response causes bronchoconstriction, but as the inflammation persists, permanent damage occurs, causing bronchiectasis (**fig 1**). *Symptoms:* wheeze, cough, sputum (plugs of mucus containing fungal hyphae, see p440), dyspnoea, and 'recurrent pneumonia'. *Investigations:* CXR (transient segmental collapse or consolidation, bronchiectasis); *Aspergillus* in sputum; positive *Aspergillus* skin test and/or *Aspergillus*-specific IgE RAST (radioallergosorbent test); positive serum precipitins; eosinophilia; raised serum IgE. *Treatment:* prednisolone 30–40mg/24h PO for acute attacks; maintenance dose 5–10mg/d. Sometimes itraconazole is used in combination with corticosteroids. Bronchodilators for asthma. Sometimes bronchoscopic aspiration of mucous plugs is needed.

3 *Aspergilloma (mycetoma):* A fungus ball within a pre-existing cavity (often caused by TB or sarcoidosis). It is usually asymptomatic but may cause cough, haemoptysis (may be torrential), lethargy ± weight loss. *Investigations:* CXR (round opacity within a cavity, usually apical); sputum culture; strongly positive serum precipitins; *Aspergillus* skin test (30% +ve). *Treatment* (only if symptomatic). Consider surgical excision for solitary symptomatic lesions or severe haemoptysis. Oral itraconazole and other antifungals have been tried with limited success. Local instillation of amphotericin paste under CT guidance yields partial success in carefully selected patients, eg in massive haemoptysis.

4 *Invasive aspergillosis: Risk factors:*[27] immunocompromise, eg HIV, leukaemia, burns, Wegener's (p728), and SLE, or after broad-spectrum antibiotic therapy. *Investigations:* sputum culture; BAL; biopsy; serum precipitins; CXR (consolidation, abscess). Early chest CT and serial serum measurements of galactomannan (an *Aspergillus* antigen) may be helpful. Diagnosis may only be made at lung biopsy or autopsy. *Treatment:* Voriconazole is superior to IV amphotericin.[28] Alternatives: IV miconazole or ketoconazole (less effective). *Prognosis:* 30% mortality.

5 *Extrinsic allergic alveolitis (EAA)* may be caused by sensitivity to *Aspergillus clavatus* ('malt worker's lung'). Clinical features and treatment are as for other causes of EAA (p188). Diagnosis is based on a history of exposure and presence of serum precipitins to *A. clavatus*. Pulmonary fibrosis may occur if untreated.

Using amphotericin B Test dose: 1mg in 20mL 5% dextrose IV over 20–30min. Observe closely for the next ½h for signs of anaphylaxis (shock, swelling, wheeze etc). There are various formulations. Consult *BNF*. *Do not give any other drug in the same IVI.* SE: anaphylaxis; serious nephrotoxicity; fever; rash; anorexia; nausea; D&V; headache; myalgia; arthralgia; anaemia; $\downarrow K^+$; $\downarrow Mg^{2+}$; hepatotoxicity; arrhythmias; hearing loss; diplopia; seizures; neuropathy; phlebitis. *Monitor* U&E *daily*. *AmBisome*® (liposomal amphotericin) has fewer SEs, but is expensive; it is indicated in systemic or deep mycoses where nephrotoxicity precludes conventional amphotericin; IV initial test dose: 1mg over 10min, then 1mg/kg/d, as a single IVI dose; gradually↑ if needed to 3mg/kg/d (max 5mg/kg/d).[29] Alternatives: *Abelcet*® and *Amphocil*®.

Other fungal infections *Candida* and *Cryptococcus* may cause pneumonia in the immunosuppressed (see p440).

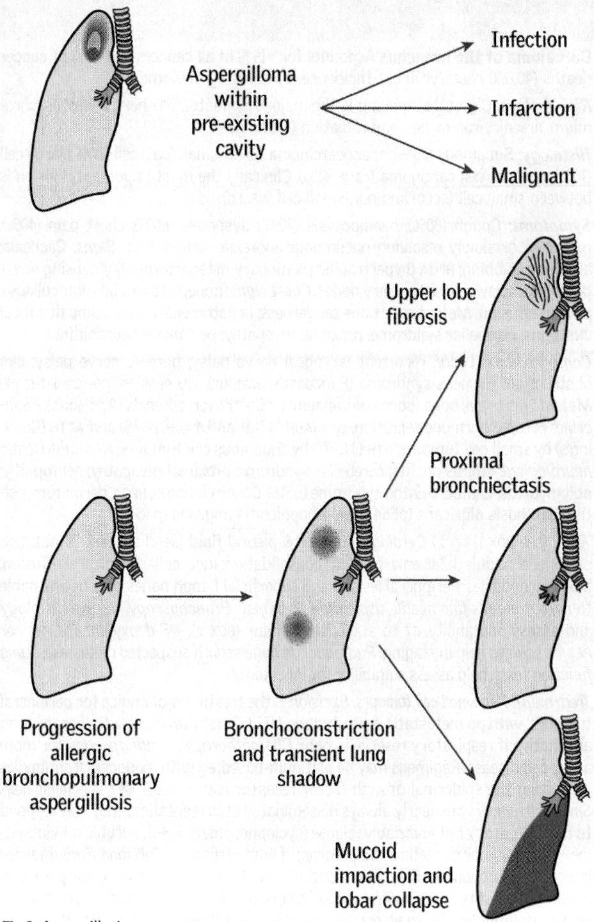
Aspergilloma
within
pre-existing
cavity
Infection
Infarction
Malignant
Upper lobe
fibrosis
Proximal
bronchiectasis
Progression of
allergic
bronchopulmonary
aspergillosis
Bronchoconstriction
and transient lung
shadow
Mucoid
impaction and
lobar collapse

Fig 1. Aspergillosis.

Carcinoma of the bronchus Accounts for ≈19% of all cancers and 27% of cancer deaths (40,000 cases/yr in UK). Incidence is increasing in women.

Risk factors: Cigarette smoking is the major risk factor. Others: asbestos, chromium, arsenic, iron oxides, and radiation (radon gas).

Histology: Squamous (35%); adenocarcinoma (27%); small (oat) cell (20%); large cell (10%); alveolar cell carcinoma (rare, <1%). Clinically the most important division is between small cell (SCLC) and non-small cell (NSCLC).

Symptoms: Cough (80%); haemoptysis (70%); dyspnoea (60%); chest pain (40%); recurrent or slowly resolving pneumonia; anorexia; weight loss. *Signs:* Cachexia; anaemia; clubbing; HPOA (hypertrophic pulmonary osteoarthropathy, causing wrist pain); supraclavicular or axillary nodes. *Chest signs:* none, or: consolidation; collapse; pleural effusion. *Metastases:* bone tenderness; hepatomegaly; confusion; fits; focal CNS signs; cerebellar syndrome; proximal myopathy; peripheral neuropathy.

Complications: Local: recurrent laryngeal nerve palsy; phrenic nerve palsy; SVC obstruction; Horner's syndrome (Pancoast's tumour); rib erosion; pericarditis; AF. *Metastatic:* brain; bone (bone pain, anaemia, ↑Ca^{2+}); liver; adrenals (Addison's). *Endocrine:* ectopic hormone secretion, eg SIADH (↓Na^+ and ↑ADH, p678) and ACTH (Cushing's) by small cell tumours; PTH (↑Ca^{2+}) by squamous cell tumours. *Non-metastatic neurological:* confusion; fits; cerebellar syndrome; proximal myopathy; neuropathy; polymyositis; Lambert-Eaton syndrome (p516). *Other:* clubbing, HPOA, dermatomyositis; acanthosis nigricans (p564); thrombophlebitis migrans (p564).

Tests: (see BOX 1, **fig 1**) *Cytology:* sputum & pleural fluid (send at least 20mL). *CXR:* peripheral nodule; hilar enlargement; consolidation; lung collapse; pleural effusion; bony secondaries. Peripheral lesions and superficial lymph nodes may be amenable to *percutaneous fine needle aspiration* or *biopsy*. *Bronchoscopy:* to give histology and assess operability. *CT* to stage the tumour (BOX 2). *^{18}F-deoxyglucose PET*[1] *or PET/CT scan* to help in staging. *Radionuclide bone scan:* if suspected metastases. *Lung function tests*: help assess suitability for lobectomy.

Treatment: Non-small cell tumours: Excision is the treatment of choice for peripheral tumours, with no metastatic spread: stage I/II (~25%). *Curative radiotherapy* is an alternative if respiratory reserve is poor. *Chemotherapy ± radiotherapy* for more advanced disease. Regimens may be platinum-based, eg with monoclonal antibodies targetting the epidermal growth factor receptor (cetuximab). Get specialist help. ***Small cell tumours*** are nearly always disseminated at presentation. They may respond to *chemotherapy* but invariably relapse (cyclophosphamide + doxorubicin + vincristine + etoposide; **or** cisplatin ±*radiotherapy* if limited disease). ***Palliation:** Radiotherapy* is used for bronchial obstruction, SVC obstruction, haemoptysis, bone pain, and cerebral metastases. *SVC stent* + radiotherapy and dexamethasone for SVC obstruction. *Endobronchial therapy:* tracheal stenting, cryotherapy, laser, brachytherapy (a radioactive source is placed close to the tumour). *Pleural drainage/pleurodesis* for symptomatic pleural effusions. *Drugs:* analgesia; steroids; antiemetics; cough linctus (codeine); bronchodilators; antidepressants.

Prognosis: Non-small cell: 50% 2yr survival without spread; 10% with spread. *Small cell:* median survival is 3 months if untreated; 1-1½yrs if treated.

Prevention: Quit smoking, p87. Prevent occupational exposure to carcinogens.

Other lung tumours *Bronchial adenoma:* Rare, slow-growing. 90% are carcinoid tumours; 10% cylindromas. ℞: surgery. ***Hamartoma:*** Rare, benign; CT: lobulated mass ±flecks of calcification; ?excise to exclude malignancy. ***Mesothelioma*** (p192).

1 PET= positron emission tomography

Nodule in the lung on a CXR

Malignancy (1° or 2°)	Arterio-venous malformation
Abscesses (p164)	Encysted effusion (fluid, blood, pus)
Granuloma	Cyst
Carcinoid tumour	Foreign body
Pulmonary hamartoma	Skin tumour (eg seborrhoeic wart)

TNM staging for non-small cell lung cancer

Primary tumour (T)	
TX	Malignant cells in bronchial secretions, no other evidence of tumour
TIS	Carcinoma *in situ*
T0	None evident
T1	≤3cm, in lobar or more distal airway
T2	>3cm and >2cm distal to carina *or* any size if pleural involvement *or* obstructive pneumonitis extending to hilum, but not all the lung
T3	Involves the chest wall, diaphragm, mediastinal pleura, pericardium, or <2cm from, but not at, carina
T4	Involves the mediastinum, heart, great vessels, trachea, oesophagus, vertebral body, carina, *or* a malignant effusion is present
Regional nodes (N)	
N0	None involved (after mediastinoscopy)
N1	Peribronchial and/or ipsilateral hilum
N2	Ipsilateral mediastinum or subcarinal
N3	Contralateral mediastinum or hilum, scalene, or supraclavicular
Distant metastasis (M)	
M0	None
M1	Distant metastases present

Stages

Occult	**I**	**II**	**IIIa**	**IIIb**	**IV**
TX N0 M0	TIS/T1/T2 N0 M0	T1/T2 N1 M0 *or* T3 N0 M0	T3 N1 M0 *or* T1–3 N2 M0	T1–4 N3 M0 *or* T4 N0–2 M0	T1–4 N0–3 M1

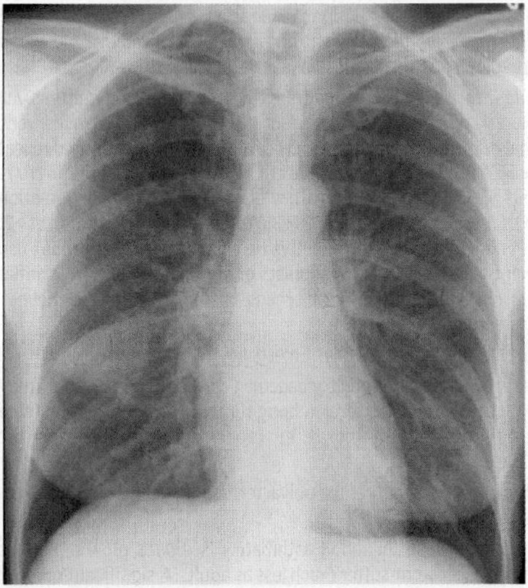

Fig 1. A wedge-shaped density in the middle lobe (a secondary). Also note a coin lesion at the right costophrenic angle. The sharp upper boundary of the middle lobe triangular mass is the middle lobe fissure. The right hilar structures are enlarged by metastases within the hilar lymph nodes.

Courtesy of Janet E. Jeddry, Yale Medical School.

Asthma[33]

Asthma affects 5–8% of the population. It is characterized by recurrent episodes of dyspnoea, cough, and wheeze caused by reversible airways obstruction. Three factors contribute to airway narrowing: *bronchial muscle contraction*, triggered by a variety of stimuli; *mucosal swelling/inflammation*, caused by mast cell and basophil degranulation resulting in the release of inflammatory mediators; *increased mucus production*.

Symptoms Intermittent dyspnoea, wheeze, cough (often nocturnal) and sputum. Ask specifically about:
Precipitants: Cold air, exercise, emotion, allergens (house dust mite, pollen, fur), infection, smoking and passive smoking;[34] pollution, NSAIDs, β-blockers,
Diurnal variation in symptoms or peak flow. Marked morning dipping of peak flow is common and can tip the balance into a serious attack, despite having normal peak flow (**fig 1**) at other times.
Exercise: Quantify the exercise tolerance.
Disturbed sleep: Quantify as nights per week (a sign of severe asthma).
Acid reflux: 40–60% of those with asthma have reflux; treating it improves spirometry—but not necessarily symptoms.[35]
Other atopic disease: Eczema, hay fever, allergy, or family history?
The home (especially the bedroom): Pets? Carpet? Feather pillows or duvet? Floor cushions and other 'soft furnishings'?
Job: If symptoms remit at weekends or holidays, work may provide the trigger (15% of cases are work-related—more for paint sprayers, food processors, welders, and animal handlers).[36] Ask the patient to measure his peak flow at intervals at work and at home (at the same time of day) to confirm this (see **fig 2**).
Days per week off work or school.

Signs Tachypnoea; audible wheeze; hyperinflated chest; hyperresonant percussion note; diminished air entry; widespread, polyphonic wheeze. ***Severe attack:*** inability to complete sentences; pulse >110bpm; respiratory rate >25/min; PEF 33–50% of predicted. ***Life-threatening attack:*** silent chest; cyanosis; bradycardia; exhaustion; PEF <33% of predicted; confusion; feeble respiratory effort.

Tests *Acute attack:* PEF, sputum culture, FBC, U&E, CRP, blood cultures. ABG analysis usually shows a normal or slightly reduced P_aO_2 and low P_aCO_2 (hyperventilation). If P_aO_2 normal but the patient is hyperventilating, watch carefully and repeat the ABG a little later. ►*If P_aCO_2 is raised, transfer to high-dependency unit or ITU for ventilation*, as this signifies failing respiratory effort. CXR (to exclude infection or pneumothorax). ***Chronic asthma:*** PEF monitoring (p156): a diurnal variation of >20% on ≥3d a wk for 2wks. Spirometry: obstructive defect (↓FEV_1/FVC, ↑RV p156); usually ≥15% improvement in FEV_1 following β_2 agonists or steroid trial. CXR: hyperinflation. Skin-prick tests may help to identify allergens. Histamine or methacholine challenge. *Aspergillus* serology.

Treatment Chronic asthma (p174). Emergency treatment (p820).

Differential diagnosis Pulmonary oedema ('cardiac asthma'); COPD (may co-exist); large airway obstruction (eg foreign body, tumour); SVC obstruction (wheeze/dyspnoea not episodic); pneumothorax; PE; bronchiectasis; obliterative bronchiolitis (suspect in elderly).

Associated diseases Acid reflux; polyarteritis nodosa (PAN, p558); Churg-Strauss syndrome (p558); ABPA (p168).

Natural history Most childhood asthmatics (see *OHCS* p164) either grow out of asthma in adolescence, or suffer much less as adults. A significant number of people develop chronic asthma late in life.

Mortality Death certificates give a figure of 2000/yr (UK): more careful surveys more than halve this figure. 50% are >65yrs old.

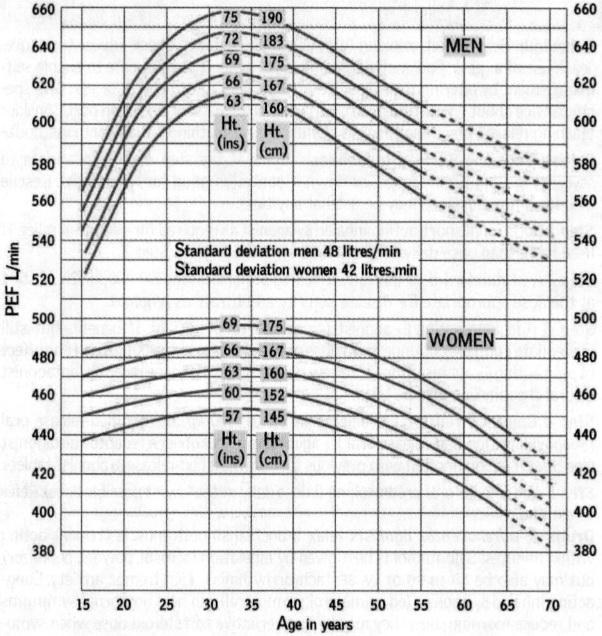

Fig 1. Normal peak expiratory flow (PEF)

Data from Nunn, AJ, Gregg, I. New regression equations for predicting peak expiratory flow in adults. BMJ 1989;298:1068-70.

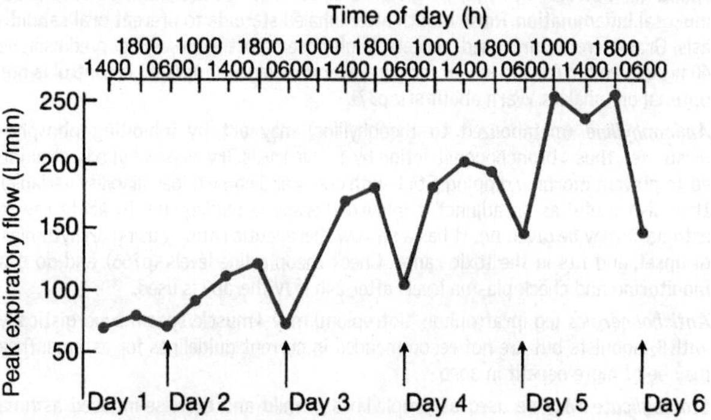

Fig 2. Examples of serial peak flow charts

Behaviour Help to quit smoking (p87). Avoid precipitants. Check inhaler technique. Teach use of a peak flow meter to monitor PEF twice a day. Educate to enable self-management by altering their medication in the light of symptoms or PEF. Give specific advice about what to do in an emergency; provide a written action plan. Consider teaching relaxed breathing to avoid dysfunctional breathing[38] (Papworth method).[1]

British Thoracic Society guidelines[39] Start at the step most appropriate to severity; moving up if needed, or down if control is good for >3 months. Rescue courses of prednisolone may be used at any time.

Step 1 Occasional short-acting inhaled **β_2-agonist** as required for symptom relief. If used more than once daily, or night-time symptoms, go to Step 2.

Step 2 Add standard-dose inhaled steroid, eg **beclometasone** 100-400µg/12h, or start at the dose appropriate for disease severity, and titrate as required.

Step 3 Add long-acting β_2-agonist (eg **salmeterol** 50µg/12h). If benefit—but still inadequate control—continue and ↑dose of **beclometasone** to 400µg/12h. If no effect of long acting β_2-agonist stop it. Review diagnosis. Leukotriene receptor antagonist or oral theophylline may be tried.

Step 4 Consider trials of: **beclometasone** up to 1000µg/12h; modified-release oral **theophylline**; modified-release oral **β_2-agonist**; oral leukotriene receptor antagonist (see below), in conjunction with previous therapy. Modified-release β_2 agonist tablets.

Step 5 Add regular oral **prednisolone** (1 dose daily, at the lowest possible dose). Refer to asthma clinic.

Drugs ***β_2-adrenoceptor agonists*** relax bronchial smooth muscle (↑cAMP), acting within minutes. Salbutamol is best given by inhalation (aerosol, powder, nebulizer), but may also be given PO or IV. SE: tachyarrhythmias, ↓K^+, tremor, anxiety. Long-acting inhaled β_2-agonist (eg salmeterol, formoterol) can help nocturnal symptoms and reduce morning dips. They may be an alternative to ↑steroid dose when symptoms are uncontrolled; doubts remain over whether they are associated with an increase in adverse events.[40] SE: as salbutamol, paradoxical bronchospasm.[41]

Corticosteroids are best inhaled to minimize systemic effects, eg beclometasone via spacer (or powder), but may be given PO or IV. They act over days to ↓bronchial mucosal inflammation. Rinse mouth after inhaled steroids to prevent oral candidiasis. Oral steroids are used acutely (high-dose, short courses, eg prednisolone 40mg/24h PO for 7d) and longer term in lower dose (eg 5-10mg/24h) if control is not optimal on inhalers. Warn about SEs: p371.

Aminophylline (metabolized to theophylline) may act by inhibiting phosphodiesterase, thus ↓bronchoconstriction by ↑cAMP levels. Try as prophylaxis, at night, PO, to prevent morning dipping. Stick with one brand name (bioavailability variable). It is also useful as an adjunct if inhaled therapy is inadequate. In acute severe asthma, it may be given IVI. It has a narrow therapeutic ratio, causing arrhythmias, GI upset, and fits in the toxic range. Check theophylline levels (p766), and do ECG monitoring and check plasma levels after 24h if IV therapy is used.

Anticholinergics (eg ipratropium, tiotropium) may ↓muscle spasm synergistically with β_2-agonists but are not recommended in current guidelines for asthma. They may be of more benefit in COPD.

Cromoglicate May be used as prophylaxis in mild and exercise-induced asthma (always inhaled), especially in children. It may precipitate asthma.

Leukotriene receptor antagonists (eg montelukast, zafirlukast) block the effects of cysteinyl leukotrienes in the airways by antagonising the $CystLT_1$ receptor.

Anti-IgE monoclonal antibody Omalizumab[42] may be of use in highly selected patients with persistent allergic asthma. Given as a subcutaneous injection every two to four weeks depending on dose. Specialists only.

1 Integrated breathing and relaxation training (Papworth method) is psychological *and* physical: patients learn to drop their shoulders, relax their abdomen, and breathe calmly and appropriately.

Doses of some inhaled drugs used in bronchoconstriction

	Inhaled aerosol	Inhaled powder	Nebulized *(supervised)*
Salbutamol			
Dose example:	100–200μg/6h	200–400μg/6h	2.5–5mg/6h
Airomir® is a CFC-free example of a breath-actuated inhaler			
Terbutaline			
Single dose		500μg[1]	2.5mg/mL
Recommended regimen		500μg/6h	5–10mg/6–12h
Salmeterol			
Dose/puff	25μg	50μg	—
Recommended regimen	50–100μg/12h	50–100μg/12h	—
Ipratropium bromide (COPD)			
Dose/puff	20μg	40μg	250μg/mL
Recommended regimen	20–40μg/6h	40–80μg/6h	250–500μg/6h
Steroids			
(Clenil Modulite®=beclometasone; Pulmicort®=budesonide;[1] Flixotide®=fluticasone)			
Fluticasone (Flixotide®)			
Doses available/puff	50, 100μg & 250μg & 500μg	As for aerosol	250μg/mL
Recommended regimen	100–250μg/12h	100–250μg/12h max 1mg/12h	0.5–2mg/12h
Clenil Modulite®			
Doses available/puff	50 & 100μg 250μg	—	—
Recommended regimen	100μg/12h ↓ 200μg/12h ↓ 250μg/12h ↓ 500–1000μg/12h		

►Prescribe beclometasone by brand name, and state that a CFC-free inhaler should be dispensed. This is because, dose for dose, Qvar® is twice as potent as the other available CFC-free brand (Clenil Modulite®).

Any dose ≥250μg ≈ significant steroid absorption: carry a steroid card; this recommendation is being widened, and lower doses (beclometasone) are now said to merit a steroid card (manufacturer's information).

1 Available as a Turbohaler®; Autohalers® are an alternative (breath-actuated) and don't need breathing coordination, eg Airomir (salbutamol) & Qvar® (beclometasone). Accuhalers deliver dry powders (eg Flixotide®, Serevent®).

Systemic absorption (via the throat) is less if inhalation is through a **large-volume device**, eg Volumatic® or AeroChamber Plus® (for Airomir & Qvar) devices. The latter is more compact. Static charge on some devices reduces dose delivery, so wash in water before dose; leave to dry (don't rub). It's pointless to squirt many puffs into a device: it is best to repeat single doses, and be sure to inhale *as soon as the drug is in the spacer*. SE: local (oral) candidiasis (p230); ↑rate of cataract if lifetime dose ≥2g beclometasone.

Chronic obstructive pulmonary disease (COPD)

Definitions COPD is a common progressive disorder characterized by airway obstruction (FEV_1 <80% predicted; FEV_1/FVC <0.7; see p156 and TABLE below) with little or no reversibility. It includes chronic bronchitis & emphysema. Usually patients have *either* COPD *or* asthma, not both: COPD is favoured by: • Age of onset >35yrs • Smoking (passive or active) or pollution related[44] • Chronic dyspnoea • Sputum production • Minimal diurnal or day-to-day FEV_1 variation. **Chronic bronchitis** is defined *clinically* as cough, sputum production on most days for 3 months of 2 successive yrs. Symptoms improve if they stop smoking. There is no excess mortality if lung function is normal. **Emphysema** is defined *histologically* as enlarged air spaces distal to terminal bronchioles, with destruction of alveolar walls.

Prevalence 10–20% of the over-40s; 2.5×10^6 deaths/yr worldwide.[45]

Pink puffers and blue bloaters (ends of a spectrum) *Pink puffers* have ↑alveolar ventilation, a near normal P_aO_2 and a normal or low P_aCO_2. They are breathless but are not cyanosed. They may progress to type 1 respiratory failure (p180). *Blue bloaters* have ↓alveolar ventilation, with a low P_aO_2 and a high P_aCO_2. They are cyanosed but not breathless and may go on to develop cor pulmonale. Their respiratory centres are relatively insensitive to CO_2 and they rely on hypoxic drive to maintain respiratory effort (p180)→*supplemental oxygen should be given with care.*

Symptoms Cough; sputum; dyspnoea; wheeze. **Signs** Tachypnoea; use of accessory muscles of respiration; hyperinflation; ↓cricosternal distance (<3cm); ↓expansion; resonant or hyperresonant percussion note; quiet breath sounds (eg over bullae); wheeze; cyanosis; cor pulmonale.

Complications Acute exacerbations ± infection; polycythaemia; respiratory failure; cor pulmonale (oedema; JVP↑); pneumothorax (ruptured bullae); lung carcinoma.

Tests *FBC:* PCV↑. *CXR:* Hyperinflation (>6 anterior ribs seen above diaphragm in mid-clavicular line); flat hemidiaphragms; large central pulmonary arteries; ↓peripheral vascular markings; bullae. *ECG:* Right atrial and ventricular hypertrophy (cor pulmonale). *ABG:* P_aO_2 ↓ ± hypercapnia. *Lung function* (p156p159): obstructive + air trapping (FEV_1 <80% of predicted—see p156, FEV_1:FVC ratio <70%, TLC↑, RV↑, DLCO↓ in emphysema—see p158). Learn how to do spirometry from an experienced person: ensure *maximal* expiration of the full breath (it takes ≥4sec; it's *not* a quick puff out). *Trial of steroids:* See BOX.

Treatment *Chronic stable:* see BOX; ››*Emergency* ℞: p822. Offer *smoking cessation advice* with cordial vigour (p87). BMI is often low: *diet advice ± supplements*[46] *may* help, p586. *Mucolytics* (*BNF* 3.7) may help chronic productive cough (NICE).[47] Disabilities may cause serious, treatable *depression;* screen for this (p11). *Respiratory failure:* p180. *Flu and pneumococcal vaccinations:* p402.

Long-term O₂ therapy (LTOT): An MRC trial showed that if P_aO_2 was maintained ≥8.0kPa for 15h a day, 3yr survival improved by 50%. UK DOH guidelines suggest LTOT should be given for: **1** Clinically stable non-smokers with P_aO_2 <7.3kPa—despite maximal ℞. These values should be stable on two occasions >3 wks apart. **2** If P_aO_2 7.3–8.0 *and* pulmonary hypertension (eg RVH; loud S_2) + cor pulmonale. **3** O_2 can also be prescribed for terminally ill patients.

Predicted FEV_1 (Caucasian ♂; litres, ↓level in other races)[1]										♀									
Height cm	*150*	*155*	*160*	*165*	*170*	*175*	*180*	*185*	*190*	*195*	*145*	*150*	*155*	*160*	*165*	*170*	*175*	*180*	*185*	*190*
♂ *Age (yr)*	2.5	2.8	3.0	3.2	3.5	3.7	3.9	4.1	4.4	4.6	2.1	2.2	2.3	2.5	2.6	2.7	2.9	3.0	3.1	3.3
25	2.9	3.2	3.4	3.7	4.0	4.2	4.3	4.7	5.0	5.3	2.6	2.7	2.9	3.0	3.1	3.3	3.4	3.5	3.7	3.8
30	2.8	3.1	3.3	3.6	3.8	4.1	4.3	4.6	4.9	5.1	2.5	2.6	2.8	2.9	3.0	3.2	3.3	3.4	3.6	3.7
40	2.5	2.8	3.0	3.3	3.6	3.8	4.1	4.3	4.6	4.9	2.3	2.4	2.5	2.7	2.8	3.0	3.0	3.2	3.3	3.5
50	2.2	2.5	2.8	3.0	3.3	3.5	3.8	4.0	4.3	4.6	2.1	2.2	2.3	2.5	2.6	2.7	2.9	3.0	3.1	3.3
60	2.0	2.2	2.5	2.8	3.0	3.3	3.5	3.8	4.0	4.3	1.7	2.0	2.1	2.3	2.4	2.5	2.7	2.8	2.9	3.1
70	1.7	2.0	2.2	2.5	2.7	3.0	3.3	3.5	3.8	4.0	1.6	1.8	1.9	2.1	2.2	2.3	2.5	2.6	2.7	2.9
80	1.4	1.7	2.0	2.2	2.5	2.7	3.0	3.3	3.5	3.8	1.4	1.6	1.7	1.9	2.0	2.1	2.2	2.4	2.5	2.7

Data from www.nationalasthma.org.au/publications/spiro/appc.html#Mean

1 African FEV_1 is 10–15% lower; Chinese: 20% lower; Indian: 10% lower; NB: PEF varies little between groups.

British Thoracic Society (BTS)/NICE COPD guidelines

Assessment of COPD Spirometry; bronchodilators may slightly improve FEV_1
Trial of oral steroids; look for >15% ↑ in FEV_1
CXR: ?bullae ?other pathology
Arterial blood gases: hypoxia ?hypercapnia

Severity of COPD

Mild	FEV_1 50–80% of predicted
Moderate	FEV_1 30–49% of predicted
Severe	FEV_1 <30% of predicted

Treating stable COPD

- *General*: Stop smoking, encourage exercise, treat poor nutrition or obesity, influenza and pneumococcal vaccination, pulmonary rehabilitation/palliative care. NIPPV: see p797. **NB:** air travel is risky if FEV_1 <50% or P_aO_2 <6.7kPa.
- *Mild*: Antimuscarinic, eg **ipratropium** or β_2 agonist inhaled PRN.
- *Moderate*: Regular anticholinergic eg **ipratropium** or **tiotropium** or long-acting inhaled β_2 agonist (LABA), eg **salmeterol** + inhaled corticosteroids, eg **beclometasone,** especially if FEV_1 <50% and ≥2 exacerbations/yr (Seretide® combines the latter 2).[1] Symbicort® is **budesonide + formoterol.** 49
Oral **theophylline** (p174) has a role.
- *Severe*: LABA + inhaled steroid + anticholinergic. refer to specialist. Consider steroid trial and home nebulizers.
- *Pulmonary hypertension*: Assess the need for LTOT (see p176). Treat oedema with diuretics.

More advanced COPD

- ►Pulmonary rehabilitation is *greatly* valued by patients.
- Consider LTOT if P_aO_2 <7.3kPa (see OPPOSITE). Also theophylline (do blood levels).
- Indications for surgery: recurrent pneumothoraces; isolated bullous disease; lung volume reduction surgery (selected patients). Some centres also offer NIV to a small number of suitable patients, in severe disease.
- Assess home set-up and support needed. Treat depression (p11).

Indications for specialist referral

- Uncertain diagnosis, or suspected severe COPD, or a rapid decline in FEV_1.
- Onset of cor pulmonale.
- Bullous lung disease (to assess for surgery).
- Assessment for oral corticosteroids, nebulizer therapy, or LTOT.
- <10 pack-years smoking (=PYS =the number of packs/day × years of smoking) or COPD in patient <40yrs (eg is the cause α_1-antitrypsin deficiency? p264).
- Symptoms disproportionate to lung function tests.
- Frequent infections (to exclude bronchiectasis).

Steroid trial

30mg **prednisolone**/24h PO for 2wks. If FEV_1 rises by >15%, the COPD is 'steroid responsive' and benefit may be had by using long-term inhaled corticosteroids (p167). If this doesn't achieve the post-prednisolone FEV_1, request expert help. **NB:** NICE says that 'reversibility testing is not necessary as a part of the diagnostic process or to plan initial therapy with bronchodilators or corticosteroids. It may be unhelpful or misleading because: **1** Repeated FEV_1 measurements can show small spontaneous fluctuations; **2** Results of a reversibility tests on different occasions can be inconsistent and not reproducible; **3** Over-reliance on a single reversibility test may be misleading unless the change in FEV_1 is >400 mL. **4** Definition of a significant change is arbitrary; **5** Response to long-term therapy is not predicted by acute reversibility testing.'

1 Cochrane meta-analyses (2007) of trials (including TORCH) favour steroids + LABA *vs* either alone. LABA alone may ↑exacerbation rates, but no excess hospitalisations or mortality; steroid inhalers alone are associated with ↑mortality (by 33%) compared with steroids + LABA. Steroid inhalers may ↑risk of pneumonia, but when combined with LABA, advantages outweigh disadvantages.

Acute respiratory distress syndrome (ARDS)

ARDS, or acute lung injury, may be caused by direct lung injury or occur secondary to severe systemic illness. Lung damage and release of inflammatory mediators cause increased capillary permeability and non-cardiogenic pulmonary oedema, often accompanied by multiorgan failure.

Causes *Pulmonary:* Pneumonia; gastric aspiration; inhalation; injury; vasculitis (p558); contusion. *Other:* Shock; septicaemia; haemorrhage; multiple transfusions; DIC (p346); pancreatitis; acute liver failure; trauma; head injury; malaria; fat embolism; burns; obstetric events (eclampsia; amniotic fluid embolus); drugs/toxins (aspirin, heroin, paraquat).

Clinical features Cyanosis; tachypnoea; tachycardia; peripheral vasodilatation; bilateral fine inspiratory crackles.

Investigations FBC, U&E, LFT, amylase, clotting, CRP, blood cultures, ABG. CXR shows bilateral pulmonary infiltrates. Pulmonary artery catheter to measure pulmonary capillary wedge pressure (PCWP).

Diagnostic criteria One consensus requires these 4 to exist: **1** Acute onset. **2** CXR: bilateral infiltrates. **3** Pulmonary capillary wedge pressure (PCWP) <19mmHg or a lack of clinical congestive heart failure. **4** Refractory hypoxaemia with P_aO_2 : FiO_2 <200 for ARDS. Others include total thoracic compliance <30mL/cm H_2O.

Management Admit to ITU; give supportive therapy; treat the underlying cause.

- *Respiratory support* In early ARDS, continuous positive airway pressure (CPAP) with 40–60% oxygen may be adequate to maintain oxygenation. But most patients need mechanical ventilation. Indications for ventilation: P_aO_2: <8.3kPa despite 60% O_2; P_aCO_2: >6kPa. The large tidal volumes (10–15mL/kg) produced by conventional ventilation plus reduced lung compliance in ARDS may lead to high peak airway pressures ± pneumothorax. A low-tidal-volume, pressure-limited approach, with either low or moderate high positive end-expiratory pressure (PEEP) improves outcome.
- *Circulatory support* Invasive haemodynamic monitoring with an arterial line and Swan-Ganz catheter aids the diagnosis and may be helpful in monitoring PCWP and cardiac output. A conservative fluid management approach improves outcome. Maintain cardiac output and O_2 delivery with inotropes (eg dobutamine 2.5–10μg/kg/min IVI), vasodilators, and blood transfusion. Consider treating pulmonary hypertension with low-dose (20–120 parts per million) nitric oxide, a pulmonary vasodilator. Haemofiltration may be needed in renal failure and to achieve a negative fluid balance.[50]
- *Sepsis* Identify organism(s) and treat accordingly. If clinically septic, but no organisms cultured, use empirical broad-spectrum antibiotics (p161). Avoid nephrotoxic antibiotics.
- *Other:* Nutritional support: enteral is best: p586 & p588, with high fat, antioxidant formulations. Steroids protect those at risk of fat embolization and with pneumocystosis and may improve outcome in subacute ARDS. Their role in established ARDS is controversial.[51,52]

Prognosis Overall mortality is 50%–75%. Prognosis varies with age of patient, cause of ARDS (pneumonia 86%, trauma 38%), and number of organs involved (3 organs involved for >1wk is 'invariably' fatal).

Risk factors for ARDS

Sepsis	Massive transfusion
Hypovolaemic shock	Burns (p858)
Trauma	Smoke inhalation (p859)
Pneumonia	Near drowning
Diabetic ketoacidosis	Acute pancreatitis
Gastric aspiration	DIC (p346)
Pregnancy	Head injury
Eclampsia	ICP↑
Amniotic fluid embolus	Fat embolus
Drugs/toxins	Heart/lung bypass
Paraquat, heroin, aspirin	Tumour lysis syndrome (p526)
Pulmonary contusion	Malaria

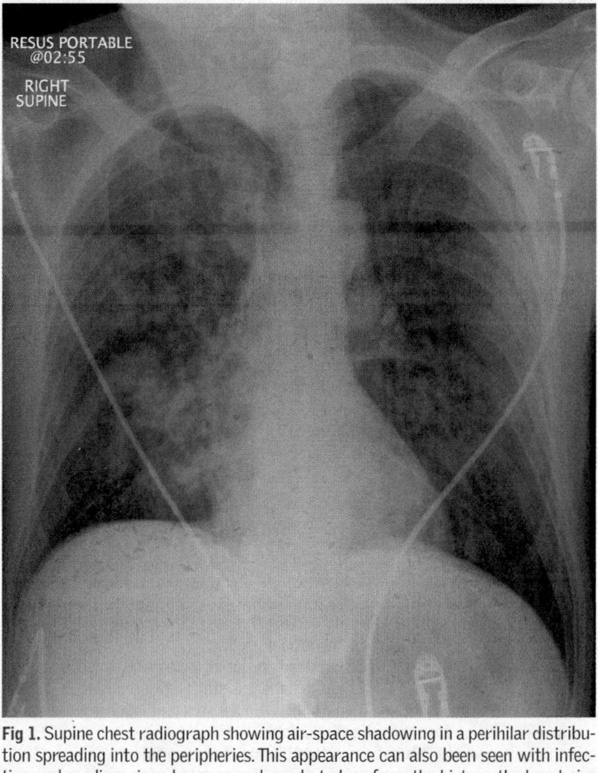

Fig 1. Supine chest radiograph showing air-space shadowing in a perihilar distribution spreading into the peripheries. This appearance can also been seen with infection and cardiogenic pulmonary oedema, but clues from the history, the heart size and lack of pleural effusions can suggest ARDS over the latter. Remember though, that this is a supine projection—the patient is lying flat with the X-ray beam AP—causing the cardiac shadow to be artificially enlarged and pleural effusions to level out on the posterior chest wall so they will not obscure the costophrenic angles unless very large.

Image courtesy of Nottingham University Hospitals NHS Trust Radiology Department

Respiratory failure occurs when gas exchange is inadequate, resulting in hypoxia. It is defined as a P_aO_2 <8kPa and subdivided into 2 types according to P_aCO_2 level.

Type I respiratory failure: defined as hypoxia (P_aO_2 <8kPa) with a normal or low P_aCO_2. It is caused primarily by ventilation/perfusion (V/Q) mismatch, e.g.:

- Pneumonia
- Pulmonary oedema
- PE
- Asthma
- Emphysema
- Fibrosing alveolitis
- ARDS (p178)

Type II respiratory failure: defined as hypoxia (P_aO_2 <8kPa) with hypercapnia (P_aCO_2 >6.0kPa). This is caused by alveolar hypoventilation, with or without V/Q mismatch. Causes include:

- *Pulmonary disease:* asthma, COPD, pneumonia, pulmonary fibrosis, obstructive sleep apnoea (OSA, p194).
- *Reduced respiratory drive:* sedative drugs, CNS tumour or trauma.
- *Neuromuscular disease:* cervical cord lesion, diaphragmatic paralysis, poliomyelitis, myasthenia gravis, Guillain-Barré syndrome.
- *Thoracic wall disease:* flail chest, kyphoscoliosis.

Clinical features are those of the underlying cause together with symptoms and signs of hypoxia, with or without hypercapnia.

Hypoxia: Dyspnoea; restlessness; agitation; confusion; central cyanosis. If longstanding hypoxia: polycythaemia; pulmonary hypertension; cor pulmonale.

Hypercapnia: Headache; peripheral vasodilatation; tachycardia; bounding pulse; tremor/flap; papilloedema; confusion; drowsiness; coma.

Investigations are aimed at determining the underlying cause:

- Blood tests: FBC, U&E, CRP, ABG.
- Radiology: CXR.
- Microbiology: sputum and blood cultures (if febrile).
- Spirometry (COPD, neuromuscular disease, Guillain-Barré syndrome).

Management depends on the cause:

Type I respiratory failure

- Treat underlying cause.
- Give oxygen (35–60%) by facemask to correct hypoxia.
- Assisted ventilation if P_aO_2 <8kPa despite 60% O_2.

Type II respiratory failure the respiratory centre may be relatively insensitive to CO_2 and respiration could be driven by hypoxia.

- Treat underlying cause.
- Controlled oxygen therapy: start at 24% O_2. ►*Oxygen therapy should be given with care.* Nevertheless, don't leave the hypoxia untreated.
- Recheck ABG after 20min. If P_aCO_2 is steady or lower, increase O_2 concentration to 28%. If P_aCO_2 has risen >1.5kPa and the patient is still hypoxic, consider a respiratory stimulant (eg doxapram 1.5–4mg/min IVI) or assisted ventilation (eg NIPPV, p823, ie non-invasive positive pressure ventilation).
- If this fails, consider intubation and ventilation, if appropriate.

Administering oxygen

Oxygen is usually given via a facemask or nasal cannulae. It is good practice to prescribe it—this avoids inadvertent administration of too much or too little. Titrate the amount guided by the SaO_2: aim for ~ 94-98% (or 88-92% if, or at risk of, hypercapnia); and the clinical condition of the patient. Humidification is only required for longer-term delivery of O_2 at high flow rates, tracheostomies, but may ↑ expectoration in bronchiectasis. ►Be careful in those with COPD (p822).

Nasal cannulae: preferred by patients, but O_2 delivery is relatively imprecise and may cause nasal soreness. The flow rate (1-4L/min) roughly defines the concentration of O_2 (24-40%). May be used to maintain SaO_2 when nebulizers need to be run using air eg COPD.

Simple face mask: delivers a variable amount of O_2 depending on the rate of inflow. Far less precise than venturi masks - so don't use if hypercapnia or type 2 respiratory failure. Risk of CO_2 accumulation (within the mask and so in inspired gas) if flow rate <5L/min.

Venturi mask: provide a precise % of O_2 (FiO_2) at high flow rates.
Colour codes:

24%	BLUE
8%	WHITE
5%	YELLOW
40%	RED
60%	GREEN

Start at 24-28% in COPD.

Non-rebreathing mask: these have a reservoir bag and deliver high concentrations of O_2 (60-90%), determined by the inflow (10-15L/min) and the presence of flap valves on the side. They are commonly used in emergencies, but are imprecise and should be avoided in those requiring controlled O_2 therapy.

Promoting oxygenation Other ways to ↑ oxygenation to reach the target SaO_2 (this should be given as a number on the drug chart):

- Treat anaemia (transfuse if essential)
- Improve cardiac output (treat heart failure)
- Chest physio to improve ventilation/perfusion mis-match.

When to consider ABG (arterial blood gas) measurement

- Any unexpected deterioration in an ill patient. (Technique: see p785).
- Anyone with an acute exacerbation of a chronic chest condition.
- Anyone with impaired consciousness or impaired respiratory effort.
- Signs of CO_2 retention, eg bounding pulse, drowsy, tremor (flapping), headache.
- Cyanosis, confusion, visual hallucinations (signs of P_aO_2↓; S_AO_2 is an alternative)
- To validate measurements from transcutaneous pulse oximetry (p156).

Pulmonary embolism (PE)

Causes PEs usually arise from a venous thrombosis in the pelvis or legs. Clots break off and pass through the veins and the right side of the heart before lodging in the pulmonary circulation. Rare causes include: right ventricular thrombus (post-MI); septic emboli (right-sided endocarditis); fat, air, or amniotic fluid embolism; neoplastic cells; parasites.

Risk factors
- Recent surgery, especially abdominal/pelvic or hip/knee replacement
- Thrombophilia, eg antiphospholipid syn. (p368)
- Leg fracture
- Prolonged bed rest/reduced mobility
- Malignancy
- Pregnancy/postpartum; Pill/HRT
- Previous PE

Clinical features These depend on the number, size, and distribution of the emboli; small emboli may be asymptomatic, whereas large emboli are often fatal.
Symptoms: Acute breathlessness, pleuritic chest pain, haemoptysis; dizziness; syncope. Ask about risk factors (above), past history or family history of thromboembolism. *Signs:* Pyrexia; cyanosis; tachypnoea; tachycardia; hypotension; raised JVP, pleural rub; pleural effusion. Look for signs of a cause, eg deep vein thrombosis.

Tests
- FBC, U&E, baseline clotting, D-dimers (BOX).
- ABG may show a $\downarrow P_aO_2$ and a $\downarrow P_aCO_2$.
- CXR may be normal, or show oligaemia of affected segment, dilated pulmonary artery, linear atelectasis, small pleural effusion, wedge-shaped opacities or cavitation (rare).
- ECG may be normal, or show tachycardia, right bundle branch block, right ventricular strain (inverted T in V_1 to V_4). The classical SI QIII TIII pattern (p92) is rare.

►Further investigations are shown on p828; see also BOX, p753.

Treatment ►►See p828. Anticoagulate with LMW heparin (p828). Start warfarin (p344). Stop heparin when INR is >2 and continue warfarin for a minimum of 3 months (see p345); aim for an INR of 2-3. Thrombolysis for massive PE (50mg bolus of alteplase). Consider placement of a *vena caval filter* in patients who develop emboli despite adequate anticoagulation (NB increased risk if placed without concomitant anticoagulation).

Prevention Give heparin (eg dalteparin 2500U/24h SC) to all immobile patients. Prescribe compression stockings and encourage early mobilization. Stop HRT and the Pill pre-op (if reliable with another form of contraception). If past or family history of thromboembolism, consider investigation for thrombophilia (p368).

Pneumothorax

Management ►►p824.

Causes Often spontaneous (especially in young thin men) due to rupture of a subpleural bulla. Other causes: asthma; COPD; TB; pneumonia; lung abscess; carcinoma; cystic fibrosis; lung fibrosis; sarcoidosis; connective tissue disorders (Marfan's sy., Ehlers-Danlos sy.), trauma; iatrogenic (subclavian CVP line insertion, pleural aspiration or biopsy, transbronchial biopsy, percutaneous liver biopsy, +ve pressure ventilation).

Clinical features *Symptoms:* There may be no symptoms (especially if fit, young and small pneumothorax) or there may be sudden onset of dyspnoea and/or pleuritic chest pain. Patients with asthma or COPD may present with a sudden deterioration. Mechanically ventilated patients may present with hypoxia or an increase in ventilation pressures. *Signs:* Reduced expansion, hyper-resonance to percussion and diminished breath sounds on the affected side. *With a tension pneumothorax, the trachea will be deviated away from the affected side.* See X-ray p763.

►►**Managing a tension pneumothorax** See p824. Placing a chest drain, ►►p780.

Investigating suspected PE

Diagnosis of PE is improved by adopting a stepwise approach, combining an objective probability score, with subsequent investigations, as follows.

Assess the clinical probability of a PE: many systems exist and are usually based around elements drawn from the history and clinical examination

Scoring system for investigation of suspected DVT*

Feature	Score
Active cancer, or treatment within 6 months	1
Paralysis, paresis, or recent plaster immobilization of lower limbs	1
Recently bed-ridden (>3 days) or major surgery (< 4weeks)	1
Localized tenderness along venous system	1
Entire leg swollen	1
Calf circumference >3cm more than other side, 10cm below tibial tuberosity	1
Pitting oedema > than in asymptomatic leg	1
Collateral superficial veins	1
Alternative diagnosis as likely, or more likely, than DVT	-2
Total score: 0=low probability; 1–2 moderate probability; ≥3 high probability	

*Adapted from Wells et al. *Lancet* 1997 350 1795

D-dimers: only perform in those patients **without** a high probability of a PE. A negative D-dimer test effectively excludes a PE in those with a low or intermediate clinical probability, and imaging is NOT required. However, a positive test does not prove a diagnosis of a PE, and imaging is required.

Imaging: The conventional 1st-line, if the CXR is normal, was a V/Q *scan* (p158, p752 & p828; look for perfusion defects with no corresponding ventilation defects). If 'normal', a PE is reliably excluded. If non-diagnostic, further imaging is required, but may give some false positives. The recommended 1st-line imaging modality is now CT pulmonary angiography (**CTPA**), which can show clots down to 5th-order pulmonary arteries (after the 4th branching). This may also be useful for subjects with indeterminate isotope scans. Bilateral leg ultrasound (or rarely venograms) may also be sufficient to **confirm**, but not exclude, a PE in patients with a co-existing clinical DVT.

Pleural effusion

Definitions A pleural effusion is fluid in the pleural space. Effusions can be divided by their protein concentration into *transudates* (<25g/L) and *exudates* (>35g/L), see BOX. Blood in the pleural space is a *haemothorax*, pus in the pleural space is an *empyema*, and chyle (lymph with fat) is a *chylothorax*. Both blood and air in the pleural space is called a *haemopneumothorax*.

Causes *Transudates* may be due to ↑venous pressure (cardiac failure, constrictive pericarditis, fluid overload), or hypoproteinaemia (cirrhosis, nephrotic syndrome, malabsorption). Also occur in hypothyroidism and Meigs' syndrome (right pleural effusion and ovarian fibroma). ***Exudates*** are mostly due to increased leakiness of pleural capillaries secondary to infection, inflammation, or malignancy. Causes: pneumonia; TB; pulmonary infarction; rheumatoid arthritis; SLE; bronchogenic carcinoma; malignant metastases; lymphoma; mesothelioma; lymphangitis carcinomatosis.

Symptoms Asymptomatic—or dyspnoea, pleuritic chest pain.

Signs *Decreased expansion; stony dull percussion note; diminished breath sounds* occur on the affected side. Tactile vocal fremitus and vocal resonance are ↓ (inconstant and unreliable). Above the effusion, where lung is compressed, there may be *bronchial breathing*. With large effusions there may be *tracheal deviation* away from the effusion. Look for aspiration marks and signs of associated disease: malignancy (cachexia, clubbing, lymphadenopathy, radiation marks, mastectomy scar); stigmata of chronic liver disease; cardiac failure; hypothyroidism; rheumatoid arthritis; butterfly rash of SLE.

Tests *CXR:* Small effusions blunt the costophrenic angles, larger ones are seen as water-dense shadows with concave upper borders. A completely horizontal upper border implies that there is also a pneumothorax. (See **fig 1**; **figs 1&2**,p737).

Ultrasound is useful in identifying the presence of pleural fluid and in guiding diagnostic or therapeutic aspiration.

Diagnostic aspiration: Percuss the upper border of the pleural effusion and choose a site 1 or 2 intercostal spaces below it (don't go too low or you'll be in the abdomen!). Infiltrate down to the pleura with 5-10mL of 1% lidocaine. Attach a 21G needle to a syringe and insert it just above the upper border of an appropriate rib (avoids neurovascular bundle). Draw off 10-30mL of pleural fluid and send it to the lab for *clinical chemistry* (protein, glucose, pH, LDH, amylase), *bacteriology* (microscopy and culture, auramine stain, TB culture), *cytology* and, if indicated, *immunology* (rheumatoid factor, ANA, complement).

Pleural biopsy: If pleural fluid analysis is inconclusive, consider parietal pleural biopsy with an Abrams' needle. See p778 for details. Thoracoscopic or CT-guided pleural biopsy increases diagnostic yield (by enabling direct visualization of the pleural cavity and biopsy of suspicious areas).

Management is of the underlying cause.

- ***Drainage*** If the effusion is symptomatic, drain it, repeatedly if necessary. Fluid is best removed slowly (≤2L/24h). It may be aspirated in the same way as a diagnostic tap, or using an intercostal drain (see p780).
- ***Pleurodesis*** with tetracycline, bleomycin, or talc may be helpful for recurrent effusions. Thorascopic talc pleurodesis is most effective for malignant effusions. Empyemas (p164) are best drained using a chest drain, inserted under ultrasound or CT guidance.
- ***Intra-pleural streptokinase*** Of no benefit.
- ***Surgery:*** Persistent collections and increasing pleural thickness (on ultrasound) requires surgery.[56]

Pleural fluid analysis

Gross appearance	*Cause*
Clear, straw-coloured	Transudate, exudate
Turbid, yellow	Empyema, parapneumonic effusion[1]
Haemorrhagic	Trauma, malignancy, pulmonary infarction
Cytology	
Neutrophils ++	Parapneumonic effusion, PE
Lymphocytes ++	Malignancy, TB, RA, SLE, sarcoidosis
Mesothelial cells ++	Pulmonary infarction
Abnormal mesothelial cells	Mesothelioma
Multinucleated giant cells	RA
Lupus erythematosus cells	SLE
Clinical chemistry	
Protein <25g/L	Transudate
>35g/L	Exudate
25–35g/L	If pleural fluid protein/serum protein >0.5, effusion is an exudate
Glucose <3.3mmol/L	Empyema, malignancy, TB, RA, SLE
pH <7.2	Empyema, malignancy, TB, RA, SLE
LDH↑ (pleural:serum >0.6)	Empyema, malignancy, TB, RA, SLE
Amylase↑	Pancreatitis, carcinoma, bacterial pneumonia, oesophageal rupture
Immunology	
Rheumatoid factor	RA
Antinuclear antibody	SLE
Complement levels↓	RA, SLE, malignancy, infection

1 Inflammation of the pleura caused by pneumonia may lead to infected pleural fluid (empyema); if it is not infected, the term parapneumonic effusion is used.

Sarcoidosis

A multisystem granulomatous disorder of unknown cause. Prevalence highest in Northern Europe, eg UK: 10-20/10^5 population. Usually affects adults aged 20-40yrs, more common in women. AfroCaribbeans are affected more frequently and more severely than Caucasians, particularly by extra-thoracic disease. Associated with HLA-DRB1 and DQB1 alleles.

Clinical features In 20–40%, the disease is discovered incidentally, after a routine CXR, and is thus asymptomatic. ***Acute sarcoidosis*** often presents with erythema nodosum (**fig 1**, p564)[1] ± polyarthralgia. It usually resolves spontaneously.

Pulmonary disease 90% have abnormal CXRs with bilateral hilar lymphadenopathy (**BHL, fig 1**) ± pulmonary infiltrates or fibrosis; see below for staging. *Symptoms:* Dry cough, progressive dyspnoea, ↓exercise tolerance and chest pain. In 10-20% symptoms progress, with concurrent deterioration in lung function.

Non-pulmonary signs are legion: lymphadenopathy; hepatomegaly; splenomegaly; uveitis; conjunctivitis; keratoconjunctivitis sicca; glaucoma; terminal phalangeal bone cysts; enlargement of lacrimal & parotid glands (**fig 5** on p349); Bell's palsy; neuropathy; meningitis; brainstem and spinal syndromes; space-occupying lesion; erythema nodosum (**fig 1**, p564); lupus pernio; subcutaneous nodules; cardiomyopathy; arrhythmias; hypercalcaemia; hypercalciuria; renal stones; pituitary dysfunction.

Tests *Blood:* ↑ESR, lymphopenia, LFT↑, serum ACE↑ in ~60% (nonspecific), ↑Ca^{2+}, ↑immunoglobulins. ***24h urine:*** Ca^{2+}↑. ***Tuberculin skin test*** is -ve in two-thirds; ***CXR*** is abnormal in 90%: *Stage 0:* normal. *Stage 1:* BHL. *Stage 2:* BHL + peripheral pulmonary infiltrates. *Stage 3:* peripheral pulmonary infiltrates alone. *Stage 4:* progressive pulmonary fibrosis; bulla formation (honeycombing); pleural involvement. ***ECG*** may show arrhythmias or bundle branch block. ***Lung function tests*** may be normal or show reduced lung volumes, impaired gas transfer, and a restrictive ventilatory defect. ***Tissue biopsy*** (lung, liver, lymph nodes, skin nodules, or lacrimal glands) is diagnostic and shows non-caseating granulomata. ***Kveim tests*** are now obsolete.

Bronchoalveolar lavage (BAL) shows ↑lymphocytes in active disease; ↑neutrophils with pulmonary fibrosis.

Ultrasound may show nephrocalcinosis or hepatosplenomegaly.

Bone X-rays show 'punched out' lesions in terminal phalanges.

CT/MRI may be useful in assessing severity of pulmonary disease or diagnosing neurosarcoidosis. ***Ophthalmology assessment*** (slit lamp examination, fluorescein angiography) is indicated in ocular disease.

Management[57] ►*Patients with BHL alone don't need treatment as most recover spontaneously.* ***Acute sarcoidosis:*** Bed rest, NSAIDs.

Indications for corticosteroids:

- Parenchymal lung disease (symptomatic, static, or progressive)
- Uveitis
- Hypercalcaemia
- Neurological or cardiac involvement.

Prednisolone (40mg/24h) PO for 4-6 wks, then ↓dose over 1yr according to clinical status. A few patients relapse and may need a further course or long-term therapy.

Other therapy: In severe illness, IV **methylprednisolone** or immunosuppressants (**methotrexate**, **hydroxychloroquine**, **ciclosporin**, **cyclophosphamide**) may be needed. Anti-TNFα therapy may be tried in refractory cases, or lung transplantation.

Prognosis 60% of patients with thoracic sarcoidosis resolve over 2yrs. 20% respond to steroid therapy; in the rest, improvement is unlikely despite therapy.

1 A detailed history and exam (including for synovitis) + CXR, 2 ASO-titres & a tuberculin skin test is usually enough to diagnose erythema nodosum: R Pugol 2000 *Arthr Rheu* **43** 584

2 ACE is also ↑ in: hyperthyroidism, Gaucher's, silicosis, TB, hypersensitivity pneumonitis, asbestosis, pneumocystosis. ACE levels may help monitor sarcoidosis activity. ↑ACE levels in CSF help diagnose CNS sarcoidosis (when serum ACE-i may be normal). ACE is *lower* in: Caucasians; and anorexia.

Causes of BHL (bilateral hilar lymphadenopathy)

- Sarcoidosis
- Infection eg TB, mycoplasma
- Malignancy, eg lymphoma, carcinoma, mediastinal tumours
- Organic dust disease, eg silicosis, berylliosis
- Extrinsic allergic alveolitis
- Histocytosis X

Differential diagnosis of granulomatous diseases

Infections	Bacteria	TB, leprosy, syphilis
		Cat scratch fever
	Fungi	*Cryptococcus neoformans*
		Coccidioides immitis
	Protozoa	Schistosomiasis
Autoimmune	Primary biliary cirrhosis	
	Granulomatous orchitis	
Vasculitis (p558)	Giant cell arteritis	
	Polyarteritis nodosa	
	Takayasu's arteritis	
	Wegener's granulomatosis	
Organic dust disease	Silicosis, berylliosis	
Idiopathic	Crohn's disease	
	de Quervain's thyroiditis	
	Sarcoidosis	
Extrinsic allergic alveolitis		
Histiocytosis X		

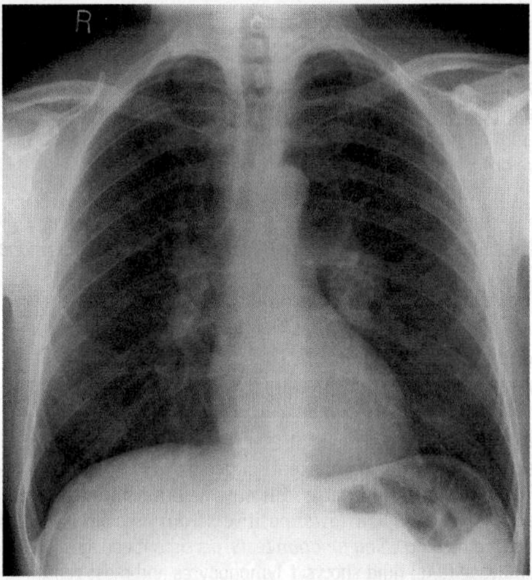

Fig 1. PA chest radiograph showing bilateral hilar lymphadenopathy. The important differentials for this appearance are: sarcoidosis, TB, lymphoma, pneumoconioses and metastatic disease. This patient has sarcoidosis but there are no other stigmata (such as the presence of infiltrates, fibrosis and honeycombing) on this image.

Image courtesy of Norfolk and Norwich University Hospitals NHS Trust Radiology Department

Interstitial lung disease (ILD)

This is the generic term used to describe a number of conditions that primarily affect the lung parenchyma in a diffuse manner. They are characterized by chronic inflammation and/or progressive interstitial fibrosis, and share a number of clinical and pathological features. See BOX and **fig 1**.

Clinical features Dyspnoea on exertion; non-productive paroxysmal cough; abnormal breath sounds; abnormal CXR or high resolution CT; restrictive pulmonary spirometry with a reduced DLCO (p158).

Pathological features Fibrosis and remodelling of the interstitium; chronic inflammation; hyperplasia of type II epithelial cells or type II pneumocytes.

Classification The ILDs can be broadly grouped into three categories:

Those with known cause, eg
- Occupational/environmental, eg asbestosis, berylliosis, silicosis, cotton workers' lung (byssinosis).
- Drugs, eg nitrofurantoin, bleomycin, amiodarone, sulfasalazine, busulfan
- Hypersensitivity reactions, eg extrinsic allergic alveolitis
- Infections, eg TB, fungi, viral

Those associated with systemic disorders, eg
- Sarcoidosis
- Rheumatoid arthritis
- SLE, systemic sclerosis, mixed connective tissue disease, Sjögren's syndrome
- Ulcerative colitis, renal tubular acidosis, autoimmune thyroid disease

Idiopathic, eg
- Idiopathic pulmonary fibrosis (IPF)/cryptogenic fibrosing alveolitis (p190)
- Cryptogenic organizing pneumonia
- Lymphocytic interstitial pneumonia

Extrinsic allergic alveolitis (EAA)

In sensitized individuals, inhalation of allergens (fungal spores or avian proteins) provokes a hypersensitivity reaction. In the acute phase, the alveoli are infiltrated with acute inflammatory cells. With chronic exposure, granuloma formation and obliterative bronchiolitis occur.

Causes
- Bird-fancier's and pigeon-fancier's lung (proteins in bird droppings).
- Farmer's and mushroom worker's lung (*Micropolyspora faeni, Thermoactinomyces vulgaris*).
- Malt worker's lung (*Aspergillus clavatus*).
- Bagassosis or sugar workers' lung (*Thermoactinomyces sacchari*).

Clinical features *4–6h post-exposure:* Fever, rigors, myalgia, dry cough, dyspnoea, crackles (no wheeze). *Chronic:* Increasing dyspnoea, weight↓, exertional dyspnoea, Type I respiratory failure, cor pulmonale.

Tests *Acute:* Blood: FBC (neutrophilia); ESR↑; ABGs; positive serum precipitins (indicate exposure only). *CXR:* upper-zone mottling/consolidation; hilar lymphadenopathy (rare). *Lung function tests:* reversible restrictive defect; reduced gas transfer during acute attacks. *Chronic: Blood tests:* positive serum precipitins. *CXR:* upper-zone fibrosis; honeycomb lung. *Lung function tests:* persistent changes (see above). Bronchoalveolar lavage (BAL) fluid shows ↑ lymphocytes and mast cells.

Management *Acute attack:* Remove allergen and give O_2 (35–60%), then: Oral prednisolone (40mg/24h PO), followed by reducing dose.

Chronic: Avoid exposure to allergens, or wear a face mask or +ve pressure helmet. Long-term steroids often achieve CXR and physiological improvement. Compensation (UK Industrial Injuries Act) may be payable.

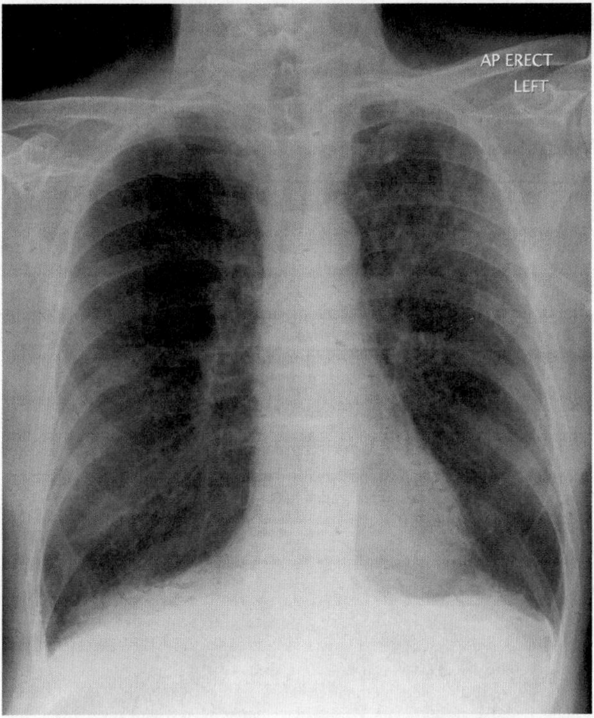

Fig 1. AP chest radiograph showing air-space shadowing in the left upper zone (compare the relative lucency with the right upper zone). Although this appearance often represents infection (ie pneumonia), it is nonspecific. Important differentials to remember for this distribution of shadowing include lymphoma, alveolar cell carcinoma (both to be considered if not resolving in appearance on follow-up imaging), and haemorrhage.

Image courtesy of Nottingham University Hospitals NHS Trust Radiology Department

Causes of fibrotic shadowing on a CXR

Upper zone	Mid zone	Lower zone
• TB • Extrinsic allergic alveolitis • Ankylosing spondylitis • Radiotherapy • Sarcoidosis, histoplasmosis	• Progressive massive fibrosis (PMF)	• Idiopathic pulmonary fibrosis • Asbestosis

Idiopathic pulmonary fibrosis (IPF)

This is a type of idiopathic interstitial pneumonia. Inflammatory cell infiltrate and pulmonary fibrosis of unknown cause (also known as cryptogenic fibrosing alveolitis). The commonest cause of interstitial lung disease.

Symptoms Dry cough; exertional dyspnoea; malaise; weight↓; arthralgia.

Signs Cyanosis; finger clubbing; fine end-inspiratory crepitations.

Complications Respiratory failure; increased risk of lung cancer.

Tests *Blood:* ABG (P_aO_2↓; P_aCO_2↑); CRP↑; immunoglobulins↑; ANA (30% +ve), rheumatoid factor (10% +ve). *CXR:* (**fig 1**) Lung volume↓; bilateral lower zone reticulo-nodular shadows; honeycomb lung (advanced disease). CT shows similar changes to the CXR but is more sensitive and is an essential tool for diagnosis. *Spirometry:* Restrictive (p156); ↓transfer factor. *BAL* (bronchoalveolar lavage) may indicate activity of alveolitis: lymphocytes↑ (good response/prognosis) or neutrophils and eosinophils↑ (poor response/prognosis). *⁹⁹TCm-DTPA scan:* (diethylene-triamine-penta-acetic acid) may reflect disease activity. *Lung biopsy* may be needed for diagnosis.[59] The histological changes observed on biopsy are referred to as *usual interstitial pneumonia* (UIP).

Management Best supportive care: oxygen, pulmonary rehabilitation, opiates, palliative care input. It is strongly recommended that high-dose steroids are **NOT** used except where the diagnosis of IPF is in doubt. All patients should be considered for current clinical trials **lung transplantation.**[60]

Prognosis 50% 5yr survival rate (range 1-20yrs).

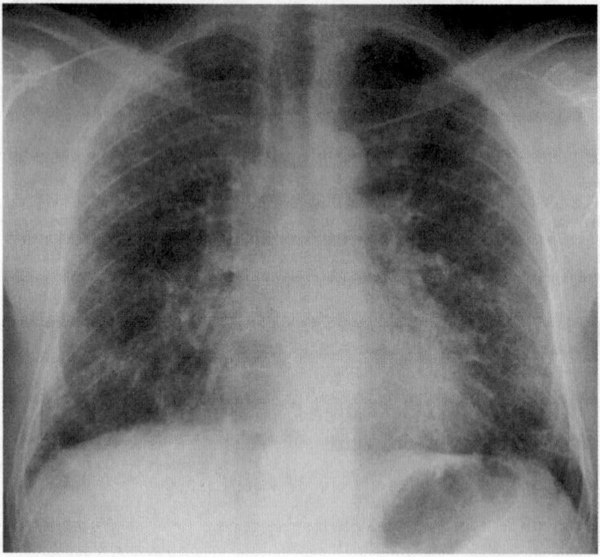

Fig 1. Interstitial lung disease due to idiopathic pulmonary fibrosis (a similar appearance to the interstitial oedema of moderate left heart failure, but without a big heart).

Courtesy of Prof P Scally

Coal worker's pneumoconiosis (CWP) A common dust disease in countries that have or have had underground coal-mines. It results from inhalation of coal dust particles (1.5–2.5μm in diameter) over 15–20yrs. These are ingested by macrophages which die, releasing their enzymes and causing fibrosis.

Clinical features: Asymptomatic, but co-existent chronic bronchitis is common. CXR: many round opacities (1–10mm), especially in upper zone.

Management: Avoid exposure to coal dust; treat co-existing chronic bronchitis; claim compensation (in the UK via the Industrial Injuries Act).

Progressive massive fibrosis (PMF) is due to progression of CWP, which causes progressive dyspnoea, fibrosis, and, eventually, cor pulmonale. CXR: upper-zone fibrotic masses (1–10cm).

Management: Avoid exposure to coal dust; claim compensation (as above).

Caplan's syndrome is the association between rheumatoid arthritis, pneumoconiosis, and pulmonary rheumatoid nodules.

Silicosis is caused by inhalation of silica particles, which are very fibrogenic. A number of jobs may be associated with exposure, eg metal mining, stone quarrying, sandblasting, and pottery/ceramic manufacture.

Clinical features: Progressive dyspnoea, ↑incidence of TB, CXR shows diffuse miliary or nodular pattern in upper and mid-zones and egg-shell calcification of hilar nodes. Spirometry: restrictive ventilatory defect.

Management: Avoid exposure to silica; claim compensation (as above).

Asbestosis is caused by inhalation of asbestos fibres. Chrysotile (white asbestos) is the least fibrogenic—crocidolite (blue asbestos) is the most fibrogenic. Amosite (brown asbestos) is the least common and has intermediate fibrogenicity. Asbestos was commonly used in the building trade for fire proofing, pipe lagging, electrical wire insulation, and roofing felt. Degree of asbestos exposure is related to degree of pulmonary fibrosis.

Clinical features: Similar to other fibrotic lung diseases with progressive dyspnoea, clubbing, and fine end-inspiratory crackles. Also causes pleural plaques, ↑risk of bronchial adenocarcinoma and mesothelioma.

Management: Symptomatic. Patients are often eligible for compensation through the UK Industrial Injuries Act.

Malignant mesothelioma is a tumour of mesothelial cells that usually occurs in the pleura, and rarely in the peritoneum or other organs. It is associated with occupational exposure to asbestos but the relationship is complex. 90% report previous exposure to asbestos, but only 20% of patients have pulmonary asbestosis. The latent period between first exposure and development of the tumour may be up to 45yrs.

Clinical features: Chest pain, dyspnoea, weight loss, finger clubbing, recurrent pleural effusions. Signs of metastases: lymphadenopathy, hepatomegaly, bone pain/tenderness, abdominal pain/obstruction (peritoneal malignant mesothelioma).

Tests: CXR or CT: pleural thickening/effusion. Bloody pleural fluid.

Diagnosis is made on histology, following a pleural biopsy—obtained at thoracoscopy. Often the diagnosis is only made post-mortem.

Management: Pemetrexed (Alimta®) + cisplatin chemotherapy can improve survival. Surgery is hard to evaluate (few randomized trials). Radiotherapy is controversial.

Prognosis is poor (especially without treatment), eg <2yrs.

Coal worker's pneumoconiosis (CWP) A common dust disease in countries that have or have had underground coal-mines. It results from inhalation of coal dust particles (1-3μm in diameter) over 15-20yrs. These are ingested by macrophages which die, releasing their enzymes and causing fibrosis.

Clinical features: Asymptomatic, but co-existing chronic bronchitis is common. CXR: many round opacities (1-10mm), especially upper zone.

Management: Avoid exposure to coal dust; treat co-existing chronic bronchitis; claim compensation (in the UK, *via* the Industrial Injuries Act).

Progressive massive fibrosis (PMF) is due to progression of CWP, which causes progressive dyspnoea, fibrosis, and eventually, cor pulmonale. CXR: upper-zone fibrotic masses (1-10cm).

Management: Avoid exposure to coal dust; claim compensation (as above).

Caplan's syndrome is the association between rheumatoid arthritis, pneumoconiosis, and pulmonary rheumatoid nodules.

Silicosis (see **fig 1**) is caused by inhalation of silica particles, which are very fibrogenic. A number of jobs may be associated with exposure, eg metal mining, stone quarrying, sandblasting, and pottery/ceramic manufacture.

Clinical features: Progressive dyspnoea, ↑incidence of TB, CXR shows diffuse miliary or nodular pattern in upper and mid-zones and egg-shell calcification of hilar nodes. Spirometry: restrictive ventilatory defect.

Management: Avoid exposure to silica; claim compensation (as above).

Asbestosis is caused by inhalation of asbestos fibres. Chrysotile (white asbestos) is the least fibrogenic—crocidolite (blue asbestos) is the most fibrogenic. Amosite (brown asbestos) is the least common and has intermediate fibrogenicity. Asbestos was commonly used in the building trade for fire proofing, pipe lagging, electrical wire insulation, and roofing felt. Degree of asbestos exposure is related to degree of pulmonary fibrosis.

Clinical features: Similar to other fibrotic lung diseases with progressive dyspnoea, clubbing, and fine end-inspiratory crackles. Also causes pleural plaques, ↑risk of bronchial adenocarcinoma and mesothelioma.

Management: Symptomatic. Patients are often eligible for compensation through the UK Industrial Injuries Act.

Malignant mesothelioma is a tumour of mesothelial cells that usually occurs in the pleura, and rarely in the peritoneum or other organs. It is associated with occupational exposure to asbestos but the relationship is complex.[61] 90% report previous exposure to asbestos, but only 20% of patients have pulmonary asbestosis. The latent period between exposure and development of the tumour may be up to 45yrs.

Clinical features: Chest pain, dyspnoea, weight loss, finger clubbing, recurrent pleural effusions. Signs of metastases: lymphadenopathy, hepatomegaly, bone pain/tenderness, abdominal pain/obstruction (peritoneal malignant mesothelioma).

Tests: CXR/CT: pleural thickening/effusion. Bloody pleural fluid.

Diagnosis is made on histology, following a pleural biopsy—Abrams' needle (p778), thoracoscopy. Often the diagnosis is only made post-mortem.

Management: **Pemetrexed** (Alimta®) + **cisplatin** chemotherapy can improve survival.[62] Surgery is hard to evaluate (few randomized trials). Radiotherapy is controversial.

Prognosis is poor (especially without pemetrexed, eg <2yrs). >650 deaths/yr in UK.

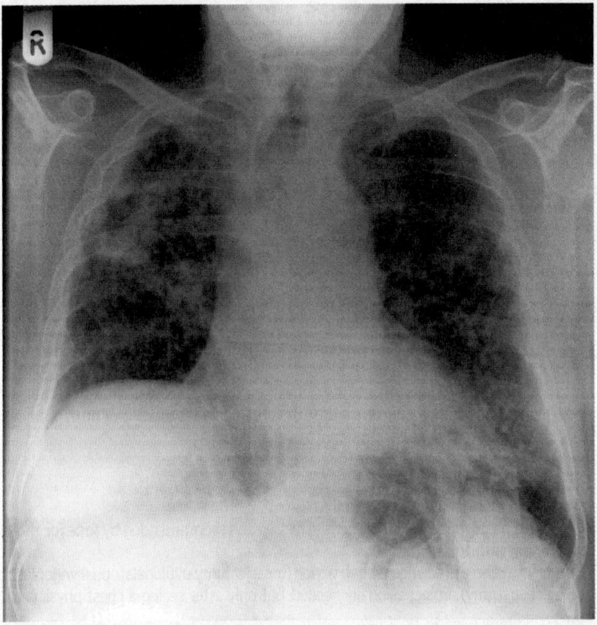

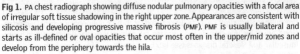

Fig 1. PA chest radiograph showing diffuse nodular pulmonary opacities with a focal area of irregular soft tissue shadowing in the right upper zone. Appearances are consistent with silicosis and developing progressive massive fibrosis (PMF). PMF is usually bilateral and starts as ill-defined or oval opacities that occur most often in the upper/mid zones and develop from the periphery towards the hila.

Image courtesy of Derby Hospitals NHS Foundation Trust Radiology Department

Obstructive sleep apnoea syndrome

This disorder is characterized by intermittent closure/collapse of the pharyngeal airway causing apnoeic episodes during sleep. These are terminated by partial arousal.

Clinical features The typical patient is a obese, middle-aged man who presents because of snoring or daytime somnolence. His partner often describes apnoeic episodes during sleep.

- Loud snoring
- Daytime somnolence
- Poor sleep quality
- Morning headache
- Decreased libido
- Cognitive performance↓

Complications Pulmonary hypertension; Type II respiratory failure (p180). Sleep apnoea is also reported as an independent risk factor for hypertension.[63]

Investigations Simple studies (eg pulse oximetry, video recordings) may be all that are required for diagnosis. Polysomnography (which monitors oxygen saturation, airflow at the nose and mouth, ECG, EMG chest and abdominal wall movement during sleep) is diagnostic. The occurrence of 15 or more episodes of apnoea or hypopnoea during 1h of sleep indicates significant sleep apnoea.

Management[64]

- Weight reduction
- Avoidance of tobacco and alcohol
- CPAP via a nasal mask during sleep is effective and recommended by NICE for those with moderate to severe disease.[65]
- Surgery to relieve pharyngeal obstruction (tonsillectomy, uvulopalatopharyngoplasty, or tracheostomy) are occasionally needed, but only after seeing a chest physician.

Cor pulmonale

Cor pulmonale is right heart failure caused by chronic pulmonary arterial hypertension. Causes include chronic lung disease, pulmonary vascular disorders, and neuromuscular and skeletal diseases (see BOX).

Clinical features Symptoms include dyspnoea, fatigue, or syncope. Signs: cyanosis; tachycardia; raised JVP with prominent *a* and *v* waves; RV heave; loud P_2, pansystolic murmur (tricuspid regurgitation); early diastolic Graham Steell murmur; hepatomegaly and oedema.

Investigations *FBC:* Hb and haematocrit↑ (secondary polycythaemia). *ABG:* hypoxia, with or without hypercapnia. *CXR:* enlarged right atrium and ventricle, prominent pulmonary arteries (see **fig 1**). *ECG:* P pulmonale; right axis deviation; right ventricular hypertrophy/strain.

Management

- *Treat underlying cause*—eg COPD and pulmonary infections.
- *Treat respiratory failure*—in the acute situation give 24% oxygen if P_aO_2 <8kPa. Monitor ABG and gradually increase oxygen concentration if P_aCO_2 is stable (p180). In COPD patients, long-term oxygen therapy (LTOT) for 15h/d increases survival (p176). Patients with chronic hypoxia when clinically stable should be assessed for LTOT.
- *Treat cardiac failure* with diuretics such as furosemide, eg 40-160mg/24h PO. Monitor U&E and give amiloride or potassium supplements if necessary. Alternative: spironolactone.
- Consider *venesection* if haematocrit >55%.
- Consider *heart-lung transplantation* in young patients.

Prognosis Poor. 50% die within 5yrs.

Causes of cor pulmonale

Lung disease
- Asthma (severe, chronic)
- COPD
- Bronchiectasis
- Pulmonary fibrosis
- Lung resection

Pulmonary vascular disease
- Pulmonary emboli
- Pulmonary vasculitis
- Primary pulmonary hypertension
- ARDS (p170)
- Sickle-cell disease
- Parasite infestation

Thoracic cage abnormality
- Kyphosis
- Scoliosis
- Thoracoplasty

Neuromuscular disease
- Myasthenia gravis
- Poliomyelitis
- Motor neuron disease

Hypoventilation
- Sleep apnoea
- Enlarged adenoids in children

Cerebrovascular disease

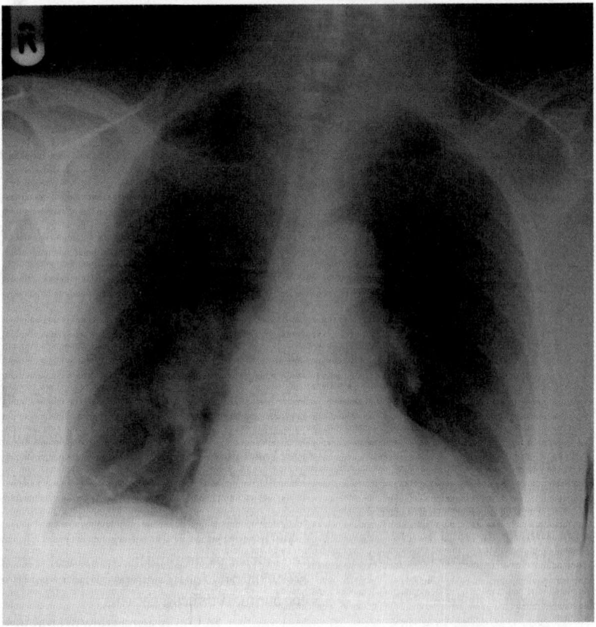

Fig 1. PA chest radiograph showing enlarged pulmonary arteries from pulmonary artery hypertension. When caused by interstitial lung disease and leading to right heart failure, this would be termed cor pulmonale. No signs of interstitial lung disease are identifiable in this image.

Image courtesy of Derby Hospitals NHS Foundation Trust Radiology Department

Contents

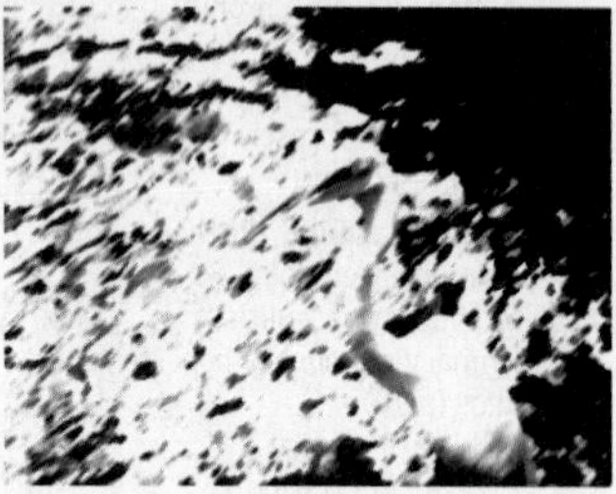

Fig 1. In German, **Gestalt** means both *the whole* form (as being more than the sum of its parts) and *the pattern*. A gestalt has come to mean (in WH Auden's words)[1] the place where indiscrete perceptions and extensions meet and new meanings are created. The ideal endocrinologist is a master of gestalt pattern-recognition (myxoedema, acromegaly, and the rest—see p 197). On viewing the above, he or she sees the dots and the bird, but does not get *too* carried away by filling in the gaps.[2]

Nor is he or she put off by missing or paradoxical data (eg *increase* in weight in thyrotoxicosis, seen in up to 30%).[3]

Egrets of course tend to nest together, and it is a common endocrine occurrence to find hypothyroidism nested inside hypopituitarism, or autoimmune diabetes nested within Addison's disease. So always ask yourself "What else is being revealed?" and "What else is being concealed?"—think (if you dare) of those ruptured ectopic pregnancies which conceal thyrotoxic storms[4] and how your antenatal β-blockers mask a phaeochromocytoma until parturition engenders its eruption. Prepare your mind not with our single images of endocrinopathies but with entire galleries.

With **inverse gestalt** we deconstruct an all too familiar picture into its component dots to see what new forms emerge: a useful method for our most difficult patients..

Image courtesy of Louis Vinke

Relevant pages in other chapters:
Diabetic ketoacidosis (►►p842); hypoglycaemia (►►p844); surgery and diabetes (p590); the eye in diabetes (*OHCS* p446); thyroid emergencies (►►p844); thyroid lumps (p602); Addison's disease, thyroid disease, and surgery (p593); Addisonian crisis and hypopituitary coma (►►p846); phaeochromocytoma emergencies (►►p846).

The endocrinology of food behaviour, mood, and obesity:
Cholecystokinin, GLP-1, ghrelin, and peptide YY etc: *OHCS* p530.

In dermatology (endocrine control of sebocytes via CRH): *OHCS* p583.

In pregnancy: Thyroid disease: *OHCS* p25; diabetes in pregnancy: *OHCS* p24.

In childhood: Childhood diabetes: *OHCS* p186; thyroid problems: *OHCS* p182.

We thank Dr Stephen Gilbey who is our Specialist Reader for this chapter.

The essence of endocrinology—for scientists

- Define a syndrome, and match it to a gland malfunction.
- Measure the gland's output in the peripheral blood. Define clinical syndromes associated with too much or too little secretion (*hyper-* and *hypo*-syndromes, respectively; *eu-* means normal, neither ↑ nor ↓, as in *euthyroid*). Note factors that may make measurement variable, eg diurnal release of cortisol.
- If suspecting hormone deficiency, test by stimulating the gland that produces it (eg short ACTH stimulation test or *Synacthen*® test in Addison's). If the gland is not functioning normally, there will be a blunted response to stimulation.
- If suspecting hormone excess, test by inhibiting the gland that produces it (eg dexamethasone suppression test in Cushing's). If there is a hormone secreting tumour then this will fail to suppress via normal feedback mechanisms.
- Find a way to image the gland. NB: non-functioning tumours or 'incidentalomas' may be found in health, see p216. Imaging alone does not make the diagnosis.
- Aim to halt disease progression; diet and exercise can stop progression of impaired fasting glucose to frank diabetes.[5] For other glands, halting progression will depend on understanding autoimmunity, and the interaction of genes and environment. In thyroid autoimmunity (an archetypal autoimmune disease), it is possible to track interactions between genes and environment (eg smoking and stress) via expression of immunologically active molecules (HLA class I & II, adhesion molecules, cytokines, CD40, and complement regulatory proteins).[6]

Endocrinologists love this reductionist approach, but have been less successful at understanding ***emergent phenomena***—those properties and performances of ours which cannot be predicted from full knowledge of our perturbed parts.[7] We understand the diurnal nature of cortisol secretion, for example, but the science of relating this to dreams, the consolidation of memory, and the psychopathology of families and other groups (such as the endocrinology ward round you may be about to join) is in its infancy.[8] But as doctors we are steeped in the hormonal lives of patients (as they are in ours)—and we may as well start by recognising this now.

The essence of endocrinology—for those doing exams

"What's wrong with *him*?" your examiner asks, baldly. While you apologise to the patient for this rudeness by asking: "Is it alright if we speak about you as if you weren't here?" think to yourself that if you were a betting man or woman you would wager that the diagnosis will be endocrinological. In no other discipline are *gestalt* impressions so characteristic. To get good at recognizing these conditions, spend time in endocrinology out-patients and looking at collections of clinical photographs. Also, specific cutaneous signs are important, as follows.

Thyrotoxicosis: Hair loss; pretibial myxoedema (confusing term, p210); onycholysis (nail separation from the nailbed); bulging eyes (exophthalmos/proptosis).

Hypothyroidism: Hair loss; eyebrow loss; cold, pale skin; characteristic face. You might, perhaps *should*, fail your exam if you blurt out "Toad-like face".

Cushing's syndrome: Central obesity and wasted limbs (='lemon on sticks'); moon face; buffalo hump; supraclavicular fat pads; striae.

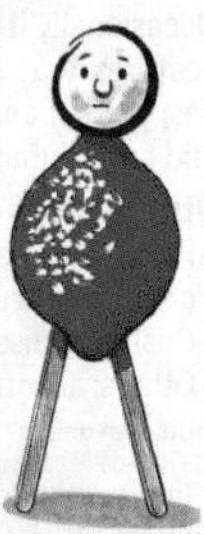

Addison's disease: Hyperpigmentation (face, neck, palmar creases).

Acromegaly: Acral (distal) + soft tissue overgrowth; big jaws (macrognathia), hands and feet; the skin is thick; facial features are coarse.

Hyperandrogenism (♀): Hirsutism; temporal balding; acne.

Hypopituitarism: Pale or yellow tinged thinned skin, resulting in fine wrinkling around the eyes and mouth, making the patient look older.

Hypoparathyroidism: Dry, scaly, puffy skin; brittle nails; coarse hair.

Pseudohypoparathyroidism: Short stature, short neck & short 4th & 5th metacarpals.

DM results from lack or reduced effectiveness of endogenous insulin. Hyperglycaemia is one aspect of a far-reaching metabolic derangement, which causes serious microvascular (retinopathy, nephropathy, neuropathy) or macrovascular problems: stroke, renovascular disease, limb ischaemia—and above all heart disease: most people having an MI will have some derangement of glucose control. *So think of DM as a vascular disease:*[1] when meeting a diabetic person we all should be in a state of acute anxiety until we know for sure that BP is well-controlled (≪145/80mmHg). What does 'we all' mean? Diabetes is the archetype of a universal disease (world-wide prevalence: >240 million, and rising): we all have it or know someone who has it, and *so we are all responsible for its treatment and prevention*—and patients ('peer advisers') have an important role in teaching each other:[9] there are not enough doctors (let alone diabetologists) to manage it alone. It is a community enterprise.

Type 1 DM Usually juvenile onset but may occur at *any* age. ***Cause:*** Insulin deficiency from autoimmune destruction of insulin-secreting pancreatic β cells. Patients must have insulin, and are prone to ketoacidosis and weight loss. It is associated with other autoimmune diseases (>90% carry HLA DR3 ± DR4). Concordance is only ~30% in identical twins, indicating environmental influence. 4 genes are important—one (6q) determines islet sensitivity to damage (eg from viruses or cross-reactivity from cows' milk-induced antibodies). Latent autoimmune diabetes of adults (LADA) is a form of type 1 DM, with slower progression to insulin dependence in later life.

Type 2 DM (formerly non-insulin-dependent DM, NIDDM) appears to be prevalent at 'epidemic' levels in many places, mainly due to changes in lifestyle, but also because of better diagnosis and improved longevity.[10] Higher prevalence occurs in Asians, men, and the elderly (up to 18%).[11] Most are over 40yrs, but teenagers are now getting type 2 DM (*OHCS* p156). ***Cause*** ↓Insulin secretion ± ↑insulin resistance. It is associated with obesity, lack of exercise, calorie and alcohol excess.[12] ≥80% concordance in identical twins, indicating stronger genetic influence than in type 1 DM. Typically progresses from a preliminary phase of impaired glucose tolerance (IGT) or impaired fasting glucose (IFG), see BOX. (►This a unique window for lifestyle intervention.) Maturity onset diabetes of the young (MODY) is a rare autosomal dominant form of type 2 DM affecting young people with a +ve family history (*OHCS* p187).

Diagnosis of diabetes mellitus: WHO criteria (rather arbitrary![2])

- Symptoms of hyperglycaemia (eg polyuria, polydipsia, unexplained weight loss, visual blurring, genital thrush, lethargy) **AND** raised venous glucose detected once—fasting ≥7mmol/L or random ≥11.1mmol/L **OR**
- Raised venous glucose on 2 separate occasions—fasting ≥7mmol/L, random ≥11.1mmol/L or oral glucose tolerance test (**OGTT**)—2h value ≥11.1mmol/L.

If in doubt, do an OGTT: is 2h glucose level >11.1mmol/L. ***How to do a 2h OGTT:***
- Fast overnight. Give 75g of glucose in 300mL water to drink in the morning.
- Measure venous plasma glucose before and 2h after the drink.

HbA1c (≥6.7%), capillary glucose and glycosuria are less reliable.

Occasionally it may be difficult to differentiate whether a patient has type 1 or 2 DM. Features that suggest type 1 DM include weight loss; persistent hyperglycaemia despite diet and medications; presence of autoantibodies: islet cell antibodies (ICA) and anti-glutamic acid decarboxylase (GAD) antibodies; ketonuria on urine dipstick.

Other causes of DM ►Steroids; anti-HIV drugs; newer antipsychotics; thiazides.[13]
- Pancreatic: pancreatitis; surgery (where >90% pancreas is removed); trauma; pancreatic destruction (haemochromatosis, cystic fibrosis); pancreatic cancer.
- Cushing's disease; acromegaly; phaeochromocytoma; hyperthyroidism; pregnancy.
- Others: acanthosis nigricans; congenital lipodystrophy; glycogen storage diseases.

1 Chicken or egg? Most type II diabetes-associated genes have a function in the vasculature, and stress in β-cells can result from vascular defects in the pancreas, so maybe vascular events trigger DM.
2 These values reflect economic and political realities: biological realities are different: risk of DM retinopathy relates to glucose levels >5.6mmol/L, for example. But defining DM as >5.6 would cost £billions. To be useful, normal values need individualizing according to BMI, lipids, smoking & BP etc: see p765.

Other categories of dysglycaemia and diabetes mellitus

Impaired glucose tolerance (IGT) Fasting plasma glucose <7mmol/L and OGTT (oral glucose tolerance) 2h glucose ≥7.8mmol/L but <11.1 mmol/L.

Impaired fasting glucose (IFG) Fasting plasma glucose ≥6.1mmol/L but <7mmol/L (WHO criteria). Do an OGTT to exclude DM. The cut-off point is somewhat arbitrary: Americans use 5.55mmol/L (100mg/dL) and 4.8 is the cut-off in Israel.[14] [15] IGT and IFG denote different abnormalities of glucose regulation (post-prandial and fasting). There may be lower risk of progression to DM in IFG than IGT. Manage both with lifestyle advice (exercise & diet, p87) + annual review. Incidence of DM if IFG and HbA1c at high end of normal (5.5-6.4%) is ~25%.[16] Giving those with heart failure and IFG ACE-i drugs prevents progress to DM (3% *vs* 48% over 3yrs).[17]

Gestational diabetes (*OHCS* p24) 4% of pregnancies. Risk ↑ if: aged over 25; family history +ve; weight ↑; non-Caucasian; HIV+ve).[18] Distinguish gestational impaired glucose tolerance (GIGT) from gestational DM (GDM) using the same diagnostic values as above. Problems with GDM: ↑birthweight; neonatal hypoglycaemia; sacral agenesis. Glucose tolerance changes during pregnancy. At ≥6wks postpartum, do a further 75g OGTT. Even if -ve, 50% will eventually go on to develop DM.

Type 1 versus type 2 diabetes mellitus

	Type 1 DM	Type 2 DM
Epidemiology	Often starts before puberty	Older patients (usually)
Genetics	HLA D3 and D4 linked	No HLA association
Cause	Autoimmune β cell destruction	Insulin resistance/β cell dysfunction
Presentation	Polydipsia, polyuria, weight ↓, ketosis	Asymptomatic/complications, eg MI

►Not all new-onset DM in older people is type 2: if ketotic ± a poor response to oral hypoglycaemics (and patient is slim or has a family or personal history of autoimmunity), think of latent autoimmune diabetes in adults (LADA) and measure islet cell antibodies.[19]

Screening for diabetes? ►30% of diabetes is undiagnosed![20]

►Whenever you have a needle in a vein, do a blood glucose (unless recently done); note if fasting or after food. This is non-systematic, but better than urine tests (too many false -ves). Better still may be systematic screening. In one UK primary care trial, 5% of those screened aged 40-69 had new diabetes. Risk ↑ if:[21] ♂; waist circumference ↑, BP ↑ or triglycerides ↑. NB: screening inevitably causes anxiety.[22]

Insulin resistance and the metabolic syndrome

Mechanisms of insulin resistance:

- Obesity may cause insulin resistance by ↑ rate of release of non-esterified fatty acids causing post-receptor defects in insulin's action.
- Mutation of genes encoding insulin receptors.
- Circulating autoantibodies to the extracellular domain of the insulin receptor.

Risk of insulin resistance ↑ if:
• Metabolic syndrome
• Obese
• Asians¹
• TB drugs; SSRIs[23] [24]
• Pregnancy
• Acromegaly; Cushing's
• Renal failure
• Cystic fibrosis
• Polycystic ovary (*OHCS* p252)
• Werner's syn. (*OHCS* p655)

Metabolic syndrome (syndrome X) comprises central obesity,[1] hypertension, hyperglycaemia, dyslipidaemia (↑triglycerides, ↓HDL) from interaction of genes and sedentary overnutrition perpetuated by social norms. ~20% are affected.[USA DATA] [25] Presence of mild inflammation makes it different from simple obesity.[26] ***Possible consequences:*** Vascular events (MI); DM; neurodegeneration;[27] microalbuminuria;[28] gallstones;[29] cancers (eg pancreas);[30] fertility problems ♂&♀ ℞: Exercise (Tai Chi is validated);[31] statins,[32] weight ↓ ± Mediterranean (?ketogenic) diet,[33] antihypertensives, hypoglycaemics (metformin ± glitazones, p200).[34] Explain that benefits are more than simply chemical: there is an intriguing two-way interaction between depression and insulin resistance:[35] ►Wise doctors and nurses will use this fact and work on many different levels to lead patients out of illness into health. Examples are motivational therapy and weekly phone interventions.[36]

1 In Gujaratis, Punjabis, Sri Lankans, Pakistanis & Bangladeshis have a low threshold for diagnosing obesity (BMI >23) and for vigorous intervention. ►**Waist circumference reference intervals:** p205.

Be holistic: address *all* vascular risk factors. Obsessive focusing on achieving normoglycaemia may be harmful,[37 38] eg if it detracts from biopsychosocial health (p9) and quitting smoking.[etc] Aim for ***structured*** education and motivation from an interdisciplinary team of doctors, specialist nurses, dieticians (BOX 1), chiropodists, and fellow patients (peer advisers). Maybe you skimmed over the last phrase rushing to get to the meat of the topic? Slow down...reflect on the implications that randomized trials show that group learning from fellow patients is better at lowering HbA1c than well-run diabetic clinics:[39] we doctors are not all that important![40]

Individualized care Educate/negotiate on target HbA1c (eg 6.5%), capillary glucose analysis, exercise, diet: p236—saturated fats↓, sugar↓, starch-carbohydrate↑, moderate protein.[41] Foods made just for diabetics are *not* needed. Give smoking cessation, foot-care (p204), & pre-conception advice (*OHCS* p24). One could regard bariatric surgery as a cure for diabetes in selected patients.[42] Care during pregnancy is best shared with an interested obstetrician and diabetologist (*OHCS* p24). Advise informing driving licence authority and not to drive if hypoglycaemic spells (p153; loss of awareness of hypoglycaemia may lead to a loss of driving licence; permanent if HGV).

Drugs Start a statin[1] (p109) & control BP[2] (p134). *Type 1 DM:* BOX 2. *Type 2 DM:* start a
• ***biguanide*** **(metformin)** at once (European & USA advice)[43] to ↑ insulin sensitivity & help weight. *SE:* nausea; diarrhoea; abdominal pain; *not* hypoglycaemia. Avoid if eGFR ≲36mL/min[44] (∵ lactic acidosis). *Dose:* 1.5g of modified-release version after food.[45] Stop if: tissue hypoxia (eg MI, sepsis); and morning before GA and contrast medium containing iodine (restart when renal function OK).[46] If HbA1c ≳7% 16wks later, add a
• ***sulfonylurea*** to ↑insulin secretion; eg **gliclazide MR** 30mg with breakfast; max 120 mg/d. *SE:* hypoglycaemia (monitor glucose); it ↑weight, so sitagliptin, below, is a good alternative here if BMI ≳35 or hypoglycaemia is an issue. If at 6mths, HbA1c ≳7.4%
• ***insulin*** may be needed (BOX 2), eg Novorapid® >6U just before or after main meals, ***or*** a
• ***glitazone*** to ↑ insulin sensitivity; SE: hypoglycaemia, fractures, fluid retention, LFT↑ (do LFT every 8wks for 1yr, stop if ALT up >3-fold). CI: past or present CCF; osteoporosis; monitor weight, and stop if ↑ or oedema. Example: **pioglitazone** 15–45mg/24h.[47] It replaces either metformin or sulfonylurea. It is occasionally used with insulin. ***Others:***
• ***sulfonylurea receptor binders*** **(nateglinide)**: ↑β-cell insulin release. 60mg PO ½h before meals, eg tds, ↑dose as needed.[48] Alternative: **repaglinide**. They target post-prandial hyperglycaemia ($t_{½}$ is short[49]—metformin works mostly on fasting glucose). They have a role in those with irregular mealtimes if glycaemic control is poor.[50]
• ***glucagon-like peptide (GLP) analogues*** Incretins are gut peptides that work by augmenting insulin release: 2 drug classes exploit them: ***GLP-1 analogues***—**exenatide** 5μg SC bd ¼h before meals (>6h apart; avoid if eGFR <30; ↑after >4wks to 10μg bd—and *DPP-4 inhibitors* (dipeptidyl peptidase 4 breaks down GLP-1, **sitagliptin; vilagliptin**). They may be an alternative to insulin (if eGFR >50), eg if obese (they ↓ appetite).[51]
• ***α-glucosidase inhibitors*** **(acarbose)** ↓breakdown of starch to sugar (an add-on drug, often disappointing!), 50mg chewed at start of each meal. Start once daily; max 200mg/8h. SE: wind (less if *slow* dose build-up), abdominal distension/pain, diarrhoea.

Monitoring glucose control: 1 Fingerprick glucose if type 1 DM (and some type 2).[3]
2 Glycated haemoglobin (HbA1c (DCCT/IFCC, p700)) relates to mean glucose level over previous 8wks (RBC ½-life). Targets are negotiable, eg 6.5–7.4% (depends on patient's wish and arterial risk, eg past MI or stroke). If at risk from the effects of hypoglycaemia, eg elderly patients prone to falls, consider less tight control. Also in one good study very tight control increased all-cause mortality.[52] Complications rise with rising HbA1c, so *any* improvement helps. *Fructosamine* (glycated plasma protein) reflects control over 3wks (helps fine tune ℞, eg in pregnancy; also use in haemoglobinopathies).
3 Be sure to ask about hypoglycaemic attacks (and whether symptomatic). Hypoglycaemic awareness may diminish if control is too tight, or with time in type 1 DM, due to ↓glucagon secretion. It may return if control is loosened.

1 **Simvastatin** 40mg nocte; if triglyceride >4.5mmol/L: **Bezalip**® 200mg/8h (+**Omacor**® omega 3 if still ↑)
2 Target BP <140/80mmHg; 130/80 if: stroke, MI, retinopathy, microalbuminuria (℞ **ARB** or **ACE-i**, p123)
3 Fingerprick glucose if: on insulin; to inform about hypoglycaemia; intercurrent illness (glucose may be ↑↑)

What is the best diet for obese patients with type 2 diabetes?

Dietary carbohydrate is a big determinant of postprandial glucose levels, and we know that low-carbohydrate diets improve glycaemic control. How do low-carbohydrate, ketogenic diets (<20g of carbohydrate daily; LCKD) compare with low-glycaemic index, reduced-calorie diet (eg 500kcal/day deficit from weight maintenance diet)? In one randomized study over 24 weeks, LCKD had greater improvements in HbA1c (-1.5% *vs* -0.5%), weight (-11kg *vs* -7kg), and HDL. Diabetes drugs were reduced or eliminated in 95% of LCKD *vs* 62% of LGID participants.[53] NB: effects on renal function and mortality are unknown so these diets remain controversial.

Using insulin

▸▸Ketoacidosis p842; HONK p844

For good control, it is *vital* to educate to self-adjust doses in the light of exercise, fingerprick glucose, and calorie intake. Ensure: • Phone support (trained nurse 7/24) • Dose titration to target—eg by 2-4U steps • Can modify diet wisely and avoid binge drinking (danger of delayed hypoglycaemia) • Partner can abort hypoglycaemia: sugary drinks; GlucoGel® PO if coma (no risk of aspiration).

NB: fingerprick glucoses *before* a meal inform about long-acting insulin doses; those done *after* meals inform about the dose of short-acting glucose.

Subcutaneous insulins are short-, medium-, or long-acting. Strength: 100U/mL.

1 Ultra-fast acting (Humalog®; Novorapid®); inject at start of meal, or just after (unless sugar-laden)—helps match what is actually eaten (*vs* what is planned).[54]
2 Isophane insulin (awkward, variable peak at 4-12h): favoured by NICE (it's cheap!).
3 Pre-mixed insulins, with ultra-fast component (eg NovoMix® 30). 30% short acting / 70% long-acting
4 Long-acting recombinant human insulin analogues (***insulin glargine***, eg 0.4U/kg/d) are used at bedtime in type 1 or 2 DM.[55] There is no awkward peak, so good if nocturnal hypoglycaemia is an issue.[56] Caution if considering pregnancy. Molecular modification ensures it's soluble at acid pH, but precipitates in subcutaneous tissue, and is slowly released. ***Insulin detemir*** (eg 0.5U/kg/d) is similar and has a role in intensive insulin regimens for type 2 overweight diabetics.[57,58,59]

Common insulin regimes ►*Plan the regime to suit the lifestyle, not vice versa.* Disposable pens (FlexPen® ?more accurate than SoloStar®[60]): dial dose; insert needle 90° to skin. Vary injection site (outer thigh/abdomen); change needle daily.

- 'BD biphasic régime': twice daily premixed insulins by pen (eg Novomix 30®)—useful in type 2 DM or type 1 with regular lifestyle.
- 'QDS regime': before meals ultra-fast insulin + bedtime long-acting analogue: useful in type 1 DM for achieving a flexible life-style (eg for adjusting doses with size of meals, or exercise).
- Once-daily before-bed long-acting insulin: a good initial insulin regimen when switching from tablets in type 2 DM. Typical dose to work up to (slowly!): ≥1U/24h for every unit of body mass index in adults. Consider retaining metformin (±pioglitazone) if needed for tight control and patient is unable to use BD regime.

Dose adjustment for normal eating (DAFNE): Multidisciplinary teams promoting autonomy can save lives. DAFNE found that training in flexible, intensive insulin dosing improved glycaemic control as well as wellbeing.[61] It is resource intensive.

Subcutaneous insulin dosing during intercurrent illnesses (eg influenza)

- Illness often increases insulin requirements despite reduced food intake.
- Maintain calorie intake, eg using milk.
- Check blood glucose ≥4 times a day and look for ketonuria. Increase insulin doses if glucose rising. Advise to get help from a specialist diabetes nurse or GP if concerned (esp. if glucose levels are rising or ketonuria). One option is 2-hourly Novorapid® insulin (eg 6-8U) preceded by a fingerprick glucose check.
- Admit if vomiting, dehydrated, ketotic (▸▸p842), a child, or pregnant.

Prospective studies show that good control of hyperglycaemia is key to preventing complications in type 1 and 2 DM. Don't treat in isolation: assess *global* vascular risk, eg: BP, cholesterol,[1] obesity and smoking. ►*Focus on education and lifestyle advice* (eg exercise to ↑insulin sensitivity), healthy eating, and weight reduction—p236; NICE comments that drugs such as orlistat have a role if weight loss of >2.5kg has been achieved by lifestyle advice and BMI >28kg/m². ►*Find out what problems are being experienced* (eg glycaemic control, morale, erectile dysfunction—p222).

Assess vascular risk: *BP* (BOX). Target is <140/<80mmHg (or <125/<75 with renal disease: ↑creatinine, microalbuminuria—see below, or dipstick proteinuria). BP control is critical for preventing macrovascular disease and mortality. Discuss ***smoking*** and offer referral to cessation services. Check ***plasma lipids*** (see below).

Look for complications • Check injection sites for infection or lipohypertrophy (fatty change): advise on rotating sites of injection if present.

- ***Vascular disease*** Chief cause of death. MI is 4-fold commoner in DM and is more likely to be 'silent'). Stroke is twice as common. Women are at high risk—DM removes the vascular advantage conferred by the female sex. Address other risk factors—diet, smoking, hypertension (p87). Suggest a statin (eg simvastatin 40mg nocte) for all, even if no overt IHD, vascular disease, or microalbuminuria. Fibrates are useful for ↑triglycerides & ↓HDL (p704). Aspirin 75mg reduces vascular events (if past stroke or MI) and is good as statin co-therapy (safe to use in diabetic retinopathy; use in primary prevention is disappointing, at least at 100mg/day).
- ***Nephropathy*** (p309) Microalbuminuria is when urine dipstick is -ve for protein but the urine albumin:creatinine ratio (UCR) is ≥30mg/mmol (p771) reflecting early renal disease and ↑vascular risk. If UCR >30, inhibiting the renin-angiotensin system, even if BP is normal, protects the kidneys, eg the A2A blocker (p309) candesartan 8-32mg/d decreases albumin excretion by up to 60%; if given with ACE-i (p109, dual blockade), further reductions are possible. Spironolactone may also help. Refer if UCR >70 ± GFR falling by >5mL/min/1.73m²/yr.
- ***Diabetic retinopathy*** Blindness is *preventable. Arrange annual fundoscopy or retinal photography for all patients.* Refer to an ophthalmologist if pre-proliferative changes or if any uncertainty at or near the macula (the only place capable of 6/6 vision). ►Pre-symptomatic screening enables laser photocoagulation to be used, aimed to stop production of angiogenic factors from the ischaemic retina. Indications: maculopathy or proliferative retinopathy. See **figs 1-4**.
  - ***Background retinopathy:*** Microaneurysms (dots), haemorrhages (blots) & hard exudates (lipid deposits). Refer if near the macula, eg for intravitreal triamcinolone.
  - ***Pre-proliferative retinopathy:*** Cotton wool spots (eg infarcts), haemorrhages, venous beading. These are signs of retinal ischaemia. Refer to a specialist.
  - ***Proliferative retinopathy:*** New vessels form. Needs urgent referral.
  - ***Maculopathy:*** (hard to see in early stages). Suspect if acuity↓. Prompt laser, intravitreal steroids or anti-angiogenic agents may be needed in macular oedema.

  Pathogenesis: Capillary endothelial change → vascular leak → microaneurysms → capillary occlusion → local hypoxia + ischaemia → new vessel formation. High retinal blood flow caused by hyperglycaemia (& BP↑ & pregnancy) triggers this, causing capillary pericyte damage. Microvascular occlusion causes ***cotton wool spots*** (± ***blot haemorrhages*** at interfaces with perfused retina). ***New vessels*** form on the disc or ischaemic areas, proliferate, bleed, fibrose, and can detach the retina. Aspirin[1] (2mg/kg/d) may prevent it: there is no evidence that it ↑ bleeding.
- ***Cataracts:*** May be juvenile 'snowflake' form, or 'senile'—which occur earlier in diabetic subjects. Osmotic changes in the lens induced in acute hyperglycaemia reverse with normoglycaemia (so wait before buying glasses).
- ***Rubeosis iridis:*** New vessels on iris: occurs late and may lead to glaucoma.
- ***Metabolic complications:*** p842. ***Diabetic feet:*** p204. ***Neuropathy:*** p204.

1 As DM has so many vascular events, give a statin (p704) if LDL >3mmol/L **or** BP >140. Even consider a statin *whatever* the pre-treatment cholesterol; discuss with your patient. Lindholm 2003 *Lancet* **361** 2000

Controlling BP in those with diabetes—3 typical scenarios

1 BP <145/80 mmHg and no microalbuminuria and 10yr coronary event risk (CER10, p664) ≤15%: simply check BP every 6 months, or more often.
2 BP ≥140/80 and <160/100 and CER10 >15%, but no microalbuminuria: start an antihypertensive (NICE recommends ACE-i, ARB, or a thiazide). Target BP <140/80 (negotiate with patient). For doses and discussion, see p134.
3 BP ≥140/80 and microalbuminuria is present: ensure ACE-i or A2A are part of the approach (contraindications: p109). Target BP: <125/75 (if patient willing).

The role of aspirin prophylaxis (75mg/d PO) is uncertain in DM with hypertension.[1]

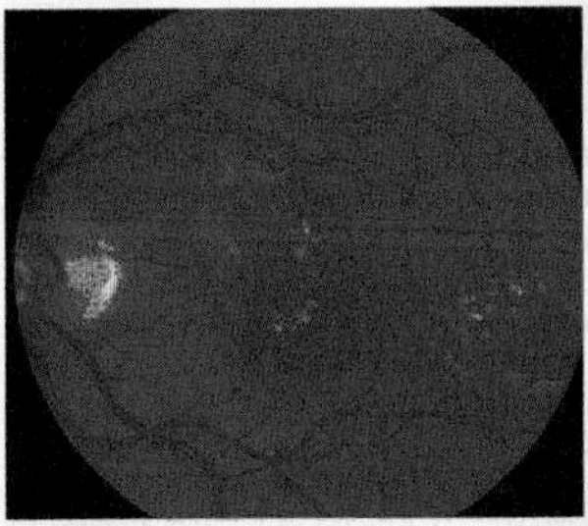

Fig 1. Background retinopathy, with micro-aneurysms and hard exudates.[70]

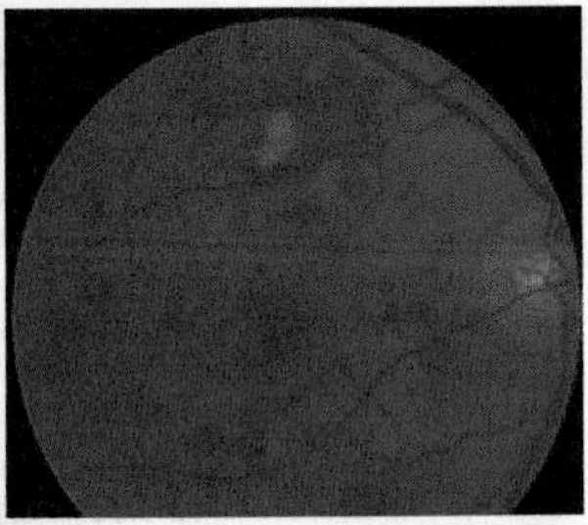

Fig 2. Pre-proliferative retinopathy, with haemorrhages and a cotton-wool spot.

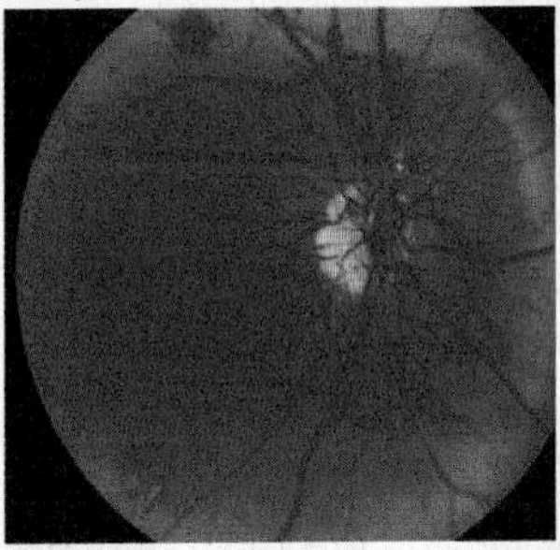

Fig 3. Proliferative retinopathy, with new vessel formation and haemorrhages.[71]

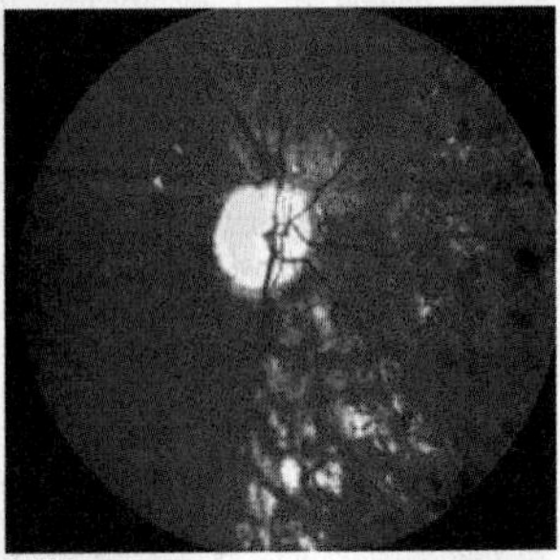

Fig 4. Scars from previous laser photocoagulation.[72]

Figs 1,3 & 4 courtesy of Prof J Trobe; fig 2 ©OTM (OUP)

Improving quality of life: going beyond the pleasures of the flesh

"I cannot eat what I want because of your pitiful diet. Sex is out because diabetes has made me impotent. Smoking is banned, so what's left? I'd shoot myself if only I could see straight." Start by acknowledging your patient's distress. Don't shrug it off—but don't take it at face value, either. Life may be transformed by cataract surgery, sildenafil (unless contraindicated, p222), dietary negotiation, and sport (it needn't be shooting). Take steps to simplify care. Stop blood glucose self-monitoring if it's achieving nothing (constant prickings are known to ↓ quality of life).[73] Even if all these interventions fail, you have one trump card up your sleeve: "Let's both try to find one new thing of value before we next meet—and compare notes". This opens the way to vicarious pleasure: a whole new world.

1 Aspirin ↓ leucocyte adhesion in diabetic retinal capillaries and ↓ expression of integrins on leucocytes and it ↓nitric oxide synthetase (eNOS) levels and ↓vasoactive cytokine tumour necrosis factor, known to be raised in diabetic retinopathy but benefits are hard to prove, and harm is possible.

►Amputations are common (100/week[UK])[74]—and preventable: *good care saves legs.* ►Refer *early* to high-quality interdisciplinary foot care services, which integrate podiatry, imaging, vascular surgery, and skilled optimization of diabetic care.

Signs Examine feet regularly. Distinguish between ischaemia (critical toes ± absent dorsalis pedis pulses) and peripheral neuropathy (injury or infection over pressure points, eg the metatarsal heads). In practice, many have both.

Neuropathy: Sensation↓ in 'stocking' distribution (test sensation with a 10g monofilament fibre applied with just sufficient force to bend it), absent ankle jerks, neuropathic deformity: pes cavus, claw toes, loss of transverse arch, rocker-bottom sole. Sensory loss is patchy, so examine all areas using a monofilament.

Ischaemia: If the foot pulses cannot be felt, do Doppler pressure measurements. Any evidence of neuropathy or vascular disease raises risk of foot ulceration. *Educate* (daily foot inspection—eg with a mirror so the sole can be fully inspected; comfortable shoes—ie very soft leather, increased depth, cushioning insoles/trainers; weight-distributing cradles; no barefoot walking,[75] no corn-plasters). *Regular chiropody* to remove callus, as haemorrhage and tissue necrosis may occur below, leading to ulceration. *Treat fungal infections* (p440). *Surgery* (including endovascular angioplasty balloons, stents, and subintimal recanalization) has a role. Get advice.[76]

Absolute indications for surgery:
• Abscess or deep infection
• Spreading anaerobic infection
• Gangrene/rest pain
• Suppurative arthritis

Foot ulceration Typically painless, punched-out ulcer (**fig 1**) in an area of thick callus ± superadded infection. Causes cellulitis, abscess ± osteomyelitis. *Assess degree of:* **1** Neuropathy (clinically). **2** Ischaemia (clinically + Doppler ± angiography). **3** Bony deformity, eg Charcot joint (clinically + x-ray). See **fig 2**. **4** Infection (swabs, blood culture, x-ray for osteomyelitis, probe ulcer to reveal depth).

Management: Regular chiropody to remove callus. Relieve high-pressure areas with bed rest ± therapeutic shoes (Pressure Relief Walkers® may be as good as total contact casts[77]); metatarsal head surgery may be needed. If there is cellulitis, admit for IV antibiotics. Common organisms: staphs, streps, anaerobes. Start with **benzylpenicillin** 1.2g/6h IV and **flucloxacillin** 1g/6h IV ± **metronidazole** 500mg/8h IV, refined when microbiology results are known. IV insulin and **fenofibrate** improve healing. Get surgical help. The degree of peripheral vascular disease, general health, and patient request will determine whether local excision and drainage, vascular reconstruction, and/or amputation (and how much) is appropriate.

Diabetic neuropathies: Symmetric sensory polyneuropathy: ('glove & stocking' numbness, tingling, and pain, eg worse at night). ℞: (in order) **paracetamol**→ tricyclic (**amitriptyline** 10–25mg nocte; gradually↑to 150mg)→ **gabapentin** (p508)[78]→**capsaicin cream** (counter-irritant)→**baclofen** (GABA agonist),[79] → **SSRI** (don't stop last 2 sudden-ly).[80] **Avoiding weight-bearing** helps.[81] Shock-like lancinating pains respond better to **anticonvulsants** (p496: gabapentin, carbamazepine, pregabalin, topiramate, lamotrigine).[82]

Mononeuritis multiplex: (eg III & VI cranial nerves) Treatment: hard! If sudden or severe, immunosuppression may help (corticosteroids, IV immunoglobulin, ciclosporin).[83]

Amyotrophy: Painful wasting of quadriceps and other pelvifemoral muscles. Use electrophysiology to show eg lumbosacral radiculopathy, plexopathy, or proximal crural neuropathy.[84] Natural course: variable with gradual but often incomplete improvement. IV immunoglobulins have been used.[85]

Autonomic neuropathy: (p509) Postural BP drop; ↓cerebrovascular autoregulation; gastroparesis; urine retention; erectile dysfunction (ED); diarrhoea. The latter may respond to **codeine phosphate** (the lowest dose to control symptoms, eg 15mg/8h PO). Gastroparesis (early satiety, post-prandial bloating, nausea/vomiting) is diagnosed by gastric scintigraphy with a ^{99}technetium-labelled meal.[86] It may respond to anti-emetics, or **tetracycline** if there is bacterial overgrowth. Postural hypotension may respond to **fludrocortisone** 50–300µg/24h PO (SE: oedema, ↑BP).

Preventing loss of limbs: primary or secondary prevention?

Traditionally prevention involves foot care advice in diabetic clinics (eg "Don't go bare-foot"), promoting euglycaemia and normotension.[1] But despite this, the sight of a diabetic patient minus one limb is not rare, and must prompt us to redouble our commitment to primary prevention, ie stopping those at risk from ever getting diabetes. In one prospective study of those with impaired glucose tolerance (IGT) and other risk factors, after 3 years, the incidence of diabetes per 100 person-years was 5 in those receiving simple exercise and diet advice, 8 in a group given metformin, and 11 in the placebo group. Advice and metformin decreased incidence of diabetes by 58% (NNT ≈7) and 31% (NNT ≈14), respectively, compared with placebo.[87] One vital group to focus on are those with the metabolic syndrome.[2]

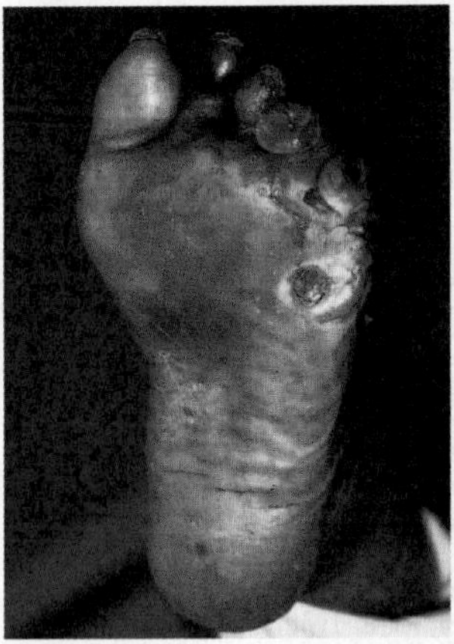

Fig 1. Gangrene (toes 2, 4 & 5). After amputation, (eg forefoot/Syme's, or above or below knee, depending on Doppler), even the least self-pitying are entitled to a period of narcissistic grief: "I begin again to walk, on crutches. What nuisance, what fatigue, what sadness, when I think about all my ancient travels, and how active I was just 5 months ago! Where are the runnings across mountains, the walks, the deserts, the rivers, and the seas? And now, the life of a legless cripple. For I begin to understand that crutches, wooden and articulated legs, are a pack of jokes...Goodbye to family, goodbye to future! My life is gone, I'm no more than an immobile trunk".[88] Arthur Rimbaud

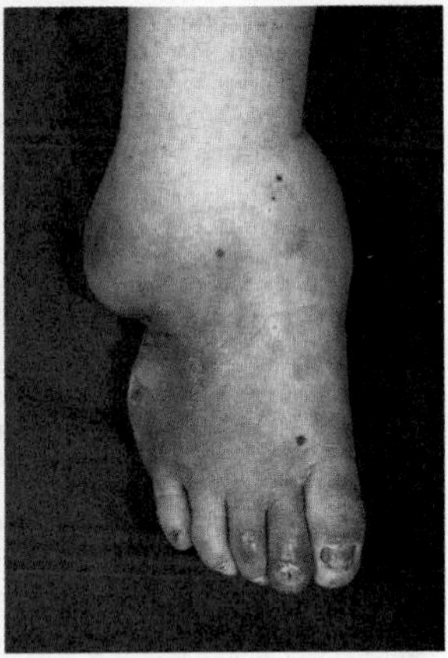

Fig 2. Charcot (neuropathic) joint, caused by loss of pain sensation, leading to ↑mechanical stress (unimpeded by pain) and repeated joint injury. Swelling, instability and, eventually, deformity, have developed. ►Early recognition is vital (cellulitis or osteomyelitis are often misdiagnosed) Treatment: offload all weight (bed rest or non-weight-bearing crutches); immobilisation by a total contact cast until oedema and local warmth reduce and bony repair is complete (≥8wks). Bisphosphonates may help.[89] Charcot joints are also seen in tabes dorsalis, spina bifida, syringomyelia, and leprosy. X-ray: p540. Figs 1 & 2 ©OUP/*OTM*.

1 HbA_{1c} ≤7% (+bands at 8% & 9% too) & BP ≤145/85 are current UK GP targets (GPs get a substantial quality payment if most have an HbA_{1c} ≤7% and 60% have BP ≤145/85 (≤140/85 if eGFR <50)); for non-diabetic hypertensives, the target BP is ≤150/90mmHg in 70%. Targets exist for cholesterol, smoking, etc; see *OHCS* p471 for details of the largest public health results-driven intervention ever.

2 **Metabolic syndrome** is central obesity or BMI >30 **plus any 2 of:** • Triglycerides ≥1.7mmol/L • HDL <1.03 • BP ≥130/85mmHg • Fasting glucose ≥5.6mmol/L or type 2 DM. There is also insulin resistance, but it is hard to measure, and is not part of the operational definition (nor is a glucose tolerance test essential). See K Alberti 2006 *Diabetic Medicine* 23 469-80

Waist circumference for central obesity

Europeans	♂ ≥94cm;	♀ ≥80cm
South (S) Asians	♂ ≥90cm;	♀ ≥80cm
Chinese	♂ ≥90cm;	♀ ≥80cm
Japanese	♂ ≥85cm;	♀ ≥90cm

S & Central Americans use S Asian *pro tem*
Africans + Middle East use European *pro tem*

►This is the commonest endocrine emergency—see p844. Prompt diagnosis and treatment is essential—brain damage & death can occur in severe prolonged cases.

Definition Plasma glucose ≤3mmol/L. Threshold for symptoms varies. See BOX.

Symptoms • *Autonomic*—Sweating, anxiety, hunger, tremor, palpitations, dizziness. • *Neuroglycopenic*—Confusion, drowsiness, visual trouble, seizures, coma. Rarely focal symptoms, eg transient hemiplegia. Mutism, personality change, restlessness and incoherence may lead to misdiagnosis of alcohol intoxication or even psychosis.[90]

Two types: 1 Fasting hypoglycaemia *Causes:* The chief cause is insulin or sulfonylurea treatment in a known diabetic eg with ↑activity, missed meal, accidental or non-accidental overdose. In a *non-diabetic* adults you must **EXPLAIN** the mechanism:

Exogenous drugs, eg *insulin, oral hypoglycaemics* (p 200). Does she have access to these (diabetic in the family)? Body-builders may misuse insulin to help stamina.[91] Also: *alcohol*, eg a binge with no food; *aspirin poisoning;* ACE-*i; β-blockers; pentamidine; quinine sulfate; aminoglutethamide*; insulin-like growth factor.[92]
Pituitary insufficiency.
Liver failure, plus some rare inherited enzyme defects.
Addison's disease.
Islet cell tumours (insulinoma, see below) and immune hypoglycaemia (eg anti-insulin receptor antibodies in Hodgkin's disease).
Non-pancreatic neoplasms, eg fibrosarcomas & haemangiopericytomas.

Diagnosis and investigations (see BOX 2)
- Document hypoglycaemia by taking fingerprick (on filter-paper at home for later analysis) during attack and lab glucose if in hospital (monitors are often not reliable at low readings). • Take a drug history and exclude liver failure.
- 72h fasting may be needed (monitor closely). Take blood samples for glucose, insulin, C-peptide and plasma ketones if symptomatic.

Interpreting results
- Hypoglycaemic hyperinsulinaemia (HH): *Causes:* Insulinoma, sulfonylureas, insulin injection (no detectable C-peptide—only released with endogenous insulin); non-insulinoma pancreatogenous hypoglycaemia syndrome, mutation in the insulin-receptor gene. Congenital HH is caused by mutations in genes involved in insulin secretion (ABCC8, KCNJ11, GLUD1, CGK, HADH, SLC16A1, HNF4A, ABCC8 & KCNJ11).[93]
- Insulin low or undetectable, no excess ketones. *Causes:* Non-pancreatic neoplasm; anti-insulin receptor antibodies.
- Insulin↓, ketones↑. *Causes:* Alcohol, pituitary insufficiency, Addison's disease.

2 Post-prandial hypoglycaemia May occur after gastric/bariatric surgery ('dumping', p624), and in type 2 diabetes. *Investigation:* Prolonged OGTT (5h, p198).

Treatment ►►See p844. Treat with oral sugar, and a long-acting starch (eg toast); If cannot swallow, 25–50mL 50% glucose IV (via large vein with 0.9% saline flush to prevent phlebitis) or glucagon 1mg IM if no IV access (short duration of effect so repeat after 20min and *follow with oral carbohydrate*). If episodes are often, advise many small high-starch meals. If post-prandial glucose↓, give slowly absorbed carbohydrate (high fibre). In diabetics, rationalise insulin therapy (p201).

Insulinoma This often benign (90–95%) pancreatic islet cell tumour is sporadic or seen with MEN-1 (p215). It presents as fasting hypoglycaemia, with Whipple's triad: **1** Symptoms associated with fasting or exercise **2** Recorded hypoglycaemia with symptoms **3** Symptoms relieved with glucose. ***Screening test:*** Hypoglycaemia + plasma insulin↑ during a long fast. ***Suppressive tests:*** Give IV insulin and measure C-peptide. Normally exogenous insulin suppresses C-peptide production, but this does not occur in insulinoma. ***Imaging:*** CT/MRI ± endoscopic pancreatic US ± IACS (see BOX 2; all fallible, so don't waste too much time before proceeding to intra-operative visualization[94] ± intra-operative ultrasound).[95] ^{18}F-L-3,4-dihydroxyphenylalanine PET-CT can help guide laparoscopic surgery.[96] ***Treatment:*** Excision. ***Nesidioblastosis***: see BOX 2. If this doesn't work, options are: ↑diet, diazoxide, dextrose IVI, enteral feeding, everolimus.[97]

The definition of hypoglycaemia is context-dependent

Because the brain stops working if plasma glucose levels get too low we are all nervous of levels ≤3mmol/L. But some people can walk around quite happily at this level. So what is definitely abnormal? A rule such as *'Any plasma glucose <1.7mmol/L'* constitutes hypoglycaemia may be true (a normal neonate may descend to this level but no further during the 1st day of life: even so—he or she needs feeding urgently)—but it is not a very helpful rule if the context is a fingerprick glucose on someone having seizures. Here it is better to rephrase the question: "***In this ill patient when can I be sure that a low glucose is not contributing to their illness***?" The answer may be 4mmol/L, allowing for inaccuracy in fingerprick blood glucose levels (NB: whole blood glucose is 10-15% < plasma glucose.)[98] If <4, you may be wise to treat (p844)—just in case.

A different context is a call from the lab to say that a glucose is 2.50mmol/L. Contact the patient, who may be up and about and happy; confirm that they are not on any hypoglycaemic agents. Have they binged on alcohol in the 24h before the test? Skipped meals? Could this low glucose be a sign of an illness such as an insulinoma? Unlikely, but possible. Keep an open mind; let the GP know. Explain about signs of hypoglycaemia and to see a doctor if such signs occur. Consider further tests (p 206) eg dotted about the day to catch other episodes of hypoglycaemia. Be more inclined to investigate if the effects of even mild hypoglycaemia might be disastrous (eg in pilots) or if there are unexplained symptoms.

When should I investgate borderline hypoglycaemia? Whipple answered the question thus (*Whipple's triad*): symptoms or signs of hypoglycemia + ↓plasma glucose + resolution of those symptoms or signs after plasma glucose raises.[99]

First thoughts in proven hypoglycaemia Exclude drugs, critical illnesses, hormone deficiencies, and non-islet cell tumours. If none of these, diagnosis narrows to accidental, surreptitious/malicious hypoglycemia, or endogenous hyperinsulinism (if the latter, do insulin, C-peptide, proinsulin, β-hydroxybutyrate, and circulating oral hypoglycaemic agents during hypoglycemia). Measure insulin antibodies.

Pursuing a voyage to the islets of Langerhans to the bitter end

A 50-year-old had episodic early-morning sweats and tremors and was found to have hyperinsulinaemic hypoglycaemia. Selective intra-arterial calcium infusions (IACS) showed a 2-fold increase in insulin secretion after infusion of the splenic and superior mesenteric arteries,[100] so setting the stage for 'hunt the insulinoma'.

But cross-sectional imaging and endoscopic ultrasound were normal. At laparotomy, no lesion was found despite mobilisation of the pancreas, or during intra-operative ultrasound. "Time to sew up and go home?" "No!" said the surgeon "I'm going to do a distal pancreatectomy". Histology showed no discrete insulinoma, but diffuse islet cell hyperplasia (**nesidioblastosis**).[101] How much pancreas to resect? Too little and nothing is gained: too much spells pancreatic endocrine disaster. Luckily the surgeon guessed right, and the patient was cured by the procedure.[102]

Physiology (fig 1) The hypothalamus secretes thyrotropin-releasing hormone (TRH), a tripeptide, that stimulates production of thyroid-stimulating hormone (TSH,=thyrotropin), a glycoprotein, from the anterior pituitary. TSH increases production and release of thyroxine (T_4) & triiodothyronine (T_3) from the thyroid, which exert -ve feedback on TSH production. The thyroid produces mainly T_4, which is 5-fold less active than T_3. 85% of T_3 is formed from peripheral conversion of T_4. Most T_3 and T_4 in plasma is protein bound, eg to thyroxine-binding globulin (TBG). The unbound portion is the active part. T_3 and T_4 ↑cell metabolism, via nuclear receptors, and are thus vital for growth and mental development. They also ↑catecholamine effects.

Thyroid hormone abnormalities are usually due to problems in the thyroid gland itself, and rarely caused by the hypothalamus or the anterior pituitary.

Basic tests Free T_4 & T_3 are more useful than total T_4 & T_3 as the latter are affected by TBG. Total T_4 and T_3 are ↑ when TBG is ↑ and *vice versa*. TBG is ↑ in pregnancy, oestrogen therapy (HRT, oral contraceptives) and hepatitis. TBG is ↓ in nephrotic syndrome and malnutrition (both from protein loss), drugs (androgens, corticosteroids, phenytoin), chronic liver disease and acromegaly. TSH is very useful:

- ***Hyperthyroidism suspected:*** Ask for T_3, T_4, and TSH. In hyperthyroidism, all will have ↓TSH (except for the rare phenomenon of a TSH-secreting pituitary adenoma). Most have raised T_4, but ~1% have only raised T_3.
- ***Hypothyroidism suspected or monitoring replacement ℞:*** Ask for only T_4 and TSH. T_3 does not add any extra information. TSH varies through the day: trough at 2PM; 30% higher during darkness, so during monitoring, try to do at the same time.

↑TSH, ↓T_4	Hypothyroidism
↑TSH, normal T_4	Treated hypothyroidism or subclinical hypothyroidism (p213)
↑TSH, ↑ T_4	TSH secreting tumour or thyroid hormone resistance
↑TSH, ↑ T_4 and ↓T_3	Slow conversion of T_4 to T_3 (deiodinase deficiency; euthyroid hyperthyroxinaemia[1]) or thyroid hormone antibody artefact.[103,104]
↓TSH, ↑ T_4 or ↑T_3	Hyperthyroidism
↓TSH, normal T_4 & T_3	Subclinical hyperthyroidism
↓TSH, T_4↓	Central hypothyroidism (hypothalamic or pituitary disorder)
↓TSH, ↓ T_4 & ↓ T_3	Sick euthyroidism (below) or pituitary disease
Normal TSH, abnormal T_4	Consider changes in thyroid-binding globulin, assay interference, amiodarone, or pituitary TSH tumour

Sick euthyroidism: In any systemic illness, TFTs may become deranged. The typical pattern is for 'everything to be low'. The test should be repeated after recovery.
Assay interference is caused by antibodies in the serum, interfering with the test.

Other tests • *Thyroid autoantibodies:* Antithyroid peroxidase (TPO; formerly called microsomal) antibodies or antithyroglobulin antibodies may be increased in autoimmune thyroid disease: Hashimoto's or Graves' disease. If +ve in Graves', there is an increased risk of developing hypothyroidism at a later stage.

- *TSH receptor antibody:* May be ↑ in Graves' disease (useful in pregnancy).
- *Serum thyroglobulin:* Useful in monitoring the treatment of carcinoma (p602), and in detection of factitious (self-medicated) hyperthyroidism, where it is low.
- *Ultrasound:* This distinguishes cystic (usually, but not always, benign) from solid (possibly malignant) nodules. If a solitary (or dominant) large nodule, in a multinodular goitre, do a fine-needle aspiration to look for thyroid cancer; see **fig 2**, p603.
- *Isotope scan:* (^{123}Iodine, ^{99}technetium pertechnetate, etc; see fig 3, p 752). Useful for determining the cause of hyperthyroidism and to detect retrosternal goitre, ectopic thyroid tissue or thyroid metastases (+ whole body CT). If there are suspicious nodules, the question is: does the area have increased (hot), decreased (cold), or the same (neutral) uptake of isotope as the remaining thyroid (see **fig 2**)? Few neutral and almost no hot nodules are malignant. 20% of 'cold' nodules are malignant. Surgery is most likely to be needed if: • Rapid growth • Compression signs • Dominant nodule on scintigraphy • Nodule ≥3cm • Hypo-echogenicity.[105] See also p752.

1 In 'consumptive hypothyroidism' deiodinase activity is ↑↑; suspect if thyroxine doses have to be ↑↑.

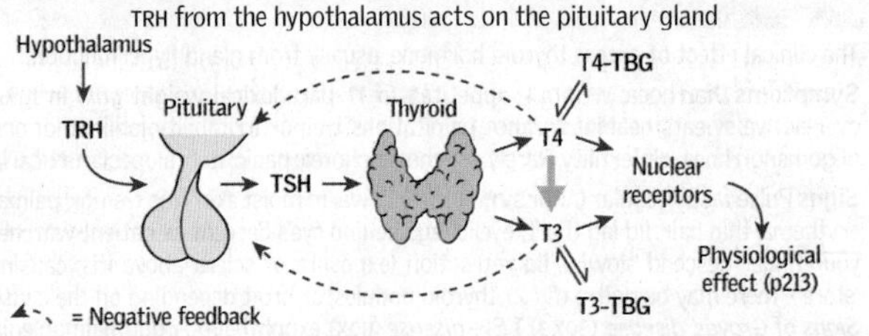

Fig 1. Pathways involved in thyroid function.

Screen the following for abnormalities in thyroid function:

- Patients with atrial fibrillation
- Patients with hyperlipidaemia (4–14% have hypothyroidism)
- Diabetes mellitus—on annual review
- Women with type 1 DM during 1st trimester and post delivery (3-fold rise in incidence of postpartum thyroid dysfunction)
- Patients on amiodarone or lithium (6 monthly)
- Patients with Down's or Turner's syndrome, or Addison's disease (yearly)

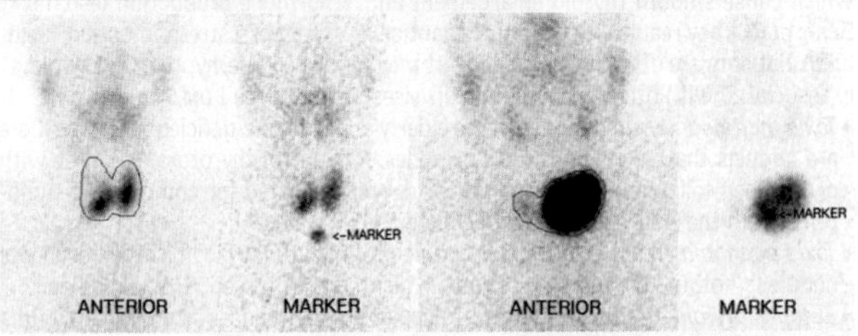

Fig 2. The images are with and without markers placed over the sternal notch. We can see on the left that the nodule is metabolically inactive ('cold'). The hot nodule (right pair) is a very avid nodule causing background thyroid suppression. Image courtesy of Dr Y. T. Huang.

The clinical effect of excess thyroid hormone, usually from gland hyperfunction.

Symptoms Diarrhoea; weight↓; appetite↑ (if ↑↑, paradoxical weight *gain* in 10%); over-active; sweats; heat intolerance; palpitations; tremor; irritability; labile emotions; oligomenorrhoea ±infertility. Rarely psychosis; chorea; panic; itch; alopecia; urticaria.

Signs Pulse fast/irregular (AF or SVT; VT rare);[107] warm moist skin; fine tremor; palmar erythema; thin hair; lid lag (**fig 1;** eyelid lags behind eye's descent as patient watches your finger descend slowly); lid retraction (exposure of sclera above iris; causing 'stare'). There may be goitre (**fig 2**); thyroid nodules; or bruit depending on the cause. ***Signs of Graves' disease:*** (BOX 3) **1** *Eye disease* (BOX): exophthalmos, ophthalmoplegia. **2** *Pretibial myxoedema:* oedematous swellings above lateral malleoli: the term *myxoedema* is confusing here **3** *Thyroid acropachy:* extreme manifestation, with clubbing, painful finger and toe swelling, and periosteal reaction in limb bones.[108]

Tests TSH↓ (suppressed), T_4 & T_3↑. There may be mild normocytic anaemia, mild neutropenia (in Graves'),[109] ESR↑, Ca^{2+}↑, LFT↑. ***Also:*** Check thyroid autoantibodies. Isotope scan if the cause is unclear, to detect nodular disease or subacute thyroiditis. If ophthalmopathy, test visual fields, acuity, and eye movements (see BOX 1).

Causes • ***Graves' disease:*** Prevalence: 0.5% (~⅔ of cases of hyperthyroidism). ♀:♂ ≈9:1. Typical age: 40–60yrs (younger if maternal family history). Cause: circulating IgG autoantibodies binding to and activating G-protein-coupled thyrotropin receptors, which cause smooth thyroid enlargement and ↑ hormone production (esp. T_3).[110] Scan: p603. They react with orbital autoantigens.[111] Triggers: stress; infection; childbirth. Patients are often hyperthyroid but may be, or become, hypo- or euthyroid. It is associated with other autoimmune diseases: vitiligo, type 1 DM, Addison's.

- ***Toxic multinodular goitre:*** Seen in the elderly and in iodine-deficient areas.[112] There are nodules that secrete thyroid hormones. ℞: Control thyrotoxicosis first with drugs, then follow with radioiodine. Surgery is indicated for compressive symptoms from the enlarged thyroid (dysphagia or dyspnoea).[113]
- ***Toxic adenoma:*** There is a solitary nodule producing T_3 & T_4. On isotope scan, the nodule is 'hot' (p208), and the rest of the gland is suppressed. ℞: Radioiodine.
- ***Ectopic thyroid tissue:*** Metastatic follicular thyroid cancer,[114] choriocarcinoma (*OHCS* p264) or struma ovarii: ovarian teratoma with thyroid tissue.
- ***Exogenous:*** Iodine excess, eg food contamination, contrast media (►►thyroid storm, p844, if already hyperthyroid).[115] Levothyroxine excess causes ↑T_4, ↓T_3, ↓thyroglobulin.
- ***Others:* 1 *Subacute de Quervain's thyroiditis:*** Self-limiting post-viral with painful goitre, T°↑ ± ↑ESR. Low isotope uptake on scan. ℞: NSAIDs. **2 *Drugs:*** Amiodarone (p212), lithium (hypothyroidism more common).[116] **3** Postpartum **4** *TB* (rare).[117]

Treatment

1 ***Drugs:*** β-blockers (eg **propranolol** 40mg/6h) for rapid control of symptoms. ***Antithyroid medication:*** 2 strategies (equally effective):[118] **A)** ***Titration*** eg **carbimazole** 20–40mg/24h PO for 4wks, reduce according to TFTs every 1–2 months. **B)** *Block-replace:* Give carbimazole + thyroxine simultaneously (less risk of iatrogenic hypothyroidism). In Graves', maintain on either regime for 12–18 months then withdraw. ~50% will relapse, requiring radioiodine or surgery. Carbimazole SE: agranulocytosis (↓↓neutrophils, can lead to dangerous sepsis; rare (0.03%); warn to stop and get an urgent FBC if signs of infection, eg T°↑, sore throat/mouth ulcers.

2 ***Radioiodine (*** ^{131}I ***):*** Most become hypothyroid post-treatment. There is no evidence for ↑cancer, birth defects or infertility in women. CI: pregnancy, lactation. Caution in active hyperthyroidism as risk of thyroid storm (p845).

3 ***Thyroidectomy:*** Carries a risk of damage to recurrent laryngeal nerve (hoarse voice) and hypoparathyroidism. Patients may become hypo- or hyperthyroid.

4 ***In pregnancy and infancy:*** Get expert help. See *OHCS* p25 & *OHCS* p182.

Complications Heart failure (thyrotoxic cardiomyopathy, ↑ in elderly),[119] angina, AF (seen in 10–25%: control hyperthyroidism and warfarinize if no contraindication), osteoporosis, ophthalmopathy, gynaecomastia. ►►Thyroid storm (p845).

Thyroid eye disease

This is seen in 25–50% of people with Graves' disease. The main known risk factor is smoking. The eye disease may not correlate with thyroid disease and the patient can be euthyroid, hypothyroid, or hyperthyroid at presentation. Eye disease may be the first presenting sign of Graves' disease, and can also be worsened by treatment, typically with radioiodine (usually a transient effect). Retro-orbital inflammation and lymphocyte infiltration results in swelling of the orbit.

Symptoms Eye discomfort, grittiness, tear production↑, photophobia, diplopia, acuity↓, afferent pupillary defect (p79) may mean optic nerve compression: ►*Seek expert advice at once as decompression may be needed.* Nerve damage does not necessarily go hand-in-hand with protrusion. Indeed, if the eye cannot protrude for anatomical reasons, optic nerve compression is more likely—a paradox!

Signs Exophthalmos—appearance of protruding eye; proptosis—eyes protrude beyond the orbit (look from above in the same plane as the forehead); conjunctival oedema; corneal ulceration; papilloedema; loss of colour vision. Ophthalmoplegia (especially of upward gaze) occurs due to muscle swelling and fibrosis.

Tests Diagnosis is clinical. CT/MRI of the orbits may reveal enlarged eye muscles.

Management Get specialist help. Treat hyper- or hypothyroidism. Advise to stop smoking as this worsens prognosis.[120] Most have mild disease that can be treated symptomatically (artificial tears, sunglasses, avoid dust, elevate bed when sleeping to ↓periorbital oedema). Diplopia may be managed with a Fresnel prism stuck to one lens of a spectacle (aids easy changing as the exophthalmos changes).

In more severe disease with ophthalmoplegia or gross oedema, try high-dose steroids (IV methylprednisolone is better than prednisolone 100mg/day PO)[121]—decreasing according to symptoms. Surgical decompression is used for severe sight-threatening disease, or for cosmetic reasons once the activity of eye disease has reduced (via an inferior orbital approach, using space in the ethmoidal, sphenoidal, and maxillary sinuses). Eyelid surgery may improve cosmesis and function. Orbital radiotherapy can be used to treat ophthalmoplegia but has little effect on proptosis. ***Future options:*** Anti-TNFα antibodies (eg infliximab).

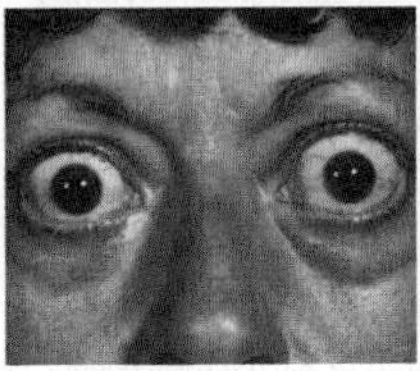

Fig 1. Thyroid eye disease: lid retraction causing a 'staring' appearance.

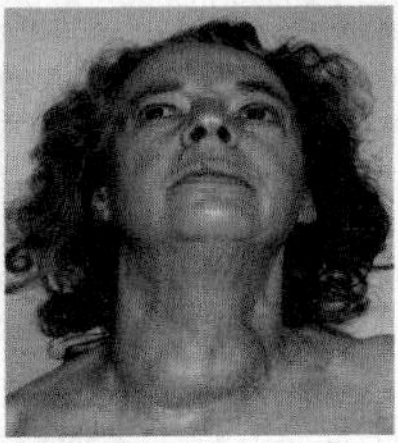

Fig 2. Goitre

Causes of goitre

Diffuse
- Physiological, or
- Graves' disease
- Hashimoto's thyroiditis
- Subacute (de Quervain's) thyroiditis (painful)

Nodular
- Multinodular goitre
- Adenoma
- Carcinoma

Manifestations of Graves' disease—and pathophysiology

Pituitary	Suppressed THS	↓Expression of thyrotropin β subunit[et al]
Heart	↑Rate; ↑contractility	↑Serum atrial natriuretic peptide[et al]
Liver	↑Peripheral T_3; LDL↓ (p704)	↑Type 1 5'-deiodinase; LDL receptors
Bone	↑Bone turnover; osteoporosis	↑Osteocalcin; ↑alk phos; ↑urinary N-telopeptide
Genital ♂	↓Libido; erectile dysfunction	↑Sex hormone globulin; ↓testosterone
Genital ♀	Irregular menses	Oestrogen antagonism
Metabolic	↑Thermogenesis; ↑O_2 use	↑Fatty acid oxidation; ↑Na-K ATPase
White fat	↓Fat mass	↑Adrenergic-mediated lipolysis
CNS basal ganglia	Stiff person syndrome (rare)[1]	Antibodies to glutamic acid decarboxylase[122] [123]
Muscle	Proximal myopathy	↑Sarcoplasmic reticulum Ca^{2+}-activated ATPase
Thyroid	↑Secretion of T_3 & T_4	↑Type 2 5'-deiodinase activity in thyroid[124]

1 Emotional or tactile stimuli cause spasms; seen in any autoimmune state (eg type 1 DM); Rx: baclofen ± IV Ig.

This is the clinical effect of thyroid hormone lack. It is common (4/1000/yr). If treated, prognosis is excellent; untreated it is disastrous (eg heart disease, dementia*etc*). ►*As it is insidious, both you and your patient may not realize anything is wrong*, so be alert to subtle, nonspecific symptoms, particularly in women ≥40yrs old (♀:♂ ≈6:1).

Symptoms Tired; sleepy, lethargic; mood↓; cold-disliking; weight↑; constipation; menorrhagia; hoarse voice; ↓memory/cognition; dementia; myalgia; cramps; weakness.

Signs BRADYCARDIC; reflexes relax slowly; ataxia (cerebellar); dry thin hair/skin; yawning/drowsy/coma (p844); cold hands ± T°↓; ascites ± non-pitting oedema (lids; hands; feet) ± pericardial or pleural effusion; round puffy face/double chin/obese; defeated demeanour; immobile ± ileus; CCF. Also: neuropathy; myopathy; goitre (some causes). See **fig 1**.

Diagnosis (p208) ►Have a low threshold for doing TFTs! TSH↑ (eg ≥4mU/L);[1] T4↓ (in rare secondary hypothyroidism: T4↓ & TSH↓ or ↔ due to lack from the pituitary, p224). Cholesterol & triglyceride↑; macrocytosis (less often normochromic anaemia too).

Autoimmune causes of primary hypothyroidism

- *Primary atrophic hypothyroidism:* ♀:♂ ≈6:1. Common. Diffuse lymphocytic infiltration of the thyroid, leading to atrophy, hence no goitre.
- *Hashimoto's thyroiditis:* Goitre due to lymphocytic and plasma cell infiltration. Commoner in women aged 60–70yrs. May be hypothyroid or euthyroid; rarely initial period of hyperthyroid ('Hashitoxicosis'). Autoantibody titres are very high.

Both are seen with other autoimmune diseases (type 1 DM, Addison's & PA, p328).

Other causes ►World-wide the chief cause is *iodine deficiency*. Others:

- *Post-thyroidectomy or radioiodine treatment.*
- *Drug-induced:* Antithyroid drugs, amiodarone, lithium, iodine.
- *Subacute thyroiditis:* Temporary hypothyroidism after hyperthyroid phase.

Secondary hypothyroidism Not enough TSH (∵ hypopituitarism, p224); very rare.

Hypothyroidism's associations Turner's & Down's syndromes, cystic fibrosis, primary biliary cirrhosis, ovarian hyperstimulation (*OHCS* p311);[125] POEMs syndrome—**p**olyneuropathy, **o**rganomegaly, **e**ndocrinopathy, **m**-protein band (plasmacytoma) + skin pigmentation/tethering. ***Genetic:*** Dyshormonogenesis: genetic (often autosomal recessive) defect in hormone synthesis, eg Pendred's syndrome (with deafness): there is ↑uptake on isotope scan, which is displaced by potassium perchlorate.

Pregnancy problems Eclampsia, anaemia, prematurity, ↓birthweight, stillbirth, PPH.

Treatment

- *Healthy and young:* Levothyroxine (T4), 50–100µg/24h PO; review at 12wks. Adjust 6 weekly by clinical state and to normalize but not suppress TSH (keep TSH >0.5mU/L). Thyroxine's $t_{½}$ is ~7d, so wait ~4wks before checking TSH to see if a dose change is right. NB: small changes in serum free T4 have a logarithmic effect on TSH.[126] Once normal, check TSH yearly. Enzyme inducers (p702) ↑metabolism of levothyroxine.
- *Elderly or ischaemic heart disease:* Start with 25µg/24h; ↑dose by 25µg/4wks according to TSH (►cautiously, as thyroxine may precipitate angina or MI).
- *If diagnosis is in question and T_4 already given:* Stop T4; recheck TSH in 6 weeks.

Amiodarone is an iodine-rich drug structurally like T_4; 2% of users will get significant thyroid problems from it. Hypothyroidism can be caused by toxicity from iodine excess (T_4 release is inhibited). Thyrotoxicosis may be caused by a destructive thyroiditis causing hormone release. Here, radioiodine uptake can be undetectable and if this is the case, glucocorticoids may help. Get expert help. Thyroidectomy may be needed if amiodarone cannot be discontinued.[127] $T_{½}$ of amiodarone ≈80d, so problems persist after withdrawal. If on amiodarone, check TFTs 6-monthly.

1 ►*Treat the patient not the blood level!* No exact cut-off in TSH can be given partly because risk of death from heart disease mirrors TSH ***even when in the normal range*** in women. Risk ≈1.4 if TSH 1.5–2.4 *vs* 1.7 if TSH 2.5–3.5. If TSH >3.65 and possibly symptomatic, a low dose of levothyroxine may be tried. Monitor symptoms, TSH & T_4 carefully. Over-exposure to thyroxine may cause osteoporosis ± AF.

Why are symptoms of thyroid disease so various, and so subtle?

Almost all our cell nuclei have receptors showing a high affinity for T_3: that known as TRα-1 is abundant in muscle and fat; TRα-2 is abundant in brain; and TRβ-1 is abundant in brain, liver, and kidney. These receptors, via their influence on various enzymes, affect the following processes:

- The metabolism of substrates, vitamins, and minerals.
- Modulation of all other hormones and their target-tissue responses.
- Stimulation of O_2 consumption and generation of metabolic heat.
- Regulation of protein synthesis, and carbohydrate and lipid metabolism.
- Stimulation of demand for co-enzymes and related vitamins.

Subclinical thyroid disease

Suspect if TSH >4mU/L (or perhaps <3.65[128]) with normal T_4 & T_3, and no obvious symptoms.[129] It is common: ~10% of those >55yrs have ↑TSH. Risk of progression to frank hypothyroidism is ~2%, and increases as TSH↑; risk doubles if thyroid peroxidase antibodies are present, and is also increased in men. ***Management:***

- Confirm that raised TSH is persistent (recheck in 2-4 months).
- Recheck the history: if any non-specific features (eg depression), discuss benefits of treating (p212) with the patient: maybe they will function better.
- Have a low threshold for carefully supervised treatment as your patient may not be so asymptomatic after all, and cardiac deaths *may* be prevented.[130] [131] [132] [133] [134] [135] Treat if: **1** TSH ≥10mu/L **2** +ve thyroid autoantibodies **3** Past (treated) Graves' **4** Other organ-specific autoimmunity (type 1 DM, myasthenia, pernicious anaemia, vitiligo), as they are more likely to progress to clinical hypothyroidism.[136] ***If TSH 4–10, and vague symptoms***, treat for 6 months—only continue if symptoms improve (or the patient is trying to conceive).[137] If the patient does not fall into any of these categories, monitor TSH yearly.
- Risks from well-monitored treatment of subclinical hypothyroidism are small (but there is an ↑risk of atrial fibrillation and osteoporosis if over-treated).

Subclinical hyperthyroidism occurs when TSH↓, with normal T_4 and T_3. There is a 41% increase in relative mortality from all causes versus euthyroid control subjects—eg from AF and osteoporosis.[138] ***Management:***[139]

- Confirm that suppressed TSH is persistent (recheck in 2-4 months).
- Check for a non-thyroidal cause: illness, pregnancy, pituitary or hypothalamic insufficiency (suspect if T_4 or T_3 are at the lower end of the reference range), use of TSH suppressing medication, eg thyroxine, steroids.
- If TSH <0.1, treat on an individual basis, eg with symptoms of hyperthyroidism, AF, unexplained weight loss, osteoporosis, goitre.
- Options are carbimazole or propylthiouracil—or radioiodine therapy.
- If no symptoms, recheck 6 monthly.

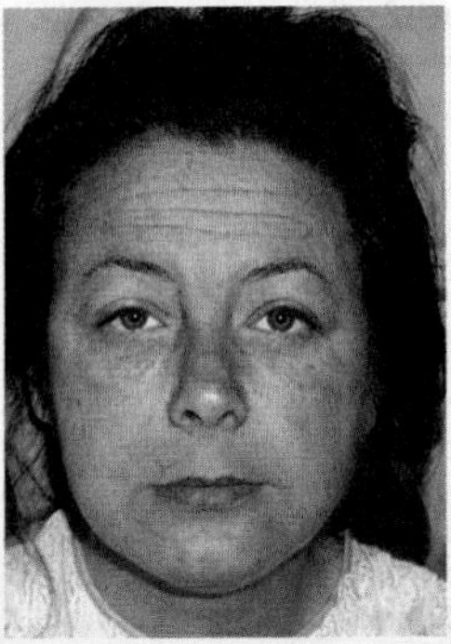

Fig 1. Facial appearance in hypothyroidism. Look for: pallor; coarse, brittle, diminished hair (scalp, axillary, and pubic); dull or blank expression lacking sparkle; coarse features; puffy lids. These signs are subtle: ►have a low threshold for measuring TSH (in yourself, your friends, and your patients). *Clinical Skills:* Oxford Core Text, 404, OUP.

Parathyroid hormone (PTH) is normally secreted in response to low ionised Ca^{2+} levels, by 4 parathyroid glands situated posterior to the thyroid (p670). The glands are controlled by -ve feedback via Ca^{2+} levels. PTH acts by: • ↑Osteoclast activity releasing Ca^{2+} & PO_4^{3-} from bones • ↑Ca^{2+} & ↓PO_4^{3-} reabsorption in the kidney • Active 1,25dihydroxy-vitamin D_3 production is ↑. Overall effect is ↑Ca^{2+} and ↓ PO_4^{3-}.

Primary hyperparathyroidism *Causes:* ~80% solitary adenoma, ~20% hyperplasia of all glands, <0.5% parathyroid cancer. *Presentation:* Often 'asymptomatic' (►***not in retrospect***!)[140], with ↑Ca^{2+} on routine tests. Signs relate to: **1** ↑Ca^{2+} (p690): weak, tired, depressed, thirsty, dehydrated-but-polyuric; also renal stones, abdominal pain, pancreatitis, and ulcers (duodenal:gastric≈7:1). **2** Bone resorption effects of PTH can cause pain, fractures, and osteopenia/osteoporosis. **3** BP↑: ►so check Ca^{2+} in ***everyone*** with hypertension.[141] *Association: MEN-1* (BOX 1). *Tests:* Ca^{2+}↑ & PTH↑ or inappropriately normal (other causes of this: thiazides, lithium, familial hypocalciuric hypercalcaemia, tertiary hyperparathyroidism). Also PO_4^{3-}↓ (unless in renal failure), alk phos↑ from bone activity, 24h urinary Ca^{2+}↑. *Imaging: osteitis fibrosa cystica* (due to severe resorption; rare) may show up as subperiosteal erosions, cysts, or brown tumours of phalanges ± acro-osteolysis (**fig 1**) ± 'pepper-pot' skull. *DEXA* (p697; for osteoporosis, p696).[142] ℞: If mild: advise ↑fluid intake to prevent stones; avoid thiazides + high Ca^{2+} & vit D intake; see 6-monthly. Excision of the adenoma or of all 4 hyperplastic glands prevents fractures and peptic ulcers.[143] *Indications:* high serum or urinary Ca^{2+}, bone disease, osteoporosis, renal calculi, ↓renal function, age ≤50yrs.[144] *Complications:* Hypoparathyroidism, recurrent laryngeal nerve damage (∴ hoarse), symptomatic Ca^{2+}↓ (hungry bones syndrome; check Ca^{2+} daily for ≥14d post-op). Pre-op ultrasound & MIBI scan (**fig 1**, p725) may localise an adenoma; intra-operative PTH sampling is used to confirm removal.[145] *Recurrence:* ~8% over 10yrs.[146] **Cinacalcet** (a 'calcimimetic') ↑ sensitivity of parathyroid cells to Ca^{2+} (∴ ↓PTH secretion); monitor Ca^{2+} within 1 week of dose changes; SE: myalgia; testosterone↓.[147]

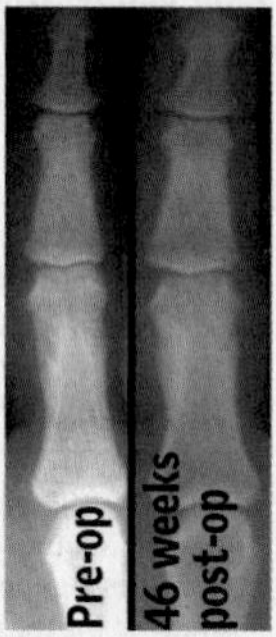

Fig 1. Acro-osteolysis. ©Dr Ian Maddison myweb.lsbu.ac.uk

Secondary hyperparathyroidism Ca^{2+}↓, PTH↑ (appropriately). *Causes:* ↓vit D intake, chronic renal failure. ℞: Correct causes. Phosphate binders (Ca^{2+}-free, eg **lanthanum**, are good but costly);[148] **vit D**; **cinacalcet** if PTH ≥85pmol/L and parathyroidectomy tricky.[149]

Tertiary hyperparathyroidism Ca^{2+}↑, ↑↑PTH (inappropriately). Occurs after prolonged secondary hyperparathyroidism, causing glands to act autonomously having undergone hyperplastic or adenomatous change. This causes Ca^{2+}↑ from ↑↑secretion of PTH unlimited by feedback control. Seen in chronic renal failure.

Malignant hyperparathyroidism Parathyroid-related protein (PTHrP) is produced by some squamous cell lung cancers, breast and renal cell carcinomas. This mimics PTH resulting in Ca^{2+}↑ (PTH is ↓, as PTHrP is not detected in the assay).

Hypoparathyroidism

Primary hypoparathyroidism PTH secretion is ↓ due to gland failure. *Tests:* Ca^{2+}↓, PO_4^{3-}↑ or ↔, alk phos ↔. *Signs:* Those of hypocalcaemia, p692 ± autoimmune co-morbidities (BOX 2). *Causes:* Autoimmune; congenital (Di George synd., *OHCS* p642). ℞: **Ca^{2+} supplements** + **calcitriol** (or **synthetic PTH** /12h SC: it prevents hypercalciuria).[150]

Secondary hypoparathyroidism Radiation, surgery (thyroidectomy, parathyroidectomy), hypomagnesaemia (magnesium is required for PTH secretion).

Pseudohypoparathyroidism Failure of target cell response to PTH. *Signs:* Short metacarpals (esp. 4th and 5th, **fig 2**), round face, short stature, calcified basal ganglia (**fig 3**), IQ↓. *Tests:* Ca^{2+}↓, ↑PTH, alk phos ↔ or ↑. ℞: As for 1° hypoparathyroidism.

Pseudopseudohypoparathyroidism The morphological features of pseudohypoparathyroidism, but with normal biochemistry. The cause for both is genetic.[151]

Multiple endocrine neoplasia (MEN types 1, 2a, and 2b)

In MEN syndromes there are functioning hormone-producing tumours in multiple organs (they are inherited as autosomal dominants).[152] They comprise: • MEN-1 & 2 • Neurofibromatosis (p518) • Von Hippel-Lindau & Peutz-Jeghers syndromes (p726 & p722)[153] • Carney complex (spotty skin pigmentation, schwannomas, myxoma of skin, mucosa, or heart, especially atrial myxoma), and endocrine tumours: eg pituitary adenoma, adrenal hyperplasia, and testicular tumour.[154]

MEN-1 Parathyroid hyperplasia/adenoma (~95%; most ↑Ca^{2+}).
Pancreas endocrine tumours (70%)—**gastrinoma** (p730) or **insulinoma** (p206), or, rarely, **somatostatinoma** (DM+steatorrhoea+gallstones/cholangitis), **VIPoma** (p246), or **glucagonomas** (±glucagon syndrome: migrating rash; glossitis; cheilitis, **fig 2** p321; anaemia; weight↓; plasma glucagon↑; glucose↑).[155]
Pituitary prolactinoma (~50%) or GH secreting tumour (acromegaly: p226); also, adrenal and carcinoid tumours are associated.

The MEN-1 gene is a tumour suppressor gene. Menin, its protein, alters transcription activation.[156] Many are sporadic, presenting in the 3rd–5th decades.

MEN-2a Thyroid: Medullary thyroid carcinoma (seen in ~100%, p602).
Adrenal: Phaeochromocytoma (~50%, usually benign and bilateral).
Parathyroid hyperplasia (~80%, but less than 20% have ↑Ca^{2+}).[157] [158]

MEN-2b[159] has similar features to MEN2a plus mucosal neuromas and Marfanoid appearance (p720), but no hyperparathyroidism.[160] Mucosal neuromas consist of 'bumps' on: lips, cheeks, tongue, glottis, eyelids, and visible corneal nerves.[161]

The gene involved in MEN-2a and b is the *ret* proto-oncogene, a receptor tyrosine kinase. Tests for *ret* mutations are revolutionizing MEN2 treatment by enabling a prophylactic thyroidectomy to be done before neoplasia occurs, usually before 3 yrs of age.[162] **NB:** *ret* mutations rarely contribute to sporadic parathyroid tumours.

Autoimmune polyendocrine syndromes[163]

Autoimmune disorders cluster into two defined syndromes:

Type 1: Autosomal recessive, rare.
Cause: Mutations of AIRE (Auto ImmuneREgulator) gene on chromosome 21.
Features: • Addison's disease • Chronic mucocutaneous candidiasis • Hypoparathyroidism. Also associated with hypogonadism, pernicious anaemia, autoimmune primary hypothyroidism, chronic active hepatitis, vitiligo, alopecia.

Type 2: HLA D3 and D4 linked, common. *Cause:* Polygenic.
Features: • Addison's disease • Type 1 diabetes mellitus (in 20%).
• Autoimmune thyroid disease—hypothyroidism or Graves' disease.
Also associated with primary hypogonadism, vitiligo, alopecia, pernicious anaemia, chronic atrophic gastritis, coeliac disease, dermatitis herpetiformis.

This is all rather MRCP-exam-ish: learn if you want, but... you don't have to be a good swot to be a good doctor.

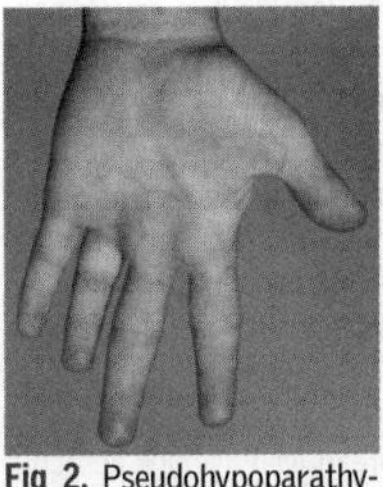

Fig 2. Pseudohypoparathyroidism: short 4th & 5th metacarpals.

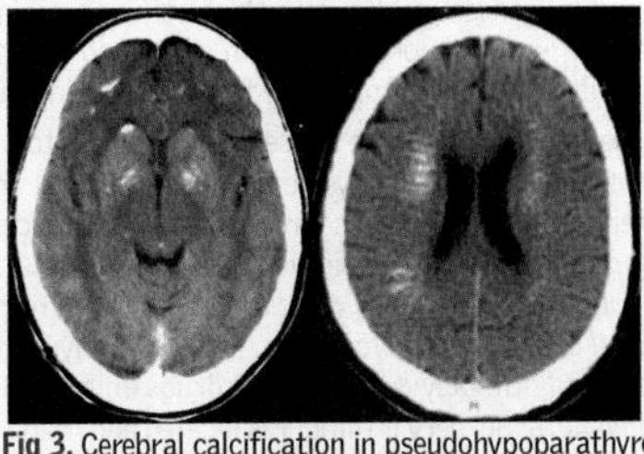

Fig 3. Cerebral calcification in pseudohypoparathyroidism: periventricular (left) and basal ganglia (right).[164]
Figure 3 courtesy of Professor Peter Scally.

These 2 topics are heavy on detail! But don't forget *all* about hyperparathyroidism: ►it's the best cause of a high Ca^{2+} and ►surgery can ***transform*** a life even if Ca^{2+} only slightly raised.[165] Also, MEN *is* important...►it's the most treatable form of pancreatic neoplasia.

Physiology The adrenal cortex produces steroids: **1** *Glucocorticoids* (eg cortisol), which affect carbohydrate, lipid and protein metabolism, **2** *Mineralocorticoids*, which control sodium and potassium balance (eg aldosterone, p682), and **3** *Androgens*, sex hormones which have weak effect until peripheral conversion to testosterone and dihydrotestosterone. Corticotropin-releasing factor (CRF) from the hypothalamus stimulates ACTH secretion from the pituitary, which in turn stimulates cortisol and androgen production by the adrenal cortex. Cortisol is excreted as urinary free cortisol and various 17-oxogenic steroids.

Cushing's syndrome This is the clinical state produced by chronic glucocorticoid excess + loss of the normal feedback mechanisms of the hypothalamo-pituitary-adrenal axis and loss of circadian rhythm of cortisol secretion (normally highest on waking). The chief cause is oral steroids. Endogenous causes are rare: 80% are due to ↑ACTH;[166] of these a pituitary adenoma (Cushing's disease) is the commonest cause.

1 ACTH-dependent causes: (↑ACTH)

- ***Cushing's disease*** Bilateral adrenal hyperplasia from an ACTH-secreting pituitary adenoma (usually a microadenoma, p226). ♀:♂>1:1. Peak age: 30–50yrs. A low-dose dexamethasone test (BOX) leads to no change in plasma cortisol, but 8mg may be enough to more than halve morning cortisol (as occurs in normals).[167]
- ***Ectopic ACTH production*** Especially small cell lung cancer and carcinoid tumours, p278. Specific features: pigmentation (due to ↑↑ACTH), hypokalaemic metabolic alkalosis (↑↑cortisol leads to mineralocorticoid activity), weight loss, hyperglycaemia. Classical features of Cushing's are often absent. Dexamethasone even in high doses (8mg) fails to suppress cortisol production.
- ***Rarely: Ectopic CRF production***—some thyroid (medullary) and prostate cancers.

2 ACTH-independent causes: (↓ACTH due to -ve feedback)

- ***Adrenal adenoma/cancer*** (may cause abdo pain ± virilization in ♀, p222). Because the tumour is autonomous, dexamethasone in any dose will not suppress cortisol.
- ***Adrenal nodular hyperplasia*** (no dose of dexamethasone suppresses cortisol)[168]
- ***Iatrogenic*** Pharmacological doses of steroids (common).
- ***Rarely: Carney complex*** p215. ***McCune–Albright syndrome*** See *OHCS* p650.

Symptoms Weight↑; mood change (depression, lethargy, irritability, psychosis); proximal weakness; gonadal dysfunction (irregular menses; hirsutism; erectile dysfunction); acne; recurrent Achilles tendon rupture; occasionally virilization if ♀.

Signs Central obesity; plethoric, moon face; buffalo neck hump; supraclavicular fat distribution; skin & muscle atrophy; bruises; purple abdominal striae (**fig 1**); osteoporosis; BP↑; glucose↑; infection-prone; poor healing. Signs of the cause (eg abdo. mass).

Tests Random plasma cortisols may mislead, as illness, time of day, and stress (eg venepuncture) influences results. Also, don't rely on imaging to localise the cause: non-functioning 'incidentalomas' occur in ~5% on adrenal CT and ~10% on pituitary MRI. MRI detects only ~70% of pituitary tumours causing Cushing's (many are too small).

Treatment Depends on the cause. • ***Iatrogenic:*** Stop medications if possible.

- ***Cushing's disease:*** Selective removal of pituitary adenoma (trans-sphenoidally). Bilateral adrenalectomy if source unlocatable, or recurrence post-op (complication: *Nelson's syndrome*: ↑skin pigmentation due to ↑↑ACTH from an enlarging pituitary tumour, as adrenalectomy removes -ve feedback; responds to pituitary radiation).
- ***Adrenal adenoma or carcinoma:*** Adrenalectomy: 'cures' adenomas but rarely cures cancer. Radiotherapy & adrenolytic drugs (mitotane) follow if carcinoma.
- ***Ectopic ACTH:*** Surgery if tumour is located and hasn't spread. Metyrapone, ketoconazole and fluconazole ↓cortisol secretion pre-op or if awaiting effects of radiation. Intubation + mifepristone (competes with cortisol at receptors) + etomidate (blocks cortisol synthesis) may be needed, eg in severe ACTH-associated psychosis.[169]

Prognosis Untreated Cushing's has ↑ vascular mortality.[170] Treated, prognosis is good (but myopathy, obesity, menstrual irregularity, BP↑, osteoporosis, subtle mood changes and DM often remain—so follow up carefully, and manage individually).[171]

Investigating suspected Cushing's syndrome[172]

First, confirm the diagnosis (a raised plasma cortisol), then localize the source on the basis of laboratory testing. Use imaging studies to confirm the likely source.

1st-line *Overnight dexamethasone suppression test* is a good outpatient test. Give dexamethasone 1mg PO at midnight; do serum cortisol at 8AM. If normal, this high dose of steroid causes -ve feedback, ↓ACTH and ↓cortisol secretion to <50nmol/L. In Cushing's syndrome, there is no cortisol suppression. False -ve rate: <2%; false +ves: 2% normal, 13% obese and 23% of inpatients. *NB:* false +ves (*pseudo-Cushing's*) are seen in depression, obesity, alcohol excess, and inducers of liver enzymes (↑ rate of dexamethasone metabolism, eg phenytoin, phenobarbital, rifampicin, p702). *24h urinary free cortisol* (normal: <280nmol/24 h) is an alternative.

2nd-line tests, if above abnormal: *48h dexamethasone suppression test:* Give dexamethasone 0.5mg/6h PO for 2d. Measure cortisol at 0 and 48h (last test at 6h after last dose). Again, in Cushing's syndrome, there is a failure to suppress cortisol. *Midnight cortisol:* Needs admission (unless salivary cortisol is used[173]). Often inaccurate due to difficulties in measurement. Normal circadian rhythm (cortisol *lowest* at midnight, *highest* early morning) is lost in Cushing's syndrome. Midnight blood, via a cannula during sleep, shows cortisol ↑ in Cushing's).

Localization tests (where is the lesion?) If the above are +ve—*Plasma ACTH: If ACTH is undetectable*, an adrenal tumour is likely → CT adrenal glands. If no mass, proceed to *adrenal vein sampling* or *adrenal scintigraphy* (radiolabelled cholesterol derivative). ***If ACTH is detectable***, distinguish a pituitary cause from ectopic ACTH production by the following: *High-dose dexamethasone suppression test:* Give dexamethasone 2mg/6h PO for 2d. Measure plasma and urinary cortisol at 0 and 48h. Complete or partial suppression indicates Cushing's disease as the pituitary retains some feedback control. An ectopic source is not under feedback control. **Or** *corticotropin releasing hormone test:* 100µg ovine or human CRH IV.[174] Measure cortisol at 120min. Cortisol rises with pituitary disease but not with ectopic ACTH production. CRH is corticotropin-releasing hormone.

If tests indicate that cortisol responds to manipulation, Cushing's disease is likely. Image the pituitary (MRI). If no mass is seen, *bilateral inferior petrosal sinus* blood *sampling* may help in confirming a pituitary adenoma, where the sinuses are sampled for ACTH release from the pituitary.

If tests indicate that cortisol does not respond to manipulation, hunt for the source of ectopic ACTH—eg IV contrast CT of chest, abdomen & pelvis[175] ± MRI of neck, thorax and abdomen, eg for small ACTH secreting carcinoid tumours.

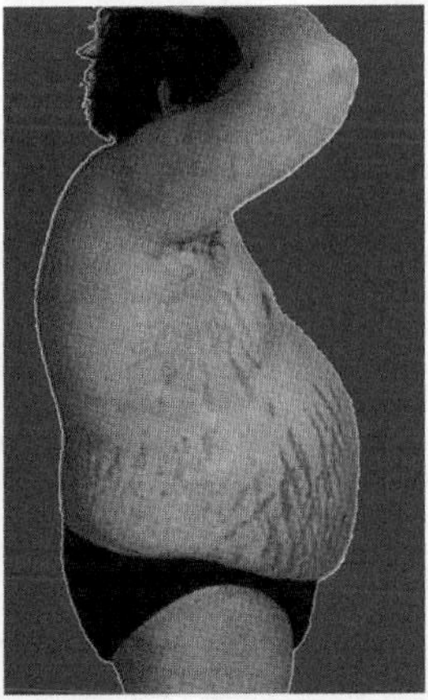

Fig 1. Hypercortisolism weakens skin; even normal stretching (or the pressure of obesity, as here) can make its elastin break—and on healing we see these depressed purple scars (striae), like flecks of puckered crêpe paper. Cortisone or rapid growth contributes to striae in other contexts: pregnancy; adolescence (eg in the 'love-handle' area); weight lifting; sudden-onset obesity, or from strong steroid creams. Striae mature into silvery crescents looking like the underside of willow leaves. Unsightly immature striae may be improved by YAG lasers.[176]

Addison's disease (adrenal insufficiency)

⏩Anyone on prednisolone for long enough to suppress the pituitary-adrenal axis, or who has overwhelming sepsis, or has metastatic cancer may suddenly develop adrenal insufficiency with deadly hypovolaemic shock.[177] ⏩See p846.

Primary adrenocortical insufficiency (Addison's disease) is rare (~0.8/100,000), but can be fatal. Destruction of the adrenal cortex leads to glucocorticoid (cortisol) and mineralocorticoid (aldosterone) deficiency (see **fig 1**). Signs are capricious: it is *'the unforgiving master of non-specificity and disguise'*.[178] You may diagnose a viral infection or anorexia nervosa in error (K^+ is ↓ in the latter but ↑ in Addison's).

Cause 80% are due to autoimmunity in the UK.[1] ***Other causes:*** TB (commonest cause worldwide), adrenal metastases (eg from lung, breast, renal cancer), lymphoma,[179] opportunistic infections in HIV (eg CMV, *Mycobacterium avium*, p411); adrenal haemorrhage (⏩Waterhouse–Friederichsen syndrome p728; antiphospholipid syndrome; SLE)[180], congenital (late-onset congenital adrenal hyperplasia).

Symptoms Often diagnosed late: lean, tanned, tired tearful ± weakness, anorexia, dizzy, faints, flu-like myalgias/arthralgias. *Mood:* depression, psychosis,[181] low self-esteem.[2] *GI:* nausea/vomiting, abdominal pain, diarrhoea/constipation. *Think of Addison's in all with unexplained abdominal pain or vomiting.*[182] Pigmented palmar creases & buccal mucosa (↑ACTH; cross-reacts with melanin receptors). Postural hypotension. Vitiligo. ⏩*Signs of critical deterioration* (p846): Shock (↓BP, tachycardia), T°↑, coma.

Tests Na^+↓ & K^+↑ (due to ↓mineralocorticoid), glucose ↓ (due to ↓cortisol). Also: uraemia, Ca^{2+}↑, eosinophilia, anaemia. **Δ:** *Short ACTH stimulation test (Synacthen® test):* Do plasma cortisol before and ½h after tetracosactide (Synacthen®) 250µg IM. Addison's is excluded if 2nd cortisol >550nmol/L. Steroid drugs may interfere with assays: ask lab. **NB:** in pregnancy and contraceptive pill, cortisol levels may be reassuring but falsely↑, due to ↑cortisol-binding globulin. *Also* • *ACTH:* In Addison's, 9AM ACTH is ↑ (>300ng/L: inappropriately high). It is low in secondary causes (see below). • *21-Hydroxylase adrenal autoantibodies:* +ve in autoimmune disease in >80% • *Plasma renin & aldosterone:* To assess mineralocortocoid status. *AXR/CXR:* Any past TB, eg upper zone fibrosis or adrenal calcification? If no autoantibodies, consider further tests (eg adrenal CT) for TB, histoplasma, or metastatic disease.[183]

Treatment Replace steroids: ~15–25mg *hydrocortisone* daily, in 2–3 doses, eg 10mg on waking, 5mg lunchtime.[184] Avoid giving late (may cause insomnia). Mineralocorticoids to correct postural hypotension, Na^+↓, K^+: *fludrocortisone* PO from 50–200µg daily. Adjust both on clinical grounds. If there is a poor response, suspect an associated autoimmune disease[1] (check thyroid, do coeliac serology: p280).[185]

Steroid use: Warn against abruptly stopping steroids. Emphasize that prescribing doctors/dentists/surgeons *must* know of steroid use: give *steroid card*, advise wearing a bracelet declaring steroid use. Add 5–10mg hydrocortisone to daily intake before strenuous activity/exercise. Double steroids in febrile illness, injury or stress. Give out syringes and in-date IM hydrocortisone, and show how to inject 100mg IM if vomiting prevents oral intake (seek medical help; admit for IV fluids if dehydrated).

Follow-up Yearly (BP, U&E); watch for autoimmune diseases (pernicious anaemia *et al*).[1]

Prognosis (treated) Adrenal crises and infections do cause excess deaths: mean age at death for men is ~65yrs (11yrs < estimated life expectancy; women lose ~3yrs).[186]

Secondary adrenal insufficiency The commonest cause is iatrogenic, due to long term steroid therapy leading to suppression of the pituitary-adrenal axis. This only becomes apparent on withdrawal of the steroids. Other causes are rare and include hypothalamic-pituitary disease leading to ↓ACTH production. Mineralocorticoid production remains intact, and there is no hyperpigmentation as ↓ACTH.

1 Autoimmune polyglandular syndromes types 1–4: **1** Monogenic syndrome (AIRE gene on chromosome 21); signs: candidiasis, hypoparathyroidism+Addison's. **2** (Schmidt syndrome) adrenal insufficiency+ autoimmune thyroid disease ± DM ± pleuritis/pericarditis **3** Autoimmune thyroid disease + other autoimmune conditions but *not* Addison's. **4** Autoimmune combinations not included in 1-3 above.
2 Adrenal destruction also causes depletion of adrenal androgens. These may have an effect on quality of life. However, studies on replacement of dehydroepiandosterone (DHEA), a precursor of sex hormone synthesis, in adrenal failure have been inconclusive.

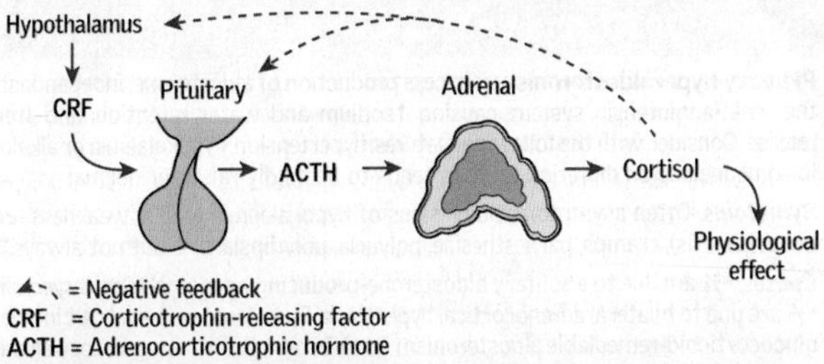

Fig 1. Pathways involved in adrenal function.

Excerpt from the notes of Miss E.L.R., 92 days before her death from undiagnosed Addison's disease. From the Coroner's Court...

"Typical day—wakes up at 11.30, still feels tired, then will have some breakfast and usually fall asleep on the couch. The most energy req. activity in last 1 month is—cooking herself a pasta meal. Then, totally exhausted will sleep more in pm, then eat some dinner. Goes to bed at 11pm—latest. Not able to concentrate...Used to weigh 45kg. Now weighs 42kg." 187

Placed on a page about Addison's disease, we might think there are sufficient clues to raise the suspicion of Addison's (even though her electrolytes were not particularly awry, and her pigmentation was barely perceptible). But change the context to our last busy clinic. We are a little distracted. The memory of Addison's is fading. Who among us will hear the alarm bell ring?

Hyperaldosteronism

Primary hyperaldosteronism is excess production of aldosterone, independent of the renin-angiotensin system, causing ↑sodium and water retention, and ↓renin release. Consider with the following features: hypertension, hypokalaemia or alkalosis in someone not on diuretics. Sodium tends to be mildly raised or normal.

Symptoms: Often asymptomatic or signs of hypokalaemia (p688): weakness (even quadriparesis), cramps, paraesthesiae, polyuria, polydipsia. BP↑ but not always.[188]

Causes: ~⅔ are due to a solitary aldosterone-producing adenoma[1] (***Conn's syndrome***). ~⅓ are due to bilateral adrenocortical hyperplasia. Rare causes: adrenal carcinoma or glucocorticoid-remediable aldosteronism (**GRA**). In GRA, the ACTH regulatory element of the 11β-hydroxylase gene fuses to the aldosterone synthase gene, increasing aldosterone production, and bringing it under the control of ACTH.

Tests: (see BOX) U&E (ideally not on diuretics, hypotensives, steroids, K^+, or laxatives for 4wks). Do not rely on a low K^+, as >20% are normokalaemic. For GRA (suspect if there is a family history of early hypertension), genetic testing is available. NB: renal artery stenosis is a more common cause of refractory ↑BP and ↓K^+ (p308).

Treatment: • *Conn's:* Laparoscopic adrenalectomy. Spironolactone (max 300mg/24h PO) for 4wks pre-op controls BP & K^+. 6-monthly imaging detects recurrence.[189]
- *Hyperplasia:* Treated medically: spironolactone, amiloride, or eplerenone (a newer selective aldosterone receptor antagonist, which doesn't cause gynaecomastia).
- *GRA*: dexamethasone 1mg/24h PO for 4wks, normalizes biochemistry but not always BP. If BP is still ↑, use spironolactone as an alternative. • *Adrenal carcinoma:* Surgery ± post-operative adrenolytic therapy with mitotane—prognosis is poor.

Secondary hyperaldosteronism Due to a high renin from ↓renal perfusion, eg in renal artery stenosis, accelerated hypertension, diuretics, CCF or hepatic failure.

Bartter's syndrome This is a major cause of congenital (autosomal recessive) salt wasting—via a sodium and chloride leak in the loop of Henle via a defective channel. Presents in childhood with failure to thrive, polyuria and polydipsia. BP is *normal*. Sodium loss leads to volume depletion, causing ↑renin and aldosterone production, leading to hypokalaemia and metabolic alkalosis, ↑urinary K^+ and Cl^-. ***Treatment:*** K^+ replacement, NSAIDs (to inhibit prostaglandins), and ACE-i.

Phaeochromocytoma

These are rare catecholamine-producing tumours. They arise from sympathetic paraganglia cells (=phaeochrome bodies), which are collections of adrenaline-secreting chromaffin cells. They are usually found within the adrenal medulla. Extra-adrenal tumours (paragangliomas) are rarer, often found by the aortic bifurcation (the organs of Zuckerkandl). Phaeochromocytomas *roughly* follow the 10% rule: 10% are malignant, 10% are extra-adrenal, 10% are bilateral, and 10% are familial. They are a dangerous but treatable cause of hypertension (in <0.1%).

Associations ~90% are sporadic; 10% are part of hereditary cancer syndromes (p215), eg thyroid, MEN-2a and 2b, neurofibromatosis, von Hippel-Lindau syndrome.[190]

Classic triad Episodic headache, sweating, and tachycardia (±BP↑, ↓ or ↔, BOX 2).[191]

Tests WCC↑ • Plasma + 3×24h urines for free metadrenaline & normetadrenaline (better than catecholamines & vanillylmandelic acid[192,193]) ± clonidine suppression test if borderline. • *Localization:* Abdominal CT/MRI, or meta-iodobenzylguanidine (MIBG—chromaffin-seeking isotope) scan (can find extra-adrenal tumours, p753).

Treatment ***Surgery***, α- & β-blockade pre-op: phenoxybenzamine (α-blocker) is used *before* β-blocker to avoid crisis from unopposed α-adrenergic stimulation. *Consult the anaesthetist.* ***Post-op:*** Do 24h urine metadrenalines 2wks post-op, monitor BP (risk of BP↓↓). ►►***Emergency ℞:*** p846. If malignant, chemotherapy or therapeutic radiolabelled MIBG may be used.[194] ***Follow-up:*** Lifelong: malignant recurrence may present late.[195]

1 Tumours from the zona glomerulosa, zona fasciculata, or zona reticularis associate with syndromes of ↑ mineralocorticoids, glucocorticoids, or androgens respectively, usually; remember 'GFR≈miner GA'.

Hypertension: a common context for hyperaldosteronism tests

Think of Conn's in these contexts: • Hypertension associated with hypokalaemia • Refractory hypertension, eg despite ≥3 antihypertensive drugs • Hypertension occurring before 40yrs of age (especially in women).[196]

The approach to investigation remains controversial. The **aldosterone/renin ratio** (ARR) is a good initial screening test. It is ideally measured when the patient has been upright or sitting for 2h, as posture affects results. Antihypertensives should be withheld for 2 weeks (spironolactone for 6 weeks) if possible. α-blockers can be used to control hypertension, as they do not affect the test. A raised ratio ie ↑aldosterone and ↓renin, indicates hyperaldosteronism. Additional **suppression tests** are done in some centres with fludrocortisone or saline, to test their ability to suppress aldosterone production.

Further investigation is needed to differentiate the cause of hyperaldosteronism. One method is to assess the effect of posture. Renin, aldosterone and cortisol are measured after the patient has been lying overnight, then repeated after being upright for 4 hours. Renin production increases on standing, causing ↑aldosterone production. This is exaggerated in bilateral hyperplasia, but there is no effect in Conn's, as aldosterone production is autonomous.

CT or **MRI** of the adrenals is done to localise the cause. This should be done after hyperaldosteronism is proven, due to the high number of adrenal incidentalomas. If imaging shows a unilateral adenoma, surgical excision is indicated. If no nodules or bilateral nodules are seen, a **trial of glucocorticoids** (eg dexamethasone) may be used to test for GRA. In GRA, dexamethasone causes ↓ACTH production by negative feedback, and therefore ↓aldosterone production.

If the above are inconclusive, **adrenal vein sampling** may be done (venous blood is sampled from both adrenals). If one side reveals increased aldosterone production compared with the other, an adenoma is likely. **Adrenal scintigraphy** is an alternative, where increased unilateral uptake of the isotope indicates adenoma.

Features of phaeochromocytoma (often episodic and often vague)

Try to diagnose before death: suspect if BP hard-to-control, accelerating or episodic.

- *Heart:* Pulse↑; palpitations/VT; dyspnoea; faints; angina; MI/LVF; cardiomyopathy.[1]
- *CNS:* Headache; visual disorder; dizziness; tremor; numbness; fits; encephalopathy; Horner's syndrome (paraganglioma) subarachnoid/intraventricular haemorrhage.
- *Psychological:* Anxiety; panic; hyperactivity; confusion; episodic psychosis.
- *Gut:* D&V, abdominal pain over tumour site;[197] mass; mesenteric vasoconstriction.
- *Others:* Sweats/flushes; heat intolerance; pallor; T°↑; backache; haemoptysis.

Symptoms may be precipitated by straining, exercise, stress, abdominal pressure, surgery, or by agents such as β-blockers, IV contrast agents, or the tricyclic you so kindly prescribed, thinking that the patient's bizarre symptoms were only explicable by psychopathology, such as depression. The site of the phaeochromocytoma may determine precipitants, eg if pelvic, precipitants include sexual intercourse, parturition, defecation, and micturition. Adrenergic crises may last minutes to days. Suddenly patients feel "as if about to die"—and then get better, or go on to develop a stroke or cardiogenic shock. On examination, there may be no signs, or hypertension ± signs of heart failure/cardiomyopathy (±paradoxical shock, similar to Takosubo's),[1] episodic thyroid swelling, glycosuria during attacks, or terminal haematuria from a bladder phaeochromocytoma.

1 *Takotsubo cardiomyopathy* (=stress- or catecholamine-induced cardiomyopathy/broken heart syndrome) may cause sudden chest pain mimicking MI, with ↑ST segments, and its signature apical ballooning on echo (also ↓ ejection fraction) occurring during catecholamine surges. It is a cause of MI in the presence of normal arteries. The stress may be medical (HAH482) or psychological.

Hirsutism is common (10% of women) and usually benign. It implies hair growth in women, in the male pattern. Causes are familial, idiopathic or are due to ↑ androgen secretion by the *ovary* (eg polycystic ovarian syndrome, ovarian cancer, *OHCS* p281), the *adrenal gland* (eg late-onset congenital adrenal hyperplasia, *OHCS* p250, Cushing's syndrome, adrenal cancer), or *drugs* (eg steroids). ***Polycystic ovarian syndrome (PCOS)*** causes secondary oligo- or amenorrhoea, infertility, obesity, acne & hirsutism (*OHCS* p252). Ultrasound: bilateral polycystic ovaries. Blood tests: ↑testosterone (if ≥6nmol/L, look for an androgen-producing adrenal or ovarian tumour), ↓sex-hormone binding globulin, ↑LH:FSH ratio (not consistent), TSH, lipids. Metformin may restore cycles and fertility, and helps insulin resistance (consider OGTT, p199). Address any feelings on lack of conformity to society's perceived norms of feminine beauty.[198] A multifaceted approach helps distress and improves sexual self-worth.

Management: What else is going on in her life that makes it worse *now*? Be supportive!
- Local measures: Shaving; laser photoepilation; wax; creams, eg **eflornithine**, or electrolysis (expensive/time-consuming, but effective); bleach (1:10 hydrogen peroxide).
- Oestrogens help, so consider the combined Pill (*OHCS* p302)—Yasmin® is one choice as its progestogen, **drospirenone**, is an anti-mineralocorticoid).[199] If no real help after 6–8 months, try Dianette® (its anti-androgen is **cyproterone acetate**; it's not licensed as a simple contraceptive. SE: depression.[200]
- **Metformin** & **spironolactone** are sometimes tried.[201] NNT 2-5 Healthy eating is important.
- **Clomifene** is used for infertility (a fertility expert should prescribe).

Virilism Onset of amenorrhoea, clitoromegaly, deep voice, temporal hair recession + hirsutism. Look for an androgen-secreting adrenal or ovarian tumour.

Gynaecomastia (ie abnormal amount of breast tissue in men; may occur in normal puberty). Oestrogen/androgen ratio↑ (*vs* galactorrhoea in which prolactin is↑). ***Cause:*** Hypogonadism (see BOX), liver cirrhosis (oestrogens↑), hyperthyroidism, tumours (oestrogen-producing eg testicular, adrenal; HCG-producing eg testicular, bronchial); drugs: oestrogens, spironolactone, digoxin, testosterone, marijuana; if stopping is impossible, consider testosterone if hypogonadism ± anti-oestrogen (tamoxifen).[202]

Erectile dysfunction (ED=impotence) Erections result from nitric oxide (NO) induced cyclic guanosine monophosphate (cGMP) build-up. cGMP-dependent protein kinase activates large-conductance, Ca^{2+}-activated K^+ channels so hyperpolarizing and relaxing vascular and trabecular smooth muscle cells, allowing engorgement.[203]

ED is common after 50yrs, and often multi-factorial. A psychological facet is common (esp. if ED occurs only in some situations, if onset coincides with stress, and if early morning 'incidental' erections still occur: these also persist in early organic disease). ***Organic causes:*** The big 3: smoking, alcohol and diabetes (∵ endothelial dysfunction +autonomic neuropathy). Also: ***Endocrine***: hypogonadism, hyperthyroidism, ↑prolactin; ***Neurological:*** cord lesions, MS, autonomic neuropathy; ***Pelvic surgery*** eg bladder-neck, prostate; ***radiotherapy***; ***atheroma***; ***renal*** or ***hepatic failure***; ***prostatic hyperplasia***; ***penile anomalies*** eg post-priapism, or Peyronie's (p722); ***Drugs:*** Digoxin, β-blockers, diuretics, antipsychotics, antidepressants, oestrogens, finasteride, narcotics.

Workup: After a full sexual & psychological history do: U&E, LFT, glucose, TFT, LH, FSH, lipids, testosterone, prolactin ± Doppler. Is penile arterial pressure enough for inflow? Is penile sensation OK (if not, ?CNS problem). Is the veno-occlusive mechanism OK?

℞: • Treat causes • Counselling • Oral phosphodiesterase (PDE5) inhibitors ↑cGMP. Erection isn't automatic (depends on erotic stimuli). **Sildenafil** (Viagra®) 25–100mg ½–1h pre-sex (food & alcohol upset absorption).[204] [205] ***SE:*** headache (16%); flushing (10%); dyspepsia (7%); stuffy nose (4%); transient blue-green tingeing of vision (inhibition of retinal PDE6).[206] ***CI:*** See BOX. **Tadalafil** (Cialis®; long $t_{½}$) 10–20mg ½–36h pre-sex. Don't use >once daily. SE: headache, dyspepsia, myalgia; ?no visual SEs. **Vardenafil** (Levitra® 5–20mg).[207] • Vacuum aids (ideal for penile rehabilitation after radical prostatectomy),[208] intracavernosal injections, transurethral pellets, and prostheses (inflatable or malleable; partners may receive unnatural sensations).[209] • Corpus cavernosum tissue engineering (eg on acellular collagen scaffolds) is in its infancy.[210]

Contraindications[ci]/cautions to Viagra® and other oral ED agents

- Concurrent use of nitrates[ci]
- BP↑↑ or systolic ≤90mmHg[ci] arrhythmia
- Degenerative retinal disorders,[ci] eg retinitis pigmentosa (for sildenafil)
- Unstable angina[ci] Stroke <6mths ago[ci]
- Myocardial infarction <90d ago[ci]
- Bleeding; peptic ulcer (sildenafil)
- Marked renal or hepatic impairment

Other cautions ►Angina (especially if during intercourse).
- Peyronie's disease or cavernosal fibrosis.
- Risk of priapism (sickle-cell anaemia, myeloma, leukaemia).
- Concurrent complex antihypertensive regimens.
- Dyspnoea on minimal effort (sexual activity may be unsupportable).

Use in coronary artery disease has been a question, but is probably OK.[211]

Interactions: Nitrites[ci]; cytochrome P450 (CYP3A) inducers: macrolides, protease inhibitors, theophyllines, azole antifungals, rifampicin, phenytoin, carbamazepine, phenobarbital, grapefruit juice (↑bioavailability). Caution if α-blocker use; avoid vardenafil with type 1A (eg quinidine; procainamide) and type 3 antiarrhythmics (sotalol; amiodarone)—as well as nitrates as above.[212]

When does a lifestyle malcontent become a disease?

"When should health providers pay for erectile treatment?" In the UK, the NHS will pay (endorse 'SLS'/ selected list substances on prescription) if ED is causing *severe* distress[2] or a MINIBOX context applies.

It is easy to criticise politicians who produce these arbitrary-looking criteria by recourse to clever counterexamples, but they need our support because they are making rationing (which is an inescapable fact of clinical life) *overt, open, available to scrutiny,* and *rational modification.* All too often rationing is covert, and nobody takes responsibility for it.

Free ED treatment if:[NHS]
- Prostatectomy
- Prostate cancer
- Diabetes mellitus
- Dialysis/renal transplant
- Spinal cord/pelvic injury
- Radical pelvic surgery[1]
- Parkinson's disease; MS
- Spina bifida
- Single gene CNS disease
- Poliomyelitis + after-effects

Free Viagra® for all? Given that WHO defines health as ***complete*** physical, mental and social wellbeing (a state presumably only experienced during sexual intercourse), surely free access to Viagra® *et al* is what every health system should endorse as its top priority? This is exactly what Mexico City enacted in 2008[213] for men over 70. It is not reported what their partners felt about this initiative.

You can only avoid politics if you avoid life.

Male hypogonadism

Hypogonadism is failure of testes to produce testosterone, sperm, or both. Features: small testes, ↓libido, erectile dysfunction, loss of pubic hair, ↓muscle bulk, ↑fat, gynaecomastia, osteoporosis; mood↓. If prepubertal: ↓virilization; incomplete puberty; eunuchoid body; reduced secondary sex characteristics. Causes:

Primary hypogonadism is due to testicular failure, eg from • Local trauma, torsion, chemotherapy/irradiation • Post-orchitis eg mumps, HIV, brucellosis, leprosy • Renal failure, liver cirrhosis or alcohol excess (toxic to Leydig cells). • Chromosomal abnormalities eg Klinefelter's syndrome (47XXY)—delayed sexual development, small testes and gynaecomastia. Anorchia is rare.

Hypogonadism secondary to: ↓Gonadotropins (LH & FSH), eg from • Hypopituitarism • Kallman's syndrome—isolated gonadotropin releasing hormone deficiency, often with anosmia and colour blindness • Systemic illness (eg COPD; HIV; DM) • Laurence-Moon-Biedl & Prader-Willi syndromes (*OHCS* p648 & p652) • Age.

℞: (p224) If total testosterone ≤8nmol/L, on 2 mornings (or <15 if LH↑ too) and muscle bulk↓, testosterone may help,[214] eg 1% dermal gel[215] [216] (Testogel®). Heart,[217] bladder & sexual function may perk up in age-related hypogonadism.[218] Beware medicalizing aging! CI: Ca^{2+}↑; nephrosis; prostate, breast♂ or liver ca. Monitor PSA.

1 Success for reversing ED post-op is only 43% *vs* 85% in those with neurological conditions.
2 Criteria include marked disruption to relationships or mood, judged by a certified prescriber

Hypopituitarism entails ↓secretion of anterior pituitary hormones. (**figs 1, 2**)They are affected in this order: growth hormone (GH), gonadotropins: follicle-stimulating hormone (FSH) and luteinizing hormone (LH), prolactin (PRL), thyroid-stimulating hormone (TSH), and adrenocorticotrophic hormone (ACTH). Panhypopituitarism is deficiency of all anterior hormones, usually caused by irradiation, surgery, or pituitary tumour.

Causes are at 3 levels: **1** ***Hypothalamus:*** Kallman's syndrome (p223), tumour, inflammation, infection (meningitis, TB), ischaemia. **2** ***Pituitary stalk:*** Trauma, surgery, mass lesion (craniopharyngioma, p226), meningioma, carotid artery aneurysm. **3** ***Pituitary:*** Tumour, irradiation, inflammation, autoimmunity,[1] infiltration (haemochromatosis, amyloid, metastases), ischaemia (pituitary apoplexy, p226; DIC;[2] Sheehan's syndrome[3]).

Features are due to: **1 Hormone lack:** • ***GH lack:*** Central obesity, atherosclerosis, dry wrinkly skin, strength↓, balance↓, wellbeing↓, exercise ability↓, cardiac output↓, osteoporosis, glucose↓.219 • ***Gonadotropin (FSH; LH) lack:*** ♀: Few, scant, or no menses (oligomenorrhoea or amenorrhoea), fertility↓, libido↓, osteoporosis, breast atrophy, dyspareunia. ♂: Erectile dysfunction, libido↓, muscle bulk↓, hypogonadism (↓hair, all over; small testes; ejaculate volume↓; spermatogenesis↓). • ***Thyroid lack:*** As for hypothyroidism (p212). • ***Corticotropin lack:*** As for adrenal insufficiency (p218). NB: no ↑skin pigmentation as ↓ACTH. • ***Prolactin lack:*** Rare: absent lactation.

2 Cause: eg pituitary tumour (p226), causing mass effect, or hormone secretion with ↓secretion of other hormones—eg prolactinoma, acromegaly, rarely Cushing's.

Tests (The triple stimulation test is now rarely done.)

- ***Basal tests:*** LH & FSH (↓ or ↔), testosterone or oestradiol (↓); TSH (↓ or ↔), T_4 (↓); prolactin (may be ↑, from loss of hypothalamic dopamine that normally inhibits its release), insulin-like growth factor-1 (IGF-1; ↓—used as a measure of GH axis, p230), cortisol (↓). Also do U&E (Na^+↓ from dilution), Hb↓ (normochromic, normocytic).
- ***Dynamic tests:*** **1** Short Synacthen® test: (p218) to assess the adrenal axis.220
  2 Insulin tolerance test (ITT): Done in specialist centres to assess the adrenal and GH axes. *CI:* epilepsy, heart disease, adrenal failure. Consult lab first. It involves IV insulin to induce hypoglycaemia, causing stress to ↑cortisol and GH secretion. It is done in the morning (water only taken from 22:00h the night before). Have 50% glucose & hydrocortisone to hand and IV access. Glucose must fall below 2.2mmol/L and the patient should become symptomatic when cortisol and GH are taken. Normal: GH >20mU/L, and peak cortisol >550nmol/L.
  3 Arginine + growth hormone releasing hormone test.
  4 Glucagon stimulation test are alternatives when ITT is contraindicated.
- ***Investigate cause:*** MRI scan to look for a hypothalamic or pituitary lesion.

Treatment involves hormone replacement and treatment of underlying cause.

- ***Hydrocortisone*** for secondary adrenal failure (p218).
- ***Thyroxine*** if hypothyroid (p212, but TSH is useless for monitoring).
- Hypogonadism (for symptoms and to prevent osteoporosis). ♂: Options include ***testosterone enanthate*** 250mg IM every 3 weeks, daily topical gels or buccal mucoadhesive tablets. Patches and gels are also used.[4] ♀: (*premenopausal*) ***Oestrogen:*** Transdermal oestradiol patches, oestradiol implants or contraceptive pill (exceeds replacement needs) ± ***testosterone*** or ***dehydroepiandrosterone*** (DHEA, in hypoandrogenic women; a small amount may improve wellbeing and sexual function,221 and help bone mineral density and lean body mass). ***Gonadotropin*** therapy is needed to induce fertility in both men and women.
- Growth hormone (BOX). Refer to an endocrinologist for insulin tolerance testing.

1 Autoimmune hypophysitis (=inflamed pituitary) mimics pituitary adenoma. It may be triggered by pregnancy or immunotherapy blocking CTLA-4. No pituitary autoantigen is yet used diagnostically.
2 Snake bite is a common cause in India (eg when associated with acute renal failure).
3 Sheehan's syndrome is pituitary necrosis after postpartum haemorrhage.
4 Testogel® (50mg testosterone in 5g of gel) is applied in a thin film. 100mg/d may be needed (approach by 25mg increments). Use on clean, dry, healthy skin (shoulders, arms abdomen), as soon as sachet is opened. Allow to dry for 5min. Wash hands after use, avoid shower/bath for at least 6h. Avoid skin contact with gel sites to prevent testosterone transfer to others (esp pregnant women and children).

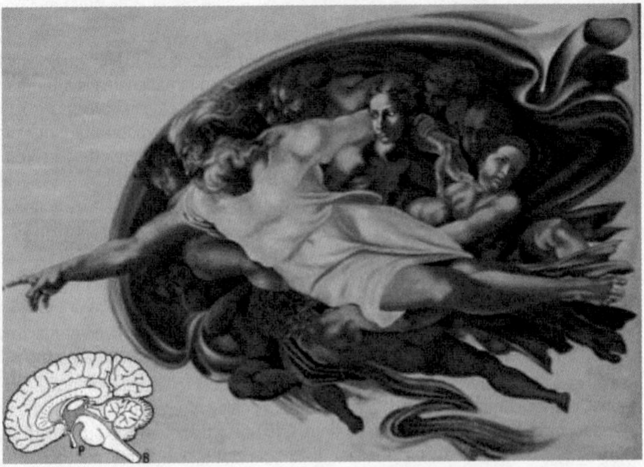

Fig 1. Neuroendocrinology: emotions ⇄ thoughts ⇄ actions. As Michelangelo foretold (in his *Creation of Adam*) 'all gods and demons that have ever existed are within us as possibilities, desires, and ways of escape'.[222] Within the dark red vault of our skull we see human and god-like forms reaching out, as thoughts escape into actions—with legs extending into our brainstem (B) and a fist is pushing from our hypothalamus into the pituitary stalk (P).[223] Frank Lynn Meshberger Above the pituitary we have thoughts, ideas, impulses, and neurotransmitters. Below we have hormones. Between is the realm of neuroendocrinology—the neurosecretory cells which turn emotions into the releasing factors for the pituitary hormones (fig 2). Image courtesy of Gary Bevans.

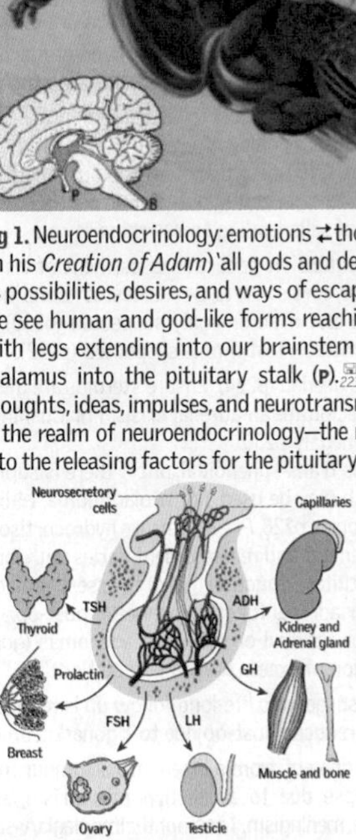

Fig 2. Neuroregulation and integration of endocrine axes makes us who we are—and who we are and what we do feeds back into our hormonal milieu.[224] [225] Multifactorial disruptions within the growth hormone (GH), luteinizing hormone (LH)-testosterone, adrenocorticotropin (ACTH)-cortisol and insulin axes play a major role in healthy maturation and ageing. But it is a truism to say that good health depends on the right balance and feedback loops. The myth of the pituitary as the 'conductor of the orchestra' is exploded by the placenta—that maverick organ with its heavy metal drowning out anything that the pituitary can do (p231).[226]

Using somatropin (GH) in those >25yrs old (see nice.org.uk)

Somatotropin addresses problems of ↑fat mass, ↓bone mass, ↓lean body mass (muscle bulk), ↓exercise capacity and problems with heat intolerance. **NB**: increased abdominal fat results in reduced insulin sensitivity and dyslipidaemia.

Somatropin uses DNA technology to mimic human GH. It can be used in known GH deficiency, eg peak GH response of <9mU/L (3ng/mL) during ITT—if there is impaired quality of life and treatment for other pituitary deficiencies is under way.[227]

Self-injection 0.15–0.3mg/d; needs lessen with age. Dose titration (1st 3 months of therapy) is done by an endocrinologist. *SE:* oedema, carpal tunnel syndrome, myalgia, CCF, BP↑, ICP↑ (rare). IGF-1 levels rise with GH replacement. ↑IGF-1 is linked with ↑risk of neoplasia.[228] *CI:* malignancy, pregnancy, renal transplant.

Somatropin can be stopped after 9 months if quality of life scores do not improve by 7 points or more. *Using GH in children:* See *OHCS* p180.

Pituitary tumours

Pituitary tumours (almost always benign adenomas) account for 10% of intracranial tumours (see **figs 1 & 2**). They may be divided by size: a microadenoma is a tumour <1cm across, and a macroadenoma is >1cm. There are 3 histological types.

1 *Chromophobe*—70%. Many are non-secretory,[1] some cause hypopituitarism. Half produce prolactin (PRL); a few produce ACTH or GH. Local pressure effect in 30%.
2 *Acidophil*—15%. Secrete GH or PRL. Local pressure effect in 10%.
3 *Basophil*—15%. Secrete ACTH. Local pressure effect rare.

Classification by hormone secreted (may be revealed by immunohistology)			
PRL only (→prolactinoma)	35%	ACTH (→Cushing's disease)	7%
GH only (→acromegaly)	20%	LH/FSH/TSH	≥1%[2] 229
PRL and GH	7%	No obvious hormone	30%

Symptoms are caused by pressure, hormones (eg galactorrhoea), or hypopituitarism (p224). FSH-secreting tumours can cause macro-orchidism in men, but are rare.

Features of local pressure Headache, visual field defects (bilateral temporal hemianopia, due to compression of the optic chiasm), palsy of cranial nerves III, IV, VI (pressure or invasion of the cavernous sinus; **fig 3**). Also, diabetes insipidus (DI) (p232; more likely from hypothalamic disease); disturbance of hypothalamic centres of T°, sleep, and appetite; erosion through floor of sella leading to CSF rhinorrhoea.

Tests MRI defines intra- and supra-sellar extension; accurate assessment of visual fields; screening tests: PRL, IGF-1 (p230), ACTH, cortisol, TFTs, LH/FSH, testosterone in ♂, short Synacthen® test. Glucose tolerance test if acromegaly suspected (p230). If Cushing's suspected, see p217. Water deprivation test if DI is suspected (p232).

Treatment Start hormone replacement as needed (p224). Ensure steroids are given before levothyroxine, as thyroxine may precipitate an adrenal crisis. For Cushing's disease see p217, prolactinoma p228, acromegaly p230.

- ***Surgery*** **(fig 4)**: Most pituitary surgery is trans-sphenoidal, but if there is suprasellar extension, a trans-frontal approach may be used. For prolactinoma, 1st-line treatment is medical with a dopamine agonist, p228. *Pre-op:* Ensure hydrocortisone 100mg IV/IM. Subsequent cortisol replacement and reassessment varies with local protocols: get advice. *Post-op:* Retest pituitary function (p224) to assess replacement needs. Repeating dynamic tests for adrenal function ≥6 weeks post-op.
- ***Radiotherapy:*** (eg stereotactic) Good for residual or recurrent adenomas (good rates of tumour control and normalization of excess hormone secretion). 230

Post-op Recurrence may occur late after surgery, so life-long follow up is required. Fertility should be discussed: this may be reduced post-op due to ↓ gonadotropins.

Pituitary apoplexy Rapid pituitary enlargement from a bleed into a tumour may cause mass effects, cardiovascular collapse due to acute hypopituitarism, and death. 231 Suspect if acute onset of headache, meningism, ↓GCS, ophthalmoplegia/visual field defect, especially if there is a known tumour (may present like subarachnoid haemorrhage). ℞: Urgent steroids (hydrocortisone 100mg IV) and meticulous fluid balance ± cabergoline (dopamine agonist, if prolactinoma) ± surgery; find the cause, eg a predisposition to thrombosis, from antiphospholipid syndrome. 232

Craniopharyngioma Not strictly a pituitary tumour: it originates from Rathke's pouch so is situated between pituitary and the 3rd ventricle floor. They are rare, but are the commonest childhood intracranial tumour. Over 50% present in childhood with growth failure; adults may present with amenorrhoea, ↓libido, hypothalamic symptoms (eg diabetes insipidus, hyperphagia, sleep disturbance) or tumour mass effect, see above. ***Tests:*** CT/MRI (calcification in 50%, may also be seen on skull XR). ***Treatment:*** Surgery ± post-op radiation; test pituitary function post-op.

1 If <1cm, usually 'incidentaloma'; most non-functioning macroadenomas are revealed by mass effect and/or hypopituitarism. Here, recurrence after surgery is common, so follow carefully with MRIs.
2 Sensitive methods of TSH measurement have improved recognition of TSH-secreting tumours. These are now more frequently found at microadenoma stage, medially located, and *without* associated hormone hypersecretion. In these tumours, somatostatin analogues (p230) are very helpful.

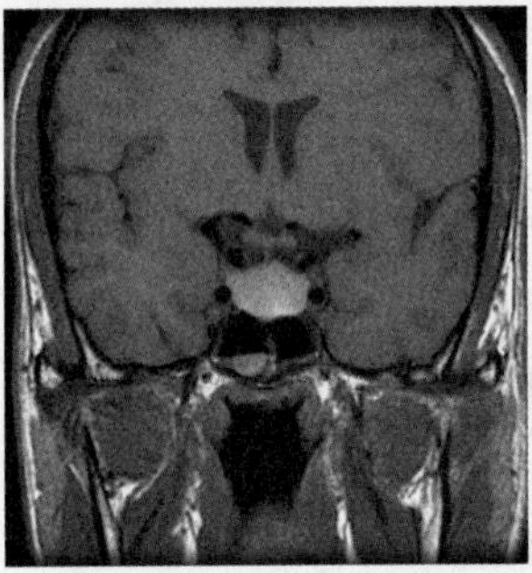

Fig 1. Sagittal T1 weighted MRI of the brain (no gadolinium contrast) showing a lesion in the pituitary fossa, most likely a haemorrhagic pituitary adenoma. Differential diagnosis includes a Rathke's cleft cyst.

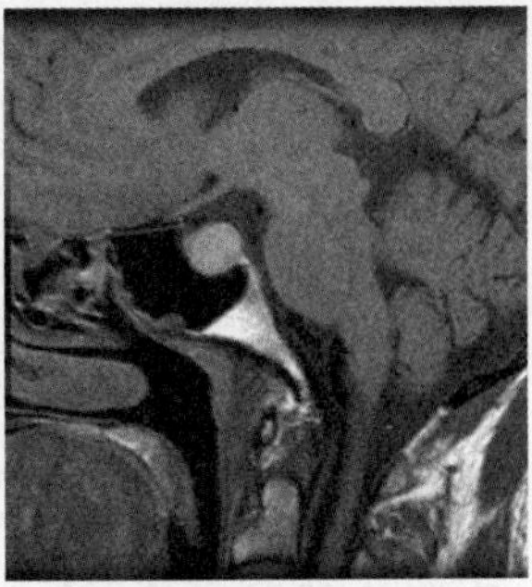

Fig 2. Coronal T1 weighted MRI of the brain (no gadolinium contrast) showing a lesion in the pituitary fossa. (see fig 1).

Figs 1 & 2 Courtesy of Norwich Radiology Dept.

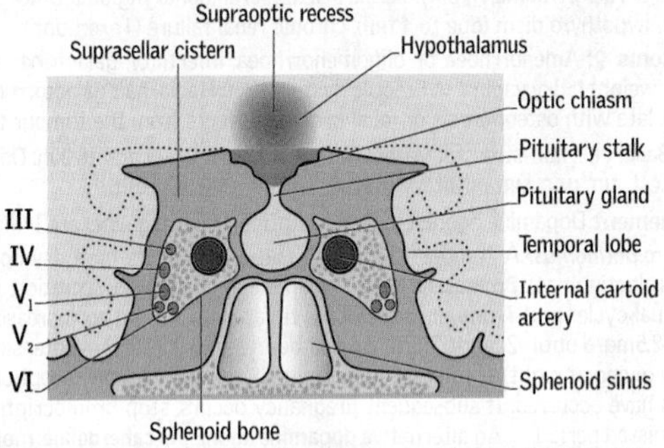

Fig 3. The pituitary gland's relationships to cranial nerves III, IV, V, & VI.

Courtesy of *Oxford Handbook Of Endocrinology & Diabetes*, 101, OUP.

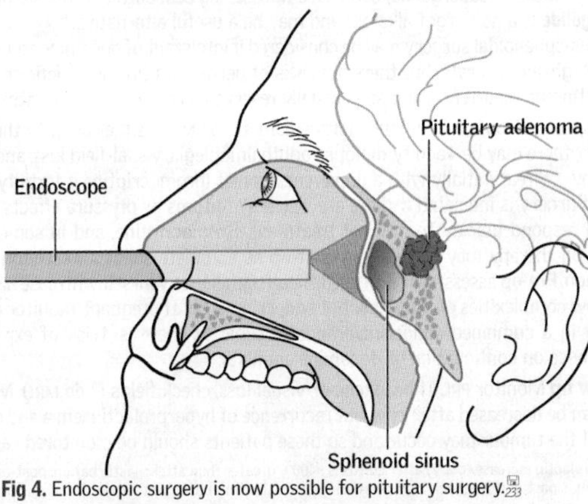

Fig 4. Endoscopic surgery is now possible for pituitary surgery. 233

Hyperprolactinaemia

This is the commonest hormonal disturbance of the pituitary. It presents earlier in women (menstrual disturbance) but later in men (eg with erectile dysfunction and or mass effects). Prolactin stimulates lactation.*et al* [1,2] Raised levels lead to hypogonadism, infertility & osteoporosis, by inhibiting secretion of gonadotropin releasing hormone (hence ↓LH/FSH & ↓testosterone or oestrogen).

Causes of raised plasma prolactin (PRL; >390mU/L) PRL is secreted from the anterior pituitary and release is inhibited by dopamine produced in the hypothalamus. Hyperprolactinaemia may result from **1** Excess production from the pituitary, eg prolactinoma. **2** Disinhibition, by compression of the pituitary stalk, reducing local dopamine levels or **3** Use of a dopamine antagonist. A PRL of 1000-5000mU/L may result from any, but >5000 is likely to be due to a prolactinoma, with macroadenomas (>10mm) having the highest levels, eg 10,000-100,000.

- ***Physiological:*** Pregnancy; breastfeeding; stress. (Acute rises occur post-orgasm).[1]
- ***Drugs (most common cause):*** Metoclopramide; haloperidol; α-methyldopa; oestrogens; ecstasy/MDMA;[2] antipsychotics (a reason for 'non-compliance': *sustained* hyperprolactinaemia may cause ↓libido, anorgasmia, and erectile dysfunction).[234]
- ***Diseases:*** *Prolactinoma:* micro- or macroadenoma; *Stalk damage:* pituitary adenomas, surgery, trauma; *Hypothalamic disease:* craniopharyngioma, other tumours; *Other:* hypothyroidism (due to ↑TRH), chronic renal failure (↓excretion).

Symptoms ♀: Amenorrhoea or oligomenorrhoea; infertility; galactorrhoea. Also: libido↓, weight↑, dry vagina. **♂:** Erectile dysfunction, ↓facial hair, galactorrhoea. May present late with osteoporosis or local pressure effects from the tumour (p226).

Tests Basal PRL: non-stressful venepuncture between 09.00 and 16.00h. Do a pregnancy test, TFT, U&E. MRI pituitary if other causes are ruled out.

Management Dopamine agonists (bromocriptine or cabergoline) are 1st line.

Microprolactinomas: A tumour <10mm on MRI (~25% of us have asymptomatic microprolactinomas). **Bromocriptine**, a dopamine agonist, ↓PRL secretion, restores menstrual cycles and ↓tumour size. Dose is titrated up: 1.25mg PO; increase weekly by 1.25-2.5mg/d until ~2.5mg/12h. SE: nausea, depression, postural hypotension (minimise by giving at night). If pregnancy is planned♀, use barrier contraception until 2 periods have occurred. If subsequent pregnancy occurs, stop bromocriptine after the 1st missed period.[235] An alternative dopamine agonist is **cabergoline**: more effective and fewer SE, but there is less data on safety in pregnancy. NB: ergot alkaloids (bromocriptine & cabergoline) can cause fibrosis (eg echocardiograms are needed). **Quinagolide** is a non-ergot alkaloid and may be a useful alternative.

Trans-sphenoidal surgery may be considered if intolerant of dopamine agonists. It has a high success rate, but there are risks of permanent hormone deficiency and prolactinoma recurrence, and so is usually reserved as a second-line treatment.

Macroprolactinomas: A tumour >10mm diameter on MRI. As they are near the optic chiasm, there may be ↓acuity, diplopia, ophthalmoplegia, visual-field loss, and optic atrophy.[236] Treat initially with a dopamine agonist (bromocriptine if fertility is the goal). Surgery is indicated if there are visual symptoms or pressure effects which fail to respond quickly to medical treatment. Bromocriptine, and in some cases radiation therapy, may be required post-op as complete surgical resection is uncommon. Pre-op assessment is often difficult: familiarize yourself with case histories to show complexities of this aspect of endocrinology.[3] If pregnant, monitor closely ideally in a combined endocrine/antenatal clinic as there is ↑risk of expansion. Get advice on continuation of dopamine agonists.

Follow up Monitor PRL. If headache or visual loss, check fields (? do MRI). Medication can be decreased after 2yrs, but recurrence of hyperprolactinaemia and expansion of the tumour may occur, and so these patients should be monitored carefully.

1 The prolactin increase (♂&♀) after coitus is ~400% greater than after masturbation; post-orgasmic prolactin is part of a feedback loop decreasing arousal by inhibiting central dopaminergic processes. The size of post-orgasmic prolactin increase is a neurohormonal index of sexual satisfaction.

2 MDMA also ↑oxytocin; prolactin+oxytocin are thought to mediate post-orgasmic wellbeing.

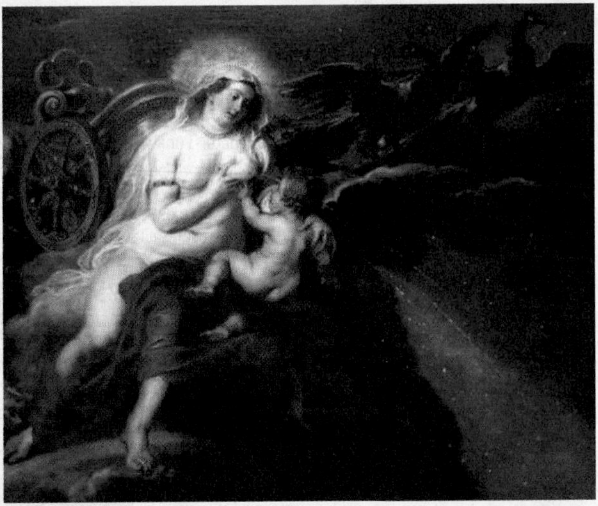

Fig 1. Galactorrhoea can be prolific enough to create medium-sized galaxies (bottom right). In the *Birth of the Milky Way* (Courtesy of the Prado Museum[237]) Hera is depicted by Rubens in her chariot, being drawn through the night sky by ominous black peacocks. Between journeys, she enjoyed discussing difficult endocrinological topics with her husband Zeus (who was also her brother), such as whether women or men find sexual intercourse more enjoyable. Hera inclined to the latter—and it is on this flimsy evidence, and her gorgeous galactorrhoea, that we diagnose her hyperprolactinaemia (which is known to decrease desire, lubrication, orgasm, and satisfaction).[238] In the end, this issue was settled, in favour of Zeus's view, by Tiresias, who had unique insight into this intriguing question: every time this soothsayer saw two snakes entwined, (s)he changed sex, so coming to know a thing or two about gender and pleasure. This is a primordial example of an 'N of 1' trial, where the subject is his or her own control. Generalizability can be a problem with this methodology.

Image courtesy of the Prado Museum

3 A 46yr-old lady had galactorrhoea for 7yrs, and a ↑prolactin (3133mU/L) and intact pituitary function with no eye signs. MRI showed 1.9cm pituitary tumour + extra-sellar extension. Is transsphenoidal resection needed for a presumed macroadenoma with hyperprolactinaemia, or a dopamine-agonist trial? *Possible answer:* try drugs, and monitor MRI if initial prolactin ≥2000mU/L.

Acromegaly

This is due to ↑secretion of GH (growth hormone) from a pituitary tumour (99%) or hyperplasia, eg via ectopic GH-releasing hormone from a carcinoid tumour. ♀:♂ ≈1:1. Incidence:[UK] 3/million/yr.[239] ~5% are associated with MEN-1 (p215). GH stimulates bone & soft tissue growth through ↑secretion of insulin-like growth factor-1 (IGF-1).

Symptoms Acroparaesthesia (*akron*=extremities); amenorrhoea; libido↓; headache; ↑sweating; snoring; arthralgia; backache; **fig 1**: "My rings don't fit, nor my old shoes, and now I've got a wonky bite (malocclusion) and curly hair. I put on lots of weight, all muscle and looked good for awhile; now I look so haggard".[240] [241]

Signs (BOX) often predate diagnosis by >4yrs. If acromegaly occurs before bony epiphyses fuse (rare), gigantism occurs.

Complications (may present with CCF[242] or ketoacidosis).[243]

- Impaired glucose tolerance (~40%), DM (~15%).[244]
- Vascular: BP↑, left ventricular hypertrophy (±dilatation/CCF), cardiomyopathy, arrhythmias. There is ↑risk of ischaemic heart disease and stroke (?due to ↑BP ± insulin resistance and GH-induced increase in fibrinogen and decrease in protein S).[245]
- Neoplasia: colon cancer risk↑; colonoscopy may be needed.[246]

Acromegaly in pregnancy (Subfertility is common) Pregnancy may be normal; signs & chemistry may remit.[247] Monitor glucose.

Tests ↑Glucose, ↑Ca^{2+} & ↑PO_4^{3-}.[248] *GH:* Don't rely on random GH as secretion is pulsatile and during peaks acromegalic and normal levels overlap. GH also ↑ in: stress, sleep, puberty, and pregnancy. Normally GH secretion is inhibited by high glucose, and GH hardly detectable. In acromegaly GH release fails to suppress.

- If basal serum GH is >0.4µg/L (1.2mIU/L) and/or if IGF-I↑ (p224), an oral glucose tolerance test (OGTT) is needed. 2000 *Consensus statement* If the lowest GH value during OGTT is above 1µg/L (3mIU/L), acromegaly is confirmed. With general use of very sensitive assays, it has been said that this cut-off be decreased to 0.3µg/L (0.9mIU/L).[249] *Method:* Collect samples for GH glucose at: 0, 30, 60, 90, 120, 150min. Possible false +ves: puberty, pregnancy, hepatic and renal disease, anorexia nervosa, and DM.
- MRI scan of pituitary fossa. • Look for hypopituitarism (p224).
- Visual fields and acuity. • ECG, echo. Old photos if possible.

Treatment Aim to correct (or prevent) tumour compression by excising the lesion, and to reduce GH and IGF-I levels to at least a 'safe' GH level of <2µg/L (<6mIU/L).[250] A 3-part strategy: **1** Trans-sphenoidal surgery is often 1st-line. **2** If surgery fails to correct GH/IGF-I hypersecretion, try somatostatin analogues (SSA) and/or radiotherapy, SSA being generally preferred. Example: **octreotide** (Sandostatin Lar®, given monthly IM), or **lanreotide** (Somatuline LA®). SE: pain at the injection site; gastrointestinal: abdominal cramps, flatulence, loose stools, ↑gallstones; impaired glucose tolerance. **3** The GH antagonist **pegvisomant** (recombinant GH analogue) is used if resistant or intolerant to SSA. It suppresses IGF-1 to normal in 90%, but GH levels may rise; rarely tumour size increases, so monitor closely. *Radiotherapy:* If unsuited to surgery or as adjuvant; may take years to work. *Follow-up:* Yearly GH, IGF-1 ±OGTT; visual fields; vascular assessment. BMI; photos (**fig 2,3**).

Prognosis May return to normal (any excess mortality is mostly vascular). 16% get diabetes with SSAs *vs* ~13% after surgery.[251]

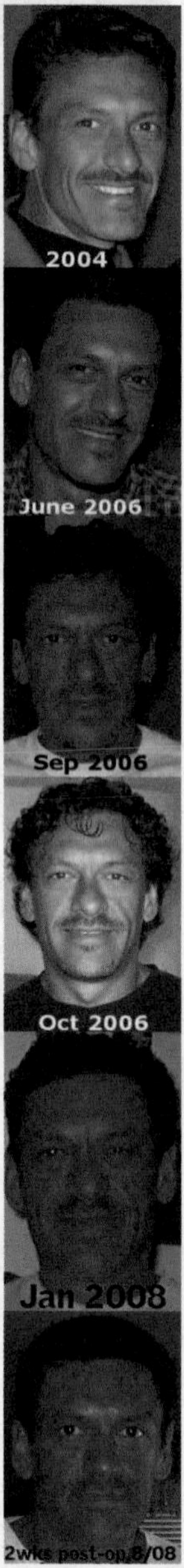

Fig 1. Acromegaly. Courtesy of Omar Rio[252]

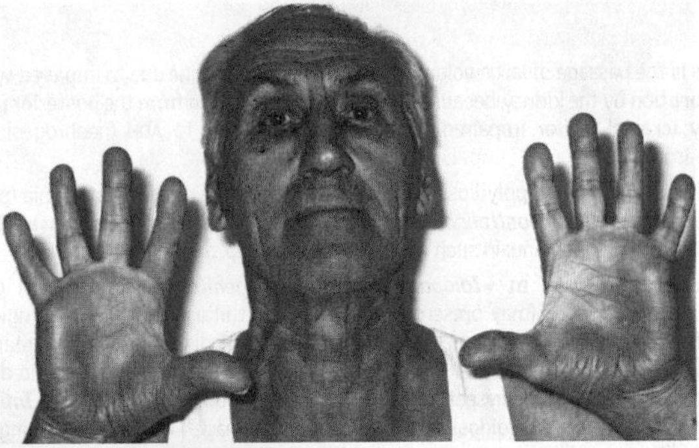

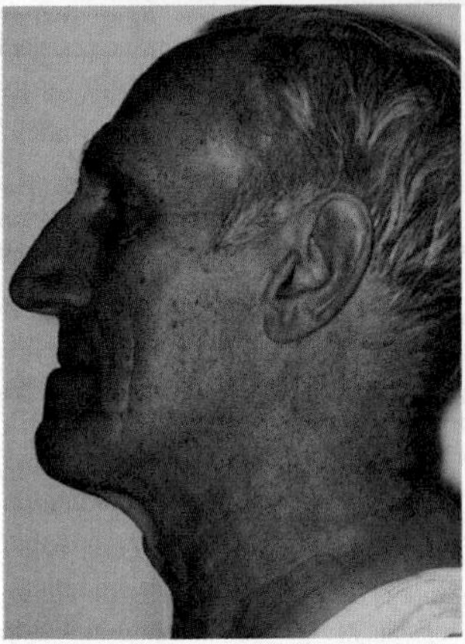

Signs of acromegaly

- ↑Growth of hands (**fig 2**; may be spade-like), jaw (**fig 3**) & feet (sole may encroach on the dorsum)[253]
- Coarsening face; wide nose
- Big supraorbital ridges
- Macroglossia (big tongue)
- Widely spaced teeth
- Puffy lips, lids, & skin (oily & large-pored); also skin tags
- Scalp folds (*cutis verticis gyrata*; ∵ expanding but tethered skin)
- Skin darkening (**fig 2**)
- Acanthosis nigricans (**fig 6**, p565)
- Laryngeal dyspnoea (fixed cords)
- Obstructive sleep apnoea
- Goitre (↑ thyroid vascularity)[254]
- Proximal weakness + arthropathy
- Carpal tunnel signs in 50%, p507
- Signs from any pituitary mass: hypopituitarism ± local mass effect (p226; vision↓; hemianopia); fits.[255]

Figs 2 & 3. Coarsening of the face & ↑growth of hands and mandible (prognathism).[256]

Dysmorphia,[1] personal identity, and acromegaly

We might have devoted this box to a grotesque homunculus depicting the signs of acromegaly: all disconnected lips, hands, feet, brows, and noses. But our integrative ethics disallow this, and ask us instead to see if acromegaly can reveal something universal about our patients and ourselves. What is it like to feel in the grip of some 'alien puberty' or 'empty pregnancy'? These analogies are physiological as well as metaphorical.[2,3] The changes of acromegaly are not so insidious that the patient thinks all is fine: there is often partial knowledge and a few dark thoughts on looking into the mirror. Even when we lay our lives end-to-end for inspection (**fig 1**), changes are subtle. It can take the observations of others to force us to come face-to-face with the truth of our new unfolding self. In one patient the comment was "So are you pregnant again?" "Why do you ask?" "Because your nose is as big as it was when you were last pregnant". So here we have the well-known 'physiological acromegaly of pregnancy'[2] predating the pathological, as the carnival of personal identity moves from helter-skelter to roller-coaster.

1 Morpheus, the god of sleep, has the ability to take on any human form, and to appear in dreams.
2 GH variants made by the placenta rise exponentially until 37wks' gestation; pituitary GH gradually drops to near-undetectable levels. 'Gestational acromegaly' probably develops to foster fetoplacental growth; its side effects include facial oedema, carpal tunnel symptoms, and nose enlargment.
3 Puberty sees GH- and gonad-mediated rises in bone and muscle mass + other 'acromegalic' effects.

Diabetes insipidus (DI)

This is the passage of large volumes (>3L/day) of dilute urine due to impaired water resorption by the kidney, because of reduced ADH secretion from the posterior pituitary (cranial DI), or impaired response of the kidney to ADH (nephrogenic DI). See **fig 1**.

Symptoms Polyuria; polydipsia; dehydration; symptoms of hypernatraemia (p686). ***Polydipsia can be uncontrollable and all-consuming***, with patients drinking anything *and everything* to hand: in such cases, if beer is on tap, disaster will ensue! 257

Causes of cranial DI • *Idiopathic* (≤50%) • *Congenital:* defects in ADH gene, DIDMOAD[1] • *Tumour* (may present with DI + hypopituitarism) craniopharyngioma, metastases, pituitary tumour • *Trauma:* temporary if distal to pituitary stalk as proximal nerve endings grow out to find capillaries in scar tissue and begin direct secretion again • Hypophysectomy • Autoimmune hypophysitis (p224) 258 • *Infiltration:* histiocytosis, sarcoidosis[2] • *Vascular:* Haemorrhage[3] • *Infection:* meningoencephalitis.

Causes of nephrogenic DI • Inherited • *Metabolic:* Low potassium, high calcium • *Drugs:* lithium, demeclocycline • Chronic renal disease • Post-obstructive uropathy.

Tests U&E, Ca^{2+}, glucose (exclude DM), serum and urine osmolalities. Serum osmolality estimate $\approx 2\times(Na^+ + K^+)$ + urea + glucose (all in mmol/L). Normal plasma osmolality is 285–295mOsmol/kg, and urine can be concentrated to more than twice this concentration. Significant DI is excluded if urine to plasma (U:P) osmolality ratio is more than 2:1, provided plasma osmolality is no greater than 295mOsmol/kg. In DI, despite raised plasma osmolality, urine is dilute with a U:P ratio <2. In primary polydipsia there may be dilutional hyponatraemia—and as hyponatraemia may itself cause mania, 259 be cautious of saying "It's water intoxication from psychogenic polydipsia".

Diagnosis The ***water deprivation test*** aims to test the ability of kidneys to concentrate urine for diagnosis of DI, and then to localise the cause. See BOX.
NB: it is often difficult to differentiate primary polydipsia from partial DI. OTM4 3.207

ΔΔ: DM; diuretics or lithium use; ***primary polydipsia***—this causes symptoms of polydipsia & polyuria with dilute urine. Its cause is poorly understood;[4] it may be associated with schizophrenia or mania (±Li^+ therapy 260), or, rarely, hypothalamic disease (neurosarcoid; tumour; encephalitis; brain injury; HIV encephalopathy). 261 As part of this syndrome, the kidneys may lose their ability to fully concentrate urine, due to a wash-out of the normal concentrating gradient in the renal medulla.

Treatment *Cranial DI:* Find the cause—MRI (head); test anterior pituitary function (p224). Give desmopressin, a synthetic analogue of ADH (eg Desmomelt® tablets).
Nephrogenic: Treat the cause. If it persists, try bendroflumethiazide 5mg PO/24h. NSAIDs lower urine volume and plasma Na^+ by inhibiting prostaglandin synthase: prostaglandins locally inhibit the action of ADH. 262

▸▸Emergency management • Do urgent plasma U&E, and serum and urine osmolalities. Monitor urine output carefully and check U&E twice a day initially.
- IVI to keep up with urine output. If severe hypernatraemia, do not lower Na^+ rapidly as this may cause cerebral oedema and brain injury. If Na^+ is ≥170, use 0.9% saline initially—this contains 150mmol/L of sodium. Aim to reduce Na^+ at a rate of less than 12mmol/L per day. Use of 0.45% saline can be dangerous.
- Desmopressin 2µg IM (lasts 12–24h) may be used as a therapeutic trial.

1 DIDMOAD is a rare autosomal recessive disorder: **D**iabetes **I**nsipidus, **D**iabetes **M**ellitus, **O**ptic **A**trophy and **D**eafness (also known as Wolfram's syndrome).

2 Suspect neurosarcoidosis if CSF protein↑ (seen in 34%), facial nerve palsy (25%), CSF pleocytosis (23%), diabetes insipidus (21%), hemiparesis (17%), psychosis (17%), papilloedema (15%), ataxia (13%), seizures (12%), optic atrophy (12%), hearing loss (12%), or nystagmus (9%).

3 Sheehan's syndrome is pituitary infarction from shock, eg postpartum haemorrhage. It's rare.

4 Most of us could drink 20L/d and not be hyponatraemic; some get hyponatraemic drinking 5L/d; they may have **P**sychosis, **I**ntermittent hyponatraemia, and **P**olydipsia (PIP syndrome), ?from ↑intravascular volume leading to ↑atrial natriuretic peptide, p131, hence natriuresis & hyponatraemia).

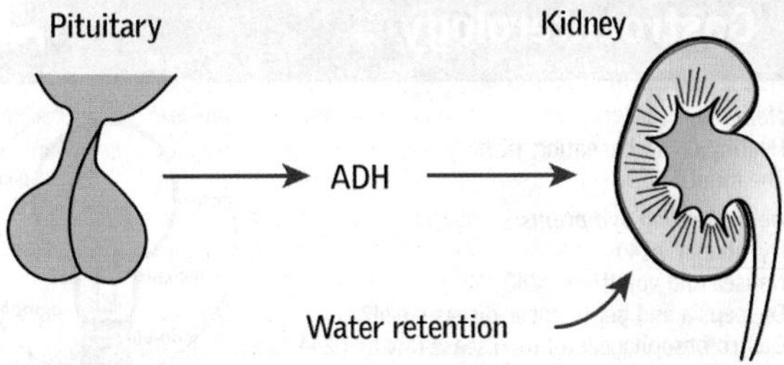

Fig 1. Pathway of renal regulation. ADH=antidiuretic hormone=ADV=antidiuretic vasopressin=arginine vasopressin=AVP. The essential role of ADH V2 and AQP2 (aquaporin 2) receptors in water homeostasis is clear now we know that mutations in their genes cause nephrogenic diabetes insipidus such that the kidney is unable to concentrate urine in response to ADH. 263

The 8-hour water deprivation test

The purpose of this test is to see if the kidneys persist in producing dilute urine despite dehydration, and then to localise the cause. Do not do the test before establishing that urine volume is >3L/d (output less than this with normal plasma Na^+ and osmolality excludes significant disturbance of water balance).

- Stop test if urine osmolality >600mOsmol/kg in Stage 1 (DI is excluded).
- Free fluids until 07.30. Light breakfast at 06.30, no tea, no coffee, no smoking.

Stage 1 Fluid deprivation (0–8h): For diagnosis of DI. Start at 08.00.

- Empty bladder, then no drinks and only dry food.
- Weigh hourly. If >3% weight lost during test, order urgent serum osmolality. If >300mOsmol/kg, proceed to Stage 2. If <300, continue test.
- Collect urine every 2 hours; measure its volume and osmolality.
- Venous sample for osmolality every 4 hours.
- Stop test after 8h (16.00) if urine osmolality >600mOsmol/kg (ie normal).

Stage 2 Differentiate cranial from nephrogenic DI.

- Proceed if urine still dilute—ie urine osmolality <600mOsmol/kg.
- Give desmopressin 2μg IM. Water can be drunk now.
- Measure urine osmolality hourly for the next 4 hours.

Interpreting the water deprivation test	
Normal	Urine osmolality >600mOsmol/kg in Stage 1 U:P ratio >2 (normal concentrating ability).
Primary polydipsia	Urine concentrates, but less than normal, eg >400–600mOsmol/kg.
Cranial DI	Urine osmolality increases to >600mOsmol/kg *after* desmopressin (if equivocal an extended water deprivation test may be tried (no drinking from 18:00 the night before)).
Nephrogenic DI	No increase in urine osmolality after desmopressin.

Contents

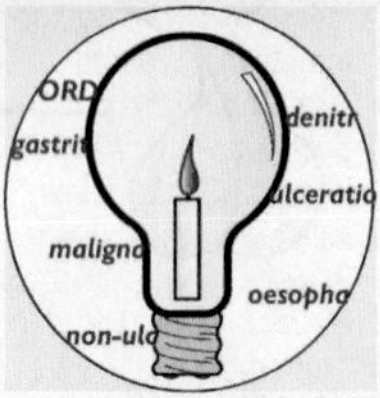

Fig 1. What shall be our guiding light through the twists and turns of the tunnelous GI tract? Perhaps more so than in any field, GI symptoms can be vague and nonspecific (eg dyspepsia, p234), often leaving us with little choice but turn to invasive procedures, which we know are not without risk (p256). Yet if we leave pathology in the dark, be it benign or malignant, we may be doing a disservice. But not every symptom needs illuminating by a scan or gadget:

- ►Get used to listening to patients' stories;
- ►Get good at dealing with uncertainty, and
- ►Know that in time you will learn the right level of illumination to use to reveal the subtle nuances and shades of gastrointestinal phenomena.

Relevant pages in other chapters: *Signs & symptoms:* Abdominal distension (p57); epigastric pain (p57); flatulence (p58); guarding (p62); heartburn (p244); hepatomegaly (p63); LIF and LUQ pain (p57); palmar erythema (p33); rebound tenderness (p62); regurgitation (p59); RIF pain (p57); RUQ pain (p57); skin discolouration (p28); splenomegaly (p606); tenesmus (p59); vomiting (p56); waterbrash (p606); weight loss (p29). *Surgical topics:* Contents to *Surgery* (p566). *Haematology:* Iron-deficiency anaemia (p320). *Infections:* Viral hepatitis (p406). *Radiology:* The plain abdominal film (AXR) (p740); radiological GI procedures (p756) *Emergencies:* Upper GI bleeding (p830); acute liver failure (p806).

We thank Simon Campbell (Consultant Gastroenterologist, Manchester Royal Infirmary), who is our Specialist Reader for this chapter.

Lumen

We learn about gastroenterological diseases as if they were separate entities, independent species collected by naturalists, each kept in its own dark matchbox—collectors' items collecting dust in a desiccated world on a library shelf. But this is not how illness works. Otto had diabetes, but refused to see a doctor until it was far advanced, and an amputation was needed. He needed looking after by his wife Aurelia. But she had her children Warren and Sylvia to look after too. And when Otto was no longer the bread-winner, she forced herself to work as a teacher, an accountant, and at any other job she could get. Otto's illness manifested in Aurelia's duodenum—as an ulcer. The gut often bears the brunt of other people's worries. Inside every piece of a gut is a lumen[1]—the world is in the gut, and the gut is in the world. But the light does not always shine. So when the lumen filled with Aurelia's blood, we can expect the illness to impact on the whole family. Her daughter knows where blood comes from ('straight from the heart... pink fizz'). After Otto died, Sylvia needed long-term psychiatric care, and Aurelia moved to be near her daughter. The bleeding duodenal ulcer got worse when Sylvia needed electroconvulsive therapy. The therapy worked and now, briefly, Sylvia, before her own premature death, is able to look after Aurelia, as she prepares for a gastrectomy.

The story of each illness told separately misses something; but even taken in its social context, this story is missing something vital—the poetry, in most of our patients lived rather than written—tragic, comic, human, and usually obscure—but in the case of this family not so obscure. Welling up, as unstoppable as the bleeding from her mother's ulcer, came the poetry of Sylvia Plath.[2]

1 *Lumen* is Latin for light (hence its medical meaning of a tubular cavity open to the world at both ends), as well as being the SI unit of light flux falling on an object—ie the power to transilluminate. All doctors have this power, whether by insightfully interpreting patients' lives and illnesses to them, or by acts of kindness—even something so simple as bringing a cup of tea.

2 ...*And here you come, with a cup of tea*
Wreathed in steam.
The blood jet is poetry,
There is no stopping it.
You hand me two children, two roses. Sylvia Plath; *Kindness*; Collected Poems; 1981; Faber
source: katemoses.com/books/w_chronology.html

'There's a lot of people in this world who spend so much time watching their health that they haven't the time to enjoy it.' Josh Billings (1818–85).

There are no good or bad **foods**, and no universally good or bad **diets**. We must not consider diet independently of desired lifestyle; and don't assume we all want to be thin, healthy, and live for ever. If we are walking to the South Pole, our bodies need as much energy-rich fat as possible. But if we are sedentary, the converse may ***not*** be true. After decades of research, we still don't know who should eat what, or when. Are 3 meals a day healthier than 1? Is fat harmful if weight is normal? Is a balanced diet (see BOX 1) best? Should we eat 3, 5, 7, or 9 fruits daily? (one recommendation for men, but some studies find no benefit beyond 3).[2] Are green vegetables (or yellow?) better than fruits? (maybe, for preventing diabetes).[3]

The traditional answer to these questions (the more fruit the better) may be wrong because of complex interactions between eating and health. All diets have unintended consequences: eg the 'good' antioxidant epicatechin (a flavonoid) in dark chocolate is annulled by taking milk at the same time.[4] Randomized trials show Atkins-type diets (low in carbohydrate ∴ ↑fat & ↑protein) improve lipid profiles and insulin resistance (possible SEs of renal problems and ↑Ca^{2+} excretion[5,6] may have been over-played,[7] but note that bowel flora is changed in a way which is ?carcinogenic).[8] To complicate matters, diet is also confounded by lifestyle—while some studies show vegetarians may be less likely to die from ischaemic heart disease,[MET 9] is this effect because vegetarians in the UK are more likely to be non-smokers?[10] Do vitamin/antioxidant supplements help? β-carotene and vitamins A & E may *increase* mortality.[11, 47 trials]

Current recommendations must take into account 3 facts:

- Obesity is an escalating epidemic costing health services as much as smoking—1 in 4 adults in the UK are now classified as obese.[12]
- Diabetes mellitus is burgeoning: in some places prevalence is >7% (p198).
- Past advice has not changed eating habits in large sections of the population.

Advice is likely to focus on the following

Body mass index (BMI): see BOX 3; aim for 20–25; ie **eat less**. Controlling quantity may be more important than quality. In hypertension, eating the 'right' things lowered BP by 0.6mmHg, but controlling weight (*OHCS* p530) caused a 3.7mmHg reduction in 6 months in one RCT.[13]

Oily fish: Rich in omega-3 fatty acid (eg mackerel, herring, pilchards, salmon—but benefits are not fully substantiated).[14] If tinned fish, avoid those in unspecified oils. Nuts are also valuable: walnuts lower total cholesterol and have one of the highest ratios of polyunsaturates to saturates (7:1). Soya protein lowers cholesterol, low-density lipoproteins, and triglycerides.

Refined sugar: (See BOX 2 for its deleterious effects.) Use fruit to add sweetness. Have low-sugar drinks: a 330mL can of non-diet carbonated soft drink can have up to 10 teaspoons (40g) of refined sugar. Don't add sugar to drinks or cereals. (In a thin, active, elderly, normoglycaemic person, sugar may be no great evil.)

Eat enough fruit and fibres: See BOX 2 and ***reduce salt intake***.

Enjoy moderate alcohol use (adults): ♀: ≤14U/wk; ♂: ≤21U/wk (higher levels are controversial)—taken regularly, not in binges. Alcohol inhibits platelet aggregation and is an antioxidant (∴ cardioprotective). There is no evidence that spirit or beer drinkers should switch to wine. There is evidence that the benefit accrues **only** to those whose LDL cholesterol is ≥5.25mmol/L.[15]

►***Avoid this diet if:*** • <5yrs old • Need for low residue (eg Crohn's, UC, p274) or special diet (coeliac disease, p280) • Weight loss is expected. ***Emphasis may be different in:*** Dyslipidaemia (p704); DM (p198); obesity; constipation (p248); liver failure (p258); chronic pancreatitis (p280); renal failure (less protein); BP↑.[16]

Difficulties It is an imposition to ask us to change our diet (children often refuse point-blank); a more subtle approach is to take a food we enjoy (crisps) and make it healthier (eg low-salt crisps made from jacket potatoes and fried in sunflower oil).

Traditional low-fat nutritional advice: the balance of good health

A low-fat diet may not only be for the sake of good health, as it can also help control symptoms, eg as in gallstone disease, and while it is unrealistic to expect all our patients' troubles to drift away as the weight comes off, we can offer the incentive of an improvement in both symptoms and health as encouragement.

Starchy foods Bread, rice, pasta, potatoes, etc. form the main starch energy source (wholemeal/unprocessed is recommended).

Fibre (Mainly non-starch polysaccharide (NSP) the preferred term) 14g/1000kcal is recommended for children and adults. Fibre is claimed to ↓risk of vascular disease, diabetes, breast cancer,[17] and obesity—as well as constipation and piles. Soluble fibre improves insulin sensitivity (non-diabetics and diabetics). If obese, fibre supplements may aid weight loss.[18] Prebiotic fibres might enhance immunity.[19] ↑Fluid intake with diets high in NSP, eg 8 cups (1-2½ pints) daily. Warn about bulky stools. NSP can ↓Ca^{2+} and iron absorption, so restrict main intake to 1 meal a day.

Fruit and vegetables eg >6 pieces of fruit (with skins)[20] or portions of pulses, beans, or lightly cooked greens per day (aims to ↓vascular and cancer deaths).[21]

Meat and alternatives Meat should be cooked without additional fat. Lower fat alternatives, such as white meat (poultry, without skin), white fish, and vegetable protein sources (eg pulses, soya) are encouraged.

Dairy foods Low-fat semi-skimmed milk/yoghurt; edam or cottage cheese.

Fat and sugary foods Avoiding extra fat in cooking is advised ('grill, boil, steam, or bake, but don't fry'). Fatty spreads (eg butter) are kept to a minimum and snack foods (crisps, sweets, biscuits, or cake) are avoided.

Losing weight—why and how?

The risks of too much sugar Excess sugar causes caries, diabetes, obesity—which itself contributes to osteoarthritis, cancer,[22] hypertension,[23] and ↑oxidative stress—so raising cardiovascular mortality[24] and much more.

Losing weight Motivational therapy. Consider referral to a dietician—a needs-specific diet may be best. In conjunction with exercise and diet strategies, targeted weight-loss can also be achieved successfully with psychotherapy.[25]

Drugs for obesity? The most desirable treatment for obesity is still primary prevention, but pharmacotherapy does work.[26] *Orlistat* lowers fat absorption (hence SE of oily faecal incontinence). *Sibutramine* increases post-ingestive satiety (SE hypertension and tachycardia; monitor BP, eg 2-weekly for ≥3 months)—see *OHCS* p530.[1]

Surgery for obesity? See p593.

Calculating BMI

BMI is calculated as (weight in kg)/(height in m)^2

BMI	State	Some implications within the categories
<18.5	Underweight	<17.5 is one of the criteria for anorexia nervosa
18.5-25	Target	
25-30	Overweight	Weight loss should be considered
30-40	Obesity	>32 is unsuitable for day-case general surgery
>40	Extreme/morbid obesity	>40 is an indication for bariatric surgery

►Caveats: BMI does not take into account the distribution of body fat, and is harder to interpret for children and adolescents. **Waist circumference** >94cm in men and >80cm in women reflects omental fat and correlates better with risk than does BMI. For ethnic variations, see p205.

1 Research continues into the hormones involved in obesity—eg the satiety-inducing **leptin** and the hunger-inducing **ghrelin**.

Leucoplakia (fig 1) is an oral mucosal white patch that will not rub off and is not attributable to any other known disease. It is a premalignant lesion, with a transformation rate, which ranges from 0.6% to 18%.[28] Oral hairy leucoplakia is a shaggy white patch on the side of the tongue seen in HIV, caused by EBV. ►When in doubt, refer all intra-oral white lesions (see BOX).

Aphthous ulcers (fig 2) 20% of us get these shallow, painful ulcers on the tongue or oral mucosa that heal without scarring. ***Causes of severe ulcers:*** Crohn's & coeliac disease; Behçet's (p708); trauma; erythema multiforme; lichen planus; pemphigus; pemphigoid; infections (herpes simplex, syphilis, Vincent's angina, p726). ℞: ***Minor ulcers:*** avoid oral trauma (eg hard toothbrushes or foods such as toast) and acidic foods or drinks. ***Hydrocortisone*** lozenges held on the ulcer may help, as may ***tetracycline*** or antimicrobial mouthwashes (eg chlorhexidine). ***Severe ulcers:*** Possible therapies include systemic corticosteroids (eg oral ***prednisolone*** 30-60 mg/d PO for a week) or thalidomide (absolutely contraindicated in pregnancy).[29] ►Biopsy any ulcer not healing after 3 weeks to exclude malignancy; refer to an oral surgeon if uncertain.

Candidiasis (thrush; fig 3) causes white patches or erythema of the buccal mucosa. Patches may be hard to remove and bleed if scraped. ***Risk factors:*** Extremes of age; DM; antibiotics; immunosuppression (long-term corticosteroids, including inhalers; cytotoxics; malignancy; HIV). ℞: ***Nystatin*** suspension 100,000U (1mL swill & swallow/6h) or ***amphotericin*** lozenges. ***Fluconazole*** for oropharyngeal candidiasis.

Cheilitis (angular stomatitis) Fissuring of the mouth's corners is caused by denture problems, candidiasis (above), or deficiency of iron or riboflavin (vitamin B_2).

Gingivitis Gum inflammation ± hypertrophy occurs with poor oral hygiene, drugs (phenytoin, ciclosporin, nifedipine), pregnancy, vitamin C deficiency (scurvy, p278), acute myeloid leukaemia (p350), or Vincent's angina (p726).

Microstomia (fig 4) The mouth is too small, eg from thickening and tightening of the perioral skin after burns or in epidermolysis bullosa (destructive skin and mucous membrane blisters ± ankyloglossia) or systemic sclerosis (p554).

Oral pigmentation Perioral brown spots characterize Peutz-Jeghers' (p722). Pigmentation anywhere in the mouth suggests Addison's disease or drugs (eg antimalarials). Consider malignant melanoma. ***Telangiectasia:*** Systemic sclerosis; Osler-Weber-Rendu syndrome (p722). ***Fordyce glands*** (creamy yellow spots at the border of the oral mucosa and the lip vermilion) are sebaceous cysts, common and benign. *Aspergillus niger* colonisation may cause a black tongue.

Teeth (fig 5) A blue line at the gum-tooth margin suggests lead poisoning. Prenatal or childhood tetracycline exposure causes a yellow-brown discolouration.

Tongue This may be furred or dry (xerostomia) in dehydration, if on tricyclics, etc.,[1] after radiotherapy, in Crohn's disease, Sjögren's (p724) and Mikulicz's syndrome.[30] ***Glossitis*** means a smooth, red, sore tongue, eg caused by iron, folate, or B_{12} deficiency (**fig 1**, p321). If local loss of papillae leads to ulcer-like lesions that change in colour and size, use the term **geographic tongue** (harmless migratory glossitis).
Macroglossia: The tongue is too big. Causes: myxoedema; acromegaly; amyloid. A *ranula* is a bluish salivary retention cyst to one side of the frenulum, named after the bulging vocal pouch of frogs' throats (genus *Rana*).
Tongue cancer typically appears on its edge as a raised ulcer with firm edges and environs. Main risk factors are smoking and alcohol.[2] Examine under the tongue and ask patient to deviate his extended tongue sideways. Spread: anterior ⅓ of the tongue drains to the submental nodes; middle ⅓ to the submandibular nodes; posterior ⅓ to the deep cervical nodes (see BOX, p600). ***Treatment:*** Radiotherapy or surgery. 5yr survival (early disease): 80%. ►When in doubt, refer tongue ulcers.

1 Drugs causing xerostomia: ACE-i, antidepressants; antihistamines; antipsychotics; antimuscarinics/anticholinergics; bromocriptine; diuretics; loperamide; nifedipine; opiates; prazosin; prochlorperazine, etc.
2 Betel nut (*Areca catechu*) chewing, common in South Asia, may be an independent risk factor.

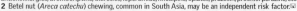

White intra-oral lesions

- Idiopathic keratosis
- Leucoplakia
- Lichen planus
- Poor dental hygiene
- Candidiasis
- Squamous papilloma
- Carcinoma
- Hairy oral leucoplakia
- Lupus erythematosus
- Smoking
- Aphthous stomatitis
- Secondary syphilis

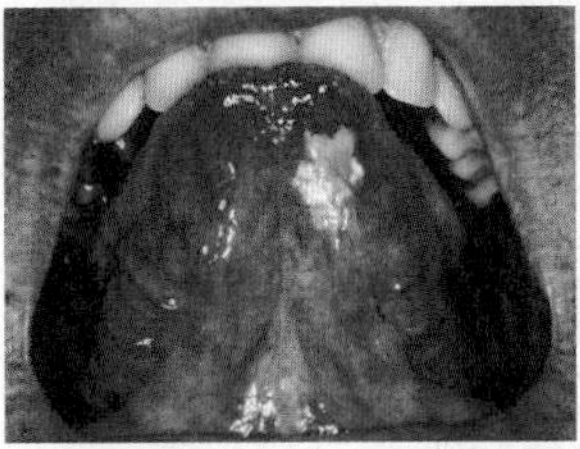

Fig 1. Leucoplakia on the underside of the tongue. It is important to refer leucoplakia because it is premalignant.

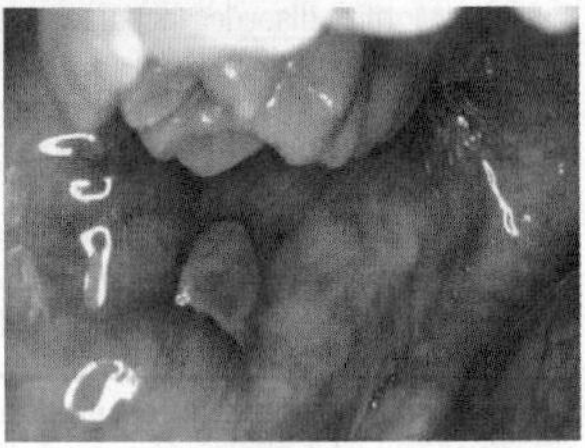

Fig 2. An aphthous ulcer inside the cheek. The name is tautological: *aphtha* in Greek means ulceration.

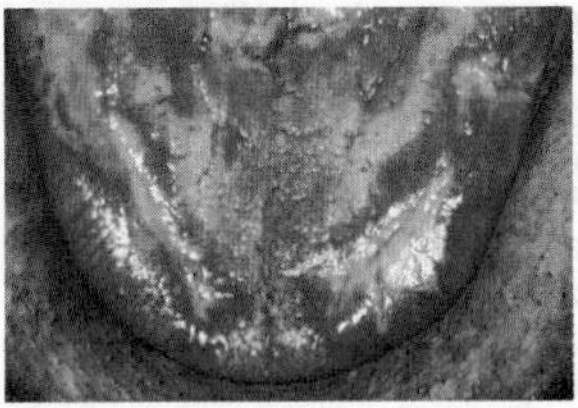

Fig 3. White fur on an erythematous tongue caused by oral candidiasis. ►Oropharyngeal candidiasis in an apparently fit patient may suggest underlying HIV infection.

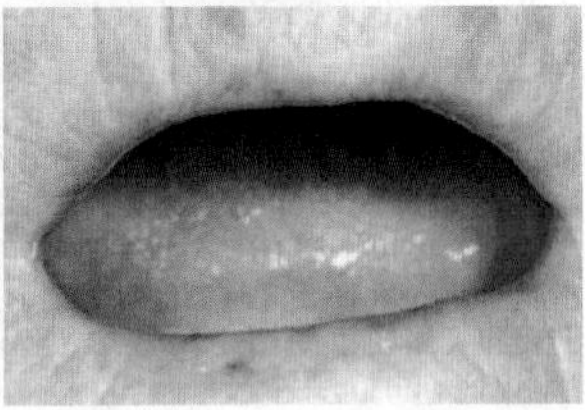

Fig 4. Microstomia (small, narrow mouth), eg from hardening of the skin in scleroderma which narrows the mouth. It is cosmetically and functionally disabling.[37]

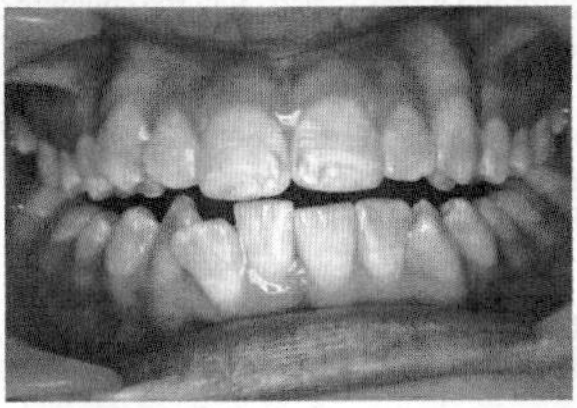

Fig 5. White bands on the teeth can be caused by excessive fluoride intake.

Dysphagia

Dysphagia is difficulty in swallowing and always needs investigating urgently to exclude malignancy (unless of short duration, and associated with a sore throat).

Causes Oral, pharyngeal, or oesophageal? Mechanical or motility related? (see BOX 1)

Clinical features There are 5 key questions to ask:

1 Was there difficulty swallowing solids **and** liquids from the start?
  Yes: Motility disorder (achalasia, neurological), or pharyngeal causes.
  No: Solids **then** liquids: suspect a stricture (benign or malignant).

2 Is it difficult to make the swallowing movement?
  Yes: Suspect bulbar palsy, especially if he coughs on swallowing.

3 Is swallowing painful (odynophagia)?
  Yes: Suspect cancer, oesophageal ulcer or spasm.

4 Is the dysphagia intermittent or is it constant and getting worse?
  Intermittent: Suspect oesophageal spasm.
  Constant and worsening: Suspect malignant stricture.

5 Does the neck bulge or gurgle on drinking?
  Yes: Suspect a pharyngeal pouch (see **fig 1**, p621).

Signs Is the patient cachectic or anaemic? Examine the mouth; feel for supraclavicular nodes (left supraclavicular node = Virchow's node—suggests intra-abdominal malignancy); look for signs of systemic disease, eg systemic sclerosis, CNS disease.

Investigations FBC (anaemia); U&E (dehydration); CXR (mediastinal fluid level, absent gastric bubble, aspiration). Upper GI endoscopy (±biopsy) is usually the 1st line investigation. Barium swallow (**fig 1**) ± video fluoroscopy is useful to diagnose high dysphagia or dysmotility (eg achalasia). Further investigations: oesophageal manometry (if normal barium swallow); ENT opinion if suspected pharyngeal cause.

Specific conditions *Oesophagitis* p244. ***Diffuse oesophageal spasm*** causes intermittent dysphagia ± chest pain. Barium swallow: abnormal contractions, eg corkscrew oesophagus.[1] ***Achalasia:*** The lower oesophageal sphincter fails to relax (due to degeneration of the myenteric plexus) causes dysphagia, regurgitation, substernal cramps, and ↓weight. Barium swallow: dilated tapering oesophagus. Treatment: endoscopic balloon dilatation, or Heller's cardiomyotomy—then proton pump inhibitors (PPIs, p244). Botulinum toxin injection is an alternative if unsuitable for an invasive procedure.[32] Calcium channel blockers and nitrates also relax the sphincter. Longstanding achalasia is a risk factor for oesophageal cancer. ***Benign oesophageal stricture:*** Caused by gastro-oesophageal reflux disease (GORD, p244), corrosives, surgery, or radiotherapy. Treatment: endoscopic balloon dilatation. ***Oesophageal cancer:*** (p620). Associations: ♂, GORD,[33] tobacco, alcohol, Barrett's oesophagus (p708), achalasia, tylosis (palmar hyperkeratosis), Paterson-Brown-Kelly (Plummer-Vinson) syndrome (post-cricoid dysphagia, upper oesophageal web + iron-deficiency).

Nausea and vomiting

(See BOX 2; causes: p56)

Tests *Bloods:* FBC, U&E, LFT, Ca^{2+}, glucose, and amylase. *ABG:* A metabolic (hypochloraemic) alkalosis from loss of gastric contents (pH >7.45, ↑HCO_3^-) indicates severe vomiting. Request a plain *AXR* if suspected bowel obstruction—see p740 for AXR findings in obstruction. Consider upper GI endoscopy (p256) if persistent vomiting. Consider head CT to rule out ↑ ICP. Identify and **treat the underlying cause** if possible.

Treatment See TABLE. Try to use pre-emptive therapy, eg pre-operatively for post-op symptoms. Try the oral route first (if feasible). Roughly ⅓ of patients with nausea need a 2nd-line anti-emetic, so be prepared to prescribe more than one on occasions, but avoid drugs in pregnancy and children. Give IV fluids with K^+ replacement if severely dehydrated or nil-by-mouth, and monitor electrolytes and fluid balance.

1 Non-propulsive contractions manifest as tertiary contractions or '**corkscrew oesophagus**' and suggest a motility disorder and may lead to impaired acid clearance. Symptoms and radiology may not correlate. *Nutcracker oesophagus* denotes distal peristaltic contractions >180mmHg. It can cause pain, eg relieved by nitrates, sublingual ***nifedipine***, or the smooth muscle relaxant ***sildenafil*** (p316).

Causes of dysphagia

Mechanical block
- Malignant stricture (**fig 1**)
  - Oesophageal cancer
  - Gastric cancer
  - Pharyngeal cancer
- Benign strictures
  - Oesophageal web or ring p240
  - Peptic stricture
- Extrinsic pressure
  - Lung cancer
  - Mediastinal lymph nodes
  - Retrosternal goitre
  - Aortic aneurysm
  - Left atrial enlargement
- Pharyngeal pouch

Motility disorders
- Achalasia
- Diffuse oesophageal spasm
- Systemic sclerosis (p554)
- Myasthenia gravis (p516)
- Bulbar palsy (p511)
- Pseudobulbar palsy (p511)
- Syringobulbia (p520)
- Bulbar poliomyelitis (p432)
- Chagas' disease (p438)

Others
- Oesophagitis (p244)
  - Infection (*Candida*, HSV)
  - Reflux oesophagitis
- Globus hystericus

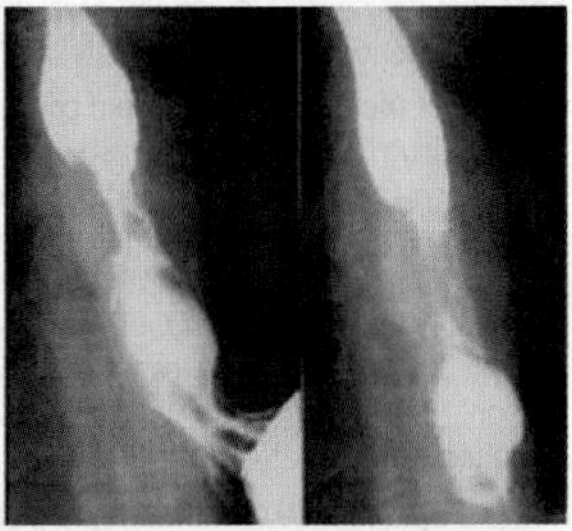

Fig 1. A malignant lower oesophageal stricture shown on barium swallow. The shouldered edges of the stricture produce an 'apple core' effect with an irregular mucosal pattern. On video fluoroscopy there would be no peristalsis visible in this segment. A benign stricture would have a more funnelled appearance with a normal mucosal pattern. Note the normal but similar appearance of the gastro-oesophageal junction inferiorly. Courtesy of Dr Stephen Golding

Ad nauseam...

Jumping into the sea is a certain cure for seasickness. John Ruskin (1819-1900)

Nausea is often described by patients as their worst symptom when they are unwell (especially by those enduring palliative care). It can be an equally difficult symptom to help control. Not all anti-emetics will work for everyone, so it is worthwhile persevering with your options to help alleviate such a disparaging and sometimes intractable symptom, since not everyone is able to jump ship so easily.

Remembering your anti-emetics

One way of recalling anti-emetics involves using (simplified) pharmacology.

Receptor	Antagonist	Dose	Notes
H_1	*Cyclizine*	50mg/8h PO/IV/IM	GI causes
	Cinnarizine	30mg/8h PO	Vestibular disorders
D_2	*Metoclopramide*	10mg/8h PO/IV/IM	GI causes; also prokinetic
	Domperidone	60mg/12h PR 20mg/6h PO	Also prokinetic
	Prochlorperazine	12.5mg IM; 5mg/8h PO	Vestibular/GI causes
	Haloperidol	1.5mg bd PO	Chemical causes, eg opioids
$5HT_3$	*Ondansetron*	4mg/8h IV	Doses can be much higher for eg emetogenic chemotherapy
Others	*Hyoscine hydrobromide*	200–600μg SC/IM	Antimuscarinic ∴ also antispasmodic and antisecretory (don't prescribe with a prokinetic)
	Dexamethasone	6-10mg/d PO/SC	Unknown mode of action; an adjuvant
	Midazolam	2-4mg/d IV	Unknown action; anti-emetic effect outlasts sedative effect[34]

►All anti-dopaminergics can cause dystonias and oculogyric crisis, especially in younger patients.

Dyspepsia is a non-specific group of symptoms related to the upper GI tract.

Non-specific symptoms Epigastric pain eg related to hunger, eating specific foods, or time of day; may be associated with bloating ± fullness after meals; heartburn (retrosternal pain with demonstrable acid reflux). **Alarm** symptoms: **A**naemia (iron deficiency); **l**oss of weight; **a**norexia; **r**ecent onset of progressive symptoms; **m**elaena or haematemesis; **s**wallowing difficulty. **Signs** Tender epigastrium (non-specific). Any abdominal mass; supraclavicular nodes ± hepatomegaly?

Managing new dyspepsia See flowchart/NICE advice. *If ≤55yrs old* test for *Helicobacter pylori*;[1] treat if +ve.[2] 'Test & treat' is more effective at reducing symptoms and recurrence than acid suppression alone (eg lansoprazole 30mg/24h PO for 4wks; SE: D&V, GI infections, oedema, bronchospasm, Stevens–Johnson syndrome/epidermal necrolysis, alopecia, photosensitivity, interstitial nephritis, LFT↑, agranulocytosis).[35] When choosing anti-acid ℞, PPIs are better than H_2-receptor antagonists (H_2RA) at controlling symptoms in uninvestigated dyspepsia. The most accurate non-invasive test for *H. pylori* is the ^{13}C breath test (TABLE). ►*If ≥55* (and **new** dyspepsia not accounted for by NSAID use and persisting for >4–6 weeks) **or** *alarm symptoms*, refer for urgent endoscopy (p256). Platelets↑, ESR↑ ± LFT↑ suggest organic causes.[36]

Duodenal ulcers (DU) are 4-fold commoner than GU. *Major risk factors: H. pylori* (~90%); drugs (aspirin; NSAIDs; steroids). *Minor:* ↑Gastric acid secretion; ↑gastric emptying (↓duodenal pH); blood group O; smoking. The role of stress is controversial. *Symptoms:* Epigastric pain typically before meals or at night, relieved by eating, or drinking milk. 50% are asymptomatic; others experience recurrent episodes. *Signs:* Epigastric tenderness. *Diagnosis:* Upper GI endoscopy (stop PPI 2wks before), see **fig 1**, p255. Test for *H. pylori*. Measure gastrin concentrations whilst off PPIs if Zollinger-Ellison syndrome (p730) is suspected. **ΔΔ:** Non-ulcer dyspepsia; duodenal Crohn's; TB; lymphoma; pancreatic cancer (p276).

Gastric ulcers (GU) occur mainly in the elderly, on the lesser curve. Ulcers elsewhere are more often malignant. *Risk factors: H. pylori* (~80%); smoking; NSAIDs; reflux of duodenal contents; delayed gastric emptying; stress, eg neurosurgery (Cushing's ulcers) or burns (Curling's ulcers). *Symptoms:* Asymptomatic or epigastric pain (related to meals ± relieved by antacids) ± weight↓. *Tests:* Upper GI endoscopy to exclude malignancy (stop PPI >2wks before, see FLOWCHART); take multiple biopsies from the ulcer's rim & base (histology, *H. pylori*) and brushings (cytology).

Treating peptic ulcers *Lifestyle* Avoid food that worsens symptoms; stop smoking (smoking slows healing in GU and ↑relapse rates in DU). *H. pylori eradication:* Triple therapy is 80–85% effective at eradication.[1] *Drugs to reduce acid:* PPIs are the most effective, eg *lansoprazole* 30mg/24h PO for 4 (DU) or 8 (GU) weeks. H_2RAs may have a place for individual responders, eg *ranitidine* 300mg each night PO for 8 weeks. *NSAID-associated ulcers:* Stop NSAID if possible. PPIs are the most effective drugs for treatment and prevention of GI ulcers and bleeding in patients on antiplatelet therapy. Misoprostol has ↑side effects and sucralfate and H_2 blockers are not adequately effective.[37] If symptoms persist, re-endoscope, recheck for *H. pylori*, and reconsider the differential diagnosis. *Surgery:* p626.

Complications Bleeding ►►(p252), perforation ►►(p608), malignancy, gastric outflow↓.

Functional (non-ulcer dyspepsia) Treatment is difficult and often unsatisfactory. *H. pylori* eradication (only after a +ve result) may be beneficial,[38] but long-term effects of such a strategy are unknown (SE include ↑reflux). There is limited supporting evidence in favour of treating with PPIs or psychotherapy. Treatments with antacids, antispasmodics, bismuth, H_2 blockers, misoprostol, prokinetic agents, sucralfate, or tricyclic antidepressants has uncertain or no supporting evidence.[39]

1 *H. pylori* is the commonest bacterial pathogen found worldwide (>50% of the world population over 40yrs has it). It's a **class I carcinogen** causing chronic gastritis, duodenal/gastric ulcers & gastric cancer, and may be associated with coronary artery disease, stroke, vitamin B12 and iron deficiency.

Why do we use the ¹³C breath test to detect *Helicobacter*?

Of all the non-invasive tests, the ¹³C breath test is the most accurate.

Test		Sensitivity	Specificity
Invasive	CLO test	95%	95%
	Histology	95%	95%
	Culture	90%	100%
Non-invasive	¹³C breath test	95%	95%
	Stool antigen	95%	94%
	Serology	92%	83%

Differential diagnosis of dyspepsia

- Non-ulcer dyspepsia
- Oesophagitis/ GORD
- Duodenal/gastric ulcer
- Gastric malignancy
- Duodenitis
- Gastritis

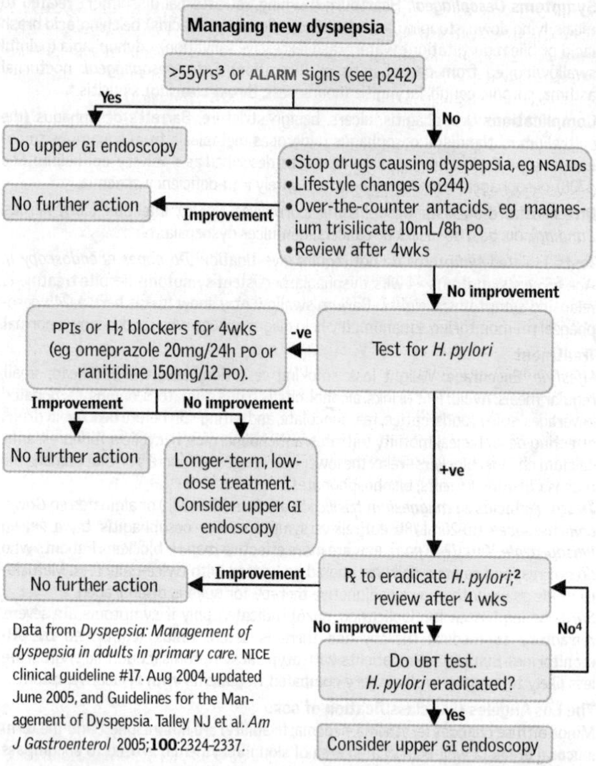
Managing new dyspepsia
>55yrs³ or ALARM signs (see p242)
Yes
No
Do upper GI endoscopy
• Stop drugs causing dyspepsia, eg NSAIDs
• Lifestyle changes (p244)
• Over-the-counter antacids, eg magnesium trisilicate 10mL/8h PO
• Review after 4wks
No further action
Improvement
No improvement
PPIs or H2 blockers for 4wks (eg omeprazole 20mg/24h PO or ranitidine 150mg/12 PO).
-ve
Test for H. pylori
Improvement
No improvement
No further action
Longer-term, low-dose treatment. Consider upper GI endoscopy
+ve
No further action
Improvement
℞ to eradicate H. pylori;²
review after 4 wks
No improvement
No⁴
Do UBT test.
H. pylori eradicated?
Yes
Consider upper GI endoscopy

Data from *Dyspepsia: Management of dyspepsia in adults in primary care*. NICE clinical guideline #17. Aug 2004, updated June 2005, and Guidelines for the Management of Dyspepsia. Talley NJ et al. *Am J Gastroenterol* 2005;**100**:2324-2337.

Why not start everyone on a PPI straight away? Simple measures are safer (more and more PPI SE are reported). Also, PPIs & ranitidine cause false -ve breath tests and antigen tests: stop for >2wks before (>4wks for bismuth & antibiotics).[40] ►See NICE.

2 *H. pylori* eradication (NICE/*BNF*): **either** PAC500 regimen (full dose **PPI**, **amoxicillin** 1g, **clarithromycin** 500mg) bd **or** PMC250 (full dose **PPI**, **metronidazole** 400mg, **clarithromycin** 250mg) bd for 7d. PPIs: **omeprazole** 20mg/12h; **lansoprazole**: 30mg/12h; PPI alternative: **ranitidine bismuth citrate** 400mg/12h. **Resistant cases: tripotassium dicitratobismuthate** (De Noltab® 2 bd ½h ac) + PPI + 2 antibiotics for 14d. Bismuth causes black stools: warn the patient! NB: you may need to continue the PPI if the ulcer is large or bleeds.
3 Some experts recommend endoscopy if >45yrs old
4 Don't treat +ve cases of *H. pylori* more than twice. If still +ve, do endoscopy.

GORD is common. A current definition of the disorder is 'a condition which develops when the reflux of stomach contents causes troublesome symptoms (ie at least two heartburn episodes per week) and/or complications'.[41] Dysfunction of the lower oesophageal sphincter predisposes to the gastro-oesophageal reflux of acid. If reflux is prolonged or excessive, it may cause oesophagitis (**fig 1**), benign oesophageal stricture, or Barrett's oesophagus (**fig 2** and p708). Several factors may predispose patients to pathological reflux, including hiatus hernia (see below), lower oesophageal sphincter hypotension, loss of oesophageal peristaltic function, abdominal obesity, gastric acid hypersecretion, delayed gastric emptying, overeating,[42] smoking; alcohol, pregnancy, surgery in achalasia, drugs (tricyclics, anticholinergics, nitrates), systemic sclerosis, *Helicobacter pylori*?[1]

Symptoms *Oesophageal:* Heartburn (burning, retrosternal discomfort related to meals, lying down, stooping, and straining, relieved by antacids); belching; acid brash (acid or bile regurgitation); waterbrash (excessive salivation); odynophagia (painful swallowing, eg from oesophagitis or ulceration). ***Extra-oesophageal:*** nocturnal asthma, chronic cough, laryngitis (hoarseness, throat clearing), sinusitis.[43]

Complications Oesophagitis, ulcers, benign stricture, Barrett's oesophagus (the epithelium of the distal oesophagus undergoes metaplasia from squamous to columnar type. Endoscopic appearance can be described as a 'velvety' epithelium. See p708), oesophageal adenocarcinoma, and rarely iron-deficiency anaemia.

Differential diagnosis Oesophagitis (corrosives, NSAID); infection (CMV, herpes, *Candida*); DU; gastric ulcers or cancers; non-ulcer dyspepsia.

Tests Isolated symptoms do not require investigation. ***Do upper GI endoscopy if:*** Age >55yrs; symptoms >4 wks; dysphagia; persistent symptoms despite treatment; relapsing symptoms; weight↓. Barium swallow may show hiatus hernia. 24h oesophageal pH monitoring ±manometry help diagnose GORD when endoscopy is normal.

Treatment

Lifestyle: **Encourage:** Weight loss; smoking cessation; raise the bed head; small, regular meals. **Avoid:** Hot drinks, alcohol, citrus fruits, tomatoes, onions, carbonated beverages, spicy foods, coffee, tea, chocolate, and eating <3h before bed. Avoid drugs affecting oesophageal motility (nitrates, anticholinergics, tricyclic antidepressants, calcium channel blockers—relax the lower oesophageal sphincter) or that damage the mucosa (NSAIDs, K^+ salts, bisphosphonates).

Drugs: Antacids eg ***magnesium trisilicate mixture*** (10mL/8h) or alginates eg ***Gaviscon Advance***® (10-20mL/8h PO) relieve symptoms. For oesophagitis, try a PPI eg ***lansoprazole*** 30mg/24h PO.[44] PPIs are more effective than H_2 blockers. Patients who do not respond to once-daily PPI should be treated with twice-daily PPIs. Metoclopramide as monotherapy or adjunctive therapy for GORD is discouraged.[45]

Surgery: (eg Nissen fundoplication, p626) Indicated only if symptoms are severe, refractory to medical therapy **and** there is severe reflux (confirmed by pH-monitoring). Symptoms in patients with atypical symptoms (cough, laryngitis) are less likely to improve with surgery compared to patients with typical symptoms.

The Los Angeles (LA) classification of GORD

Minor diffuse changes (erythema, oedema; friability) are not included, and the term **mucosal break** (a well-demarcated area of slough/erythema) is used to encompass the old terms erosion and ulceration. There are 4 grades:[46]

1 ≥1 mucosal break(s)<5mm long not extending beyond 2 mucosal fold tops.
2 Mucosal break >5mm long limited to the space between 2 mucosal fold tops.
3 Mucosal break continuous between the tops of 2 or more mucosal folds but which involves less than 75% of the oesophageal circumference.
4 Mucosal break involving ≥75% of the oesophageal circumference.

1 The role of *H. pylori* in GORD is still not yet established, with the evidence pointing both ways.

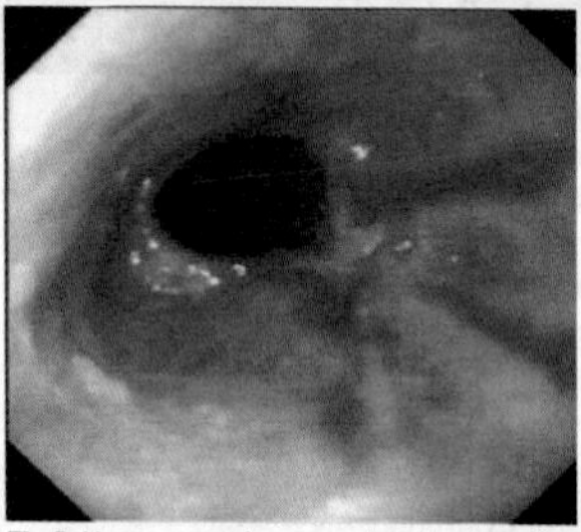

Fig 1. Upper GI endoscopy showing longitudinal mucosal breaks in severe oesophagitis.

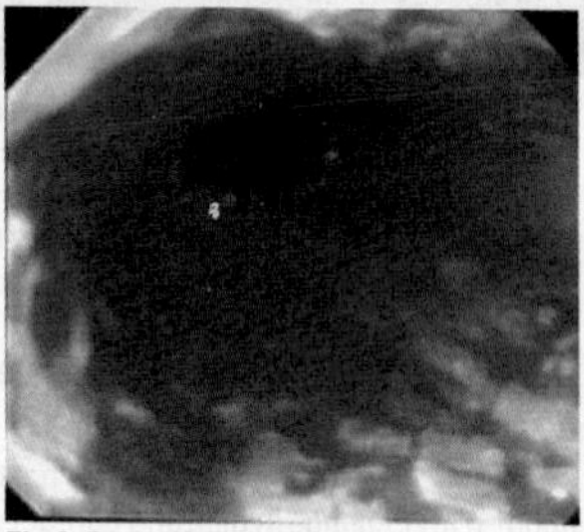

Fig 2. Barrett's oesophagus.

Figs 1 & 2 courtesy of Dr A Mee

Hiatus hernia

Sliding hiatus hernia (80%) is where the gastro-oesophageal junction slides up into the chest—see BOX. Acid reflux often happens as the lower oesophageal sphincter becomes less competent in many cases.

Rolling hiatus hernia (20%) is where the gastro-oesophageal junction remains in the abdomen but a bulge of stomach herniates up into the chest alongside the oesophagus—see BOX and **fig 3**. As the gastro-oesophageal junction remains intact, gross acid reflux is uncommon.

Clinical features Common: 30% of patients >50yrs, especially obese women. 50% have symptomatic gastro-oesophageal reflux.

Imaging Barium swallow is the best diagnostic test; upper GI endoscopy visualizes the mucosa (?oesophagitis) but cannot reliably exclude a hiatus hernia.

Treatment: Lose weight. Treat reflux symptoms. Surgery indications: intractable symptoms despite aggressive medical therapy, complications (see above). It is advised to repair rolling hiatus hernia prophylactically (even if asymptomatic) as it may strangulate, which needs prompt surgical repair (which has a high mortality and morbidity rate).

Hiatus hernia—sliding and rolling

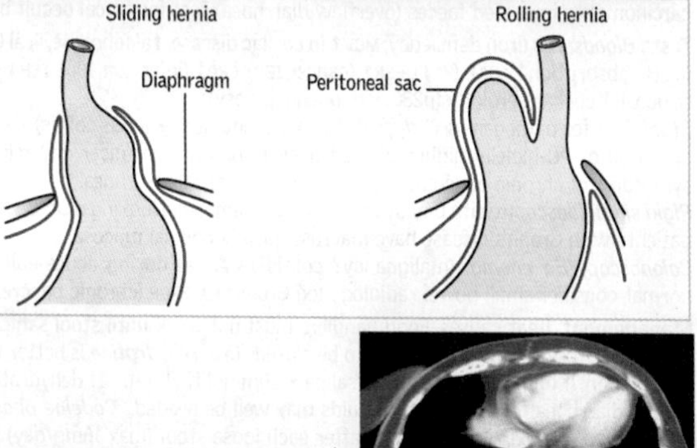

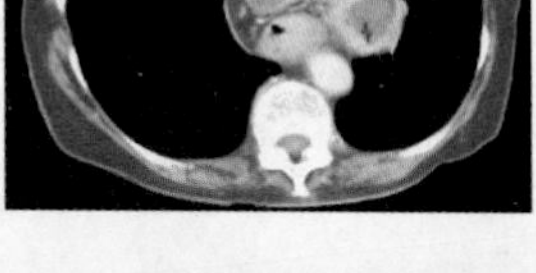

Fig 3. CT chest with IV contrast showing the rolling components of a hiatus hernia anterior to the oesophagus. Between the oesophagus and the vertebral column on the left hand side, is the aorta.

Image courtesy of Dr Stephen Golding.

Traveller's diarrhoea: p377

Diarrhoea means increased stool water (hence ↑stool volume, eg >200mL daily), and this increases stool frequency and the passage of liquid stool. If it is the stool's fat content which is increased, use the term **steatorrhoea** (=pale, malodorous stool that is difficult to flush away, p280). Distinguish both from faecal urgency (which suggests rectal pathology eg cancer, UC).[47]

Common causes
• Gastroenteritis
• Viral
• Bacterial
• Parasites/protozoa
• IBS (p276)
• Drugs (see below)
• Colorectal cancer
• Ulcerative colitis (UC)
• Crohn's disease
• Coeliac disease
Less common causes
• Microscopic colitis[1]
• Chronic pancreatitis
• Bile salt malabsorption
• Thyrotoxicosis
• Laxative abuse
• Lactose intolerance
• Ileal/gastric resection
• Overflow diarrhoea
• Bacterial overgrowth
• *C. difficile* (BOX)
Rare causes
• Autonomic neuropathy
• Addison's disease
• Ischaemic colitis
• Amyloidosis
• Tropical sprue
• Gastrinoma
• VIPoma[2]
• Carcinoid syndrome
• Medullary thyroid CA
• Pellagra

Clinical features Take a detailed history: (is he a chef?)
Acute or chronic? If acute suspect gastroenteritis. Ask about travel, change in diet, and contact history. Chronic diarrhoea alternating with constipation suggests irritable bowel (p248). Anorexia, weight↓, nocturnal diarrhoea & anaemia suggest an organic cause.
Bloody diarrhoea: Campylobacter, Shigella, Salmonella, E. coli, amoebiasis, UC, Crohn's disease, colorectal cancer (p618), colonic polyps, pseudomembranous colitis, ischaemic colitis (p488).
Fresh PR bleeding: See p631.
Mucus occurs in IBS(p276), colorectal cancer, and polyps.
Pus suggests IBD (inflammatory bowel disease), diverticulitis, or a fistula/abscess.
Large bowel symptoms: Watery stool ± blood or mucus; pelvic pain relieved by defecation; tenesmus; urgency.
Small bowel symptoms: periumbilical (or RIF) pain not relieved by defecation; watery stool or steatorrhoea.
Non-GI causes: Antibiotics; PPIs; cimetidine; propranolol, cytotoxics; NSAIDs; digoxin; alcohol; laxative abuse; **medical conditions:** thyrotoxicosis; autonomic neuropathy; Addison's disease; carcinoid syndrome.

Examination Look for weight↓, clubbing, anaemia, oral ulcers (p238), rashes and abdominal scars. Assess severity of dehydration (dry mucous membranes, ↓skin turgor and capillary refill >2s). **Feel** for an enlarged thyroid or an abdominal mass. Do a rectal examination for masses (eg rectal carcinoma) or impacted faeces (overflow diarrhoea). Test for faecal occult blood.

Tests *Bloods:* FBC (iron deficiency; MCV↑ in coeliac disease, ↑alcohol use, ileal Crohn's (as B_{12} absorption↓); U&E (K^+↓); ESR↑ (cancer, IBD); CRP↑ (infection, IBD). TSH↓ (thyrotoxicosis); coeliac serology (p280 ± duodenal biopsy).
Stool: Test for pathogens & *C. difficile* toxin (pseudomembranous colitis). Faecal fat excretion or ^{13}C-hiolein (highly labelled triolein) breath test (nicer and reliable) if symptoms of chronic pancreatitis, malabsorption, or steatorrhoea.[48]
Rigid sigmoidoscopy: with biopsy of normal and abnormal looking mucosa: ~15% of patients with Crohn's disease have macroscopically normal mucosa.
Colonoscopy/Ba enema: (malignancy? colitis?) ►Avoid during acute episode. If normal, consider small bowel radiology (eg Crohn's) ± ERCP (chronic pancreatitis).

Management Treat causes. Food handlers must not work until stool samples are -ve. If an outbreak, wards may need to be closed. *Oral rehydration* is better than IV rehydration; if impossible, give 0.9% saline + 20mmol K^+/L IVI. ►If dehydrated and bloody diarrhoea for >2 weeks, IV fluids may well be needed. *Codeine phosphate* 30mg/6h PO or *loperamide* 2mg PO after each loose stool (max 16mg/day) reduce stool frequency.[49] Avoid antibiotics except in infective diarrhoea causing systemic illness (see FLOWCHART)—because of the risk of developing antibiotic resistance.

1 Think of this in any chronic diarrhoea; do biopsy (may be +ve on normal looking colonic mucosa—reported as 'lymphocytic' or 'collagenous' colitis). Prognosis: good. *Budesonide* is 1st-line, followed by a 5-aminosalycilic acid agent (p265), *bismuth subsalicylate* (eg Pepto-Bismol®), or *loperamide*.
2 Vasoactive intestinal polypeptide-secreting tumour; suspect if K^+↓ & acidosis; Ca^{2+}↑; Mg^{2+}↓.

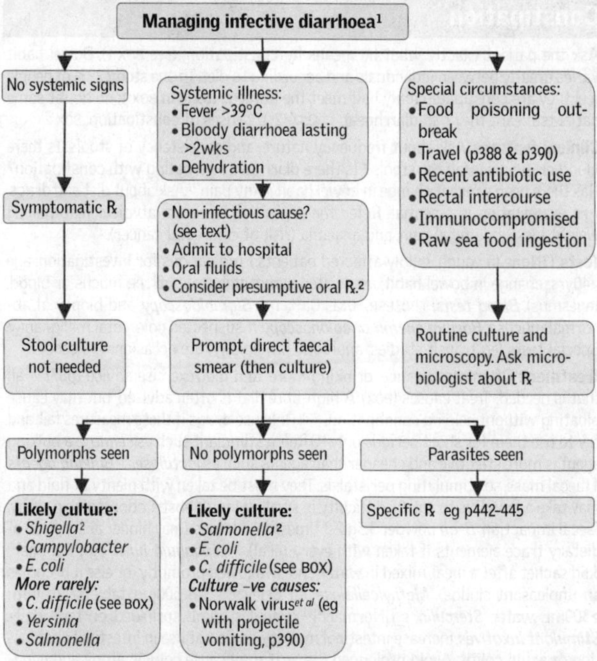

Clostridium difficile: the cause of pseudomembranous colitis

C. difficile, is a Gram +ve 'superbug' whose spores are contagious (faecal-oral or from the environment, where spores can live for ages and are hard to eradicate).

Signs: T°↑; colic; mild diarrhoea—or serious bloody diarrhoea with systemic upset—CRP↑↑, WCC↑, albumin↓, and colitis (with yellow adherent plaques on inflamed non-ulcerated mucosa—the pseudomembrane) and multi-organ failure.

Asymptomatic carriage: 1-3% of all adults. ***Risk factors:*** Age↑; in hospital; bed occupancy >80%; antibiotic use (esp. broad-spectrum or IV). ***Deaths:*** 6500/yr[uk].

Toxins: Tissue culture, ELISA, and PCR help defect *C. difficile* toxins (CDT). Some strains produce no toxin and are non-pathogenic; most produce toxins A *and* B. Some strains are hypervirulent, eg NAP1/027.

℞: Stop the causative antibiotic (if possible). Treatment is not usually needed if asymptomatic (use of antibiotics for *C. difficile* is controversial). If symptomatic, give **metronidazole** 400mg/8h PO for 10d. (**vancomycin** 125mg/6h PO is better in severe disease; if complications, up to 2g/day).[50]

►Urgent colectomy may be needed if toxic megacolon, LDH↑, or if deteriorating.

Recurrent disease: Repeat metronidazole once only (overuse causes irreversible neuropathy). NB: probiotics may prevent recurrences (*Saccharomyces boulardii* 500mg/12h, unless immunosuppressed or CVP line *in situ*). Administration of stools (via NGT or colonoscope) from healthy subjects may have a role.[51]

Preventing spread: Meticulous cleaning, use of disposable gloves, not using rectal thermometers, hand-washing, and ward protocols (eg 'bare below elbows').

1 Be aware of your local pathogens, and be prepared to close wards and hospitals if contagion is afoot.
2 Prompt specific ℞: eg ciprofloxacin 500mg/12h po for 6d may be needed before sensitivities are known.

Constipation

Ask the patient exactly what he means by 'constipation' (see BOX 1). Bowel habit varies greatly between individuals and according to diet. In one study, 29% of people feel they are constipated (only half meet the Rome criteria in BOX 1; no doubt some patients meant they had diarrhoea).[52] ♀:♂≈2:1. Causes of constipation: BOX 2.

Clinical features Ask about frequency, nature, and consistency of stools. Is there blood or mucus in/on the stools? Is there diarrhoea alternating with constipation? Has there been a recent change in bowel habit? Any pain?[1] Ask about diet and drugs. ►**PR examination** is essential. Refer the patient if there are atypical features, eg weight loss, abdominal pain, and anaemia (risk of colorectal cancer).

Tests (?None in young, mildly affected patients.) Indications for investigation: age >40yrs; change in bowel habit; associated symptoms (weight↓, PR mucus or blood, tenesmus). ***Blood tests:*** FBC, ESR, U&E, Ca^{2+}, TFT. ***Sigmoidoscopy*** and biopsy of abnormal mucosa. ***Barium enema*** or ***colonoscopy*** if suspected colorectal malignancy. Special tests (eg transit studies; anorectal physiology) are occasionally needed.

Treatment Often reassurance, drinking more, and diet/exercise advice (p87) is all that is needed. Treat causes (BOX). A high-fibre diet is often advised, but may cause bloating without helping constipation.[53] ►Only use drugs if these measures fail, and try to use them for short periods only.[2] Often, a stimulant such as *senna* ± a bulking agent is more effective and cheaper than agents such as *lactulose*.[54] ***Bulking agents*** ↑faecal mass, so stimulating peristalsis. They must be taken with plenty of fluid and may take a few days to act. CI: difficulty in swallowing; GI obstruction; colonic atony; faecal impaction. ***Bran*** powder 3.5g 2-3 times/d with food (may hinder absorption of dietary trace elements if taken with every meal).[55] ***Ispaghula husk***, eg 1 Fybogel® 3.5g sachet after a meal, mixed in water and swallowed promptly (or else it becomes an unpleasant sludge). ***Methylcellulose***, eg Celevac® 3-6 500mg tablets/12h with ≥300mL water. ***Sterculia***, eg Normacol® granules, 10mL sprinkled on food daily. ***Stimulant laxatives*** increase intestinal motility, so do not use in intestinal obstruction or acute colitis. Avoid prolonged use as it **may** cause colonic atony and hypokalaemia (but there are no good long-term data). Abdominal cramps are an important SE. Pure stimulant laxatives are ***bisacodyl*** tablets (5-10mg at night) or suppositories (10mg in the mornings) and ***senna*** (2-4 tablets at night). ***Docusate sodium*** and ***danthron***[3] (=dantron) have stimulant and softening actions. ***Glycerol*** suppositories act as a rectal stimulant. ***Sodium picosulfate*** (5-10mg up to 12h beforehand) is useful for rapid bowel evacuation prior to procedures. ***Stool softeners*** are particularly useful when managing painful anal conditions eg fissure. ***Arachis oil*** enemas lubricate and soften impacted faeces. ***Liquid paraffin*** should not be used for a prolonged period (SE: anal seepage, lipoid pneumonia, malabsorption of fat-soluble vitamins). ***Osmotic laxatives*** retain fluid in the bowel. ***Lactulose***, a semisynthetic disaccharide, produces osmotic diarrhoea of low faecal pH that discourages growth of ammonia-producing organisms. It is useful in hepatic encephalopathy (initial dose: 30-50mL/12h). SE: bloating, so its role in treating constipation is limited. ***Magnesium salts*** (eg magnesium hydroxide; magnesium sulfate) are useful when rapid bowel evacuation is required. ***Sodium salts*** (eg Microlette® and Micralax® enemas) should be avoided as they may cause sodium and water retention. ***Phosphate enemas*** are useful for rapid bowel evacuation prior to procedures.

What if laxatives don't help? A multi-disciplinary approach with behaviour therapy, psychological support, habit training ± sphincter-action biofeedback may help. $5HT_4$ agonists, which induce peristalsis by systemic rather than luminal means, are under trial (*tegaserod* and *prucalopride*: neither currently licensed in UK).[56]

1 *Levator ani syndrome:* recurrent chronic rectal pain without detectable organic cause. Pain is typically worse on walking and may be brought on by defecation. It may be reproduced by coccygeal traction (on PR) with a specific trigger point on the levator muscle.
2 Risks of laxative abuse are overemphasized ('cathartic colon' is a questionable entity); stimulant laxatives may be used chronically on those who do not respond to bulk or osmotic laxatives alone.
3 **Danthron** causes colon & liver tumours in animals, so reserve use for the very elderly or terminally ill.

A definition of constipation

Infrequent bowel movements (≲3 times weekly), or passing stools less often than the person's own normal habit, or with difficulty, straining, or pain.

Making constipation glamorous

The best way to make something glamorous is to associate it with somewhere beautiful, immortal, and seductive, so now we have the famous Rome criteria—named after 'the eternal city'.

The Rome criteria

Constipation: the presence of ≥2 symptoms during bowel movements (BMs):

- Straining for ≥25% of BMs
- Lumpy or hard stools in ≥25% of BMs
- Sensation of incomplete evacuations for ≥ 25% BMs
- Sensation of anorectal obstruction or blockage for ≥25% of BMs
- Manual manoeuvres to facilitate at least 25% of BMs (eg digital evacuation, support of the pelvic floor)
- Fewer than 3 BMs per week

Chronicity entails constipation for the last 90 days, with onset ≥6 months ago.

Rome feeds anal fixations[57]

►Applying the Rome criteria teaches us to be obsessive about our bowels—a prime example of medicalizing our way into two diseases for the price of one—or, quite often, none, as it is possible to be healthy and pass stools only weekly.

As well as moving beyond the traditional oral, anal and phallic stages of development, we propose that doctors must also move beyond their stage of obsessive counting, before they can be of real service to their patients.[58]

All roads lead away from Rome

Most people declaring themselves to be constipated do so in flagrant disregard of the Rome criteria,[59] perhaps on the grounds that you cannot tell someone they are not hungry just because they eat more than 2 meals a day.

Furthermore, the highest prevalence of constipation is in nursing homes, the one place where Rome cannot penetrate very far as the inmates tend to be too cognitively challenged to report sensations of anal blockage etc.[60]

Causes of constipation

General

- Poor diet ± lack of exercise
- Poor fluid intake/dehydration
- Irritable bowel syndrome
- Old age
- Post-operative pain
- Hospital environment (↓privacy, having to use a bed pan)
- Distant, squalid, or fearsome toilets

Anorectal disease (esp. if painful)

- Anal fissure (p632) or stricture
- Rectal prolapse
- Proctalgia fugax (p632)
- Mucosal ulceration/neoplasia
- Levator ani syndrome[1]

Intestinal obstruction

- Colorectal carcinoma (p618)
- Strictures (eg Crohn's disease)
- Pelvic mass (eg fetus, fibroids)
- Diverticulosis (rectal bleeding is a commoner presentation)
- Pseudo-obstruction (p613)

Metabolic/endocrine

- Hypercalcaemia (p690)
- Hypothyroidism (rarely *presents* with constipation)
- Hypokalaemia (p688)
- Porphyria
- Lead poisoning

Drugs (pre-empt by diet advice)

- Opiates (eg morphine, codeine)
- Anticholinergics (eg tricyclics)
- Iron
- Some antacids, eg with aluminium
- Diuretics, eg furosemide
- Calcium channel blockers

Neuromuscular (slow transit from decreased propulsive activity)

- Spinal or pelvic nerve injury (eg trauma, surgery)
- Aganglionosis (Chagas' disease, Hirschsprung's disease)
- Systemic sclerosis
- Diabetic neuropathy

Other causes

- Chronic laxative abuse (rare—diarrhoea is commoner)
- Idiopathic slow transit
- Idiopathic megarectum/colon
- Psychological, associated with depression or abuse as a child.

NB: constipation is unlikely to be the sole symptom of serious disease, so be reassuring (if PR, ESR & TSH are ↔).

Jaundice (**icterus**) refers to yellow pigmentation of skin, sclerae, and mucosae due to ↑plasma bilirubin (visible at >35μmol/L—not always easy to spot when mild). Jaundice is classified by the site of the problem (pre-hepatic, hepatocellular, or cholestatic/obstructive) or by the type of circulating bilirubin (conjugated or unconjugated). **Kernicterus** is seen in infants with unconjugated hyperbilirubinaemia and involves deposition of unbound bilirubin in the basal ganglia, which can cause **opisthotonus**.

Unconjugated hyperbilirubinaemia:
As unconjugated bilirubin is water insoluble, it does not enter urine, resulting in unconjugated (acholuric) hyperbilirubinaemia.
Overproduction: haemolysis; ineffective erythropoiesis.
Impaired hepatic uptake: drugs (contrast agents, rifampicin), congestive cardiac failure.
Impaired conjugation: glucuronyl transferase deficiency (Gilbert's, p714, & Crigler-Najjar syndromes, p710).
Physiological neonatal jaundice is caused by a combination of the above mentioned mechanisms (bilirubin production is ↑ due to short lifespan of RBCs, and bilirubin conjugation is not completely developed).

Conjugated hyperbilirubinaemia:
Hepatocellular dysfunction: There is hepatocyte damage, usually with some cholestasis. *Causes:* Viruses: hepatitis (p406, eg A, B, C, etc.), CMV (p404), EBV (p401); drugs (see TABLE); alcoholic hepatitis; cirrhosis (see BOX); liver metastases/abscess; haemochromatosis; autoimmune hepatitis (AIH); septicaemia; leptospirosis; α_1-antitrypsin deficiency (p264); Budd-Chiari (p710); Wilson's disease (p269); failure to excrete conjugated bilirubin (Dubin-Johnson, p712, and Rotor syndromes, p724); right heart failure; toxins, eg carbon tetrachloride; fungi (*Amanita phalloides*, **fig 2**).
Impaired hepatic excretion: Primary biliary cirrhosis, primary sclerosing cholangitis, extrinsic compression of the bile duct, drug-induced cholestasis (see BOX), common bile duct gallstones; pancreatic cancer, lymph nodes at the porta hepatis, drugs for cholangiocarcinoma, choledochal cyst, biliary atresia, Mirrizi's syndrome (obstructive jaundice from common bile duct compression by a gallstone impacted in the cystic duct, often associated with cholangitis). As conjugated bilirubin is water-soluble, it is excreted in urine, making it dark. Less conjugated bilirubin enters the gut and the faeces become pale. When severe, it can be associated with an intractable pruritus which is best treated by relief of the obstruction.

Clinical features *Ask* about blood transfusions, intravenous drug use, body piercing, tattoos, sexual activity, travel abroad, jaundiced contacts, family history, alcohol consumption, and **all** medications (eg old drug charts; GP records). *Examine* for signs of chronic liver disease (p260), hepatic encephalopathy (p259), lymphadenopathy, hepatomegaly, splenomegaly, ascites and a palpable gall bladder (which in conjunction with painless jaundice suggests a cause other than gallstones—Courvoisier's 'law'). Pale stools with dark urine ≈ cholestatic jaundice.

Tests See p260 for screening tests in suspected liver disease.[1] *Urine:* Bilirubin is absent in pre-hepatic causes, hence 'acholuric' jaundice; urobilinogen is absent in obstructive jaundice. *Haematology:* FBC, clotting, blood film, reticulocyte count, Coomb's test. *Biochemistry:* U&E, LFT[1] (bilirubin, ALT, AST, alk phos, γ-GT, total protein, albumin).[61] *Ultrasound:* Are the bile ducts dilated >6mm (obstruction—see **fig 3**, p281)? Are there gallstones, hepatic metastases or a pancreatic mass? *ERCP* (p756) if bile ducts are dilated and LFT not improving. *MRCP* (p757) or endoscopic ultrasound (EUS) if conventional ultrasound shows gallstones but no definite common bile duct stones. Perform a *liver biopsy* (p256) if the bile ducts are normal. Consider abdominal *CT* or *MRI* if abdominal malignancy is suspected clinically.

1 Albumin & INR are the best indicators of hepatic synthetic function. ↑Transaminases (ALT, AST) indicate hepatocyte damage. ↑Alk phos is typical of obstructive jaundice, but also occurs in hepatocellular jaundice, malignant infiltration, pregnancy (placental isoenzyme), Paget's disease, and childhood (bone isoenzyme).

The pathway of bilirubin metabolism

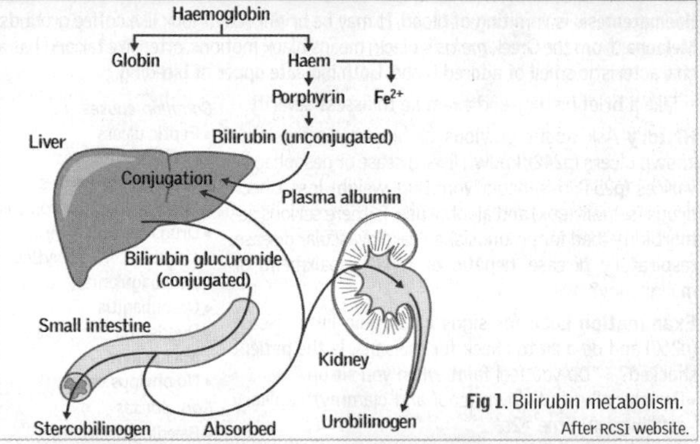

Fig 1. Bilirubin metabolism.
After RCSI website.

Bilirubin metabolism

Bilirubin is formed from the breakdown of haemoglobin (**fig 1**). Bilirubin metabolism has three steps: hepatic uptake, conjugation, and excretion. In the liver, bilirubin is conjugated with glucuronic acid by hepatocytes, making it water soluble. Conjugated bilirubin is secreted into the bile and passes out into the gut. Some is taken up again by the liver (via the enterohepatic circulation) and the rest is converted to urobilinogen by gut bacteria. Urobilinogen is either reabsorbed and excreted by the kidneys, or converted to stercobilin, which colours faeces brown.

Causes of jaundice in a previously stable patient with cirrhosis

- Sepsis (esp. UTI, pneumonia, or peritonitis)
- Malignancy: eg hepatocellular carcinoma
- Alcohol; drugs (BOX 3)
- GI bleeding

Look for signs of decompensation: ascites; dilated abdominal veins; neurological upset; peripheral oedema.

Drug-induced jaundice

1 Haemolysis	• Antimalarials (eg dapsone)	
2 Hepatitis	• Paracetamol overdose (p856) • Isoniazid, rifampicin, pyrazinamide • Monoamine oxidase inhibitors	• Sodium valproate • Halothane • Statins
3 Cholestasis	• Flucloxacillin (may be weeks after ℞) • Fusidic acid, co-amoxiclav, nitrofurantoin • Steroids (anabolic; the Pill)	• Sulfonylureas • Prochlorperazine • Chlorpromazine

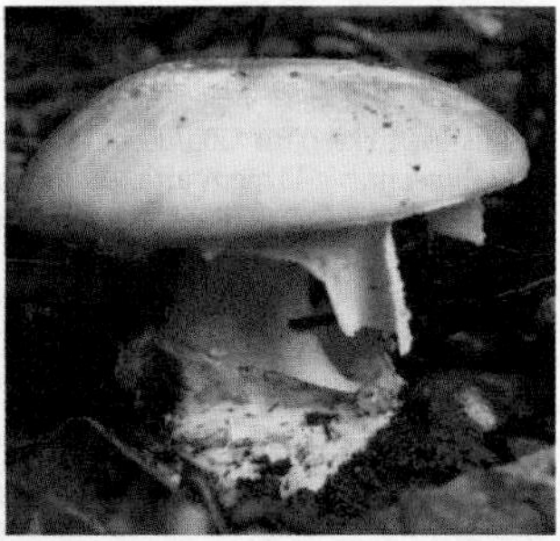

Fig 2. 62 *Amanita phalloides* (Latin for 'phallic toadstool'; also known as the 'death cap') is a lethal cause of jaundice. It is the most toxic mushroom known. After ingestion (its benign appearance is confusing), amatoxins induce hepatic necrosis eg with liver failure. Some have been treated successfully by transplantation. ©Ian Herriott. NB: don't use this image for identification!

Haematemesis is vomiting of blood. It may be bright red or look like coffee grounds. **Melaena** (from the Greek *melas* = black) means black motions, often like tar, and has a characteristic smell of altered blood. Both indicate upper GI bleeding.

►Take a brief history and examine to assess severity.

Common causes
• Peptic ulcers
• Mallory-Weiss tear
• Oesophageal varices
• Gastritis/gastric erosions
• Drugs (NSAIDs, aspirin, steroids, thrombolytics, anticoagulants)
• Oesophagitis
• Duodenitis
• Malignancy
• No obvious cause
Rare causes
• Bleeding disorders
• Portal hypertensive gastropathy
• Aorto-enteric fistula[1]
• Angiodysplasia
• Haemobilia
• Dieulafoy lesion[2]
• Meckel's diverticulum
• Peutz-Jeghers' syndrome
• Osler-Weber-Rendu synd.

History Ask about previous GI bleeds; dyspepsia or known ulcers (p242); known liver disease or oesophageal varices (p254); dysphagia; vomiting; weight loss. Check drugs (see MINIBOX) and alcohol use. Is there serious co-morbidity (bad for prognosis), eg cardiovascular disease, respiratory disease, hepatic or renal impairment, or malignancy?

Examination Look for signs of chronic liver disease (p260) and do a PR to check for melaena. Is the patient shocked? ►"Do you feel faint when you sit up?"

- Peripherally shut down (cool and clammy); capillary refilling (CR) time >2s.
- ↓GCS (may be tricky to assess in decompensated liver disease) or signs of encephalopathy (p259).
- Poor urine output, eg <25mL/h or <½mL/kg/h.
- Tachycardic (pulse >100bpm, and JVP not raised).
- Hypotensive (systolic BP <100mmHg)
- Postural drop in BP (>20mmHg systolic).
- Calculate the ***Rockall risk score*** (see TABLE 1).

Acute management (see p830). In summary:

►►Protect airway and give high-flow oxygen.

►►Insert 2 large-bore (14–16G) IV cannulae and take blood for FBC (an early Hb may be normal because haemodilution has not yet taken place), U&E (↑urea out of proportion to creatinine is indicative of a massive blood meal), LFT, clotting, and cross-match 4–6 units (give 1 unit per g/dL <14g/dL).

►►Give IV fluids (p831) to restore intravascular volume while waiting for blood to be crossmatched.[63] In a dire emergency—ie haemodynamically deteriorating despite fluid resuscitation measures—give group O Rh-ve blood.

►►Insert a urinary catheter and monitor hourly urine output.

►►Organize a CXR, ECG, and check ABG.

►►Consider a CVP line to monitor and guide fluid replacement.

►►Transfuse (with crossmatched blood) until haemodynamically stable.

►►Correct clotting abnormalities (***vitamin** K*, FFP, platelets).

►►Monitor pulse, BP, and CVP (keep >5cmH$_2$0) at least hourly until stable.

►►Arrange an urgent ***endoscopy***, preferably at a dedicated endoscopy unit.[★][64,65]

►►Inform surgeons of all severe bleeds on admission.

Further management

- Re-examine after 4h and give FFP if >4 units transfused.
- Monitor pulse, BP, CVP, and urine output hourly; ↓frequency to 4hrly if haemodynamically stable.
- Transfuse to keep Hb >10g/dL; always keep 2 units of blood in reserve.
- Give *omeprazole* 40 mg IV **after** endoscopy (reduces risk of rebleeding and need for surgery, but not mortality, in peptic ulcer bleeding).[66]
- Check FBC, U&E, LFT, and clotting daily.
- Keep nil by mouth for 24h. Allow clear fluids after 24h and light diet after 48h, as long as there is no evidence of rebleeding (BOX and p254).

►►See p254 for additional management in suspected variceal bleeding.

1 A patient with an aortic graft repair and upper GI bleeding is considered to have an aorto-enteric fistula until proven otherwise: CT abdomen is usually required as well as endoscopy.

2 A Dieulafoy lesion is the rupture of an unusually big arteriole, eg in the fundus of the stomach.

Rockall risk-scoring for upper GI bleeds

	0 pts	1 pt	2 pts	3 pts
Pre-endoscopy				
Age[I]	<60yrs	60–79yrs	≥80yrs	
Shock: systolic BP pulse rate[I]	BP >100mmHg <100/min	BP >100mmHg Pulse >100/min	BP <100mmHg	
Comorbidity[I]	Nil major	Cardiac failure Ischaemic heart disease	Renal failure Liver failure	Metastases
Post-endoscopy				
Diagnosis[F]	Mallory–Weiss tear; no lesion; no sign of recent bleeding	All other diagnoses	Upper GI malignancy	
Signs of recent haemorrhage on endoscopy[F]	None, or dark red spot		Blood in upper GI tract; adherent clot; visible vessel	

I These criteria make up the initial Rockall score, which is a more reliable predictor of mortality in peptic ulcer bleeding than the final score.[67]
F Added to the initial score, these criteria make up the final Rockall score.

Prediction of rebleeding and mortality from the Rockall score[68]

Rockall scores help predict risk of rebleeding and mortality after upper GI bleeding.[69] An initial score >6 is said to be an indication for surgery, but decisions relating to surgery are rarely taken on the basis of Rockall scores alone (p254).

Score	Mortality: Initial score	Mortality: Final score (after endoscopy)
0	0.2%	0%
1	2.4%	0%
2	5.6%	0.2%
3	11.0%	2.9%
4	24.6%	5.3%
5	39.6%	10.8%
6	48.9%	17.3%
7	50.0%	27.0%
8+	-	41.1%

Management of peptic ulcer bleeds based on endoscopic findings

High-risk[70]

Active bleeding or nonbleeding visible vessel

Admit the patient to a monitored bed or ICU and perform endoscopic haemostasis. Start an IVI PPI (omeprazole 80mg bolus dose plus continuous infusion at 8mg/h) for 72h. H_2 blockers, somatostatin, or octreotide have no role. If haemodynamically stable start oral intake of clear liquids 6h after endoscopy. Change to oral PPI after completion of IV therapy. Initiate treatment if positive for *H. pylori*.

Adherent clot

Do endoscopic removal of adherent clot, followed by endoscopic haemostasis, then treat as above.

Low-risk

Flat, pigmented spot or clean base

There is no need for endoscopic haemostasis. Consider early hospital discharge after endoscopy if the patient has an otherwise low clinical risk and safe home environment. Treat with a PPI. Initiate oral intake with a regular diet 6h after endoscopy in stable patients. Initiate treatment if positive for *H. pylori* (p243).

Endoscopy should be arranged after resuscitation, within 4h of a suspected variceal haemorrhage, or when bleeding is ongoing within 24h of admission. It can identify the site of bleeding, be used to estimate the risk of rebleeding, and to administer treatment, preferably 2 of: eg ***adrenaline***, sclerotherapy, variceal banding (**fig 2**, p255) or argon plasma coagulation (for superficial lesions).[71] *Endoscopic signs associated with risk of rebleeding:* active arterial bleeding (80% risk); visible vessel (50% risk); adherent clot/black dots (30% risk).

Rebleeding 40% of rebleeders die of complications. Identify high-risk patients (TABLE, p253) and monitor closely for signs of rebleeding. IVI of ***omeprazole*** has a preventive role. Get help; **inform a surgeon at once if:** • Haematemesis with melaena • ↑Pulse rate • ↓CVP (assess via JVP or CVP line) • ↓BP • ↓Urine output.

Indications for surgery (p638) ►Contact the surgical team at the onset
- Severe bleeding or bleeding despite transfusing 6U if >60yrs (8U if <60yrs)
- Active or uncontrollable bleeding at endoscopy—or rebleeding.
- Initial Rockall score ≥3 or final Rockall score >6 (but see TABLE 2, p253).

Varices Portal hypertension causes dilated collateral veins (varices) at sites of portosystemic anastomosis. Varices most commonly occur in the lower oesophagus, but may also be found in the stomach around the umbilicus (*caput medusae* is rare) and in the rectum. Varices develop in patients with cirrhosis once portal pressure (measured by hepatic venous pressure gradient) is >10mmHg; if >12mmHg variceal bleeding may develop—associated with a mortality of 30–50% per episode.[72]

Other causes of portal hypertension *Pre-hepatic:* Portal vein thrombosis; splenic vein thrombosis. *Intra-hepatic:* Cirrhosis (80% in UK); schistosomiasis (commonest worldwide); sarcoidosis; myeloproliferative diseases; congenital hepatic fibrosis. *Post-hepatic:* Budd–Chiari syndrome (p710); right heart failure; constrictive pericarditis; veno-occlusive disease. *Risk factors for variceal haemorrhage:* ↑Portal pressure, variceal size, endoscopic features of the variceal wall (eg haematocystic spots) and Child–Pugh score ≥8 (see TABLE, p261).[73]

Suspect varices as a cause of GI bleeding if there is alcohol abuse or cirrhosis. Look for signs of chronic liver disease, encephalopathy, splenomegaly, ascites, hyponatraemia, coagulopathy and thrombocytopenia.

Prophylaxis *Primary* Without treatment ~30% of cirrhotic patients with varices bleed—reducible to 15% by: **1** Non-selective β-blockade (propranolol 40–80mg/12h PO) **2** Repeat endoscopic banding ligation. One recent study showed that banding had significantly better outcome than β-blocker therapy in patients with cirrhosis.[74] Endoscopic sclerotherapy is not used as complications (eg stricturing) may outweigh benefits.[75] *Secondary* After an initial variceal bleed, risk of further bleeding is high—80% will rebleed within 2 years. Options are 1 and 2 as above + transjugular intrahepatic portosystemic shunting (TIPSS)[1] for varices resistant to banding or surgical shunts if TIPSS is impossible for technical reasons. Endoscopic banding may be better than sclerotherapy (lower bleeding rates and fewer complications).[76]

Acute variceal bleeding Get help at the bedside from your senior.
- ▸▸Resuscitate until haemodynamically stable (do not give 0.9% saline).
- ▸▸Correct clotting abnormalities with ***vitamin K*** and FFP.
- ▸▸Start IVI of ***terlipressin*** 2mg bolus, then 1–2mg/4h for ≤3d; relative risk of death ↓ by 34%).[77] Somatostatin analogues are alternatives (less used in the UK).[78,79]
- ▸▸Endoscopic banding (p255, **fig 2**) or sclerotherapy should be tried (banding may be impossible because of limited visualization).
- ▸▸If bleeding uncontrolled, a Minnesota tube or Sengstaken–Blakemore tube (see BOX) should be placed by someone with experience; get an anaesthetist's help.

1 TIPSS works by shunting blood away from the portal circulation through an artificial side-to-side portosystemic anastomosis created in the liver; also used in uncontrolled variceal haemorrhage.

Balloon tamponade with a Sengstaken-Blakemore tube

In life-threatening variceal bleeding, this can buy time to arrange transfer to a specialist liver centre or for surgical decompression. It uses balloons to compress gastric and oesophageal varices. Before insertion, inflate balloons with a measured volume (120-300mL) of air giving pressures of 60mmHg (check with a sphygmomanometer).

- Deflate, and clamp exits.
- Pass the lubricated tube (try to avoid sedation) and inflate the gastric balloon with the predetermined volume of air. Cooling the tube beforehand probably doesn't make it any easier to pass.[80]

►Check position with a portable X-ray before inflating the oesophageal balloon.

- Check pressures (should be 20-30mmHg greater than on the trial run). This phase of the procedure is dangerous: do not over-inflate the balloon because of the risk of oesophageal necrosis or rupture.
- Tape to patient's forehead to ensure the gastric balloon impacts gently on the gastro-oesophageal junction.
- Place the oesophageal aspiration channel on continuous low suction and arrange for the gastric channel to drain freely.
- Leave *in situ* until bleeding stops. Remove after <24h.

Various other techniques of insertion may be used, and tubes vary in structure. **►Do not try to pass one yourself if you have no or little experience:** ask an expert; if unavailable, transfer urgently to a specialist liver centre.

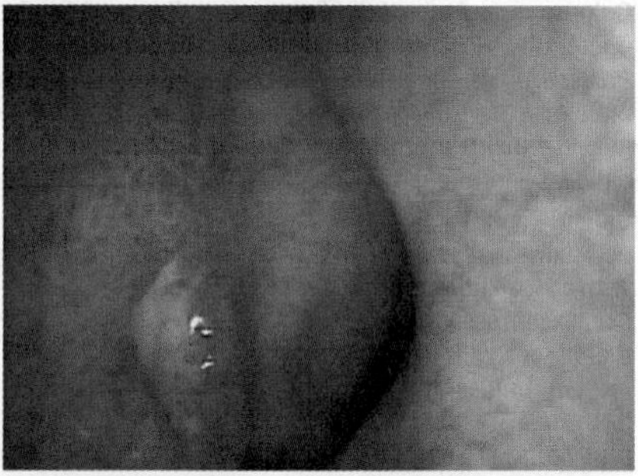

Fig 1. Upper GI endoscopy image of a duodenal ulcer. See p234 for the topic of peptic ulceration and 'Lumen' BOX, p227, for possible enlightenment.
Image courtesy of Dr Jon Simmons

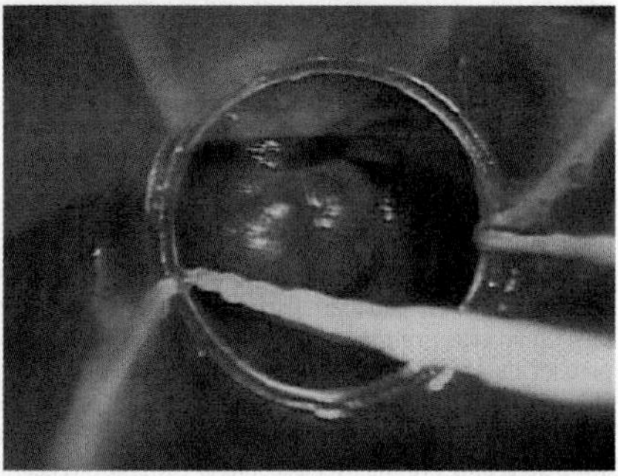

Fig 2. Upper GI endoscopy image of variceal banding. The technique involves sucking up a varix into the transparent banding chamber, then placing an elastic band around the varix. After a few days the banded varix starts to slough, leaving behind scar tissue in a shallow ulcer. See also p254.
Image courtesy of Dr Jon Simmons

►Consent is required for all these interventions and procedures—see p570.

Upper GI endoscopy *Indications:* See TABLE 1. *Pre-procedure:* Stop anti-acid therapy for 2 weeks beforehand if possible—these mask diagnosis of up to ~30% of adenocarcinomas. Nil by mouth for 4h beforehand. Advise the patient not to drive for 24h if sedation is being given. Arrange follow-up. ***Procedure:*** Sedation may be given (eg *midazolam* 1-5mg IV; monitor O_2 saturation with a pulse oximeter). The pharynx is sprayed with local anaesthetic and a flexible endoscope is passed. Continuous suction must be available to prevent aspiration. ***Complications:*** Transient sore throat; amnesia following sedation; perforation (<0.1%); cardiorespiratory arrest (<0.1%).

Duodenal biopsy is the gold standard for diagnosing coeliac disease (p280). It is also useful in investigating unusual causes of malabsorption, eg giardiasis, lymphoma, Whipple's disease, amyloid, or microscopic colitis (p246).

Sigmoidoscopy views the rectum + sigmoid to splenic flexion. Rigid or flexible sigmoidoscopy should precede barium enema in suspected colorectal cancer. Flexible sigmoidoscopes gain better access than rigid ones (→splenic flexure), but ~25% of colon cancers are still out of reach. It can be used therapeutically (±insertion of a flatus tube) for decompression of sigmoid volvulus (see BOX, p613). ***Preparation:*** Give a ***phosphate enema.*** ***Procedure:*** PR examination is performed first. Do biopsies—macroscopic appearances may be normal in some diseases, eg IBD, amyloidosis, microscopic colitis.

Colonoscopy *Indications:* See TABLE 2. ***Preparation:*** Prescribe ***sodium picosulfate*** (Picolax®) 1 sachet for the morning and afternoon of the day before the procedure. ***Procedure:*** PR examination is performed first. Sedation (monitor O_2 saturation with a pulse oximeter) and analgesia are given before a flexible colonoscope is passed and guided around the colon. ***Complications:*** Abdominal discomfort; incomplete examination; perforation (0.1%); haemorrhage after biopsy or polypectomy. See **figs 2-6**.

Capsule endoscopy *Indications:* Assessment of small bowel disease esp. in Crohn's (after excluding strictures with a small bowel contrast study or patency capsule) or obscure/occult GI bleeding. Also now able to image the oesophagus, despite quick transit time.[82] ***Pre-procedure:*** Clear fluids only the evening before and then nil by mouth as for colonoscopy. ***Procedure:*** A pill-sized capsule (**fig 1**) transmits video images via radiowaves to pads on the skin. Information is stored in a device worn on the belt. Normal activity can take place during the examination. ***Complications:*** Capsule retention (occurs in 1%: endoscopic or surgical removal is required); obstruction (usually in the terminal ileum or site of a stricture); incomplete examination (eg battery failure, slow transit, achalasia). ***Disadvantages:*** No therapeutic intervention and gives poor localisation of lesions; misses 16% of colon cancers.

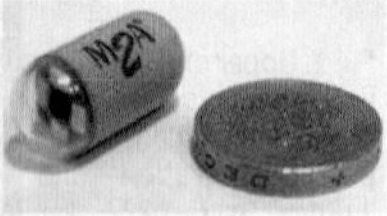

Fig 1. The size of a capsule (£1 coin for scale).[81] ©St Mark's Hospital Endoscopy Unit

Liver biopsy This may be done percutaneously (if clotting is normal) or via the transjugular route with FFP cover. ***Indications:*** Abnormal LFT, chronic viral hepatitis; alcoholic hepatitis; autoimmune hepatitis (AIH); suspected cirrhosis; suspected carcinoma; biopsy of hepatic lesions; investigation of PUO. Now usually performed with US/CT guidance. ***Pre-procedure:*** Nil by mouth for 8h. Check clotting (INR <1.5) and platelet count (>100 × 10^9/L). Prescribe analgesia. ***Procedure:*** Sedation may be given. If not done under US guidance, the liver borders are percussed out and where there is dullness in the mid-axillary line in expiration, local anaesthetic (*lidocaine* 2%) is infiltrated down to the liver capsule. Breathing is rehearsed and a needle biopsy is taken with the breath held in expiration. Afterwards the patient lies on the right side for 2h, then in bed for 4h while regular pulse and BP observations are taken. ***Complications:*** Local pain; pneumothorax; bleeding (<0.5%); death (<0.1%).

Endoscopy images: See www.gastrosource.com/kisweb/atlas.htm and figs 2-6.

Indications for upper GI endoscopy

Diagnostic indications	Therapeutic indications
Haematemesis	Treatment of bleeding lesions
Dyspepsia (>55yrs old p242)	Variceal banding and sclerotherapy
Gastric biopsy (?cancer)	Stricture dilatation
Duodenal biopsy	Palliation, eg stent insertion, laser therapy
Persistent vomiting	Argon plasma coagulation for suspected
Iron-deficiency anaemia	vascular abnormality

Indications for colonoscopy

Diagnostic indications	Therapeutic indication
Rectal bleeding—when settled, if acute	Polypectomy
Iron-deficiency anaemia	Angiodysplasia (argon plasma photocoagulation)
Persistent diarrhoea	
Biopsy of lesion seen on barium enema	Decompression
Assessment or suspicion of IBD	Pseudo-obstruction
Colon cancer surveillance	Volvulus

Streptococcus bovis SBE (the cancer is the portal of entry)

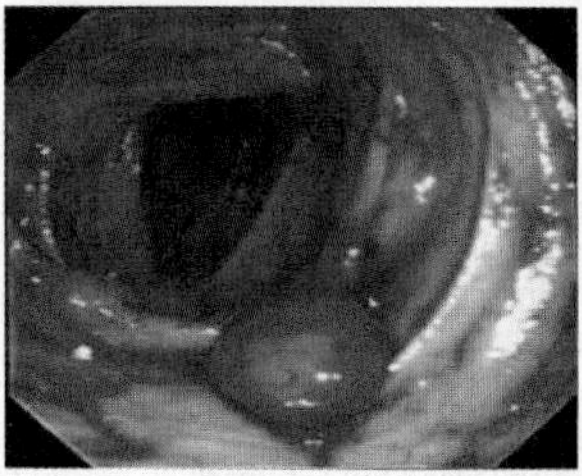

Fig 2. Colonoscopy image of a large colonic polyp. An advantage of colonoscopy over barium enema is the ability to perform biopsy or intervention at the same time—in this case, polypectomy.

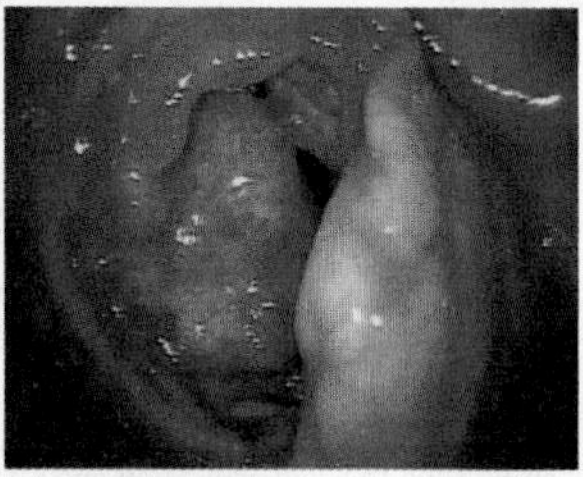

Fig 3. Colonoscopy image of a colonic adenocarcinoma—see p618. Compared with a colonic polyp (**fig 2**), the carcinoma is irregular in shape and colour, larger and more aggressive.

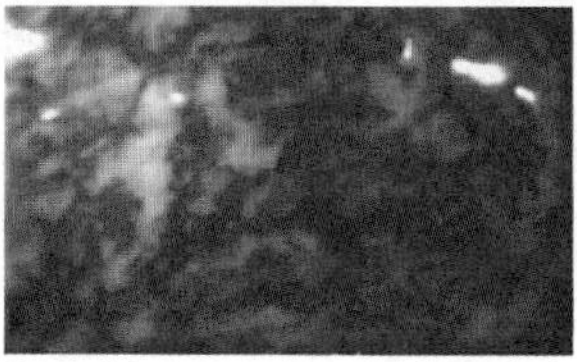

Fig 4. Colonoscopy image of the colonic mucosa in active ulcerative colitis (p272). Mucosa is red, inflamed and friable (bleeds on touching). If severe, there may be mucopurulent exudate, mucosal ulceration, and spontaneous bleeding. In quiescent disease there may only be a distorted or absent mucosal vascular pattern.

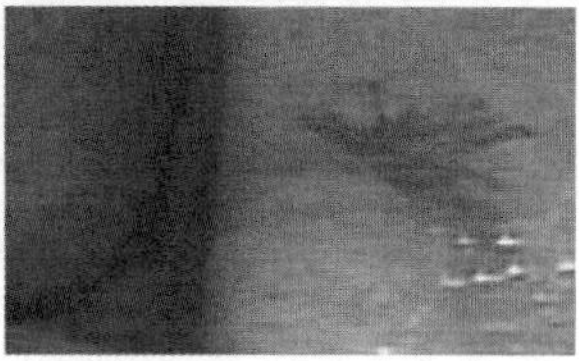

Fig 5. Colonoscopy image of a small angiodysplasia lesion in the colonic mucosa. Argon plasma coagulation is a common treatment for this condition—see p630.

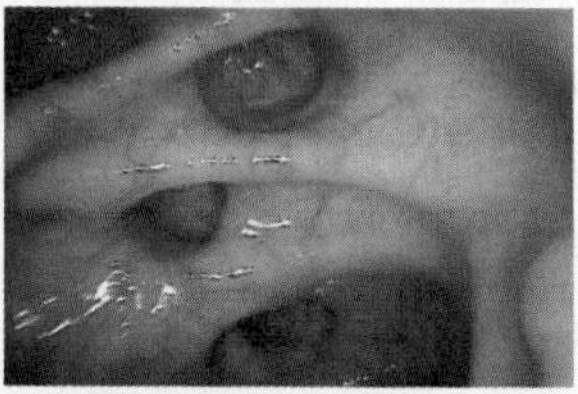

Fig 6. Colonoscopy image showing diverticulosis of the colon. Navigating safely through the colon, avoiding the false lumina of the diverticula, can be a challenge. Endoscopy is avoided if the diverticula are acutely inflamed in diverticulitis because of the risk of perforation. See p630 for the topic of diverticular disease.

Figs 2 & 4 courtesy of Dr Anthony Mee
Figs 3, 5 & 6 courtesy of Dr J Simmons

Definitions Liver failure may occur suddenly in the previously healthy liver: **acute hepatic failure**. More commonly it occurs as a result of decompensation of chronic liver disease = **acute-on-chronic hepatic failure. Fulminant hepatic failure** is a clinical syndrome resulting from massive necrosis of liver cells leading to severe impairment of liver function: **hyperacute** = encephalopathy (BOX 1) within 7d of onset of jaundice; **acute** = within 8–28d; **subacute** = within 5–26 weeks. There is decreasing risk of cerebral oedema as the onset of encephalopathy is increasingly delayed.

Causes *Infections:* Viral hepatitis (esp B, C, CMV), yellow fever, leptospirosis. ***Drugs:*** Paracetamol overdose, halothane, isoniazid. ***Toxins:*** *Amanita phalloides* mushroom (**fig 2**, p251), carbon tetrachloride. ***Vascular:*** Budd–Chiari synd. (p710), veno-occlusive disease. ***Others:*** Alcohol, primary biliary cirrhosis, haemochromatosis, autoimmune hepatitis, α_1-antitrypsin deficiency, Wilson's disease, fatty liver of pregnancy (*OHCS* p26), malignancy, HELLP syndrome (Haemolysis, Elevated Liver enzymes and Low Platelets; it is usually associated with pre-eclampsia; see *OHCS* p26).

Signs Jaundice, hepatic encephalopathy (see BOX 2), *fetor hepaticus* (smells like pear drops), asterixis (p50), constructional apraxia (can he draw a 5-pointed star?). Signs of chronic liver disease (p260) suggest acute-on-chronic hepatic failure.

Tests *Blood:* FBC (?infection,[1] ?GI bleed), U&E,[2] LFT, clotting (↑PT/INR), glucose, paracetamol level, hepatitis, CMV & EBV serology, ferritin, α_1-antitrypsin, caeruloplasmin, autoantibodies (p555). ***Microbiology:*** Blood culture; urine culture; ascitic tap for MC+S of ascites—neutrophils >250/mm³ indicates spontaneous bacterial peritonitis (p260). ***Radiology:*** CXR; abdominal ultrasound; Doppler flow studies of the portal vein (& hepatic vein in suspected Budd–Chiari syndrome, p710). ***Neurophysiology:*** EEG, evoked potentials (and neuroimaging) have a limited role.[83]

Management ►► Beware sepsis, hypoglycaemia, GI bleeds (varices) and encephalopathy:
- Nurse with a 20° head-up tilt in ITU. Protect the airway with intubation and insert an NG tube to avoid aspiration and remove any blood from stomach.
- Insert urinary and central venous catheters to assess fluid status.
- Monitor T°, respirations, pulse, BP, pupils, urine output hourly. Daily weights.
- Check FBC, U&E (BOX 2), LFT, and INR daily.
- 10% dextrose IV, 1L/12h to avoid hypoglycaemia. Do blood glucose every 1–4h.
- Treat the cause, if known (eg GI bleeds, sepsis, paracetamol poisoning, p856). N-acetylcysteine probably does not help in non-paracetamol liver failure.[84]
- If malnourished, get dietary help because good nutrition ↓ mortality (eg diet rich in carbohydrate- and protein-derived calories, preferably orally).[85] Give thiamine and folate supplements.
- Haemofiltration or haemodialysis, if renal failure develops (see BOX 2).
- Avoid sedatives or other drugs with hepatic metabolism (see BOX 3 and *BNF*), but treat seizures with ***lorazepam***.[86]
- Consider PPI as prophylaxis against stress ulceration eg ***omeprazole*** 40mg/d IV/PO.
- Liaise early with nearest transplant centre regarding appropriateness—see BOX 4.

Treat complications *Bleeding:* *Vitamin K* 10mg/d IV for 3d, platelets, FFP + blood as needed ± endoscopy. ***Infection:*** Until sensitivities are known, give *ceftriaxone* 1–2g/24h IV. ► Avoid *gentamicin* (↑risk of renal failure). ***Ascites:*** Fluid restriction, low-salt diet, daily weights, diuretics (see p260). ***Hypoglycaemia:*** Check blood glucose regularly and give 50mL of 50% glucose IV if levels fall below 2mmol/L or symptomatic. ***Encephalopathy:*** Avoid sedatives; 20° head-up tilt in ITU; *lactulose* 30–50ml/8h PO + regular enemas to ↓numbers of nitrogen-forming bowel organisms. Aim for 2–4 soft stools/d. ***Cerebral oedema:*** Give 20% *mannitol* IV; hyperventilate.

Prognosis Poor prognostic factors: grade III or IV encephalopathy, age >40yrs, albumin <30g/L, ↑INR, drug-induced liver failure, late-onset hepatic failure worse than fulminant failure. 65% survival post-transplantation.

1 Neutrophilic leucocytosis need not mean a secondary infection: alcoholic hepatitis may be the cause.
2 Urea is synthesized in the liver, so is a poor test of renal function in liver failure; use creatinine instead.

Hepatic encephalopathy

As the liver fails, nitrogenous waste (as ammonia) builds up in the circulation and passes to the brain, where astrocytes clear it (by processes involving the conversion of glutamate to glutamine). This excess glutamine causes an osmotic imbalance and a shift of fluid into these cells—hence cerebral oedema.[87]

Grade I	Altered mood/behaviour; sleep disturbance (eg reversed sleep pattern)
Grade II	Increasing drowsiness; confusion, slurred speech
Grade III	Stupor; incoherence; restlessness, significant confusion
Grade IV	Coma

►Rule out other causes of reduced consciousness when considering hepatic encephalopathy, eg sepsis, trauma, hypoglycaemia, and seizure activity.

What is hepatorenal syndrome (HRS)?

HRS is defined as renal failure in patients with advanced chronic liver disease. Suspect HRS in any patient with liver failure and signs and symptoms of pre-renal uraemia (p298), who does not respond to volume replacement therapy. ►It is important to make the diagnosis only after other causes of renal impairment have been excluded. HRS is not well understood; however, the initial event seems to be splanchnic arterial vasodilatation, followed by renal vasoconstriction. *Other signs:* ↓effective circulatory volume, (↓venous return and cardiac output),[88] ↓GFR, and **normal** renal histology. Raised neuropeptide Y (NPY) and activation of the renin-angiotensin-aldosterone axis occur, further worsening renal vasoconstriction. ADH levels also ↑ in an attempt to restore intravascular volume. Two types of HRS are described: **HRS 1** is a rapidly progressive deterioration in circulatory and renal function (median survival <2wks); **HRS 2** is a more steady deterioration (median survival ~6 months). Other factors in cirrhosis may contribute to poor renal function (p261). ***Treatment*** is IV *albumin* + arterial vasocontrictors eg, *terlipressin*, to replenish the depleted volume. Haemodialysis (as supportive therapy) and TIPSS (p254) may be needed. Liver transplantation is treatment of choice, even after improvement in renal function, since prognosis is so poor.[89]

Prescribing in liver failure

Avoid opiates, diuretics (↑risk of encephalopathy), oral hypoglycaemics, and saline-containing IVIs. *Warfarin* effects are enhanced. ***Hepatotoxic drugs include:*** Paracetamol, methotrexate, phenothiazines, isoniazid, azathioprine, oestrogen, 6-mercaptopurine, salicylates, tetracycline, mitomycin.

King's College Hospital[UK] criteria for liver transplantation

Paracetamol liver failure
- Arterial pH <7.3 24h after ingestion

Or all of the following:
- Prothrombin time (PT) >100s
- Creatinine >300μmol/L
- Grade III or IV encephalopathy

Non-paracetamol liver failure
- PT >100s

Or 3 out of 5 of the following:
1. Drug-induced liver failure
2. Age <10 or >40yrs old
3. >1wk from 1st jaundice to encephalopathy
4. PT >50s
5. Bilirubin ≥300μmol/L[90]

Fulfilment of the criteria is a good predictor of poor outcome in acute liver failure, but failure to meet the criteria does not predict survival. Transplantation is either **cadaveric** (heart-beating or non-heart-beating)[1] or from **live donors** (right lobe). Gaining **valid consent** from the donor is difficult (see BOX, p571). See also BOX, p263 for indications in chronic disease.

1 There has been a renewed interest and ↑ in the number of non-heart-beating cadaveric donors.

Cirrhosis (Greek *kirrhos* = yellow) implies irreversible liver damage. Histologically, there is loss of normal hepatic architecture with bridging fibrosis and nodular regeneration.

Causes Most often chronic alcohol abuse, HBV, and HCV infection. Others: see BOX 1.

Signs May be none (just ↑LFT) or decompensated end-stage liver disease. ***Chronic liver disease:*** Leuconychia: white nails with lunulae undemarcated, from hypoalbuminaemia; Terry's nails—white proximally but distal ⅓ reddened by telangiectasias;[91] clubbing; palmar erythema; hyperdynamic circulation; Dupuytren's contracture; spider naevi (**fig 1**); xanthelasma; gynaecomastia; atrophic testes; loss of body hair; parotid enlargement; hepatomegaly, or small liver in late disease.

Complications ***Hepatic failure:*** Coagulopathy (↓factors II, VII, IX, & X causes ↑INR); encephalopathy—ie liver flap (asterixis) + confusion/coma; hypoalbuminaemia (oedema, leuconychia); sepsis (pneumonia; septicaemia); spontaneous bacterial peritonitis (SBP); hypoglycaemia. ***Portal hypertension:*** Ascites (**fig 2**); splenomegaly; portosystemic shunt including oesophageal varices (± life-threatening upper GI bleed) and *caput medusae* (enlarged superficial periumbilical veins). ***HCC:*** ↑risk.

Tests ***Blood:*** LFT: ↔ or ↑bilirubin, ↑AST, ↑ALT, ↑alk phos and ↑γGT. Later, with loss of synthetic function, look for ↓albumin ± ↑PT/INR. ↓WCC and ↓platelets indicate hypersplenism. ***Find the cause:*** Ferritin, iron/total iron-binding capacity (p262); hepatitis serology; immunoglobulins (p266); autoantibodies (ANA, AMA, SMA, p555); α-fetoprotein (p270); caeruloplasmin in patients <40yrs old (p269); α_1-antitrypsin (p264). ***Liver ultrasound + duplex*** may show a small liver or hepatomegaly, splenomegaly, focal liver lesion(s), hepatic vein thrombus, reversed flow in the portal vein, or ascites. ***MRI:*** Caudate lobe size↑, smaller islands of regenerating nodules, and the presence of the right posterior hepatic notch are more frequent in alcoholic cirrhosis than in virus-induced cirrhosis.[92] MRI scoring systems based on spleen volume, liver volume, and presence of ascites or varices/collaterals can quantify severity of cirrhosis in a way that correlates well with Child grades (see BOX 2).[93] ***Ascitic tap*** should be performed and fluid sent for urgent MC+S—neutrophils $>250/mm^3$ indicates spontaneous bacterial peritonitis (see below for treatment). ***Liver biopsy*** (p256) confirms the clinical diagnosis.

Management ***General:*** Good nutrition is vital. Alcohol abstinence (p282); *baclofen* 10mg/8h PO helps cravings (p455, start with 5mg)[94] and is not contra-indicated in cirrhosis, unlike naltrexone (avoid in hepatorenal syndrome). Avoid NSAIDs, sedatives, and opiates. ***Colestyramine*** helps pruritus (4g/12h PO, 1h after other drugs). Consider ultrasound ± α-fetoprotein every 3–6 months to screen for HCC, p270.[95] ***Specific: Interferon-α*** (± ***ribavirin***) improves LFT and may slow development to HCC in HCV-induced cirrhosis (p406). High-dose ***ursodeoxycholic acid*** in PBC (p266) may normalise LFT, but may have no effect on disease progression.[96] ***Penicillamine*** for Wilson's disease (p269). ***Ascites:*** Bedrest, fluid restriction (<1.5L/d), low-salt diet (40–100mmol/d). Give ***spironolactone*** 100mg/24h PO; ↑dose every 48h, to 400mg/24h—it counters deranged renin-angiotensin-aldosterone (RAA) axis. Chart daily weight and aim for weight loss of ≤½kg/d. If response is poor, add in ***furosemide*** ≤120mg/24h PO; do U&E (watch Na^+) often. Therapeutic paracentesis with concomitant albumin infusion (6–8g/L fluid removed) may be tried. ***Spontaneous bacterial peritonitis (SBP):*** ►Must be considered in any patient with ascites who deteriorates suddenly (may be asymptomatic). Common organisms are *E. coli*, *Klebsiella*, and streps.[97] ℞: eg ***cefotaxime*** 2g/6h or ***tazocin®*** 4.5g/8h (see datasheet) for 5d or until sensitivities known (+ ***metronidazole*** 500mg/8h IV if recent instrumentation to ascites). Give prophylaxis for high-risk patients (↓albumin, ↑PT/INR, low ascitic albumin) or those who have had a previous episode: eg ***norfloxacin*** 400mg PO daily. ***Renal failure:*** See BOX 3.

Prognosis Overall 5yr survival is ~50%. Poor prognostic indicators: encephalopathy; serum Na^+ <110mmol/L; serum albumin <25g/L; ↑INR.

Liver transplantation is the only definitive treatment for cirrhosis (p263). This increases 5yr survival from ~20% in end-stage disease to ~70%.[98]

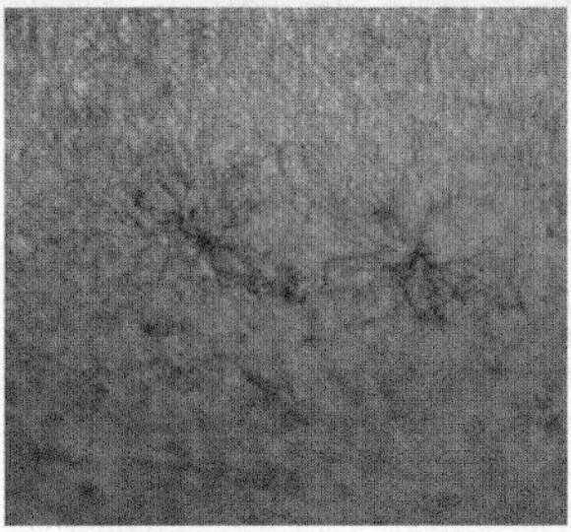

Fig 1. Spider naevi. These consist of a central arteriole, from which numerous vessels radiate (like the legs of a spider). These fill from the centre as opposed to telangiectasias that fill from the edge. They occur most commonly in skin drained by the superior vena cava. Up to 5 are said to be normal (they are common in young ♀). Causes include liver disease, contraceptive steroids, and pregnancy (ie changes in oestrogen metabolism).[99]

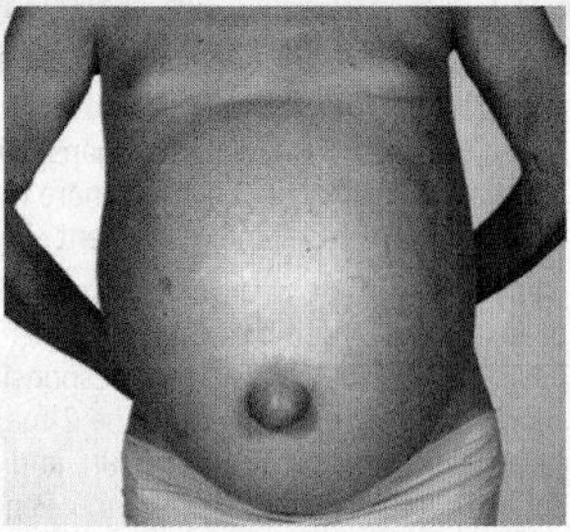

Fig 2. Gross ascites. Note the umbilical hernia (p615) and a mild degree of gynaecomastia. There are veins visible on the anterior abdominal wall, though they are not in the pattern of *caput medusae*.[100]

Causes of cirrhosis

- Chronic alcohol abuse
- Non-alcoholic steatohepatitis (NASH)
- Chronic HBV or HCV infection[1]
- Autoimmune disease: PBC (p266); PSC (p267); AIH (p268)
- Genetic disorders: haemachromatosis (p262); α_1-antitrypsin deficiency (p264); Wilson's disease (p269)
- Others: can be cryptogenic in up to 20%; Budd-Chiari syndrome (p710, hepatic vein thrombosis)
- Drugs: eg amiodarone, methyldopa, methotrexate

Child-Pugh grading of cirrhosis and risk of variceal bleeding

Grade A = 5–6, grade B = 7–9, grade C >10. Risk of variceal bleeding is much higher if score is >8. The grading can also be used to predict mortality and quantify need for liver transplantation (p263). NB: all such scoring systems come with the 'non-parametric health warning', see p10.

	1 point	**2 points**	**3 points**
Bilirubin (μmol/L)	<34	34-51	>51
Albumin (g/L)[101]	>35	28-35	<28
Prothrombin time (seconds > normal)	1-3	4-6	>6
Ascites	none	slight	moderate
Encephalopathy (p251)	none	1-2	3-4

Cirrhosis and deteriorating renal function

In cirrhosis, reduced hepatic clearance of immune complexes leads to their trapping in the kidney (∴ IgA nephropathy ± hepatic glomerulosclerosis). HCV can cause cryoglobulinaemia ± membranoproliferative glomerulonephritis; HBV may cause membranous nephropathy ± PAN. Membranoproliferative glomerulonephritis can occur in α_1-antitrypsin deficiency.[102] See p259 for hepatorenal syndrome.

1 Clues as to which patients with chronic HCV will get cirrhosis: platelet count ≤140 x 10^9/L, globulin/albumin ratio ≥1, and AST/ALT ratio ≥1—100% +ve predictive value but lower sensitivity (~30%).

Hereditary haemochromatosis (HH)

This is an inherited disorder of iron metabolism in which ↑ intestinal iron absorption leads to deposition in multiple organs (joints, liver, heart, pancreas, pituitary, adrenals and skin). Middle-aged males are more frequently and severely affected than women, in whom the disease tends to present ~10yrs later (menstrual blood loss is protective).

Genetics HH is one of the commonest inherited diseases in those of Northern European (especially Celtic) ancestry (carrier rate of ~1 in 10 and a frequency of homozygosity of ~1:200–400). The gene responsible for most HH is called HFE, found on the short arm of chromosome 6. The 2 major mutations are termed C282Y and H63D. C282Y accounts for 60–90% of HH, and H63D accounts for 3–7%, with compound heterozygotes accounting for 1–4%. Penetrance is unknown but is <100%.[103]

Clinical features Asymptomatic early on—then tiredness, arthralgia (MCP and large joints) and impotence. Later: slate-grey skin pigmentation; DM ('bronze diabetes' due to iron deposition in pancreas); signs of chronic liver disease (p260); hepatomegaly; cirrhosis; dilated cardiomyopathy; hypogonadism (p224) from pituitary dysfunction↓ or via cirrhosis (not from testicular iron deposition); associated osteoporosis.[104] Other endocrinopathies include hyporeninaemic hypoaldosteronism.[105] Some patients are susceptible to certain bacterial infections (eg *Yersinia enterocolitica* liver abscess).

Tests *Blood:* ↑LFT, ↑serum ferritin; ↑serum iron; ↓TIBC; transferrin saturation >80%.[1] HFE genotyping. Blood glucose (?DM). ***Joint x-rays*** may show chondrocalcinosis. ***Liver biopsy:*** Perl's stain quantifies iron loading[2] and assesses disease severity. ***MRI*** can be used to estimate hepatic iron loading. Do ***ECG*** & ***ECHO*** if you suspect cardiomyopathy.

Management *Venesect* ~1 unit/wk, until mildly iron-deficient. Iron will continue to accumulate, so maintenance venesection is needed for life (1U every 2–3 months). Aim to maintain haematocrit <0.5, serum ferritin <100µg/L, TIBC >50µmol/L, and transferrin saturation <40%. ***Other monitoring:*** Diabetes (p198). HbA_{1c} levels may be falsely low as venesection reduces the time available for Hb glycosylation.[106] ***Over-the-counter self-medication:*** Make sure that vitamin preparations etc. contain no iron. ***Dietary intake:*** Maintaining a well-balanced low-iron diet may help. Drinking tea, coffee or red wine with meals reduces iron absorption, but fruit and fruit juice (high in vitamin C) and white wine increase absorption. ***Screening:*** serum ferritin and genotype. Screen 1st-degree relatives of affected patients by genetic testing even if they are asymptomatic and have normal LFTs (in young people LFT may be normal).[107] Prevalence of iron overload in asymptomatic C282Y homozygotes is ≤4.5 per 1000 persons screened. How many will go on to develop iron overload is unknown.

Prognosis Venesection returns life expectancy to normal if non-cirrhotic and non-diabetic. Arthropathy may improve or worsen. Gonadal failure is irreversible. In non-cirrhotic patients, venesection may improve liver histology. ►Cirrhotic patients have >10% chance of developing HCC. Sources vary on the exact risk: some authorities quote 30%, others 22%.[108] One cause of variability is varying co-factors: age over 50yrs ↑risk by 13-fold; being HBsAg +ve by 5-fold and alcohol abuse by 2-fold.[109]

Secondary haemochromatosis may occur in any haematological condition where many transfusions (~40L in total) have been given.[110] To reduce need for transfusions, find out if the haematological condition responds to erythropoietin or marrow transplantation before irreversible effects of iron overload become too great. See iron management in thalassaemia, p336.

1 In heterozygotes, biochemical tests may be normal or show mild ↑ in transferrin saturation or ferritin.

2 The HII aims to separate HH from other causes of hepatic siderosis (eg HBV; alcoholic cirrhosis). It is less used now that genotyping is available. HII in µmol iron/gram liver/year = [iron concentration (µg iron per gram dry weight of liver)/55.846 (atomic weight of Fe)]/patient's age. HII >1.9 in a non-cirrhotic liver strongly suggests HH. ►*Caveats*: • ~7% of those with HH have a HII <1.9. Using a threshold hepatic iron concentration of 71µmol/g as well as HII can detect most of these. • Cirrhotic livers can rapidly accumulate iron in non-HH liver disease making HII >1.9. Some say that an HII cut-off of ~4.2 is best in diagnosing HH in cirrhotics. • Iron is not uniformly distributed in the liver (sampling variation). • Correlation among HII, phenotypic HH, & genotypic HH is not 100%.

A bit about iron metabolism

The average adult absorbs 1-1.5mg of iron per day from a typical Western diet containing 12-20mg of iron. Red meats, liver, seafoods, enriched breakfast cereals and pulses and even some spices (eg paprika) are particularly iron-rich. Most dietary iron is Fe^{3+}, which is reduced by low gastric pH and ascorbic acid (vitamin C) to better-absorbed Fe^{2+}. Absorption occurs mainly in the duodenum and jejunum, though very small amounts are absorbed in the stomach and ileum. Regulation of iron levels (by an unknown mechanism) is based mainly on absorption, while iron excretion is in the form of uncontrolled shedding of the gut lining.[111] The majority (60-70%) of body iron circulates in haemoglobin, though it is also found in myoglobin, bound to enzymes and proteins (such as the β-globulin, transferrin), in mitochondria, and in hepatocytes—as ferritin and haemosiderin. Iron requirements are greater for women (menstrual loss), when growing, in pregnancy and in chronic infection.

In HH the total body iron is up to 10-fold that of a normal person, with loading found particularly in the liver and pancreas (×100). Hepatic disease classically starts with fibrosis, progressing to cirrhosis as a late feature.

Liver transplantation in chronic liver disease

The first ever liver transplantation was performed by Starzl in Denver, USA, in 1963. The first in the UK was in 1968 at Addenbrooke's Hospital, Cambridge.[112] Between 1996 and 2000 there were ~3,400 liver transplants performed in the UK and Ireland. The limiting step for the procedure is often the waiting-list for a donor organ (live or cadaveric—see p259). The indications for transplantation in chronic disease (see TABLE) are generally because of advanced cirrhosis (p260), the grading of which has been used as a selection criterion.[1]

Indications	Contraindications
• Advanced cirrhosis secondary to:	• Extrahepatic malignancy
• Alcoholic liver disease	• Multiple primary or secondary tumours
• Hepatitis B & C	• Severe cardiorespiratory disease
• PBC (p266)	• Systemic sepsis
• AIH (p268)	• HIV infection
• Wilson's disease	• Non-compliance with drug therapy
• α_1-antitrypsin deficiency	
• PSC (p267)	
• Hepatocellular cancer (1 nodule <5cm or 2-3 nodules <3cm)	

The post-operative period involves 12-24h on ITU, with enteral feeding starting as soon as possible and close monitoring of LFT. Immunosuppressant protocols usually involve a combination of ***ciclosporin*** or ***tacrolimus*** together with ***azathioprine*** or ***mycophenolate mofetil*** and ***prednisolone***. Hyperacute rejection is a result of ABO incompatibility. Acute rejection (T-cell mediated) occurs in about 50% at 5-10 days, with the patient feeling unwell and developing pyrexia and tender hepatomegaly—it can usually be managed by increasing or altering the immunosuppressant regimen. Other complications include sepsis (especially Gram -ve), hepatic artery thrombosis, CMV infection, chronic rejection (at 6-9 months), disease recurrence,[113] and very rarely, graft-*versus*-host disease.[114] The average patient survival at 1yr is ~80% (5yr survival 60-90%), though this varies between different patients with different diseases. Poor pre-transplant renal function has been identified as a predictor of poor outcome.[115] (See also BOX, Indications for transplantation in acute liver failure, p259.)

1 The incredibly difficult selection of patients for liver transplantation can also be made according to the Model for End-stage Liver Disease (MELD).

The glycoprotein α_1-antitrypsin is one of a family of **ser**ine **p**rotease **in**hibitors (deficiency is called a '**serpin**opathy') controlling inflammatory cascades. It is synthesized in the liver, making up 90% of serum α_1-globulin on electrophoresis (p701). α_1-antitrypsin deficiency is the chief genetic cause of liver disease in children. In adults, its lack causes emphysema in ~75% (the role of α_1-antitrypsin in the lung is to protect against tissue damage from neutrophil elastase—a process that is also induced by cigarette smoking, p176), chronic liver disease and HCC (p270). *Other associations:* Asthma, pancreatitis, gallstones, Wegener's (p728). *Prevalence:* ~1:4000.

Genetics The gene for this autosomal recessive disorder is found on chromosome 14; carrier frequency of 1:10. Genetic variants are typed by electrophoretic mobility as **medium** (M), **slow** (S), or **very slow** (Z). S and Z types are due to single amino acid substitutions at positions 264 and 342, respectively. These result in ↓production of α_1-antitrypsin (S=60%, Z=15%). The normal genotype is PiMM, the homozygote is PiZZ; heterozygotes are PiMZ & PiSZ (at low risk of developing liver disease).

The patient Symptomatic patients usually have the PiZZ genotype: dyspnoea from emphysema; cirrhosis; cholestatic jaundice. Cholestasis often remits in adolescence.

Tests Serum α_1-antitrypsin (α1AT) levels↓. *Liver biopsy:* (p256) Periodic acid Schiff (PAS) +ve; diastase-resistant globules. *Phenotyping* by isoelectric focusing requires expertise to distinguish SZ and ZZ phenotypes. *Prenatal diagnosis* is possible by DNA analysis of chorionic villus samples obtained at 11-13wks' gestation. DNA tests are likely to find greater use in the future. Measuring lung density with *CT* may be better than lung function tests at predicting disease progression and mortality.[116]

Management Mostly supportive for emphysema and liver complications. Quit smoking. Consider **augmentation therapy** with *α_1-antitrypsin* pooled from human plasma if FEV_1<80% of predicted and if not smoking (120mg/kg IV every 2wks is conveniently self-given via SC intravenous injection port systems. It is very expensive!) Plasma levels of >0.7g/L are considered protective. *Liver transplantation* (p259) is treatment of choice in decompensated cirrhosis.

Prognosis Male gender and obesity may predispose to advanced liver disease.[117] Emphysema is the cause of death in most, liver disease in ~5%. In adults, cirrhosis ± HCC affect 25% of α_1-antitrypsin-deficient adults >50yrs.

Screening tests for chronic liver disease

- HBV, & HCV serology—see p406.
- Iron studies for haemochromatosis: ↑ferritin, ↑iron, ↓TIBC: see p262.
- α_1-antitrypsin deficiency (plasma for genetics): see above.
- Wilson's disease: ↓serum copper, ↓caeruloplasmin– see p269.
- PBC: ↑AMA, see p266.
- PSC: ANA, AMA & ANCA may be +ve, see p267.
- AIH: ↑ANA + ↑ASMA; ↑IgG, see p268.
- Check all immunoglobulins: IgA (↑ in alcoholic liver disease); IgG (↑ in AIH) & IgM (↑ in PBC).
- HCC: ↑α-fetoprotein, see p270.
- Conjugated and unconjugated bilirubin (for Gilbert's).

Approach to abnormal liver function tests (LFTs)

Abnormal LFT can be found in ~17% of the asymptomatic general population. However, remember that a normal LFT does not exclude liver disease.

Tests of hepatocellular injury or cholestasis

Aminotransferases (AST, ALT) are released in the bloodstream after hepatocellular injury. ALT is more specific for hepatocellular injury (but also expressed in kidney and muscle). AST is also expressed in the heart, skeletal muscle, and RBCs.[118]

Alkaline phosphatase may originate from the placenta, kidney, intestine, and WCC. Some physiological conditions can also ↑ alk phos (eg adolescence, pregnancy).[119] *Gamma-glutamyltransferase (GGT)* is present in renal tubules, the liver, pancreas, and intestine.

Tests of hepatic function: Serum albumin, serum bilirubin, PT.

Hepatocellular predominant liver injury High levels of AST and ALT are usually observed which prompts further evaluation without delay.

Alcoholic liver disease: AST/ALT ratio is typically 2:1 or more. When the history is not reliable, normal alk phos, ↑GGT and macrocytosis suggest this condition.[120]

Acute viral hepatitis: AST & ALT raised. Bilirubin may be normal. NB: AST may be ↑↑, p407 & p283.

Chronic viral hepatitis (especially if full hepatitis C and B viruses) is one of the most common causes of abnormal LFT worldwide.

Autoimmune hepatitis (AIH) occurs mainly in young and middle-aged females with concomitant autoimmune disorders (eg rheumatological diseases, autoimmune thyroiditis).[121]

Fatty infiltration of the liver is probably the most common cause of mild abnormality of LFT in the general population. Risk factors for non-alcoholic fatty liver disease (steatohepatitis): obesity, DM, and ↑lipids. This is a diagnosis of exclusion. One study found that in 83% of patients with elevated AST and ALT whose serum evaluation was otherwise negative, liver biopsy revealed steatosis of no prognostic significance or steatohepatitis. In 10% of the patients, however, liver biopsy was normal—a reminder that, at times, mildly elevated transaminase levels do not represent any underlying pathology.[122] Although imaging techniques (US, CT, or MRI) are suggestive of the disease, liver biopsy is the only means able to diagnose the disease accurately.[123] [124]

Ischaemic hepatitis can be seen in conditions when effective circulatory volume is low (eg MI, hypotension, haemorrhage). AST and ALT are ↑, as well as LDH.[125]

Toxic hepatitis: paracetamol overdose is the cause of more than half of the cases with acute liver failure in the UK. As there are no specific serological tests to identify drug-induced hepatic toxicity, taking a thorough history is vital.

Cholestasis predominant liver injury

AST and ALT are mildly elevated. Alk phos and GGT levels are also high.

Management For each specific diagnosis, manage accordingly. If the patient is asymptomatic and all the initial evaluations are negative, try a period of lifestyle modification: give help for reducing weight and alcohol use (p282 & *OHCS* p513); control DM and hyperlipidaemia, and stop potentially hepatotoxic medications.

Follow up Repeat tests after 6 months. If abnormalities persist do US. Abdominal CT also has a role. If the diagnosis is not apparent from the US, further testing is suggested, eg: α_1-antitrypsin levels, serum caeruloplasmin (Wilson's disease), antigliadin and antiendomysial antibody (coeliac disease), ANA and ASMA (AIH). The decision on liver biopsy needs to be made on an individual basis.[126]

Primary biliary cirrhosis (PBC)

PBC associations
Thyroid disease
Rheumatoid arthritis
Sjögren's syndrome
Keratoconjunctivitis sicca
Systemic sclerosis
Renal tubular acidosis
Membranous glomerulonephritis

Interlobular bile ducts are damaged by chronic granulomatous inflammation causing progressive cholestasis, cirrhosis, and portal hypertension. ***Cause:*** Possibly an autoimmune response triggered by environmental factors, with genetic predisposition thought to be of importance. ♀:♂≈9:1. ***Prevalence:*** ≤4/100,000. ***Peak presentation:*** ~50yrs old.

Clinical features Often asymptomatic and diagnosed after finding ↑alk phos on routine LFT. Lethargy and pruritus may occur, and can precede jaundice by months to years. ***Signs:*** Jaundice; skin pigmentation; xanthelasma (p704); xanthomata; hepatomegaly; and splenomegaly. ***Complications:*** Osteoporosis is common. Malabsorption of fat-soluble vitamins (A, D, K) due to cholestasis and ↓ bilirubin in the gut lumen results in osteomalacia and coagulopathy. Other complications include: portal hypertension; ascites; variceal haemorrhage; hepatic encephalopathy; HCC (p270). See MINIBOX for associations.

Tests *Blood tests:* ↑Alk phos, ↑γGT, and mildly ↑AST and ALT; late disease: ↑bilirubin, ↓albumin, ↑prothrombin time. 98% are antimitochondrial antibody (AMA) M_2 subtype +ve (highly specific). Other autoantibodies (p555) may occur in low titres (see BOX). Immunoglobulins are ↑ (especially IgM). TSH and cholesterol may be ↑. ***Radiology:*** US to exclude extrahepatic cholestasis. ***Liver biopsy:*** Granulomas around the bile ducts, progressing to cirrhosis.[1]

Treatment *Symptomatic:* Pruritus: try ***colestyramine*** 4–8g/24h PO; ***naltrexone*** and ***rifampicin*** may also help. Diarrhoea: ***codeine phosphate***, eg 30mg/8h PO. Osteoporosis prevention: p696. ***Specific:*** Fat-soluble vitamin prophylaxis: vitamin A, D, and K. Consider high dose ***ursodeoxycholic acid (UDCA)***, 10–15mg/kg/d in 2–4 divided doses. One review claimed that it had a marginal therapeutic effect with improvement of ascites, jaundice and LFT, but no long-term effect on mortality or need for liver transplantation, though others have suggested a trend towards improved survival and a lower transplantation rate. A main benefit was the paucity of SE.[127] ***Liver transplantation*** (p263) is the last recourse for patients with end-stage disease (eg bilirubin >100µmol/L) or intractable pruritus. Recurrence in the graft has been histologically estimated at 17% after ~5 years, and although graft failure can occur as a result of recurrence, this is rare and not predictable.

Prognosis Once jaundice develops, survival is <2yrs. In one study, at 2yrs post-transplant, predicted survival without transplant was 55% and actual survival was 79%. At 7yrs, these figures were 22% and 68%, respectively.[128]

Testing for autoantibodies—entering a minefield?

The conditions in the next few pages all include the measurement of autoantibodies—with their varying sensitivities and specificities—as part of an investigative work-up. But dare we tread our way precariously through this dangerous minefield scattered with duds and tripwires, just to reach the other side in some degree of greater diagnostic certainty? Although we do measure some autoantibodies in the routine screen for suspected liver disease (p264), just how far should we go into this minefield with our patients before we think about the consequences? The best approach is most likely a combination of experience, close attention to the latest medical evidence, and individual circumstances.

1 Hepatic granulomas are not specific to PBC as they are also found in sarcoidosis, tuberculosis, schistosomiasis, brucellosis, parasitic infection and drug reactions.

Primary sclerosing cholangitis (PSC)

PSC is a disorder of unknown cause characterized by non-malignant non-bacterial inflammation, fibrosis, and strictures of the intra- and extrahepatic bile ducts. It most commonly occurs in men, especially those who suffer from ulcerative colitis[1] (hence the implication of immunological mechanisms).

Associations with PSC
Ulcerative colitis[1]
HLA-A1, B8, & DR3
Crohn's disease (much rarer)
HIV infection

The patient Chronic biliary obstruction and secondary biliary cirrhosis lead to liver failure and death (or transplantation) over ~10yrs. *Symptoms:* Patients may be asymptomatic and found incidentally after finding alk phos↑ on LFT; or else symptoms may fluctuate, eg jaundice; pruritus; abdominal pain; fatigue. *Signs:* Jaundice; hepatomegaly; portal hypertension. *Complications:* Bacterial cholangitis; cholangiocarcinoma (20–30% ► checking LFT, cancer markers, eg CA19-9, and radiological follow-up is needed); ↑risk of colorectal cancer. 30% of patients in some series had an overlap syndrome with type 1 AIH (p268).[2] See MINIBOX for associations.

Tests *Blood:* ↑Alk phos initially followed by ↑bilirubin; hypergammaglobulinaemia; AMA negative, but ANA, SMA, & ANCA may be +ve, see p555. *ERCP* (see **fig 1**) is needed to distinguish between large duct and small duct disease. It shows multiple strictures of the biliary tree with a characteristic 'beaded' appearance. *MRCP* (see **fig 2**) is cost effective and accurate in diagnosis compared with ERCP. *Liver biopsy* shows a fibrous, obliterative cholangitis.

Management There is no curative medical therapy and liver transplant is the only effective treatment. *Drugs: Colestyramine* 4–8g/24h PO for pruritus (*naltrexone* and *rifampicin* may also help). *Ursodeoxycholic acid* improves cholestasis but has no clear clinical effects.[129] Antibiotics for bacterial cholangitis. *Endoscopic stenting* helps symptomatic dominant strictures. Yearly *ultrasound* screening may help detect cholangiocarcinoma, with cholecystectomy advocated for gallbladder polyps. *Liver transplantation* (p259) is indicated in end-stage disease. Recurrence occurs in up to 30%; 5yr graft survival is >60%. Prognosis is worse for those with concomitant IBD, as 5–10% develop colorectal cancer post-transplant.[130] Do *colonoscopy screening* yearly in UC because of the higher risk of colorectal cancer.

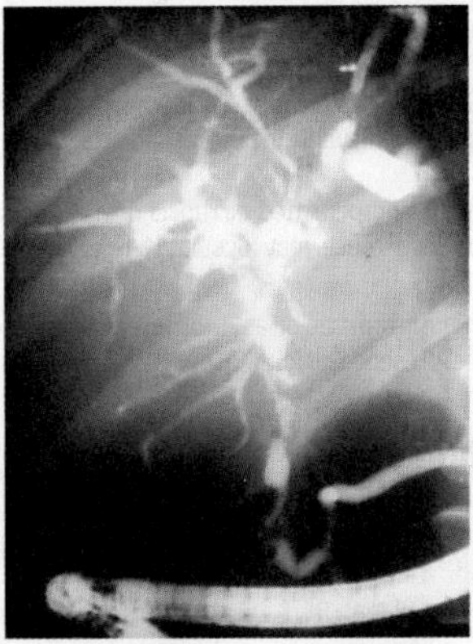

Fig 1. ERCP showing the features of PSC.

Figure courtesy of Dr Anthony Mee.

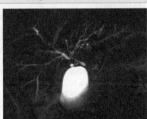

Fig 2. MRCP showing features of PSC. The intrahepatic ducts show multifocal strictures. (MRCP = magnetic resonance cholangiopancreatography.)

Figure courtesy of Norwich Radiology Department.

1 3% of those with UC have PSC, but 80–100% of those with PSC have UC/Crohn's associated with PSC has a higher rate of backwash ileitis and rectal sparing—it may be a distinct IBD-phenotype.

2 Do anti-mitochondrial, anti-nuclear, anti-smooth muscle, anti-liver kidney microsomal type 1, anti-liver cytosol type 1, perinuclear anti-neutrophil nuclear, & anti-soluble liver antigen antibodies.

An inflammatory liver disease of unknown cause[1] characterized by suppressor T-cell defects with autoantibodies directed against hepatocyte surface antigens. Three types have been distinguished by the presence of circulating autoantibodies (see TABLE). AIH predominantly affects young and middle-aged women. 25% present with acute hepatitis and signs of autoimmune disease, eg fever, malaise, urticarial rash, polyarthritis, pleurisy, pulmonary infiltration, or glomerulonephritis. The remainder present insidiously or are asymptomatic and diagnosed incidentally with signs of chronic liver disease. Amenorrhoea is common and disease tends to attenuate during pregnancy. *Complications:* Those associated with cirrhosis (p260) and drug therapy.

Tests Abnormal LFT (AST, ALT, serum bilirubin and alk phos are ↑ in most patients), hypergammaglobulinaemia (especially IgG), +ve autoantibodies (ANA, SMA, or LKM1). Other autoantibodies, eg anti-soluble liver antigen (SLA) and antimeasles virus may be seen. Anaemia, WCC↓, and platelets↓ indicate hypersplenism. ***Liver biopsy*** (p256): mononuclear infiltrate of portal and periportal areas & piecemeal necrosis, fibrosis, or cirrhosis. ***MRCP*** (p267) helps exclude PSC if alk phos disproportionately↑.

Diagnosis depends on excluding other diseases as there is no pathognomonic sign or laboratory test. There is genuine overlap with other chronic liver disease: eg PBC (p266), PSC (p267) and chronic viral hepatitis.[131] Diagnostic criteria exist but are not fully validated (eg the revised IAHG system).[2]

Types of autoimmune hepatitis

Type I	Affects adults or children (bimodal distribution) Anti-smooth muscle antibodies (ASMA) positive in 80%[132] Antinuclear antibody (ANA) positive in 10% Hypergammaglobulinaemia (IgG)
Type II	Affects mainly girls and young women More commonly progresses to cirrhosis Anti-liver/kidney microsomal type 1 (LKM1) antibodies
Type III	Affects adults and is clinically indistinguishable from type I Antibodies against soluble liver antigen or liver-pancreas antigen

Management

Immunosuppressant therapy: ***Prednisolone*** 30mg/d PO for 1 month; ↓by 5mg a month to a maintenance dose of 5-10mg/d PO. Corticosteroids can sometimes be stopped after 2yrs but relapse occurs in 50–86%. ***Azathioprine*** (50-100mg/d PO) may be used as a steroid-sparing agent. Remission is achievable in 80% of patients within 3yrs. 10- and 20yr survival rates are >80%.[133]

Liver transplantation (p263) is indicated for decompensated cirrhosis or if there is failure to respond to medical therapy, but recurrence may occur. It is effective (actuarial 10yr survival is 75%).

Prognosis appears not to matter whether symptomatic or asymptomatic at presentation (10yr survival ~80% for both). The presence of cirrhosis at presentation reduces 10yr survival from 94% to 62%.[134]

Associations of autoimmune hepatitis

• Pernicious anaemia	• Autoimmune haemolysis
• Ulcerative colitis	• Diabetes mellitus
• Glomerulonephritis	• PSC
• Autoimmune thyroiditis	• HLA A1, B8, & DR3 haplotype

1 Hepatotropic viruses (eg measles, herpes viruses) and some drugs appear to trigger AIH in genetically predisposed individuals exposed to a hepatotoxic *milieu intérieur*. Viral interferon can inactivate cytochrome P-450 enzymes (∴ ↓ metabolism of ex- or endogenous hepatotoxins). Putative examples of exogenous agents: monosodium glutamate (MSG; E621) and aspartame (E951), which, if regularly consumed in excess, may promote formation of salt bridges between amino acids. These compounds then act as autoantigens causing CD4 T-helper cell activation.

2 International Autoimmune Hepatitis Group (revised) 1999.

Wilson's disease/hepatolenticular degeneration

Wilson's disease is a rare inherited disorder with toxic accumulation of copper (Cu) in the liver and CNS (especially basal ganglia, eg globus pallidus hypodensity ± putamen cavitation) due to failure of biliary copper excretion. It is treatable, so screen all young patients with cirrhosis. ***Prevalence:*** 3:100,000.

Genetics

It is an autosomal recessive disorder of a gene on chromosome 13 that codes for a copper transporting ATPase, ATP7B. Many mutations are known (>200) with HIS1069GLU being the commonest in European populations.

Pathophysiology

Total body copper content is ~100-150mg, with an average intake of 1-5mg/day, which is absorbed in the proximal small intestine. In the liver, copper is incorporated into caeruloplasmin. In Wilson's disease, intestinal copper absorption and transport into the liver are intact, while copper incorporation into caeruloplasmin in hepatocytes and its excretion into bile are impaired. Therefore, copper accumulates in liver, and later in other organs.

Clinical features

Children usually present with ***liver disease*** (hepatitis, cirrhosis, fulminant liver failure); young adults often start with ***CNS signs:*** psychiatric problems are common. Also: tremor; dysarthria, dysphagia; dyskinesias; dystonias; purposeless stereotyped movements (eg hand clapping); dementia; parkinsonism; micrographia; ataxia/clumsiness. ***Affective features:*** Depression/mania; labile emotions; libido↑↓; personality change. ►Ignoring these may cause years of needless misery. ***Cognitive/behavioural:*** Memory↓; quick to anger; slow to solve problems; IQ↓; delusions; mutism. ***Kayser–Fleischer rings:*** Copper deposits in iris (Descemet's membrane; see **fig 1** *OHCS* p448—pathognomonic but not invariable; may need slit lamp to see). ***Also:*** Haemolysis; blue lunulae (nails); polyarthritis; hypermobile joints; grey skin; abortions; hypoparathyroidism.

Tests 24h urinary copper excretion is high (>100µg/24h, normal <40µg), while serum copper and caeruloplasmin levels are usually low. ***Falsely low caeruloplasmin:*** Protein-deficiency states (eg nephritic syndrome, malabsorption). ***Falsely high caeruloplasmin:*** caeruloplasmin is an 'acute phase reactant', and may be high during inflammation, eg infection, pregnancy. Molecular genetic testing can confirm the diagnosis. ***Liver biopsy:*** ↑Hepatic copper content. ***MRI:*** Basal ganglia degeneration (± fronto-temporal, cerebellar, and brainstem atrophy).[135]

Management

Diet: Avoid eating foods with a high copper content (eg liver, chocolate, nuts, mushrooms, legumes, and shellfish). Copper content of atypical water sources (eg well water) should be analysed. ***Drugs:*** Lifelong *penicillamine* (500mg/6–8h PO for 1yr, maintenance 0.75-1g/d). SE: nausea, rash, WCC↓, Hb↓, platelets↓ haematuria, nephrosis, lupus. Monitor FBC & urinary Cu and protein excretion. Say 'report sore throat, T°↑, or bruising at once' in case WCC/platelets↓↓. Stop if WCC <2.5×10⁹/L or platelets falling (or <120×10⁹/L). Alternative: *Trientine dihydrochloride* 600mg/6-12h PO (SE: rash; sideroblastic anaemia). ***Liver transplantation*** (p263) if severe liver disease. ***Screen siblings*** as asymptomatic homozygotes need treating.

Prognosis: Pre-cirrhotic liver disease is reversible, though neurological damage is less so. There are no clear clinical prognostic indicators.[136] Death occurs from liver failure, variceal haemorrhage (p254), or infection.

The commonest (90%) liver tumours are secondary (metastatic) tumours, eg from breast, bronchus, or the gastrointestinal tract (see TABLE 1). Primary hepatic tumours are much less common and may be benign or malignant (see TABLE 2).

Symptoms Fever, malaise, anorexia, weight↓, RUQ pain (∵ liver capsule stretch). Jaundice is late, except with cholangiocarcinoma. Benign tumours are often asymptomatic. Tumours may rupture causing intraperitoneal haemorrhage.

Signs Hepatomegaly (smooth, or hard and irregular, eg metastases, cirrhosis, HCC). Look for signs of chronic liver disease (p260) and evidence of decompensation (jaundice, ascites). Feel for an abdominal mass. Listen for a bruit over the liver (HCC).

Tests ***Blood:*** FBC, clotting, LFT, hepatitis serology, α-fetoprotein (↑ in 50-80% of HCC, though it is a poor prognostic indicator,[137] and may be normal if tumour <3cm). ***Imaging:*** US **(fig 1)** or CT to identify lesions and guide diagnostic biopsies. MRI is better for distinguishing benign from malignant lesions. ERCP (p756) and biopsy should be performed for suspected cholangiocarcinoma. ***Liver biopsy*** (p256) may achieve a histological diagnosis; ►careful multidisciplinary discussion is required if potentially resectable, as seeding along the biopsy tract can occur. Other investigations for metastases (eg CXR, mammography, endoscopy, colonoscopy, CT, MRI, marrow biopsy) are tailored according to the suspected primary.

Liver metastases signify advanced disease. Treatment and prognosis vary with the type and extent of primary tumour. Chemotherapy may be effective (eg lymphomas, germ cell tumours). Small, solitary metastases may be amenable to resection (eg colorectal carcinoma).[138] In most, treatment is palliative. ***Prognosis:*** <6 months.

Hepatocellular carcinoma (HCC) A malignant tumour of hepatocytes, accounting for 90% of primary liver cancers. Common in China & sub-Saharan Africa (40% of cancers), rare in the West (~2% of cancers). ***Causes:*** Viral hepatitis (persistent HCV or HBV, especially if >2.3×10^4 virions/mL; see p406);[1] cirrhosis (alcohol, haemochromatosis, PBC); aflatoxin; parasites (*Clonorchis sinensis*) and anabolic steroids. ***Management:*** Resection of solitary tumours <3cm diameter improves 3yr survival rate (59% from 13%), though ~50% have recurrence by 3yrs. Applying the Milan criteria for liver transplantation gives a 5yr survival rate of 70%.[2] Chemotherapy, percutaneous ablation, and tumour embolization are also options.[139] ***Prognosis:*** Often <6 months, with a 95% 5yr mortality. Fibrolamellar HCC, which occurs in children/young adults, has a better prognosis (60% 5yr survival). ***Prevention*** is vital. ►Ensure HBV vaccination (see BOX). ►Don't reuse needles. ►Screen blood products. ►Reduce exposure to aflatoxins (anti-humidity measures such as sun-drying to ↓spread of this common fungal contaminant in stored maize); this is most important for those who harbour HBV (risk is highly synergistic).[140] ***Screening*** using ultrasound and α-fetoprotein levels needs further evaluation as its impact on survival is unproven.[141]

Cholangiocarcinoma = biliary tree malignancy; ~10% of liver primaries. ***Causes:*** Flukes (*Clonorchis,* p445) in the East; PSC (screening by CA19-9 may be helpful, p267); congenital biliary cysts; biliary-enteric drainage surgery;[142] N-nitroso toxins.[143] ***The patient:*** Fever, abdominal pain (±ascites), malaise, ↑bilirubin; ↑↑alk phos. ***Pathology:*** Usually slow-growing. Most are distal extrahepatic or perihilar. ***Management:*** 70% are unsuitable for surgical resection. Of those that are, 76% recur. **Surgery:** eg major hepatectomy + extrahepatic bile duct excision + caudate lobe resection. 5yr survival is ~30%.[144] Specific post-op complications include liver failure, bile leak and GI bleeding.[145] **Palliative stenting** of an obstructed extrahepatic biliary tree, percutaneously or via ERCP (p756), improves quality of life. ***Prognosis:*** ~5 months.

Benign tumours ***Haemangiomas*** are the commonest benign liver tumours. They are often an incidental finding on ultrasound or CT scan (see **fig 1**) and do not require treatment. Biopsy should be avoided! ***Adenomas*** are common. Causes: Anabolic steroids, the oral contraceptive pill; pregnancy. Only treat if symptomatic, or >5cm.

1 2.3×10^4 virions/mL by PCR is a low level, so almost all are at risk.

2 Milan criteria for liver transplantation in HCC: 1 nodule <5cm or 2-3 nodules <3cm.

Primary liver tumours

Malignant*	Benign
HCC	Cysts
Cholangiocarcinoma	Haemangioma
Angiosarcoma	Adenoma
Hepatoblastoma	Focal nodular hyperplasia
Fibrosarcoma	Fibroma
Leiomyosarcoma	Leiomyoma

*Prognosis—regardless of type—is poor.

Origins of secondary liver tumours

Common in ♂	Common in ♀	Less common (either sex)
Stomach	Breast	Pancreas
Lung	Colon	Leukaemia
Colon	Stomach	Lymphoma
	Uterus	Carcinoid tumours

Prevention of hepatitis B, hepatitis B-associated cirrhosis, chronic hepatitis, and hepatic neoplasia

Use hepatitis B vaccine, Engerix B®, 1mL into deltoid; repeat at 1 & 6 months (child: 0.5mL × 3 into the anterolateral thigh). ***Indications:*** Everyone (WHO advice, even in areas of 'low' endemicity).[146] This strategy is expensive, but not as expensive as trying to rely on the ultimately unsuccessful strategy of vaccinating at-risk groups—health workers (eg GPs, dentists, nurses, etc.), IV drug users, sexual adventurers, male or immigrant prostitutes (homo- or heterosexual), those on haemodialysis, and the sexual partners of known HB_e antigen +ve carriers. The immunocompromised and others may need further doses. Serology helps time boosters and finds poor or non-responders (correlates with older age, smoking, and ♂ sex). ►**Know your own antibody level!**

Anti-HBS (IU/L)	Actions and comments—UK advice (USA advice is different)
>1000	Good level of immunity; retest in ~4yrs.
100-1000	Good level of immunity; if level approaches 100, retest in 1yr.
<100	Inadequate; give booster and retest.
<10	Non-responder; give booster and retest; if <10 get consent to check hepatitis B status: HBsAg +ve means chronic infection; anti-HB core +ve represents past infection and immunity.

NB: protective immunity begins about 6 weeks after the 1st immunizing dose, so it is inappropriate if exposure is recent; here, specific anti-hepatitis B immunoglobulin is the best option if not already immunized.

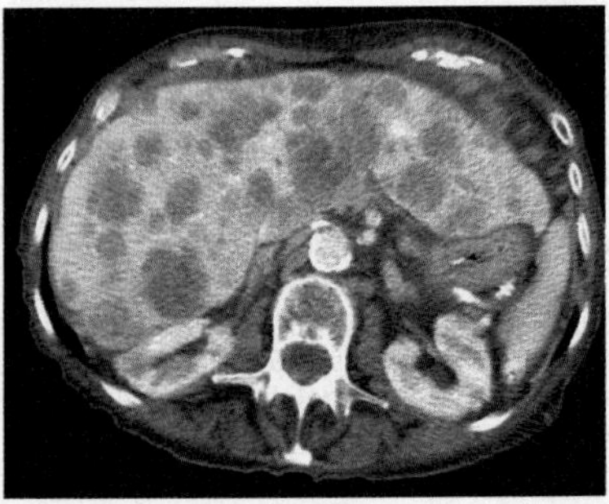

Fig 1. Axial CT of the liver after IV contrast showing multiple round liver lesions of varying size, highly suggestive of hepatic metastasis.

Courtesy of Norwich Radiology Dept

UC is a relapsing and remitting inflammatory disorder of the colonic mucosa. It may affect just the rectum (proctitis, as in ~50%) or extend proximally to involve part of the colon (left-sided colitis, in ~30%) or the entire colon (pancolitis, in ~20%). It 'never' spreads proximal to the ileocaecal valve (except for backwash ileitis). ***Cause:*** Unknown;[1] there is some genetic susceptibility. ***Pathology:*** Hyperaemic/ haemorrhagic granular colonic mucosa ± pseudopolyps formed by inflammation. Punctate ulcers may extend deep into the lamina propria—inflammation is normally not transmural. Mucosal disease differentiates it from Crohn's disease. ***Histology:*** See biopsy, below. ***Prevalence:*** 100-200/100,000. ***Incidence:*** 10-20/100,000/yr. ♀:♂ >1:1. Most present aged 15-30yrs. UC is 3-fold as common in non-smokers (the opposite is true for Crohn's disease)—symptoms may relapse on stopping smoking.

Symptoms Gradual onset of diarrhoea (± blood and mucus). Crampy abdominal discomfort is common; bowel frequency is related to severity of disease (see TABLE). Systemic symptoms are common during attacks, eg fever, malaise, anorexia, weight↓. Urgency and tenesmus occur with rectal disease.

Signs May be none. In acute, severe UC there may be fever, tachycardia, and a tender, distended abdomen. ***Extraintestinal signs:*** Clubbing; aphthous oral ulcers; erythema nodosum (p275); pyoderma gangrenosum; conjunctivitis; episcleritis; iritis; large joint arthritis; sacroiliitis; ankylosing spondylitis; fatty liver; PSC (p267); cholangiocarcinoma; nutritional deficits; amyloidosis.[147]

Tests ***Blood:*** FBC, ESR, CRP, U&E, LFT, and blood cultures. ***Stool MC+S*** and ***CDT*** (p247) to exclude infections (*C. difficile, Salmonella, Shigella, Campylobacter, E. coli, amoebae*). *AXR:* No faecal shadows; mucosal thickening/islands (**fig 4**, p740); colonic dilatation (below). ***Erect CXR:*** Perforation. ***Sigmoidoscopy:*** Inflamed, friable mucosa. ***Rectal biopsy:*** Inflammatory infiltrate; goblet cell depletion; glandular distortion; mucosal ulcers; crypt abscesses. ***Barium enema:*** ►**Never do a barium enema during a severe acute attack or as a diagnostic test.** ***Colonoscopy*** shows disease extent and allows biopsy (**fig 4**, p256). See also BOX 2.

Assessing severity in UC: the Truelove and Witts criteria

Parameter	Mild	Moderate	Severe
Motions/day	<4	4-6	>6
Rectal bleeding	Small	Moderate	Large
Temperature at 6AM (p24)	Apyrexial	37.1-37.8°C	>37.8°C
Pulse rate (beats/min)	<70	70-90	>90
Haemoglobin	>11g/dL	10.5-11g/dL	<10.5g/dL
ESR	<30mm/h		>30mm/h

Complications ►Perforation and bleeding are 2 serious dangers, also:
- Toxic dilatation of colon (mucosal islands, colonic diameter >6cm).
- Venous thrombosis: Give prophylaxis to all inpatients (p344).[148]
- Colonic cancer: risk ≈15% with pancolitis for 20yrs; surveillance colonoscopy may be used (eg 2-4yearly), but proving this saves lives has been difficult.[149] [150]

Inducing remission *Mild UC:* If <4 motions/d and the patient is well, give ***prednisolone*** (eg 20-40mg/d PO) + ***mesalazine***, eg Pentasa® (MR 500mg tabs; up to 1g/6h) or Asacol MR (4.8g/day).[151] For mild distal disease use twice-daily steroid foams PR (eg ***hydrocortisone*** as Colifoam®), or ***prednisolone*** 20mg **retention enemas** (Predsol®). If symptoms improve, ↓steroids gradually (there should be at least a 5-ASA foam enema superior to steroid suppository). If no improvement after 2wks, treat as moderate UC.

Moderate UC: If 4-6 motions/d, but otherwise well, give oral ***prednisolone*** 40mg/d for 1wk, then 30mg/d for 1wk, then 20mg for 4 more weeks + a 5-aminosalycilic acid (5-ASA) + and twice-daily steroid enemas.[2] If improving, ↓steroids gradually. If no improvement after 2 weeks, treat as a severe UC.

1 UC & Crohn's *may* involve adhesin-expressing strains of *E. coli* capable of inducing interleukin-8 production and transepithelial migration of WBCs—see OTM 2.613.

2 *Budesonide* (Entocort) enemas, 1 nocte, may have fewer SEs ∵ ↓suppression of plasma cortisol.

Severe UC: If systemically unwell and passing >6 motions/d, admit for:

- Nil by mouth and IV maintenance hydration (eg 1L of 0.9% saline + 2L dextrose-saline/24h, + 20mmol K^+/L; less if elderly).
- ***Hydrocortisone*** 100mg/6h IV.
- Rectal steroids, eg ***hydrocortisone*** 100mg in 100mL 0.9% saline/12h PR.
- Monitor T°, pulse, and BP—and record stool frequency/character on a stool chart.
- Twice-daily exam: document distension, bowel sounds and tenderness.
- Daily FBC, ESR, CRP, U&E ± AXR.
- Consider the need for blood transfusion (if Hb <10g/dL). Parenteral nutrition is only very rarely required (eg if severely malnourished).
- If improving in 5d, transfer to ***prednisolone*** PO (40mg/24h) with a 5-ASA (below, eg ***sulfasalazine*** 500mg/6h) to maintain remission.
- If on day 3 CRP >45 or stool frequency >6, consider ***ciclosporin/infliximab***/surgery.

Topical therapies Proctitis may respond to ***suppositories*** (*prednisolone* 5mg or *mesalazine*, eg Asacol® 250mg/8h or Pentasa® 1g at bedtime). Topical 5-ASAs work better than topical steroids.[152] Procto-sigmoiditis may respond to ***foams*** PR (20mg Predfoam®/12–24h or 5-ASA, eg Asacol® 1g/d); disposable applicators aid accurate delivery. Retention enemas may be needed in left-sided colitis.

Indications for surgery
Perforation
Massive haemorrhage
Toxic dilatation
Failure to respond to medical therapy

Surgery ~20% will require surgery at some stage. *Procedures:* Proctocolectomy + terminal ileostomy (may be possible to retain the ileocecal valve, and hence reduce liquid loss);[153] colectomy with later ileo-anal pouch. *Surgical mortality:* 2–7%, ↑ to 50% if perforation. Pouchitis can be successfully treated with antibiotics (eg ***metronidazole*** + ***ciprofloxacin*** for 2wks) and immunosuppressants.[154]

Novel therapies A short course of *ciclosporin* (eg 2mg/kg IV per day; unlicensed indication) may help obtain remission quickly in patients with steroid-refractory UC, although it is markedly nephrotoxic and not suitable for long courses (►monitor levels, do U&E, LFT and BP often—stop if raised and get expert help).[155] Short-term response to *ciclosporin* is generally good (>75%) but long-term remission is disappointing. *Infliximab* (see p275) may be effective as rescue therapy in UC, though evidence is scarce.[156]

Maintaining remission All *5-ASAs* ↓relapse rate from 80% to 20% at 1yr—examples are *sulfasalazine*, *mesalazine*, and *olsalazine*.[1] Maintenance continues for life. *Sulfasalazine* (500mg/6h PO) is 1st-line. SEs relate to sulfapyridine intolerance (headache, nausea, anorexia, malaise). Other SEs: T°↑, rash, haemolysis (►monitor FBC), hepatitis, pancreatitis, paradoxical worsening of colitis, and reversible oligospemia.[157] ***Newer 5-ASAs*** (eg *mesalazine* 400–800mg/8h PO or *olsalazine* 500mg/12h PO) are just as effective at maintaining remission, have fewer SEs, but are more expensive. They are indicated in *sulfasalazine* intolerance and young men in whom fertility is a concern (less effect on sperm).[158] *Azathioprine* (2–2.5mg/kg/d PO after food) is indicated as a steroid-sparing drug in those with steroid side effects or those who relapse quickly if steroids are reduced.[159] Treat for several months, and monitor FBC every 4–6wks.

Patients with 'indeterminate colitis'

This is a diagnosis for when IBD has been fully investigated and cannot be definitely labelled as UC or Crohn's disease. It tends to resemble UC more than Crohn's disease, and some cases may be due to lack of recognition of unusual variants of UC that involve transmural inflammation or skip lesions. Regarding surgical management, it is probably appropriate to perform colectomy + pouch formation, if indicated (see MINIBOX), though pouch failure rate is higher than in UC.[160]

1 **Sulfasalazine** is a 5-aminosalicylic acid (5-ASA, the active ingredient) + sulfapyridine (carries 5-ASA to the colon, where it is cleaved off), **mesalazine is** 5-ASA and **olsalazine** is a dimer of 5-ASA that is also cleaved in the colon. Rare hypersensitivity reactions: worsening colitis, pancreatitis, pericarditis, nephritis.

Crohn's disease[1] is a chronic inflammatory GI disease characterized by transmural granulomatous inflammation. It may affect any part of the gut from mouth to anus, but favours the terminal ileum (in 50%) and proximal colon. Unlike UC, there is unaffected bowel between areas of active disease (skip lesions). *Cause:* Unknown.[2] Mutations of the NOD2/CARD15 gene ↑risk. *Prevalence:* 50–100/100,000. *Incidence:* 5–10 per 100,000/yr. *Associations:* Altered cell-mediated immunity. Smoking ↑risk ×3–4 and NSAIDs may exacerbate disease.

Symptoms Diarrhoea, abdominal pain, and weight loss are common (failure to thrive in children). Fever, malaise, anorexia occur with active disease.

Signs Aphthous ulcerations; abdominal tenderness; right iliac fossa mass; perianal abscesses/fistulae/skin tags; anal/rectal strictures. *Extraintestinal signs:* Clubbing, erythema nodosum (**fig 1**), pyoderma gangrenosum, conjunctivitis, episcleritis, iritis, large joint arthritis, seronegative spondyloarthropathy (sacroiliitis, ankylosing spondylitis), fatty liver, PSC (p267—colonic disease only), cholangiocarcinoma, renal stones,[3] osteomalacia, malnutrition, amyloidosis.

Complications Small bowel obstruction; toxic dilatation (colonic diameter >6cm, toxic dilatation is rarer than in UC); abscess formation (abdominal, pelvic, or ischiorectal); fistulae (present in ~10%), eg colovesical (bladder), colovaginal, perianal, enterocutaneous; perforation; rectal haemorrhage; colonic carcinoma.

Tests *Blood:* FBC, ESR, CRP, U&E, LFT, blood culture. Serum iron, B_{12}, and red cell folate if anaemia. *Markers of activity:* Hb↓; ↑ESR; ↑CRP; ↑WCC; ↓albumin. *Stool MC + S* and *CDT* (p247) to exclude infectious diarrhoea (*C. difficile, Salmonella, Shigella, Campylobacter, E. coli*). Do *sigmoidoscopy + rectal biopsy* if the mucosa looks normal (20% have microscopic granulomas). *Small bowel enema* detects ileal disease. *Capsule endoscopy* (p256) also has an important and growing role in assessing small bowel disease. *Barium enema* (rarely used) may show cobblestoning, 'rose thorn' ulcers, and colon strictures with rectal sparing. *Colonoscopy* (**fig 2**) is preferred to barium enema to assess disease extent. *MRI* can assess pelvic disease and fistulae (as good as EUA). Small bowel *MRI* can assess disease activity and show site of strictures.

Management Severity is harder to assess than in UC, but T°↑; pulse↑; ↑ESR; ↑CRP; ↑WCC; ↓albumin reflect severity and merit admission. *Mild attacks:* Patients are symptomatic but systemically well. *Prednisolone* 30mg/d PO for 1wk, then 20mg/d for 1 month. See in clinic every 2–4 weeks. If symptoms resolve, ↓prednisolone by 5mg every 2–4 weeks; stop steroids when parameters are normal (see also BOX).

Severe attacks: Admit for IV steroids, nil by mouth, and IV hydration (eg 1L 0.9% saline + 2L dextrose-saline/24h, + 20mmol K^+/L, less if elderly). Then:

- *Hydrocortisone* 100mg/6h IV.
- Treat rectal disease: steroids (eg *hydrocortisone* 100mg in 100mL 0.9% saline/12h PR).
- *Metronidazole* 400mg/8h PO, or 500mg/8h IV, helps (esp. in perianal disease or superadded infection). SEs: alcohol intolerance; irreversible neuropathy.
- Monitor T°, pulse, BP, and record stool frequency/character on a stool chart.
- Physical examination daily. Daily FBC, ESR, CRP, U&E, and plain AXR.
- Consider need for blood transfusion (if Hb <10g/dL) and parenteral nutrition.
- If improving after 5d, transfer on to oral *prednisolone* (40mg/d).
- If no response (or deterioration) during IV therapy, consider CT abdomen to exclude collections, and seek surgical advice.

Perianal disease occurs in about 50%. MRI and examination under anaesthetic (EUA) are an important part of assessment. Treatment includes oral antibiotics, immunosuppressant therapy ± *infliximab*, and local surgery ± seton insertion. 161

1 Burrill B. Crohn was a US gastroenterologist (1884–1983). The original paper was penned in 1932.

2 **Environmental agents** are implicated. **Genetics:** Colon involvement goes with ↑CARD15 gene expression in macrophages & intestinal epithelial cells. **Dysregulated immune responses** might be primary or from infecting gut commensals, eg *Mycobacterium avium paratuberculosis*; *E. coli* adhesins, p272, may have a role.

3 Malabsorption of fat → Ca^{2+} binds fat left in lumen (saponification) → oxalate free to be absorbed (normally binds Ca^{2+} in lumen & excreted in stool) → renal excretion of oxalate → hyperoxaluria & renal stones.

Additional therapies in Crohn's disease

Azathioprine (AZA) (2-2.5mg/kg/d PO) is effective therapy and useful as a steroid-sparing agent, eg for those with steroid side effects or if experiencing multiple/rapid relapses. It takes 6-10 weeks to work.[162] Protocols are changing because steroids are so disappointing in the long term, and ***early combined immunosuppression*** (azathioprine + infliximab ± steroids) may have a role in the *initial* management—as well as later; see below; get expert advice.[163]

Sulfasalazine Efficacy of 5-ASA in Crohn's is unproven but high-dose PENTASA post-op in patients with ileal resection may ↓recurrent disease.

Elemental diets (eg E028®) are made by mixing single amino acids and are antigen free. They are not as good as steroids at inducing remission in active disease but do have a beneficial effect.[164] A **low residue diet** may help control disease activity, though diet alone is not effective at inducing remission.

Methotrexate A large RCT recommended 25mg IM weekly for induction of remission and complete withdrawal from steroids in patients with refractory Crohn's disease. NNT ≈ 5—see p671. There was no evidence for lower doses, and no substantial SE were found.[165] Methotrexate is contraindicated in pregnancy.

Surgery 50-80% need ≥1 operation in their life. In the severely affected, it can become a devastating cycle of deterioration. Indications for surgery:

- Failure to respond to drugs (most commonly)
- Intestinal obstruction (from strictures), perforation, fistulae, or abscesses.

Surgery is never curative. The aims are **1** to defunction (rest) distal disease eg with a temporary ileostomy or **2** limited resection of the worst areas—short bowel syndrome can be a complication (p582).[166] <1m of small bowel in the absence of a colon may require regular parenteral nutrition (p588). Bypass and pouch surgery is **not** done in Crohn's (∵ ↑risk of recurrence).

TNFα inhibitors TNFα plays an important role in pathogenesis of Crohn's disease, therefore TNFα inhibitors eg *infliximab* and *adalimumab* (Humira) can ↓disease activity. They counter neutrophil accumulation and granuloma formation, activates complement, and cause cytotoxicity to CD4+ T-cells, thus clearing cells driving the immune response. Response may be short-lived, but it may be repeated at 8 wks. Trials have also shown it to be effective as maintenance therapy.[167] CI: Sepsis, ↑LFT >3-fold above top end of normal, concurrent *ciclosporin* or *tacrolimus*. SE: rash. Avoid in people with known underlying malignancy.[168] TB may reactivate when on infliximab, so screen the patients before starting the treatment (CXR, PPD). Cost per QALY: (see p10) £6700 (higher in fistulizing Crohn's).[169] According to SONIC trial, combined AZA and infliximab can ↑ efficacy of ℞ at 12 months, but there are long-term safety issues (eg hepatosplenic T cell lymphomas).

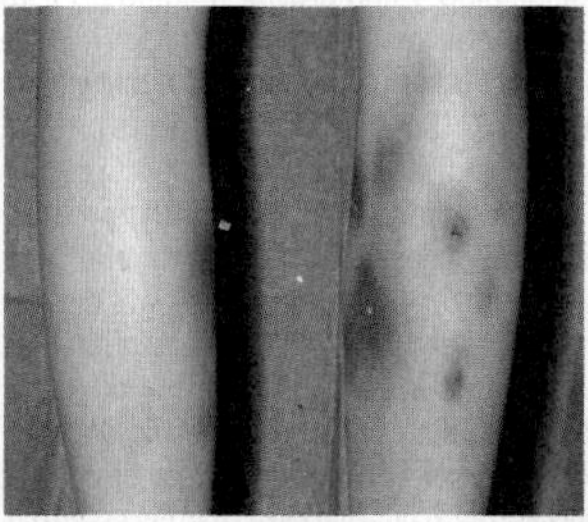

Fig 1. Erythema nodosum is a non-GI sign of Crohn's & UC. These painful purplish nodules usually occur over the shins. They regress after a few weeks, leaving a bruised appearance. Other causes include sarcoidosis, drugs, streptococcal infection, and TB.

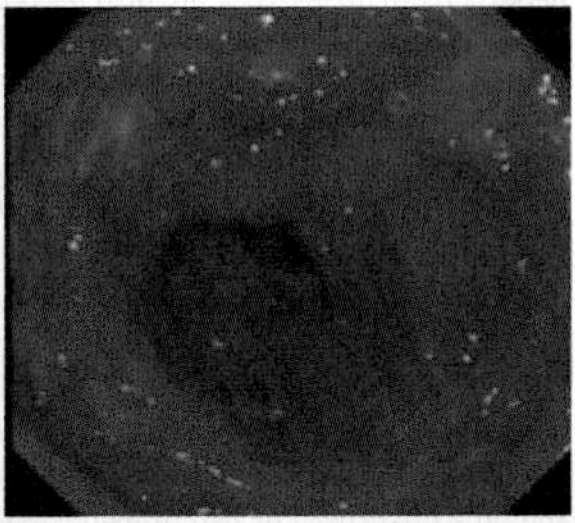

Fig 2. Colonoscopy image showing deep fissured ulcers of the colonic mucosa in Crohn's disease.

Image courtesy of Dr A Mee

Irritable bowel syndrome (IBS)

IBS denotes a mixed group of abdominal symptoms for which no organic cause can be found. Most are probably due to disorders of intestinal motility or enhanced visceral perception (the 'brain-gut' axis: see BOX). Several diagnostic criteria exist that evaluate symptoms and their duration (eg Manning, Rome II/III),[170] [171] but they are not always helpful in practice because of complex interactions between IBS and chronic pain syndromes (BOX).[172] *Prevalence:* 10–20%; age at onset: ≤40yrs; ♀:♂ ≥2:1.

Diagnosis Only diagnose IBS if abdominal pain (or discomfort) is either relieved by defecation *or* associated with altered stool form or bowel frequency (constipation and diarrhoea may alternate) *and* there are ≥2 of: urgency; incomplete evacuation; abdominal bloating/distension; mucous PR; worsening of symptoms after food. Other symptoms: nausea, bladder symptoms, backache. Symptoms are chronic (>6 months), and exacerbated by stress, menstruation, or gastroenteritis (typical post-infection IBS). *Signs:* Examination is often normal, but general abdominal tenderness is common. Insufflation of air during sigmoidoscopy (*not* usually needed) may reproduce the pain. ***Markers suggesting a disease other than IBS:*** Age >40yrs (esp male); history <6 months; anorexia; weight↓; waking at night with pain/diarrhoea; mouth ulcers; abnormal CRP, ESR, Hb, coeliac serology. ►Investigate PR bleeding urgently. **Management** See BOX.

Carcinoma of the pancreas

Epidemiology: ≤2% of all malignancy; ~6500 deaths/yr (UK). UK incidence is rising. *Typical patient:* ♂ >60yrs old. *Risk factors:* Smoking, alcohol, carcinogens, DM, chronic pancreatitis, and possibly a high fat diet. *Pathology:* Mostly ductal adenocarcinoma (metastasize early; present late). 60% arise in the pancreas head, 25% in the body, 15% tail. A few arise in the ampulla of Vater (ampullary tumour) or pancreatic islet cells (insulinoma, gastrinoma, glucagonomas, somatostatinomas (p215), VIPomas); both have a better prognosis. *Genetics:* ~95% have mutations in the KRAS2 gene.

Symptoms & signs Tumours in the head of the pancreas present with **painless obstructive jaundice**. 75% of tumours in the body and tail present with epigastric pain (radiates to back and relieved by sitting forward). Either may cause anorexia, weight loss, diabetes or acute pancreatitis. *Rarer features:* Thrombophlebitis migrans (eg an arm vein becomes swollen and red, then a leg vein); Ca^{2+}↑; marantic endocarditis; portal hypertension (splenic vein thrombosis); nephrosis (renal vein metastases). *Signs:* Jaundice + palpable gall bladder (Courvoisier's 'law': see p250); epigastric mass; hepatomegaly; splenomegaly; lymphadenopathy; ascites.

Tests *Blood:* Cholestatic jaundice. CA 19-9↑ (p538) is non-specific, but may help assess prognosis. *Imaging:* US or CT can show a pancreatic mass ± dilated biliary tree ± hepatic metastases. They are also used to guide biopsy and provide staging prior to surgery/stent insertion. Compared to MRI and CT, EUS (endoscopic sonography) is the most accurate diagnostic and staging technique.[173] ERCP (p756) shows the biliary tree anatomy and may localize the site of obstruction. **℞:** Most ductal carcinomas present with metastatic disease; <10% are suitable for radical surgery. *Surgery:* Consider pancreatoduodenectomy (Whipple's, p279) if fit and the tumour <3cm with no metastases. Post-op morbidity is high (mortality <5% in experienced hands) and non-curative resections confer no survival benefit. *Post-op chemotherapy* delays disease progression. *Palliation of jaundice:* Endoscopic or percutaneous stent insertion may help jaundice and anorexia. Rarely, palliative bypass surgery is done for duodenal obstruction or unsuccessful ERCP. *Pain relief:* Disabling pain may need big doses of opiates (p576), or radiotherapy. Coeliac plexus infiltration with alcohol may be done at the time of surgery, or percutaneously. Referral to a palliative care team is essential.

Prognosis Dismal. Mean survival <6 months. 5yr survival: <2%. Overall 5yr survival after Whipples' procedure (p279) 5–14%. Prognosis is better if: tumour <3cm; no nodes involved; -ve resection margins at surgery; ampullary or islet cell tumours.

Management of IBS (mostly in primary care) NICE 2008

Make a *positive* diagnosis (see IBS, p276) but also 'exclude' other diagnoses, so:
- If the history is classic, FBC, ESR, CRP, LFT & coeliac serology (p280) is sufficient.
- If ≥60yrs or **any** marker or organic disease (T° ↑, blood PR, weight ↓): colonoscopy.
- Have a low threshold for referring if family history of ovarian or bowel cancer.
- If diarrhoea is prominent, do: LFT; stool culture; B12/folate; antiendomysial antibodies (coeliac, p280); TSH; consider referral ± barium follow-through (if symptoms suggest small bowel disease) ± rectal biopsy.

Further investigation should be guided by symptoms and include:
- Upper GI endoscopy (dyspepsia, reflux) or small bowel radiology (Crohn's).
- Duodenal biopsy (coeliac disease), eg if antiendomysial antibodies +ve.
- Giardia tests, p436 (it often triggers IBS; anti-parasitic ℞ may not help).173
- ERCP (p756, eg chronic pancreatitis) or MRCP, p267 if active pancreatitis.
- Transit studies and anorectal physiological studies—rarely used.

Refer if: 1 Diagnosis unsure 2 If changing symptoms in 'known IBS' 3 *To surgeon* if rectal mucosal prolapse 4 *To dietician* if food intolerance 5 *To counsellor* if marked stress or depression is (seen in ≥50%) 6 *To gynaecologist* if cyclical pain, dyspareunia, or dysmenorrhoea; ►endometriosis (*OHCS* p288) often mimics IBS 7 *To dermatologist* if co-existing atopy (IBS is 3-fold more common in atopy).174 8 *To yourself* (wearing a different hat) or *pain clinic* if overlapping chronic pain syndromes (fibromyalgia; chronic fatigue, chronic pelvic pain) or detrusor problems.

℞ Rarely 50% successful, so ***be pragmatic***. ►Forge a ***therapeutic alliance*** with your patient.175 ***Explanation*** and ***reassurance*** are vital as is ***interdisciplinary teamwork*** (interdisciplinary implies a harmonized approach—not just multidisciplinary with each of the above specialists ploughing their own furrow).176
- *Food intolerance:* Exclusion diets may be tried (difficult; may lead to obsessions) Try limiting cereals high in bran, and whole grains such as brown rice). In a few, fructose intolerance is part of the problem.177 Drink plenty (8 cups/d; but limit tea, coffee, alcohol and fizzy drinks).178 Probiotics *may* help: once-daily *Bacillus coagulans* GBI-30, *B. infantis* 35624, *E. coli* DSM17252, and *L. acidophilus*-SDC 2012, 2013 can help pain & bloating.179 180 181
- *Constipation* (p248): ↑ fibre intake slowly (can paradoxically worsen flatulence/ bloating; avoid insoluble fibre, such as bran). Fybogel® (***ispaghula***) or Celevac® (***methylcellulose***; start with 3-6 tabs/12h with >300mL fluid) have non-fermentable fibre—and are better than ***lactulose*** which ferments (↑ gas production is hard to distinguish from bloating).182 *Diarrhoea:* Try avoiding sorbitol (artificial sweetener); try a bulking agent ± ***loperamide*** 2mg after each loose stool; max 16mg/d; SE: colic, nausea, dizziness, constipation, bloating, ileus. Bismuth, eg De-Nol® 120mg/8h PO, has been tried (SE: dark stools).183
- *Colic/bloating:* Antispasmodics: ***mebeverine*** 135mg/8h PO (available over the counter); ***alverine citrate*** 60-120mg/8h PO; ***dicycloverine*** 10-20mg/8h PO).
- *Dyspeptic symptoms:* May respond to ***metoclopramide*** or antacids.
- *Psychological therapy:* Emphasize positive aspects and prognosis: in 50% symptoms go or improve after 1 year; <5% worsen. Symptoms are still troublesome in the rest at 5yrs. Tricyclics are often helpful, eg ***amitriptyline*** 10-50mg at night (SE: constipation, dry mouth, etc).184 185 Cognitive-behavioural therapy (*OHCS* p372), and gut-focus hypnotherapy[1] all have roles. Explain that all forms of stress (sexual, physical, or verbal abuse) perpetuate IBS.

The future Interest is being expressed in modulating the brain-gut axis by neurotransmitter manipulation. *Visceral hypersensitivity:* Those with IBS have lower visceral pain thresholds. Use of amitriptyline and SSRIs is now advocated.

1 12wks of hypnosis helps abnormal sensory perception: ►Do not think of hypnosis as dubious; it is a neat way to influence the brain-gut axis, reducing doctor dependency and stopping patients from being patients (passive recipients of suffering). Benefits may last ≥5yrs.

 (also see TABLE, p281)

Nutritional disorders

►Always consider that more than one nutritional disorder is likely to be present.

Scurvy is due to lack of vitamin C.[1] Is the patient poor, pregnant, or on an odd diet? *Signs:* **1** Listlessness, anorexia, cachexia (p29). **2** Gingivitis, loose teeth, and foul-breath (halitosis). **3** Bleeding from gums, nose, hair follicles, or into joints, bladder, gut. **4** Muscle pain/weakness. **5** Oedema.[186][187] *Diagnosis:* No test is completely satisfactory. WBC ascorbic acid↓. ℞: Dietary education; ***ascorbic acid*** ≥250mg/24h PO.

Beriberi There is heart failure with general oedema (wet beriberi) or neuropathy (dry beriberi) due to lack of vitamin B_1 (thiamine). For treatment and diagnostic tests, see Wernicke's encephalopathy (p728).

Pellagra = lack of nicotinic acid. Classical triad: **d**iarrhoea, **d**ementia, **d**ermatitis (Casal's necklace) ± neuropathy, depression, insomnia, tremor, rigidity, ataxia, fits. It may occur in carcinoid syndrome and anti-TB drugs (isoniazid). It is endemic in China and Africa. ℞: Education, electrolyte replacement, ***nicotinamide*** 100mg/4h PO.[188] See BOX.

Xerophthalmia This vitamin A deficiency syndrome is a major cause of blindness in the Tropics. Conjunctivae become dry and develop oval or triangular spots (Bitôt's spots). Corneas become cloudy and soft. See *OHCS* p450. Give ***vitamin A*** 200,000 units stat PO, repeat in 24h and a week later (halve dose if <1yr old; quarter if <6 months old); ►get special help if pregnant: vitamin A embryopathy must be avoided. Re-educate and monitor diet.

Carcinoid tumours

A diverse group of tumours of enterochromaffin cell (neural crest) origin, by definition capable of producing 5HT. Common sites: appendix (45%), ileum (30%) or rectum (20%).[2] They also occur elsewhere in the GI tract, ovary, testis, and bronchi. 80% of tumours >2cm across will metastasize (ie consider all as malignant). *Symptoms & signs:* Initially few. GI tumours can cause appendicitis, intussusception, or obstruction. Hepatic metastases may cause RUQ pain. Tumours may secrete bradykinin, tachykinin, substance P, VIP, gastrin, insulin, glucagon, ACTH (∴ Cushing's syndrome), parathyroid, and thyroid hormones. 10% are part of MEN1 syndrome (p215) and 10% occur with other neuroendocrine tumours.[189]

Carcinoid syndrome occurs in ~5% and implies hepatic involvement. *Symptoms and signs:* Bronchoconstriction; paroxysmal flushing especially in upper body (± migrating weals); diarrhoea; CCF (tricuspid incompetence and pulmonary stenosis from 5HT-induced fibrosis). *CNS effects:* Many, eg **enhanced** ability to learn new stimulus-response associations.[190] ►*Carcinoid crisis:* (see EMERGENCY BOX).

Diagnosis 24h urine 5-hydroxyindoleacetic acid↑ (5HIAA, a 5HT metabolite; levels change with drugs and diet: discuss with lab). If liver metastases are not found, try to find the primary (CXR; chest/pelvis MRI/CT). *New tests:* Plasma chromogranin A (reflects tumour mass);[191] ^{111}Indium octreotide scintigraphy (octreoscan);[192] positron emission tomography (p752) techniques are also being developed.

Treatment *Carcinoid syndrome: **Octreotide*** (somatostatin analogue) blocks release of tumour mediators and counters peripheral effects. Alternative: lanreotide. Effects lessen over time. Other options: ***loperamide*** or ***cyproheptadine*** for diarrhoea;[193] ***interferon-α*** as add-in therapy with ***octreotide***.[194] *Tumour therapy:* Resection is the only cure for carcinoid tumours (**fig 1**), so it is vital to find the primary site (see above). At surgery the tumours have an intense yellow appearance. Procedures depend on site, eg rectal carcinoid tumours <1cm can be resected endoscopically.[195] Surgical debulking (eg enucleating), embolization, or radiofrequency ablation of hepatic metastases can ↓symptoms. Give ***octreotide*** cover to avoid precipitating a massive carcinoid crisis. *Median survival:* 5–8yrs (~3yrs if metastases are present, but may be up to 20yrs; so beware of giving up too easily, even in metastatic disease).[196]

1 The link of diet (oranges and lemons) with the symptoms of 'the scurvy' is accredited to the naval surgeon James Lind, as described in his *Treatise* of 1753.

2 Some are never clinically detected: 1 in 300 autopsies have a small bowel carcinoid tumour.

Food mountains, the pellagra paradox, and the sorrow that weeping cannot symbolize[1]

'The sweet smell is a great sorrow on the land. Men who can graft the trees and make the seed fertile and big can find no way to let the hungry people eat their produce... The works of the roots of the vines, of the trees, must be destroyed to keep up the price...

There is a crime here that goes beyond denunciation. There is a sorrow here that weeping cannot symbolize. There is a failure here that topples all our success. The fertile earth, the straight tree rows, the sturdy trunks, and the ripe fruit. And children dying of pellagra must die because a profit cannot be taken from an orange. And coroners must fill in the certificates—died of malnutrition—because the food must rot, must be forced to rot.

The people come with nets to fish for potatoes in the river, and the guards hold them back; they come in rattling cars to get the dumped oranges, but the kerosene is sprayed. And they stand still and watch the potatoes float by, listen to the screaming pigs being killed in a ditch and covered with quicklime, watch the mountains of oranges slop down to a putrefying ooze; and in the eyes of the people there is a failure; and in the eyes of the hungry there is a growing wrath. In the souls of the people the grapes of wrath are filling and growing heavy, growing heavy for the vintage.'

How do John Steinbeck's grapes grow in our 21st century soil? Too well; a double harvest, it turns out, as not only is much of the world starving, amid plenty (for those who can pay) but there is a new 'sorrow in our land that weeping cannot symbolize': pathological 'voluntary' **self-starvation**, again amid plenty, in pursuit of the body-beautiful according to images laid down by media gods. If gastroenterologists had one wish it might not be the ending of all their diseases, but that humankind stand in a right relationship with Steinbeck's fertile earth, his straight trees, his sturdy trunks, and his ripe fruit.

Whipple's procedure

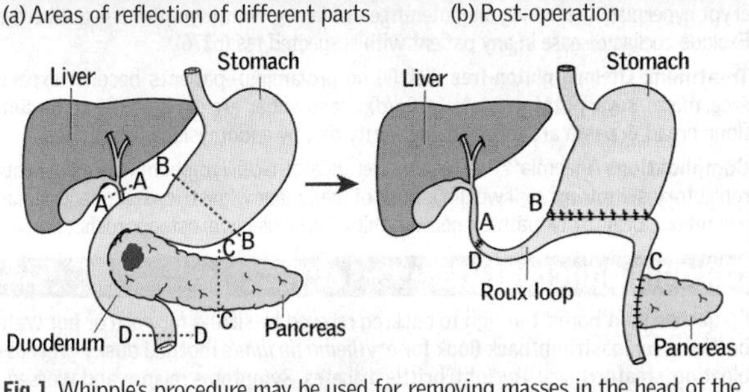

Fig 1. Whipple's procedure may be used for removing masses in the head of the pancreas—typically from pancreatic carcinoma, or rarely, a carcinoid tumour. 197

Carcinoid crisis

When a tumour outgrows its blood supply or is handled too much during surgery, mediators flood out. There is life-threatening vasodilatation, hypotension, tachycardia, bronchoconstriction and hyperglycaemia. It is treated with high-dose *octreotide*, supportive measures and careful management of fluid balance (ie a central line is needed—see p789 for insertion technique).

1 J Steinbeck *The Grapes of Wrath*, chapter 25.

Causes—see BOX 1

Symptoms Diarrhoea; ↓weight; lethargy; steatorrhoea (stool fat↑; hard to flush away).

Deficiency signs Anaemia (↓Fe, B_{12}, folate); bleeding disorders (↓vit K); oedema (↓protein); metabolic bone disease (↓vit D); neurological features, eg neuropathy.

Tests FBC (↓ or ↑MCV); ↓Ca^{2+}; ↓Fe; ↓B_{12} + folate; ↑INR; lipid profile; coeliac tests (below). *Stool:* Sudan stain for fat globules; stool microscopy (infestation); α1AT (p642), elastase. *Barium follow-through:* Diverticula; Crohn's; radiation enteritis. *Breath hydrogen analysis:* for bacterial overgrowth. Take samples of end-expired air; give glucose; take more samples at ½h intervals; ↑exhaled hydrogen = overgrowth. *Endoscopy + small bowel biopsy, ERCP:* (p756) biliary obstruction; chronic pancreatitis. **Causes** See BOX. **Tropical malabsorption** (*Giardia, Cryptosporidium parvum, Isospora belli, Cyclospora cayetanensis*, microsporidia.) *Tropical sprue:* Villous atrophy+malabsorption occurring in the Far and Middle East and Caribbean—the cause is unknown. *Tetracycline* 250mg/6h PO + *folic acid* 15mg/d PO + optimum nutrition may help. 198

Coeliac disease

►Suspect this in all those with diarrhoea + weight loss or anaemia. This is a T-cell mediated autoimmune disease of the small bowel in which prolamin (alcohol-soluble proteins in wheat, barley, rye ± oats) intolerance causes villous atrophy and malabsorption.[1] *Associations:* HLA DQ2 in 95%; the rest are DQ8; autoimmune disease; dermatitis herpetiformis. *Prevalence:* 1 in 300-1500 (more common in Irish). Occurs at any age (peaks in infancy and 50-60yrs). ♀:♂ >1:1. There is a 10% prevalence in 1st degree relatives and a 30% relative risk for siblings.

Presentation: Steatorrhoea; diarrhoea; abdominal pain; bloating; nausea + vomiting; aphthous ulcers, angular stomatitis; weight↓; fatigue; weakness; iron-deficiency anaemia; osteomalacia; failure to thrive (children). ⅓ are asymptomatic.

Diagnosis Antibodies: α-gliadin, transglutaminase & anti-endomysial—an IgA antibody, 95% specific unless patient is IgA-deficient. Duodenal biopsy done at endoscopy (p256—as good as jejunal biopsy if ≥4 taken): subtotal villous atrophy, ↑ intra-epithelial WBCs + crypt hyperplasia, **reversing** on gluten-free diet (along with ↓symptoms & antibodies). Exclude coeliac disease in any patient with suspected IBS (p276).

Treatment Lifelong gluten-free diet (ie no prolamins)—patients become experts. Rice, maize, soya, potatoes, oats (≤50g/d), 199 and sugar are OK. Gluten-free biscuits, flour, bread, & pasta are prescribable. Verify diet by endomysial antibody tests.

Complications Anaemia; 2° lactose-intolerance; GI T-cell lymphoma (rare; suspect if refractory symptoms or ↓weight); ↑risk of malignancy (gastric, oesophageal, bladder, breast, brain); myopathies; neuropathies; hyposplenism; osteoporosis.

Chronic pancreatitis

Epigastric pain 'bores' through to back, eg relieved by sitting forward or hot water bottles on epigastrium/back (look for *erythema ab igne*'s mottled dusky greyness); bloating; steatorrhoea; ↓weight; brittle diabetes. Symptoms relapse and worsen.

Causes: Alcohol; rarely: familial; cystic fibrosis; haemochromatosis; pancreatic duct obstruction (stones/tumour); ↑PTH; congenital (*pancreas divisum*). **Tests** *Ultrasound* (eg pseudocyst, p639) ± *CT* (pancreatic calcifications confirm the diagnosis), *MRCP* + *ERCP* (risks acute attack); *AXR:* speckled pancreatic calcification; ↑glucose; breath tests eg ^{13}C-hiolien. 200 **Treatment** *Drugs:* Give analgesia (coeliac-plexus block may give brief relief); 201 *lipase*, eg Creon®; fat-soluble vitamins (eg Multivite®). Insulin needs may be high or variable (beware hypoglycaemia). *Diet:* No alcohol; low fat may help. Medium-chain triglycerides (MCT oil®) may be tried (no lipase needed for absorption, but diarrhoea may be worsened). *Surgery:* For unremitting pain; narcotic abuse (beware of this); weight↓: eg pancreatectomy or pancreaticojejunostomy (a duct drainage procedure). **Complications** Pseudocyst; diabetes; biliary obstruction; local arterial aneurysm; splenic vein thrombosis; gastric varices; pancreatic carcinoma.

Causes of gastrointestinal malabsorption

Common in the UK
- Coeliac disease
- Chronic pancreatitis
- Crohn's disease

Rarer
- ↓*Bile:* PBC; ileal resection; biliary obstruction; colestyramine.
- *Pancreatic insufficiency:* Pancreatic cancer; cystic fibrosis.
- *Small bowel mucosa:* Whipple's disease (p730); tropical sprue; radiation enteritis; small bowel resection; brush border enzyme deficiencies (eg lactase insufficiency); drugs (metformin, neomycin, alcohol); amyloid (p364).
- *Bacterial overgrowth:* Spontaneous (esp. in elderly); in jejunal diverticula; post-op blind loops. PPI treatment and DM are also risk factors. Try *metronidazole* 400mg/8h PO or *oxytetracycline* 250mg/6h.
- *Infection:* Giardiasis; diphyllobothriasis (B_{12} malabsorption); strongyloidiasis.
- *Intestinal hurry:* Post-gastrectomy dumping; post-vagotomy; gastrojejunostomy.

Deficiency syndromes and the sites of nutrient absorption

Nutrient	Site of absorption	Deficiency syndrome
Vitamin		
A^F	Small intestine	Xerophthalmia (p278)
B_1 (thiamine)	Small intestine	Beriberi (p278); Wernicke's encephalopathy (p728)
B_2 (riboflavin)	Proximal small intestine	Angular stomatis; cheilitis (p238)
B_6 (pyridoxine)	Small intestine	Polyneuropathy
B_{12}	Terminal ileum	Macrocytic anaemia (p326); neuropathy; glossitis
C	Proximal ileum	Scurvy (p278)
D^F	Jejunum as free vitamin	Rickets (p698); osteomalacia (p698)
E^F	Small intestine	Haemolysis; neurological deficit
K^F	Small intestine	Bleeding disorders (p328)
Folic acid	Jejunum	Macrocytic anaemia (p326)
Nicotinamide	Jejunum	Pellagra (p278)
Mineral		
Calcium	Duodenum + jejunum	p690
Copper	Stomach + Jejunum	Menkes' kinky hair syndrome
Fluoride	Stomach	Dental caries
Iodide	Small intestine	Goitre; cretinism
Iron	Duodenum + jejunum	Microcytic anaemia (p320)
Magnesium	Small intestine	p692
Phosphate	Small intestine	Osteoporosis; anorexia; weakness
Selenium	Small intestine	Cardiomyopathy (p693)
Zinc	Jejunum	Acrodermatitis enteropathica; poor wound healing

F = fat-soluble vitamin, thus deficiency is likely if there is fat malabsorption.

1 Infectious aetiological agents have been implicated: eg *Candida albicans* could be one trigger. HWP1 has amino acid sequences identical to coeliac disease-related α-gliadin T-cell epitopes.

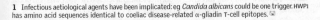

Alcoholism

An alcoholic is one whose repeated drinking leads to harm in his work or social life. It is common (~25%), ranging from binge drinking to heavy daily intake, and is usually tied in with other life or health issues. Other addictions may also be involved. ►Denial is a leading feature of alcoholism, so be sure to question relatives. Benefits of low dose alcohol (eg <20U/wk in men, <15U/wk in women, see p236) are unproven.

CAGE questions Ever felt you ought to cut down on your drinking? Have people annoyed you by criticizing your drinking? Ever felt bad or guilty about your drinking? Ever had an eye-opener to steady nerves in the morning? CAGE (yes to ≥2) is quite good at detecting alcohol abuse and dependence (sensitivity 43-94%; specificity 70-97%),[202] but accuracy does change according to background population. There are several other screening methods: eg TWEAK (see BOX 1); AUDIT.[203]

Organs affected (►Don't forget the risk of trauma whilst intoxicated.)[204]
The liver: Normal in 50%; γGT↑ or ↑↑ (but may be ↑ in any condition that causes liver inflammation, eg AIH (p268), HBV). *Fatty liver:* Acute and reversible, but may progress to cirrhosis if drinking continues (also seen in obesity, DM, and with amiodarone). *Alcoholic hepatitis:* see BOX 2 & 3. 80% progress to cirrhosis (hepatic failure in 10%). *Cirrhosis* (p260): 5yr survival is 48% if drinking continues (if not, 77%). *Biopsy:* Mallory bodies ± neutrophil infiltrate (can be indistinguishable from NASH, p261).
CNS: Poor memory/cognition: multiple high-potency vitamins IM may reverse it; cortical atrophy; retrobulbar neuropathy; fits; falls; wide-based gait neuropathy; confabulation; Korsakoff's (p718) ± Wernicke's encephalopathy (p728).
GI tract: Obesity; diarrhoea; gastric erosions; peptic ulcers; varices (p254); pancreatitis (acute and chronic); carcinoma; oral mucosal lesions.
Blood: MCV↑; anaemia from: marrow depression, GI bleeding, alcoholism-associated folate deficiency, haemolysis; sideroblastic anaemia. See p320.
Heart: Arrhythmias; BP↑; cardiomyopathy; sudden death in binge drinkers.

Withdrawal starts 10-72h after last drink. *Signs:* Pulse↑; BP↓; tremor; confusion; fits; hallucinations (*delirium tremens*)—may be visual or tactile, eg animals crawling all over skin. Consider it in any new (≤3d) ward patient with acute confusion.

Alcohol contraindications Driving; hepatitis; cirrhosis; peptic ulcer; drugs (eg antihistamines, metronidazole); carcinoid; pregnancy (fetal alcohol syndrome—IQ↓, short palpebral fissure, absent philtrum, and small eyes).

Management *Alcohol withdrawal:* Admit; do BP + TPR/4h. Beware BP↓. For the 1st 3d give generous ***chlordiazepoxide***, eg 10-50mg/6h PO, weaning over 7-14d (see TABLE 2); alternative: ***diazepam***; the once-preferred ***clomethiazole*** readily causes addiction. Vitamins may be needed (p728). ***Prevention:*** (*OHCS* p513): Alcohol-free beers; low-risk drinking (see below), remembering that there are no absolutes and that risk is a continuum. *1U≈9g ethanol≈1 spirits measure ≈1glass wine≈½pint beer.* ***Treating established alcoholics*** may be rewarding, particularly if they really want to change. If so, **group therapy** or **self-help** (eg 'Alcoholics Anonymous') may be useful—especially if self-initiated and determined. Encourage the will to change. ***Suggest:*** **1** Graceful ways of declining a drink, eg "I'm seeing what it's like to go without for a bit". **2** not buying him- or herself a drink when it is his/her turn. **3** "Don't lift your glass to your lips until after the slowest drinker in your group takes a drink". **4** "Sip, don't gulp". Give follow-up and encouragement.

Relapse 50% will relapse soon after starting treatment. ***Acamprosate*** (p455)[205] may help intense anxiety, insomnia, and craving. CI: pregnancy, severe liver failure, creatinine >120μmol/L. SE: D&V, libido ↑ or ↓; dose example: 666mg/8h PO if >60kg and <65yrs old.[206] It should be started as soon as acute withdrawal is complete and continued for ~1yr. ***Disulfiram*** can be used to treat chronic alcohol dependence. It causes acetaldehyde build-up (like metronidazole) with extremely unpleasant effects to **any** alcohol ingestion—eg flushing, throbbing headache, palpitations. Care must be taken to avoid alcohol (eg toiletries, food, medicines) since severe reactions can occur. ►Confer with experts if drugs are to be used.

TWEAK screening questions[207]

• Have you an increased tolerance of alcohol?	2 points
• Do you worry about your drinking?	2 points
• Have you ever had alcohol as an eye-opener in the morning?	1 point
• Do you ever get amnesia after drinking alcohol?	1 point
• Have you ever felt the need to c(k)ut down on your drinking?	1 point

A score of ≥2 suggests an alcohol problem. It may be more sensitive than the CAGE questionnaire in some populations (eg pregnant women).[208]

Patterns of lab tests in alcoholic and other liver disease

	AST	ALT	AST : ALT	MCV
Alcoholic liver disease	↑↑	↑	>2	↑↑
Hepatitis C (HCV)	↑ or ↔	↑↑	<1*	↔
Non-alcoholic fatty liver disease	↑	↑↑	<1	↑ or ↔

*ratio may reverse if cirrhosis develops. See p742 for reference intervals.

Managing alcoholic hepatitis [209 210]

Clinical picture TPR↑; anorexia; D&V; tender hepatomegaly ± jaundice; bleeding; ascites. *Bloods:* WCC↑; INR↓; AST↑; MCV↑; urea↑. ►Severe hepatitis is indicated by jaundice, encephalopathy and coagulopathy.

- Majority of patients must be hospitalised.
- Screen for infections ± ascitic fluid tap and treating for SBP (p260).
- Stop alcohol consumption: for withdrawal symptoms, if *chlordiazepoxide* by the oral route is impossible, try *lorazepam* IM.
- High-dose B vitamins IV as *Pabrinex®*—1 pair of ampoules in 50mL 0.9% saline IVI over ½h; (see Datasheet)—have resuscitation equipment to hand.
- Optimize nutrition (35–40kcal/kg/d non-protein energy). Use ideal body weight for calculations, eg if malnourished.
- A low-protein diet *should not* be given even if severe encephalopathy is present. Give 1.5g/kg/d of protein. This prevents encephalopathy, sepsis, and some deaths.
- Daily weight; LFT; U&E; INR. If creatinine↑, get help with this—HRS (p259). Na^+↓ is common, but water restriction may make matters worse.

Give steroids to patients with a Maddrey score >32 and/or encephalopathy (Maddrey Discriminant Factor (DF) = (4.6 × PT-control time) + [bilirubin] (in μmol/L)). ►exclude sepsis before initiation of steroids: eg prednisolone 40mg/d for 5d tapered off over 3 weeks. The DF score roughly reflects mortality, see below. *Prognosis:* Mild episodes often resolve with no affect on mortality. Severe hepatitis can have a 30d mortality of 50%, reduced to 5% if only mild. ►At 1 year after an admission for alcoholic hepatitis, 40% are dead, a sobering thought.

An example of a chlordiazepoxide-reducing regimen

Day	AM	noon	PM	At night	total/d
1	20mg	20mg	20mg	20mg	80mg
2	20mg	15mg	15mg	20mg	70mg
3	15mg	15mg	15mg	15mg	60mg
4	15mg	10mg	10mg	15mg	50mg
5	10mg	10mg	10mg	10mg	40mg
6	10mg	5mg	5mg	10mg	30mg
7	5mg	5mg	5mg	5mg	20mg
8	5mg	-	-	5mg	10mg
9	-	-	-	5mg	5mg
10	-	-	-	-	discontinue

►*Caveats:* doses may need to be higher for the 1st few days for severe withdrawal; there may still be mild withdrawal symptoms at day 3. Have a 5mg dose written for PRN use.

7 Renal medicine

Contents

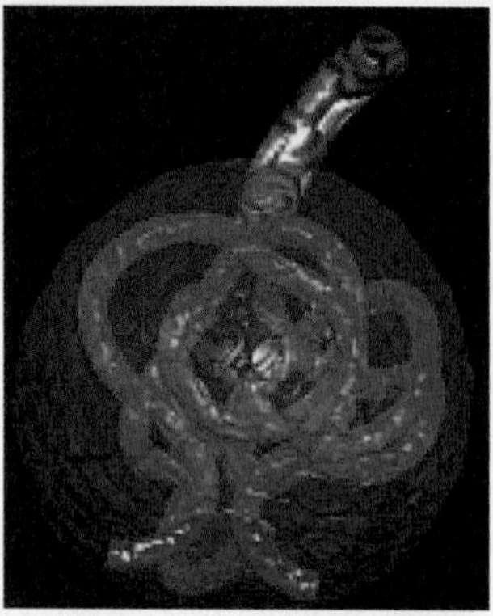

Fig 1. Electron microscope image of arterioles in a glomerulus. (Courtesy of Dr Roger Wagner) Its shape reminds us of the explosive ethical and biological controversies in renal medicine:
- How to estimate glomerular filtration rates reliably (p683)
- Withdrawing dialysis at life's end (p304)
- Managing consent in kidney donors (p305)
- How to pay for new cancer drugs (p10)
- In choosing who gets which renal service, who is more equal than whom? (p315)

Relevant pages in other chapters: Symptoms and signs: Frequency (p64); loin pain (p57); oedema (p29); oliguria (p65); polyuria (p65).

Surgery: Renal & urological ca (p646); urinary retention (p644); incontinence (p650).
Clinical chemistry: Kidney function (p682); ►Creatinine clearance and eGFR (p683); Urate and the kidney (p694).
Emergencies: Management of acute renal failure: p848.

Also: Vasculitis (p558); polyarteritis nodosa (p558); urological cancers (p646); genitourinary TB (p293); immunosuppressives (p370); biochemistry of renal function (p682); electrolyte physiology (p688); Na^+ (p666 & p686); K^+ (p688); calcium (p690); urate and the kidney (p694); osteomalacia (p698); urinary tract imaging (p758); catheters (p776).

In OHCS: Gynaecological urology (*OHCS* p306); bacteriuria and pyelonephritis in pregnancy (*OHCS* p28); obstetric causes of acute tubular necrosis (*OHCS* p28); chronic renal disease in pregnancy (*OHCS* p28); UTI in children (*OHCS* p174); urethral valves (*OHCS* p132); horseshoe kidney (*OHCS* p132); ectopic kidney (*OHCS* p132); hypospadias (*OHCS* p132); Wilms' nephroblastoma (*OHCS* p133); renal failure in children (*OHCS* p176); nephritis and nephrosis in children (*OHCS* p178); Potter's syndrome (*OHCS* p132).

We thank Dr Andrew Mooney who is our Specialist Reader for this chapter.

Renal disease typically presents with one or more of rather a short list of clinical syndromes—listed from 1 to 7 below. One underlying pathology may have a variety of clinical presentations, and vice versa.

1 *Proteinuria:* Normal protein excretion is <150mg/day, as the glomerular basement membrane prevents passage of high-molecular-weight proteins (eg albumin) into urine. Heavy proteinuria (>3g/d) is almost always a sign of glomerular disease.

2 *Haematuria:* Blood in the urine may arise from anywhere in the renal tract. Take haematuria seriously, as it may be the only sign of GU malignancy (esp if >40yrs old and a smoker). However, in the majority of cases it has a benign cause (eg infection, renal stones). The question of who to refer haematuria patients to (urologist or nephrologist) is answered on p286.

3 *Renal pain and dysuria:* **Renal pain** is usually a dull and constant and in the loin. It may be due to renal obstruction (look for swelling ± tenderness), pyelonephritis, acute nephritic syndrome, polycystic kidneys, or renal infarction. **Renal (ureteric) colic** is severe waxing and waning loin pain radiating to groin or thigh, eg with fever and vomiting. It is caused by a renal stone, clot, or a sloughed papilla. **Urinary frequency** with **dysuria** (pain on voiding) suggests a UTI.

4 *Oligiuria and polyuria:* **Oliguria** is a urine output of <0.5mL/kg/hr. *Pathological causes*: renal perfusion↓, renal parenchymal disease, renal tract obstruction. **Polyuria** is the voiding of abnormally high volumes of urine, usually from high fluid intake—or diabetes mellitus, diabetes insipidus (p232), hypercalcaemia, renal medulla disorders (urine concentration is impaired), and SVT (p120).

5 *Acute renal failure (ARF)* is significant decline in renal function occurring over hours or days, detected by a rising plasma creatinine (± oliguria). ARF usually occurs secondary to a circulatory dysfunction (hypotension, hypovolaemia, sepsis) or urinary obstruction. Primary renal disease is a less common cause.

6 *Chronic renal failure (CRF)* **or chronic kidney disease (CKD)** is defined as irreversible, substantial, and long-standing loss of renal function. It is classified according to glomerular filtration rate (GFR): see p683. There is often a poor correlation between symptoms and severity of renal disease. Progression may be so insidious that patients attribute symptoms to age or a minor illnesses. **Some guidelines advise nephrology referral if CKD stage ≥3** (p300),[2] ie GFR <60mL/min, *if other features are present:* • GFR is falling progressively • Microscopic haematuria • Urine protein:creatinine ratio (PCR)↑, p286 • Unexplained anaemia, hyperkalaemia, or calcium or phosphate imbalance • Suspected systemic illness (eg SLE) • BP uncontrolled despite taking 3 drugs. Refer *urgently* if GFR 15–29 (same-day if <15) even if *no* other features present.

7 *Silence:* Serious renal failure may cause **no symptoms at all**. This is why we do U&Es before surgery and other major interventions. The silence of renal disease creeps up on us (doctors and patients)—with uncanny stealth which is as alarming as the image in **fig 2**—'Silence', by Tiago Phelipe. This picture serves to remind us not to dismiss odd chronic symptoms such as fatigue or 'not being quite with it'—without doing a blood test. *Microalbuminuria* is a famously silent harbinger of serious renal and cardiovascular risk. It is described on p314. In one study, 30% of those with type 2 diabetes mellitus died within ~5 years of developing microalbuminuria. This is partly preventable by use of ACE-i.

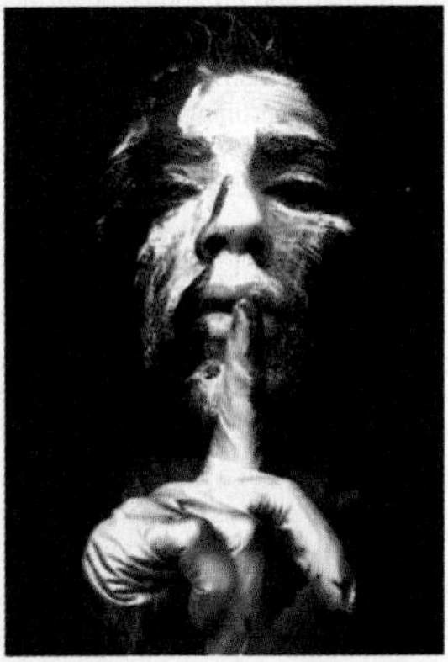

Fig 2. Silence. Courtesy of Tiago Phelipe.

Examine mid-stream urine (MSU) whenever you suspect renal disease.

Haematuria Blood in the urine may arise from anywhere in the renal tract. It may be *macroscopic* (visible to the naked eye) or *microscopic* (found on dipstick testing or presence of ≥3 RBCs per high-power field on microscopic evaluation of urinary sediment. Always confirm by repeating the test).[3] It may also happen after viral diseases or vigorous exercise. *Renal causes:* Neoplasia, glomerulonephritis (often IgA nephropathy, p294), tubulointerstitial nephritis, polycystic kidney, papillary necrosis, infection (pyelonephritis), trauma. *Extrarenal:* Calculi, infection (cystitis, prostatitis, urethritis), neoplasia (bladder, prostate, urethra), trauma (eg from catheter).
Management: Take a thorough history:
Painless haematuria is more ominous, eg bladder or other GU cancer or glomerulonephritis (GN). Some drugs can cause haematuria: eg, captopril, cephalosporins, ciprofloxacin, furosemide, NSAIDs, aspirin.[4] Assess BP, urine MC&S, FBC, ESR, CRP, clotting, RBC morphology, proteinuria, U&E, GFR, risk factors for renal tract cancer (smoking, compound analgesic use, industrial toxin exposure, age >50 years). *Others:* AXR/KUB, p640 (stones), urine cytology.
Haematuria + dysuria is usually from a UTI. • Isolated microscopic haematuria, age <40 years-old, no proteinuria, normal GFR: 'observe and review' may be sufficient. • Haematuria and proteinuria, RBC casts, dysmorphic cells or ↓GFR: this often indicates serious renal disease. Do renal ultrasound (US) and refer to a nephrologist. A kidney biopsy may be needed • Haematuria and cancer risk factor (eg age >50): do renal US ±IVP (intravenous pyelography) and refer to a urologist.[5] US does not expose patients to IV contrast media; however, subtle findings in the renal collecting system may be difficult to detect by US.[6] Not all women with recurrent UTI + haematuria need cystoscopy, but have a good reason *not* to do cystoscopy (Reynard's rule).[7]

Proteinuria Normal protein excretion is <150mg/d, consisting of <30mg/d of albumin. This may rise to ~300mg/d—eg orthostatic proteinuria (related to posture), during fever, or after exercise. ***Causes:*** Glomerular or tubular disease (eg *nephrotic syndrome,* p512), DM, amyloidosis. ↑BP, interstitial nephritis, heavy metals, multiple myeloma (though dipsticks do not detect light chains), pregnancy, CCF. Dipstick detects albumin and is less sensitive to globulins or Bence-Jones proteins. The sulfosalicylic acid turbidity test qualitatively screens for proteinuria and has greater sensitivity for Bence Jones proteins.[8] *Estimation of proteinuria:* 24h urine collection for protein and creatinine quantifies proteinuria *if* collected accurately: spot tests for urine albumin:creatinine ratio or urine protein : creatinine index are much easier and provide reasonably accurate information (albumin:creatinine ratio is preferred to protein:creatinine ratio, esp in diabetics[9]). ***Microalbuminuria:*** Ultra-sensitive dipsticks are now available to measure microalbuminuria (albumin excretion 30-300mg/24h). ***Causes:*** DM, ↑BP, minimal change GN.

Other substances:

Glucose DM, low renal threshold, pregnancy, sepsis, renal tubular damage. ***Ketones:*** Starvation, ketoacidosis. ***Leucocytes:*** UTI, vaginal discharge. ***Nitrites:*** UTI, high-protein meal. ***Bilirubin:*** Obstructive jaundice. ***Urobilinogen:*** Pre-hepatic jaundice. ***Specific gravity:*** Normal range: 1.000-1.030 (useful to assess degree of proteinuria or haematuria). ***pH:*** Normal range: 4.5-8 (acid-base balance: p684).

Microscopy Put a drop of fresh urine (MSU or suprapubic aspirate) on a microscope slide, cover with a coverslip and examine under low (×100) and high (×400) power for leucocytes, red cells, bacteria, casts and crystals. If renal disease is suspected, a centrifuged urine should be examined. See p290 for more details and images.

24h urine for Na^+, K^+, Ca^{2+}, urea, creatinine ± protein excretion. Take blood simultaneously for creatinine to calculate creatinine clearance (p683; eGFR may mislead).

Urinalysis

Using dipsticks Store dipsticks in a closed container in a cool, dry place, not refrigerated. If improperly stored, or past expiry date, do not use. For urine tests, dip the dipstick briefly in urine, run edge of strip along container and hold strip horizontally. **Read at the specified time**—check instructions for the type of stick. For haematuria, proteinuria, etc., see p286.

Urine specific gravity (SG) can be measured by dipstick. It is not a good measure of osmolality. Causes of low SG (<1.003): diabetes insipidus, renal failure. Causes of high SG (>1.025): diabetes mellitus, adrenal insufficiency, liver disease, heart failure, acute water loss. Hydrometers underestimate SG by 0.001 per 3°C above 16°C.

Sources of error in interpreting dipstick results

Bilirubin: False +ve: phenothiazines. False -ve: urine not fresh, rifampicin.

Urobilinogen: False -ve: urine not fresh. Normally present in urine due to metabolism of bilirubin in the gut by bacteria and subsequent absorption. Excess may give a false +ve test for prophobilinogen.

Ketones: L-dopa affects colour (can give false +ve). 3-hydroxybutyrate gives a false negative result.

Blood:
False-positive dipstick haematuria: haemoglobinuria, dehydration, myoglobinuria (eg in rhabdomyolysis), porphyria, phenindione, phenolphthalein, or contamination with menstrual blood.
False-negative: low urinary pH, air-exposed dipsticks.

Urine glucose: Depends on test. Pads with glucose oxidase are not affected by other reducing sugars (unlike Clinitest®) but can give false +ve to peroxide, chlorine; and false -ve with ascorbic acid, salicylate, L-dopa.

Protein:
False positive: urine pH>7.5; concentrated urine; gross haematuria; presence of penicillin, sulphonamides, pus, semen or vaginal secretions.
False negative: dilute urine; non-albumin urinary proteins.

Blood glucose: Sticks use enzymatic method and are glucose specific. A major source of error is applying too little blood (a large drop to cover the pad is necessary), and poor timing. Reflectance meters increase precision but introduce new sources of error.

Adrift on the miraculous stream [10]

Only doctors, toddlers and poets have the earthiness to enjoy unselfconsciously the act and organs of micturition. James Joyce, for example, explicitly associates micturition with poetic creativity.[11] His most amusing book, *Finnegans Wake*, is a (mid-) stream-of-consciousness poem, born of a primordial lad wetting his widdle into rivering waters.[1] But most patients are far more furtive in bringing to us their offerings of gold, amber, and straw. So offer a hand to get the sample right:

- Aim to get a sample from the middle contents of your bladder (waste the 1st bit).
- Women: hold open your labia. Men: roll back your foreskin: it will not be needed.
- Pass some urine into the toilet.
- Then, without hesitation, deviate the stream into the sterile bottle provided.
- No touching the voided sample or the mouth of the bottle.
- Don't be too overflowing or too mean (but a little tiddle is better than nothing).
- If it all goes wrong, or the voiding is null, have a drink, and start again.

1 "Before he fell hill he filled heaven: a stream, alplapping streamlet, coyly coiled um, cool of her curls: We were but thermites then, wee, wee...If Dann's dane, Ann's dirty, if he's plane she's purty, if he's fane, she's flirty, with her auburnt streams, and her coy cajoleries, and her dabblin drolleries, for to rouse his rudderup, or to drench his dreams". *Finnegans Wake.*

Carbonic anhydrase inhibitors: eg *Acetazolamide*. They inhibit the action of carbonic anhydrase in the proximal convoluted tubule. *Effects:* The major renal effect is bicarbonate excretion. *Clinical use:* Reducing intra-ocular pressure (treatment of glaucoma), prevention of high altitude (acute mountain) sickness (by inducing CNS, acidosis and hyperventilation). *Side effects:* Drowsiness, paraesthesias. Alkalinisation of urine may cause precipitation of calcium salts and formation of renal stones. Patients with hepatic impairment may develop hepatic encephalopathy. They can also cause hyperkalaemic metabolic acidosis.

Loop diuretics eg *furosemide, torasemide, bumetanide*. They inhibit the co-transport of $Na^+/K^+/2Cl^-$ in the thick ascending limb of the loop of Henle. Diuresis usually occurs about 4h after a dose. *Effects:* Massive NaCl excretion. Calcium excretion is also increased. *Clinical use:* Treatment of oedema (heart failure, ascites) and, particularly, acute pulmonary oedema. They can also be used in treating severe hypercalcaemia. *Side effects:* Hypokalaemic metabolic alkalosis (because of K^+ and H^+ excretion), hypovolaemia, ototoxicity, allergic reactions.

Thiazide diuretics eg ***bendroflumethiazide, chlortalidone, cyclopenthiazide, indapamide, metolazone***. Their action begins within 1-2 hours after oral use, and lasts for 12-24 hours. They inhibit NaCl transport in distal convoluted tubule. *Effects:* Moderate sodium and chloride excretion. They result in low urine calcium by increasing urinary calcium resorption (the opposite effect of loop diuretics). *Clinical use:* Hypertension, chronic therapy for oedematous conditions (eg heart failure). They can also control chronic renal stone formation because of their ability to decrease urine calcium concentrations. *Side effects:* Hyponatraemia, K^+ wasting, hyperglycaemia, increased serum lipid and uric acid levels (thiazide diuretics are contra-indicated in gout).

Potassium-sparing diuretics *Spironolactone* and *eplerenone* are aldosterone antagonists. *Amiloride* and *triamterene* block sodium channels in collecting tubules. *Effects:* they increase sodium excretion and decrease K^+ and H^+ excretion. *Clinical use:* they are usually used to control the K^+ wasting caused by chronic therapy with loop diuretics or thiazides. Spironolactone and eplerenone have significant long-term benefits in aldosteronism (↑ serum aldosterone, which occurs in cirrhosis and heart failure). *Side effects:* Hyperkalaemia, anti-androgenic effects (eg gynaecomastia) especially with spironolactone.

Osmotic diuretics: *Mannitol* is freely filtered at the glomerulus but poorly reabsorbed from the tubule. Therefore, it remains in the lumen and holds water by osmotic effect. *Effects:* Mannitol can reduce brain volume and intracranial pressure by osmotically extracting water from the tissue into the blood. *Clinical use:* Haemolysis, rhabdomyolysis, reducing intra-ocular and intra-cranial pressures. *Side effects:* ↓Na^+, pulmonary oedema, headache, nausea, vomiting.

1 Principle source: Katzung & Trevor's Pharmacology: Examination & Board Review (7th Ed). Authors: Trevor AJ, Katzung BG and Masters SB. McGraw-Hill Medical. 2004.

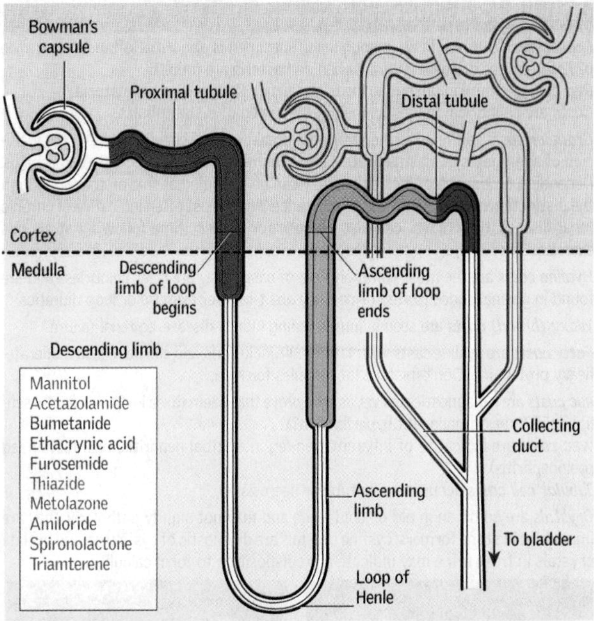

Fig 1. The nephron and major transport mechanisms in it.

Proximal convoluted tubule This segment reabsorbs amino acids, glucose, and numerous cations. It is also responsible for 60-70% of the total reabsorption of Na^+. Bicarbonate is reabsorbed by means of the enzyme carbonic anhydrase; this process can be inhibited by carbonic anhydrase inhibitors (eg acetazolamide). Some drugs that are used in treating gout affect uric acid transport in this segment.

Thick ascending limb of the loop of Henle $Na^+/K^+/2Cl^-$ co-transporter (which is the target of loop diuretics) acts in this segment. It is also a major site of calcium and Mg reabsorption. 20-30% of the filtered sodium is reabsorbed in this segment.

Distal convoluted tubule 5-8% of sodium reabsorption occurs in this segment. Calcium is also reabsorbed in this segment under the control of PTH.

Cortical collecting tubule In this segment Na^+ is reabsorbed accompanied by an equivalent excretion of K^+ or H^+ ions into urine. Therefore this segment is the main site of urine acidification and K^+ excretion. This is also the site of action of the potassium-sparing diuretics.

Leucocytes: >10/mm^3 in an unspun urine specimen is abnormal, often from UTI, see p292 for causes of sterile pyuria (when no bacteria are found).
Red cells: >2/mm^3 in unspun urine is abnormal. *Causes:* See haematuria.
Casts are cylindrical bodies formed in the lumen of distal tubules.

Granular casts can result either from the breakdown of cellular casts or the inclusion of aggregates of plasma proteins (eg albumin) or immunoglobulin light chains. Depending on the size of inclusions, they can be classified as fine or coarse, though the distinction has no diagnostic significance. While most often indicative of chronic renal disease, these casts can also be seen for a short time following strenuous exercise.

Hyaline casts are the most common type of casts. They are clear, colourless and are found in normal concentrated urine. They are ↑ in fever, exercise or loop diuretics.

Waxy (broad) casts are seen in longstanding kidney disease, eg renal failure.

Fatty casts are hyaline casts with fat globule inclusions, and can be seen in moderate-heavy proteinuria. Don't mistake fat globules for RBCs.

RBC casts are a diagnostic marvel, as they *prove* that haematuria is glomerular (vasculitis (p558), GN, or malignant hypertension?).
WBC casts are indicative of inflammation (eg interstitial nephritis) or infection (eg pyelonephritis).
Tubular cell casts occur in acute tubular necrosis.

Crystals are common in old or cold urine and may not signify pathology. They are important in stone formers: cystine crystals are diagnostic of cystinuria, and oxalate crystals in fresh urine may indicate a predisposition to form calculi.

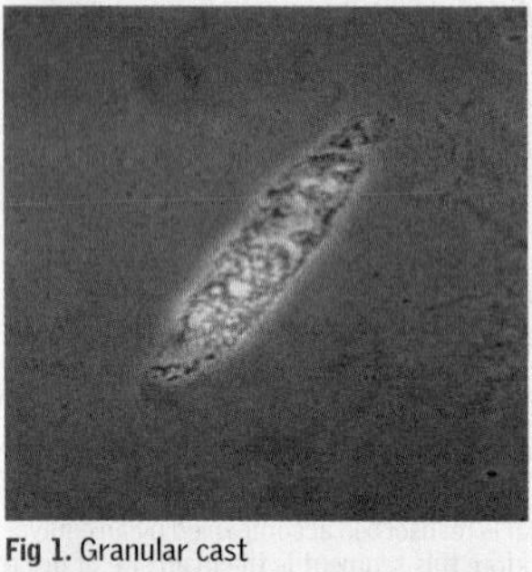

Fig 1. Granular cast

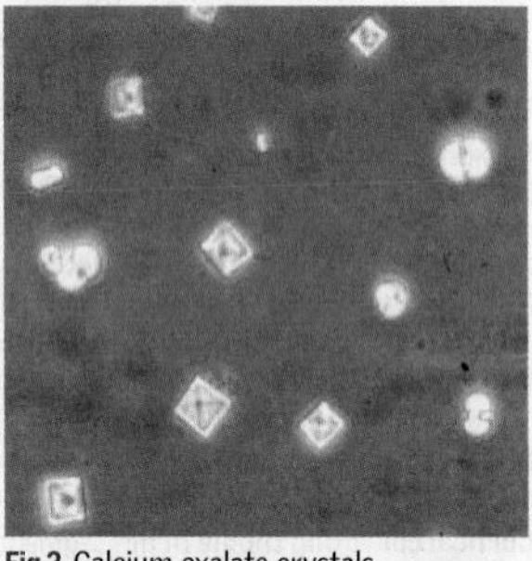

Fig 2. Calcium oxalate crystals

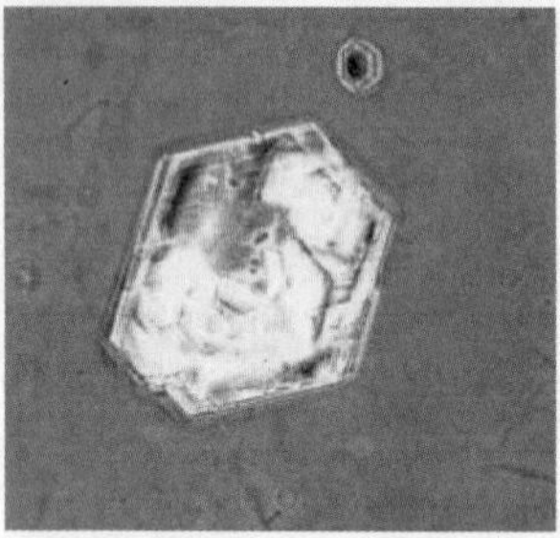

Fig 3. Cystine crystals

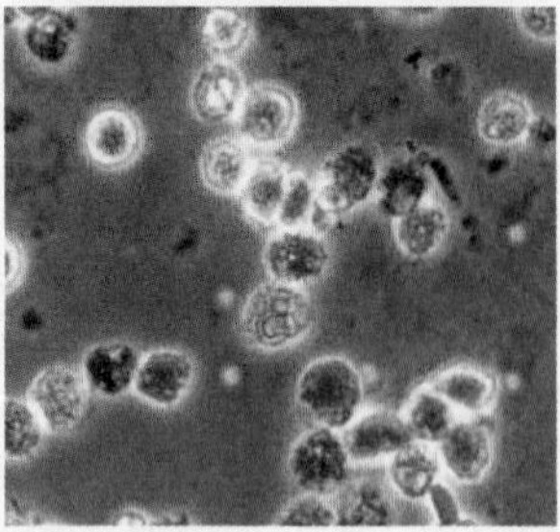

Fig 4. White cells

Figures 1-12 reproduced from Davison et al, *Oxford Textbook of Clinical Nephrology*, 3rd edition, with permission from Oxford University Press.

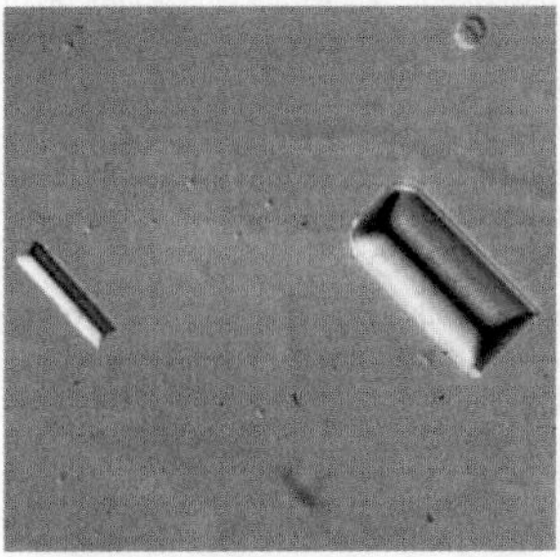

Fig 5. Triple phosphate crystals

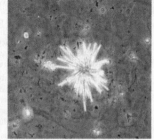

Fig 6. Calcium phosphate crystals

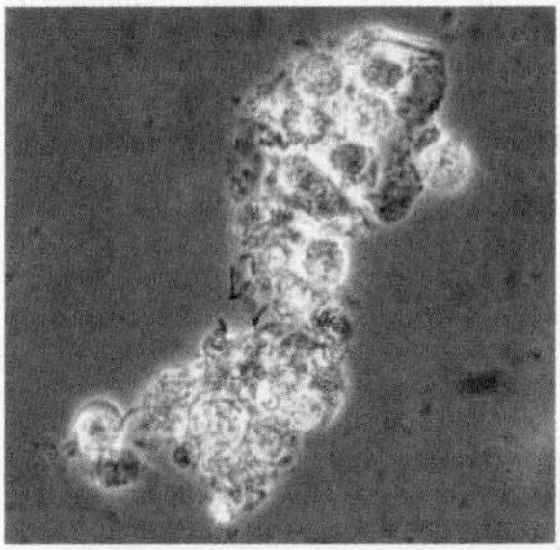

Fig 7. White cell cast

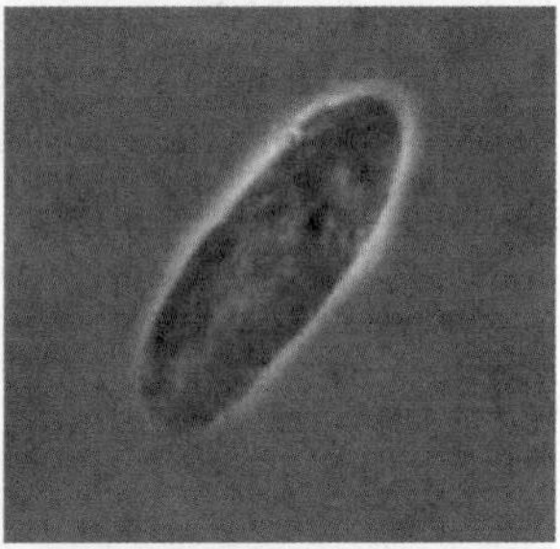

Fig 8. Hyaline cast

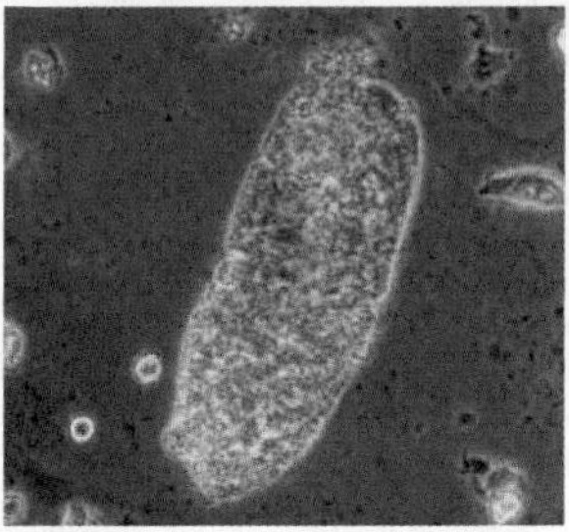

Fig 9. Waxy cast

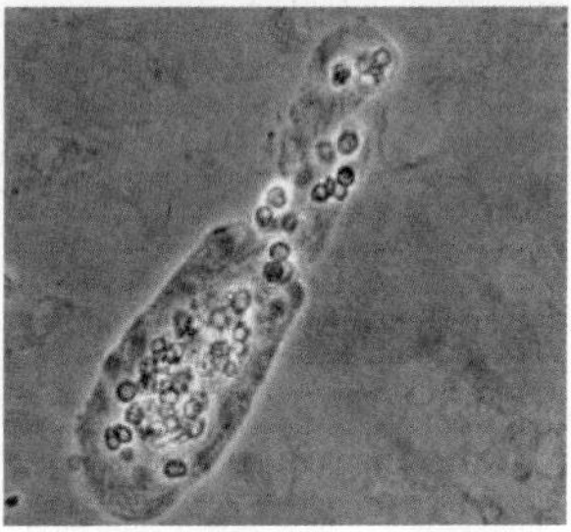

Fig 10. Red cell cast

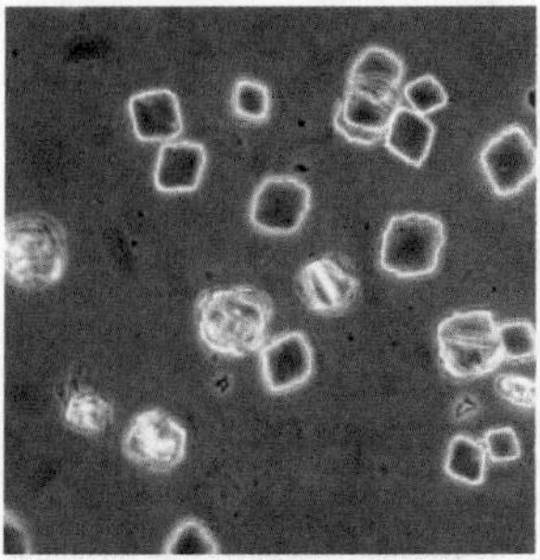

Fig 11. Uric acid crystals

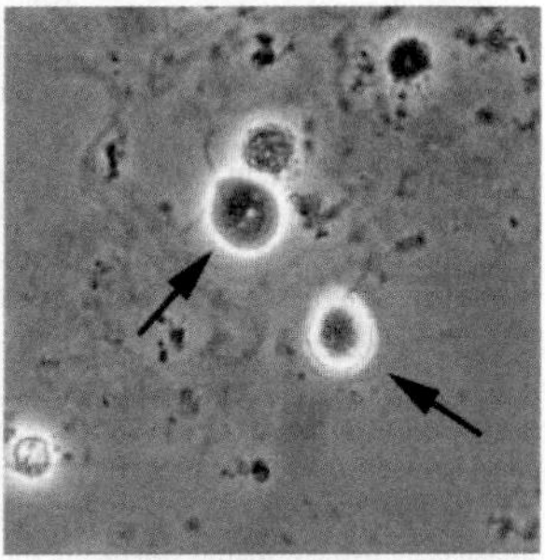

Fig 12. *Trichomonas vaginalis*

Definitions Bacteriuria: Bacteria in the urine; may be asymptomatic or symptomatic. **UTI:** The presence of a pure growth of >10^5 organisms per mL of fresh MSU. Lower UTI: urethra (**urethritis**), bladder (**cystitis**), prostate (**prostatitis**). Upper UTI: renal pelvis (**pyelonephritis**). Up to ⅓ of women with symptoms have bacteriuria; (=**abacterial cystitis** or the **urethral syndrome**).

Classification: UTIs may be **uncomplicated** (normal renal tract and function) or **complicated** (abnormal renal/GU tract, voiding difficulty/outflow obstruction ↓renal function, impaired host defences, or virulent organism eg *Staph. aureus*). A **recurrent** UTI is a further infection with a new organism. A **relapse** is a further infection with the same organism. For urethritis, see p418.

Risk factors ♀, sexual intercourse, exposure to spermicide in ♀ (by diaphragm or condoms), pregnancy, menopause; ↓*host defence* (immunosuppression, DM); *urinary tract*: obstruction (p642), stones, catheter, malformation. **NB:** in pregnancy, UTI is common and often asymptomatic, until serious pyelonephritis, premature delivery (± fetal death) supervenes, so do routine dipstix in pregnancy. Urine in catheterized bladders is almost always infected—MSUs and ℞ are pointless unless the patient is ill.

Organisms *E. coli* is the main organism (>70% in the community but ≤41% in hospital). Also *Staphylococcus saprophyticus, Proteus mirabilis*. Rarer: *Enterococcus faecalis, Klebsiella, Enterobacter* and *Acinetobacter* species, *Pseudomonas aeruginosa, Serratia marascens, Candida albicans,* and *Staph. aureus*.

Symptoms *Acute pyelonephritis:* High fever, rigors, vomiting, loin pain and tenderness, oliguria (if acute renal failure).

Cystitis: Frequency, dysuria, urgency, strangury, haematuria, suprapubic pain.

Prostatitis: Flu-like symptoms, low backache, few urinary symptoms, swollen or tender prostate on PR. Treatment: see p647.

Signs Fever, abdominal or loin tenderness, foul-smelling urine. Occasionally distended bladder, enlarged prostate. **NB:** see *Vaginal discharge*, p418.

Tests If symptoms are present, dipstick the urine; treat empirically if nitrites or leucocytes are +ve while awaiting sensitivities on an MSU. If dipstick is -ve, consider sending an MSU for lab MC&S to confirm this. Send a lab MSU anyway if male, a child (*OHCS* p174; do ultrasound), pregnant, immunosuppressed or ill. A pure growth of >10^5 organisms/mL is diagnostic. If <10^5 organisms/mL and pyuria (eg >20 WBCs/mm^3), the result may still be significant. Cultured organisms are tested for sensitivity to a range of antibiotics (p378). Do fasting glucose & PSA (wait 6 mo, as UTI causes false +ves).

Causes of sterile pyuria: ►TB

- Treated UTI <2 weeks prior
- Inadequately treated UTI
- Appendicitis
- Calculi; prostatitis
- Bladder tumour
- UTI with fastidious culture requirement
- Papillary necrosis (eg DM or analgesic excess)
- Tubulointerstitial nephritis
- Polycystic kidney
- Chemical cystitis (eg cyclophosphamide)

Blood tests: FBC, U&E, CRP, and blood cultures eg if systemically unwell ('urosepsis'). *Ultrasound or IVU/cystoscopy:* Consider for UTI in children; men; if failure to respond to treatment; recurrent UTI (>2/year); pyelonephritis; unusual organism; persistent haematuria. IVU: see p758. NB: in one study on men, ultrasound combined with plain XR of kidneys, ureters and bladder (KUB) was as effective as IVU in detecting urinary tract abnormalities, and avoided exposure to IV contrast.[12]

Prevention of UTI Drink more water. Antibiotic prophylaxis, continuously or postcoital, ↓UTI rates in females with many UTIs. Self-treatment with a single antibiotic dose as symptoms start is an option. Drinking 200–750ml of cranberry or lingo berry juice a day, or taking cranberry concentrate tablets, ↓risk of symptomatic recurrent infection in women by 10–20%[13] (may inhibit adherence of bacteria to bladder uroepithelial cells; avoid if taking warfarin). There is no evidence that postcoital voiding, or pre-voiding, or advice on wiping patterns in females is of benefit.[14]

Features of genitourinary tuberculosis

None is specific, so have a high index of suspicion (esp. if HIV+ve), look for a high ESR/CRP, and find out about past lung TB (but often there is no past history of this). In one study of 100 males with GU TB 67% of symptoms appeared acutely.[15]

- Dysuria (eg in 50% of those with prostate TB)
- Flank pain (59%; a cold abscess in the flank is a rare presentation)
- Perineal pain (40%)
- Mycobacteriuria 38% (early morning sample)
- Scrotal fistula 12%
- Leucocytes in urine 85% , eg 'sterile pyuria'; (78% in prostatic secretions)
- Haematuria in 53%

What is the predictive value of urinary symptoms and dipstick for diagnosing UTI?

This is a controversial area, with a meta-analysis on 70 studies concluding that in the general population, a combination of negative nitrite and leucocyte tests on dipstick was sufficient to rule out UTI.[MET 16]

However, a recent small prospective study (n=59) showed that although a negative dipstick test accurately predicted the absence of UTI according to urine culture, treating these patients with trimethoprim still reduced symptoms of dysuria, suggesting that the cause in these patients may be infection not detected by current urine dipstick or culture techniques.[17]

Managing UTI

►Drink plenty of fluids; urinate often (don't 'hold on').

Management of bacterial UTI in adult non-pregnant women

- Consider empirical treatment in otherwise healthy women who present with lower UTI: trimethoprim 200mg/12h PO or nitrofurantroin for 3–6 days (if normal renal function). Alternative: cefalexin 1g/12h (if eGFR >40). 2nd line: co-amoxiclav PO (7d course). The latter 2 may cause problems with *C. difficile*. If there is no response, do a urine culture.
- In case of vaginal itch or discharge consider other diagnoses and do a pelvic exam.
- In non-pregnant women with upper UTI, take a urine culture and treat with cefuroxime 1.5g/8h IV then oral × 7d course (or ciprofloxacin for 7 days if it is not severe). Avoid nitrofurantroin as it does not achieve effective concentrations in blood. Resistance to trimethoprim is also very common. Non-pregnant women with asymptomatic bacteriuria do not need antibiotics. Screening for and treatment of asymptomatic bacteriuria is not recommended in non-pregnant, premenopausal women.

Managing bacterial UTI in pregnant women Get expert help. Any bacteriuria (symptomatic or asymptomatic) should be treated with an antibiotic, and urine culture should be repeated at each antenatal visit.

Managing bacterial UTI in adult men

- Take UTI in men seriously as it often results from an anatomical or functional anomaly. Therefore, all men with symptoms of upper UTI, recurrent UTI or who fail to respond to antibiotic therapy, should be referred to a urologist. Also consider prostatitis, epididymitis and chlamydial infection.
- Bacterial UTI in men may need a two-week course of a quinolone, such as levofloxacin (if no response, think of prostatitis and treat for 4 weeks).
- Antibiotic therapy of asymptomatic bacteriuria in elderly men (>65yrs old) is not recommended, as it does not reduce morbidity or mortality while it increases the risk of adverse events such as rashes or GI problems.

Glomerulonephritis (GN)

Features GN is a common cause of ESRF[1] in adults, along with diabetes and hypertension. They are a group of disorders where damage to the glomerular filtrating apparatus causes a leak of protein ± blood into the urine, depending on the disease. Patients may be asymptomatic or present with haematuria (may be microscopic, ± red cell casts, p286), proteinuria, renal failure, or hypertension.

Tests *Blood:* FBC, U&E, LFT, ESR, CRP; immunoglobulins, electrophoresis, complement (C3, C4); autoantibodies (p555): ANA, ANCA, anti-dsDNA, anti-GBM; blood culture, ASOT, HBsAg, anti-HCV (p406). ***Urine:*** RBC casts, MC&S, Bence-Jones protein. ***24 urine:*** protein. Many experts now recommend using a spot (preferably early morning) urine sample for a protein:creatinine ratio or an albumin:creatinine ratio as these tests are less prone to error, give quicker results, and have been shown to be as accurate as 24 hour urine collections.[19] ***CXR, renal ultrasound ± renal biopsy*** (p758).

Nephrotic syndrome (p296)

Nephritic syndrome: Patients present with haematuria with RBC casts ± dysmorphic RBCs, proteinuria, ↑BP, and progressive oliguria and renal impairment.

General management ►Refer to a nephrologist. Keep BP ≤130/80, or ≤125/75 if proteinuria >1g/d. Include an ACE-i or ARA; in a recent study, a combination of both was better in preventing progression to renal failure in proteinuria.[20]

• ***IgA nephropathy (Berger's disease):*** Commonest GN in the developed world. Most present with **macro- or microscopic haematuria**; occasionally nephritic syndrome (haematuria + RBC casts). ***Typical patient:*** Young ♂ with episodic macroscopic haematuria, occurring a few days after URTI eg pharyngitis. Recovery is often rapid between attacks. There is ↑IgA, possibly due to infection, which forms immune complexes and deposits in mesangial cells. ***Renal biopsy:*** Mesangial proliferation, immunofluorescense shows deposits of IgA and C3. ***℞:*** General measures. Role of immunosuppression is not certain; however, steroids may ↓proteinuria and slow down the decline of renal function. Cyclophosphamide may also be effective in some patients with rapidly deteriorating renal function.[21] ***Prognosis:*** Worse if ↑BP, male, proteinuria or renal failure at presentation. 20% of adults develop ESRF over ~20yrs.

• ***Systemic lupus erythematous (SLE):*** ~1/3 of patients with SLE will have evidence of renal involvement with vascular, glomerular, and tubulointerstitial damage.

• ***Anti-glomerular basement membrane (GBM) disease*** **(figs 1 & 2)**: Also known as Goodpasture's disease, this is caused by the development of auto-antibodies to type IV collagen, an essential component of the GBM. Type IV collagen is also found in the lung and haemoptysis may also be a feature, especially in smokers. Young males are most commonly affected, but it can occur at any age or in any gender. Patients present with macroscopic haematuria, progressing rapidly to oliguria. Renal failure may occur within days of onset of symptoms. If treatment (plasma exchange, corticosteroids ± cytotoxics) is started early, the disease can be cured and relapses are rare.[22]

• ***Proliferative GN*** is classified histologically: focal, diffuse, or mesangiocapillary GN. The chief cause is post-streptococcal GN (a diffuse proliferative GN), occurring 1-12 weeks after a sore throat or skin infection. A streptococcal antigen is deposited on the glomerulus (**fig 3**), causing a host reaction and immune complex formation. *Presentation:* Usually **nephritic syndrome**. ***Renal biopsy:*** Inflammatory reaction affecting mesangial and endothelial cells, IF: IgG and C3 deposits (in a typical case of post-streptococcal GN, there is no need for renal biopsy). ***Serology:*** ↑ASOT; ↓C3. *Treatment:* Supportive: >95% recover renal function.

• ***Henoch–Schönlein purpura (HSP)*** is a systemic variant of IgA nephropathy, causing a small vessel vasculitis. ***Features:*** Purpuric rash on extensor surfaces (typically on the legs), flitting polyarthritis, scrotal and scalp swelling, abdominal pain (GI bleeding) and nephritis. ***Diagnosis:*** Usually clinical. Confirmed with positive IF for

1 *Abbreviations:* ANA=antinuclear antibody; ASOT=anti-streptolysin O titre; BM=basement membrane (glomerular); EM=electron microscope; ESRF=end-stage renal failure; HCV=hepatitis C virus; IF=immunofluorescence. Commonest presentations are in **bold**.

IgA and C3 in skin or renal biopsy (identical to IgA nephropathy). *Treatment:* Same as IgA nephropathy. *Prognosis:* 15% nephritic patients → ESRF; if both nephritic & nephrotic syndrome, 50% →ESRF.

• ***Rapidly progressive GN (RPGN)*** The most aggressive GN, with potential to cause ESRF over days. There are different causes; all have the biopsy finding of crescents affecting most glomeruli (a proliferation of parietal epithelial cells and macrophages in Bowman's capsule). RPGN is classified pathologically into 3 categories: 23

1 Immune complex disease (~45% of cases): post-infectious (endocarditis, shunt nephritis), multi-system disease (SLE), IgA nephropathy, Henoch-Schönlein purpura.
2 Pauci-immune disease (~50% of cases, 80-90% ANCA +ve): Wegener's granulomatosis (C-ANCA +ve, p728), microscopic polyangiitis (P-ANCA +ve), Churg-Strauss, p710.
3 Anti-GBM antibody disease (~3%, 10-40% ANCA +ve): Goodpasture's disease, p715.

Clinically: Signs of **renal failure**. There may be features of the individual systemic disease (eg fever, malaise, myalgia, weight loss, haemoptysis). Massive pulmonary haemorrhage is the most common cause of death in ANCA +ve patients. *Treatment:* Aggressive immunosuppression with high-dose corticosteroids and cyclophosphamide, with plasma exchange to remove existing antibodies. *Prognosis:* Poor if initial serum creatinine >600μmol/L. Below this, ~80% have some improvement of renal function with treatment.

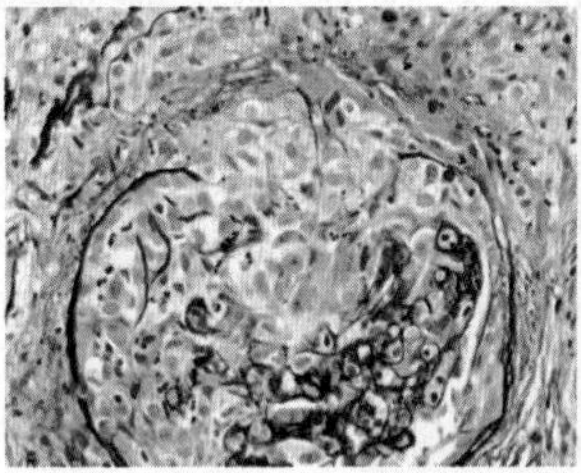

Fig 1. Crescentic GN: a proliferation of epithelial cells and macrophages with rupture of Bowman's capsule, in this patient caused by anti-glomerular basement membrane (Goodpasture's) disease.

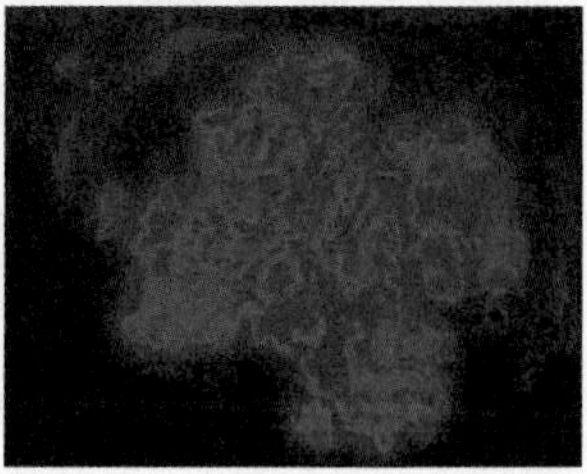

Fig 2. Immunofluorescence for IgG, showing linear staining for glomerular basement, characteristic of anti-glomerular basement membrane (Goodpasture's) disease.

Figures 1 & 2 courtesy of Dr Ian Roberts

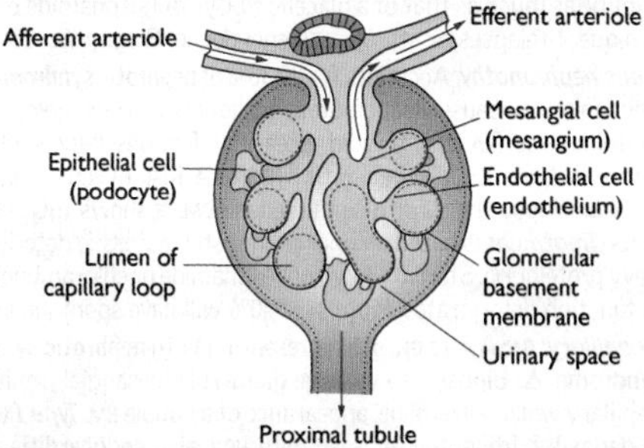

Fig. 3 A normal glomerulus. Blood is filtered from the capillary lumen, through the fenestrated endothelial layer, glomerular basement membrane and the epithelial cell layer. The juxtaglomerular apparatus is the region of the nephron where the afferent arteriole comes into direct contact with the distal convoluted tubule. It regulates filtrate formation and systemic blood pressure (renin-angiotensin-aldesterone system, p682)

►*If there is oedema, dipstick an MSU for protein to avoid missing this vital diagnosis.*

Definition Nephrotic syndrome is a triad of proteinuria (>3g/24h, or a spot urine protein:creatinine ratio of >300-350mg/mmol), hypoalbuminaemia (albumin <25g/L), and oedema. Severe hyperlipidaemia (total cholesterol >10mmol/L) is often present.[24] It was thought that protein loss caused ↓serum albumin, resulting in ↓plasma oncotic pressure and oedema. But plasma oncotic pressure is unchanged, and oedema is now thought to be from Na^+ retention in the extracellular compartment and molecular changes in the capillary barrier.

Clinical features Ask about acute or chronic infections, drugs, allergies, systemic symptoms (vasculitis, p558; malignancy). ***Signs:*** Oedema: typically pitting and dependent (↑ with gravity). It occurs periorbitally (tissue resistance is low here), and peripherally in limbs—genital oedema, ascites and anasarca[1] develop later. BP↑ or ↔. **ΔΔ:** CCF (↑JVP, pulmonary oedema, *mild* proteinuria) or liver disease (↓albumin).

Complications ↑***Susceptibility to infection:*** Infection (eg cellulitis, *Streptococcus* infections and spontaneous bacterial peritonitis) happens in up to 20% of adult patients because of ↓serum IgG, ↓complement activity, and ↓T cell function (due in part to loss of immunoglobulin in urine and also to immunosuppressive treatments). ***Thromboembolism:*** (up to 40%): eg DVT/PE, renal vein thrombosis. This hypercoagulable state is partly due to ↑clotting factors & platelet abnormalities. ***Hyperlipidaemia:*** ↑cholesterol and triglycerides, thought to be due to hepatic lipoprotein synthesis in response to low oncotic pressure.

Tests As for GN (p294); check cholesterol. ***Renal biopsy:*** Do in all adults. In children (*OHCS* p178) most have minimal change GN, so a course of steroids is usually tried initially. Biopsy is reserved for those whose proteinuria has not reduced after 1 month, or if features suggest another cause, eg age <1yr, family history, extrarenal disease (eg arthritis, rash, anaemia), renal failure, haematuria.

• ***Minimal change glomerulonephritis (MCGN):*** Commonest cause of **nephrotic syndrome** in children (76%, and 20% of nephrotic adults). It is thought to be T-lymphocyte mediated, and may rarely present with haematuria or ↑BP. ***Associations:*** Hodgkin's lymphoma, drugs (eg NSAIDs). ***Tests:*** *Selective* proteinuria: only smaller proteins leaked eg albumin. ***Renal biopsy:*** Normal on light microscopy (hence the name); EM: fusion of podocytes. **℞:** 95% of children and 70% of adults undergo remission with steroids, but are prone to relapse (some RCTs have shown that the effect of steroids might be as much as that of a placebo[25]). Cyclophosphamide or ciclosporin are used if frequent relapses or steroid SE/dependence. ***Prognosis:*** ~1% → ESRF.

• ***Membranous nephropathy:*** Accounts for 20-30% of **nephrotic syndrome** in adults; 2-5% in children. Unknown cause. ***Associations:*** Malignancy, drugs (gold, penicillamine, captopril), autoimmune (RA, SLE, thyroid disease), infections (HBV, syphilis, leprosy, filiariasis). ***Presentations:*** Usually **nephrotic syndrome**. Risk of renal vein thrombosis (p297). ***Diagnosis:*** Biopsy shows diffuse thickened GBM: IF shows IgG and C3 subepithelial deposits. ***Treatment*** is based on poor prognostic factors: ie deteriorating renal function, heavy proteinuria. Steroids + cyclophosphamide or chlorambucil are considered if renal function deteriorates. ***Prognosis:*** 40% will have spontaneous remission.

• ***Mesangiocapillary: GN:*** A rare GN, often presenting with **nephrotic syndrome**, ~30% nephritic syndrome. **Δ:** Biopsy shows large glomeruli: mesangial proliferation and thickened capillary walls → 'tramline' appearance of a double BM. ***Type I*** (subendothelial immune deposits): Idiopathic or seen with HCV, also endocarditis, visceral abscess, infected arteriovenous shunts, HBV. ↓C4 levels (*classical* complement activation); ***Type II*** (intramembranous deposits): sometimes with partial lipodystropy (gaunt facial appearance). ↓serum C3 and +ve C3 nephritic factor (*alternative* complement activation) **℞:** None proven of benefit so far; steroids are used in children, and use of anti-CD20 (Rituximab) therapy has been reported.[26] ***Prognosis:*** 50% develop ESRF. It can recur in transplants.

1 ↑Fluid in organs and cavities with severe oedema (+ tissue hardening). Anasarca also occurs in: CCF, liver failure, protein-losing enteropathy, fetal hydrops, capillary leak syndrome with monoclonal gammopathy.

• *Focal segmental glomerulosclerosis* (FSGS) may be primary (idiopathic) or secondary (vesicoureteric reflux, IgA nephropathy, Alport's syndrome (*OHCS* p638), vasculitis (p558), sickle-cell disease, heroin use). HIV is associated with a subtype. ***Presentations:*** Usually **nephrotic syndrome or proteinuria**. ~50% have impaired renal function. ***Renal biopsy:*** Some glomeruli have scarring of certain segments (ie *focal sclerosis*). IF (immunofluorescence): IgM and C3 deposits in affected areas. ***R̷:*** Responds to corticosteroids in ~30%. Cyclophosphamide or ciclosporin are considered if steroid-resistant. ***Prognosis:*** 30-50% → ESRF. It recurs in 20-50% of transplanted kidneys, which may respond to plasma exchange.

• *Thin basement membrane nephropathy* Genetic cause, autosomal dominant: **persistent microscopic haematuria**, rarely minor proteinuria. ***Diagnosis:*** Renal biopsy: thin glomerular BM on electron microscopy (EM). ***Prognosis:*** Usually benign. Small risk of CRF, preceded by ↑BP and proteinuria—monitor 1-2 yearly.

General measures ►Monitor U&E, BP, fluid balance and weight regularly. The underlying cause should be treated as appropriate (eg GN, see p294).

- The cause of the oedema is Na^+ retention; therefore the key to treatment is to create a -ve Na^+ balance. Aim for Na^+ intake <3 g/day, and fluid intake ~1.5 L/day.
- In adults, diuretics are often used, eg furosemide 80-250mg/24h PO ± metolazone or spironolactone, with monitoring of U&E. Aim ~0.5-1kg/day loss.
- Proteinuria is an independent risk factor for cardiovascular disease. ACE-I or A2A are the mainstay of treatment. They ↓proteinuria.
- Treat infections promptly. Pneumococcal vaccinations are recommended. The role of antibiotic prophylaxis is not clear.[27]
- Muscle wasting is a major problem in severe nephrotic syndrome. However, the optimal protein intake for such patients is not clear. A low-protein diet runs the risk of negative nitrogen balance and malnutrition and so is not recommended.[28]
- Treating the underlying cause of nephrotic syndrome will improve or resolve the hyperlipidaemia in most cases. If persistent, treat with a statin (p704).
- Avoid prolonged bed rest. Give prophylactic anticoagulation if immobile, and also if serum albumin is < 20g/l and proteinuria is within the nephrotic range.[29]
- Treat hypertension (p134). If proteinuria>1g/24h, target BP is 125/75.[30] ACE-i or ARA should be used 1st line. Address other risk factors such as smoking, exercise, diet.

Renal vein thrombosis can occur in nephrotic syndrome due to hypercoagulable state (esp. in membranous nephropathy). ***Other causes:*** Invasion by renal cell cancer, thrombophilia. ***Signs:*** Often asymptomatic, but may present with loin pain, haematuria, palpable kidney, sudden deterioration in renal function, or with pulmonary embolism. ***Diagnosis:*** Doppler ultrasound, CT **(fig 1)**, MRI or renal angiography (venous phase). ***R̷:*** Anticoagulate with warfarin for 3-6 months (or until albumin >25g/L) if no contraindications. Target INR is 2-3.

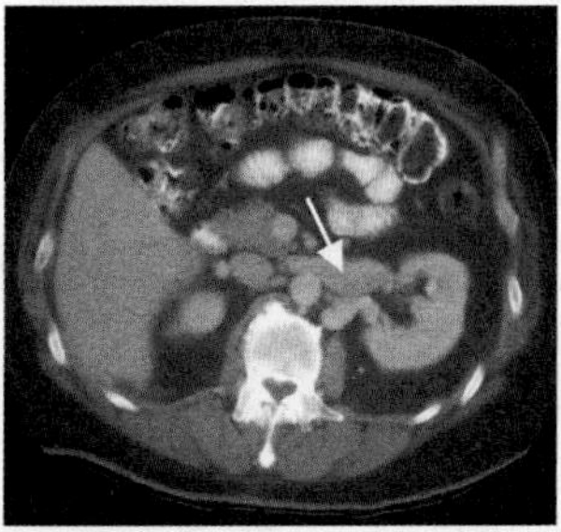

Fig 1. Renal vein thrombus.

Reproduced with permission from Lalani, Kanne, Hatfield, et al. RadioGraphics 2004;24: 1069-1086.

Definition A significant deterioration in renal function occurring over hours or days, clinically manifesting as an abrupt and sustained rise in serum urea and creatinine. It might be asymptomatic, but oliguria (urine volume <400mL/24h) is common. Life threatening consequences include volume overload, K^+↑, and metabolic acidosis. ARF may arise as an isolated problem; more commonly it occurs in the setting of circulatory disturbance, eg severe illness, sepsis, trauma, or surgery—or in the context of nephrotoxic drugs. ARF is common esp in patients with DM, ↑BP, and the elderly.

Causes NB: pre-renal failure and acute tubular necrosis (ATN) account for >80%.
1 ***Pre-renal*** (40-70% of cases): Due to renal hypoperfusion eg hypovolaemia, sepsis (causing systemic vasodilatation), CCF, cirrhosis, renal artery stenosis, NSAIDs or ACE-i (these interfere with renal blood flow). 2 ***Intrinsic*** (10-50% of cases): ATN is damage to the renal tubular cells, caused by *ischaemia* (with causes of renal hypoperfusion as above) or *nephrotoxins* (p307): often due to drugs (aminoglycosides, amphotericin B, tetracyclines), radiological contrast agents, uric acid crystals, haemoglobinuria (in rhabdomyolysis), or myeloma. Recovery of renal function usually occurs within weeks, although mortality remains ~50%. Others: *Vascular:* vasculitis, malignant ↑BP, cholesterol emboli, HUS, TTP (p308); GN; interstitial nephritis (p306); hepatorenal syndrome. 3 ***Post-renal:*** (10% of cases); Due to urinary tract obstruction.

Assessment ►Make sure you know about the renal effects of *all* drugs taken.

1 ***Is the renal failure acute or chronic?*** Suspect chronic renal failure if: History of comorbidity eg DM, ↑BP, long duration of symptoms, previously abnormal blood tests (GP records, laboratory results). Small kidneys on US (<9cm), with ↑ echogenicity. The *presence* of anaemia, Ca^{2+}↓ or PO_4^{3-}↑ may not help to distinguish ARF from CRF, as these can occur within days, but their *absence* suggests ARF.

2 ***Is there urinary tract obstruction?*** Obstruction should always be considered as a cause of ARF because it is reversible and prompt treatment prevents permanent renal damage. It should be suspected in patients with a single functioning kidney, or in those with history of renal stones, BPH, or previous pelvic/retroperitoneal surgery. Examine for a palpable bladder, pelvic or abdominal masses, or an enlarged prostate. Complete anuria suggests renal tract obstruction and is unusual in ARF. Renal US is the preferred method to detect dilatation of the renal pelvis and calyces, although obstruction may be present without dilatation, esp in malignancy.

3 ***Is there a rare cause of ARF?***—eg glomerulonephritis. These are usually associated with haematuria or proteinuria, and warrant urgent renal referral for consideration of a renal biopsy and treatment.

Tests • ***Blood tests:*** U&E (►►beware K^+↑), FBC, LFT, clotting, CK, ESR, CRP. Consider ABG, blood cultures, and also hepatitis serology if dialysis is considered. If the cause is unclear, consider: serum immunoglobulins, electrophoresis, complement levels (C3/C4), autoantibodies (ANA, ANCA, anti-dsDNA, anti-GBM—p294 & p555) and ASOT. • ***Urine:*** *Dipstick* for leucocytes, nitrite, blood, protein, glucose. *Microscopy* for RBC, WBC, crystals, casts. *Culture* and *sensitivity*. *Chemistry:* U&E, creatinine, osmolality, Bence-Jones protein. • ***CXR:*** Pulmonary oedema? • ***ECG:*** Signs of hyperkalaemia? • ***Renal ultrasound:*** Renal size or obstruction?

Distinguishing pre-renal failure and ATN

	Pre-renal	*ATN*
Urine Na (mmol/L)	<20	>40
Urine osmolarity (mosm/L)	>500	<350
Urine/plasma urea	>8	<3
Urine/plasma creatinine ratio (index)	>40	<20
Fractional Na excretion (%)	<1	>2

In pre-renal failure, urine is concentrated and sodium is reabsorbed by working tubular cells. This fails to happen in ATN. **NB:** values are influenced by diuretics and pre-existing disease, and they do not predict prognosis.

Acute renal failure (ARF): management

►*Enlist specialist help.* While awaiting this, make sure that recent U&E and urine microscopy results are to hand. Treat the treatable: [31]

- Identify and correct pre-renal and post-renal factors. If shock is the cause (↓intravascular volume, *below*), use protocol on p805.
- Urgent US scan (today); you *must* check for a palpable bladder, but its absence does not rule out obstruction.
- Find and treat exacerbating factors: eg hypovolaemia, sepsis, BP⇈.
- Stop nephrotoxic drugs—eg NSAIDs, ACE-i, gentamicin, vancomycin, amphotericin. Stop metformin if creatinine is >150mmol/L, see p200.
- Signs of vasculitis? Nosebleed, haematuria, rash, ESR/CRP↑? do autoantibodies.

NB: Assessing signs of ↓intravascular volume can be difficult: look for ↓urine volume, invisible JVP, poor tissue turgor, ↓BP, ↑pulse. When in doubt, consider inserting a CVP line to measure the venous pressure. Signs of fluid overload: gallop rhythm on cardiac auscultation, ↑BP, ↑JVP, lung crepitations, peripheral oedema.

Monitoring Consider transfer to HDU or ICU. Pulse, BP, CVP, & urine output hourly (insert a urinary catheter). Daily fluid balance + weight chart. Match input to loss (urine, vomit, diarrhoea, drains) + 500mL for insensible loss (more if T°↑).

- Correct volume depletion with intravenous fluid—colloid, saline, or blood (only if hyperkalaemia is not a problem) as appropriate.
- If the patient is septic, take appropriate cultures and treat empirically with antibiotics (p161). Remove any potential sources of sepsis when no longer required, eg IV or urinary catheters.
- Re-check if any nephrotoxic drugs; adjust doses of renally excreted drugs (p301).
- Nutrition is vital: aim for normal calorie intake (more if catabolism↑↑, eg burns, sepsis) and protein ~0.5g/kg/d. If oral intake is poor, consider nasogastric nutrition early (parenteral if NGT impossible, p588).

Treat complications *Hyperkalaemia* may cause arrhythmias or cardiac arrest. *ECG changes* (in order): Tall 'tented' T waves; small or absent P wave; increased PR interval; widened QRS complex; 'sine wave' pattern; asystole. ECG p689. ℞:

►►Intravenous **calcium:** 10mL of 10% calcium gluconate IV via a big vein over 2min, repeated as necessary until ECG improves. This is cardioprotective.

►►Intravenous **insulin + glucose:** see p849. Insulin stimulates intracellular uptake of K^+, lowering serum K^+ by 1-2mmol/L over ~60min. Check capillary glucose ~30min after giving insulin.

►►**Salbutamol** 5mg nebulizer. ►►Consider **calcium resonium,** 15g/8h, p849, PO or PR to bind K^+ in the gut. This works over a longer period. SE: constipation.

►►**Haemodialysis** or haemofiltration is usually required if anuric.

Pulmonary oedema (p812): ►►Sit up and give high-flow **oxygen** by face mask.

►►Venous vasodilator, eg **morphine** 2.5mg IV (+**metoclopramide** 10mg IV).

►►**Furosemide** 120-250mg IV over 1 hour (larger doses are needed in renal failure).

►►If no response, urgent **haemodialysis** or haemofiltration is necessary.

►►Consider continuous positive airways pressure **ventilation** (CPAP) therapy.

►►Consider **venesection** (100-200mL) if the patient is *in extremis*.

►►Intravenous **nitrates** also have a role (see p813).

Bleeding: Impaired haemostasis due to ↑urea may be compounded by the precipitating cause. Give PPIs or H_2 antagonist. In case of active bleeding give:

- Fresh frozen plasma & platelets as needed—if there are clotting problems.
- Blood transfusion to maintain Hb >10g/dL and haematocrit >30%.
- Desmopressin (p338) to ↑factor VIII activity, normalizing bleeding time.

Indications for acute dialysis • Refractory pulmonary oedema • Persistent hyperkalaemia (K^+ >7mmol/L) • Severe metabolic acidosis (pH<7.2 or base excess <10) • Uraemic encephalopathy • Uraemic pericarditis (pericardial rub).

Prognosis Worse if oliguric. Mortality depends on the cause: burns (80%); trauma/surgery (60%); medical illness (30%); obstetric/poisoning (10%).

Chronic renal failure (CRF)

Definition Kidney damage for ≥3 months based on findings of abnormal structure or function **or** GFR <60 mL/min/ 1.73 m^2 for >3 months with or without evidence of kidney damage. Classification: 5 stages (BOX). Symptoms usually only occur once stage 4 is reached (GFR <30). End-stage renal failure (ESRF) is defined as GFR <15 mL/min/1.73 m^2 **or** need for renal replacement therapy (dialysis or transplant).[32]

Causes *Common:* BP↑ and DM. *Also:* Glomerulonephritis, renovascular disease, pyelonephritis, polycystic disease, BPH, interstitial nephritis, analgesic nephropathy, renal stones. *Rare:* Myeloma, amyloidosis, SLE, scleroderma, vasculitis (p558), HUS (p308), nephrocalcinosis, gout, renal tumour, Alport's syndrome, Fabry's disease (p712).

History Ask about: past UTI, known ↑BP, DM, family history. Take a careful drug history. Any fatigue, weakness, anorexia, vomiting, metallic taste, pruritus, restless legs, bone pain, impotence/infertility? Symptoms are common when urea is >40mmol/L. Dyspnoea, ankle swelling (fluid overload?).

Screening: High-risk groups should be screened for CRF: DM, ↑BP, age >60, recurrent UTIs, urinary obstruction, or a systemic illness that affects the kidneys (eg SLE), cardiovascular disease (IHD, CCF, peripheral vascular disease and cerebral vascular disease), structural renal tract disease, renal stones, BPH, family history of stage 5 CRF or hereditary kidney disease, opportunistic detection of haematuria or proteinuria. *Signs:* Pallor, yellow skin pigmentation, brown nails, purpura, bruising, excoriation, BP↑, cardiomegaly, pericardial rub, pleural effusion, pulmonary or peripheral oedema, proximal myopathy (+ cause eg DM: peripheral neuropathy, retinopathy). Later if untreated: arrhythmias, encephalopathy, seizures, and coma.

Tests • *Blood:* Hb↓ (normochromic, normocytic), ESR, U&E (↑urea, ↑creatinine), glucose (DM); ↓Ca^{2+}, ↑PO_4^{3-}, ↑alk phos (renal osteodystrophy); ↑PTH (hyperparathyroidism, p214). • *Urine:* MC&S, dipstick, 24h urinary protein. • *Imaging: Renal ultrasound:* renal size is usually small, eg <9cm, but may be normal or large with CRF in DM, polycystic kidney disease, amyloidosis, myeloma, systemic sclerosis, asymmetric renal vascular disease. Consider *DTPA scan*, p190. *CXR:* Cardiomegaly, pleural/pericardial effusions or pulmonary oedema. *Bone X-rays* may show renal osteodystrophy. • *Renal biopsy* should be considered if the cause is unclear and there are normal-sized kidneys.

Classifying renal impairment in chronic kidney disease (CKD)[33]

This is based on presence of kidney damage and GFR, irrespective of diagnosis.[1]

Stage	GFR (mL/min)	Notes
1	>90	Normal or ↑GFR with other evidence of renal damage*
2	60–89	Slight ↓GFR with other evidence of renal damage*
3 A	45–59	Moderate ↓GFR with or without evidence of other renal damage*
3 B	30–44	
4	15–29	Severe ↓GFR with or without evidence of renal damage*
5	<15	Established renal failure

*Proteinuria, haematuria, or evidence of renal disease. One reason to classify renal impairment is to motivate secondary prevention, eg to 'mandate' ACE-i or ARB if BP >140/85 especially if proteinuria is present or stage ≥3.

Problems using MDRD formula to grade renal disease by eGFR (p683):

- The MDRD formula was validated for patients with established renal failure: its use for screening general populations is questionable.
- Most elderly people (~56%[34]) are in ≥stage 3 by eGFR, but this may not progress much or impinge on their health. Labelling them may do harm.[35] Stage 3 is now divided into stage 3a and 3b (eGFR 30–45).[36]
- eGFR is very dependent on diet (too pessimistic if recent meat meal).
- The formula is less accurate the milder the CKD. In one non-peer-reviewed study using ^{51}Cr-EDTA measured GFR (n=178), only 79% were correctly placed in stage 3, and 59% in stage 2.[37] ►Remember that the eGFR is only a screening test and, especially in mild renal impairment, may err on the side of pessimism.

1 Based on **k**idney **d**isease **o**utcomes **q**uality **i**nitiative **c**hronic **k**idney **d**isease (K/DOQI CKD) classification

Monitoring renal function

Some patients with CRF lose renal function at a constant rate. Creatinine is made at a fairly constant rate and rises on a hyperbolic curve as renal function declines, so the reciprocal creatinine plot is a straight line, parallel to the fall in GFR. This is used to monitor renal function and to predict need for dialysis—but there is much individual variation in progression, so the plot is of limited use.[38] Rapid decline in renal function greater than that expected may be due to: infection, dehydration, uncontrolled ↑BP, metabolic disturbance (eg Ca^{2+}↑), obstruction, nephrotoxins (eg drugs). Intervention at this point may delay ESRF. Registry data show the mean estimated GFR at which dialysis is commenced is ~8mL/min.

Background decline may be retardable by using ACE-i or A2A (angiotensin-II antagonists).

Why does falling GFR matter? 2 answers: **1** Good renal function is essential for an optimum *milieu intérieur.* **2** A falling GFR is an *independent* risk factor for cardiovascular disease; ►***this is the chief cause of death from renal failure.***

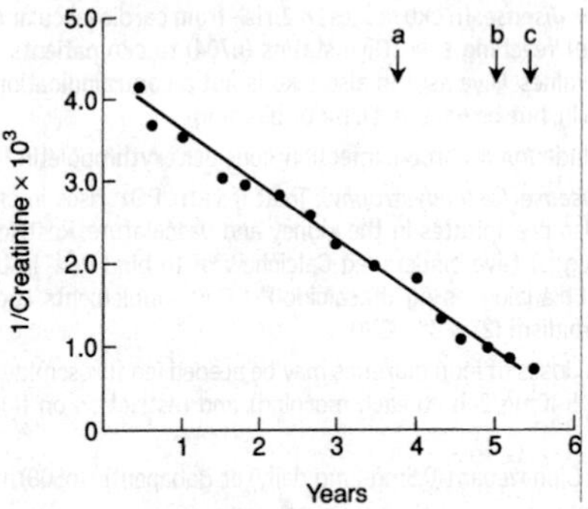

Fig 1. Plot of reciprocal plasma creatinine (μmol/L) against time in a patient with adult polycystic kidney disease. The letters represent life events: (a) work promotion, (b) arterio-venous fistula, and (c) haemodialysis.

GFR is usually given as mL/min/1.73m². 1.72m² is the surface area of the average person; this is roughly proportional to renal mass. So a small person (say, surface area 1.6m²) should have their GFR multiplied by ~1.72/1.6. Beware spurious accuracy!

Prescribing in renal failure

Relate dose modification to GFR, and the extent to which a drug is renally excreted. This is significant for aminoglycosides (gentamicin, p767), cephalosporins, and a few other antibiotics (p378–p381), heparin, lithium, opiates, and digoxin. ►Never prescribe in renal failure before checking how its administration should be altered. Loading doses (eg digoxin) should not be changed. If the patient is on dialysis (peritoneal or haemodialysis), dose modification depends on how well it is eliminated by dialysis. Consult the drug's *Data Sheet* or the pharmacist. Dosing should be timed around dialysis.

Nephrotoxic drugs: Reduce the dose (the dose adjustment factor, DAF, reflects the fraction excreted unchanged in the urine—*F*). $DAF = 1/(F(k_f - 1) + 1)$, where the k_f is the relative kidney function = creatinine clearance/120. The usual dose (but not the loading dose) should be *divided* by the DAF. In only a few drugs is *F* big enough to be important, as below.

Aminoglycosides	0.9	Cephalosporins	1.0
Lithium	1.0	Sulfamethoxazole	0.3–0.5
Digoxin	0.75	Procainamide	0.6
Ethambutol	0.7	Tetracycline	0.4–0.6

Chronic renal failure (management)[39]

►*Refer early to a nephrologist.* Treat reversible causes: relieve obstruction, stop nephrotoxic drugs, deal with Ca^{2+}↑ and cardiovascular risk. An independent, graded association exists between a reduced GFR and the risk of death, cardiovascular events, and hospitalization. These findings highlight the clinical and public health importance of chronic renal insufficiency.[40]

Lifestyle advice: CKD patients should take exercise, achieve a healthy weight and stop smoking. Match dietary and fluid intake with excretion. Na^+ restriction: helps control BP and prevent oedema. A moderate protein diet is recommended (dietary protein restriction is thought by some experts to slow down the progression of disease, but beware of protein-calorie malnutrition). K^+ restriction only if hyperkalaemia; HCO_3^- supplements to correct acidosis

↑*BP:* Even a small BP drop may save significant renal function.[41] Target BP is <140/85 (<130/80 if diabetic or >1g proteinuria/d).[42] In diabetic kidney disease, even with normal BP, treat with an ACE-i or ARA.[43]

Cardiovascular disease: In CKD stages 1 & 2, risk from cardiovascular death is higher than the risk of reaching ESRF. Give statins (p704) to CKD patients irrespective of baseline lipid values. Give aspirin also (CKD is not a contraindication to the use of low-dose aspirin, but beware of ↑ risk of bleeding).

Anaemia: Exclude IDA & chronic infection; consider erythropoietin.[1]

Renal bone disease (osteodystrophy): Treat if ↑PTH. PO_4^{3-} rises in CRF, which ↑PTH further, and also precipitates in the kidney and vasculature. Restrict dietary PO_4^{3-} (milk, cheese, eggs). Give binders (eg Calcichew®)[2] to bind PO_4^{3-} in the gut to ↓ its absorption. Vit D analogues (eg alfacalcidol)[3] & Ca^{2+} supplements ↓bone disease and hyperparathyroidism (2° & 3°, p214).

Oedema: High doses of loop diuretics may be needed (eg furosemide 250mg–2g/24h ± metolazone 5–10mg/24h PO each morning), and restriction on fluid and sodium intake.

Restless legs: Clonazepam (0.5mg–2mg daily) or gabapentin (p508) may help.

Prepare for dialysis/transplantation: See p304

1 *Recombinant human erythropoietin (r-HuEPO):* darbepoetin alfa (Aranesp®) dose **if not on dialysis:** 0.75μg/kg SC every 2wks initially, then ↑ by ~25% if Hb rises by <1g/dL in 4 wks (↓by 25% if rises by >2g/dL in 4wks). Once target Hb is reached (eg 10g/dL), give twice the 2-weekly dose each month. **If on dialysis:** Give injections every 2wks, once target reached on the renal unit. Monitor BP, Hb, Fe & K^+. SureClick® prefilled 0.3mL pens contain 30, 60 or 150μg; 0.4mL pens give 40 & 80μg; 0.6mL gives 300μg. If Hb falls despite adequate Fe, B_{12} & folate, & no infection, haemolysis, or blood loss etc, suspect red cell aplasia (∵ EPO antibodies) ►**stop** ***at once***; get help. Don't exceed target Hb (IV access thrombosis; BP↑; MI).

2 Aluminium-containing agents are toxic so are rarely used now. Ca^{2+}-containing agents risk hypercalcaemia and soft tissue calcification. Sevelamer and lanthanum are newer alternatives, and do not ↑calcium.

3 Alfacalcidol & calcitriol (=1,25-dihydroxycholecalciferol) help by ↓parathyroid hormone, but greatly ↑ intestinal Ca^{2+} & PO_4^{3-} absorption and bone mineral mobilization, leading to PO_4^{3-}↑ & Ca^{2+}↑ (risks vascular calcification). New vit D analogues (eg paricalcitol weekly IV) retain suppressive action on PTH & gland growth, but have less effect on Ca^{2+} & PO_4 absorption, and help cardiovascular status.

Renal biopsy

Most acute renal failure is due to pre-renal causes or acute tubular necrosis, and recovery of renal function typically occurs over the course of a few weeks. Renal biopsy should be performed only if knowing histology will influence management. Once chronic renal failure is established, the kidneys are small, there is a higher risk of bleeding from biopsy, and the results are usually unhelpful.

Indications for renal biopsy:

- Unexplained acute renal failure or chronic renal insufficiency (p298)
- Acute nephritic syndromes
- Unexplained proteinuria and haematuria
- Previously identified and treated lesions to plan future therapy
- Systemic diseases associated with kidney dysfunction, such as systemic lupus erythematosus (SLE), Goodpasture's syndrome, and Wegener's granulomatosis, to confirm the extent of renal involvement and to guide management
- Suspected transplant rejection, to differentiate it from other causes of acute renal failure (p305)
- To guide treatment.[44]

Pre-procedure: Check FBC, clotting, group & save. Obtain written informed consent. Ultrasound (if only 1 kidney, risk is magnified). Stop aspirin 1 week and warfarin at least 2 days in advance.

Contraindications: • Abnormal clotting • Hypertension >160/>90mmHg • Single kidney (except for renal transplants) • Chronic renal failure with small kidneys (<9cm) • Uncooperative patient • Horseshoe kidney • Renal neoplasms.

Procedure: Biopsy is done under ultrasound guidance with the patient lying in the prone position and the breath held. Samples should be sent to histology. A clear indication on the request form of why the test has been done, eg exclude amyloidosis, will help in the selection of special stains, immunofluorescence and use of electron microscopy.

Post-procedure: Bed rest for a minimum of 6hrs. Monitor pulse, BP, symptoms, and urine colour. Bleeding is the main complication; most occurs within 8hrs, although it may be delayed by up to 72hrs. Macroscopic haematuria occurs in ~10%, although blood transfusion is only needed in ~1-2%. Aspirin or warfarin can be restarted the next day if uncomplicated.

Optimal timing to start dialysis is widely debated; guidelines suggest starting when GFR <15mL/min with symptoms,[45] (however, UK and USA registry data show that mean GFR at start of dialysis is ~8mL/min). Early psychological preparation is vital. Medical preparation involves creating an arteriovenous fistula (p315) for haemodialysis, or inserting a Tenchkoff catheter for peritoneal dialysis. Choice of haemo- *vs* peritoneal dialysis depends on medical, social[1] and psychological factors.

Haemodialysis (HD) Blood flows on one side of a semipermeable membrane while dialysis fluid flows in the opposite direction on the other side. Solute transfer occurs by diffusion. Small solutes (eg urea) diffuse readily, while larger solutes diffuse less readily and are not cleared as effectively.[46] Ultrafiltration is the removal of excess fluid by creating -ve transmembrane pressure. *Problems:* • Disequilibration syndrome[2] • BP↓/arrhythmias • Time consuming • Access: *fistula:* thrombosis, stenosis, aneurysm, steal syndrome, ischaemia or *temporary line:* infection, blockage.

Haemofiltration Blood is filtered continuously across a highly permeable synthetic membrane, allowing removal of waste products by a process of convection. Compared with diffusion, convection removes larger solutes at almost the same rate as small solutes.[47] The ultrafiltrate is substituted with an equal volume of replacement fluid. It is more expensive and takes longer than HD, but there is less haemodynamic instability and so it is used for critically ill patients.

Peritoneal dialysis (PD) is simple to perform, requires less complex equipment than HD and is easier at home. It is useful in children, the elderly, and in those with cardiovascular disease. PD fluid is introduced into the peritoneal cavity via a Tenchkoff catheter and uraemic solutes diffuse into it across the peritoneal membrane. Ultrafiltration is achieved by adding osmotic agents, eg glucose to the dialysis fluid. *Problems:* • Peritonitis (60% *Staphylococci*, 20% Gram -ve organisms, <5% fungi) • Exit-site infection • Catheter malfunction • Loss of membrane function. • Obesity (glucose in dialysis fluid) • Hernias • Back pain. ***Continuous ambulatory peritoneal dialysis (CAPD)*** uses the smallest daily volume of dialysate fluid to prevent uraemia. 2L bags are changed 3-5 times a day to produce, with ultrafiltration, a total dialysate of 10L. ***Automated peritoneal dialysis*** uses a cycler machine to enhance solute and fluid removal. Techniques include continuous cyclic peritoneal dialysis (CCPD), intermittent peritoneal dialysis (IPD), night intermittent peritoneal dialysis (NIPD), and tidal intermittent peritoneal dialysis (TIPD).

Complications: Annual mortality is ~20%. ***Cardiovascular disease***, eg IHD, cardiac failure and stroke are much commoner in dialysis patients and are a major cause of mortality. ↑ BP persists in 25-30% of patients on HD. ***Anaemia*** is common. ℞: erythropoietin (± haematinic supplements). ***Protein-calorie malnutrition*** is common in HD and is associated with ↑morbidity and mortality. ***Bleeding tendency*** is due to platelet dysfunction. Acute bleeding is treated with desmopressin and transfusion, as necessary. ***Renal bone disease:*** high bone turnover, renal osteodystrophy and osteitis fibrosa (due to ↑ PTH). ℞: alfacalcidol, Ca^{2+} supplements, and PO_4 binders (p302). ***Infection:*** Uraemia causes granulocyte dysfunction. Sepsis-related mortality is 100- to 300-fold greater in dialysis patients than general population. ***β_2-microglobulin amyloidosis*** is due to amyloid which accumulates in long-term dialysis patients: it may cause carpal tunnel syndrome, arthralgia, and fractures. ***Acquired renal cysts*** occur years after dialysis and may present with haematuria or malignant transformation. ***Malignancy*** is commoner in dialysis patients; this may be related to the cause, eg urothelial tumours in analgesic nephropathy.

Stopping dialysis Dialysis exerts a big toll on quality of life, and it may all become too much, eg if very old[48] or there is comorbidity (eg psychiatric or mobility issues[1]). 8-20% of deaths in dialysis patients are due to its withdrawal.[49] ►Good palliation allows a good death and mitigates discomfort caused by uraemia: • Respiratory distress: morphine • Myoclonic jerks: clonazepam • Hallucinations: haloperidol ± midazolam • Secretions: hyoscine. *Doses:* p438. Good communication in the renal team, well-rehearsed protocols, and living wills help the big ethical dilemma.[50]

Renal transplantation

This is the treatment of choice for end-stage renal failure (ESRF). Each patient requires careful assessment and consideration of the advantages and disadvantages of dialysis *vs* transplantation.

Assessment *Note the following:* Virology status: CMV, Hep B & C, HIV, EBV, varicella-zoster. These may cause severe disease while immunocompromised. Note if there is existing urine output, and cardiovascular disease. Previous TB may reactivate so isoniazid and pyridoxine prophylaxis is given to proven cases and high-risk groups. ABO blood group and tissue typing for HLA is required.
Make sure pre-op potassium is controlled. If not, dialysis may be needed.

Contraindications Active infection, Ca, severe heart disease or comorbidity.

Types of graft >6000 are waiting in the UK, often in vain, for a transplant. *Cadaveric donor* grafts are obtained from a brainstem-dead donor with supported circulation and ventilation. *Non-heart beating donor* grafts are retrieved from patients without an active circulation, and hence rapid retrieval is needed to minimise ischaemia. Success rates from these is approaching that of cadaveric grafts. *Living related donor* (LRD) grafts offer the advantages of an optimally timed surgical procedure, HLA haplotype matching, and improved graft survival. *Live unrelated donation* has become increasingly common between spouses or friends who satisfy the complex rules of ULTRA.[3] Consent is problematic.

Immunosuppressants Most regimes involve **1** Ciclosporin or tacrolimus, **2** azathioprine or mycophenolate ± **3** Prednisolone. Pre-op anti-interleukin-2 receptor antibodies (eg basiliximab) reduce rates of early rejection.

Complications *Post-op:* Bleed, thrombosis, infection, urinary leaks, oliguria.

Acute rejection: (<6 months) This is characterized by rising serum creatinine ± fever and graft pain. Graft biopsy shows an immune cell infiltrate and tubular damage. ℞: High-dose IV methylprednisolone. Resistant cases require anti-thymocyte globulin (ATG).

Chronic rejection: (>6 months). It is now called interstitial fibrosis plus tubular atrophy (IFTA). Presents with a gradual rise in serum creatinine and proteinuria. Graft biopsy shows vascular changes, fibrosis, and tubular atrophy. It is not responsive to ↑immunosuppression.

Ciclosporin/tacrolimus toxicity: Acute: afferent arteriole vasoconstriction, causing ↓renal blood flow and ↓GFR. *Chronic:* tubular atrophy and fibrosis.

Infection: Often community-acquired infections or those related to ↓T-cell immunity (∵ immunosuppression), eg skin infections (fungi, warts, HSV, zoster) and opportunists (TB, fungi, *Pneumocystis carinii* pneumonia, CMV).

Malignancy: Immunosuppression causes ↑risk of neoplasia 5-fold and ↑ infection with viruses of malignant potential (EBV, HBV, HHV-8: p716). Typical tumours: skin (basal & squamous) cancer, lymphoma (EBV-related), anogenital cancer.

Atheromatous vascular disease: This is commoner in transplant patients than in the general population and is a leading cause of death.

Hypertension: This occurs in >50% of transplant patients and may be due to diseased native kidneys, immunosuppressant drugs or dysfunction in the graft. Management is along standard lines (p134).

Prognosis 1yr graft survival: HLA identical 95%; 1 mismatch 90-95%; complete mismatch 75-80%. Average *half-life* of cadaveric grafts is ~10yrs, 20yrs for HLA-identical living related donor grafts—this is increasing.

1 Home haemodialysis gets over some problems with dialysis. Consider in all needing dialysis if: • Willing to learn • Stable on dialysis • Space for the equipment • No precluding concomitant disease • Good vascular access, ie fistula • There is a carer to assist (get their *informed* consent).
2 Characterised by nausea, vomiting, headache, altered consciousness, and rarely seizures or coma, owing to rapid changes in plasma osmolality and cerebral oedema, occurring on initial dialysis.
3 The Unrelated Live Transplant Regulatory Authority: http://www.advisorybodies.doh.gov.uk/ultra.

Tubulointerstitial nephritis: Inflammation of the renal interstitium may be acute or chronic. ***Acute tubulointerstitial nephritis*** is mediated by an immune reaction to medications, infections and other causes. **Drugs:** NSAIDs, ***antibiotics:*** cephalosporins, penicillins, sulphonamides, rifampicin; *diuretics:* furosemide, thiazides; also allopurinol, cimetidine, amphotericin; **infections:** *Staphylococci*, *Streptococci*, *Brucella*, *Leptospira*, hantaviruses; **immune disorders** eg SLE, glomerulonephritis—or *no* obvious cause. ***Features:*** May present with renal impairment, ↑BP, or ARF. Systemic symptoms eg fever, rash, arthralgia, with eosinophilia, uveitis, and ↑IgE. *Diagnosis:* Renal biopsy: infiltration of the renal interstitium and tubules with T lymphocytes, macrophages, and plasma cells. Urinary eosinophils may be seen. ℞: Stop any cause. ARF: p298. Prednisolone 1mg/kg is used, but has not been studied in a randomised trial. *Prognosis:* Most have full recovery of renal function. ***Chronic tubulointerstitial nephritis (CIN)*** results from many disorders, leading to extensive fibrosis and tubular loss on renal biopsy. Patients present with CRF. *Causes:* chronic pyelonephritis often with reflux nephropathy, sickle-cell disease, lead or cadmium intoxication.

Balkan nephropathy is a form of CIN causing progressive renal impairment to ESRF. It is endemic in areas along the River Danube. Environmental and genetic factors are thought to be important. ***Clinical features:*** First appear at 30-50 yrs of age: anaemia, glycosuria, aminoaciduria, coppery-yellow pigmentation of the palms and soles, β_2-microglobinuria. Patients are usually normotensive and without oedema; ↑ BP only develops with ESRF.[52] There is an ↑ risk of urothelial tumours, reported in up to 40%.[53]

Analgesic nephropathy is associated with the prolonged, heavy ingestion of compound analgesics, especially those containing caffeine (as it leads to habituation), NSAIDs, paracetamol, and phenacetin (now withdrawn), leading to interstitial nephritis and papillary necrosis. There is often a history of chronic pain. ***Signs:*** slowly progressive CRF. Urinalysis may be normal or may reveal sterile pyuria and/or mild proteinuria (<1.5 g/day). ↑BP and anaemia are common in moderate to advanced disease; proteinuria >3.5 g/day can also occur at this time. Renal colic and haematuria can result from a sloughed papilla. ***Tests:*** IVU has ↓ sensitivity and can be nephrotoxic. CT without contrast is more sensitive.[54] Biopsy shows CIN. ℞: Stop analgesics, antibiotics for infection. Sudden flank pain should prompt an ultrasound or IVU to look for obstruction from a sloughed papilla. There is an ↑ risk of urothelial tumours.

Urate nephropathy ***Acute crystal nephropathy:*** acute oliguric or anuric renal failure due to uric acid precipitation within the tubules. It is most often due to overproduction of uric acid in patients with lymphoma, leukaemia, or a myeloproliferative disease, particularly after chemotherapy has induced rapid cell lysis.[55] The renal parenchyma appears bright on US. Plasma urate is often markedly raised ± urinary birefringent crystals on microscopy (p290, **fig 6**). ℞: p346: keep well hydrated, allopurinol pre-chemotherapy, urinary alkalinization with sodium bicarbonate (as uric acid is more soluble in alkaline urine). ***Chronic urate nephropathy:*** Whether chronic hyperuricaemia (eg with gout) leads to renal failure is debated. This does, however, occur in Lesch-Nyhan syndrome.[1] ℞: allopurinol. ***Uric acid calculi***, see p640.

Hypercalcaemia is associated with the following renal diseases: nephrogenic diabetes insipidus (p232), renal calculi (p640) and nephrocalcinosis: diffuse renal parenchymal calcification, often asymptomatic, causing progressive renal impairment. Nephrocalcinosis is seen in hypercalcaemia (eg malignancy, hyperparathyroidism, myeloma, sarcoidosis, vit D intoxication) or RTA type 1 (p310). ***Tests:*** AXR for renal calculi/nephrocalcinosis. ℞: Treat cause.

Radiation nephritis is renal impairment following radiotherapy and occurs acutely (<1 year) or can have a chronic onset (years later). ***Signs:*** ↑BP, proteinuria, progression to CRF. Biopsy shows interstitial fibrosis. ℞: Strict BP control, nil specific. *Prevention:* during radiotherapy, ensure adequate shielding (or exclusion) of renal areas.

1 An X-linked disorder due to hypoxanthine-guanine phosphoribosyltransferase deficiency, leading to ↑uric acid, and mental retardation, involuntary movement, self-mutilation, gout and renal failure.

Nephrotoxins

Many agents may be toxic to the kidneys and cause acute renal failure (ARF), usually by direct acute tubular necrosis, or by causing interstitial nephritis.

Exogenous nephrotoxins include:

- Analgesics (NSAIDs)
- Antimicrobials (gentamicin, sulphonamides, tetracycline, vancomycin, amphotericin, aciclovir)
- Radio-contrast media (see below)
- Anaesthetic agents (methoxyflurane, enflurane)
- Chemotherapeutic agents (cisplatin)
- ACE-i and ARAs (angiotensin II receptor antagonists)
- Immunosuppressants (ciclosporin, methotrexate)
- Heavy metal poisoning (mercury, lead, cadmium, arsenic, bismuth)
- Organic solvents (ethylene glycol, carbon tetrachloride)
- Insecticides, herbicides, *Amanita* mushrooms, snake venom

Endogenous nephrotoxins include:
Pigments: eg *haemoglobinuria* in haemolysis: p330, *myoglobin*—see below.
Crystals: eg urate. • Proteins: eg immunoglobulin light chains in myeloma.

Aminoglycosides (gentamicin, amikacin, and streptomycin) are well-recognized nephrotoxins. The typical picture is of mild non-oliguric renal failure, 1-2wks into therapy. Risk is ↑by old age, renal hypoperfusion, pre-existing renal impairment, high dosage or prolonged treatment, and co-administration of other nephrotoxins. Recovery may be delayed or incomplete. Single bolus doses of aminoglycosides can be as effective as multiple doses in treating infection and less nephrotoxic.

Radiocontrast nephropathy is a very common cause of iatrogenic ARF with IV contrast radiological studies. Risk factors are diabetes mellitus, high doses of contrast medium, hypovolaemia, other nephrotoxic agents, and pre-existing renal impairment. Prevention is key: stop nephrotoxic agents peri-procedure, and pre-hydrate with IV 0.9% sodium chloride in patients with risk factors. Acetylcysteine or IV sodium bicarbonate may be used. ►Follow local protocols and inform radiology, who may use less nephrotoxic contrast.

Rhabdomyolysis results from skeletal muscle breakdown, with release of its contents into the circulation, including myoglobin, K^+, PO_4^{3-}, urate and creatine kinase (CK). Complications include ↑K^+ and ARF: myoglobin is filtered by the glomeruli and precipitates, obstructing renal tubules. ***Causes:*** Many, including *post-ischaemia*; eg embolism, clamp on artery during surgery, *trauma:* prolonged immobilisation (eg after falling), burns, crush injury, excessive exercise, uncontrolled seizures; *drugs and toxins:* statins, fibrates, alcohol, ecstasy, heroin, snake bite, carbon monoxide, neuroleptic malignant syndrome (p855); *infections:* Coxsackie, EBV, influenza; *metabolic:* K^+↓, PO_4^{3-}↓, myositis, malignant hyperpyrexia (p574); *inherited muscle disorders:* McArdle's disease (p718), Duchenne's muscular dystrophy (p514). ***Clinical features:*** Often of the cause, with muscle pain, swelling, tenderness, and red-brown urine. ***Tests:*** Plasma CK >1000iu/L (often >10000iu/L). MI must be excluded as a cause (CK-MB <5%). Visible myoglobinuria (tea- or cola-coloured urine) occurs when urinary myoglobin exceeds 250µg/ml (normal <5ng/ml), corresponding to the destruction of > 100g of muscle.[56] Urine is +ve for blood on dipstick but *without* RBCs on microscopy. Confirmed by +ve urinary myoglobin. Others: K^+↑, PO_4^{3-}↑↑, Ca^{2+}↓ (enters muscle), urate↑. ARF occurs 12-24 hours later, and DIC is associated (p346). Compartment syndrome can result from muscle injury. ***Treatment:*** Urgent treatment for hyperkalaemia (p849). IV fluid rehydration is a priority to prevent ARF: maintain urine output at 300mL/h until myoglobinuria has ceased, initially up to 1.5L fluid/h may be needed. If oliguric, CVP monitoring is useful to prevent fluid overload. IV sodium bicarbonate is used to alkalinize urine to pH >6.5, to stabilise a less toxic form of myoglobin. Dialysis may be needed. Full renal recovery is likely.

Hypertension may be a cause or consequence of renal disease. *Essential hypertension* (p132) The extent to which renal impairment develops in mild-moderate hypertension is debated. *Accelerated (malignant) hypertension* is characterized by a severe increase in BP, grade III or IV hypertensive retinopathy (p562) and renal failure. ℞: p134. *Pre-eclampsia:* OHCS p48. ↑BP + proteinuria + oedema in 2nd/3rd trimester. Proteinuria is due to glomerular endothelial cell swelling. ARF may result. **Renal diseases causing hypertension** are the commonest cause of secondary hypertension. Most renal diseases are associated with ↑BP; commonly: diabetic nephropathy, glomerulonephritis, chronic interstitial nephritis, polycystic kidneys or renovascular disease.

Renovascular disease (See **fig 1**)
This is stenosis of the renal artery or one of its branches. *Causes:* Atherosclerosis (in 80%: >50yrs, arteriopaths: often co-existent IHD, stroke or peripheral vascular disease), fibromuscular dysplasia (10%, younger ♀). Rarer: Takayasu's arteritis, antiphospholipid syndrome, post-renal transplant, thromboembolism, external mass compression. *Clinically:* ↑BP resistant to treatment; worsening renal function after ACE-i/ARA in bilateral renal artery stenosis; 'flash' pulmonary oedema: sudden onset, without LV impairment on cardiac echo. Abdominal ± carotid or femoral bruits, and weak leg pulses may be found. *Tests:* US: renal size asymmetry (affected side is smaller), disturbance in renal blood flow on Doppler US. CT/MR angiography are more sensitive. Renal angiography is 'gold standard', but done after CT/MR as it is invasive. See p759. ℞: Comprehensive drug regimens, transluminal angioplasty ± stent placement or revascularisation surgery. Medical treatment and surgery have comparable outcomes regarding survival, cardiovascular events, and renal function.[57]

Haemolytic uraemic syndrome (HUS)
HUS is characterised by microangiopathic haemolytic anaemia (MAHA): intravascular haemolysis + red cell fragmentation. Endothelial damage triggers thrombosis, platelet consumption and fibrin strand deposition, mainly in the renal microvasculature. The strands cause mechanical destruction of passing red blood cells. Thrombocytopenia and ARF result. *Causes:* 90% are from *E. coli strain* O157 ('O' denotes the somatic antigen as opposed to H, the flagellar antigen). This produces a verotoxin that attacks endothelial cells. This typically affects young children in outbreaks (more common than sporadically) after eating undercooked contaminated meat. Signs: abdominal pain, bloody diarrhoea, and ARF. *Tests:* Blood film: fragmented RBC (schistocytes, p330). ↓platelets, ↓Hb. Clotting tests are normal. There may be haematuria/proteinuria. ℞: Seek expert advice. Often resolves spontaneously. Dialysis for ARF may be needed. Plasma exchange is used in severe persistent disease. *Prognosis:* Worse in non-*E. Coli* cases. Mortality 3-5%.

Thrombotic thrombocytopenic purpura (TTP)
TTP is a sextet of: **1** Fever **2** Fluctuating CNS signs (eg seizures, hemiparesis, ↓consciousness, ↓vision) **3** MAHA (severe, often with jaundice) **4** Platelets↓↓ (±mucosal bleeding) **5** Renal failure **6** Haematuria/proteinuria. Adult ♀ are chiefly affected, mortality is higher than HUS. There is a genetic or acquired deficiency of a protease that normally cleaves multimers of von Willebrand factor (vWf). Large vWf multimers form, causing platelet aggregation and fibrin deposition in small vessels, leading to microthrombi (). *Causes:* Often unknown: drugs (clopidogrel, ciclosporin), pregnancy, HIV, SLE. ►*It is a haematological emergency: get expert help. Tests:* As HUS. ℞: Urgent **plasma exchange** may be life-saving. **Steroids, IV vincristine, IV immune globulin**[58] and **splenectomy** have roles in non-responders.[59] Because thrombotic thrombocytopenic purpura is uncommon, a high index of suspicion is required for rapid diagnosis and prompt initiation of plasma-exchange treatment. ►The unexplained occurrence of thrombocytopaenia and anaemia should prompt immediate consideration of the diagnosis and evaluation of a peripheral blood smear for evidence of microangiopathic haemolytic anaemia..[60]

Diabetes mellitus (type 2) and the kidney

Diabetes is best viewed as a vascular disease—with the kidney as one of its chief targets for end-organ damage. The single most important intervention in the long-term care of DM is the control of BP, to protect the heart, the brain, and the kidney. Renal damage may be preventable. ►Everyone with type 2 DM should be tested regularly (6-monthly) for microalbuminuria (30-300mg albumin excreted per day). A convenient way to do this test is to look for an early-morning urine (EMU) albumin:creatinine ratio of >3 (using EMUs improves consistency).

Microalbuminuria gives early warning of impending renal problems and is also a strong independent risk factor for cardiovascular disease. Those who are positive should be started on an ACE-i (p109) or angiotensin-2 receptor antagonists (ARA), *irrespective* of blood pressure. ***Examples of ARA doses:*** irbesartan 150-300mg/24h PO or losartan 50mg/d PO; increase after 1 month to 100mg daily. *SE:* U&E↑ (monitor K^+ & creatinine periodically; stop if there is a rise in creatinine of >20%), flushing, myalgia, headaches, dyspepsia, cough (although commoner with ACE-i). Usually, ACE-i are first-line and ARAs for ACE-i intolerant individuals. There is currently insufficient evidence that ACE-i and ARA are of additive specific benefit in diabetic nephropathy, beyond additional antihypertensive benefit.[61] In one study, the combination of telmisartan and ramipril was associated with more adverse events without an increase in benefit.[62] ►Example of target BP in DM *if no proteinuria:* 130/80; *if microalbuminuria/proteinuria* is present, aim: 125/75mmHg.

Is microalbuminuria reversible? Answer: sometimes—and more likely if:
• Recent onset • HbA_{1c} <8% • Systolic <115mmHg • Cholesterol <5mmol/L.[1]

Cholesterol emboli

Cholesterol emboli may be released from atheromatous plaques (often aorta) which lodge in the distal microcirculation (eg renal vessels, peripheral circulation, gut) to cause ischaemia. An inflammatory response leads to fever, myalgia and ↑eosinophils. ***Risks:*** Atheroma, ↑cholesterol, aortic aneurysm, thrombolysis, arterial catheterisation eg during interventional radiological procedures. ***Signs:*** Fever, uncontrolled ↑BP, livedo reticularis (p559), oliguria, ARF, gangrene, GI bleeds. **℞:** Haemodynamic monitoring, nutritional and metabolic support, dialysis when indicated. Statins are also tried (p704); avoid anticoagulants and instrumentation. ***Prognosis:*** Often progressive and fatal; some regain renal function after dialysis.

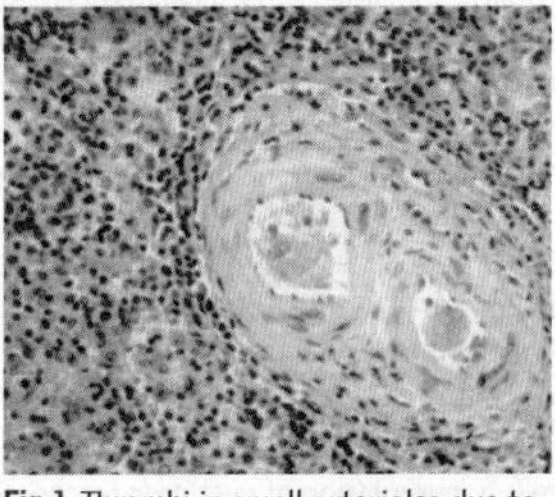

Fig 1. Thrombi in small arterioles due to fibrin &platelet deposition, characteristic of TTP.[63] Courtesy of Prof Christine Lawrence

1 Perkins B 2003 *NEJM* **348** 2285 *n*=386; Regression of microalbuminuria had a 6yr cumulative incidence of 58%. This could not be linked specifically to use of ACE-i.

 Nephrogenic diabetes insipidus p232.

Renal tubular acidosis (RTA) is a metabolic acidosis due to impaired acid secretion by the kidney. There is a hyperchloraemic metabolic acidosis with normal anion gap (p684). Type 3 RTA is a rare combination of types 1 & 2.

Type 1 (distal) RTA is due to an inability to excrete H^+ and generate acidic urine in the *distal* tubule, even in states of metabolic acidosis. It may complicate many renal disorders. *Features* include rickets (+ growth failure) or osteomalacia, due to buffering of H^+ with calcium in bone. Nephrocalcinosis with renal calculi, leading to recurrent UTIs, is due to a combination of hypercalciuria (from bone), ↓urinary citrate (reabsorbed as a buffer for H^+) and alkaline urine: all favour calcium phosphate stone formation. **Δ:** Acid load: oral ammonium chloride load is given—there is failure to lower urine pH <5.5. ℞: Oral sodium bicarbonate or citrate. Complications are from renal calculi—end-stage renal failure may result from nephrocalcinosis.

Type 2 (proximal) RTA is due to a 'bicarbonate leak': a defect in HCO_3 reabsorption in the *proximal* tubule resulting in excess HCO_3 in the urine. The tubules are able to reabsorb some HCO_3, so urine can acidify during systemic acidosis when HCO_3 level drops. Type 2 RTA is often associated with a more generalised tubular defect (Fanconi syndrome, below), and is rarer than type 1. Hypokalaemia is common, due to the osmotic diuretic effect of ↓HCO_3 reabsorption, causing ↑flow rate to distal tubule ∴ ↑K^+ excretion. *Diagnosis:* IV sodium bicarbonate load: there is a high fractional excretion of HCO_3 (>15%). *Treatment:* High doses of bicarbonate (≥10mmol/kg/d) are required (this is often intolerable).

Type 4 (hyperkalaemic) RTA is due to 'hyporeninaemic hypoaldosteronism'. Hypoaldosteronism causes hyperkalaemia and acidosis (↓K^+ and H^+ excretion). *Causes:* Mild renal impairment (eg with tubulointerstitial disease or DM), hypoadrenalism or drugs (K^+-sparing diuretics, NSAIDs, ACE-i/ARA). *Treatment:* Remove any cause. Fludrocortisone 0.1mg PO, furosemide or calcium resonium are used to control hyperkalaemia.

Fanconi syndrome The proximal tubule is responsible for reabsorption of many solutes, including 50% of filtered sodium, most bicarbonate and all filtered glucose and amino acids. Fanconi syndrome is a disturbance of proximal tubule function, with defective reabsorption of amino acids, K^+, phosphate (leading to hypophosphataemic rickets and osteomalacia), glucose (glycosuria) and bicarbonate (type 2 RTA: above). Also, there is polyuria (due to osmotic diuresis), and hypokalaemia (↑Na delivery to distal tubules leads to ↑exchange). *Causes: Idiopathic Fanconi syndrome:* No identifiable cause. Mostly sporadic, some inherited. *Features*: dehydration, failure to thrive. Vitamin D resistant rickets is typical. There may be progressive renal failure in early adulthood. *Inherited:* Errors of metabolism eg cystinosis (below), fructose intolerance, galactosaemia, glycogen storage disease, Wilson's disease (p269), tyrosinaemia, Lowe's syndrome (X-linked ♂ disorder with aminoaciduria, IQ↓, hypotonia, cataracts, abnormal skull shape and progressive renal failure, ie 'oculocerebrorenal syndrome'). *Acquired:* Tubule damage eg heavy metals (lead, mercury, cadmium, platinum, uranium), drugs (out-of-date tetracycline, iphosphamide), light chains (myeloma, amyloidosis), immunological (interstitial nephritis, transplant rejection). ℞: Remove any cause and replace losses. K^+, sodium bicarbonate, PO_4^{3-} and vitamin D supplements are used.

Cystinosis (fig 1) There is accumulation of cystine in lysosomes due to an autosomal recessive defect. Cystine deposits cause Fanconi syndrome, visual impairment, myopathy and hypothyroidism, with progression to ESRF <10yrs. ℞: As Fanconi syndrome. Oral cysteamine ↓intralysosomal cystine and delays ESRF, but is poorly tolerated. Renal cystinosis does not recur after transplant; extra-renal disease progresses.

Hereditary hypokalaemic tubulopathies *Bartter's syndrome:* p220; *Gitelman syndrome:* ↓NaCl reabsorption at the distal tubule due to an autosomal recessive mutation, causing ↑solute loss, and ↑K^+ loss due to 2° hyperaldosteronism. Also hypocalciuria and hypomagnesaemia.

Causes of renal tubular acidosis

Type 1 (distal)
- Idiopathic
- Genetic (eg Marfan's, Ehlers-Danlos syndrome)
- Autoimmune disease (eg SLE, Sjögren's, autoimmune hepatitis)
- Nephrocalcinosis (eg hypercalcaemia, medullary sponge kidney)
- Tubulointerstitial disease (eg chronic pyelonephritis, chronic interstitial nephritis, obstructive uropathy, renal transplant rejection)
- Drugs (eg lithium, amphotericin)

Type 2 (proximal)
- Idiopathic
- Fanconi syndrome
- Tubulointerstitial disease (eg myeloma, interstitial nephritis)
- Drugs (eg lead or other heavy metals, acetazolamide, out of date tetracycline)

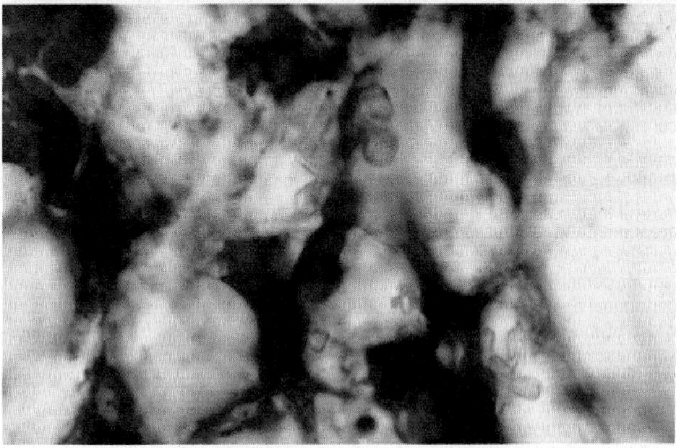

Fig 1. Cystine crystals in the bone marrow, found in cystinosis. Crystals accumulate in most tissues, especially the kidneys.[64] Courtesy of Professor Christine Lawrence

Autosomal dominant polycystic kidney disease (ADPKD) *Prevalence:* 1:1000. Genes on chromosomes 16 (PKD1) and 4 (PKD2). *Signs:* Renal enlargement with cysts, abdominal pain ± haematuria (haemorrhage into a cyst), cyst infection, renal calculi, BP↑, progressive renal failure. *Extrarenal:* liver cysts, intracranial aneurysm→SAH (subarachnoid haemorrhage, which may present with a very severe headache requiring immediate medical attention), mitral valve prolapse. ℞: Monitor U&E. ↑BP should be treated aggressively, with target levels of <130/80mmHg[65] (ACE-i are best choices). Treat infections, dialysis or transplantation for ESRF, genetic counselling. Pain may be helped by laparoscopic cyst removal or nephrectomy. ↑water intake, ↓Na^+ intake, and avoiding caffeine may also help.[66] *Screening for SAH* with magnetic resonance angiography may be done in 1st-degree relatives of those with SAH + ADPKD. Some screen with no family history, especially for certain occupations (eg pilots).

Autosomal recessive polycystic kidney disease (See **fig 1** and *OHCS* p132). Prevalence 1:40,000, chromosome 6. *Signs*: Infancy: renal cysts, congenital hepatic fibrosis.

Medullary cystic disease Inherited disorder with tubular loss and medullary cyst formation. The juvenile (autosomal recessive) form accounts for 10–20% of ESRF in children. The adult form (autosomal dominant) is rare. *Signs:* Shrunken kidneys, cysts restricted to the renal medulla, salt wasting, polyuria, polydipsia, enuresis (↓urine concentrating ability), failure to thrive, renal impairment→ ESRF.[67] *Extrarenal:* retinal degeneration, retinitis pigmentosa, skeletal changes, cerebellar ataxia, liver fibrosis.

Renal phakomatoses (neuroectodermal syndromes) *Tuberous sclerosis: OHCS* p638. A complex autosomal dominant disorder with hamartoma formation in skin, brain, eye, kidney, and heart caused by genes on chromosomes 9 (TSC1) & 16 (TSC2). *Signs* are variable: • Skin: adenoma sebaceum, angiofibromas (see images in *OHCS* p639), 'ash leaf' hypomelanic macules, shagreen patches (sacral plaques of shark-like skin), periungual fibroma • IQ↓ • Epilepsy. *Von Hippel–Lindau syndrome* (p726) is the chief cause of inherited renal cancers. *Cause:* Germline mutations of the VHL tumour-suppressor gene (also inactivated in most sporadic renal cell cancers).[68]

Alport's syndrome *OHCS* p638. *Prevalence:* 1:5000. ~85% of cases are X-linked, due to mutations in the COL4A5 gene, which encodes the α_5 chain of type IV collagen.[69] *Signs:* Haematuria, proteinuria and progressive renal insufficiency. Patients often exhibit systemic manifestations, eg sensorineural deafness and ocular defects (eg lenticonus: bulging of lens capsule seen on slit-lamp examination).[70] *Pathology:* Thickened GBM with 'splitting'. The Goodpasture's antigen is missing (hence risk of anti-GBM glomerulonephritis post-renal transplant). ℞: None specific, as for renal failure.

Fabry's disease See p712.

Hyperoxaluria *Primary hyperoxaluria* is an autosomal recessive inherited error of metabolism due to an enzyme defect. *Secondary hyperoxaluria* is due to • ↑intake eg rhubarb, spinach, tea • ↑intestinal reabsorption due to ileal disease (Crohn's, ileal by-pass), short bowel syndrome, low Ca^{2+} intake. *Signs:* Oxalate renal stones (p640), nephrocalcinosis, progressive renal failure, cardiac conduction defects, arterial disease (oxalate crystallisation), osteodystrophy. *Treatment:* High fluid intake to prevent calculi (keep urine output ~3L/day), ↓dietary oxalate, calcium supplements (binds oxalate in the gut so ↓absorption). If these do not work, pyridoxine (vitamin B_6) is used to ↓endogenous oxalate production (SE: peripheral neuropathy in high doses). Magnesium or cholestyramine are also used to ↓oxalate absorption. Hepatic transplantation may be curative in primary hyperoxaluria, and may be combined with renal transplant.

Cystinuria The commonest aminoaciduria, causing ↓tubular reabsorption of the dibasic amino acids COAL **C**ystine, **O**rnithine, **A**rginine and **L**ysine, due to an autosomal recessive defect. *Features:* Manifests with cystine renal stones (p640). *Treatment:* ↑Fluid intake to keep urine output ~3L/day; urine alkalinization with potassium citrate (↑solubility of cystine). Penicillamine is used, which binds cystine in soluble complexes. **NB:** do not confuse this condition with cystinosis (where there are no stones, p310).

Genetics: triumphs and disasters

As soon as genetics solves one problem, others appear. You might think that the application of science to medicine is an undisputed boon. Petty has provided a compelling counter-example.[71] A man with adult polycystic kidney disease due to a PKD1 mutation is in end-stage renal failure. A transplant from a matched, living, related, unaffected donor is highly desired. There are problems in his family, but he persuades his adult children to have genetic testing to see if there are eligible donors. Each is apparently happy to donate a kidney to his/her father.

A can of worms is opened when one son realizes that he is the only child who can offer a good match—and that his brother is carrying the same mutation as his estranged father (there is a 50:50 chance of passing on the PKD gene). The eligible son would rather save his kidney to help his brother than his father. Old animosities resurface, and the family is in turmoil. How will you feel if the father dies of a complication of dialysis, and both his sons feel guilty forever? We should not be too surprised at all this: often in medicine bad comes out of our good intentions. How can we make good come out of bad? By remembering this example, and not doing tests lightly, and by making genetic counselling as professional as possible, so complications can be foreseen and disasters pre-empted. Furthermore, do not have unreasonable expectations about what genetic counselling can do. The number of diseases being found to have a significant genetic component is increasing faster than geneticists can formulate rational guidelines for screening.[72]

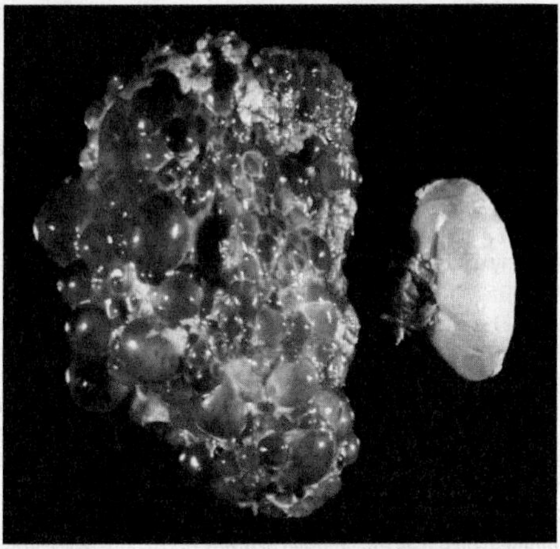

Fig 1. A polycystic kidney (left) compared with a normal sized kidney (right). The progressive increase in size often leads to abdominal discomfort, and there may be haemorrhage into a cyst causing haematuria, or infection.[73] Courtesy of the PKD Foundation

Renal manifestations of systemic disease

Amyloidosis (p364) can cause proteinuria, nephrotic syndrome or progressive renal failure. *Diagnosis:* US: large kidneys; biopsy: see p364. ***Treatment*** p364.

Diabetes This is one of the commonest causes of ESRF in the UK, accounting for ~18%. ***Pathology:*** Hyperglycaemia causes renal hyperperfusion, increasing GFR. This causes hypertrophy and ↑renal size. Mesangial hypertrophy and focal glomerulosclerosis (Kimmelstiel-Wilson lesion) occur later due to ↑glomerular pressure. This initially causes ***microalbuminuria*** (detectable on laboratory tests but not on dipstick: albuminuria 30-300mg/d), a sign of early diabetic nephropathy and a strong independent predictor of cardiovascular mortality. This progresses to proteinuria (albuminuria >300mg/d): ESRF usually occurs within 5-10 years. Diabetic retinopathy usually co-exists, and hypertension is common. It occurs in ~30%, partly due to genetic predisposition.

Type 1 ***DM nephropathy*** occurs typically 20–40yrs post-diagnosis.

Type 2 ***DM ('maturity onset') nephropathy:*** ►See p309 (BOX). >10-30% have nephropathy at diagnosis, and prevalence increases linearly with time.

Treatment: Good glycaemic control delays onset and progression of nephropathy. If microalbuminuria is present, additional important interventions to slow progression of renal disease are • BP target <125/<75 • Use of ACE-i or ARA, even if normotensive (these ↓intraglomerular pressure, p309) • Smoking cessation. Once ESRF has been reached, combined pancreas and renal transplant is possible in *selected* patients.

Infection Associated nephropathies are common causes of renal disease. ***Glomerulonephritis*** occurs with many bacterial, viral and parasitic infections, including post-streptococcal, hepatitis B or C, HIV, SBE/IE, shunt nephritis, visceral abscess, syphilis, malaria, schistosomiasis and filiariasis. ***Vasculitis*** (p558) may occur with hepatitis B or C, post-streptococcal or staphylococcal septicaemia. ***Interstitial nephritis:*** Seen with bacterial pyelonephritis, viral (CMV, HIV, hepatitis B, hantavirus), fungal and parasitic (leishmaniasis, toxoplasmosis) infections.

Malignancy ***Direct effects:*** Renal infiltration (leukaemia, lymphoma), obstruction (pelvic tumours), metastases. ***Indirect:*** Hypercalcaemia, nephrotic syndrome, acute renal failure, amyloidosis, glomerulonephritis. ***Treatment associated:*** Nephrotoxic drugs, tumour lysis syndrome, radiation nephritis.

Myeloma (p362**)** is characterized by excess production of monoclonal antibody ± light chains, which are excreted and detected in ⅔ of cases as Bence-Jones proteinuria. Myeloma kidney is due to blockage of tubules by casts, consisting of light chains. The light chains have a direct toxic effects on tubular cells, causing ATN. ***Features:*** ARF, CRF, amyloidosis (may cause proteinuria and nephrotic syndrome), hypercalcaemic nephropathy. ***Treatment:*** Ensure fluid intake of 3L/day to prevent further impairment. Dialysis may be required in ARF. It might be possible to remove light chains by plasma exchange using special filters.

Rheumatological diseases ***Rheumatoid arthritis (RA)*** NSAIDs may cause interstitial nephritis. Penicillamine and gold can cause membranous nephropathy. AA amyloidosis (p364) occurs in ~15% of RA (often asymptomatic). ***SLE*** involves the glomerulus in 40-60% of adults, causing acute or chronic disease. Proteinuria and ↑BP are common. Histological patterns range from minimal change to crescentic GN. Consider a renal biopsy if nephritic syndrome or deteriorating renal function. ℞: ACE-i if proteinuria. Corticosteroids and immunosuppressants (cyclophosphamide or mycophenolate) are used if biopsy shows aggressive GN (p556). ***Systemic sclerosis*** (p554) may affect the kidney, especially in diffuse disease. 'Renal crisis' presents with ARF + accelerated hypertension. ℞: ACE-i if ↑BP or in renal crisis. Dialysis or transplant may be required.

Hyperparathyroidism Clinical features are from hypercalcaemia: p306.

Sarcoidosis may involve the kidney, often by abnormal calcium metabolism (p186). Interstitial nephritis and rarely glomerulonephritis are also associated.

Epilogue: the man in a red canoe who saved a million lives

Mostly we commute to work each day driven by motives we would rather not look at too deeply. But one renal physician used a red canoe to commute each day from his houseboat to the hospital. He could have been a very rich man but instead Belding Scribner gave his invention away, and continued his modest existence. He invented the Scribner shunt—a **U** of teflon connecting an artery to a vein, so allowing haemodialysis to be something which could be repeated as often as needed. Before Scribner, glass tubes had to be painfully inserted into blood vessels, which would be damaged by the procedure so that haemodialysis could only be done for a few cycles. Clyde Shields was his first patient with chronic renal failure to receive the shunt—on 9 March 1960, and said that his first treatment 'took so much of the waste I'd stored up out of me that it was just like turning on the light from darkness'.[74] Scribner took something that was 100% fatal and overnight turned it into a condition with a 90% survival. In so doing he founded a branch of bioethics because not everyone could have the treatment immediately. This is the branch of ethics that is to do with who gets what—ie distributive justice. In Scribner's day, this was decided by the famous 'Life and Death Committee' which had the unenviable job of choosing who would survive by placing people in order of precedence.

Scribner has said that his inventions sprang from his empathy for patients, including himself. 'I was a sickly child' he said, and at various times he needed a heart-lung machine, a new hip, and donated corneas. He was the sort of man whose patients would inspire him to worry away at their problems during the day—and then to awake at night with a brilliant solution.

On 19 June 2003, his canoe was found afloat but empty—and like those ancient Indian burial canoes found at Wiskam which have been polished to an unimaginable lustre by the action of the shifting sands around the Island of the Dead, so we polish and cherish the image of this man who gave everything away.

Contents

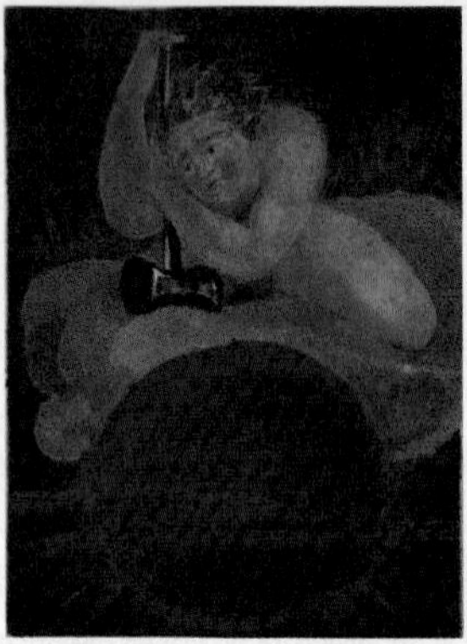

Fig 1. The old methodology: a naked haematologist works alone hammering a red cell into shape. "Every space larger than a red globule of Man's blood is visionary, and it is created by the Hammer of Los." Image from the *Song of Los*, William Blake.

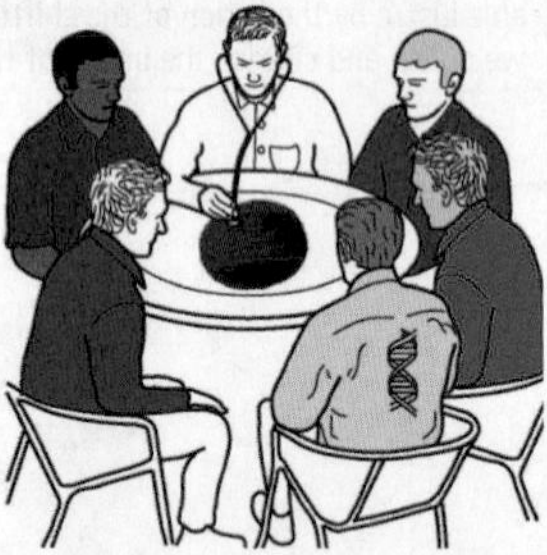

Fig 2. The new methodology: teamwork in action, as haematologist, geneticist, and lab staff deal with a troublesome spherocyte. ×3000

Relevant pages elsewhere: Haemolytic uraemic syndrome p308; thrombotic thrombocytopenic purpura p308; normal values (p769).

Read this! D Nathan *Genes, Blood, and Courage*, Harvard University Press. ISBN 0-674-34473-L Dayem Saif, a 6-year-old with a stature of a 2-year-old, has an Hb of 1.5g/dL—as low as his chance of survival with thalassaemia. This story about lab medicine and its stormy application at the bedside is *so* worth reading when feeling hemmed in by difficult patients, for it shows that there are no difficult patients, only difficult times. The book portrays the vital nature of the doctor-patient relationship, and warns us against labelling people—unless the label is a poem: Dayem is Arabic for *Immortal Sword*.

We thank Dr Drew Provan who is our Specialist Reader for this chapter.

On the taking of blood and of holidays

This is not one of those pages about how you should be kind to the patient, explain in full what you are about to do, talk him or her through venepuncture, label the bottles carefully, and make a plan for communicating the results. Be all this as it may, there is something else which needs communicating about the *act* of taking blood. It is partly to do with the fact that as blood is life, and, because, as Ruskin taught us, 'there is no wealth but life', we are led to the conclusion that what is special about taking blood is that for once *we* are being given something valuable by the patient. What is this wealth? The answer is *time*. For while the blood is flowing into our tube we cannot be disturbed. We are excused from answering our bleeps, and from making polite conversation (a few grunts in reply to patients' enquires about the colour of their blood is quite sufficient)—and we can indulge in that almost unimaginable luxury, at least as far as life on the wards is concerned, of ***reflecting on our own thoughts.*** Accepting this sacred time as a sort of hypnotic holiday is excellent. For however many nights we have been awoken, and through however many wards we have traipsed to this bedside, this little holiday will be worth an hour's sleep—if our mind is furnished and ready to empty itself of all objectivity.

The best sight in haematological practice is, during venepuncture, to appreciate those occasions when, owing to some chance characteristic of flow, the jet of blood streaming into our tube breaks up into countless globules, and before coalescing again, these globules jostle together like the overcrowded chain of events which led us to this bedside. During this time, allow your own thoughts to coalesce into a more peaceful order if you can, and let William Blake help you banish objectivity, for he knew some truths about haematology unknown to strictly rational practitioners of this art:

The Microscope knows not of this nor the Telescope: they alter
The ratio of the Spectator's Organs but leave Objects untouch'd
For every space larger than a red globule of Man's blood
Is visionary, and is created by the Hammer of Los:[1]
And every Space smaller than a Globule of Man's blood opens
Into Eternity of which this vegetable Earth is but a shadow.
The red Globule is the unwearied Sun by Los created
To measure Time and Space to mortal Men ...

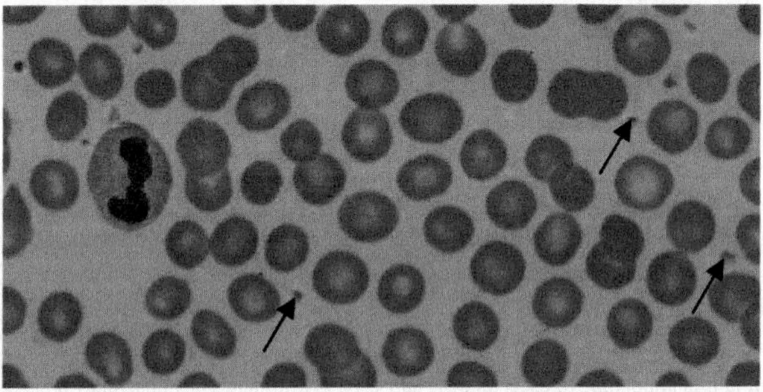

Fig 3. A normal blood film, with a neutrophil, normal red cells, and platelets (arrows).
Courtesy of Prof. Krzysztof Lewandowski

1 Los, the ***globe of fire***, is a symbol used by Blake to encompass the exultant energy of creation, the poetic imagination, and the burning brightness where all his noble images were pounded out of eternity and compounded into the most compressed verse and art we have (*see* P Ackroyd 1996 *Blake*, Minerva). These lines are from his poem *Milton*, section 29, lines 17-24, page 516 in OUP's *Blake: Complete Writings*, edited (1925-1969) by Geoffrey Keynes, the surgeon, who, incidentally, led the way to lumpectomy for breast cancer, in preference to the much-hated radical mastectomy.

Anaemia

Anaemia is defined as a low haemoglobin (Hb) concentration, and may be due either to a low red cell mass or increased plasma volume (eg in pregnancy). A low Hb (at sea level) is <13.5g/dL for men and <11.5g/dL for women. Anaemia may be due to reduced production or increased loss of RBCs and has many causes. These will often be distinguishable by history, examination, and inspection of the blood film.

Symptoms Due to the underlying cause or to the anaemia itself: fatigue, dyspnoea, faintness, palpitations, headache, tinnitus, anorexia—and angina if there is pre-existing coronary artery disease.

Signs May be absent even in severe anaemia. There may be pallor (eg conjunctivae, although this is not a reliable sign; see fig 1). In severe anaemia (Hb <8g/dL), there may be signs of a hyperdynamic circulation, eg tachycardia, flow murmurs (ejection-systolic loudest over apex), and cardiac enlargement; or retinal haemorrhages (rarely). Later, heart failure may occur: here, rapid blood transfusion may be fatal.

Types of anaemia The first step in diagnosis is to look at the mean cell volume (MCV, *normal* MCV is 76–96 femtolitres, 10^{15} fL = 1L).

Low MCV—microcytic anaemia (correlates with mean cell Hb ≤27 picograms).[4]

1 Iron-deficiency anaemia (IDA, most common cause): p320.
2 Thalassaemia (suspect if the MCV is 'too low' for the Hb level and the red cell count is ↑). In multiethnic locations whenever a microcytosis is found some labs helpfully do plasma ferritin and a high-performance liquid chromatography (HPLC) assay, using the original sequestrene blood sample.[5] This allows reporting of α-thalassaemia as the likely diagnosis if there is no iron deficiency. See p336.
3 Sideroblastic anaemia (very rare): p320.

NB: the last two are conditions where there is an accumulation of iron, and so tests will show serum iron↑, ferritin↑, and a low total iron-binding capacity (TIBC).

Normal MCV (normocytic anaemia)

1 Acute blood loss
2 Anaemia of chronic disease (or ↓MCV)
3 Bone marrow failure
4 Renal failure
5 Hypothyroidism (or ↑MCV)
6 Haemolysis (or ↑MCV)
7 Pregnancy

If WCC↓ or platelet↓, suspect marrow failure: see p358.

High MCV (macrocytic anaemia)

1 B12 or folate deficiency
2 Alcohol excess—or liver disease
3 Reticulocytosis (p322, eg with haemolysis)
4 Cytotoxics, eg hydroxycarbamide
5 Myelodysplastic syndromes
6 Marrow infiltration
7 Hypothyroidism
8 Antifolate drugs (eg phenytoin)

Haemolytic anaemias do not fit into the above classification as the anaemia may be normocytic or, if there are many young (hence larger) RBCs and reticulocytes, macrocytic (p330). Suspect if there is a reticulocytosis (>2% of RBCs; or reticulocyte count $>100\times10^9$/L), mild macrocytosis, haptoglobin↓, bilirubin↑ & urobilinogen↑. Often mild jaundice (but no bilirubin in urine as haemolysis causes pre-hepatic jaundice).

Does he need a blood transfusion? Usually No!—unless there is severe acute anaemia (one review suggests that transfusion is not essential for *most* patients unless Hb <7g/dL).[6] If there is an acute cause (eg haemorrhage with active peptic ulcer), transfusion up to 8g/dL is sometimes needed. Chronic anaemia is better tolerated, and it is important to ascertain the cause, eg in iron-deficiency anaemia, iron supplements will raise the haemoglobin in a safer and less costly way.

In severe anaemia with heart failure, transfusion is vital to restore Hb to a safe level, eg 6–8g/dL, but must be done with great care. Give packed cells *slowly* with 10–40mg furosemide IV/PO with alternate units (dose depends on previous exposure to diuretics; do not mix with blood). Check for rising JVP and basal crackles. If CCF gets worse, stop and treat. If immediate transfusion is essential, a 2–3 unit exchange transfusion can be tried, removing blood at same rate as it is transfused.

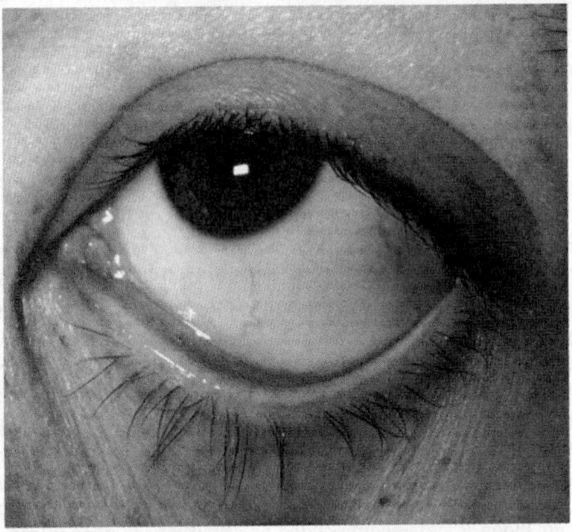

Fig 1. 'Conjunctival pallor', *the* classic sign of anaemia, is a confusing term as the conjunctiva is translucent, transmitting the colour of structures under it. The 'pallor' refers to the vasculature on the inner surface of the lid which is lacking Hb.
It is this colour 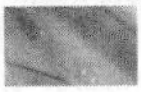 but it should be: 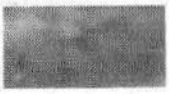

Iron-deficiency anaemia (IDA)

This is common (seen in up to 14% of menstruating women).

Causes: • Blood loss, eg menorrhagia or GI bleeding (upper p252; lower p631).
- Poor diet may cause IDA in babies or children (but rarely in adults), those on special diets, or wherever there is poverty.
- Malabsorption (eg coeliac disease) is a cause of refractory IDA.
- In the Tropics, hookworm (GI blood loss) is the most common cause.

Signs: Chronic IDA (signs now rare): koilonychia (**fig 1** and p32), atrophic glossitis, angular cheilosis (**fig 2**), and rarely, post-cricoid webs (Plummer-Vinson syndrome).

Tests: Microcytic, hypochromic anaemia with anisocytosis and poikilocytosis (**fig 3** and **4**). ↓MCV, ↓MCH & ↓MCHC. Confirmed by ferritin↓ (also serum iron↓ with ↑total iron-binding capacity—TIBC, but these are less reliable). ↑red cell protoporphyrin. **NB:** ferritin is an acute phase protein and ↑ with inflammation eg infection, malignancy. Serum transferrin receptors are also ↑ in IDA but are less affected by inflammation. If MCV↓, and good history of menorrhagia, oral iron may be started without further tests. Otherwise investigate for GI blood loss: gastroscopy, sigmoidoscopy, barium enema or colonoscopy, stool microscopy for ova if hookworm etc is a possibility. Faecal occult blood is not recommended as sensitivity is poor. ►*Iron deficiency without an obvious source of bleeding mandates a careful GI workup.*[1]

Treatment: Treat the cause. Oral iron eg ferrous sulfate 200mg/8h PO. SE: nausea, abdominal discomfort, diarrhoea or constipation, black stools. Hb should rise by 1g/dL/week, with a modest reticulocytosis (ie young RBC, p322). Continue until Hb is normal and for at least 3 months, to replenish stores. Intravenous iron is almost never needed, but may be indicated if the oral route is impossible or ineffective, eg functional iron deficiency in chronic renal failure, where there is inadequate mobilization of iron stores in response to the acute demands of erythropoietin therapy.

The usual reason that IDA fails to respond to iron replacement is that the patient has rejected the pills. Negotiate on concordance issues (p3). Is the reason for the problem GI disturbance? Altering the dose of elemental iron with a different preparation may help. There may be continued blood loss, malabsorption, anaemia of chronic disease; or there is misdiagnosis, eg when thalassaemia is to blame.

The anaemia of chronic disease

This is associated with many diseases, including chronic infection (eg TB, osteomyelitis), vasculitis, rheumatoid arthritis, malignancy, andrenal failure. There is cytokine-driven inhibition of red cell production. ***Investigations:*** Mild normocytic anaemia (eg Hb >8g/dL), ferritin normal or ↑. ***Treatment:*** Treat the underlying disease. The anaemia of renal failure is partly due to erythropoietin deficiency and recombinant erythropoietin (p302) is effective in raising the haemoglobin level (SE: flu-like symptoms, hypertension, mild rise in the platelet count). It is also effective in raising Hb and improving quality of life in those with malignant disease.[7]

Sideroblastic anaemia

Microcytic anaemia does not equal iron deficiency! 20% of older people with an MCV <75fL are not iron deficient. ►***Think of sideroblastic anaemia whenever a microcytic anaemia is not responding to iron.***[8] Do a ferritin; look at a film (hypochromia) and a marrow (**figs 5 & 6**). It is characterized by ineffective erythropoiesis, leading to ↑iron absorption, iron loading in the marrow ± haemosiderosis (endocrine, liver & heart damage due to iron deposition). It may be congenital (rare, X-linked) or acquired, eg idiopathic as one of the myelodysplastic/myeloproliferative diseases, but it can follow chemotherapy, anti-TB drugs, irradiation, alcohol or lead excess. ℞: Remove the cause. Pyridoxine may help ± repeated transfusion for severe anaemia.

1 In one study, 11% presenting to their GP with IDA had GI carcinoma. Consider both upper and lower GI investigation as in another study, 29% (n=89) had abnormalities on both.

Interpreting plasma iron studies

	Iron	TIBC	Ferritin
Iron deficiency	↓	↑	↓
Anaemia of chronic disease	↓	↓	↑
Chronic haemolysis	↑	↓	↑
Haemochromatosis	↑	↓ (or ↔)	↑
Pregnancy	↑	↑	↔
Sideroblastic anaemia	↑	↔	↑

TIBC: total iron binding capacity.

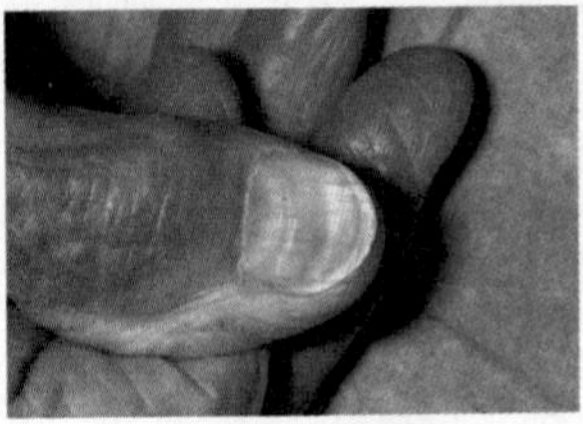

Fig 1. Koilonychia. Spoon-shaped nails, found in iron-deficiency anaemia.

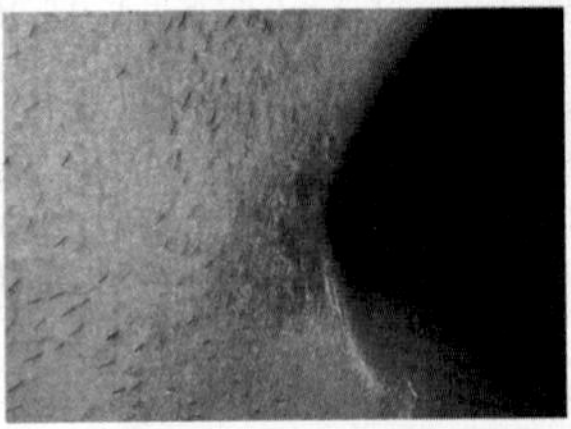

Fig 2. Angular cheilosis, ulceration at the side of the mouth, in iron deficiency. Also a feature of vitamin B_{12} and B_2 (riboflavin) deficiency, and glucgonoma (p215). [9]

Courtesy of Professor Thomas Habif

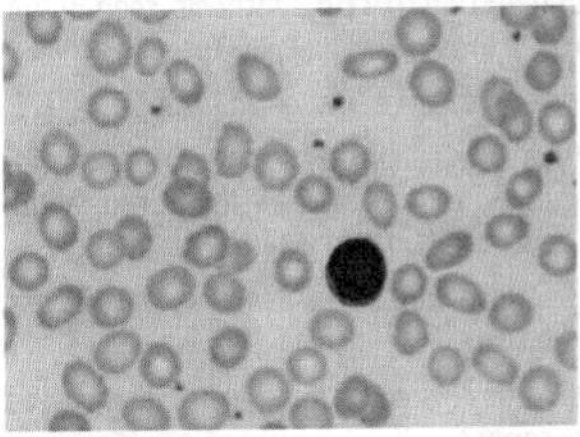

Fig 3. Microcytic hypochromic cells in iron-deficiency anaemia. [10]

Courtesy of Prof. Krzysztof Lewandowski

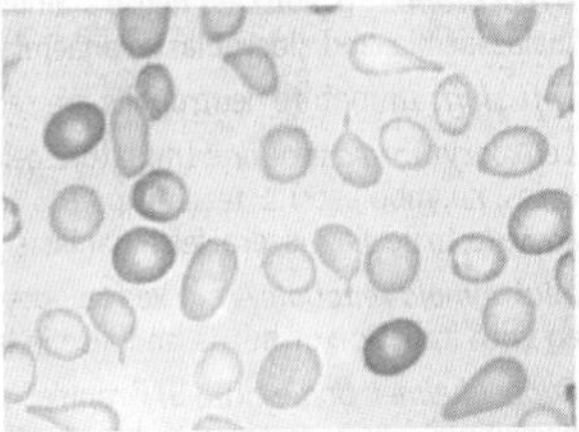

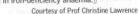

Fig 4. Poikilocytosis and anisocytosis seen eg in iron-deficiency anaemia. [11]

Courtesy of Prof Christine Lawrence

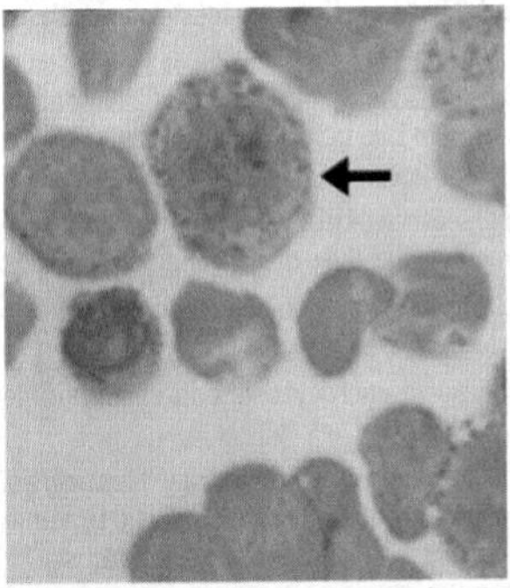

Fig 5. Pathological ring sideroblasts in the marrow, with a perinuclear ring of iron granules, found in sideroblastic anaemia. [12]

Courtesy of Prof Christine Lawrence

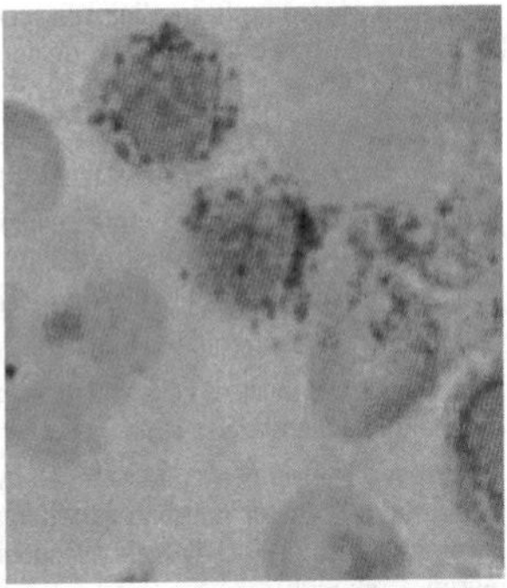

Fig 6. Two ringed sideroblasts showing how the distribution of what we take to be peri-nuclear mitochondrial ferritin can vary. [13]

Courtesy of Prof. Tangün & Dr Köroğlu. [14]

►Many haematological (and other) diagnoses are made by careful examination of the peripheral blood film. It is also necessary for interpretation of the FBC indices.

Anisocytosis is variation in RBC size, eg megaloblastic anaemia, thalassaemia, IDA.

Acanthocytes: (**fig 1**) Spicules on RBCs (∵ unstable RBC membrane lipid structure); causes: splenectomy; alcoholic liver disease; abetalipoproteinaemia; spherocytosis.

Basophilic RBC stippling: (**fig 2**) Denatured RNA found in RBCs, indicating accelerated erythropoiesis or defective Hb synthesis. Seen in lead poisoning, megaloblastic anaemia, myelodysplasia, liver disease, haemoglobinopathy, eg thalassaemia.

Blasts: Nucleated precursor cells. They are not normally in peripheral blood, but are seen in myelofibrosis, leukaemia or malignant infiltration by carcinoma.

Burr cells (echinocytes): RBC projections (less marked than in acanthocytes); **fig 3**.

Cabot rings: Seen in RBCs in: pernicious anaemia; lead poisoning; bad infections (**fig 9**).[15]

Dimorphic picture: Two populations of red cells. Seen after treatment of Fe, B12, or folate deficiency, in mixed deficiency (↓Fe with ↓B12 or folate), post-transfusion, or with primary sideroblastic anaemia, where a clone of abnormal erythroblasts produce abnormal red cells, alongside normal red cell production.

Howell–Jolly bodies: DNA nuclear remnants in RBCs, which are normally removed by the spleen (**fig 8**). Seen post-splenectomy and in hyposplenism (eg sickle-cell disease, coeliac disease, congenital, UC/Crohn's, myeloproliferative disease, amyloid). Also in dyserythopoietic states: myelodysplasia, megaloblastic anaemia.

Hypochromia: (p320). Less dense staining of RBCs due to ↓Hb synthesis, seen in IDA, thalassaemia, and sideroblastic anaemia (iron stores unusable, p320).

Left shift: Immature neutrophils are sent out of the marrow, eg in infection, p325.

Leukoerythroblastic film: Immature cells (myelocytes, promyelocytes, metamyelocytes, normoblasts) ± tear-drop RBCs from marrow infiltration/infection (malignancy; TB; brucella; visceral leishmaniasis;[16] parvovirus B19)[17]—or in UC[18] or haemolysis.

Leukaemoid reaction: A marked leucocytosis (WCC $>50\times10^9$/L). Seen in severe illness, eg with infection or burns, and also in leukaemia.

Pappenheimer bodies: (**fig 5**) Granules of siderocytes containing iron. Seen in lead poisoning, carcinomatosis, and post-splenectomy.

Poikilocytosis is variation in RBC shape, eg in IDA, myelofibrosis, thalassaemia.

Polychromasia: RBCs of different ages stain unevenly (young are bluer). This is a response to bleeding, haematinic replacement (ferrous sulfate, B12, folate), haemolysis, or marrow infiltration. Reticulocyte count is raised.

Reticulocytes: (normal range: 0.8–2%; or $<85\times10^9$/L) **fig 6**. Young, larger RBCs (contain RNA) signifying active erythropoiesis. Increased in haemolysis, haemorrhage, and if B12, iron or folate is given to marrow that lack these.

Right shift: Hypermature white cells: hypersegmented polymorphs (>5 lobes to nucleus) seen in megaloblastic anaemia, uraemia, and liver disease. See p326, **fig 1**.

Rouleaux formation: (**fig 7**) Red cells stack on each other (it causes a raised ESR; p366). Seen with chronic inflammation, paraproteinaemia and myeloma.

Spherocytes: Spherical cells found in hereditary spherocytosis and autoimmune haemolytic anaemia. See p332.

Schistocytes: Fragmented RBCs sliced by fibrin bands, in intravascular haemolysis. (p332, **fig 4**) Look for microangiopathic anaemia, eg DIC (p346), haemolytic uraemic syndrome, thrombotic thrombocytopenic purpura (TTP: p308), or pre-eclampsia.

Target cells: (also known as Mexican hat cells, **fig 8** and **fig 3**, p337) These are RBCs with central staining, a ring of pallor, and an outer rim of staining seen in liver disease, hyposplenism, thalassaemia—and, in small numbers, in IDA

Tear-drop RBCs: Seen in extramedullary haemopoiesis; see leukoerythroblastic film.

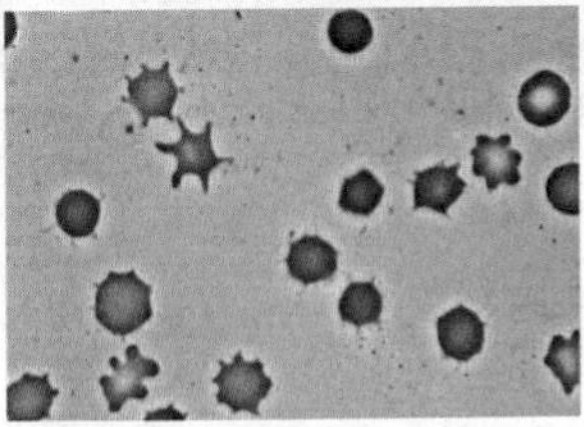

Fig 1. Acanthocytosis.

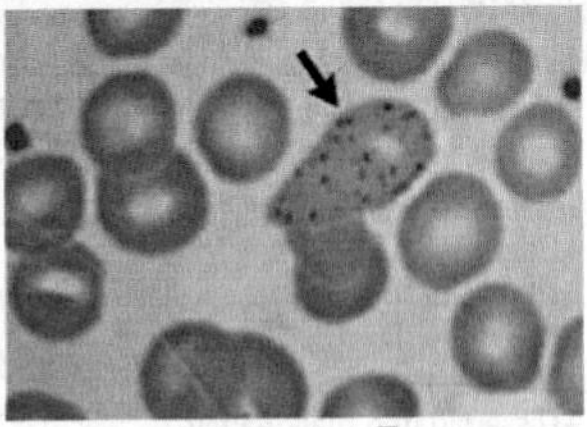

Fig 2. Basophilic stippling.

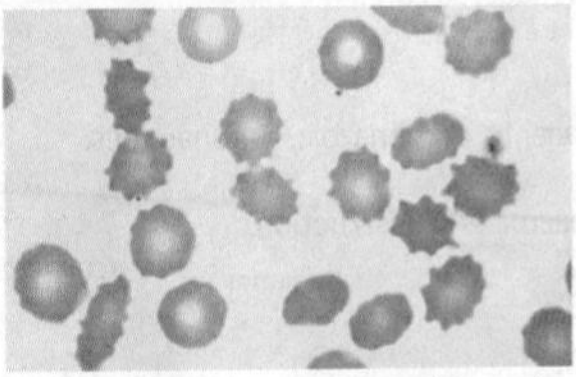

Fig 3. Burr cells: the cause may be renal or liver failure, or an EDTA storage artifact.

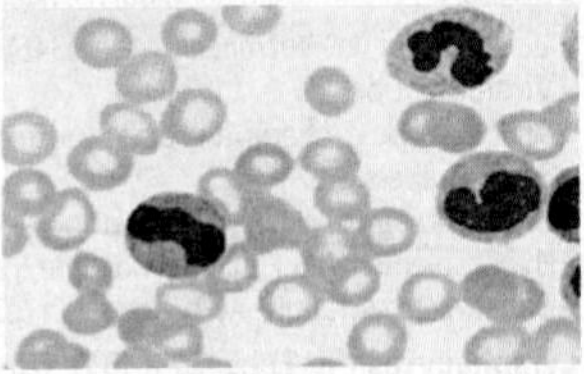

Fig 4. Left shift: presence of immature neutrophils in the blood. See p322.

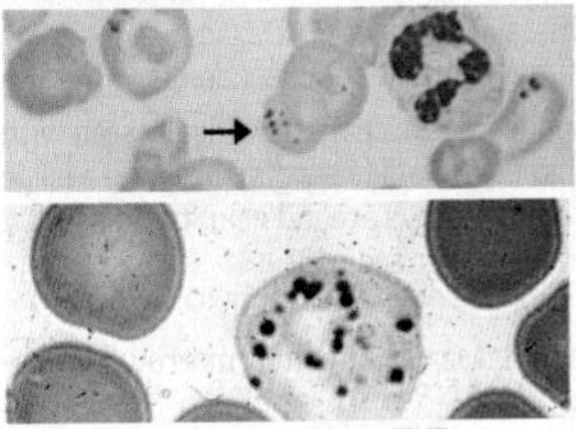

Fig 5. Pappenheimer bodies.

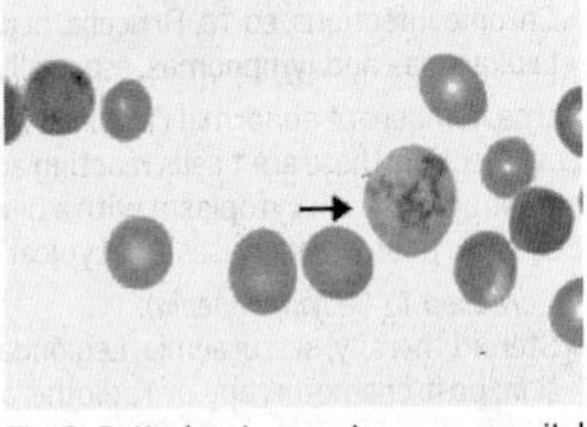

Fig 6. Reticulocytes. RNA in RBCs; supravital staining (azure B; cresyl blue) is needed.

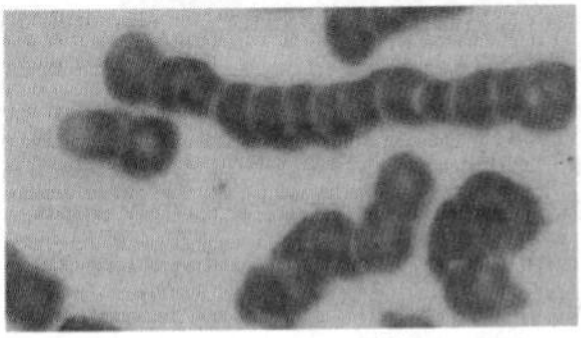

Fig 7. Rouleaux formation.

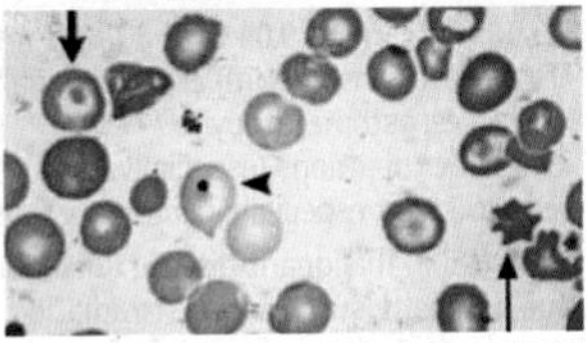

Fig 8. Film in hyposplenism: target cell (short arrow), acanthocyte (long arrow) and a Howell–Jolly body (arrow head).

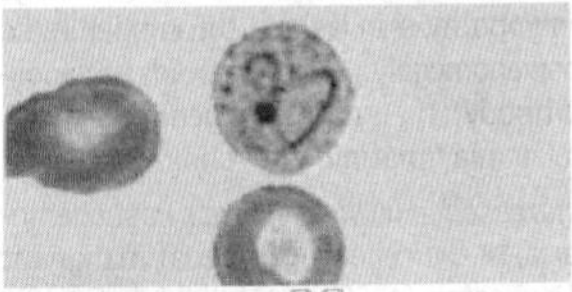

Fig 9. A Cabot ring.[1]

Figs 1, 6 & 7 ©Dr N Medeiros; figs 2 & 8 ©Prof. Barbara Bain & Massachusetts Medical Society; figs 3, 5 (top) ©Prof. Christine Lawrence; fig 4 ©Prof. Krzysztof Lewandowski; figs 5 (bottom) & 9 ©Crookston Collection.

1 Cabot 'figure-of-eight' rings may be microtubules from mitotic spindles. It is easy to confuse them with malaria parasites, p385 (especially if stippling gives a 'chromatin dot' artefact, as here). Richard Clarke Cabot (1868–1939) liked diagnostic challenges: it was he who founded the dastardly hard but beautifully presented weekly clinicopathological exercises of the Massachusetts General Hospital which have made the *New England Journal of Medicine* so famous among discerning clinical detectives. You may forget all about his rings—but not his aphorisms—for example: ►***"Before you tell the truth to the patient, be sure you know the truth, and that the patient wants to hear it."***

Neutrophils (figs 1, 6) 2–7.5 × 10^9/L (40–75% of white blood cells: but absolute values are more meaningful than percentages).

Increased in (ie ***neutrophilia***):
- Bacterial infections.
- Inflammation, eg myocardial infarction, polyarteritis nodosa.
- Myeloproliferative disorders.
- Drugs (steroids).
- Disseminated malignancy.
- Stress, eg trauma, surgery, burns, haemorrhage, seizure.

Decreased in (ie ***neutropenia***—see p346)
- Viral infections.
- Drugs, eg post-chemotherapy, cytotoxic agents, carbimazole, sulfonamides.
- Severe sepsis.
- Neutrophil antibodies (SLE, haemolytic anaemia)—↑ destruction.
- Hypersplenism, eg Felty's syndrome (p367).
- Bone marrow failure—↓ production (p358).

Lymphocytes (fig 2) 1.5–4.5 × 10^9/L (20–45%).
Increased in (ie ***lymphocytosis***):
- Acute viral infections.
- Chronic infections, eg TB, Brucella, hepatitis, syphilis.
- Leukaemias and lymphomas, especially chronic lymphocytic leukaemia.

Large numbers of abnormal ('atypical') lymphocytes are characteristically seen with EBV infection: these are T cells reacting against EBV-infected B cells. They have a large amount of clearish cytoplasm with a blue rim that flows around neighbouring RBCs. See **fig 1**, p401. Other causes of 'atypical' lymphocytes: see p401.

Decreased in (ie ***lymphopenia***):
- Steroid therapy; SLE; uraemia; Legionnaire's disease; HIV infection; marrow infiltration; post chemotherapy or radiotherapy.

T-lymphocyte subset reference values: CD4 count: 537–1571/mm^3 (low in HIV infection). CD8 count: 235–753/mm^3; CD4/CD8 ratio: 1.2–3.8.

Eosinophils (fig 3) 0.04–0.4 × 10^9/L (1–6%). [30] *Increased in* (ie ***eosinophilia***):
- Drug reactions, eg with erythema multiforme, p564.
- Allergies: asthma, atopy.
- Parasitic infections (especially invasive helminths).
- Skin disease: especially pemphigus, eczema, psoriasis, dermatitis herpetiformis.

Also seen in malignant disease (including lymphomas and eosinophilic leukaemia), PAN, adrenal insufficiency,[31] irradiation, Löffler's syndrome (p718), and during the convalescent phase of any infection.

***The hypereosinophilic syndrome* (HES)** is a severe disease of unknown cause, in which an ↑ eosinophil count (>1.5 × 10^9/L for >6 weeks) leads to end-organ damage (endomyocardial fibrosis/restrictive cardiomyopathy, skin lesions, thromboembolic disease, lung disease, neuropathy, and hepatosplenomegaly). ℞: Oral steroids ± mepolizumab (an anti-interleukin-5 monoclonal antibody). If FIP1L1-PDFRA genotype, diagnose myeloproliferative HES/eosinophilic leukaemia (imatinib is 1st choice). [32]

Monocytes (fig 4) 0.2–0.8 × 10^9/L (2–10%). *Increased in* (ie ***monocytosis***): Post chemo- or radiotherapy, chronic infections (eg malaria, TB, brucellosis, protozoa), malignant disease (including M4 and M5 acute myeloid leukaemia (p350), and Hodgkin's disease), myelodysplasia.

Basophils (fig 5) 0–0.1 × 10^9/L (0–1%). *Increased in* (ie ***basophilia***): myeloproliferative disease, viral infections, IgE mediated hypersensitivity reactions (eg urticaria, hypothyroidism), and inflammatory disorders (eg UC, rheumatoid arthritis).

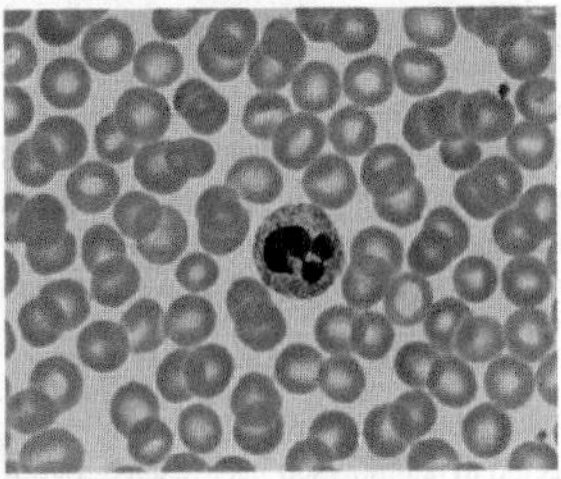

Fig 1. Neutrophil. These ingest and kill bacteria, fungi and damaged cells.[33]

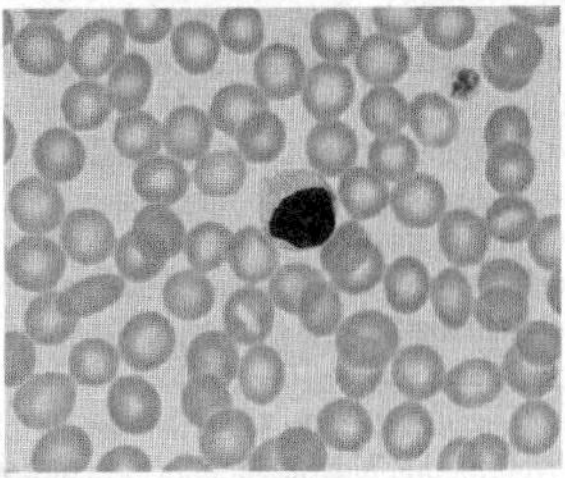

Fig 2. Lymphocyte: divided into T & B types, which have important roles in cell-mediated immunity & antibody production.[34]

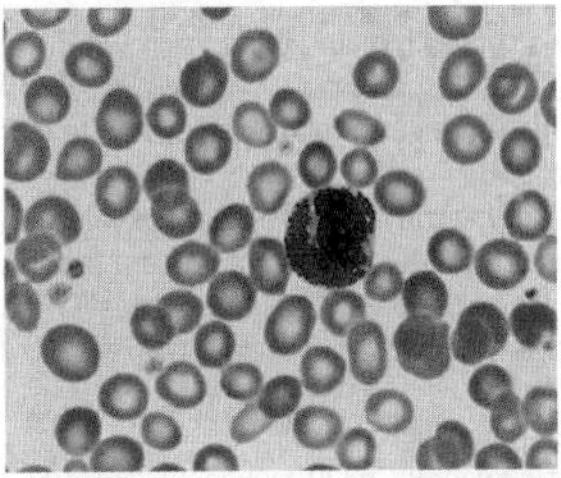

Fig 3. Eosinophil: these mediate allergic reactions, and defend against parasites.[35]

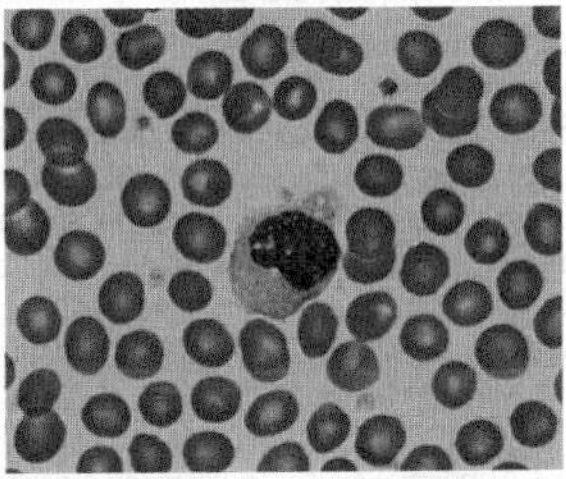

Fig 4. Monocyte: precursors of tissue macrophages.[36]

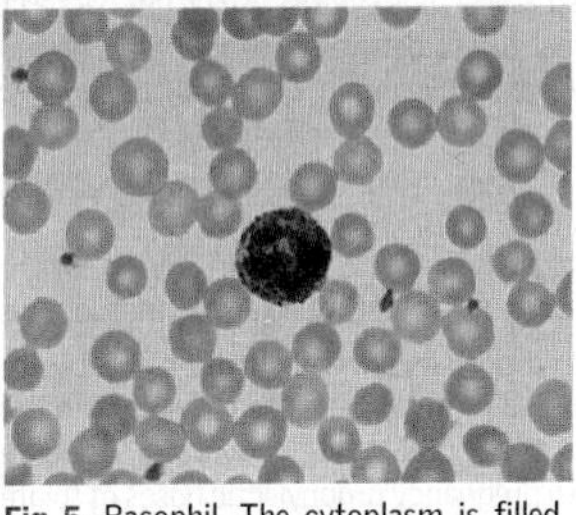

Fig 5. Basophil. The cytoplasm is filled with dark staining granules, containing histamine, myeloperoxidase and other enzymes. On binding IgE, histamine is released from the basophil.[37]

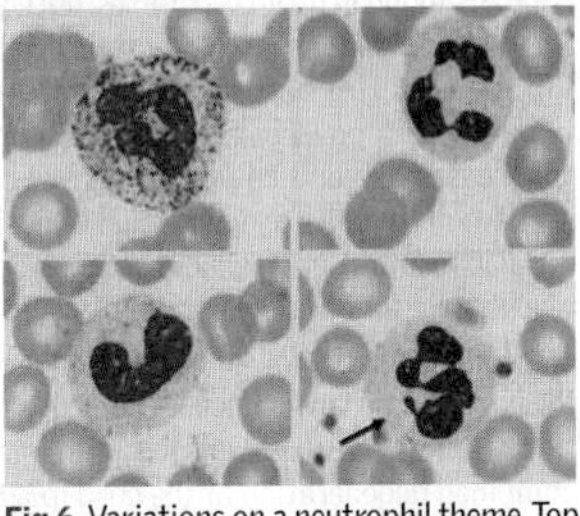

Fig 6. Variations on a neutrophil theme. Top left: 'toxic granulation': ie a neutrophil with coarse, deeply-staining granules (compare with the neutrophil to its right). This is a response to pregnancy or infection. Other neutrophil responses to infection include:

- Left shift: immature neutrophils are released with few lobes to their nuclei. A 'band form' has no lobes and may be shaped like a horse-shoe (bottom left).
- Vacuoles in the cytoplasm (the most specific sign of bacterial infection).[39]
- Döhle bodies: inconspicuous grey-blue areas of cytoplasm (residual ribosomes).

Up to 17% of neutrophils from females show a drumstick-shaped Barr body (arrow). It is the inactivated X chromosome).

Figs 1-5 courtesy of Prof. Krzysztof Lewandowski; Fig 6 Courtesy of Prof. Tangün & Dr Köroğlu.[38]

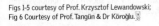

Macrocytosis (MCV >96fL) is common, often due to alcohol excess without any accompanying anaemia. Although only ~5% are due to B_{12} deficiency, pernicious anaemia is the most common cause of a macrocytic anaemia in Western countries. B_{12} and folate deficiency are megaloblastic anaemias. A megaloblast is a cell in which nuclear maturation is delayed compared with the cytoplasm. This occurs with B_{12} and folate deficiency, as they are both required for DNA synthesis.

Causes of macrocytosis

- ***Megaloblastic:*** (**fig 1**) B_{12} deficiency, folate deficiency, cytotoxic drugs.
- ***Non-megaloblastic:*** Alcohol, reticulocytosis (eg in haemolysis), liver disease, hypothyroidism, pregnancy.
- ***Other haematological disease:*** Myelodysplasia (**fig 2**), myeloma, myeloproliferative disorders, aplastic anaemia.

Tests: B_{12} and folate deficiency result in similar blood film and bone marrow biopsy appearances.
Blood film: Hypersegmented polymorphs (**fig 1**) in B_{12} and folate deficiency (target cells if liver disease; see **fig 8**, p323 & **fig 3**, p337)).
Other tests: LFT (include γGT), TFT, serum B_{12} and serum folate (or red cell folate—a more reliable indicator of folate status, as serum folate only reflects *recent* intake).
Bone marrow biopsy is indicated if the cause is not revealed by the above tests. It is likely to show one of the following four states:

1. Megaloblastic.
2. Normoblastic marrow (eg in liver disease, hypothyroidism).
3. Abnormal erythropoiesis (eg sideroblastic anaemia, p320, leukaemia, aplasia).
4. Increased erythropoiesis (eg haemolysis).

Folate is found in green vegetables, nuts, yeast & liver; it is synthesized by gut bacteria. Body stores can last for 4 months. Maternal folate deficiency causes fetal neural tube defects. It is absorbed by duodenum/proximal jejunum. ***Causes of deficiency:***

- Poor diet, eg poverty, alcoholics, elderly.
- Increased demand, eg pregnancy or ↑cell turnover (seen in haemolysis, malignancy, inflammatory disease and renal dialysis).
- Malabsorption, eg coeliac disease, tropical sprue.
- Drugs, alcohol, antiepileptics (phenytoin, valproate), methotrexate, trimethoprim.

Treatment: Assess for an underlying cause eg poor diet, malabsorption. Treat with folic acid 5mg/day PO for 4 months, ►never without B_{12} unless the patient is known to have a normal B_{12} level, as in low B_{12} states it may precipitate, or worsen, subacute combined degeneration of the cord (p328). In pregnancy prophylactic doses of folate (400µg/day) are given from conception until at least 12 wks; this helps prevent spina bifida, as well as anaemia. **NB:** if ill (eg CCF) with megaloblastic anaemia, it may be necessary to treat before serum B_{12} and folate are results are known. Do tests then treat with large doses of hydroxocobalamin, eg 1mg/48h IM—see *BNF*, with folic acid 5mg/24h PO. Blood transfusions are very rarely need, but see p318.

Folate & ischaemic heart disease Previous observational studies have indicated that higher homocysteine concentrations are associated with a greater risk of coronary heart disease. It has been suggested that folic acid supplementation may have a role in prevention of cardiac disease by lowering homocysteine levels. However, trials are disappointing (further studies awaited).[40] One meta-analysis also showed no causal relationship between high homocysteine concentrations and coronary heart disease risk in Western populations.[41]

Folate & cognition If borderline folate deficiency (as shown by ↑homocysteine), 800µg of folic acid/d for 3yrs has been found to benefit cognition.[42] the FACIT trial 2007

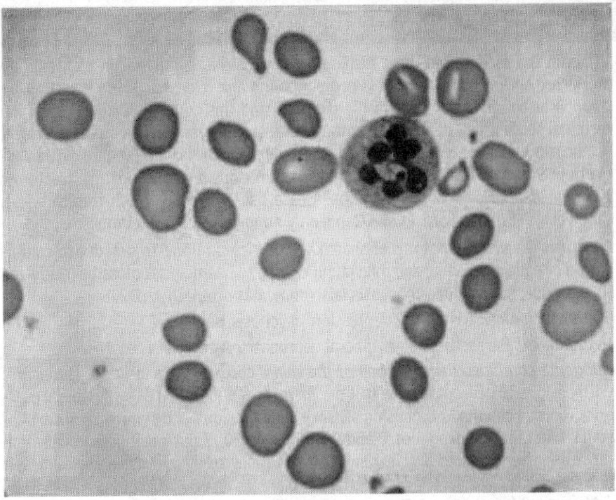

Fig 1. Megaloblastic anaemia: peripheral blood film showing many macrocytes and one hypersegmented neutrophil (normally there should be ≤5 segments).[43]

Courtesy of Professor Barbara Bain © 2005 Massachusetts Medical Society

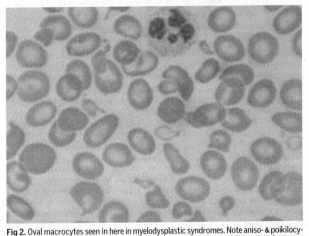

Fig 2. Oval macrocytes seen in here in myelodysplastic syndromes. Note aniso- & poikilocytosis with small fragmented cells (schistocytes). NB: B12 and folate deficiencies also cause oval macrocytes, but macrocytes caused by alcohol & liver disease are usually round.

Courtesy of Prof. Tangün & Dr Köroğlu.[44]

Vitamin B_{12} is found in meat, fish, and dairy products, but not in plants. Body stores are sufficient for 4yrs. It is protein-bound and released during digestion. B_{12} then binds to intrinsic factor in the stomach, and this complex is absorbed in the terminal ileum. In B_{12} deficiency, synthesis of thymidine, and hence DNA, is impaired, so RBC production is reduced. ***Causes of deficiency:*** • Dietary (eg vegans) • Malabsorption: *Stomach* (lack of intrinsic factor)**:** pernicious anaemia, post gastrectomy; *Terminal ileum:* ileal resection, Crohn's disease, bacterial overgrowth, tropical sprue, tapeworms (*Diphyllobothrium*) • Congenital abnormalities in metabolism.

Features *General:* Symptoms of anaemia (p318), 'lemon tinge' to skin due to combination of pallor (anaemia) and mild jaundice (due to haemolysis), glossitis (beefy-red sore tongue; fig 1), angular cheilosis (also known as stomatitis, p320).

Neuropsychiatric: Irritability, depression, psychosis, dementia.

Neurological: Paraesthesiae, peripheral neuropathy. Also:

Subacute combined degeneration of the spinal cord: Onset is insidious (*subacute*) with peripheral neuropathy due to ↓ B_{12}. There is a *combination* of symmetrical posterior (dorsal) column loss, causing sensory and LMN signs, and symmetrical corticospinal tract loss, causing motor and UMN signs (p450). Joint-position and vibration sense are often affected first leading to ataxia, followed by stiffness and weakness if untreated. The classical triad is: • Extensor plantars (UMN) • Absent knee jerks (LMN) • Absent ankle jerks (LMN). It may present with falls at night-time, due to a combination of ataxia and reduced vision, which is also seen with ↓ B_{12}. Pain and temperature sensation may remain intact even in severe cases, as the spinothalamic tracts are preserved. ►Neurological signs of B_{12} deficiency can occur without anaemia.

Pernicious anaemia (PA) This is caused by an autoimmune atrophic gastritis, leading to achlorhydria and lack of gastric intrinsic factor secretion.

Incidence 1 : 1000; ♀:♂ ≈1.6 : 1; usually >40yrs; higher incidence if blood group A.

Associations Other autoimmune diseases (p555): thyroid disease (~25%), vitiligo, Addison's disease, hypoparathyroidism. Carcinoma of stomach is ~3-fold more common in pernicious anaemia, so have a low threshold for upper GI endoscopy.

Tests • Hb↓ (3–11g/dL) • MCV↑ • WCC & platelets ↓ if severe • Serum B_{12}↓[1] • Reticulocytes ↓ or normal as production impaired • Hypersegmented polymorphs (p326) • Megaloblasts in the marrow • Specific tests for PA: **1** Parietal cell antibodies: found in 90% with PA, but also in 3–10% without. **2** Intrinsic factor (IF) antibodies: specific for pernicious anaemia, but lower sensitivity. These target B_{12} binding sites (in 50%) or ileal binding sites (in 35%).

Treatment Treat the cause if possible. If a low B_{12} is due to malabsorption, injections are required. Replenish stores with hydroxocobalamin (B_{12}) 1mg IM alternate days, eg for 2wks (or, if CNS signs, until improvement stops). Maintenance: 1mg IM every 3 months for life (child's dose: as for adult). If the cause is dietary, then oral B_{12} can be given after the initial acute course (see BOX). Initial improvement is heralded by a transient marked reticulocytosis and hence ↑MCV, after 4–5 days.

Practical hints • Beware of diagnosing PA in those under 40 yrs old: look for GI malabsorption (small bowel biopsy, p280).
- Watch for hypokalaemia as treatment becomes established.
- Transfusion is best avoided, but PA with high output CCF may require exchange transfusion (p318), after doing tests for FBC, folate, B_{12}, and marrow sampling.
- As haemopoiesis accelerates on treatment, additional iron may be needed.
- Hb rises ~1g/dL per week; WCC and platelet count should normalize in 1wk.

Prognosis Supplementation usually improves peripheral neuropathy within the first 3–6 months, but has little effect on cord signs. Patients do best if treated as soon as possible after the onset of symptoms: don't delay!

1 Plasma B_{12} levels are normal in many patients with subclinical B_{12} deficiency. See BOX.

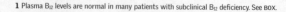

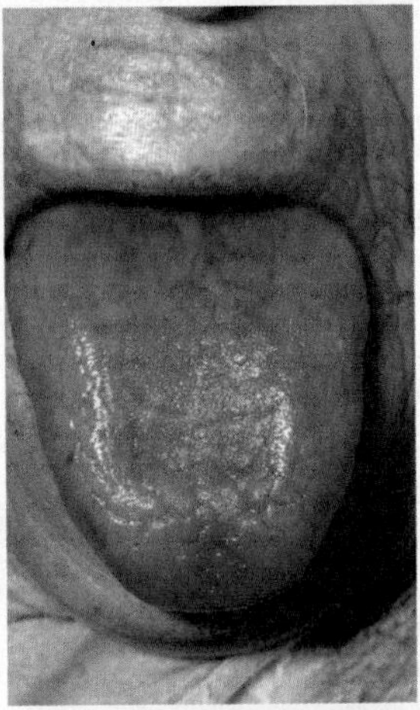

Fig 1. B12 deficiency glossitis;[45] other causes: iron (or Zn) deficiency, pellagra, contact dermatitis/specific food intolerances, Crohn's disease, drugs (minocycline, clarithromycin, some ACE-i). Glossitis may be the presenting feature of coeliac disease or alcoholism. Tongue TB: ulcers, fissure tuberculoma, or diffuse glossitis.[46]

When a low B12 is not due to pernicious anaemia

B12 deficiency is common, eg up to 15% of older people. If untreated, it can lead to megaloblastic anaemia and irreversible CNS complications. In the UK, the usual regimen is regular (eg 3-monthly) IM hydroxocobalamin (1mg). Elsewhere, ***high-dose oral B12 regimen*** (cyanocobalamin 1mg/day) is standard, less costly, and obviates the need for repeat visits to nurses. This use is not yet licensed in the UK.[47] Passive absorption of B12 occurs throughout the gut—but only 1-2% of an oral dose is absorbed this (non-terminal ileum) way. The dietary reference range is ~2μg/d.

That a low B12 is not due to PA can usually be determined by serology testing for parietal cell and intrinsic factor antibodies (but -ve in 50% of those with PA), and plasma response to oral B12, and IM B12 if no response to oral doses. The oral dose may be given as cyanocobalamin 50-150μg/daily, between meals (in the NHS, mark the prescription 'SLS', p223, to justify/communicate this special indication). This *low-dose regimen* is often sufficient for B12 deficiency of dietary origin.[48] NB: foods of non-animal origin contain no B12 unless fortified or contain bacteria. This information is important for vegans and their breastfed offspring.

Non-dietary, non-autoimmune causes of a low B12: Crohn's & coeliac disease; after gastric surgery; acid-suppressors (eg ranitidine); metformin; pancreatic insufficiency; false-low reading (seen in ≥20% so do 2 readings in isolated low B12). NB: normal serum B12 is documented in overt deficiency, which is confusing. Measuring holotranscobalamin and homocysteine or methylmalonic acid (↑ if B12 low) may be better, but have their own problems, and are non-standard tests.

NB: Schilling tests are not done as the radioisotope it uses is not available.

An approach to haemolytic anaemia[1]

Haemolysis is the premature breakdown of RBCs, before their normal life span of ~120d. It occurs in the circulation (*intravascular*) or in the reticuloendothelial system ie macrophages of liver, spleen and bone marrow (*extravascular*). In sickle-cell anaemia, lifespan may be as short as 5d. Haemolysis may be asymptomatic, but if the bone marrow does not compensate sufficiently, a haemolytic anaemia results.

An approach is first to confirm haemolysis and then find the cause—try to answer these 4 questions:

1 ***Is there increased red cell breakdown?***
- Anaemia with normal or ↑MCV.
- ↑Bilirubin: unconjugated, from haem breakdown (prehepatic jaundice).
- ↑Urinary urobilinogen (no urinary conjugated bilirubin).
- ↑Serum lactic dehydrogenase (LDH), as it is released from red cells.

2 ***Is there increased red cell production?***
- ↑Reticulocytes, causing ↑MCV (reticulocytes are large immature RBCs) and polychromasia.

3 ***Is the haemolysis mainly extra- or intravascular?***

Extravascular haemolysis may lead to splenic hypertrophy and splenomegaly. Features of intravascular haemolysis are:
- ↑Free plasma haemoglobin: released from RBCs.
- Methaemalbuminaemia: some free Hb is broken down in the circulation to produce haem and globin; haem combines with albumin to make methaemalbumin.
- ↓Plasma haptoglobin: mops up free plasma Hb, then removed by the liver.
- Haemoglobinuria: causes red-brown urine, in absence of red blood cells.
- Haemosiderinuria: occurs when haptoglobin-binding capacity is exceeded, causing free Hb to be filtered by the renal glomeruli, absorption of free Hb via the renal tubules and storage in the tubular cells as haemosiderin. This is detected in the urine in sloughed tubular cells by Prussian blue staining ~1 week after onset (implying a *chronic* intravascular haemolysis)

4 ***Why is there haemolysis?*** Causes are on p332.

History Family history, race, jaundice, dark urine, drugs, previous anaemia, travel.

Examination Jaundice, hepatosplenomegaly, gallstones (pigmented, due to ↑bilirubin from haemolysis), leg ulcers (due to poor blood flow).

Investigation FBC, reticulocytes, bilirubin, LDH, haptoglobin, urinary urobilinogen. Thick and thin films for malaria screen if history of travel. The blood film may show polychromasia and macrocytosis due to reticulocytes, or point to the diagnosis:
- Hypochromic microcytic anaemia (thalassaemia).
- Sickle cells (sickle-cell anaemia).
- Schistocytes (**fig 4**, p333; microangiopathic haemolytic anaemia).
- Abnormal cells in haematological malignancy.
- Spherocytes (hereditary spherocytosis or autoimmune haemolytic anaemia).
- Elliptocytes (**fig 7**, p333; hereditary elliptocytosis).
- Heinz bodies, 'bite' cells,[2] (glucose-6-phosphate dehydrogenase deficiency).

Further tests
- Direct antiglobulin (Coombs) *test* (DAT, **fig 1**) identifies red cells coated with antibody or complement. A +ve result indicates an immune cause of the haemolysis.
- RBC lifespan may be determined by *chromium labelling* and the major site of RBC breakdown may also be identified. This test is rarely done now.

The cause may now be obvious, but further tests may be needed. Membrane abnormalities are identified on the film and can be confirmed by *osmotic fragility* testing. *Hb electrophoresis* will detect haemoglobinopathies. *Enzyme assays* are reserved for situations when other causes have been excluded.

1 See Provan D, *Oxford Handbook of Clinical and Laboratory Investigation*, 3e, OUP.

2 On passing through the spleen, Heinz bodies may be removed, leaving an RBC with 'a bite taken out of it'. See p333 fig 2.

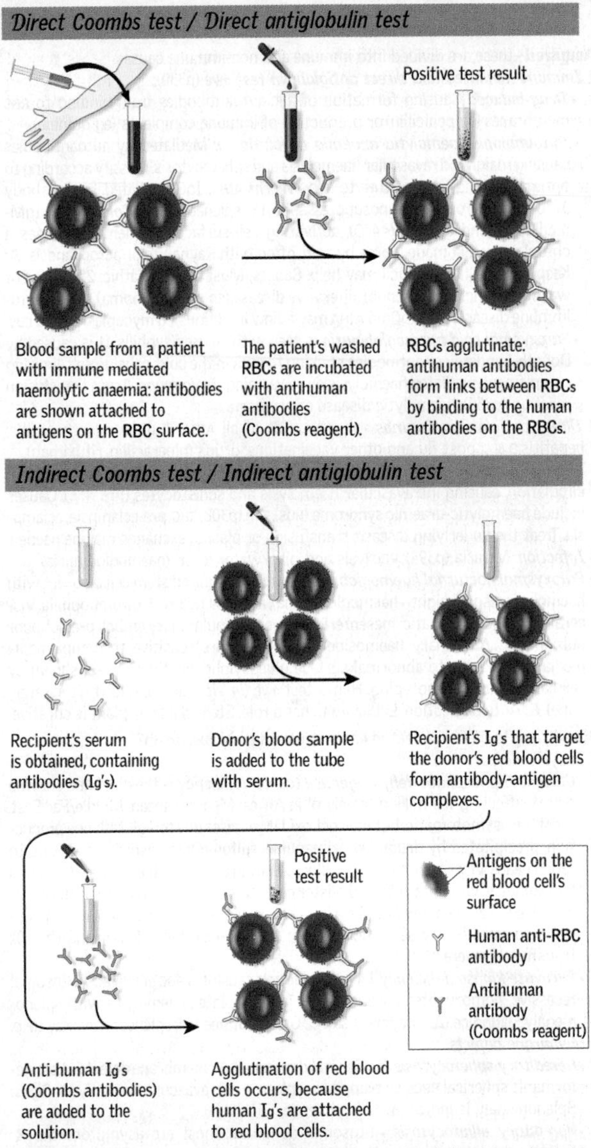
Direct Coombs test / Direct antiglobulin test
Positive test result
Blood sample from a patient with immune mediated haemolytic anaemia: antibodies are shown attached to antigens on the RBC surface.
The patient's washed RBCs are incubated with antihuman antibodies (Coombs reagent).
RBCs agglutinate: antihuman antibodies form links between RBCs by binding to the human antibodies on the RBCs.
Indirect Coombs test / Indirect antiglobulin test
Recipient's serum is obtained, containing antibodies (Ig's).
Donor's blood sample is added to the tube with serum.
Recipient's Ig's that target the donor's red blood cells form antibody-antigen complexes.
Anti-human Ig's (Coombs antibodies) are added to the solution.
Positive test result
Agglutination of red blood cells occurs, because human Ig's are attached to red blood cells.
Antigens on the red blood cell's surface
Human anti-RBC antibody
Antihuman antibody (Coombs reagent)

Fig 1. The *direct* Coombs test detects antibodies on RBCs. The *indirect* Coombs test is used in prenatal testing and before blood transfusion. It detects antibodies against RBCs that are free in serum: serum is incubated with RBCs of known antigenicity. If agglutination occurs, the indirect Coombs test is positive. With kind permission of Aria Rad.

Acquired—these are divided into immune and non-immune causes.

1 ***Immune-mediated and direct antiglobulin test +ve*** (p330):

- ***Drug-induced*** Causing formation of RBC autoantibodies from binding to RBC membranes (eg penicillin) or production of immune complexes (eg quinine).
- ***Autoimmune haemolytic anaemia (AIHA; fig 1):*** Mediated by autoantibodies causing mainly extravascular haemolysis and spherocytosis. Classify according to optimal binding temperature to RBCs: ***Warm AIHA:*** IgG-mediated, bind at body 37°C. ℞: Steroids/immunosuppressants (± splenectomy). ***Cold AIHA:*** IgM-mediated, bind at ↓T° (<4°C), activating cell-surface complement. Causes a chronic anaemia made worse by cold, often with Raynaud's or acrocyanosis. ℞: Keep warm. Chlorambucil may help. Causes: Most are idiopathic; 2° causes of warm AIHA include lymphoproliferative disease (eg CLL, lymphoma), drugs, autoimmune disease, eg SLE. Cold AIHA may follow infections, eg mycoplasma and EBV.
- ***Paroxysmal cold haemoglobinuria*** is seen with viruses/syphilis. It is caused by Donath–Landsteiner antibodies sticking to RBCs in the cold, causing self-limiting complement-mediated haemolysis on rewarming. ***Isoimmune:*** Acute transfusion reaction (p359); haemolytic disease of newborn.[50]

2 ***Direct antiglobulin/Coombs –ve AIHA:*** (2% of all AIHA) Autoimmune hepatitis; hepatitis B & C; post flu and other vaccinations; drugs (piperacillin, rituximab).[51]

3 ***Microangiopathic haemolytic anaemia (MAHA):*** A mechanical disruption of RBCs in circulation, causing intravascular haemolysis and schistocytes (**figs 4, 5**). Causes include haemolytic-uraemic syndrome (HUS), TTP (p308), DIC, pre-eclampsia, eclampsia. Treat the underlying disease; transfusion or plasma exchange may be needed.

4 ***Infection:*** Malaria (p394): RBC lysis and 'blackwater fever' (haemoglobinuria).

5 ***Paroxysmal nocturnal haemoglobinuria*** is a rare acquired stem cell disorder, with haemolysis (esp. at night→haemoglobinuria), marrow failure + thrombophilia. Visceral thrombosis (hepatic, mesenteric, CNS veins) & pulmonary emboli predict poor outcome.[52] **Δ**: Urinary haemosiderin +ve. RBCs are sensitive to complement-mediated lysis due to abnormal surface glucosylphosphatidylinositol shown by cellular immuno-phenotyping. Ham's test +ve (*in vitro* acid-induced lysis, rarely done). ℞: Anticoagulation. Eculizumab has a role. Stem cell transplant is curative.

Hereditary Is there a defect in RBC enzymes, membrane, or Hb?

1 ***Enzyme defects:***

- ***Glucose-6-phosphate dehydrogenase (G6PD) deficiency*** is the chief RBC enzyme defect, affecting 100 million mainly ♂ in Africa, Mediterranean, Middle/Far East. Most are asymptomatic, but may get oxidative crises due to ↓glutathione production, precipitated by drugs (eg primaquine, sulfonamides, aspirin), exposure to broad beans *Vicia fava* (favism), or illness. During an attack, there is rapid anaemia and jaundice, with bite cells and blister cells (**figs 2,3**) on the film. Inheritance: X-linked. **Δ**: Enzyme assay (>8wks after crisis as young RBCs may have enough enzyme so results may seem normal). ℞: Avoid precipitants (eg, henna (**fig 8**)); transfuse if severe.
- ***Pyruvate kinase deficiency*** ↓ATP production causing ↓RBC survival. Autosomal recessive; homozygotes have neonatal jaundice; later, haemolysis with splenomegaly ± jaundice. **Δ**: Enzyme assay. ℞: Often not needed; splenectomy may help.

2 ***Membrane defects***

- ***Hereditary spherocytosis*** Autosomal dominant RBC membrane defect.[53] Less deformable spherical RBCs, so trapped in spleen → extravascular haemolysis. ***Signs:*** Splenomegaly, jaundice. **Δ**: Mild anaemia. Film: **fig 6**.
- ***Hereditary elliptocytosis*** Autosomal dominant, most are asymptomatic. ℞: Folate, splenectomy is curative but reserved for severe cases. Film: **fig 7**.

3 ***Haemoglobinopathy:*** • Sickle-cell disease (p334). • Thalassaemia (p336).

Factors exacerbating haemolysis Infection leads to ↑haemolysis. The anaemia may be exacerbated by parvoviruses (*OHCS* p142), producing a cessation of marrow erythropoiesis, ie aplastic anaemia, with no reticulocyte formation (p358).

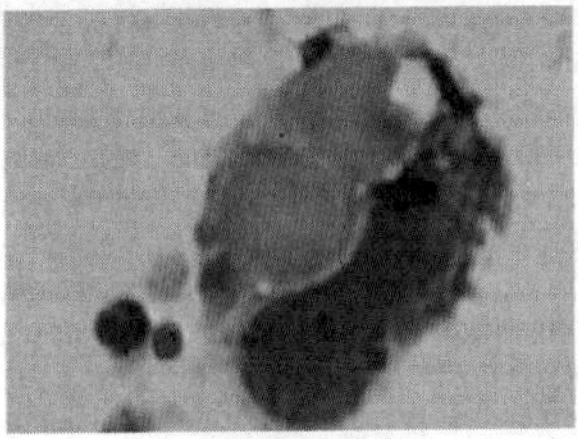

Fig 1. Autoimmune haemolytic anaemia: antibody coated red cells undergoing phagocytosis by monocytes. 54

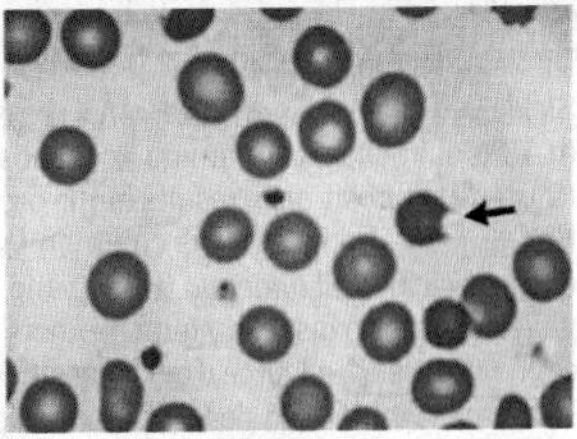

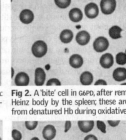

Fig 2. A 'bite' cell in G6PD, after removal of a Heinz body by the spleen; these are formed from denatured Hb during oxidative crises. 55

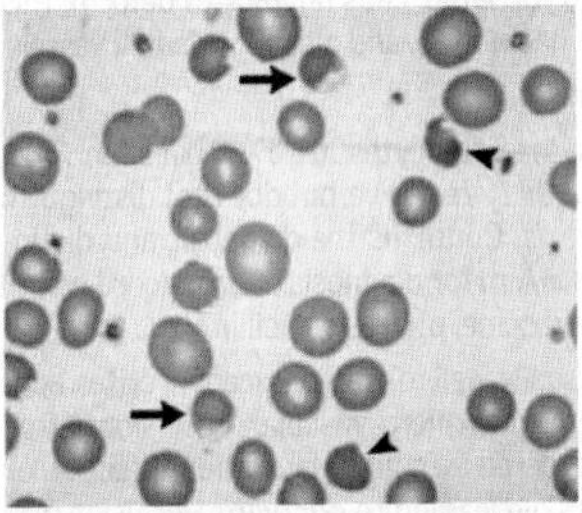

Fig 3. 'Blister' cells (arrows) in G6PD, following removal of Heinz bodies. Also contracted red cells (arrowheads). 56

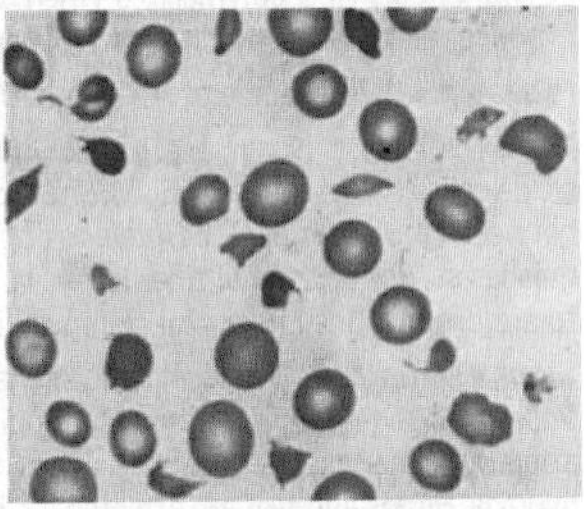

Fig 4. Microangiopathic anaemia eg from DIC: numerous cell fragments (schistocytes) are present. 57

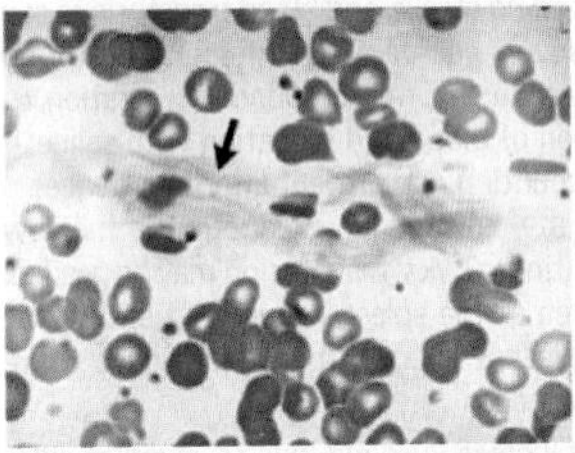

Fig 5. Fibrin strands, deposited in HUS & TTP (p308), slicing up RBCs (microangiopathy). Mechanical heart valves also slice up RBCs. 58

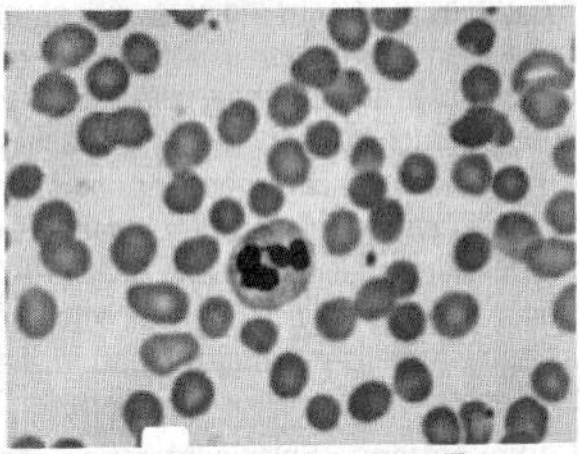

Fig 6. Hereditary spherocytosis. 59 Osmotic fragility tests: RBCs show ↑fragility in hypotonic solutions.

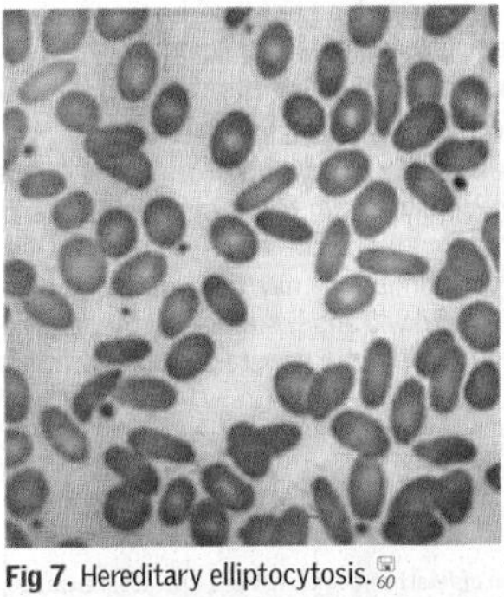

Fig 7. Hereditary elliptocytosis. 60

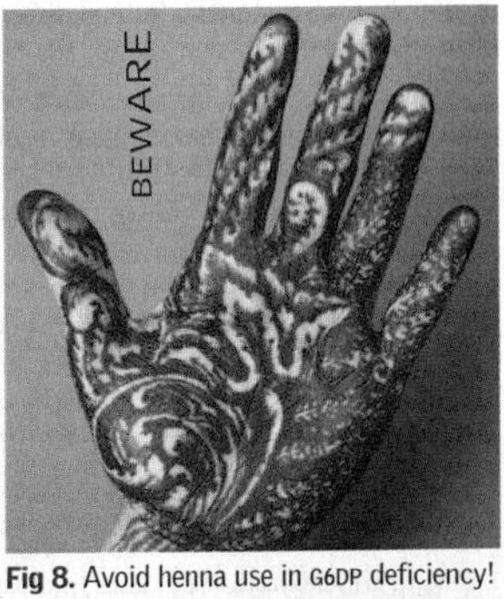

Fig 8. Avoid henna use in G6DP deficiency!

Sickle-cell anaemia is an autosomal recessive disorder causing production of abnormal β globin chains. An amino acid substitution in the gene coding for the β chain (Glu → Val at position 6) results in the production of HbS rather than HbA. HbA_2 and HbF are still produced. It is common in people of African origin. The homozygote (SS) has sickle-cell *anaemia* (HbSS), and heterozygotes (HbAS) have sickle-cell *trait*, which causes no disability (and protects from *falciparum* malaria) except in hypoxia, eg in unpressurized aircraft or anaesthesia, when vaso-occlusive events may occur, so all those of African descent need a sickle-cell test pre-op. Symptomatic sickling also occurs in heterozygotes with genes coding other Hb variants (eg HbC leading to HbSC, or β-thalassaemia trait leading to HbS/βthal).

Pathogenesis HbS polymerizes when deoxygenated, causing RBCs to deform. This produces sickle cells, which are fragile and haemolyse, and also block small vessels.

Prevalence 1:700 people of African heritage.

Tests Haemolysis is variable. Hb ≈ 6–9g/dL, ↑reticulocytes 10–20%, ↑bilirubin. *Film:* sickle cells and target cells (**fig 1**). *Sickle solubility test:* +ve, but does not distinguish between HbSS and HbAS. *Hb electrophoresis:* Confirms the diagnosis and distinguishes SS, AS states, and other Hb variants. ►Aim for diagnosis *at birth* (cord blood) to aid prompt pneumococcal prophylaxis (vaccine, p160 ± penicillin V).

Signs & symptoms Chronic haemolysis is usually well tolerated (except in crises; BOX). *Vaso-occlusive 'painful' crisis:* Common, due to micro-vascular occlusion. Often affects the marrow, causing severe pain, triggered by cold, dehydration, infection or hypoxia. Hands and feet are affected if <3yrs old leading to ***dactylitis***. Occlusion may cause ***mesenteric ischaemia***, mimicking an acute abdomen. CNS infarction occurs in ~10% of children, leading to ***stroke***, ***seizures*** or ***cognitive defects***. Transcranial Doppler ultrasonography indicates risk of impending stroke, and blood transfusions can prevent this by reducing HbS.[61] Also ***avascular necrosis*** (eg of femoral head), ***leg ulcers*** (**fig 2**) and low-flow ***priapism*** (also seen in CML, may respond to hydration, α-agonists such as phenylephrine or aspiration of blood and irrigation with saline; if for >12h prompt cavernosus-spongiosum shunting can prevent later impotence).[62]
Aplastic crisis: This is due to parvovirus B19, with sudden reduction in marrow production, especially RBCs. Usually self-limiting <2wks; transfusion may be needed.
Sequestration crisis: Mainly affects children as the spleen has not yet undergone atrophy. There is pooling of blood in the spleen ± liver, with organomegaly, severe anaemia and shock. Urgent transfusion is needed.

Complications • Splenic infarction occurs before 2yrs old, due to microvascular occlusion, leading to ↑susceptibility to infection (p367; 40% of childhood sickle deaths are caused this way; zinc supplements may help)[63][64] • Poor growth • Chronic renal failure • Gallstones • Retinal disease • Iron overload or blood-borne infection after repeated transfusion[65] • Lung damage: hypoxia→fibrosis→pulmonary hypertension, partly prevented by incentive spirometry: 10 maximal inspirations/2h.[66]

Management of chronic disease ►Get help from a haematologist.

- Hydroxycarbamide if frequent crises. Dose example: 20mg/kg/d if eGFR >60mL/min.[1]
- Splenic infarction leads to hyposplenism. Prophylaxis, in terms of antibiotics and immunization, should be given (p367).
- Febrile children risk septicaemia: repeated admission may be avoided by out-patient ceftriaxone (eg 2 doses, 50mg/kg IV on day 0 and 1). Admission may still be needed, eg if Hb <5g/dL, WCC <5 or >30 × 10^9/L, T° >40°C, severe pain, dehydration, lung infiltration. Seek expert advice.
- Bone marrow transplant can be curative, but remains controversial.

Prevention Genetic counselling; prenatal tests (*OHCS* p152–3). Parental education can help prevent 90% of deaths from sequestration crises.[67]

1 Long-term hydroxycarbamide causes ↑production of fetal haemoglobin (HbF), ↓Hb polymerization, hence fewer painful crises, chest symptoms, admissions, blood transfusions + ↓mortality by 40%. This may result from fewer episodes of marrow ischaemia and embolization. Nitric oxide is raised. NEJM 2008

Managing sickle-cell crises

►Seek expert help early.

- Give *prompt*, generous analgesia, eg IV opiates (see p576).
- Crossmatch blood. FBC, reticulocytes, blood cultures, MSU ± CXR if T° ↑ or chest signs.
- Rehydrate with IVI and keep warm. Give O_2 by mask if P_aO_2↓ or O_2 sats <95%.
- 'Blind' antibiotics (eg cephalosporin, p382) if T° >38°, unwell, or chest signs.
- Measure PCV, reticulocytes, liver, and spleen size twice daily.
- Give blood transfusion if Hb or reticulocytes fall sharply. Match blood for the blood group antigens Rh(C, D, E) and Kell, to prevent alloantibody formation. This helps oxygenation, and is as good as exchange transfusion (reserved for those who are rapidly worsening: it is a process where blood is removed and donor blood is given in stages).[69] Indications: severe chest crisis, suspected CNS event or multiorgan failure—when the proportion of HbS should be reduced to <30%.

The acute chest syndrome: Entails pulmonary infiltrates involving complete lung segments, causing pain, fever, tachypnoea, wheeze, and cough. It is serious. Incidence: ~0.1 episodes/patient/yr. 13% in the landmark Vichinsky study needed ventilation, 11% had CNS symptoms, and 9% of those over 20 years old died. Prodromal painful crisis occur ~2.5 days before any abnormalities on CXR in 50% of patients. The chief causes of the infiltrates are fat embolism from bone marrow or infection with *Chlamydia*, *Mycoplasma*, or viruses.[70] ℞: O_2, analgesia, blind antibiotics (cephalosporin + macrolide) until culture results known. Bronchodilators (eg salbutamol, p175) have proved to be effective in those with wheezing or obstructive pulmonary function at presentation. Blood transfusion (exchange if severe). *Take to ITU* if P_aO_2 cannot be kept above 9.2kPa (70mmHg) when breathing air.

Patient-controlled analgesia (example with paediatric doses) First try warmth, hydration, and oral analgesia: ibuprofen 5mg/kg/6h (codeine phosphate 1mg/kg/4–8h PO up to 3mg/kg/d may also be tried, but is less effective). If this fails, see on the ward and offer prompt morphine by IVI—eg 0.1mg/kg. Start with morphine 1mg/kg in 50mL 5% dextrose, and try a rate of 1mL/h, allowing the patient to deliver extra boluses of 1mL when needed. Do respiration and sedation score every ¼h + O_2 sats if chest/abdominal pain.[71] Liaise with the local pain service.

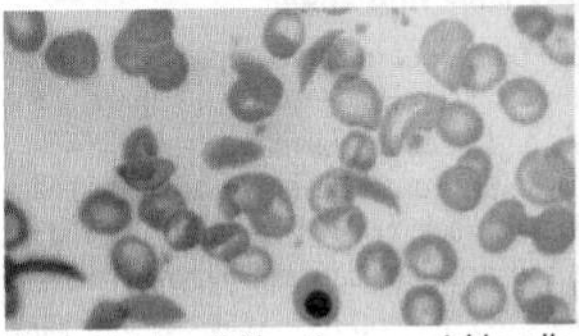

Fig 1. Sickle-cell film: there are sickle cells, target cells, and a nucleated red cell.[72]

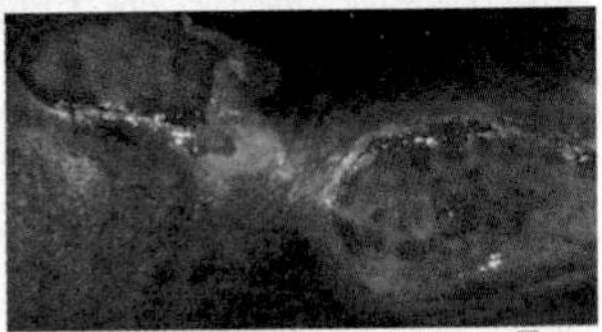

Fig 2. Leg ulcers in sickle cell disease.[73]

Figs 1 & 2 ©Prof C Lawrence.

The thalassaemias are genetic diseases of unbalanced Hb synthesis, as there is underproduction (or no production) of one globin chain (see BOX). Unmatched globins precipitate, damaging RBC membranes, causing their haemolysis while still in the marrow. They are common in areas from the Mediterranean to the Far East.

The β thalassaemias are usually caused by point mutations in β-globin genes on chromosome 11, leading to ↓β chain production (β^+) or its absence (β^0). Various combinations of mutations are possible (eg β^0/β^0, β^+/β^+, or β^+/β^0).

Tests FBC, MCV, film, iron, HbA_2, HbF, Hb electrophoresis. MRI can monitor myocardial siderosis from iron overload.[74]

β thalassaemia minor or trait (eg β/β⁺; heterozygous state): This is a carrier state, and is usually asymptomatic. Mild, well-tolerated anaemia (Hb >9g/dL) which may worsen in pregnancy. MCV <75fL, HbA_2 >3.5%, slight ↑HbF. Often confused with iron-deficiency anaemia.

β thalassaemia intermedia describes an intermediate state with moderate anaemia but not requiring transfusions. There may be splenomegaly. There are a variety of causes including mild homozygous β thalassaemia mutations, eg β^+/β^+, or co-inheritance of β thalassaemia trait with another haemoglobinopathy, eg HbC thalassaemia (1 parent has the HbC trait, and the other has β^+). Sickle-cell β^+ thalassaemia produces a picture similar to sickle-cell anaemia.

β thalassaemia major (Cooley's anaemia) denotes abnormalities in both β-globin genes, and presents in the 1st year, with severe anaemia and failure to thrive. Extramedullary haemopoiesis (RBCs made outside the marrow) occurs in response to anaemia, causing characteristic head shape, eg skull bossing (**figs 1 & 2**) and hepatosplenomegaly (also due to haemolysis). There is osteopenia (may respond to zoledronic acid).[75] Skull x-ray shows a 'hair on end' sign due to ↑marrow activity. Life-long blood transfusions are needed, with resulting iron overload/deposition seen after ~10yrs as endocrine failure (pituitary, thyroid, pancreas→diabetes mellitus), liver disease, and cardiac toxicity. The film shows very hypochromic, microcytic cells + target cells + nucleated RBCs. HbF↑↑, HbA_2 variable, HbA absent.

Treatment[76] ►Promote fitness; healthy diet. Folate (±carnitine) supplements help.[77]

- Regular (~2-4 weekly) life-long transfusions to keep Hb >9g/dL, to suppress the ineffective extramedullary haematopoiesis and to allow normal growth.
- Iron-chelators to prevent iron overload. Oral deferiprone + desferrioxamine SC twice weekly.[78] SE: pain, deafness, cataracts, retinal damage, ↑risk of *Yersinia*. Alternative: deferasirox (p334). NB: iron overload is a big problem causing hypothyroidism, hypocalcaemia,[79] hypogonadism (young men may get help from testosterone gel).[80]
- Large doses of ascorbic acid also increase urinary excretion of iron.
- Splenectomy if hypersplenism persists with increasing transfusion requirements (p367)—this is best avoided until >5yrs old due to risk of infections.
- Hormonal replacement or treatment for endocrine complications eg, diabetes mellitus, hypothyroidism. Growth hormone treatment has had variable success.[81]
- A histocompatible marrow transplant can offer the chance of a cure.[82]

Prevention Approaches include genetic counselling or antenatal diagnosis using fetal blood or DNA, then 'therapeutic' abortion.

The α thalassaemias (fig 3) There are two separate α-globin genes on each chromosome 16 ∴ there are four genes (termed αα/αα). The α thalassaemias are mainly caused by gene deletions. If all 4 α genes are deleted (--/--), death is *in utero (Bart's hydrops)*. Here, HbBarts (γ_4) is present, which is physiologically useless. HbH disease occurs if 3 genes are deleted (--/-α); there may be moderate anaemia and features of haemolysis: hepatosplenomegaly, leg ulcers and jaundice. In the blood film, there is formation of β_4 tetramers (=HbH) due to excess β chains, HbBarts, HbA and HbA_2. If 2 genes are deleted (--/αα or -α/-α), there is an asymptomatic carrier state, with ↓MCV. With one gene deleted, the clinical state is normal.

Structure of haemoglobin

The three main types of Hb in adult blood are:

Type	Peptide chains	% in adult blood	% in fetal blood
HbA	$\alpha_2\,\beta_2$	97	10–50
HbA_2	$\alpha_2\,\delta_2$	2.5	Trace
HbF	$\alpha_2\,\gamma_2$	0.5	50–90

Adult haemoglobin (HbA) is a tetramer of 2 α- and 2 β-globin chains each containing a haem group. In the first year of life, adult haemoglobin replaces fetal haemoglobin (HbF).

It might be thought that because the molecular details of the thalassaemias are so well worked out they represent a perfect example of the reductionist principle at work: find out *exactly* what is happening *within* molecules, and you will be able to explain all the manifestations of a disease. But this is not so. We have to recognize that two people with the identical mutation at their β loci may have quite different diseases. Co-inheritance of other genes and conditions (eg α thalassaemia) is part of the explanation, as is the efficiency of production of fetal haemoglobin. The reasons lie beyond simple co-segregation of genes promoting the formation of fetal Hb. The rate of proteolysis of excess α-globin chains may also be important—as may mechanisms that have little to do with genetic or molecular events. So the lesson the thalassaemias teach is more subtle than the reductionist one: it is that if you want to understand the *whole* picture, you must look at *every* level: genetic, molecular, physiological, social, and cultural. Each level influences the other, without necessarily determining them.

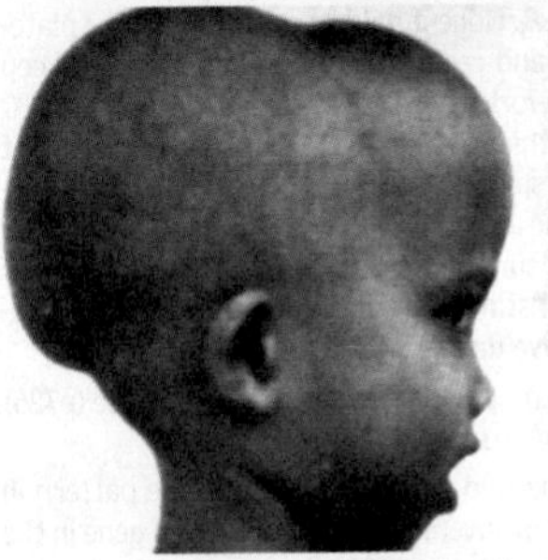

Fig 1. β thalassaemia major: bossing due to extramedullary haematopoiesis.[83]

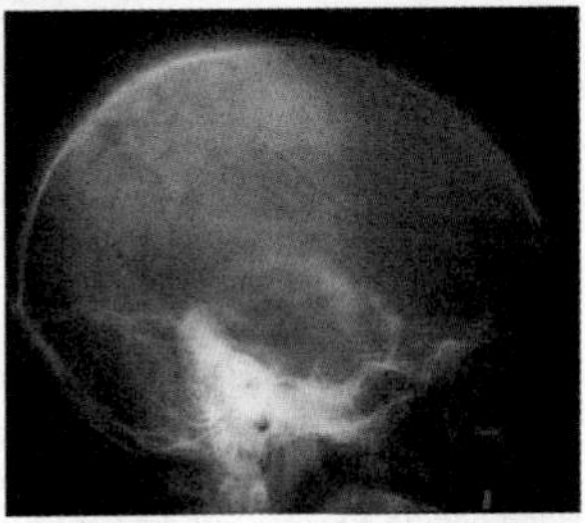

Fig 2. β thalassaemia major: skull x-ray.[84]
©Dr E van der Enden (fig 1) & Crookston collection

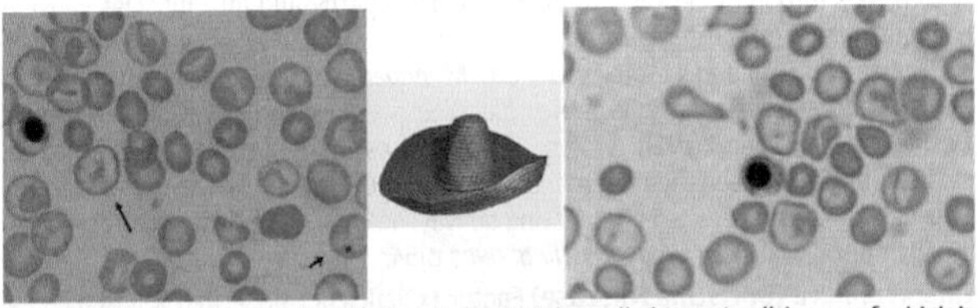

Fig 3. α thalassaemia showing Mexican hat cells (also called target cells)—one of which is arrowed on the left panel. Note also the tear-drop cell on the right panel, and the 2 normoblasts (nucleated red cells, one on each panel). The shorter arrow on the left panel points to a Howell-Jolly body. Note that the cells which are not Mexican hats are rather small (microcytic). There is also poikilocytosis (*poikilos* is Greek for varied—so this simply means that the vessels holding the haemoglobin are of varied shape).

Courtesy of Prof. Tangün & Dr Köroğlu.[85]

Bleeding disorders

After injury, 3 processes halt bleeding: vasoconstriction, gap-plugging by platelets, and the coagulation cascade (**fig 1**). Disorders of haemostasis fall into these 3 groups. The pattern of bleeding is important—vascular and platelet disorders lead to prolonged bleeding from cuts, bleeding into the skin (eg easy bruising and purpura), and bleeding from mucous membranes (eg epistaxis, bleeding from gums, menorrhagia). Coagulation disorders cause delayed bleeding into joints and muscle.

1 Vascular defects *Congenital:* Osler-Weber-Rendu syndrome (p722), connective tissue disease (eg Ehlers-Danlos syndrome *OHCS* p642, pseudoxanthoma elasticum). *Acquired:* Senile purpura, infection (eg meningococcal, measles, dengue fever), steroids, scurvy (perifollicular haemorrhages), Henoch-Schönlein purpura (p716), painful bruising syndrome—women who develop tingling under the skin followed by bruising over limbs/trunk, resolving without treatment.

2 Platelet disorders ***Decreased marrow production:*** Aplastic anaemia (p358), megaloblastic anaemia, marrow infiltration (eg leukaemia, myeloma), marrow suppression (cytotoxic drugs, radiotherapy). ***Excess destruction:*** *Immune:* Immune thrombocytopenic purpura (ITP, below), other autoimmune causes eg SLE, CLL, drugs eg heparin, viruses; *Non-immune:* DIC p346, thrombotic thrombocytopenic purpura (**TTP**) or HUS (p308), sequestration (in hypersplenism). **ITP** is caused by antiplatelet autoantibodies. It is acute (usually in children, 2wks after infection with sudden self-limiting purpura: *OHCS* p197) or chronic (seen mainly in women). Chronic ITP runs a fluctuating course of bleeding, purpura (esp. dependent pressure areas), epistaxis & menorrhagia. There is no splenomegaly. ***Tests in ITP:*** ↑megakaryocytes in marrow, antiplatelet autoantibodies often present. **℞:** None if mild. If symptomatic or platelets <20 × 10^9/L, prednisolone 1mg/kg/d, and reduce after remission; aim to keep platelets >30 × 10^9/L—takes a few days to work. If relapse, splenectomy cures ≤80%. If this fails: immunosuppression, eg azathioprine or cyclophosphamide. Platelet transfusions are not used (except during splenectomy or life-threatening haemorrhage) as these are quickly destroyed by the autoantibodies. IV immunoglobulin may temporarily raise the platelet count eg for surgery, pregnancy. Eltrombopag is a new oral thrombopoietin-receptor agonist that stimulates thrombopoiesis. ***Poorly functioning platelets:*** Seen in myeloproliferative disease, NSAIDs, and urea↑.

3 Coagulation disorders *Congenital:* Haemophilia, von Willebrand's disease (p726). *Acquired:* Anticoagulants, liver disease, DIC (p346), vitamin K deficiency.

Haemophilia A Factor VIII deficiency; inherited in an X-linked recessive pattern in 1:10,000 male births—usually due to a 'flip tip' inversion in the Factor VIII gene in the X chromosome. There is a high rate of new mutations (30% have no family history). ***Presentation*** depends on severity and is often early in life or after surgery/trauma—with bleeds into joints leading to crippling arthropathy, and into muscles causing haematomas (↑ pressure can lead to nerve palsies and compartment syndrome). ***Diagnose*** by ↑APTT and ↓factor VIII assay. ***Management:*** Seek expert advice. Avoid NSAIDs and IM injections (**fig 2**). ***Minor bleeding:*** pressure and elevation of the part. Desmopressin (0.3µg/kg/12h IVI over 20min) raises factor VIII levels, and may be sufficient. ***Major bleeds*** (eg haemarthrosis): ↑factor VIII levels to 50% of normal. ***Life-threatening bleeds*** (eg obstructing airway) need levels of 100%, eg with recombinant factor VIII. ***Genetic counselling:*** *OHCS* p154.

Haemophilia B (Christmas disease) Factor IX deficiency (inherited, X-linked recessive); behaves clinically like haemophilia A.

Acquired haemophilia is a bleeding diathesis causing big mucosal bleeds in males *and* females caused by suddenly appearing autoantibodies that interfere with factor VIII. ***Tests:*** APPT↑; VIII autoantibody↑; factor VIII activity <50%. **℞:** steroids.

Liver disease produces a complicated bleeding disorder with ↓synthesis of clotting factors, ↓absorption of vitamin K, and abnormalities of platelet function.

Malabsorption leads to less uptake of vitamin K (needed for synthesis of factors II, VII, IX, and X). Treatment is IV vitamin K (10mg) or FFP for acute haemorrhage..

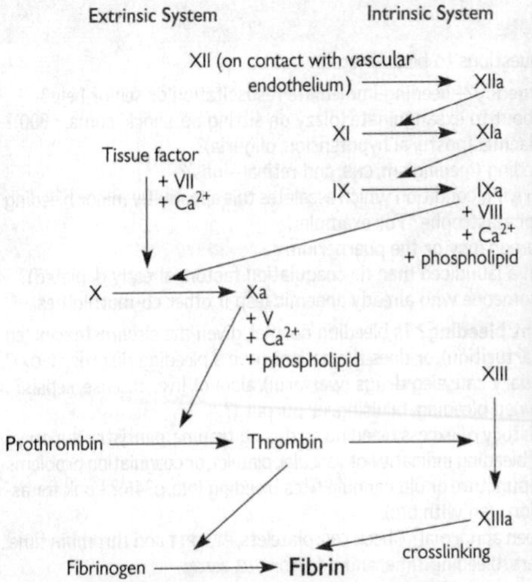

Fig 1. Intrinsic and extrinsic pathways of coagulation.

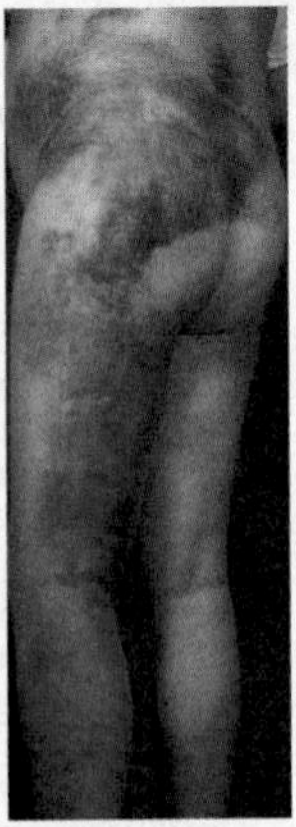

Fig 2. Mild haemophilia after an IM injection. ►Give vaccines etc SC!

Fibrinolysis

The fibrinolytic system causes fibrin dissolution and acts via the generation of plasmin. The process starts with the release of tissue plasminogen activator (t-PA) from endothelial cells, a process stimulated by fibrin formation. t-PA converts inactive plasminogen to plasmin which can then cleave fibrin, as well as several other factors. t-PA and plasminogen both bind fibrin thus localizing fibrinolysis to the area of the clot.

Mechanism of fibrinolytic agents

Alteplase (=rt-PA=Actilyse®; from recombinant DNA) is a fibrinolytic enzyme imitating t-PA, as above. Plasma $t_{½} \approx 5$min.

Streptokinase is a streptococcal exotoxin and forms a complex in plasma with plasminogen to form an activator complex, which forms plasmin from unbound plasminogen. Initially there is rapid plasmin formation which can cause uncontrolled fibrinolysis. However, plasminogen is rapidly consumed in the complex and then plasmin is only produced as more plasminogen is synthesized. The activator complex binds to fibrin, so producing some localization of fibrinolysis.

There are 3 sets of questions to be answered:

1 Is there an emergency?—needing immediate resuscitation or senior help?

- Is the patient about to exsanguinate (dizzy on sitting up, shock, coma, p800)?
- Is there hypovolaemia (postural hypotension, oliguria)?
- Is there CNS bleeding (meningism, CNS, and retinal signs)?
- Is there an underlying condition which escalates this apparently minor bleeding into an evolving catastrophe? For example:
  - Bleeding in pregnancy or the puerperium
  - GI bleeding in a jaundiced man (ie coagulation factors already depleted)
  - Bleeding in someone who already anaemic (esp if other co-morbidities).

2 Why is the patient bleeding? Is bleeding normal, given the circumstances (eg surgery, trauma, parturition), or does the patient have a bleeding disorder (BOX)?

- Is there a secondary cause eg drugs (warfarin), alcohol, liver disease, sepsis?
- Is there unexplained bleeding, bruising, or purpura?
- Past or family history of excess bleeding eg during trauma, dentistry, surgery?
- Is the pattern of bleeding indicative of vascular, platelet, or coagulation problems (p338)? Are venepuncture or old cannula sites bleeding (DIC, p346)? Look for associated conditions (eg with DIC).
- Is a clotting screen abnormal? Check FBC, platelets, PT, APTT and thrombin time. Consider D-dimers, bleeding time, and a factor VIII assay.

3 In cases of bleeding disorders, what is the mechanism? To help find the answer do FBC, film, and coagulation tests (citrate tube; false results if under-filled):

- *Prothrombin time (PT):* Thromboplastin is added to test the *extrinsic system*. PT is expressed as a ratio compared to control [International Normalized Ratio (INR), normal range = 0.9–1.2]. It tests for abnormalities in factors I, II, V, VII, X. Prolonged by: warfarin, vitamin K deficiency, liver disease, DIC.
- *Activated partial thromboplastin time (APTT):* Kaolin is added to test the *intrinsic system*. Tests for abnormalities in factor I, II, V, VIII, IX, X, XI, XII. Normal range 35–45s. Prolonged by: heparin treatment, haemophilia, DIC, liver disease.
- *Thrombin time:* Thrombin is added to plasma to convert fibrinogen to fibrin. Normal range: 10–15s. Prolonged by: heparin treatment, DIC, dysfibrinogenaemia.
- *D-dimers* are a fibrin degradation product, released from cross-linked fibrin during fibrinolysis (p339). This occurs during DIC, or in the presence of venous thromboembolism—deep vein thrombosis (DVT) or pulmonary embolism (PE). D-dimers may also be raised in inflammation, eg with infection or malignancy.
- *Bleeding time* tests haemostasis. It is done by making two small incisions into the skin of the forearm. Normal time to haemostasis: ≤10min.[87] NB: this is rarely done, as it is operator dependent; consider the PFA-100 instead (BOX 2).

Interpretation

- *Platelets:* If low, do FBC, film, clotting.
- *PT:* If long, look for liver disease or anticoagulant use.
- *APTT:* If long, consider liver disease, haemophilia (VIII or IX deficiency), or heparin.
- *Bleeding time:* Raised in von Willebrand's disease (p726), platelet disorders, and if on low- but not full-dose aspirin.[88]
- If both PT & APTT are very raised, with low platelets, and ↑D-dimers, consider DIC.

Management depends on the degree of bleeding. If shocked, resuscitate (p804). If bleeding continues in the presence of a clotting disorder or a massive transfusion, discuss the need for FFP and platelets with a haematologist. In ITP (p338), steroids ± IV immunoglobulin may be used. Especially in pregnancy (*OHCS* p88), consult an expert. Is there overdose with anticoagulants (p854)? In haemophiliac bleeds, *consult early* for coagulation factor replacement. *Never* give IM injections. Pre-op considerations: see BOX 3.

Disorder	INR	APTT	Thrombin time	Platelet count	Bleeding time	Notes
Heparin	↑	↑↑	↑↑	↔	↔	
DIC	↑↑	↑↑	↑↑	↓	↑	↑D-d, p346
Liver disease	↑	↑	↔/↑	↔/↓	↔/↑	AST↑
Platelet defect	↔	↔	↔	↔	↑(↑)	
Vit K deficiency	↑↑	↑	↔	↔	↔	
Haemophilia	↔	↑↑	↔	↔	↔	see p338
von Willebrand's	↔	↑↑	↔	↔	↑(↑)	see p726

Special tests may be available (factor assays: ►consult a haematologist).

PFA-100: an alternative to the bleeding test

The PFA-100® (Platelet Function Analyzer-100) mimics the clotting process. To do the test, a tube of fresh blood is drawn and a portion put into a test cartridge. A vacuum draws blood through a thin glass tube coated with collagen and with either adrenaline or ADP, which activates the platelets in the moving sample and promotes platelet aggregation. The time it takes for a clot to form inside the glass tube and prevent further flow is measured as a closure time (CT). An initial screen is done with collagen/adrenaline. If the CT is normal, it is unlikely that a platelet dysfunction exists. The collagen/ADP test can confirm an abnormal collagen/adrenaline test. If both are abnormal, it is likely that there is platelet dysfunction and further testing for inherited or acquired bleeding disorders is indicated. If the collagen/ADP test is normal, then the abnormal collagen/adrenaline test may be due to aspirin ingestion.[89]

Is this pre-op patient at risk of excessive bleeding?

Take a bleeding history! The more structured this is the better.[90] If excessive, prolonged, or unexplained bleeding in the past, or if on agents known to affect haemostasis, or if the liver is suspect, or there is a condition such as lupus, or if bleeding might be disastrous, further tests may be indicated after discussion with a haematologist: INR, FBC, film, aPPT, PFA-100 (see above) and von Willebrand factor (vWF: Ag). In one pre-op study the bleeding history was +ve in 11%, and tests showed impaired haemostasis in 40% of these. ~98% of these are detectable by PDA-100.[91]

►Blood should only be given if strictly necessary ***and there is no alternative.*** Outcomes are often ***worse*** after a transfusion.

- Know and use local procedures to ensure that the right blood gets to the right patient at the right time. See p569 for quantities to request.
- Take blood for crossmatching from only one patient at a time. Label immediately. This minimizes risk of wrong labelling of samples.[1]
- When giving blood, monitor TPR and BP every ½h.
- Do not use giving sets which have contained dextrose or Gelofusine®.

Group-and-save (G&S) requests Find out your local guidelines for elective surgery. Having crossmatched blood to hand may not be needed if a blood sample is already in the lab, with group determined, without any atypical antibodies (ie G&S).

Products *Whole blood:* (rarely used) Indications: exchange transfusion; grave exsanguination—use crossmatched blood if possible, but if not, use 'universal donor' group **O Rh–ve** blood, changing to crossmatched blood as soon as possible. ►Blood even <2d old has no effective platelets. ***Red cells:*** (packed to make haematocrit ~70%) Use to correct anaemia or blood loss. 1U ↑Hb by 1-1.5g/dL. In anaemia, transfuse until Hb ~8g/dL. ***Platelets:*** (p358) Not usually needed if not bleeding or count is >20 ×10⁹/L. 1U should ↑platelet count by >20 × 10⁹/L. Failure to do so suggests refractoriness—discuss with haematologist. If surgery is planned, get advice if <100 ×10⁹/L. ***Fresh frozen plasma (FFP):*** Use to correct clotting defects: eg DIC (p346); warfarin overdosage where **vitamin K** would be too slow; liver disease; thrombotic thrombocytopenic purpura (p308). It is expensive and carries all the risks of blood transfusion. Do not use as a simple volume expander. ***Human albumin solution*** is produced as 4.5% or 20% protein solution and is for use as protein replacement. 20% albumin can be used temporarily in the hypoproteinaemic patient (eg liver disease; nephrosis) who is fluid overloaded, without giving an excessive salt load. Also used as replacement in abdominal paracentesis (p779). ***Others*** Cryoprecipitate (a source of fibrinogen); coagulation concentrates (self-injected in haemophilia); immunoglobulin (*anti-D*, *OHCS* p9).

Complications of transfusion[92] ►Management of acute reactions: see BOX.

- ***Early (within 24h):*** Acute haemolytic reactions (eg ABO or Rh incompatibility); anaphylaxis; bacterial contamination; febrile reactions (eg from HLA antibodies); allergic reactions (itch, urticaria, mild fever); fluid overload; transfusion-related acute lung injury (TRALI), basically ARDS due to anti-leucocyte antibodies in donor plasma.
- ***Delayed (after 24h):*** Infections (eg viruses: hepatitis B/C, HIV; bacteria; protozoa; prions); iron overload (treatment, p336); graft-versus-host disease; post-transfusion purpura—potentially lethal fall in platelet count 5-7d post-transfusion requiring specialist treatment with IV immunoglobulin and platelet transfusions.

Massive blood transfusion This is defined as replacement of an individual's entire blood volume (>10U) within 24h. Complications: platelets↓; Ca^{2+}↓; clotting factors↓; K^{+}↑; hypothermia.

Transfusing patients with heart failure If Hb ≤5g/dL with heart failure, transfusion with packed red cells is vital to restore Hb to a safe level, eg 6-8g/dL, but must be done with great care. Give each unit over 4h with *furosemide* (eg 40mg slow IV/PO; don't mix with blood) with alternate units. Check for ↑JVP and basal lung crackles; consider CVP line. If CCF gets worse, and immediate transfusion is vital, try a 2-3U exchange transfusion, removing blood at same rate as transfused.

Autologous transfusion There is a role for patients having their own blood stored pre-op for later use. ***Erythropoietin*** (*EPO*, p302) can increase the yield of autologous blood in normal people. Intraoperative cell salvage with retransfusion is also being used more often, especially in cardiac, vascular and emergency surgery.[93] Cost-analysis shows that it may be worthwhile on an economic basis alone.[94]

1 Other methods to avoid mishaps: electronic bar code readers; bedside ABO agglutination test on a card (used in France; where this is linked with other methods, 99.65% reliability is achieved).

Transfusion reactions

All UK blood products are now leucocyte-depleted (white cells $<5\times10^6$/L) so as to reduce the incidence of complications such as alloimmunization to HLA class I antigens and febrile transfusion reactions. Does giving paracetamol and antihistamines before the transfusion prevent more serious reactions? Probably not (although some mild fevers may be prevented).[95]

Acute haemolytic reaction (eg ABO incompatibility) Agitation, T°↑ (rapid onset), ↓BP, flushing, abdominal/chest pain, oozing venepuncture sites, DIC.	STOP transfusion. Check identity and name on unit; tell haematologist; send unit + FBC, U&E, clotting, cultures, & urine (haemoglobinuria) to lab. Keep IV line open with 0.9% saline. Treat DIC (p346).
Anaphylaxis Bronchospasm, cyanosis, ↓BP, soft tissue swelling.	STOP the transfusion. Maintain airway and give oxygen. Contact anaesthetist. ▸▸See p806.
Bacterial contamination T°↑ (rapid onset), ↓BP, and rigors.	STOP the transfusion. Check identity against name on unit; tell haematologist and send unit + FBC, U&E, clotting, cultures & urine to lab. Start broad-spectrum antibiotics.
TRALI (See p342) Dyspnoea, cough; CXR 'white out'	STOP the transfusion. Give 100% O_2. ▸▸Treat as ARDS, p178. Donor should be removed from donor panel.
Non-haemolytic febrile transfusion reaction Shivering and fever usually ½–1h after starting transfusion.	SLOW or STOP the transfusion. Give an antipyretic, eg *paracetamol* 1g. Monitor closely. If recurrent, use leucocyte-depleted blood or WBC filter.
Allergic reactions Urticaria and itch.	SLOW or STOP the transfusion; *chlorphenamine* 10mg slow IV/IM. Monitor closely.
Fluid overload Dyspnoea, hypoxia, tachycardia, ↑JVP & basal crepitations.	SLOW or STOP the transfusion. Give oxygen and a diuretic, eg *furosemide* 40mg IV initially. Consider CVP line+exchange transfusion.

Blood transfusion and Jehovah's Witnesses

These patients are likely to refuse even vital transfusions on religious grounds.[1] These views must be respected, but complex issues arise if the patient is a child, or (perhaps) an adult who lives a sheltered life, and may not be able to give or withhold consent in an informed way—see p554. When in doubt, apply to the Court. Judges tend to take a narrow view on this, acting as if any immediate benefit to life must trump putative benefits in any life hereafter.[2] How can refusal be informed, it might be argued, if only the physical (and not the metaphysical) consequences of transfusion can be foreseen?

Even if metaphysical considerations are put to one side, it is a question whether giving a transfusion against consent could amount to a degrading act or torture, against which the European Convention on Human Rights gives absolute, inalienable protection. ▶Some patients may not want to forsake their principles but would not mind too much being told what to do, thereby not being the means of their child's destruction, while being true to their beliefs. It is possible to hold two incompatible beliefs at the same time.[1]

1 Accepting transfusion implies **self-expulsion** from the church, but it is no longer a '**disfellowshipping event**' with active expulsion. This tenet is based on (among others) the biblical verse "*no soul of you shall eat blood*" (Leviticus 17:12).
2 V Wason 1998 Court Order (High Court Family Division) Re L (A Minor), June 1-10.

Main indications

- *Therapeutic:* Venous thromboembolic disease: DVT and PE.
- *Prophylactic:* Prevention of DVT/PE in high-risk patients (p568), eg post-op. Prevention of stroke, eg in chronic AF or prosthetic heart valve.

Heparin *1 Low molecular weight heparin (LMWH)* Given sc. Molecular weight ~5000 Daltons (Da), eg dalteparin, enoxaparin, tinzaparin. Inactivates factor Xa (but not thrombin). T½ is 2-4-fold longer than standard heparin, and response is more predictable, and so only needs to be given once or twice daily, and no laboratory monitoring is usually required. It has replaced unfractionated heparin (UFH) as the preferred option in the prevention and treatment of venous thromboembolism and in acute coronary syndrome. See *BNF* for doses. It accumulates in renal failure: lower doses are used for prophylaxis, or UFH for therapeutic doses.

2 Unfractionated heparin (UFH) IV or SC. ~13,000Daltons. A glycosaminoglycan, which binds antithrombin (an endogenous inhibitor of coagulation), increasing its ability to inhibit thrombin, factor Xa, and IXa. Rapid onset and has a short T½. Monitor and adjust dose with APTT (p340).

SE for both: ↑Bleeding (eg at operative site, gastrointestinal, intracranial), heparin-induced thrombocytopenia (HIT), osteoporosis with long-term use. HIT and osteoporosis are less common with LMWH than UFH. Beware hyperkalaemia.

CI: Bleeding disorders, platelets $<60\times10^9$/L, previous HIT, peptic ulcer, cerebral haemorrhage, severe hypertension, neurosurgery.

Warfarin is used orally once daily as long-term anticoagulation. The therapeutic range is narrow, varying with the condition being treated (see BOX 1 and BOX 2)—and is measured as a ratio compared with the standard INR. Warfarin inhibits the reductase enzyme responsible for regenerating the active form of vitamin K, producing a state analogous to vit K deficiency. *CI:* Peptic ulcer, bleeding disorders, severe hypertension, pregnancy (teratogenic, see *OHCS* p640). Use with caution in the elderly and those with past GI bleeds. In the UK, warfarin tablets are 0.5mg (white), 1mg (brown), 3mg (blue), or 5mg (pink). ►Interactions: p768.

Others Fondaparinux is a pentasaccharide Xa inhibitor and may be used in place of LMWH for prophylaxis in certain situations. Factor Xa inhibitors (rivaroxaban and apixaban) and direct thrombin inhibitors (dabigatran) are new oral anticoagulants that do not need monitoring—but they have not yet displaced warfarin.[96]

Beginning therapeutic anticoagulation (follow local guidelines, and see *BNF*). For treatment of venous thromboembolism, LMWH or UFH are used initially, and warfarin is given in combination usually from day 1. Heparin should be continued until INR has reached target therapeutic range (see BOX 3) *and* until day 5, as warfarin has an initial prothrombotic effect.

- *LMWH* Dose according to weight (see *BNF*).

UFH IV infusion: • Give heparin 5000iu IV bolus over 30min. (10000iu in severe PE).

- Prepare syringe pump: with 0.9% saline
- Infuse heparin at a rate of 18 units/kg/h. Check APTT at 6h, aim for APTT ratio 1.5-2.5 (see BOX). Measure APTT daily or 10h after dose change.

Warfarin is given daily; start with 10mg stat at 18.00. Do INR 16h later.

- If INR <1.8 (as is likely) the 2nd dose of warfarin is 5 or 10mg at 18.00 (24h after first dose). Give the lower dose if >60yrs, liver disease, or cardiac failure. But if INR >1.8 (warfarin sensitivity; rare) give just 0.5mg.
- Do INR daily for 5d and adjust dose (see BOX—use 5mg, not 10mg dose 3 if over 60, or liver disease, or cardiac failure).
- Stop heparin after 5d and when INR >2 for 2d. Tell lab when stopped.
- Measure INR on alternate days until stable, then weekly or less often.

Antidotes If UFH overdose: stop infusion. If there is bleeding, protamine sulphate counteracts UFH: discuss with a haematologist. Warfarin: see BOX 2.

Warfarin guidelines and target levels for INR[1]

- Pulmonary embolism and DVT. Aim for INR of 2–3; 3.5 if recurrent.
- Atrial fibrillation[2]: for stroke prevention (p124). Target INR 2–3. An alternative is aspirin (but less effective), if the risk of bleeding with warfarin is high (eg falls with risk of intracranial bleed, or difficulty with monitoring).
- Prosthetic metallic heart valves: for stroke prevention. Target INR 3–4.

Duration of anticoagulation in DVT/PE
- If the cause will go away (eg post-op immobility):
  At least 6 weeks for below knee DVT.
  At least 3 months for above knee DVT or PE.
- At least 6 months if no cause found.
- Indefinitely for identified, enduring causes, eg thrombophilia (p368).

Warfarin dosage and excessive anticoagulation

Below is a guide to warfarin dosing, for target INR of 2–3:

INR	<2	2	2.5	2.9	3.3	3.6	4.1
3rd dose	10mg	5mg	4mg	3mg	2mg	0.5mg	0mg
Maintenance	≥6mg	5.5mg	4.5mg	4mg	3.5mg	3mg	*

*Miss a dose; give 1–2mg the next day (if INR >4.5, miss 2 doses).

Lower doses are given in certain groups of patients (see p334).

In cases of raised INR (see *BNF*):

INR 4.5–6	Reduce warfarin dose or omit. Restart when INR <5.
6–8	Stop warfarin. Restart when INR <5.
>8, no bleed or minor bleed	If no bleeding: stop warfarin. 0.5–2.5mg vitamin K (oral) if risk factors for bleeding. Check INR daily.
Major bleed, (including intracranial haemorrhage)	Stop warfarin. Give prothrombin complex concentrate (50units/kg; discuss with haematologist). If unavailable, give FFP (15mL/kg ≈ 1L for a 70kg man). Also give 5–10mg vitamin K IV.

Minor bleeding includes epistaxis.

Vitamin K may take several hours to work and can cause prolonged resistance when restarting warfarin, so should be avoided if possible when longterm anticoagulation is needed. Prothrombin complex concentrate contains a concentrate of factor IX, and provides a more complete and rapid reversal of warfarin than FFP.

IV heparin dosing

APTT ratio	>5	4–5	3–4	2.5–3	1.5–2.5	1.2–1.4	<1.2
Change rate (iu/h) by	-500*	-300	-100	-50	0	+200	+400

*Stop for 1 hour then recheck APTT. Reduce dose by 500iu/h and restart if <5.

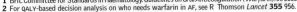

1 Brit. Committee for Standards in Haematology. *Guidelines on Oral Anticoagulation (Warfarin)*: 3e 2005.
2 For QALY-based decision analysis on who needs warfarin in AF, see R Thomson *Lancet* **355** 956.

Leukaemic patients often fall ill suddenly and deteriorate fast, so prompt treatment is vital. Major concerns are infection, bleeding and hyperviscosity (p366). Take non-specific confusion/drowsiness seriously: do blood cultures, exclude hypoglycaemia, do U&E, LFT, Ca^{2+} and clotting screen. Consider CNS bleeding—CT/MRI if any doubt. Correct haemostatic defects urgently with platelets/FFP. See p488 for delirium.

With any new patient, try to find out what the aim of treatment is: cure, or prolonging disease-free survival, or palliation of symptoms with minimal toxicity? Direct your efforts accordingly—and get help when these issues are not clear.

Neutropenic regimen (for when neutrophil count ≤1.0 × 10^9/L). ►Close liaison with a microbiologist and haematologist is vital. Abide by infection control procedures!
- Full barrier nursing if possible. Hand-washing is vital. Use a side room.
- Avoid IM injections (danger of an infected haematoma).
- Look for infection (mouth, axilla, perineum, IVI site). Take swabs.
- Check: FBC, platelets, INR, U&E, LFT. Take cultures (blood × 3—peripherally ± Hickman line; urine, sputum, stool if diarrhoea) and request a CXR.
- Wash perineum after defecation. Swab moist skin with chlorhexidine. Avoid unnecessary rectal examinations. Oral hygiene (eg hydrogen peroxide mouth washes/2h) and *Candida* prophylaxis are important (p238).
- TPR (vital signs) 4-hrly. High-calorie diet; avoid foods with high risk of microbial contamination. Vases containing cut flowers pose a *Pseudomonas* risk.

Use of antibiotics in neutropenia ►Treat any known infection promptly.
- If T° >38°C or T° >37.5°C on separate occasions, 1-2h apart, or the patient is toxic, assume septicaemia and start blind combination therapy—eg an aminoglycoside (gentamicin, p381) plus *either* ceftazidime (p379, or outside the UK, cefepime, p379) *or* piperacillin-tazobactam (p378)+vancomycin (p381) if Gram +ve organisms suspected or isolated (eg Hickman line sepsis). Check local preferences. Continue until afebrile for 72h or 5d course, and until neutrophils recover (>0.5×10^9/L). If fever persists despite antibiotics, think of CMV and fungi (eg *Candida; Aspergillus*, p440).
- Consider treatment for *Pneumocystis* (p411, eg co-trimoxazole, ie trimethoprim 20mg/kg with sulfamethoxazole 100mg/kg/day PO/IV in 2 daily doses). Remember TB!
- Genetically engineered recombinant human granulocyte-colony stimulating factor (G-CSF) stimulates neutrophil production. Follow local guidelines/expert advice.
- What about prophylaxis? Fluoroquinolones (p380) ↓mortality in acute leukaemia, high-dose chemotherapy, and for the 1st cycle of standard chemotherapy in those with solid tumours and lymphomas. Inevitably, resistance develops.[97] With monoclonal antibodies, give herpes, pneumocystis, and CMV (valganciclovir) prophylaxis.[98]

Other dangers • *Tumour lysis syndrome:* Caused by a massive destruction of cells leading to K^+↑, urate↑ and renal impairment. *Risk*↑ *if:* LDH↑, creatinine↑, urate↑, WCC >25×10^9/L.[99] *Prevention:* high fluid intake + allopurinol pre-cytotoxics. For patients at high risk of cell lysis, recombinant uricase (rasburicase) may be given. Seek advice.
- ***Hyperviscosity:*** (p366). If WCC is >100 × 10^9/L WBC thrombi may form in brain, lung, and heart (leukostasis). Avoid transfusing before lowering WCC, eg with hydroxycarbamide or leukopheresis, as viscosity rises (risk of leukostasis ↑).
- ***Disseminated intravascular coagulation*** (DIC; widespread activation of coagulation, from release of procoagulants into the circulation; **fig 1**). Clotting factors and platelets are consumed, with ↑risk of bleeding. Fibrin strands fill small vessels, haemolysing passing RBCs, and fibrinolysis is also activated. ***Causes:*** Malignancy, sepsis, trauma, obstetric events: *OHCS* p88. ***Signs:*** Bruising, bleeding anywhere (eg venepuncture sites), renal failure. ***Tests:*** Platelets↓; PT↑; APTT↑; fibrinogen↓ (correlates with severity); fibrin degradation products (D-dimers) ↑↑. Film: broken RBCs (schistocytes). ***℞:*** Treat the cause. Replace platelets if <50×10^9/L, cryoprecipitate to replace fibrinogen, FFP to replace coagulation factors. Heparin is controversial. Activated protein C reduces mortality in DIC with severe sepsis or multi-organ failure.[100] The use of all-transretinoic acid (ATRA) has significantly reduced the risk of DIC in acute promyelocytic leukaemia (the commonest leukaemia associated with DIC).

Leukaemias

These are divided into 4 main types depending on the cell line involved and the speed of disease progression:

	Lymphoid	Myeloid
Acute	Acute lymphoblastic leukaemia (ALL)	Acute myeloid leukaemia (AML)
Chronic	Chronic lymphocytic leukaemia (CLL)	Chronic myeloid leukaemia (CML)

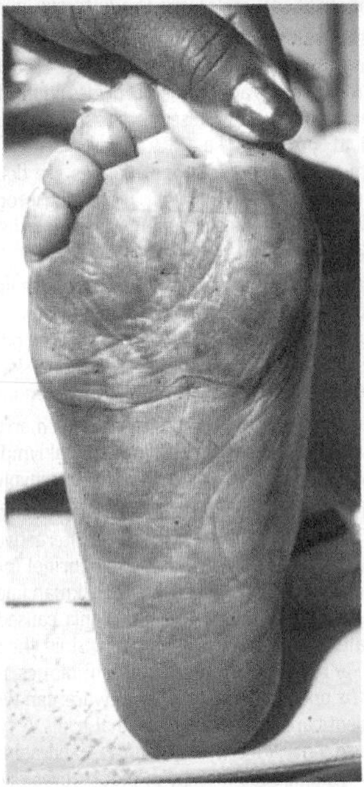

Fig 1. The appearance of DIC on the sole.[101]
Courtesy of the Crookston collection

This is a malignancy of lymphoid cells, affecting either B or T lymphocyte cell lines, arresting maturation and promoting uncontrolled proliferation of immature blast cells, with bone marrow failure and tissue infiltration. It is thought to develop from a combination of genetic susceptibility (eg with translocations, and gains and losses of whole chromosomes[1]) + an environmental trigger. Ionizing radiation, eg X-rays, during pregnancy, and Down's syndrome are important associations).[102] It is the commonest cancer of childhood, and is rare in adults. CNS involvement is common.

Classification is based on 3 systems:

1 *Morphological* The FAB system (French, American & British) divides ALL into 3 types (L1, L2, L3) by microscopic appearance. Provides limited information (**figs 1–4**).

2 *Immunological* Surface markers are used to classify ALL into:
 • Precursor B-cell ALL • T-cell ALL • B-cell ALL.

3 *Cytogenetic* Chromosomal analysis. Abnormalities are detected in up to 85%, which are often translocations. Useful for predicting prognosis, eg poor with Philadelphia chromosome (see below), and for detecting disease recurrence.

Signs and symptoms (**fig 5**) are due to:
- Marrow failure: Anaemia (↓Hb), infection (↓WCC), and bleeding (↓platelets).
- Infiltration: Hepato- and splenomegaly, lymphadenopathy—superficial or mediastinal, orchidomegaly, CNS involvement—eg cranial nerve palsies, meningism.

Common infections: Especially chest, mouth, perianal and skin. Bacterial septicaemia, zoster, CMV, measles, candidiasis, *Pneumocystis* pneumonia (p410).

Tests • Characteristic blast cells on blood film and bone marrow. WCC usually high.
- CXR and CT scan to look for mediastinal and abdominal lymphadenopathy.
- Lumbar puncture should be performed to look for CNS involvement.

Treatment ►Educate and motivate: without this, young people may shy away from the responsibilities of self-care, to their detriment.[103] Interactive video games help.[104]
- *Support:* Blood/platelet transfusion, IV fluids, allopurinol (prevents tumour lysis syndrome). Insert a subcutaneous port system/Hickman line for IV access.[105]
- *Infections:* These are dangerous, due to neutropenia caused by the disease and treatment. Immediate IV antibiotics for infection. Start the neutropenic regimen (p346): prophylactic antivirals, antifungals and antibiotics, eg co-trimoxazole to prevent *Pneumocystis* pneumonia (p346), but beware: can worsen neutropenia.
- *Chemotherapy:* Patients are entered into national trials. A typical programme is:
 Remission induction: eg vincristine, prednisolone, L-asparaginase + daunorubicin.
 Consolidation: High/medium-dose therapy in 'blocks' over several weeks.
 CNS prophylaxis: Intrathecal (or high-dose IV) methotrexate ± CNS irradiation.
 Maintenance: Prolonged chemotherapy, eg mercaptopurine (daily), methotrexate (weekly), and vincristine + prednisolone (monthly) for 2yrs. Relapse is common in blood, CNS, or testis (so examine these sites at follow-up). More details: *OHCS* p194.
- ***Matched related allogeneic marrow transplantations*** once in 1st remission is the best option in standard-risk younger adults (?too many SE if older).[106] MRC UK ALL XII [107]

Haematological remission means no evidence of leukaemia in the blood, a normal or recovering blood count, and <5% blasts in a normal regenerating marrow.

Prognosis Cure rates for children are 70–90%; for adults only 40% (higher when imatinib/rituximab, p353, are used). Poor prognosis if: adult, male, Philadelphia chromosome (p352): BCR-ABL gene fusion due to translocation of chromosomes 9 & 22, presentation with CNS signs, Hb↓[108] or WCC >100×10⁹/L or B-cell ALL. PCR is used to detect minimal residual disease, undetectable by standard means. Prognosis is poor if seen in high amounts at presentation or during remission.

Personalized treatment ►*One size does not fit all!*[109] Aim to tailor therapy to the exact gene defect, and according to individual metabolism. Monoclonal antibodies, gene-targeted retinoids, cytokines, vaccines, and T-cell infusions are relevant here.[110] Biomarkers, eg thiopurine methyltransferase, can predict toxicity from thiopurines.

1 eg t(12:21) ETV6-RUNX1, t(1;19) TCF3-PBX1, (t(9;22) BRAC-ABL1—and rearrangement of MLL.

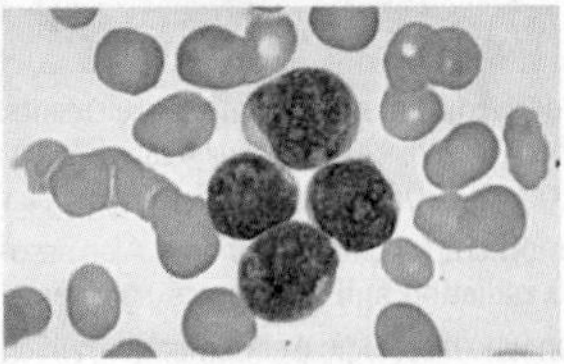

Fig 1. Blood film in ALL, L1 subtype. Small blasts with scanty cytoplasm. [111]

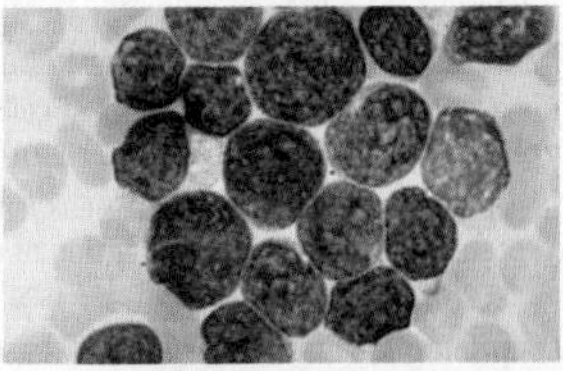

Fig 2. Bone marrow in ALL, L1 subtype. [112]

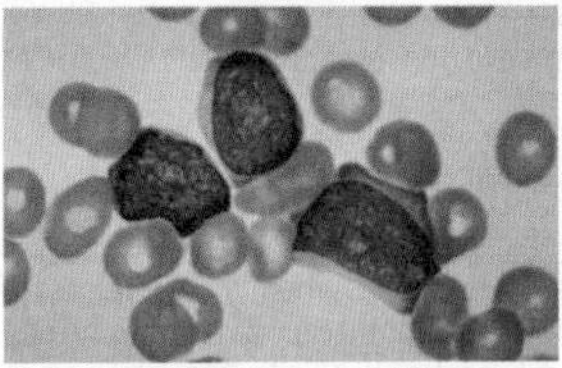

Fig 3. Blood film in ALL, L2 subtype. Larger blast cells with greater morphological variation and more abundant cytoplasm. [113]

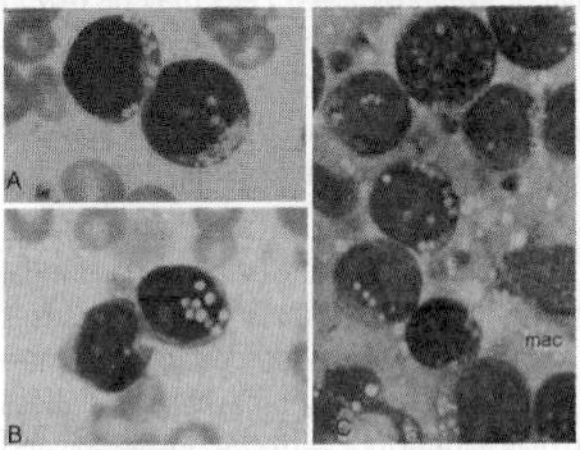

Fig 4. ALL L3. Blasts with vacuolated basophilic cytoplasm. A & B: blood films. B: lymph node (mac: macrophage). [114]

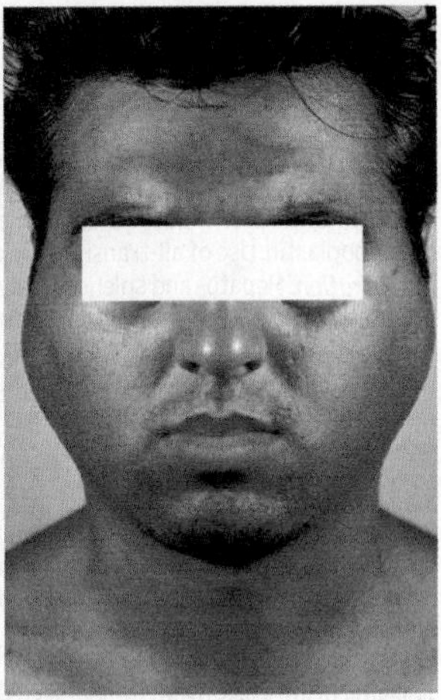

Fig 5. Bilateral parotid infiltration in ALL. [115] (Enlarged salivary glands are also seen in mumps, HIV, bulimia, myxoedema etc, p597.)

Figs 1, 2,4, and 5 courtesy of Prof. Christine Lawrence; fig 3 courtesy of Prof. Tangün & Dr Köroğlu.

Acute myeloid leukaemia (AML)

This neoplastic proliferation of blast cells is derived from marrow myeloid elements. It progresses rapidly (death in ~2 months if untreated; ~20% 3yr survival after ℞).

Incidence The commonest acute leukaemia of adults (1/10,000/yr; increases with age). AML can be a long-term complication of chemotherapy, eg for lymphoma. Also associated with myelodysplastic states (see BOX), radiation, and syndromes, eg Down's.

Morphological classification Now based on WHO histological classification, which is complex and requires specialist interpretation. It recognizes the important prognostic information from cytogenetics and molecular genetics. 5 main types:

1 AML with recurrent genetic abnormalities.
2 AML multi-lineage dysplasia (usually 2° to preexisting myelodysplastic syndrome).
3 AML, therapy related.
4 AML, other.
5 Acute leukaemias of ambiguous lineage (both myeloid and lymphoid phenotype).

Symptoms • *Marrow failure:* Symptoms of anaemia, infection or bleeding. DIC occurs in acute promyelocytic leukaemia, a subtype of AML, where there is release of thromboplastin. Use of all-transretinoic acid with chemotherapy ↓risk of DIC (p346).
• *Infiltration:* Hepato- and splenomegaly, gum hypertrophy (**fig 3**), skin involvement. CNS involvement at presentation is rare in AML.

Diagnosis WCC is often ↑, but can be normal or even low. Blast cells may be few in the peripheral blood, so diagnosis depends on bone marrow biopsy. Differentiation from ALL may be by microscopy (*see* **figs 1, 2, 4**; Auer rods are diagnostic of AML), but is now based on immunophenotyping and molecular methods. Cytogenetic analysis (eg type of mutation) affects treatment recommendations, and guides prognosis.

Complications • Infection is the major problem, related to both the disease and during treatment. Be alert to septicaemia (p346). Infections may be bacterial, fungal or viral, and prophylaxis is given for each during treatment. *Pitfalls:* AML itself causes fever, common organisms present oddly, few antibodies are made, rare organisms—particularly fungi (especially *Candida* or *Aspergillus*). • Chemotherapy causes ↑plasma urate levels (from tumour lysis)—so give allopurinol with chemotherapy, and keep well hydrated with IV fluids. • Leukostasis (p346) may occur if WCC ↑↑.

Treatment • *Supportive care* As for ALL. Walking exercises can relieve fatigue.[116 RCT]
• ***Chemotherapy*** is very intensive, resulting in long periods of marrow suppression with neutropenia + platelets↓. The main drugs used include ***daunorubicin***, and ***cytarabine***, with ~5 cycles given in 1 week blocks to achieve remission (RAS mutations occur in ~20% of patients with AML and enhance sensitivity to cytarabine).[117]
• *Bone marrow transplant (BMT)* Pluripotent haematopoietic stem cells are collected from the bone marrow. *Allogeneic* transplants from HLA-matched siblings or from matched unrelated donors (accessed via international databases) is indicated during first remission in disease with poor prognosis. The idea is to destroy leukaemic cells and the immune system by cyclophosphamide + total body irradiation, and then repopulate the marrow by transplantation from a matched donor infused IV. BMT allows the most intensive chemotherapy regimens because marrow suppression is not an issue. Ciclosporin ± methotrexate may be used to reduce the effect of the new marrow attacking the patient's body (graft *vs* host disease). *Complications:* Graft *vs* host disease (may help explain the curative effect of BMT); opportunistic infections; relapse of leukaemia; infertility. *Prognosis:* Lower relapse rates ~60% long-term survivors, but significant mortality of ~10%. *Autologous BMT* where stem cells are taken from the patient themselves, is used in intermediate prognosis disease, although some studies suggest better survival rates with intensive chemotherapy regimes. ***Autologous mobilized peripheral blood stem cell transplantation*** may offer faster haemopoietic recovery and less morbidity.[118]
• Supportive care, or lower-dose chemotherapy for disease control, may be more appropriate in elderly patients, where intensive therapies have poorer outcomes.

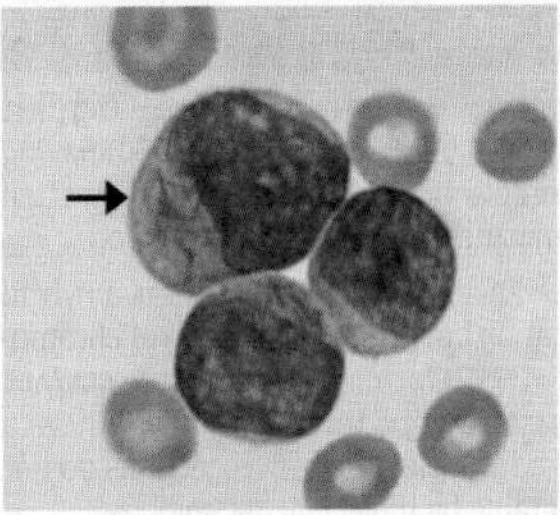

Fig 1. Auer rods (crystals of coalesced granules) found in AML myeloblast cells.[119]

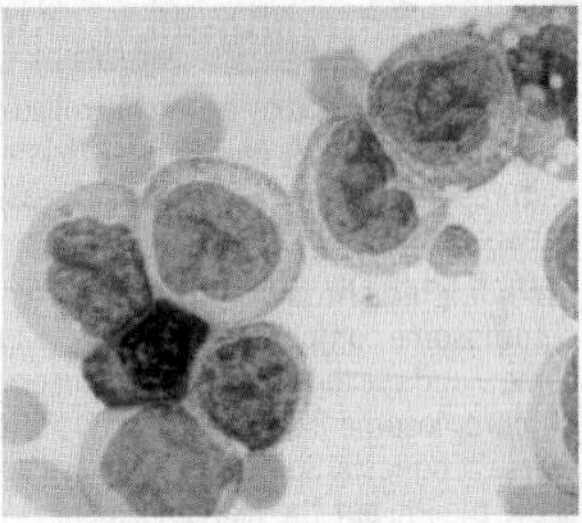

Fig 2. AML with monoblasts and myeloblasts on the peripheral blood film.[120]

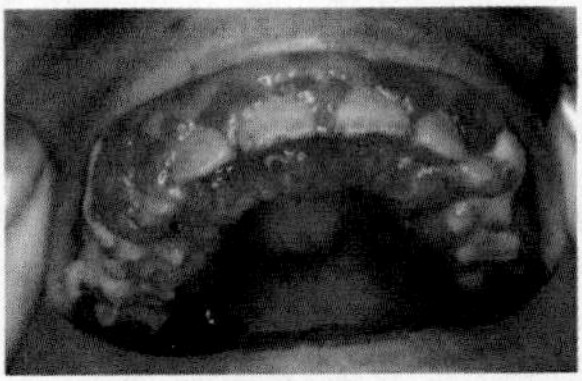

Fig 3. Gum hypertrophy in AML.[121]

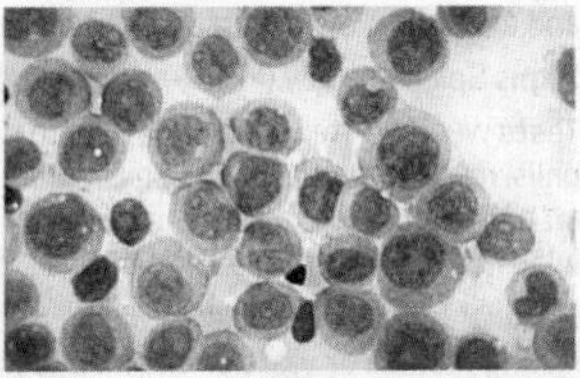

Fig 4. Marrow in AML: multiple monoblasts.[122]

Images on this page are courtesy of Professor Christine Lawrence.

Myelodysplastic syndromes (MDS, myelodysplasia)

These are a heterogeneous group of disorders that manifest as marrow failure with risk of life-threatening infection and bleeding. Most are primary disorders, but they may also develop secondary to chemotherapy or radiotherapy. 30% transform to acute leukaemia. ***Tests:*** Pancytopenia (p358), with ↓reticulocyte count. Marrow cellularity is usually increased due to ineffective haematopoiesis. Ring sideroblasts may also be seen in the marrow (**fig 5**, p321). There are different subtypes, grouped according to WHO classification.

Treatment:

- Multiple transfusions of red cells or platelets as needed
- Erythropoietin ± human granulocyte colony stimulating factor (G-CSF) may lower transfusion requirement.
- Immunosuppressives are also used, eg ciclosporin or antithymocyte globulins.
- Curative allogeneic stem cell transplantation is one option—often inappropriate owing to age-related comorbidities—most are >70yrs old.
- Thalidomide analogues such as lenalidomide have a role, eg in low-risk MDS with 5q deletions. Hypomethylating agents (eg azacytidine and decitabine) have a role in symptomatic MDS (these target epigenetic changes in MDS).

Prognosis: Median survival: from 6 months to 6 years according to disease type.

Chronic myeloid leukaemia (CML)

CML is characterized by an uncontrolled clonal proliferation of myeloid cells (**fig 2**). It accounts for 15% of leukaemias. It is a myeloproliferative disorder (p360) having features in common with these diseases eg splenomegaly. It occurs most often between 40–60yrs, with a slight male predominance, and is rare in childhood.

Philadelphia chromosome (Ph) Present in >80% of those with CML. It is a hybrid chromosome comprising reciprocal translocation between the long arm of chromosome 9 and the long arm of chromosome 22—t(9;22) forming a fusion gene BCR/ABL on chromosome 22, which has tyrosine kinase activity. Those without Ph have a worse prognosis. Some patients have a masked translocation—cytogenetics do not show the Ph, but the rearrangement is detectable by molecular techniques.

Symptoms Mostly chronic and insidious: weight↓, tiredness, fever, sweats. There may be features of gout (due to purine breakdown), bleeding (platelet dysfunction), and abdominal discomfort (splenic enlargement). ~30% are detected by chance.

Signs Splenomegaly (>75%)—often massive. Hepatomegaly, anaemia, bruising (**fig 1**).

Tests WBC ↑↑ (often >100 × 10^9/L) with whole spectrum of myeloid cells ie ↑neutrophils, myelocytes, basophils, eosinophils. Hb↓ or normal, platelets variable. Urate↑, B_{12}↑. Neutrophil alk phos score↓ (seldom performed now). Bone marrow is hypercellular. Ph found on cytogenetic analysis of blood or bone marrow.

Natural history Variable, median survival 5–6yrs. There are three phases: *chronic*, lasting months or years of few, if any, symptoms→*accelerated phase*, with increasing symptoms, spleen size, and difficulty in controlling counts→*blast transformation*, with features of acute leukaemia ± death. **Treatment** See BOX.

Chronic lymphocytic leukaemia (CLL)

Accumulation of mature B cells that have escaped programmed cell death and undergone cell-cycle arrest in the G0/G1 phase is the hallmark of CLL. It is the commonest leukaemia (>25%; incidence: ~4/100,000/yr). ♂:♀≈2:1. Mutations, trisomies and deletions (eg del17p13) influence risk; pneumonia may be a triggering event.[123]

Rai stage	**0**	Lymphocytosis alone	Median survival >13yrs
	I	Lymphocytosis + lymphadenopathy	8yrs
	II	Lymphocytosis + spleno- or hepatomegaly	5yrs
	III	Lymphocytosis + anaemia (Hb <11g/dL)	2yrs
	IV	Lymphocytosis + platelets <100 × 10^9/L	1yr

Symptoms Often none, presenting as a surprise finding on a routine FBC (eg done pre-op). May be anaemic or infection-prone. If severe: weight↓, sweats, anorexia.

Signs Enlarged, rubbery, non-tender nodes (**fig 3**). Splenomegaly, hepatomegaly.

Tests ↑Lymphocytes—may be marked (**fig 4**). Later: autoimmune haemolysis (p332), marrow infiltration: ↓Hb, ↓neutrophils, ↓platelets.

Complications 1 Autoimmune haemolysis. 2 ↑Infection due to hypogammaglobulinaemia (=↓IgG), bacterial, viral especially herpes zoster. 3 Marrow failure.

Natural history Some remain in *status quo* for years, or even regress. Usually nodes slowly enlarge (± lymphatic obstruction). Death is often due to infection (commonly pneumococcus, haemophilus, meningococcus, *Candida* or aspergillosis), or transformation to aggressive lymphoma (Richter's syndrome).

Treatment is more likely to be indicated if: • Symptomatic • Immunoglobulin genes (IGHV) are unmutated • 17p deletions (consider intensive ℞). *Fludarabine + cyclophosphamide* is better than *chlorambucil* (there is some synergism).[124] LRF CLL4 trial 2007 *Alemtuzumab* has a role.[125] [126] *Steroids* help autoimmune haemolysis. *Radiotherapy:* To relieve lymphadenopathy or splenomegaly. *Supportive care:* Transfusions, IV human immunoglobulin if recurrent infection. *Stem-cell transplant* can be tried.[127]

Prognosis ⅓ never progress; ⅓ will progress in time, and ⅓ are actively progressing. CD23 and β2 microglobulin correlate with bulk of disease and rates of progression.

Treating CML

Chemotherapy

- CML is the first example of a neoplastic disease where knowledge of the genotype has led to a rationally designed drug—imatinib (Glivec®), a specific BCR/ABL tyrosine kinase inhibitor, which has transformed therapy.128 It is more effective than the previous gold standard of α-interferon—(± cytarabine in chronic phase patients), in terms of preventing disease progression. The drug may also be effective in accelerated phase and blast crises. Imatinib gives high haematological response rates (>90%). Cytogenetic remissions are also common, but complete eradication of the Philadelphia clone, as detected by the most sensitive molecular methods, is unusual (<5% patients). SE: usually mild: nausea, cramps, oedema, skin rash, headache, arthralgia. May cause myelosuppression. Compared with α-interferon, imatinib greatly improves quality of life,129 but α-interferon may still have a role in combination therapy and in those intolerant of imatinib. NB: other more potent BCR-ABL inhibitors are available (dasatinib; nilotinib).130
- Hydroxycarbamide may still be used in patients intolerant of imatinib, or where imatinib has proved ineffective.
- Dasatinib may have a role in imatinib-resistant blast crises. Those with lymphoblastic transformation may benefit from treatment as for ALL. Treatment of myeloblastic transformation with chemotherapy rarely achieves lasting remission and allogeneic transplantation offers the only hope of long-term survival.

Stem cell transplantation Allogeneic transplantation from a HLA-matched sibling or unrelated donor is the only curative treatment but carries significant morbidity and mortality. Guidelines suggest that this approach should be used 1st line only in young patients where mortality rates are lower. Other patients should be offered imatinib. Patients are then reviewed annually to decide whether to continue imatinib, or to offer combination therapy or stem cell transplantation.

The role of autologous transplantation, if any, in CML-remains to be defined.

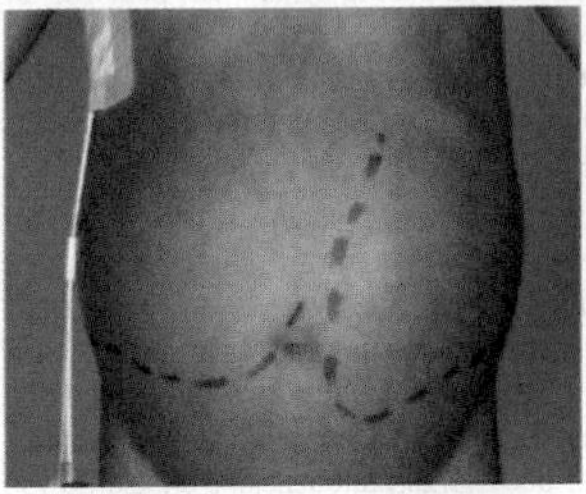

Fig 1. Hepatosplenomegaly in CML.

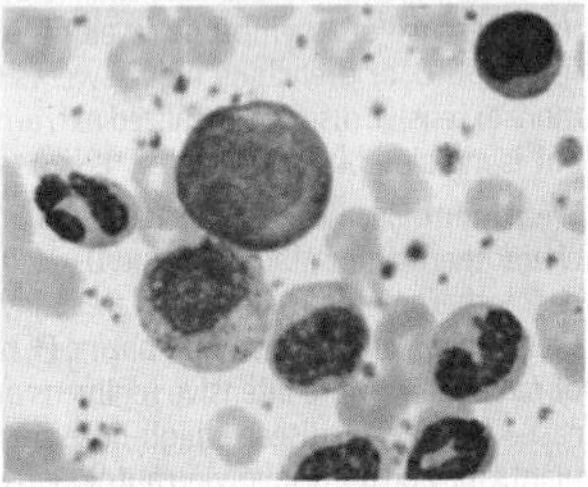

Fig 2. CML: numerous granulocytic cells at different stages of differentiation.131

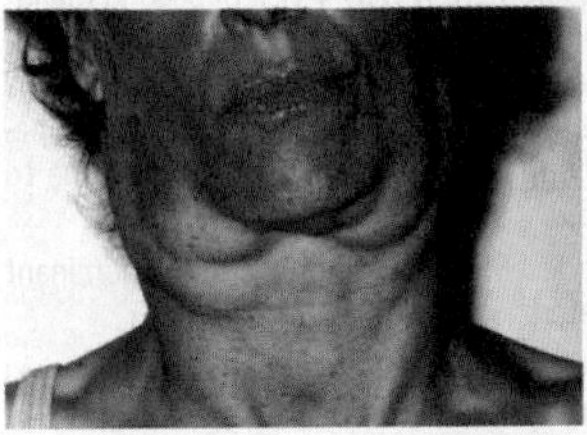

Fig 3. Bilateral cervical lymphadenopathy in CLL.

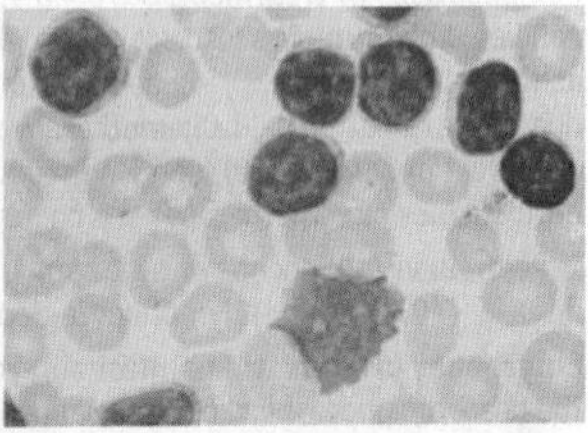

Fig 4. CLL: many lymphocytes and a 'smear' cell: a fragile cell damaged in preparation.132

Figures 2 and 4 are courtesy of Professor Christine Lawrence.

Hodgkin's lymphoma

Lymphomas are disorders caused by malignant proliferations of lymphocytes. These accumulate in the lymph nodes causing lymphadenopathy, but may also be found in peripheral blood or infiltrate organs. Lymphomas are histologically divided into Hodgkin's and non-Hodgkin's types. In Hodgkin's lymphoma, characteristic cells with mirror-image nuclei are found, called Reed–Sternberg cells (**figs 1, 2, 4**).

Hodgkin's lymphoma 2 peaks of incidence: young adults and elderly. ♂:♀ ≈2:1. Risk ↑ if: an affected sibling; EBV (p401); SLE; post-transplantation; Westernisation; 133 obese. 134

Symptoms Often presents with enlarged, painless, non-tender, 'rubbery' superficial lymph nodes, typically cervical (60–70%), also axillary or inguinal nodes (**fig 3**). The size of the nodes may increase and decrease spontaneously, and nodes can become matted. 25% have constitutional upset, eg fever, weight loss, night sweats, pruritus, and lethargy. There may be alcohol-induced lymph node pain. Mediastinal lymph node involvement can cause features due to mass effect eg bronchial or SVC obstruction (p526), or direct extension eg causing pleural effusions. *Pel-Ebstein fever* implies a cyclical fever with long periods (15–28 days) of normal or low temperature: it is, at best, rare.[1]

Signs Lymph node enlargement. Also, cachexia, anaemia, spleno- or hepatomegaly.

Tests *Tissue diagnosis* Lymph node excision biopsy if possible. Image-guided needle biopsy, laparotomy or mediastinoscopy may be needed to obtain a sample. *Bloods* FBC, film, ESR, LFT, LDH, urate, Ca^{2+}. ↑ESR or ↓Hb indicate a worse prognosis. LDH is raised as it is released during cell turnover. PET, p752 also has an uncertain role. 135

Staging (Ann Arbor system) Influences treatment and prognosis. Done by CXR, CT of thorax, abdo, pelvis ± bone marrow biopsy if B symptoms, or stage III–IV disease.

- I Confined to single lymph node region.
- II Involvement of two or more nodal areas on the same side of the diaphragm.
- III Involvement of nodes on both sides of the diaphragm.
- IV Spread beyond the lymph nodes eg liver or bone marrow.

Each stage is subdivided into '**A**'—no systemic symptoms other than pruritus; or '**B**'—presence of B symptoms: weight loss >10% in the last 6 months, unexplained fever >38°C, or drenching night sweats (requiring change of clothes). '**B**' indicates more extensive disease. Localized extra-nodal extension does not advance the stage, but is indicated by subscripted '**E**', eg **I-A$_E$**.

Treatment Chemotherapy, radiotherapy or both. Radiotherapy ± short courses of chemotherapy for stages I-A and II-A (eg with ≤3 areas involved). Longer courses of chemotherapy for II-A with >3 areas involved through to IV-B. '**ABVD**': **A**driamycin, **B**leomycin, **V**inblastine, **D**acarbazine (+ radiotherapy in younger patients) cures ~80% of patients. 136 More intensive regimens are used if poor prognosis or advanced disease.[2] In relapsed disease, high-dose chemotherapy with peripheral stem-cell transplants may be used, involving autologous (or occasionally allogeneic) transplantation of peripheral blood progenitor cells to restore marrow function after therapy. 137

Complications of treatment: See p528–9: **Radiotherapy** may ↑ risk of second malignancies—solid tumours (especially lung and breast, also melanoma, sarcoma, stomach and thyroid cancers), ischaemic heart disease, hypothyroidism and lung fibrosis due to the radiation field. **Chemotherapy SE** include myelosuppression, nausea, alopecia, infection. AML (p350), non-Hodgkin's lymphoma and infertility may be due to both chemo- or radiotherapy—see page p531.

5-year survival Depends on stage and grade: >95% in I-A lymphocyte-predominant disease; <40% with IV-B lymphocyte-depleted.

Emergency presentations Infection; SVC obstruction—JVP↑, sensation of fullness in the head, dyspnoea, blackouts, facial oedema (seek expert help; see p526).

1 Pel-Ebstein fever is dismissed by Richard Asher (*Talking Sense*), as existing only thanks to its having been exotically named (the 1885 patients of Dr P Pel had no histology, and fevers in Hodgkin's are *usually* non-specific). Another unfair reason for consigning it to myth is that the paper proving its existence and its relation to cyclical changes in node size doesn't come up in literature searches as Wilhelm *Ebstein* was spelled *Epstein* throughout.

2 eg BEACOPP (bleomycin/etoposide/doxorubicin/cyclophosphamide/vincristine/procarbazine/prednisone).

Classification *(in order of incidence)*	Prognosis
Classical Hodgkin's lymphoma	
Nodular sclerosing	Good
Mixed cellularity*	Good
Lymphocyte rich	Good
Lymphocyte depleted*	Poor

NB: nodular lymphocyte predominant Hodgkin's is recognized as a separate entity, behaving as an indolent B-cell lymphoma. **Higher incidence and worse prognosis if HIV +ve.*

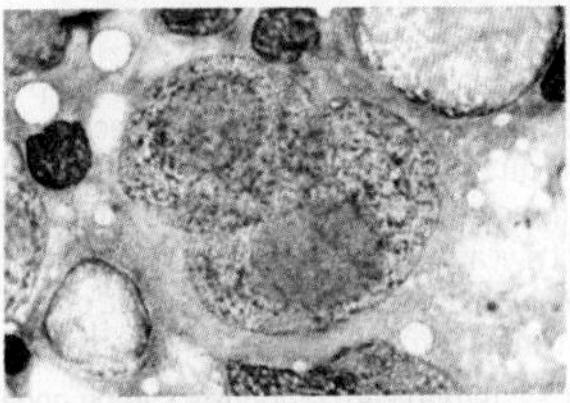

Fig 1. A Reed-Sternberg cell with 2 nuclei, characteristic of Hodgkin's lymphoma. [138]
Courtesy of Professor Christine Lawrence

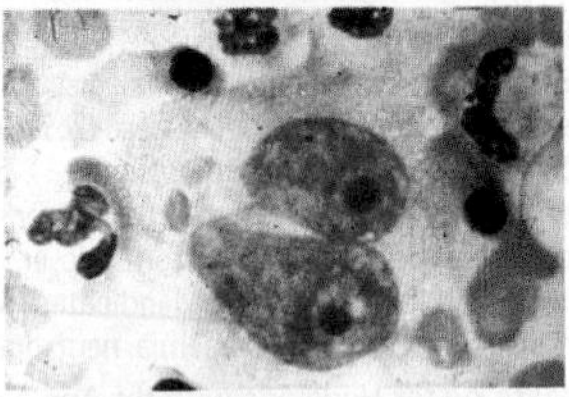

Fig 2. Another Reed-Sternberg cell. [139]
Courtesy of the Crookston collection

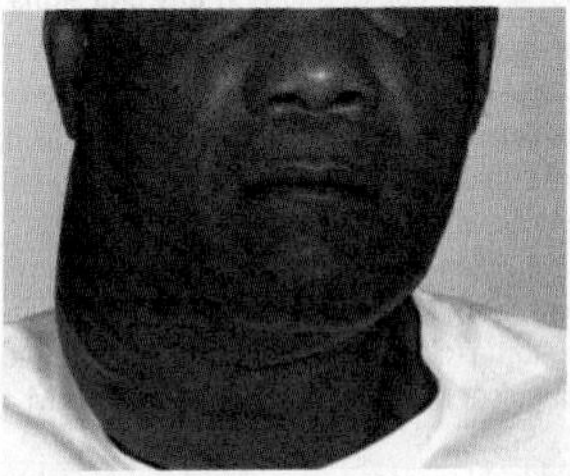

Fig 3. Cervical lymphadenopathy in Hodgkin's disease.

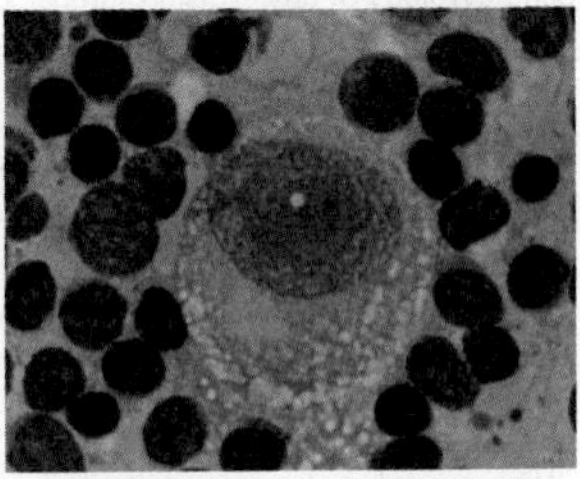

Fig 4. Mononuclear Reed-Sternberg cell in a lymph node. [140] Courtesy of Prof. Tangün & Dr Köroğlu.

Quality of life, lymphoma, and the role of expressive writing

Being treated for Hodgkin's disease is arduous. Our job is often to give encouragement—the more this is personalized for our individual patient the better.

One method is to encourage our patients to write about their experiences. In one study this gave clear-cut benefits in lymphoma patients. Participants report positive responses to writing, and post-writing half said that writing changed their thoughts about their illness in a positive way (this increased on subsequent follow-up). Textual analysis identifies themes related to experiences of positive change, transformation, and self-affirmation through reflection. [141] [142] These techniques are akin to those used in post-traumatic stress—and remind us that some of our treatments are as destabilizing to our patients as any shipwreck, rape, or earthquake. See http://my lymphomastory.com for how to avoid self-pity despite the odds. "I can whine, I can complain, I can moan, and b*tch, about all of the above, but I won't.... The true feat isn't escaping death, rather, learning how to live."

Sometimes narrating lymphoma experiences reveals bitterness, loss of control, and a feeling that life has been rendered void. [143] n=18 Here our role is to receive these negatives and to try to keep the channels of communication open, as dialogue is the only validated means of filling these voids. The need to enhance support networks and bolster social ties may trump all our pharmacological imperatives. [144]

"On prednisolone I gained 20kg and started screaming..."

This includes all lymphomas without Reed–Sternberg cells, and is a very diverse group of diseases. Most are derived from B-lymphocyte cell lines. Not all are centred on lymph nodes (extranodal tissues generating lymphoma include mucosa-associated lymphoid tissue—MALT. Gastric MALT is associated with *H. pylori*, and may regress when this is eradicated). The overall incidence of lymphoma has doubled since 1970 (to 1 : 10,000). ***Causes:*** congenital immunodeficiency, acquired immunodeficiency eg drugs, HIV infection (usually high-grade lymphoma), infection (eg HTLV-1 p346, EBV, *H. pylori*) or environmental toxins.

Signs and symptoms • Nodal disease (75% at presentation): superficial lymphadenopathy • Extranodal disease (25%) involving the oropharynx, skin (especially T-cell lymphomas—p598; *see also* **fig 3**), bone, gut, CNS, or lung. Disease of the oropharyngeal lymphoid tissue (Waldeyer's ring) causes sore throat and obstructed breathing. • Systemic symptoms—fever, night sweats, weight loss (less common than in Hodgkin's lymphoma, and indicates disseminated disease) • Pancytopenia due to marrow involvement—anaemia, neutropenia (infection) and ↓platelets (bleeding).

Tests As for Hodgkin's with the Ann Arbor system (p354). ***Diagnosis*** Lymph node biopsy. ***Bloods*** FBC, U&E, LFT, LDH. ↑LDH indicates worse prognosis as it is released with cell turnover. ***Stage*** with CT or MRI of chest, abdomen, pelvis, and marrow aspiration. Send cytology of any effusion; lumbar puncture for CSF cytology if any CNS signs.

Histology This is something of a quagmire as classification systems are complex and changing. The current classification is based on the WHO classification of lymphoid neoplasms. Discuss diagnosis and management as a multidisciplinary team, bringing together information available from clinical evaluation, histology, immunology, molecular genetics, and imaging. *Generally:*

- Low-grade lymphomas are indolent, and are often incurable and widely disseminated at presentation. Include: follicular lymphoma, marginal zone lymphoma (includes MALT lymphomas), lymphocytic lymphoma (closely related to CLL and treated similarly), lymphoplasmacytoid lymphoma (associated with production of IgM = Waldenström's macroglobulinaemia, p364). *See* **fig 4**.
- High-grade lymphomas are more aggressive, but long-term cure may be achievable. There is often a short history of rapidly enlarging lymphadenopathy with systemic symptoms. Include: Burkitt's lymphoma (childhood disease with characteristic jaw lymphadenopathy; **figs 1, 2**), lymphoblastic lymphomas (shares features with ALL), diffuse large B-cell lymphoma.

Treatment Depends on disease subtype. ***Low grade:*** If symptomless, none may be needed. Radiotherapy may be curative in localized disease. ***Chlorambucil*** is used in diffuse disease. Remission may be maintained by using ***α-interferon*** or ***rituximab*** (see below). ***Bendamustine*** is effective both with rituximab and as a monotherapy in rituximab-refractory patients.[145] ***High grade:*** (eg large B-cell lymphoma, DLBCL), **'R-CHOP' regimen**: ***Rituximab Cyclophosphamide, Hydroxydaunorubicin, vincristine*** (*Oncovin®*) and ***Prednisolone***.[1] Granulocyte colony-stimulating factors (G-CSFs) help neutropenia—eg filgrastim or lenograstim (at low doses it may be cost-effective).[146]

Survival Histology is important. Prognosis is worse if at presentation: • Age >60yrs • Systemic symptoms • Bulky disease (abdominal mass >10cm) • ↑LDH • Disseminated disease. Typical 5-yr survival for treated patients: ~30% for high-grade and >50% for low-grade lymphomas, but the picture is very variable.

1 Rituximab is indicated in CD20+ve DLBCL eg at stage II, III, or IV as well as for remission induction in relapsed stage III or IV follicular non-Hodgkin's lymphoma. It may also be used as monotherapy to maintain remission after R-CHOP or CHOP (NICE) and also indolent lymphomas such as lymphoplasmacytic lymphoma. Do not use if CHOP is contraindicated. DLBCL denotes intermediate- to high-grade lymphomas that are rapidly fatal if untreated but often respond well to intensive chemotherapy. CD20 is a surface marker expressed on most B-cell lymphomas and testing for it is routine. CD20 occurs on normal and malignant B cells, but not on precursor B cells, so obviating long-term B cell depletion. Rituximab kills CD20+ve cells by antibody-directed cytotoxicity ± apoptosis induction. It also sensitizes cells to CHOP.

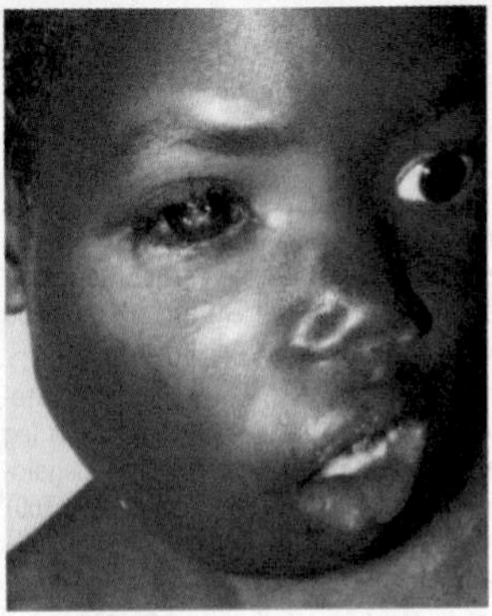

Fig 1. Burkitt's lymphoma, with characteristic jaw lymphadenopathy.[147]

Courtesy of Dr Tom D Thacher

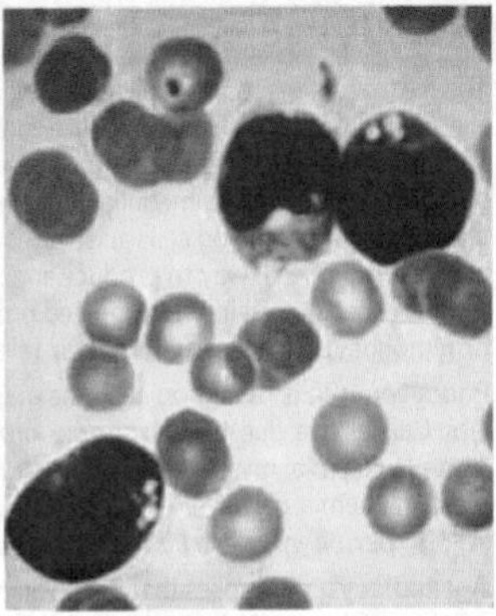

Fig 2. Burkitt's lymphoma, with 3 basophilic vacuolated lymphoma cells.[148]

Courtesy of Prof. Barbara Bain
©2005 Massachusetts Medical Society

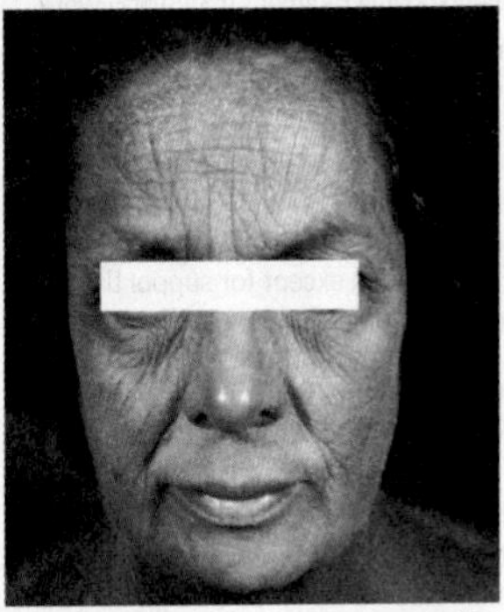

Fig 3. Cutaneous T-cell lymphoma, which has caused severe erythroderma (Sézary syndrome) in a Caucasian woman.[149]

Courtesy of Prof. Christine Lawrence

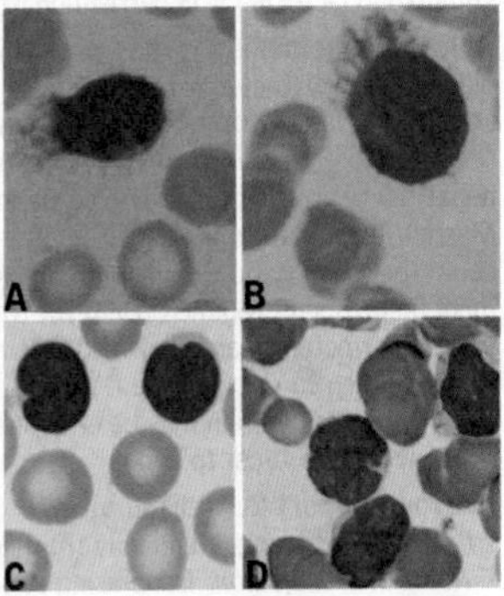

Fig 4. A & B: villous lymphocytes (splenic marginal zone lymphoma). C: 'buttock cells' with cleaved nuclei (follicular lymphoma). D: Sézary cells with convoluted nuclei.[150]

Courtesy of Prof. Tangün & Dr Köroğlu.

The marrow is responsible for haemopoiesis. In adults, this normally takes place in the central skeleton (vertebrae, sternum, ribs, skull) and proximal long bones. In some anaemias (eg thalassaemia), increased demand produces haematopoiesis beyond the marrow (extramedullary haematopoiesis), in the liver and spleen, causing organomegaly. All blood cells arise from an early pluripotent stem cell, which divides in an asymmetrical way to produce another stem cell and a progenitor cell committed to a specific cell line. Committed progenitors further differentiate into myeloid or lymphocyte lineages, before their release into the blood as mature cells.

Pancytopenia is reduction in all the major cell lines: red cells, white cells and platelets. Causes are due to **1** ↓*marrow production:* Aplastic anaemia, infiltration (eg acute leukaemia, myelodysplasia, myeloma, lymphoma, solid tumours, TB), megaloblastic anaemia, paroxysmal nocturnal haemoglobinuria (p332), myelofibrosis (p360), SLE. **2** ↑*peripheral destruction:* Hypersplenism.

Agranulocytosis implies that granulocytes (WBCs with neutrophil, basophil or eosinophil granules, **fig 1**) have stopped being made. Neutropenia (WCC $\lesssim 0.5 \times 10^9$/L) may declare itself early as a sore throat (eg 2wks after starting the drug)[151] before some fatal infection: this is why we warn patients starting drugs causing agranulocytosis[1] "Report *any* fever." (Do FBC! Look at the result!! Stop the drug!!!) Granulocyte colony stimulating factor (G-CSF) + barrier nursing + neutropenia regimens (p346) may work.[152]

Aplastic anaemia is a rare stem cell disorder leading to pancytopenia and hypoplastic marrow (the marrow stops making cells). Presents with features of anaemia (↓Hb), infection (↓WCC) or bleeding (↓platelets). ***Incidence:*** ~5 cases per million/year. ***Causes:*** Most cases are autoimmune, triggered by drugs, (viruses eg parvovirus, hepatitis) or irradiation. May also be inherited, eg Fanconi anaemia (p712). ***Tests:*** Marrow examination is needed for the diagnosis. ***Treatment:*** Support the blood count (below). Asymptomatic patients don't need much except for supportive treatment (neutropenic regimen, p346). The treatment of choice in young patients who are severely affected is an allogeneic marrow transplantation from an HLA-matched sibling, which can be curative. Otherwise, immunosuppression with ciclosporin and antithymocyte globulin may be effective, although is not curative in most. There is no clear role for G-CSF (p356).[153]

Marrow support Red cells survive for ~120d, platelets for ~8d, and neutrophils for 1–2d, so early problems are mainly from neutropenia and thrombocytopenia.

6 ***Red cell transfusion:*** Transfusing 1U should raise Hb by ~1–1.5g/dL (p342). Transfusion may drop the platelet count (you may need to give platelets before or after).

1 ***Platelets:*** Traumatic bleeds, purpura and easy bruising occur if platelets $<50 \times 10^9$/L. Spontaneous bleeding may occur if platelets $<20 \times 10^9$/L, with intracranial haemorrhage rarely. Platelets are stored at room temperature (22°C; not in the fridge). In marrow transplant or if severely immunosuppressed, platelets may need irradiation before use to prevent transfusion-associated graft-versus-host disease (GVHD). Platelets must be ABO compatible. They are not used in ITP (p338). Indications: • Platelets $<10 \times 10^9$/L • Haemorrhage (eg DIC, p346) • Before invasive procedures (eg biopsy, lumbar puncture) to increase count to $>50 \times 10^9$/L. 4U of platelets should raise the count to $>40 \times 10^9$/L in adults; check dose needed with lab.

2 ***Neutrophils:*** Use a 'neutropenic regimen' if the count $<0.5 \times 10^9$/L. See p346.

Bone marrow biopsy gives diagnostic information where there are abnormalities in the peripheral blood; it is also an important staging test in the lymphoproliferative disorders. Ideally an aspirate *and* trephine is usually from the posterior iliac crest (aspirates can be taken from the anterior iliac crest or sternum). The aspirate provides a film which is examined by microscope. The trephine is a core of bone which allows assessment of bone marrow cellularity, architecture and the presence of infiltrative disease (eg neoplasia). Coagulation disorders may need to be corrected pre-biopsy. Apply pressure afterwards (lie on that side for 1–2h if platelets are low).

1 Carbimazole, procainamide, sulfonamides, gold, clozapine, dapsone (antibody damage to stem cells).

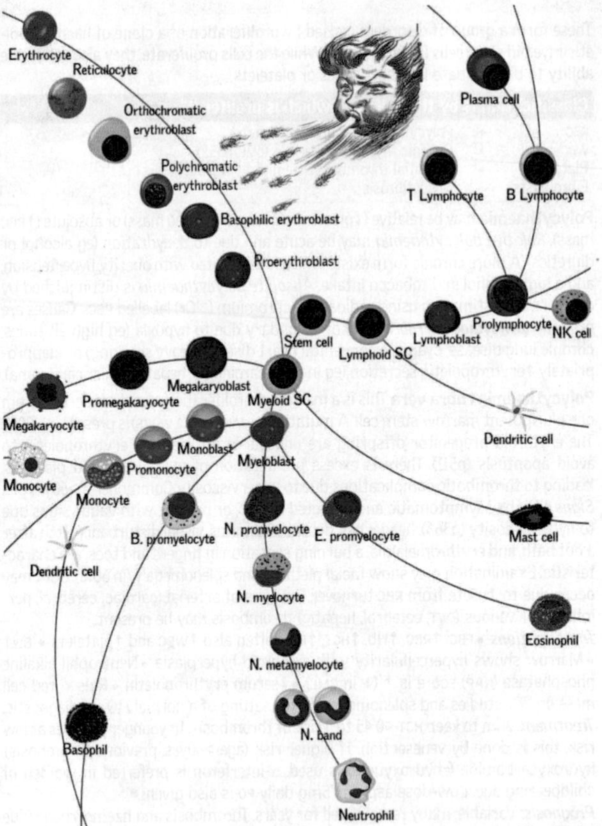

Fig 1. *Haemopoiesis and Sod's Law.* When we contemplate a diagram like this (of seemingly galactic complexity) we, being doctors, think "What can go wrong?" With a sinking feeling we realise that every arc is an opportunity for multiple disasters. Perhaps, using the Hammer of Los (p316) and our own ingenuity we might occasionally complete these pathways without Sod intervening (Sod's law states that if something can go wrong, it will—here Sod's tubercular breath is seen blowing the red cell line off course—TB is a famous cause of leukoerythroblastic anaemia). When we realise that *every day* each of us makes 175 billion red cells, 70 billion granulocytes, and 175 billion platelets[154] —we sense that Sod is smiling to himself with especial relish. *Anything* can go wrong. *Everything* can go wrong. This latter we call ***aplastic anaemia***. ***Agranulocytosis*** is when the Southerly arcs go wrong; thrombocytopenia when the West-pointing arcs go wrong. To the East we have the *lymphocytes* and their B- and T-cell complexities. ***Anaemia*** lies in the North of this diagram. And as for bleeding—how could our predecessors bear to waste a single drop of this stuff on purpose? Our minds are reeling at 175 billions red cells per day—but this is just when the system is idling. When we bleed, throughput can rise by an order of magnitude—if Sod is turning a blind eye are there are sufficient haematinics (eg iron, B12 and folate) to allow maximum haemopoiesis? Figure courtesy of Aria Rad.

The myeloproliferative disorders

These form a group of disorders caused by proliferation of a clone of haematopoietic myeloid stem cells in the marrow. While the cells proliferate, they also retain the ability to differentiate into RBCs, WBCs or platelets.

Classification is by the cell type which is proliferating		
RBC	→	Polycythaemia rubra vera (PRV)
WBC	→	Chronic myeloid leukaemia (CML, p352)
Platelets	→	Essential thrombocythaemia
Fibroblasts	→	Myelofibrosis

Polycythaemia may be relative (↓plasma volume, normal RBC mass) or absolute (↑RBC mass). *Relative polycythaemia* may be acute and due to dehydration (eg alcohol or diuretics). A more chronic form exists which is associated with obesity, hypertension, and a high alcohol and tobacco intake. *Absolute polycythaemia* is distinguished by red cell mass estimation using radioactive chromium (^{51}Cr) labelled RBCs. Causes are primary (***polycythaemia rubra vera***) or secondary due to hypoxia (eg high altitudes, chronic lung disease, cyanotic congenital heart disease, heavy smoking) or inappropriately ↑erythropoietin secretion (eg in renal carcinoma, hepatocellular carcinoma).

Polycythaemia rubra vera This is a malignant proliferation of a clone derived from one pluripotent marrow stem cell. A mutation in JAK2 (JAK2 V617F) is present in >90%. The erythroid progenitor offspring are unusual in not needing erythropoietin to avoid apoptosis (p511). There is excess proliferation of RBCs, WBCs, and platelets, leading to thrombotic complications due to hyperviscosity. Commoner if >60yrs old.
Signs May be asymptomatic and detected on FBC, or present with vague signs due to hyperviscosity (p366): headaches, dizziness, tinnitus, visual disturbance. Itch after a hot bath, and erythromelalgia, a burning sensation in fingers and toes, are characteristic. Examination may show facial plethora and splenomegaly (in 60%). Gout may occur due to ↑urate from RBC turnover. Features of arterial (cardiac, cerebral, peripheral) or venous (DVT, cerebral, hepatic) thrombosis may be present.
Investigations • FBC: ↑RCC, ↑Hb, ↑HCT, ↑PCV, often also ↑WBC and ↑platelets • B_{12}↑ • Marrow shows hypercellularity with erythroid hyperplasia • Neutrophil alkaline phosphatase (NAP) score is ↑ (↓ in CML) • ↓serum erythropoietin • Raised red cell mass on ^{51}Cr studies and splenomegaly, in the setting of a normal P_aO_2, is diagnostic.
Treatment: Aim to keep HCT <0.45 to ↓risk of thrombosis. In younger patients at low risk, this is done by venesection. If higher risk (age >60yrs, previous thrombosis), hydroxycarbamide (=hydroxyurea) is used. α-interferon is preferred in women of childbearing age. Low-dose aspirin 75mg daily PO is also given.
Prognosis: Variable, many remain well for years. Thrombosis and haemorrhage (due to defective platelets) are the main complications. Transition to myelofibrosis occurs in ~30% or acute leukaemia in ~5%. Monitor FBC every 3 months.

Essential thrombocythaemia A clonal proliferation of megakaryocytes leads to persistently ↑platelets, often >1000 × 10^9/L, with abnormal function, causing bleeding or arterial and venous thrombosis, and microvascular occlusion—headache, atypical chest pain, light-headedness, erythromelalgia (**fig 1**). Exclude other causes of thrombocytosis (see BOX). *Treatment:* Low-dose aspirin 75mg daily. Hydroxycarbamide is given to ↓platelets if >60yrs old or if previous thrombosis.

Myelofibrosis There is hyperplasia of megakaryocytes which produce platelet derived growth factor, leading to intense marrow fibrosis and myeloid metaplasia (haemopoiesis in the spleen and liver)→massive hepatosplenomegaly. ***Presentation:*** Hypermetabolic symptoms: night sweats, fever, weight loss; abdominal discomfort due to splenomegaly; or bone marrow failure (↓Hb, infections, bleeding). *Film:* Leukoerythroblastic cells (nucleated red cells, p322); characteristic teardrop RBCs (see **fig 2**). Hb↓. Bone marrow trephine for diagnosis (**fig 3**). *Treatment:* Marrow support (see p358). Allogeneic stem cell transplant may be curative in young people but carries a high risk of mortality. ***Prognosis:*** Median survival 4-5 years.

Causes of thrombocytosis

↑Platelets >450 ×10^9/L may be a reactive phenomenon, seen with many conditions including:

- Bleeding
- Infection
- Chronic inflammation, eg collagen disorders
- Malignancy
- Trauma
- Post-surgery
- Iron deficiency

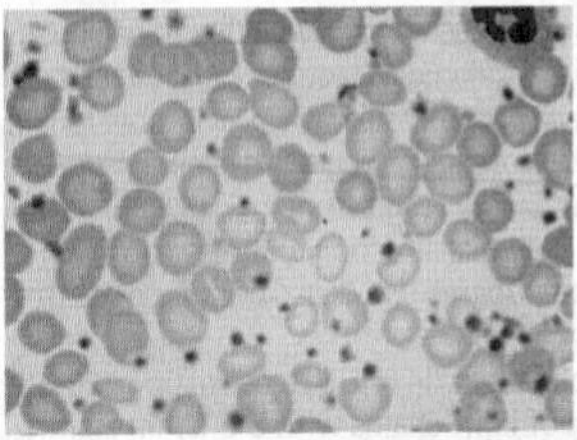

Fig 1. Essential thrombocythaemia: many platelets seen. [155] © Prof. Christine Lawrence

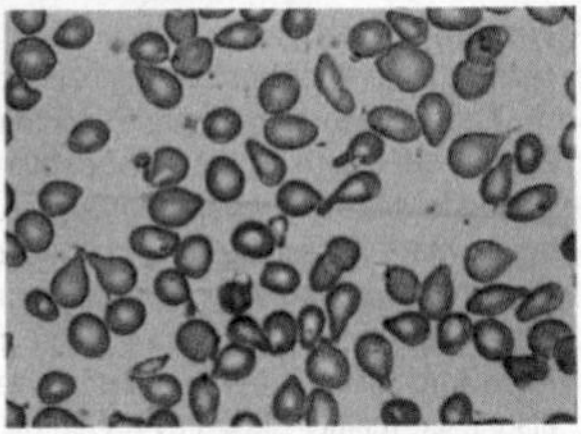

Fig 2. Tear drop cells, in myelofibrosis. [156] © Dr Nivaldo Medeiros

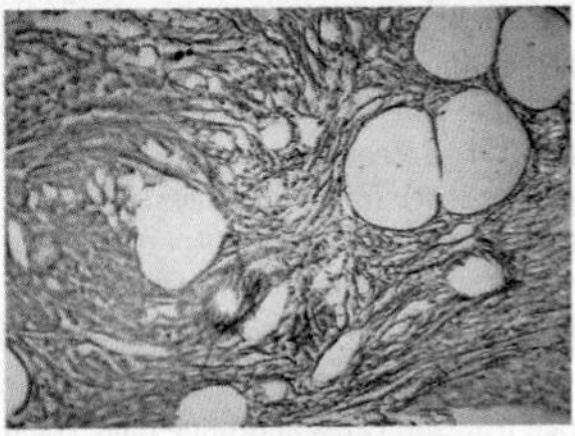

Fig 3. Marrow trephine in myelofibrosis: the streaming effect is caused by intense fibrosis. Other causes of marrow fibrosis: any myeloproliferative disorder, lymphoma, secondary carcinoma, TB, leukaemia, and irradiation. [157] ©Professor Christine Lawrence

Myeloma

Myeloma is a malignant clonal proliferation of B-lymphocyte derived plasma cells (**fig 1**). Normally many different plasma cells produce different immunoglobulins (Igs) which are polyclonal. In myeloma, a single clone of plasma cells produce identical Ig, seen as a monoclonal band, or paraprotein, on serum or urine electrophoresis (below).

Classification is based on the Ig product, which is IgG in ~⅔ and IgA in ~⅓. The small remainder are IgM or IgD. Other Ig levels are low (ie an 'immunoparesis', causing ↑susceptibility to infection. In ~⅔ of cases, urine contains Bence-Jones protein, which are free Ig light chains of kappa (κ) or lambda (λ) type, filtered by the kidney.

Incidence 5/100,000. Peak age: 70yrs. ♂:♀≈1. Afro-Caribbeans:Caucasians≈2:1.

Symptoms ►Do serum protein electrophoresis & ESR on all over 50 with back pain.

- ***Osteolytic bone lesions*** causing backache, pathological fractures (eg long bones or ribs) and vertebral collapse. ***Hypercalcaemia*** may result with symptoms (p690). Lesions are due to ↑ osteoclast activation, from signalling by myeloma cells.
- ***Anaemia, neutropenia, or thrombocytopenia*** may result from marrow infiltration by plasma cells, leading to symptoms of anaemia, infection and bleeding.
- ***Recurrent bacterial infections*** due to immunoparesis, and also because of neutropenia due to the disease and from chemotherapy.
- ***Renal impairment*** due to light chain deposition (p314 & p364) seen in up to 20% at diagnosis—mainly caused by precipitation of light chains with the Tamm-Horsfall protein in the distal loop of Henle.[158] Also, monoclonal immunoglobulins induce changes in glomeruli. A rare type of damage is deposits of light chains in the form of AL-amyloid and subsequent nephrosis[159] (and other systemic problems, p364).

Tests FBC—normocytic normochromic anaemia, film—rouleaux formation (p322), persistently ↑ESR or PV (p366), ↑urea and creatinine, ↑Ca^{2+} (in ~40%), alk phos usually normal (unless healing fracture). *See also* **figs 2-4**. ***Screening test:*** Serum & urine electrophoresis. β_2-microglobulin (as a prognostic test). ***Imaging:*** X-rays show lytic 'punched-out' lesions, eg pepper-pot skull, vertebral collapse, fractures or osteoporosis. CT or MRI may be useful to detect lesions not seen on XR. ***Diagnosis:*** see BOX.

Treatment[160] ***Supportive:*** • Bone pain should be treated with analgesia (avoid NSAIDs due to risk of renal impairment). Give all patients a ***bisphosphonate*** (clodronate, zolendronate or pamidronate), as they reduce fracture rates and bone pain. Local radiotherapy can help rapidly in focal disease. Orthopaedic procedures (vertebroplasty or kyphoplasty) may be helpful in vertebral collapse. • Anaemia should be corrected with ***transfusion***, and ***erythropoietin*** may be used. • Renal failure: Rehydrate, and ensure adequate fluid intake of 3L/day to prevent further renal impairment by light chains. Dialysis may be needed in acute renal failure • Infections: Treat rapidly with broad-spectrum antibiotics until culture results are known. Regular IV ***immunoglobulin infusions*** may be needed if recurrent.

Chemotherapy: If unsuitable for intensive ℞, ***melphalan*** + ***prednisolone*** is used. This can control disease for ~1yr, reducing paraprotein levels and bone lesions. Adding ***bortezomib*** increases the time to relapse.[161] In due course, disease may become uncontrollable and often resistant to treatment. Adding ***thalidomide*** (a teratogenic immunomodulator) improves event-free survival in the elderly.[162] SE: birth defects; drowsiness; neuropathy; neutropenia; sepsis; orthostatic hypotension; thromboembolism (aspirin, or full anticoagulation is probably wise if risk ↑, eg concurrent complex regimens, hyperviscosity, or other comorbidities).[163] In fitter people, a more vigorous approach is used (high-dose therapy and stem-cell rescue, HDT) with a **VAD** type regime: *Vincristine*, *Adriamycin* and *Dexamethasone*. Autologous stem cell transplant may then be done, which improves survival but is not curative. Allogeneic transplantation can be curative in younger patients, but carries ↑risk of mortality (~30%). Thalidomide or bortezomib may be tried in relapsed disease. NB: ***lenalidomide*** is similar to thalidomide and, being somewhat more potent, may have a role.[164]

Prognosis Median survival is 3–4 years. A raised β_2-microglobulin is associated with a worse prognosis. Death is commonly due to infection or renal failure.

Myeloma diagnostic criteria[83]

1 Monoclonal protein band in serum or urine electrophoresis
2 Increased plasma cells found on bone marrow biopsy
3 Evidence of end-organ damage from myeloma:
- Hypercalcaemia
- Renal insufficiency
- Anaemia

Bone lesions: a skeletal survey is performed after diagnosis to detect bone disease, consisting of x-rays of chest; cervical, thoracic, and lumbar spine; skull and pelvis

Causes of bone pain/tenderness

1 Trauma/fracture (steroids ↑risk)
2 Myeloma & other primary malignancy (eg solitary plasmacytoma, sarcomas)
3 Secondaries (breast, lung, prostate[etc.])
4 Osteonecrosis, eg from microemboli[1]
5 Osteomyelitis/periostitis (eg syphilis)
6 Hydatid cyst (bone is a rare site)
7 Osteosclerosis (eg from hepatitis C)
8 Paget's disease of bone
9 Sickle cell anaemia
10 Renal osteodystrophy
11 CREST syndrome/Sjögren's syndrome
12 Hyperparathyroidism. Treatment: treat the cause. NSAIDs and bisphosphonates may control symptoms.

Complications of myeloma

- *Hypercalcaemia* (p690). Occurs with active disease, eg at presentation or relapse. Rehydrate vigorously with IV saline 0.9% 4–6L/d (careful fluid balance). IV bisphosphonates, eg zolendronate or pamidronate, are useful for treating hypercalcaemia acutely.
- *Spinal cord compression* (p470 & p515). Occurs in 5% of patients with myeloma. Urgent MRI if suspected. Treatment is with dexamethasone 8–16mg/24h PO and local radiotherapy.
- *Hyperviscosity* (p366) causes reduced cognition, disturbed vision, and bleeding. It is treated with plasmapheresis to remove light chains.
- *Acute renal failure* is treated with rehydration. Urgent dialysis may be needed.

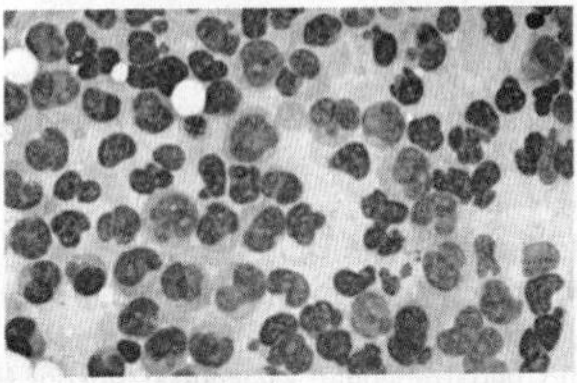

Fig 1. Myeloma bone marrow: many plasma cells with abnormal forms.[165]

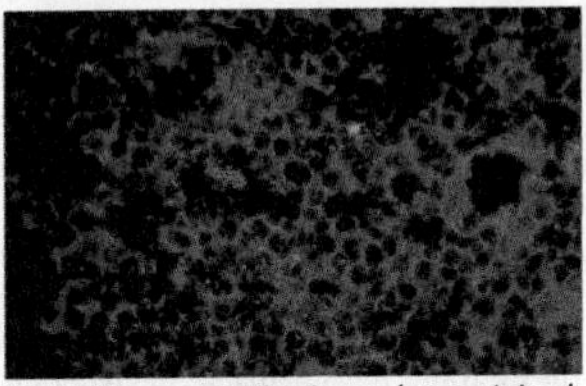

Fig 2. Marrow section in myeloma, stained with IgG kappa monoclonal antibody.[166]

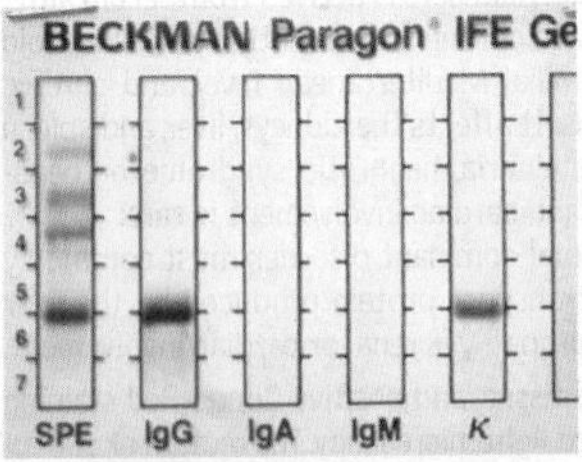

Fig 3. An IgG kappa paraprotein monoclonal band (immunofixation electrophoresis; a control sample has run on the left).[167]

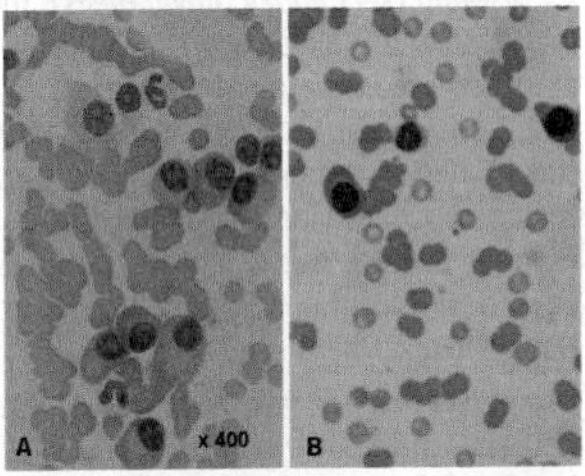

Fig 4. Plasma cells in myeloma A: marrow smear, B: peripheral smear. Note rouleaux formation of red cells (p322 & p362).

1 Avascular necrosis from sickle-cell anaemia, sepsis, antiphospholipid syndrome, fat emboli.
Figs 1-3 courtesy of Prof Christine Lawrence; fig 4 Courtesy of Prof. Tangün & Dr Köroğlu.

Paraproteinaemia

Paraproteinaemia denotes presence in the circulation of immunoglobulins produced by a single clone of plasma cells. The paraprotein is recognized as a monoclonal band (M band) on serum electrophoresis.[1] There are 6 major categories:

1 ***Multiple myeloma:*** See p362.

2 ***Waldenström's macroglobulinaemia:*** This is a lymphoplasmacytoid lymphoma producing a monoclonal IgM paraprotein. Hyperviscosity is common (p366), with CNS and ocular symptoms. Lymphadenopathy and splenomegaly are also seen. ↑ESR, with IgM paraprotein on serum electrophoresis. ℞: None if asymptomatic. Chlorambucil, fludarabine or combination chemotherapy may be used. Plasmapheresis[1] for hyperviscosity (p366).

3 ***Primary amyloidosis:*** See below.

4 ***Monoclonal gammopathy of uncertain significance*** (MGUS) is common (3% >70yrs). There is a paraprotein in the serum but no myeloma, 1° amyloid, macroglobulinaemia or lymphoma, with no bone lesions, no Bence–Jones protein and a low concentration of paraprotein, with <10% plasma cells in the marrow. Some develop myeloma or lymphoma. Refer to a haematologist (?for marrow biopsy).[168]

5 ***Paraproteinaemia in lymphoma or leukaemia:*** Eg seen in 5% of CLL.

6 ***Heavy chain disease:*** This is where neoplastic cells produce free Ig heavy chains. α chain disease is the most important, causing malabsorption from infiltration of small bowel wall. It may progress to lymphoma.

Amyloidosis[169]

This is a group of disorders characterized by extracellular deposits of a protein in abnormal fibrillar form, resistant to degradation. The following are the systemic forms of amyloidosis. Amyloid deposition is also a feature of Alzheimer's disease, type 2 diabetes mellitus and haemodialysis-related amyloidosis.

AL amyloid (primary amyloidosis): Due to clonal proliferation of plasma cells, with production of amyloidogenic monoclonal immunoglobulins. In most cases, it occurs on its own as a primary amyloidosis, with occult plasma cell proliferation. It is also seen in 15% of patients with myeloma, and smaller proportions with Waldenström's, MGUS, or lymphoma. Deposition may occur in • Kidneys: Glomerular lesions—proteinuria and nephrotic syndrome • Heart: Restrictive cardiomyopathy ('sparkling' appearance on echo), arrhythmias, angina • Nerves: Peripheral and autonomic neuropathy, carpal tunnel syndrome • Gut: Macroglossia (big tongue), malabsorption, perforation, haemorrhage, obstruction, and hepatomegaly. • Vascular: Purpura, especially periorbital—a characteristic feature (**fig 1**).

AA amyloid (secondary amyloidosis): The amyloid here is derived from serum amyloid A, an acute phase protein. It occurs with chronic inflammation in rheumatoid arthritis, inflammatory bowel disease, familial Mediterranean fever, and chronic infections—TB, bronchiectasis, osteomyelitis. It affects the kidneys, liver, and spleen (**fig 2**), and commonly presents with proteinuria, nephrotic syndrome or hepatosplenomegaly. Macroglossia is not seen, and cardiac involvement is rare.

Familial amyloidosis is a group of autosomal dominant disorder, most commonly caused by mutations in transthyretin, a transport protein produced by the liver. Usually causes a sensory or autonomic neuropathy ± renal or cardiac involvement.

Diagnosis is made with biopsy of affected tissue, and positive Congo Red staining with red-green birefringence under polarized light microscopy. The rectum or subcutaneous fat are relatively non-invasive sites for biopsy and are +ve in 80%.

℞: AA amyloidosis may improve if the primary disease is treated. AL may respond to therapy as for myeloma. Liver transplant can be curative in familial amyloidosis.

Prognosis Median survival is 1-2 years. Patients with myeloma and amyloidosis have a shorter survival than those with myeloma alone.

1 Electro*phoresis* and plasma*pheresis* look as though they should share endings, but they do not: Greek *phoros=bearing (esis=process)*, but *aphairesis* is Greek for *removal*.

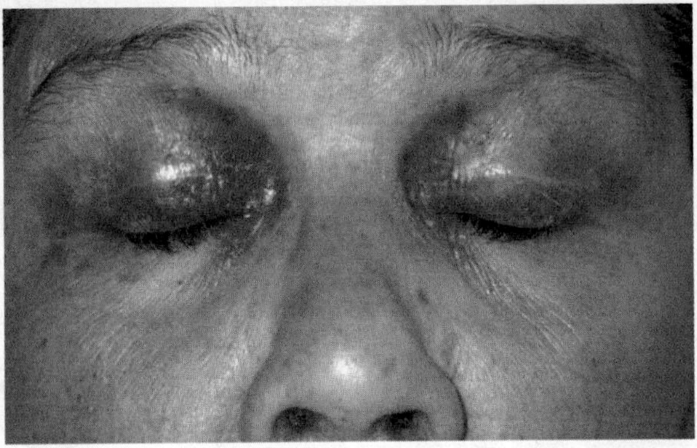

Fig 1. Periorbital purpura in amyloidosis. 170

Courtesy of Prof. Christine Lawrence

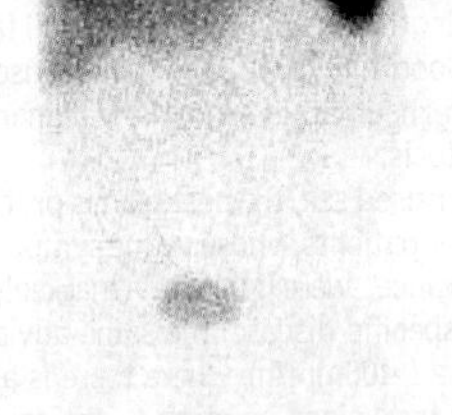

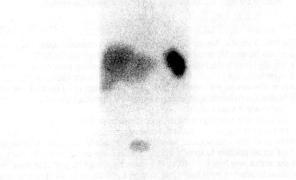

Fig 2. Areas of amyloid deposition in liver & spleen in amyloidosis (isotope scan) *Oxford Textbook of Medicine* ©OUP (with permission)

Plasma viscosity (PV)

Normal range: 1.50–1.72mPa/s.

In many labs, this has replaced the ESR, as it is less affected by anaemia and results can be produced in 15min. The PV is affected by the concentration of large plasma proteins and is raised in the same conditions as the ESR. Both PV and ESR are raised in chronic inflammation and are less affected by acute changes <24h in duration. The CRP is more sensitive in acute change (see p701).

Hyperviscosity syndrome

Blood is made to move! Our beautiful images seem to deny this, as if haematology were just a branch of histology. So what are the intrinsic disorders of flow? If blood viscosity rises there may be a few telltale signs before the quick becomes dead, eg lethargy; confusion; cognition↓; CNS disturbance; chest pain; abdominal pain; faints; visual disturbance (eg vision↓, amaurosis fugax, retinopathy—eg engorged retinal veins, haemorrhages, exudates; and a blurred disc as seen on the right). The visual symptoms ('slow-flow retinopathy') are like 'looking through a watery car windscreen' (left). Other causes of slow-flow retinopathy: carotid disease and Takayasu's disease: p726). Also spontaneous GI or GU bleeding.

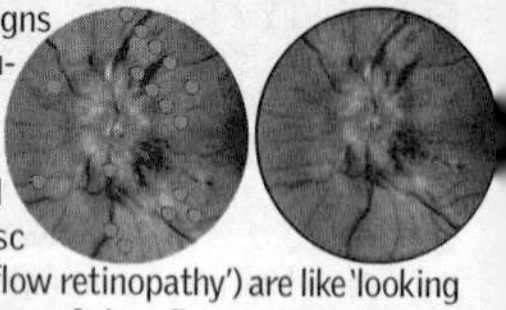

Causes of high blood viscosity: Very high red cell count (haematocrit >50, eg polycythaemia rubra vera), white cell count (>100×10⁹/L, eg leukaemia), or plasma components—usually immunoglobulins, in myeloma or Waldenström's macroglobulinaemia (p364, as IgM is larger and so ↑ viscosity more than the same amount of IgG).

Treatment: Urgent treatment is needed which depends on the cause. Venesection is done in polycythaemia. Leukopheresis in leukaemias to remove white cells. Plasmapheresis in myeloma and Waldenström's: blood is withdrawn via a plasma exchange machine, the supernatant plasma from this is discarded, and the RBCs returned to the patient after being re-suspended in a suitable medium.

Erythrocyte sedimentation rate

Normal range: ≤20mm/h.

The ESR is a sensitive but non-specific indicator of the presence of disease. It measures how far RBCs fall through a column of anticoagulated blood in 1h. It is really a length (eg 35mm in the 1st h)—not a rate.[171] If certain proteins cover red cells, these cause RBCs to stick to each other in columns so they fall faster (the same phenomenon as rouleaux on the blood film, p322). The main causes of a raised ESR are any inflammation, eg infection, rheumatoid arthritis, malignancy, myocardial infarction; or anaemia or a macrocytosis.

In those with a slightly raised ESR, the best plan is probably to wait a month and repeat it. There is a group of patients whose vague symptoms would have prompted nothing more than reassurance—were it not for a markedly raised ESR—and in whom there are no pointers to specific disease. The same advice does not hold true for those with a very high ESR (>100mm/h), where there is a 90% predictive value for disease. In practice, most have signs pointing to the cause. In one survey, serious underlying disease later found in such patients included myeloma, giant cell arteritis, abdominal aneurysm, metastatic prostatic carcinoma, leukaemia, and lymphoma. Therefore, it would be wise (after history and examination) to consider these tests: FBC, plasma electrophoresis, U&E, PSA, chest and abdominal x-rays, ± biopsy of bone marrow or temporal artery.

ESR also rises with age. A simple, reliable way[172] to allow for this is to calculate the upper limit of normal, using the Westergren method, to be (for men) age in years ÷ 2. For women, the formula is (years+10) ÷ 2. This is only a rough guide as some workers find no difference between men and women between the ages of 70 and 90yrs old.[173] NB: some conditions *lower* the ESR, eg polycythaemia (due to ↑red cell concentration), microcytosis, and sickle-cell anaemia. Even a slightly raised ESR in these patients should prompt one to ask: "*What else is the matter?*"

The spleen and splenectomy

The spleen was a mysterious organ for many years; we now know that it plays a vital immunological role by acting as a reservoir for lymphocytes, and in dealing with bacteraemias. Splenomegaly is a commonish problem and its causes are divided into *massive* (into the RIF) and *moderate*.

Causes of massive splenomegaly CML, myelofibrosis, malaria (hyperreactive malarial splenomegaly), leishmaniasis, 'tropical splenomegaly' (idiopathic—Africa, south-east Asia), and Gaucher's syndrome.

Moderate splenomegaly: See p606. • Infection (eg EBV, endocarditis, TB, malaria, leishmaniasis, schistosomiasis) • Portal hypertension (liver cirrhosis), • Haematological (haemolytic anaemia, leukaemia especially CML, lymphoma) • Connective tissue disease (RA, SLE) • Others: sarcoidosis, primary antibody deficiency (*OHCS* p198), idiopathic.

Splenomegaly can be uncomfortable and may lead to *hypersplenism:* pancytopenia as cells become trapped in the spleen's reticuloendothelial system, with symptoms of anaemia, infection, or bleeding. Splenectomy may be required if severe.

When faced with a mass in the left upper quadrant, it is vital to recognize the spleen: • Dull to percussion • It enlarges towards the RIF • It moves down on inspiration • You may feel a medial notch • 'You can't get above it' (ie the top margin disappears under the ribs). The last three features differentiate the spleen from an enlarged left kidney. Abdominal USS or CT are used to image the spleen. When hunting the cause for enlargement look for lymphadenopathy and liver disease, eg: FBC, ESR, LFT ± liver, marrow, or lymph node biopsy.

Splenectomy Main indications: splenic trauma, hypersplenism, autoimmune haemolysis: in ITP (p338) or warm autoimmune haemolytic anaemia (p332), congenital haemolytic anaemias. Splenectomy was historically performed for staging in Hodgkin's disease, but CT and MRI have replaced this role. Mobilise early post-splenectomy as transient ↑platelets predisposes to thrombi. A characteristic blood film is seen following splenectomy, with Howell–Jolly bodies, Pappenheimer bodies and target cells (see p322).

►*The main problem post-splenectomy is lifelong increased risk from infection.* The spleen contains macrophages which filter and phagocytose bacteria. Post-splenectomy infection is caused most commonly by encapsulated organisms: *Streptococcus pneumoniae*, *Haemophilus influenzae*, and *Neisseria meningitidis*. Reduce this risk by giving:[174]

1 Immunizations:
   - Pneumococcal vaccine (p160), at least 2 weeks pre-op to ensure good response, or as soon as possible after emergency splenectomy eg after trauma. Re-immunize every 5-10yrs. Avoid in pregnancy.
   - *Haemophilus influenzae* type b vaccine (Hib, see p391).
   - Meningococcal C vaccine.
   - Annual influenza vaccine (p402).

2 Life-long prophylactic oral antibiotics (phenoxymethylpenicillin). Erythromycin if penicillin allergic.

3 Patient-held cards alerting health professionals to the infection risk.

4 Pendants or bracelets to alert medical staff.

5 Advice to seek medical attention if any signs of infection.

6 Urgent hospital admission if infection develops, for treatment with broad-spectrum antibiotics.

7 If travelling abroad, warn of risk of severe malaria and advise meticulous prophylaxis, with nets, repellent, and medication.

8 The above advice also applies to hyposplenic patients, eg in sickle-cell anaemia or coeliac disease.

Thrombophilia

Thrombophilia is an inherited or acquired coagulopathy predisposing to thrombosis, usually venous: DVT or PE (venous thromboembolism: VTE). Special precautions are needed in *surgery, pregnancy*, and *enforced inactivity*. Risk is further increased by obesity, immobility, trauma (accidents or surgery), pregnancy, and malignancy. **NB:** thrombocytosis and polycythaemia may also cause thrombosis (p360). See BOX. Note only ~50% of patients with thrombosis and a +ve family history have an identifiable thrombophilia: others may have abnormalities that are as yet unidentified.

Inherited • ***Activated protein c (APC) resistance/factor v Leiden:*** Chief cause of inherited thrombophilia. Present in ~5% population, although most will not develop thrombosis. Usually associated with a single point mutation in factor v (Factor v Leiden), so that this clotting factor is not broken down by APC. Risk of venous thromboembolism (DVT or PE) is increased 5-fold in patients who are heterozygous for the mutation, and 50-fold in homozygotes. Thrombotic risk is increased in pregnancy and those on oestrogens (*OHCS* p257 & p303).

• ***Prothrombin gene mutation:*** Causes high prothrombin levels and ↑thrombosis due to down-regulation of fibrinolysis, by thrombin-activated fibrinolysis inhibitor).

• ***Protein c and protein s deficiency:*** These vitamin K-dependent factors act together to cleave and so neutralize factors v and VIII. Heterozygotes deficient for either protein risk thrombosis. Skin necrosis also occurs (esp. if on warfarin). Homozygous deficiency for either protein causes neonatal purpura fulminans—fatal, if untreated.

• ***Antithrombin deficiency:*** Antithrombin is a co-factor of heparin, and inhibits thrombin. Less common, affects 1:500. Heterozygotes' thrombotic risk is greater than protein c or s deficiency by ~4-fold. Homozygosity is incompatible with life.

Acquired Causes: '3rd generation' progesterones[1] in contraceptive Pills (see TABLE for risk of thrombosis) and the antiphospholipid syndrome (APL: p556) when serum antiphospholipid antibodies are found (lupus anticoagulant ± anticardiolipin antibody), predisposing to venous *and* arterial thrombosis, thrombocytopenia, and recurrent fetal loss in pregnancy. In most it is a primary disease, but it is also seen in SLE.

Not on Pill	5:100,000
2nd gen. Pill[1]	15:100,000
3rd gen. Pill[1]	25:100,000
Pregnancy	60:100,000

Who to investigate? Liaise with a haematologist. Do FBC, film, clotting tests: PT, thrombin time, APTT, and fibrinogen concentration ± APC resistance test, lupus anticoagulant & anticardiolipin antibodies, and assays for antithrombin and proteins c and s deficiency. Haematologists may advise DNA analysis by PCR for the Factor v Leiden mutation if the APC resistance test is +ve, and for prothrombin gene mutation. Ideally investigate while well, not pregnant, and not anticoagulated for 1 month.

Consider special tests if:
- Arterial thrombosis <50yrs (for APL)
- Venous thrombosis <40y with no risk factors
- Familial VTE or with oral contraceptives/pregnancy
- Unexplained recurrent VTE
- Unusual site, eg mesenteric or portal vein thrombosis
- Recurrent fetal loss (≥3)
- Unusual site, eg mesenteric/portal vein thrombosis
- Neonatal thrombosis

Treatment Treat acute thrombosis as standard—heparin, then warfarin to target INR of 2-3 (p345). If recurrence occurs with no other risk factors, lifelong warfarin should be considered. Recurrence whilst on warfarin should be treated by increasing target INR to 3-4. In antithrombin deficiency, high doses of heparin may be needed so liaise with a haematologist. In protein c or s deficiency, monitor treatment closely as skin necrosis may occur with warfarin.

Prevention Life-long anticoagulation is not needed if asymptomatic, but advise of ↑ risk of VTE with the Pill or HRT, and counsel as regards to the best form of contraception. Patients should also be warned of other risk factors for VTE. Prophylaxis may be needed in pregnancy, eg in antiphospholipid syndrome. Get expert help: aspirin and prophylactic heparin are used, as warfarin is teratogenic. Prophylactic SC heparin may also be indicated in high-risk situations, eg pre-surgery.

1 Desogestrel is an example. Risk of thrombosis is ~doubled with Pills containing this, *vs* levonorgestrel. Part of this effect is due to ↓ free protein S found with desogestrel (24 *vs* 33U/dL).

Other risk factors for thrombosis

Arterial	*Venous*
• Smoking	• Surgery
• Hypertension	• Trauma
• Hyperlipidaemia	• Immobility
• Diabetes mellitus	• Pregnancy, oral contraceptive pill, HRT
	• Age
	• Obesity
	• Varicose veins
	• Other conditions: heart failure, malignancy, inflammatory bowel disease, nephrotic syndrome, paroxysmal nocturnal haemoglobinuria (p332).

For thrombophilia in pregnancy, see *OHCS* p33; for anticoagulant use in pregnancy and thromboprophylaxis, see *OHCS* p16.

Immunosuppressive drugs

As well as being used in leukaemias and cancers, these are used in organ and marrow transplants, rheumatoid arthritis, psoriasis, chronic hepatitis, asthma, SLE, vasculitis (eg Wegener's, giant cell arteritis, polymyalgia, PAN), inflammatory bowel and other diseases (so this page could figure in almost any chapter).

Prednisolone Steroids can be life-saving, but bear in mind:

- Certain conditions may be made worse by steroids, eg TB, hypertension, chickenpox, osteoporosis, diabetes: here careful monitoring is needed.
- Growth retardation may occur in young patients, and the elderly frequently get more side effects from treatment.
- Interactions: [Prednisolone]↓ by antiepileptics (below) and rifampicin.
- Avoid pregnancy (may cause fetal growth retardation). If breastfeeding and prednisolone >40mg/day, see *BNF*.

Minimize side effects by using the lowest dose possible for the shortest period of time. Give doses in the morning, and alternate days if possible, to minimize adrenal suppression. Before starting long-term treatment (>3 weeks, or repeated courses) observe these guidelines:

- Explain about not stopping steroids suddenly. Collapse may result, as endogenous production takes time to restart. ►►See p846.
- Inform about the need to consult a doctor if unwell, and increase the dose of steroid at times of illness/stress (eg flu or pre-op).
- Encourage to carry a steroid card saying dose taken, and the reason.
- You *must* warn patients about the listed side effects if they are receiving long-term treatment (over 6 weeks worth): see BOX.
- Avoid over-the-counter drugs, eg NSAIDs: aspirin and ibuprofen (↑risk of DU).
- Prevent osteoporosis if long-term use (p696): exercise, bisphosphonates, calcium and vitamin D supplements, smoking cessation advice.

Do not stop long-term steroids abruptly as adrenal insufficiency may occur. Once a daily dose of 7.5mg/day of prednisolone is reached, withdrawal should be gradual. Patients on short-term treatment (<3 weeks) can be stopped immediately, unless they have had repeated courses of steroids, a history of adrenal suppression, greater than 40mg daily, or doses at night, where withdrawal should be gradual.

Azathioprine • SE: p549. • *Interactions:* mercaptopurine and azathioprine (which is metabolized to mercaptopurine) are metabolized by xanthine oxidase (XO). So azathioprine toxicity results if XO inhibitors are co-administered (eg allopurinol).

Ciclosporin This is a calcineurin inhibitor, as is tacrolimus which works in a similar way. It has an important role in reducing rejection in organ and marrow transplant. The main SE is dose-related nephrotoxicity. Doses are monitored by blood levels.

- Other SE: Gum hyperplasia, tremor, BP↑(stop if ↑↑), oedema, paraesthesiae, confusion, seizures, hepatotoxicity, lymphoma, skin cancer—avoid sunbathing.
- Monitor U&E and creatinine every 2 weeks for the first 3 months, then monthly if dose >2.5mg/kg/d (every 2 months if less than this). ►Reduce the dose if creatinine rises by >30% on 2 measurements *even if the creatinine is still in normal range.* Stop if the abnormality persists. Also monitor LFT.
- Interactions are legion: [ciclosporin]↑ by: ketoconazole, diltiazem, verapamil, the Pill, erythromycin, grapefruit juice. [ciclosporin]↓ by: barbiturates, carbamazepine, phenytoin, rifampicin. Avoid concurrent nephrotoxics: eg gentamicin. Concurrent NSAIDs augment hepatotoxicity—monitor LFT.

Methotrexate An antimetabolite. Inhibits dihydrofolate reductase, which is involved in the synthesis of purines and pyrimidines. See p549.

Cyclophosphamide An alkylating agent. SE: marrow suppression (monitor FBC), nausea, infertility, teratogenic, haemorrhagic cystitis due to an irritative urinary metabolite. There is a slight ↑risk of later developing bladder cancer or leukaemia.

Side effects of steroid use

System:	Adverse reactions:
Gastrointestinal	Pancreatitis
	Candidiasis
	Oesophageal ulceration
	Peptic ulceration
Musculoskeletal	Myopathy
	Osteoporosis
	Fractures
	Growth suppression
Endocrine	Adrenal suppression
	Cushing's syndrome
CNS	Aggravated epilepsy
	Depression; psychosis
Eye	Cataracts; glaucoma
	Papilloedema
Immune	Increased susceptibility to, and severity of infections, eg chickenpox

Steroids can also cause fever and WCC↑; steroids only rarely cause leucopenia.

Explain side effects in terms that patients understand: document this in the notes—and your plans to prevent osteoporosis if steroid use is going to be long term. Because the risks are mostly long-term, you can use your judgment about when to explain about each side effect. Because steroids can be life-threatening, explaining everything all at once in a graphic way may result in your patient being very well informed, but dead.

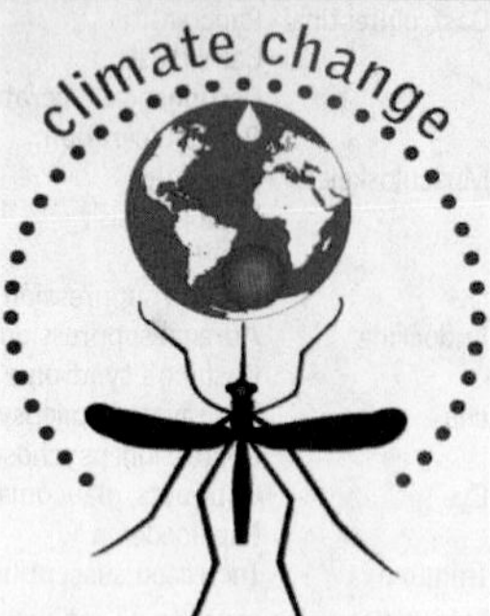

Fig 1. Don't just study pathogens! We need to understand the cultures of entire ecosystems. Interactions between pollution, global warming, poverty, and infection are often fatal: WHO estimates that our warming climate, partly caused by excess CO_2, contributes to >150,000 deaths and 5 million illnesses/yr. Global warming is extending the reach of malaria,[1] and compounds poverty, as poor areas are most vulnerable (eg access to clean water is reduced, aiding spread of mosquito-borne illness, eg malaria).[2] ►As and when the predicted 4°C rise in temperatures occurs, an extra 80 million people in Africa alone will become at risk from malaria.[3,4]

In the UK, by 2012, 3000 extra heat-related deaths/yr, 14,000 more food poisonings/yr, and 15,000 extra admissions/yr from pollution and asthma are expected[5] (and ↑ flood deaths).

Topics elsewhere: Surgical prophylaxis p572; IE, p144; pneumonia p160–6; lung abscess p164; bronchiectasis p166; lung fungi p168; UTI p292; encephalitis p834; ►►meningitis p832; septic arthritis p546. *In OHCS:* pelvic infection *OHCS* p286 & p274; prenatal & perinatal infection *OHCS* p34; measles, mumps, rubella *OHCS* p142; parvoviruses *OHCS* p142; neonatal sepsis *OHCS* p112; ill/feverish child *OHCS* p106; TB meningitis *OHCS* p204; orbital cellulitis *OHCS* p420; ophthalmic zoster *OHCS* p420; mastoiditis *OHCS* p544; sinusitis *OHCS* p558; tonsillitis *OHCS* p564; skin infections/infestations (*OHCS* p598).

1 Alternative name: Climate change, poverty and pollution.

We thank Dr Chris Conlon, our Specialist Reader, and Professor Steve Upton, of Kansas University for images from his excellent site www.k-state.edu/parasitology/625tutorials

Death by septicaemia: two views

1 "Everything is for the best in the best of all possible worlds". Candide. Voltaire
This is guaranteed (according to belief) either, in a graceful way, by God's goodness (and his always beneficent if mysterious ways) or by the messy ways of natural selection (the weak are rooted out so that the strong may flourish).

2 "Preventable death is a tragic waste for which nothing can compensate and from which we can look for no crumb of comfort." As Henry James said on learning of the death by septicaemia of the poet Rupert Brooke "I have no philosophy, nor piety, no art of reflection, no theory of compensation to meet things so hideous, so cruel, and so mad, they are just unspeakably horrible and irremediable to me and I stare at them with angry and almost blighted eyes". Henry James

We cite the infectious anger of this old Master to motivate us to do whatever it takes to stop these lives slipping through our fingers.[1] And as we look out at our burning world through his pupils we see how his *almost* blighted eyes reveal a tantalizing hint of resilience—on which we found this chapter.

UK notifiable diseases[ND] ►Inform the Consultant in Communicable Disease Control (CCDC)

Anthrax	Malaria	Rubella
Cholera	Measles	Scarlet fever
Diphtheria	Meningitis/meningococcal sepsis	Smallpox; Tetanus
Dysentery (amoebiasis, typhoid/paratyphoid)	Mumps	Tuberculosis
	Ophthalmia neonatorum	Typhus
Encephalitis	Plague	Viral haemorrhagic fevers, eg yellow fever; lassa fever
Food poisoning	Poliomyelitis	
Leprosy; Leptospirosis	Rabies; Relapsing fever	Whooping cough/pertussis

(UK Health Protection Agency www.hpa.org.uk. 020 7759 2700; webteam@hpa.org.uk)

Getting the balance right in studying infectious diseases

It is not possible for any ID chapter to be constructed so that it has the right balance throughout the world. Many of our readers come from communities where tetanus and malaria are daily problems—whereas, in UK consulting rooms, chest, GU, and ENT infections are likely to dominate.

In parts of Africa, ~70% of hospitalized patients are HIV+ve,[6] and most cannot even begin to mount an immune response to approach the classic descriptions beloved of standard textbooks (eg there is meningititis without meningism; pneumonia without fever etc), and here medicine is, it seems, no more than the pathology of immunosuppression. In Western hospital specialist ID practice, the chief problems are:

- Respiratory tract infections (p160–p168, and *Emergencies*, p826)
- Hospital-acquired infections, eg p392, p162, p420 (MRSA), p247 (*C. difficile*)
- Immunocompromise—eg HIV (p408–p415) and febrile neutropenia (p346)
- Infections associated with general surgery (p572 & p578)
- Infections in intensive care unit patients (examples on p382 & p441)
- Osteomyelitis (*OHCS* p696) and prosthetic joint infections (*OHCS* p707)
- Illness in a returning traveller (p388).

All these would be trumped by pandemic flu, if highly pathogenic (p402). But in all areas and at all times, the pitfalls are the same: not taking time to find out about your patient—where he has been, what his hobbies are (and his work), and with whom he or she has had contact. Always have a high index of suspicion for TB, and always remember that ID rarities are often very treatable.

Know your local emerging diseases (p387) and your local multi-resistant organisms; remember that it is possible to have more than one infection. ►*Two heads are better than one: so when in doubt, get help.* The best help is often from good microbiology and imaging departments. In many places these are impossible luxuries: a chest X-ray can cost more than the entire yearly health budget allocated to each patient.[7] If this is your predicament, try not to give up: bring your microscope to the bedside (p383) and campaign for better times.

1 If you feel small and insignificant in the face of this challenge, remember that the mosquito that poisoned Rupert Brooke on his way to Gallipoli in 1915 was smaller still. See also: www.survivingsepsis.org

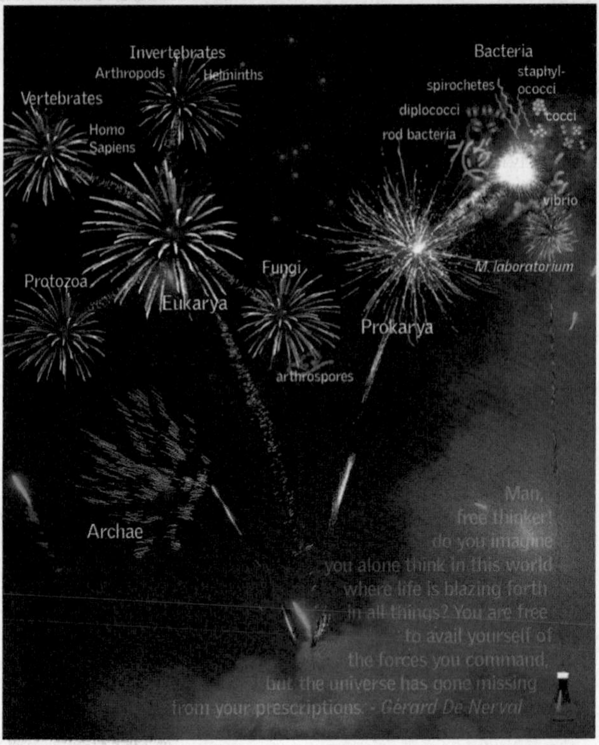

Fig 1. What is life? A thing of dynamism, fragility, beauty, danger, and evanescence, gushing forth from a single source, to be sure. But here the certainties end: what does it take to be alive? Are viruses and prions alive?[1] [8 9 10] How many branches are there on our tree?[2] [11 12 13] The harder we look, the more complexities we find. With the recent creation of synthetic bacteria (*Mycoplasma laboratorium*, seen issuing from its own domain) even the surety of a single common ancestor disappears into smoke.

Because micro-organisms get us up at night and kill our friends (p373) we think of them as bad. This is a big mistake. Kill off micro-organisms and the whole show fizzles out. Micro-organisms gave us the DNA and organelles needed for reading and digesting this page. Even killing a single pathogen might be a mistake: Sod's Law (see p359) will probably ensure that something worse will come to inhabit the vacated ecospace. So the whole affair is like one of our dear, complex geriatric patients: prod one part of her system and events ripple out in an unending stream of unintended consequences, played out under the stars (above), which themselves are evolving (p18), and which donate and receive our primordial elements (p732).

Firework photography by kind permission of David Meads.

1 If a thing is organic and converts nutrients into progeny it is alive. If not, it is either non-living, dead, dying, or male. The average mind is surprised to learn that long before birth, baby girls have their full complement of eggs for the next generation; but for biologists this fact just illustrates Aristotle's dictum that the defining essence of life is that it has a plan for its own survival and continuity.

2 Kingdoms are *not* the top categories. Think of 3 grand domains: **Archaea**, **Bacteria** (Eubacteria), and **Eucarya**. Archaea are like bacteria, having no cell nucleus or organelles, but as they have an independent evolutionary history they form a domain of their own. Eucarya have chromosomes and organelles and give rise to plants, animals, and fungi. Single-celled eukaryotes (protists) loom large in this chapter: plasmodia (malaria), trypanosoma (sleeping sickness), amoebae & giardia (p436).

Examples of pathogens from various types of bacteria

This table is not exhaustive; it is simply a guide for the forthcoming pages.

Gram-positive cocci

Staphylococci (including MRSA, p420):
- coagulase +ve, eg *Staph. aureus*
- coagulase –ve, eg *Staph. epidermidis*

Streptococci (see **fig 2** & p420):
- β-haemolytic streptococci, eg *Strep. pyogenes* Lancefield group A
- α-haemolytic streptococci
  - *Strep. mitior*
  - *Strep. pneumoniae* (pneumococcus)
  - *Strep. sanguis*
- Enterococci (non-haemolytic):
  - *Enterococcus mutans*
  - *E. faecalis* (not a typical strep)
- Anaerobic streptococci

Gram-positive bacilli (rods)

Aerobes
- *Bacillus anthracis* (anthrax: p421)
- *Corynebacterium diphtheriae* (p421)
- *Listeria monocytogenes* (p421)
- Nocardia species

Anaerobes:
- Clostridium
  - *C. botulinum* (botulism: p409)
  - *C. perfringens* (gas gangrene: p421)
  - *C. tetani* (tetanus: p424)
  - *C. difficile* (diarrhoea, p247)

Actinomyces: *Actinomyces israelii* (p421), *A. naeslundii* *A. odontolyticus*, *A. viscosus*

Intracellular bacteria: (o=obligate)

Chlamydia ° (p416, p162, *OHCS* p286)
- *C. trachomatis:* Tropical eye disease trachoma (*OHCS* p450)=serovars A–C
  - GU/cervicitis (p417)=serovars B–K[14]
  - lymphogranuloma ven. (p416)= L1-3[15]
- *Chlamydophila psittaci* (p162)
- *Chlamydophila pneumoniae* (p162)

Coxiella burnetii ° (p434)
Bartonella ° (p434)
Ehrlichia ° (p434)
Rickettsia ° (typhus, p435)
Legionella pneumophilia (p162)

Gram-negative cocci

Neisseria: *Neisseria meningitidis* (meningitis, septicaemia)
- *N. gonorrhoea* (gonorrhoea, p418)

Moraxella: *Moraxella catarrhalis* (pneumonia, p422)

Gram-negative bacilli (rods)

Enterobacteriaceae (p390 & p422):
- *Escherichia coli*
- *Shigella* species (p426)
- *Salmonella* species (p426)
- *Citrobacter freundii; C. koseri*
- *Klebsiella pneumoniae; K. oxytoca*
- *Enterobacter aerogenes; E. cloacae*
- *Serratia marascens; Proteus mirabilis*
- *Morganella morganii*
- *Providencia* species; Yersinia (*Y. pestis Y. enterocolitica, Y. paratuberculosis*)
- *Pseudomonas aeruginosa* (p422)
- *Haemophilus influenzae* (p422)
- *Brucella* species (p423)
- *Bordetella pertussis* (p422)
- *Pasteurella multocida* (p422)
- *Vibrio cholerae* (p426)
- *Campylobacter jejuni* (p390)

Anaerobes:
- *Bacteroides* (wound infections, p572)
- *Fusobacterium*
- *Helicobacter pylori* (p242)

Mycobacteria: *M. tuberculosis* TB, p398
- *M. bovis & M. leprae* (leprosy, p428)
- Atypical mycobacteria: ►Suspect if immunocompromized
- *M. avium intracellulare* (p411)
- *M. scrofulaceum, M. kansasii*
- *M. marinum*
- *M. malmoense*
- *M. xenopi, M. gordonae*
- *M. fortuitum, M. chelonae*
- *M. flavescens*
- *M. smegmatis, M. phlei*

Spirochetes (p430):
- *Treponema* (syphilis; yaws; pinta)
- *Leptospira* (Weil's dis.; canicola fever)

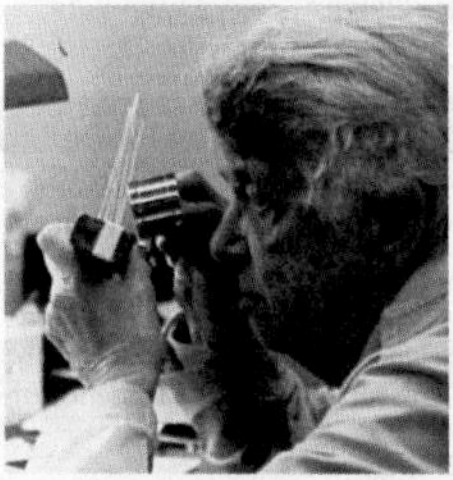

Fig 2 Streptococci are grouped by haemolytic pattern (α, β-, or non-haemolytic) or by Lancefield antigen (A-G), or by species. Rebecca Lancefield (1895-1981) is shown with her hand lens, typing streps with a variety of M protein-specific antibodies mixed with a streptococcal extract by detecting the precipitin in a pipette. Photo of Dr Lancefield courtesy of Dr V Fischetti.

DNA viruses—*A) Double-stranded DNA*	
Papovavirus	Papilloma virus: human warts JC virus: progressive multifocal leucoencephalopathy, PML
Adenovirus	>30 serotypes; 10% of viral respiratory disease 7% of viral meningitis
Human herpes viruses	Alphaherpesvirus$^{\alpha}$ (eg neurotropic) beta-$^{\beta}$ (eg epitheliotropic) and gammaherpesvirus$^{\gamma}$ (lymphotropic): • Herpes simplex virus$^{\alpha}$ (HSV) 1 & 2 (HHV-1 & HHV-2, p400) • Herpes (varicella) zoster virus$^{\alpha}$ (HHV-3, p400) • Cytomegalovirus$^{\beta}$—CMV, also called HHV-5, (p404) • Herpes virus 6$^{\beta}$ & 7$^{\beta}$ (HHV-6 & 7): roseola infantum (mild, *OHCS* p143); also post-transplant, like CMV Epstein-Barr virus (EBV) (HHV-4, p401)$^{\gamma}$ • Infectious mononucleosis (glandular fever) • Burkitt's lymphoma; nasopharyngeal carcinoma HHV-8: Kaposi's sarcoma (p716)
Pox viruses	(1) Variola: smallpox (eradicated in 1979; some stocks left) (2) Vaccinia, cowpox (3) Orf, cutaneous pustules, caught from sheep (4) Molluscum contagiosum, pearly umbilicated papules, typically seen in children or with HIV.
Hepatitis B virus	See p406
B) Single-stranded DNA	
Erythrovirus (=parvovirus)	Erythema infectiosum (fifth disease, *OHCS* p142) 'slapped cheek' appearance ± aplastic crises

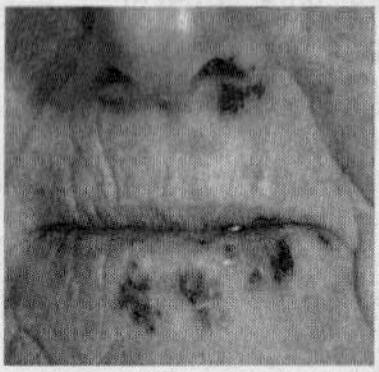

Fig 1. Oral herpes (HSV1).[16]

RNA viruses—*A) Double-stranded RNA*	
Reovirus	Eg rotavirus (p390), infantile gastroenteritis
B) Positive single-stranded RNA	
Picornavirus	**1** Rhinovirus, common cold (>90 serotypes) **2** Enteroviruses (eg echoviruses) are a leading cause of meningoencephalitis/acute flaccid paralysis.[17] **i** Coxsackie A (meningitis, gastroenteritis); Coxsackie B (pericarditis, Bornholm disease) **ii** Hepatitis A virus; **iii** Echovirus (30% of viral meningitis) **iv** Enterovirus EV71 (hand, foot & mouth disease, *OHCS* p143) **v** Poliovirus, p432
Coronavirus	Eg Urbani SARS-associated coronavirus (Dr Urbani described it and died in an outbreak in Vietnam in 2003); ►p163.
Togavirus	**1** Rubella; **2** Alphavirus; **3** Flavivirus (yellow fever, dengue, hepatitis C)
C) Negative single-stranded RNA	
Orthomyxovirus	Influenza A, B, C
Paramyxovirus	Parainfluenza, mumps, measles, respiratory syncitial virus
Arenavirus	Lassa fever, some viral haemorrhagic fevers, lymphocytic-choriomeningitis virus (LCM)
Rhabdovirus	Rabies
Bunyavirus	Some viral haemorrhagic fevers
D) Retroviruses (enveloped RNA viruses using reverse transcriptase to make DNA)	

Human immunodeficiency virus—HIV-1, HIV-2. Types A & B predominate in UK (p408)

Human T-lymphotropic virus (HTLV-I, HTLV-II). ***HTLV-I*** causes adult T-cell leukaemia/lymphoma (ATLL); a definite role in mycosis fungoides & Sézary syndrome is controversial. It is mostly asymptomatic, but 1-5% develop ATLL, a fatal expansion of virus-infected CD4+ T cells.[18] *HTLV-2* may be passed on by transfusions, injecting drug users, or sexually. It may cause tropical spastic paraparesis (p520). It is associated with ↑incidence of pneumonia and bronchitis, and arthritis.

Travel and infectious disease

Most travel-related illness is not from infections, but due to accidents, violence, MI etc. Most infections are due to ignorance or indiscretions. ►*Advice to travellers is more important than vaccination*: eg simple hygiene, malaria prophylaxis, and protective measures (eg safer sex). ***Malaria*** is a big killer; see p396 for prevention. *Rabies:* vaccinate if post-exposure vaccination is unlikely to be available (or their activities mean risk is ↑—or if they will be in a rabies area for >1month); seek immediate attention if bitten (wash the wound well); see p432. For ***cholera*** and ***traveller's diarrhoea***, see p426 & p390.[19,20]

Vaccines for travellers[21]

Routine vaccination	Selective use for travellers	Mandatory vaccination
Diphtheria, tetanus, pertussis	Meningococcal disease[3]	Yellow fever (in some countries)
Hepatitis B [1]	Hepatitis A[3]	Meningococcal disease and polio[4]
Haem. influenzae B	Cholera	
BCG[2], HPV	Japanese encephalitis[3]	
Influenza	Rabies	
MMR	Tick-borne encephalitis	
Pneumococcal disease	Typhoid fever	
Poliomyelitis	Yellow fever[3]	
Rotavirus		
Varicella		

1 Routine for certain age groups and risk factors, selective for general travellers.
2 No longer routine in most industrialized countries.
3 These vaccines are included in the routine immunization programme in several countries.
4 Required by Saudi Arabia for pilgrims; updates are available on www.who.int/wer.

If only one attendance is possible, all is not lost (make up *en route*): *malaria prophylaxis/advice:* p396. Suggested vaccines: ***Africa:*** Meningitis, typhoid, diphtheria, tetanus, polio, hepatitis A ± yellow fever. *Asia:* Typhoid, diphtheria, tetanus, polio, hepatitis A. Consider rabies and Japanese encephalitis. ***Meningitis and Hajj pilgrimage to Saudi Arabia:*** All >2yrs old *must* be vaccinated against meningococcal meningitis with quadrivalent vaccine (serogroups A, C, Y & W135); must be <3yrs ago but not within the last 10 days. If 3 months–2yrs of age, give 2 doses of the A vaccine separated by 3 months. *S. America:* Typhoid, diphtheria, tetanus, hepatitis A ± yellow fever ± rabies. ***Travel if immunocompromised:*** Avoid live vaccines. Hepatitis B vaccine: p271.

Preventing traveller's diarrhoea *Water:* If in doubt, boil all water. Chlorination is OK, but doesn't kill amoebic cysts (get tablets from pharmacies). Filter water before purifying. Distinguish between simple gravity filters and water purifiers (which also attempt to sterilize chemically). Choose a unit which is verified by bodies such as the London School of Hygiene and Tropical Medicine (eg the MASTA[22] *Travel Well Personal Water Purifier*). Make sure that all containers are disinfected. Try to avoid surface water and intermittent tap supplies. In Africa assume that all unbottled water is unsafe. With bottled water, ensure the rim is clean & dry. Avoid ice. Other water-borne diseases include schistosomiasis (p445).

Food: Hot, well-cooked food is best. Avoid salads and peel your own fruit. If you cannot wash your hands, discard the part of the food which you are holding (with bananas, careful unzipping obviates this precaution).[23]

Chemoprophylaxis: Prophylactic antibiotics are not needed in healthy people, but those eg with Crohn's/UC or immunosuppression should get prophylactic antibiotics. Bismuth salicylate can (to some extent) prevent traveller's diarrhoea. Ciprofloxacin 500mg/12h PO for 72h[24] + loperamide can give ~90% protection.

Notes
S=usually sensitive
2=S, but may be 2nd choice
? =may be resistant (esp. if hospital-acquired)
R=resistance likely
0=not appropriate
Sources: OTM & GAT (Sanford)

	Amoxicillin/ ampicillin	Cefepime[25]	Cefotaxime[26]	Ciprofloxacin	Co-amoxiclav	Colistin[27]	Erythromycin[28]	Flucloxacillin	Gentamicin	Imipenem/ meropenem	Metronidazole	Penicillin	Tetracyclines	Ticarcillin/piper-acillin/azlocillin	Trimethoprim[29]	Vancomycin/ teicoplanin
STAPH AUREUS	R	S	S	?	R	0	?	S	R	2	R	R	?	R	?	S
STREP PNEUMONIAE	?	S	?	?	?	0	?	?	R	2	R	?	?	0	?	S
STREP PYOGENESE	S	S	S	S	S	0	?	S	R	2	R	S	?	0	?	S
ENTEROCOCCUS FAECALIS	?	S	R	S	S	0	R	R	R	2	R	?	R	2	?	S
N. GONORRHOEA	?	S	S	R[30]	?	0	R[31]	0	0	2	R	?	2	0	R	0
N. MENINGITIDIS	S	S	S	S	S	0	0	0	0	2	R	S	0	0	R	R
H. INFLUENZA	?	S	S	S	?	0	?	R	0	2	R	?	S	0	S	R
E. COLI[32]	R	S	S	?	?	0	R	R	S	2	R	R	2	2R	?	R
E. COLI ESBL[33] extended spectrum beta lactamase	R	?	R	R	R	R	R	R	R	?S	R	R	R	R	R	R
KLEBSIELLA	R	S	S	S	R	2	R	R	S	2	R	R	?	2R	?	R
PROTEUS MIRABILIS	R	S	S	S	S	0	R	R	S	2	R	R	R	2R	?	R
SERRATIA SPECIES[34]	R	S	S	S	R	0	R	R	S	2	R	R	R	R	?	R
PSEUDOMONAS AERUGINOSA[35]	R	?	R	?	R	2	R	R	?	2	R	R	R	R	R	R
ACINETOBACTER BAUMANNII[36]	R	R	R	R	R	2	R	R	R[37]	p423	R	R	R	R	R	R
BACTEROIDES FRAGILIS	R	R	R	R	R	0	?	R	R	2	S	R	?	R	R	R
CLOSTRIDIUM DIFFICILE	0	0	0	0	0	0	0	0	0	0	S	0	0	0	0	S

Penicillin-based antibiotics	*Usual adult dose:*	*In renal failure:*
Amoxicillin Uses as for ampicillin but better absorbed PO. For IV therapy, use ampicillin.	250–500mg/8h PO 1g/8h in recurrent or severe pneumonia	↓Dose if cc<10 (cc=creatinine clearance, mL/min)
Ampicillin Broader spectrum than penicillin; more active against Gram -ve rods, but β-lactamase sensitive. Amoxicillin is better absorbed PO.	500mg/4–6h IM/IV Listeria: 2g/4h IVI for 10d	↓If cc <10, give doses every 12–24h
Benzylpenicillin = penicillin G Most streps, meningococcus, gonococcus, syphilis, gas gangrene, anthrax, actinomycosis, and many anaerobes.	300–600mg/6h IV, 2.4g/4h in meningitis. If dose >1.2g, inject at rate <300mg/min	Anaphylaxis risk <1:100,000; huge doses cause Na^+↑ ± fits in renal failure
Co-amoxiclav Augmentin=amoxicillin 250 or 500mg + clavulanic acid 125mg confers β-lactamase resistance so broader spectrum, but LFT may rise.	1 tab/8h PO IV form: p382. NB: May contribute to *C. diff* infections	If cc 10–50, give 1 tab/12h; if cc <10, 1 tab/24h
Flucloxacillin For Gram +ve β-lactamase producers (staphylococci).	250–500mg/6h PO ½h before food. 0.5–2g/6h IV	Dose unaltered if cc >10
Phenoxymethylpenicillin(=pen. V) Like pen. G but poorly absorbed; use as prophylaxis or to complete IV course.	250–500mg/6h PO; take ½h before food	In severe renal failure, give doses every 12h
Piperacillin Very broad spectrum including anaerobes & *Pseudomonas*. Inactive against Staphs. Reserve only for those with severe infection. May be used with aminoglycosides (but not in the same IVI).	Tazocin®= tazobactam 500mg + piperacillin 4g: dose: 4.5g/8h IV over 3–5min	Max dose of Tazocin® if eGFR <20: 4.5g/12h
Procaine penicillin (= procaine benzylpenicillin) Depot injection; good for syphilis; only available on a named patient basis in the UK.	Syphilis: p431	Dose unaltered in renal failure. Resistance in GC is a problem.[38]
Ticarcillin Very broad spectrum, eg *Pseudomonas, Proteus*. Use with an aminoglycoside; more active than azlocillin or piperacillin.	Timentin®=3g ticarcillin +200mg clavulanic acid. Dose: 3.2g/8h IV (/4h in severe infections)	If cc 10–50 dose is 1–2g/8h If cc < 10, dose is 1–2g/12h

Antibiotics: cephalosporins

Spectrum Many cephalosporins are active against staphs (including β-lactamase producers), streps (except group D, *Enterococcus faecalis & faecium*), pneumococci, *E. coli*, some *Proteus, Klebsiella, Haemophilus, Salmonella*, and *Shigella*. 2nd generation drugs (cefuroxime, cefamandole) are active against some *Neisseria* and *Haemophilus*. 3rd generation drugs (cefotaxime, ceftazidime, ceftriaxone) have better activity against Gram -ve organisms. Ceftazidime has less Gram +ve activity (esp. against *Staph aureus*) and is used in *Pseudomonas* infections.

Uses Oral cephalosporins (cefaclor, cefalexin, cefuroxime axetil) have a role in UTI, pneumonia, and otitis media, but are not 1st-line (unless penicillin-allergic; but 10% will also be cephalosporin allergic). Their major use is parenteral, eg in surgical prophylaxis or post-op infection. 3rd-generations drugs (eg ceftriaxone) may be used in septicaemia. **SEs:** Hypersensitivity; warfarin potentiation.

Antibiotic	Adult dose	Notes For body surface area calculation, see *BNF*
Cefaclor	250mg (max 1g)/8h PO	No dose change in RF
Cefalexin	500mg/8h PO; Max: 1.5g/6h PO	Max 3g/d if eGFR 40-50 (1.5g/d if eGFR 10-40; 750mg/d if eGFR <10)
Cefepime4th	1-2g/12h IVI	Good activity against *Pseudomonas*, enterobacter, other resistant Gram -ve organisms and *S. aureus*. If cc 10-50: 1-2g/12h; if cc ≤10: 1g/24h
Cefpirome4th	1-2g/12h IV over 5min	Broad spectrum, used in polymicrobial infection; pyelonephritis; pneumonia. Not for MRSA (p420) or bacteroides. Good against enterobacter.39 In renal failure, get help, eg load with 1-2g, then if: cc 20-50: 500mg-1g/12h; if cc 5-20: 500mg-1g/24h
Cefixime	Syrup: ½-1yr: 3.75mL/d 1-4yrs: 5mL/d 5-10yrs: 10mL/d Adults: 200mg/12-24h	Syrup = 100mg/5mL. Active against streps, coliforms, *Haemophilus, Proteus* and anaerobes, staphylococci, *E. faecalis*, and *Pseudomonas* are resistant. Lower dose if e GFR <20.
Cefotaxime3rd	1-2g/6-12h IV/IM; max 3g/6h (gonorrhoea: 500mg stat)	Broad spectrum for serious infections only (pneumonia, meningitis). Unreliable activity against *Pseudomonas*. If cc <10, give 2g/24h max. If cc <5 give 1g stat, then halve dose.
Cefradine	250-500mg/6h PO or 500mg-1g/12h PO or 500mg-2g/6h IM/IV	Less active than cefuroxime. Halve normal dose if eGFR 5-20.
Ceftazidime3rd	UTI: 500mg-1g/12h IM/IV Other: 1-2g/8h Max: 3g/12h if elderly Route: IV/IM but avoid IM if dose >1g	Broad spectrum, incl. most *Pseudomonas* but bad *vs* Gram +ves; for bad infections only; may help in blind ℞ of neutropenic sepsis40 (cefepime is better).41 Reduce dose if eGFR <50.
Ceftriaxone3rd	1-4g daily IM/IV over 3min; give ≤1g at each IM site. Use IVI, not IV, if dose >1g	Many Gram +ve and -ve infections. Used in meningitis (p382), pre-colonic surgery, and gonorrhoea. No activity against *Listeria*, enterococci, and *Pseudomonas*. Can use in RF if cc >10 (or limit dose to 2g/day and check levels)
Cefuroxime	250-500mg/12h PO 750mg-1.5g/8h IV/IM; Max IV: 1.5g/6h.	Broad spectrum & good Gram -ve activity. Used in: surgical prophylaxis; cholecystitis;42 post-op infections; severe pneumonia. Give per 12h if eGFR 10-20.

Abbreviations: RF = renal failure; CC= creatinine clearance; CCM = cc/1.73m² body area; 4th = 4th generation cephalosporin; not all are available in the UK; 3rd= 3rd generation. Source: *GAT* 2009.

Antibiotic (and uses)	**Adult dose**	**Notes** CC=creatinine clearance, mL/min
Amikacin See gentamicin.	7.5mg/kg/12h IV; (~50% 12–18h if cc 10–50)[3]	Resistance growing, but less common than for gentamicin
Azithromycin See clarithromycin, also good against *N. gonorrhoea*.[43]	500mg/24h PO for 3d.	SE: see erythromycin.
Chloramphenicol Rarely used 1st-line. May be used in typhoid fever & *Haemophilus* infection. Also in blind ℞ of meningitis if patient allergic to both penicillins and cephalosporins. Avoid late in lactation and pregnancy.	12.5mg/kg/6h PO or IV; 25mg/kg/6h may be used in septicaemia or meningitis	SE (rare): marrow aplasia (check FBC often), neuritis, GI upset. Avoid long or repeated courses and in liver impairment or if cc <10mL/min. *Interactions*: warfarin, rifampicin, phenytoin, sulfonylureas, phenobarbital.
Ciprofloxacin Used in adult cystic fibrosis, typhoid, *Salmonella*, *Campylobacter*, prostatitis, and serious or resistant infections. Avoid overuse.	250–750mg/12h PO 200–400mg/12h IVI over ≥½h (over 1h, if 400mg used).	Good oral anti-pseudomonal agent. β-lactamase-resistant. If eGFR <30 ↑ dose interval to /24h. SE: D&V, rash; tendon rupture (esp. if >60ys or on steroids); LFT↑. Potentiates theophylline.
Clarithromycin A macrolide, like erythromycin, used for: *S. aureus*, streptococci, *Mycoplasma*, *H. pylori*, *Chlamydia*, MAI (p411).	250–500mg/12h PO for 7–14d. *H. pylori:* 500mg/12h PO for 1wk as triple therapy (p243). MAI may need 12wks (p411) If cc 10–50 give 75%.[5]	Halve dose if eGFR <30. *Interactions:* ergot, warfarin, carbamazepine, theophyllines, zidovudine; never use with pimozide.
Clindamycin Active against Gram +ve cocci including penicillin resistant staph, and anaerobes.	150–300mg/6h PO; max 450mg/6h PO. 0.2–0.9g/8h IV or IM (by IVI only, if >600mg used)	Stop if diarrhoea occurs (pseudomembranous colitis, p247). Used in Staph. Bone/joint infection.
Co-trimoxazole Sulfamethoxazole 400mg + trimethoprim 80mg. 1st choice in *Pneumocystis jiroveci* (=*P. carinii*, p410), toxoplasmosis and nocardia. NB: can act against *S. aureus*.	960mg–1.44g/12h PO/IVI; see *Pneumocystis* (p410)	SE (mostly ∵ sulfonamide, elderly at ↑risk): jaundice; Stevens–Johnson, **fig 1** p725; marrow depression; folate↓. If eGFR 15-30, halve dose. CI: G6PD deficiency.
Doxycycline Used in travellers' diarrhoea, *Chlamydia*, leptospirosis, syphilis, and brucellosis.	200mg PO on 1st day then 100mg/24h; max 200mg/d in severe infections	As for tetracycline, but may be used in renal failure.
Erythromycin Macrolide, used in penicillin allergy. Used 1st line in atypical pneumonia, p162.	250–500mg/6h PO (≤4g/d in *Legionella*). 6.25–12.5mg/kg/6h IVI (adult and child)	SE: D&V; phlebitis in IV use. Potentiates warfarin, theophylline, ergotamine, carbamazepine.
Fusidic acid/sodium fusidate Anti-staph agent (incl. some MRSA, p420); used in osteomyelitis.	500mg/8h PO; 500mg/8h IVI over 6h if >50kg; avoid intravenous route if possible.	Combine with another anti-staphylococcal drug. SE: GI upset, reversible changes in LFTs.

Antibiotic (and uses):	Adult dose	Notes (eg use in renal failure)
Gentamicin Spectrum is wide but poor against streps & anaerobes, so use with a penicillin ± metronidazole. Synergy with ampicillin against enterococci. For serious Gram –ve infections or SBE prophylaxis.	►p766. *Once daily IV dose* over 15min: 5mg/kg[LBW] (7mg if very ill). Plasma levels *not* needed if only one stat dose used, eg in UTI.	**Avoid:** prolonged use, concurrent furosemide, use in pregnancy/myasthenia gravis. ►Do U&E often. SE: oto- and nephrotoxicity.
Imipenem (+cilastatin) Very broad spectrum: Gram +ve and –ve organisms, anaerobes and aerobes. β-lactam stable.	250–500mg/6h IVI; if cc 50–90: ¼–½g/6–8h; if 10–50: ¼g/6–12h.[8] cc <5: dialyse. High doses risk seizures.	Pregnancy/lactation: avoid. SE: fits; D&V; myoclonus, eosinophilia, WCC↓, Coombs' +ve; LFT abnormal. See package insert eg if <70kg.
Linezolid An oxazolidinone antibiotic used against MRSA, VISA, & VRE	600mg/12h PO/IVI over 1h (even if renal failure);[9] SE: D&V, gastritis, T°↑, tinnitus, neuropathy, WCC↓	May cause pancytopenia if ≥2wks use; monitor FBC. CI: BP↑↑, phaeochromocytoma, carcinoid, thyrotoxicosis
Meropenem See imipenem.	½–1g/8h IVI, max 2g/8h (1g/12h if eGFR 26-50)	Causes fewer fits than imipenem.
Metronidazole 1st choice *vs* anaerobes, *Gardnerella, Entamoeba histolytica, & Giardia lamblia;* use PO in *C. difficile.*	400mg/8h PO. PR dose: 1g/8h for 3d then 1g/12h. IVI dose: 500mg/8h for ≤10d. Pregnancy/breast-feeding: avoid high doses.	Disulfiram reaction with alcohol; interacts warfarin, phenytoin, cimetidine; care if LFT↑. SE: irreversible neuropathy (prolonged dosing).
Minocycline Spectrum is wider than tetracycline's.	100mg/12h PO	As tetracycline, but more SE (hepatitis, pneumonitis).
Nitrofurantoin UTI.	50mg/6h PO with food	CI: cc <50.
Oxytetracycline	250–500mg/6h PO	See tetracycline.
Rifampicin[UK] = rifampin[US] Mycobacteria, prophylaxis in meningitis contacts.	Dose example: 600mg x 3/wk PO before breakfast. See TB, p398	Caution in liver disease. Interferes with contraceptive pill. SE: p398.
Teicoplanin See vancomycin, but not given PO.	IV/IM: 400mg/12h for 3 doses, then 200mg/24h	If eGFR 40-60, halve dose from day 4
Tetracycline Used in chronic bronchitis; 1st line in *Chlamydia*, Lyme disease, mycoplasma, brucellosis, rickettsia.	250–500mg/6h PO 1h before food. 500–1000mg/12h IVI (not if liver disease). IV preparation not available in UK.	Avoid if <12yrs old, in pregnancy, and if cc ≤50. Absorption ↓by iron, milk, and antacids. SE: photosensitivity, D&V.
Tobramycin As gentamicin; better against *Pseudomonas.*	1mg/kg/8h IVI or slow IV/IM. Dose↓ in renal failure	Monitor levels; reduce dose if cc ≤50
Trimethoprim Used in UTI, COPD. Dose in prophylaxis: 100mg/24h PO.	200mg/12h PO (100mg/12h PO if eGFR <15)	SE: depressed marrow, D&V. cc 10-50: ½ dose after day 3. cc 10-15, ½ dose.
Vancomycin PO: *C. difficile* if severe infection (p247) or metronidazole is contra-indicated; IV: MRSA or other Gram +ve organisms (not Erysipelothrix species).	125mg/6h PO; 1g/12h IVI over 100min; do peak level 2h post-IVI, eg after dose 3; aim for <30mg/L & ≤10mg/L pre-dose 4	In renal failure, get help; nomograms are available, eg SE: renal and ototoxicity. Do not overuse (↑risk of multiple resistance).

Abbrev'ns: MRSA,p420; VISA: vancomycin-intermediate resistance *S. aureus*; VRE: vanco. resistant enterococci.

History: A good history may reveal the source of infection: ask about respiratory, GI and GU symptoms; any travel or possible immunocompromise? *Signs* (variable!) T°↑(or ↓); pulse↑; respiratory rate ↑; BP↓ (eg ≲90/70mmHg); look for localizing signs.

Tests: If time allows and not too ill, culture all possible sources before treating (blood, sputum, urine, faeces, skin/wound swabs, CSF, aspirates). Do FBC, ESR, CRP, U&E, LFT, clotting, serology, malaria film, acute phase serum. Save serum for virology (compare with convalescent sample in ~2wks), CXR, ABG if indicated. MSU/dipstick.

Prognosis: Poor if very old or young, BP↓, WCC↓, P_aO_2↓, DIC, hypothermia.

Treatment: ►►Get help (eg if you cannot get a IV access; antibiotics *must* be up and running within 1h of telltale signs of serious sepsis). Follow local guidelines. Suspect MRSA, so have a low threshold for using vancomycin (also useful if penicillin allergic). Change antibiotic in the light of sensitivities. Give drugs IV (over ≥5min) if severely ill (eg for ~2 days, then change to PO if possible). If in doubt, ask an infection specialist.

Common fatal errors: Nurses not reporting worsening vital signs; doctor not reacting, or wasting time trying in vain for IV access (p775); pharmacy slow to supply antibiotics; unsuitable antibiotic used; not acting on results of lab data.

Infection	Treatment examples (pen.=penicillin, p378)
Septicaemia (bloodstream infection)	
From urinary tract sepsis	Co-amoxiclav 1g/8h (=amoxicillin 1g+clavulanic acid 200mg) IV over 3min + gentamicin IV 5mg/kg *once daily* is typical max dose; p767
From intra-abdominal sepsis	Cefatazidime 2g/8h IM/IV + metronidazole 500mg/8h IVI
►►From meningococcal sepsis	Cefotaxime 2g/6h, p833
From skin or bone source	Flucloxacillin 1g/6h IV
Unknown cause	Co-amoxiclav 1g/8h IV+ gentamicin 5–7mg/kg IV once daily, p767 + metronidazole 500mg/8h IVI
►►With neutropenia	Tazocin® (=piperacillin 4g with tazobactam 500mg) 4.5g/8h IV over ~4min + gentamicin (as above).
Pneumonia	
Mild community-acquired	Amoxicillin 500mg/8h PO
Possible atypical pneumonia	Add erythromycin 500mg/6h PO
Severe community-acquired	Cefuroxime 1.5g/8h IV + erythromycin 12.5mg/kg/6h IV; see legionellosis, p162
Hospital-acquired	Ceftazidine (above) or Tazocin® 4.5g/8h IV
Meningitis (p832)	
Meningococcus, *Pneumococcus*[2], *Haemophilus*	►►Ceftriaxone 4g/24h IV over 3min or cefotaxime, p833 (or benzylpenicillin 1.2mg IM stat if outside hospital)
Listeria	Add ampicillin 2g/4h IVI and gentamicin, p381
If HSV encephalitis possible	Add aciclovir 10mg/kg/8h IVI (IF eGFR >50)
Endocarditis (p144)	
Empirical therapy	Vancomycin 1g/12h IV + gentamicin IV, p767
Strep. viridans	Benzylpenicillin + gentamicin IV
Enterococcus faecalis	Amoxicillin + gentamicin IV + vancomycin
Staph. aureus or *epidermidis*	Flucloxacillin + gentamicin IV
Prosthetic valve	Vancomycin + gentamicin + rifampicin
Osteomyelitis/septic arthritis	Flucloxacillin 1g/6h IV
Urinary tract infection (simple)	Trimethoprim 200mg/12h PO
Cellulitis	Flucloxacillin (p378)
Wound infection	Await swab result; if ill, flucloxacillin 1g/6h IV

Using a side-room laboratory (near-patient testing)

The main advantage of doing your own lab work is that it enables you to have intelligent chats with lab staff, and encourage their diligence (lab staff make errors out of boredom; amateurs make errors out of ignorance). The great thing is to understand the sources of error—and allow for them at the bedside.[45]

Urine Get used to microscoping your own urines. See p290. Dipstick analysis is OK but misses casts etc (p286). If dipstick +ve for leucocytes, nitrites, blood, or protein, send for culture and testing for antibiotic sensitivities. If +ve for glucose, suspect diabetes. If heavily positive for protein, check 24h collection for protein.

Blood Use universal precautions: all specimens could be HBV, HCV, or HIV +ve. To make a *thick blood film* (malaria diagnosis), use fresh whole blood: a small blob should be spread out somewhat untidily to cover ~$1cm^2$, thinly enough for watch hands to be seen through. The untidiness is helpful to the microscopist because it provides areas of varying thickness, some of which will be ideal for what is often a tricky task. Label and allow to dry. To make a *thin blood film*, put 1 drop of blood near one end of the slide. Take another slide, place its end in the drop of blood, angled at 45°. Push the slide away from you to spread the blood into a thin film (practice makes perfect!). Allow the film to dry, fix in methanol for 5s, then stain as follows.

Leishman's stain: Cover with 10 drops of Leishman's stain. After 30s add 20 drops of water. Leave for 15min. Pick up the slide with forceps (to avoid purple fingers) and rinse in fast-flowing tap water—for 1s only. Allow to dry. Now examine under oil immersion. Note red cell morphology. Do a differential white count. Polymorphs have lobed nuclei. Lymphocytes are small (just larger than red cells) and round, having little cytoplasm. Monocytes are larger than lymphocytes, but similar, with kidney-shaped nuclei. Eosinophils are like polymorphs, but have prominent pink-red cytoplasmic granules. Basophils are rare, and have blue granules. See p325 for images. Learn to use a white cell counting chamber—don't expect this to be as accurate as electronic methods.

Field's stain is easy to use and gives good (and quick) results for malaria, and allows detection of trypanosomes and filaria. Dip the slide in solution A for 5s and solution B for 3s. Dip in tap water for 5s after each staining. Stand to dry. Examine thick film for at least 5min before saying that it is negative. **NB:** ward *serology tests*, eg *Para*Sight F® are available for *P. falciparum*, but cannot replace microscopy as they are not 100% sensitive[46] and parasites are not quantified (needed to plan treatment).

Pus (Gram stain) Make a smear; fix by gentle heat. Flood slide with cresyl violet for 30s. Wash in running water. Flood with Lugol's iodine for 30s. Wash with running water. Decolourise with acetone for 1-3s until no blue colour runs out. Counterstain for 30s with neutral red or safranin. Wash and dry. Gram +ve organisms appear blue-black; Gram -ve ones look red, but are easier to miss.

Near-patient chemistry In one sense this is less taxing than the above tests—the skill lies in the people who made the reagents easy to use. A problem is quality control and the black box effect: when we put a strip into a machine, eg to measure cardiac enzymes, we cannot see the workings of the black box: it just gives a deceptively accurate-looking figure. Frequent calibration of equipment is only a partial answer to this. It is only after you have spent a long time trying to get good results from near-patient analysers, comparing paired samples with the lab, that one appreciates the reproducibility and reliability of the formal lab. ►Speed of reporting is useless if you cannot trust the results.

►Always consider this when there are evasive answers or unexplained findings, especially in younger patients. Ask direct questions: "Do you use any drugs?"; "Have you ever injected drugs? "; "Does your partner use any drugs? "; "Do you share needles? "; "Have you ever had an HIV test? "; "How do you finance your drugs?" List drugs used, and prescribed drugs, with names of prescriber.

Behavioural clues:

- Temporary resident seen by GP: "Just passing through your area".
- Demands analgesia/antiemetics. Knows pharmacopoeia well: "I just need some pethidine for my renal colic/sickle-cell crisis".
- Erratic behaviour on the ward; unexplained absences; mood swings.
- Unrousable in the mornings; agitation from day 2.
- Heavy smoking; strange smoke smells (cannabis, cocaine, heroin).

Physical clues:

- Acetone or glue smell on breath (solvent abuse).
- Small pupils (opiates), reversed by naloxone.
- Needle tracks on arms, groin, legs, between toes; IV access hard.
- Abscesses and lymphadenopathy in nodes draining injection sites.
- Signs of drug-associated illnesses (endocarditis, p144; AIDS, p410, viral hepatitis).

Common and possible presentations in drug abusers

Unconscious	p800 Benzodiazepines—if in ITU consider flumazenil 0.2mg IV over 15s then 0.1mg/min as needed, to 1mg (2mg if on ITU).
Psychosis or agitation	Ecstasy (p855), LSD, amphetamine, anabolic steroids, benzodiazepines. Haloperidol may help (p11).
Asthma or dyspnoea	Is there opiate-induced pulmonary oedema? NB: asthma may follow the smoking of heroin.
Lung abscess	Right-sided endocarditis (Staph) until proved otherwise.
PUO	Is it endocarditis, eg with no cardinal signs (p144)?
Fever/PUO/shivering/headache	Do blood cultures; start eg gentamicin (p381 & p767).
Hyperpyrexia	See phenothiazine poisoning, p855
Abscesses	If over injection site, then often of mixed organisms. Eg on injecting suspended tablets into groin.
DVT	Any compression damage (compartment syndrome)? Do CK.
Pneumonia	Pneumococcus, haemophilus, TB, pneumocystis (p410).
Tachyarrhythmia	(If young); cocaine, amphetamines, endocarditis.
Jaundice	Hepatitis A, B, or C; anabolic steroids (cholestasis).
'Glandular fever'	May be presentation of HIV seroconversion illness.
Osteomyelitis	Including spinal. *Staph. aureus*/Gram -ve organisms.
Constipation	If severe, opiate abuse may be the cause.
Blindness	Consider fungal ophthalmitis ± endocarditis.
Runny nose	Opiate withdrawal (+colic /diarrhoea, yawns, lacrimation, dilated pupils, insomnia, piloerection, myalgia, mood↓; can occur in neonates if mother is an opiate abuser); cocaine use.
Neuropathies	(and any odd CNS signs) Consider solvent abuse.
Infarctions	(eg of spinal cord, brain, heart) Suspect cocaine use.

The vocabulary of drug abusers

The first step in helping a drug abuser is to communicate. To understand what he or she is telling you, the following may be helpful.

Amphetamines	Speed; whiz; Billy; pink champagne; crystal methamphetamine = 'meth' or 'chalk'
Amyl nitrate	Goldrush; poppers; snappers
Barbiturates	Barbs; idiot pills
Cocaine	Coke; Charlie; uncle; the white; the nice; snow; rock; crack; nuggets; wash; gravel
Dihydrocodeine	DFs
Drug-induced sleep	Gauching; nodding; going on the nod
Drug intoxication	Stoned; off it; bladdered; ripped; wiped out; off my box
Heroin	Smack; the nasty; gear; brown; skag; hit; Harry; junk
Ecstasy (MDMA)	E; X; echo; disco biscuit; love drug; XTC; snow[47]
Heroin with ecstasy	Party pack (2-for-1 deal when pusher's business is low)
Filter	Bud/cigarette tip, for drawing drugs through before use
GBL (γ-butyrolactone)	Nail varnish remover (deadly if used with alcohol).
Injecting (subcutaneous/IM/failed) (subclavian)	Mainlining; hitting/jacking up; cranking; having a dig (skin popping/muscle popping/failed) (pocket shot). **NB**: febrile reaction is a 'bad hit'.[48]
Ketamine	Special K (Home Office class C drug, like cannabis); a 'K hole' is a dissociative state (hole in consciousness, p489)—may be a ketamine prelude to 'ego death'.
LSD	Acid; trips; cardboard; tabs; microdots (2mm tabs)
Marijuana	Weed; pot; draw; ganja; grass; resin; Mary; hash; skunk
Methadone	Mud; juice (implies liquid methadone)
Methylenedioxyamphetamine	MDA; snowball (like MDMA but more psychedelic)[49]
Needles	Spikes; nails (tools = syringes)
Obtaining drugs	Score (selling drugs=deal)
PCP	Angel dust; KJ; ozone; missile
Physeptone ampoules	Amps
Prostitution	Working the block/square; doing business; on the game; on the batter; flogging one's golly
Prostitute's client	Mush; punter
Shooting gallery	Supervised surroundings for injecting (conforming with some mythical British Standard of Hygiene)
Shoplifting	Grafting
Smoking heroin	Chasing the dragon (bonging=smoking cocaine)
Syringes	Works; tools (barrel of a syringe=gun)
Temazepam	Temazies
Tourniquet	Key
Wanted by police	'On me toes'; keeping head down
White heroin	China white
Withdrawing from opiates	Turkeying, clucking
Zopiclone	Zim-zims

General management of recreation drug users on the ward A non-judgemental approach will produce better cooperation and may avoid self-discharge. Establish firm rules of acceptable ward behaviour. NSAIDs are useful for pain relief. Don't prescribe benzodiazepines. Methadone may be needed if opiate addicts develop unacceptable withdrawal signs or symptoms in hospital. Get help.

Commercial sex workers need an STD screen, speculum exam (*OHCS* p242), and cervical cytology as carcinoma *in situ* is common (*OHCS* p273). Screen for syphilis (p431), HIV (p408) and hepatitis B (vaccination, p271, use gloves); give safe sex and safe injection advice. ►Liaise with community teams. See *OHCS* p362.

Contrary to Gustave Flaubert, most fevers are not caused by plums, melons, April sunshine, etc,[50] but by our immune responses to self-limiting viral infections resulting in production of interferons and cytokines. PUO in adults is defined as a temperature >38.3°C for >3wks with no obvious source despite appropriate investigations (eg after 3 days in the hospital or after 3 outpatient visits).[51] Signs of bacteraemia include confusion, renal failure, neutrophilia, ↓plasma albumin,[52] and ↑CRP, p701.

Causes[53] Infection (23%); connective tissue diseases (22%); tumours (20%); drug fever (3%); miscellaneous (14%). PUOs resist diagnosis in 25% of patients.

- ***Infections*** *Abscesses* (lung, liver, subphrenic, perinephric, pelvic); empyema; *bacteria* (*Salmonella, Brucella, Borrelia*, Leptospira, p430); rheumatic fever; SBE/IE (may be culture -ve, eg Q fever); TB (CXR may be normal, so culture sputum & urine); other *granulomas* (actinomycosis, toxoplasmosis); *parasites* (eg amoebic liver abscess, malaria, schistosomiasis, trypanosomiasis); fungi; HIV; typhus.[54] Asking "Where have you been" is vital: find an expert on that area, or else you will miss diagnoses you may have never heard of, eg melioidosis (*Burkholderia*, p447, the chief cause of fatal bacteraemic pneumonia in parts of SE Asia).
- ***Neoplasms*** Especially *lymphomas* (any pattern: Pel-Ebstein fever, p354, is rare). Occasionally *solid tumours* (GI; renal cell). Patients may be unaware of fever.
- ***Connective tissue disease*** Rheumatoid arthritis, polymyalgia rheumatica, Still's disease, giant cell arteritis, SLE, PAN, Kawasaki disease.
- ***Others*** Drugs (T°↑ may occur months after starting but remits within days of stopping; eosinophilia is a clue); pulmonary embolism; stroke; Crohn's; ulcerative colitis; sarcoid; amyloid; familial Mediterranean fever—recurrent polyserositis (peritonitis, pleurisy) + fevers, abdominal pain, and arthritis; treat with colchicine; cause: gene defect, eg at 16p13;[55] hyper IgD syndrome (periodic prolonged fevers, large joint arthritis, lymphadenopathy, abdominal pain, skin rash, and ↑IgD (>100 u/mL).[56]

Examples of intermittent fevers Always think of malaria; septicaemia (eg from diverticular disease); UTI; pelvic inflammatory disease; IE/SBE; TB; filarial fever—and rarities, eg: amyloid; *Brucella*; occult thromboembolism;[57] Castleman's disease.[58]

- ***Daily spikes:*** Abscess; TB;[59] schistosomiasis. ***Twice-daily spikes:*** Leishmaniasis.[60]
- ***Saddleback fever*** (eg fever for 7d, then normal for 3d): Colorado tick fever; Borrelia; Leptospira; dengue; Legionnaire's disease;[61] Ehrlichia[62] (p434).
- ***Longer periodicity:*** Pel-Ebstein (eg from lymphoma, p354).
- ***Remitting*** (diurnal variation, not dipping to normal): Amoebiasis; malaria; Salmonella; Kawasaki disease; CMV; TB.[63]

History Work; hobbies; sexual activities; eating raw animals; drug abuse; immunosuppression; distant travel (►p388); animal/people contacts; bites; cuts; surgery; rashes; diarrhoea; drugs (eg non-prescription); immunization; sweats; weight↓; lumps; and itching.

Examine Teeth; rectum; vagina; skin lesions; nodes; hepatosplenomegaly, p606; nails; joints; temporal arteries; retina (Roth spots, **fig 1**—caused by microinfarcts, eg from SBE/IE, hypertension, HIV, connective tissue disease, anaemia, Behçet's, viraemia, hypercoagulability).

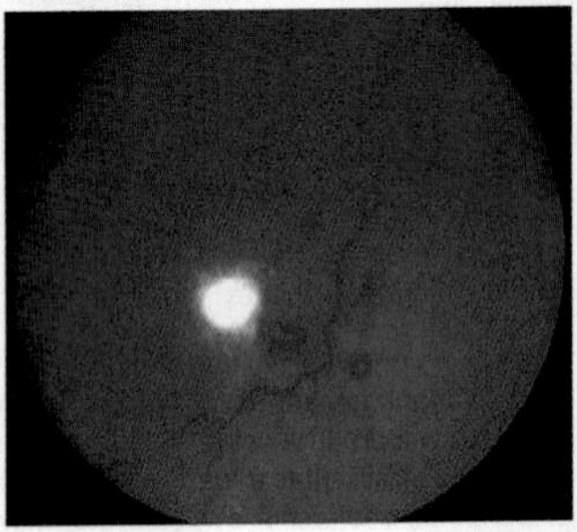

Fig 1. Roth spots. Courtesy of J Trobe.

Symptom-patterns Dialogue with experts ± decision support to diagnose fever with any other symptom. See www.emispdp.com.

New and newly re-emerging infectious diseases

Many diseases preoccupying infectious disease specialists are new or newly re-emerging: food-borne *E. coli*, waterborne *Cryptosporidium*, airborne Legionnaire's disease, blood-borne hepatitis C, and HIV have come to the fore only in the last 30 years. Why have these years been so tumultuous in the ID world? The short answer is greed and exploitation. Examples: **1** Each year we consume 4 centuries-worth of animal and plant life,[64] so promoting ecological instability. **2** Economic drive builds dams (↑breeding grounds for vectors by orders of magnitude) and forces land development, putting people closer to vectors, eg ticks, mosquitoes, and rodents. Intensive farming makes it easier for infectious agents to jump the species barrier. Viruses recently crossing species barriers to humans are hantavirus, haemorrhagic fever viruses, arboviruses, Nipah & Hendra viruses, avian influenza, monkeypox virus, SARS (p163), and CJD, p710). Consider also these 9 interacting causes:[65]

1. Famine and war (± threats of bioterrorism, eg with anthrax and smallpox). Sound vector-control practices are impossible if wars are being fought.
2. Unprecedented movements of peoples, their animals and their parasites mixing genes, cultures, customs, and behaviour, eg eating raw molluscs and crabs facilitates toxoplasma, trematode, cestode, and nematode zoonoses.
3. Microbial adaptation and change making antibiotics less successful.
4. Human susceptibility to infection (increased immunocompromise).
5. Climate change leading to shifting ecosystems and, in some places, economic disaster (p372) worsened if local populations have no immunity.
   Warmer parts of Europe (eg Italy) are now seeing tropical diseases such as Chikungunya fever (a mosquito-borne disease commoner in Africa and Asia that can cause arthritis for weeks, but is usually self-limiting).[66]
6. Human demographics (economic development and land use)—and an increasing world population (rising at ~86 million per year).
7. Tourism and commerce. West Nile virus, for example, reached New York from its ancestral home in the Middle East on a bird carried by a ship or plane.[67] With SARS, the specific tourists, businessmen, and doctors who took the virus from Hong Kong to Hanoi, Singapore, and Toronto have been identified.[68]
8. Technology and industry—easy to blame, but also part of the solution. Food security for millions living on <$1/day depends on increasing rice yields through high-tech genetic manipulation to produce insect- and saline-resistant rice. Good crops from disease-free plants mean disease-free people.
9. Breakdown of public health measures with poverty and social inequality.

Can we win against infectious diseases? No! All we can do is live with them. To help us do this in ways which are not too destructive, we need robust public health surveillance institutions, sound vector-control policies, political will, quarantine laws, and above all, openness and cooperation. SARS and its spread emphasize this in a graphic way: as the Chinese and other less-than-open societies have found out, when it comes to reporting infectious diseases, lying means dying.[1]

Winning or losing is the wrong image: infectious diseases have made us who we are. The ability of genomes to produce and emit DNA/RNA sequences allows *horizontal* transmission of genes, and is one of the main motors of evolution.[69]

Greed≈global warming≈emerging diseases≈poverty≈war

1 This led to the sacking of health ministers and more transparent reporting methods. Problems remain—eg the slow reporting in 2008 of enterovirus EV71 outbreaks—an important cause of paralysis, meningitis, brainstem encephalitis, and neurogenic pulmonary oedema/cardiogenic shock, as well as self-limiting hand foot & mouth disease (T° ↑, mouth ulcers + palm & sole vesicles).

Tropical medicine emergency advice[UK] Liverpool 0151 708 9393, London 020 7388 9600, Birmingham 0121 766 6611. **In every ill traveller, consider:**

1 *Malaria* (p394 & p396): Fever, rigors, headaches, dizziness, flu symptoms, faints, diarrhoea, thrombocytopenia. *Complications:* anaemia, renal failure, pulmonary oedema, cerebral oedema. *Diagnosis:* serial thick and thin blood films.

2 *Typhoid* (p426): Presents with fever, relative bradycardia, abdominal pains, dry cough, constipation, lymphadenopathy, headache, splenomegaly ± rose spots (rare). *Complication*: GI perforation. *Diagnosis*: blood or marrow culture.

3 *Dengue fever (DF)* (p433): Presents with fever, headache, myalgia, rash (flushing or petechial), thrombocytopenia, and leucopenia. *Diagnosis:* serology.

4 *Amoebic liver abscess* (p436): T°↑, jaundice, RUQ pain. Do ultrasound.

Examine all over: any bites/eschar, p435? Do serology, thick films & blood cultures.

►*Know your locally re-emerging diseases!* Examples: TB, Lyme disease, leptospirosis, malaria, typhus, cholera, salmonella, hepatitis A, shigella, mumps, measles, brucellosis.[70] NB: a visit to the tropics doesn't preclude mundane fevers, eg flu.

Jaundice Think of viral hepatitis, cholangitis, liver abscess, leptospirosis, typhoid, malaria, dengue fever, yellow fever, haemoglobinopathies.

Gross splenomegaly Malaria, visceral leishmaniasis (kala-azar).

Diarrhoea & vomiting (p390 & p246) *E. coli* (Travellers' diarrhoea) is commonest. Consider *Salmonella, Shigella, Campylobacter, Giardia lamblia, Vibrio cholerae*, etc. (p390). See p246 for general management. If diarrhoea prolonged, consider protozoal infection of small bowel or tropical sprue (p280). In HIV: cryptosporidia, microsporidia, and *Isospora belli* (need special stains—see **figs 1 & 2**).

Hepatosplenomegaly See p606; malaria; *Brucella*; typhoid; typhus; leishmaniasis.

Respiratory symptoms Common respiratory pathogens (p162), typhoid, *Legionella*, TB, Q fever, histoplasmosis, Löffler's (p718), HIV ± pneumocystosis. Do CXR & P_aO_2.

Arthritis Gonococcus; septicaemia; viruses (Ross river, Chikungunya).[71]

Erythema nodosum (p564) Causes: streps, TB, leprosy, fungi, Crohn's disease, ulcerative colitis, sarcoidosis, pregnancy, drugs (sulfonamides, contraceptive steroids).

Anaemia Hookworm, malaria, kala-azar, haemolysis, malabsorption.

Skin signs Scabies (itchy allergic rash + burrows, eg in finger web-spaces; p416 & *OHCS* p608), orf (pustules), molluscum contagiosum (pearly, punctate, papules), leprosy (p428, anaesthetic, hypopigmented areas), tropical ulcers, typhus ('eschar' =scab; **fig 3**), leishmaniasis (ulcers/nodules), onchocerciasis (itchy nodules), myiasis (nodules—larvae of various insects), drug reactions. Transitory migratory swellings: gnathostomiasis, Calabar swellings (loa loa, p443), urticaria, contact dermatitis.

Acute abdomen Perforating typhoid ulcer, toxic megacolon in amoebic or bacillary dysentery, sickle-cell crisis, ruptured spleen.

Rarities to consider ►Use local emergency isolation policy.
Rabies (p432) and other CNS viral infections, eg encephalitis (p466 & p834).
Yellow fever: (p432) Suspect in travellers from Africa.
Lassa fever: Occurs in Nigeria, Sierra Leone, or Liberia. *Signs:* Fever; exudative sore throat; face oedema; collapse. **Δ**: *PCR/EM;* serology. ℞: Isolate and refer.
Marburg and Ebola virus: Seen in Sudan, Zaire, Kenya. *Signs:* Fever, myalgia, D&V, pleuritic pain, hepatitis, shock, and bleeding tendency. A maculopapular rash appears on day 5-7 and desquamates in <5d. Patients may bleed from all orifices and gums.[72] **Δ**: *PCR* or electron microscopy; serology. ℞: Isolate and refer.[73]
Viruses causing haemorrhage: Dengue, Marburg, Lassa, Ebola, Crimea-Congo fever, haemorrhagic fever with renal syndrome, yellow fever. ►See p432.

►Travel details (areas visited; immunization; prophylaxis; disease exposure) are very important, even if you cannot interpret yourself, so seek expert opinion *early*.

Some typical incubation times[74]

For fever with diarrhoea: p390

Incubation times are not set in stone: expect variability.

<14 days	14 days to 6wks	>6wks
Undifferentiated fever		
Malaria	Malaria	Malaria
Typhoid	Typhoid	Hepatitis B or E
Leptospirosis	Leptospirosis	Kala-azar
Dengue fever	Hepatitis A or E	Lymphatic filariasis
Rickettsiae	Acute schistosomiasis	Schistosomiasis
Acute HIV infection	Acute HIV infection	Amoebic liver abscess
Fever with CNS signs		
Viral and bacterial meningitis and encephalitis	East African trypanosomiasis	Rabies
East African trypanosomiasis	Rabies	
Poliomyelitis		
Fever with chest signs		
Influenza	Tuberculosis	Tuberculosis
Legionellosis	Q fever	
Q fever		
Acute histoplasmosis		
SARS		

Hitch-hiking to a Fools' Paradise

We think we are absolved of thinking of tropical diseases when the answer to "Where have you been?" is "Bournemouth" and in our blinkered way we carry on in our Fools' Paradise until disaster bites. It's not just a question of forgotten holidays or amnesic stopovers. Maybe our patient is an airport baggage-handler and has been bitten by a hitch-hiking mosquito: who knows? We never will if we don't ask. Even if there has been no travel to the tropics ***global warming is ensuring that the tropics are travelling to us.*** To the first writers of medical books, Paradise was just beyond the Far East, and the world was a disc surround by oceans of blue water (**fig 1**). The world moves on, tarnished, tawdry, and trashed, and Paradise appears to be evolving with ever more serpents in the garden beguiling us with ambiguous answers to the great question: "Where have you been?"

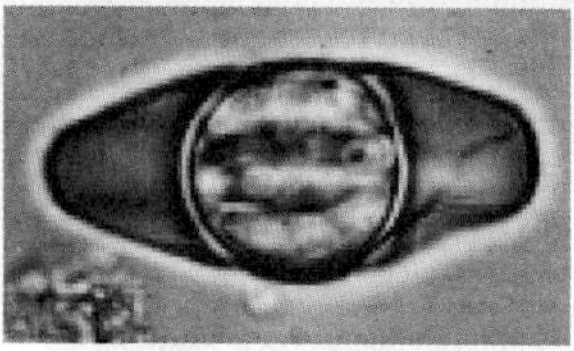

Fig 1. *Isospora belli:* a unique feature of *I. belli* oocysts is that some develop irregularly, having 1 sporocyst with 8 sporozoites.[75] Isosporiasis is an AIDS-defining illnesses (diarrhoea ± haemorrhagic colitis).

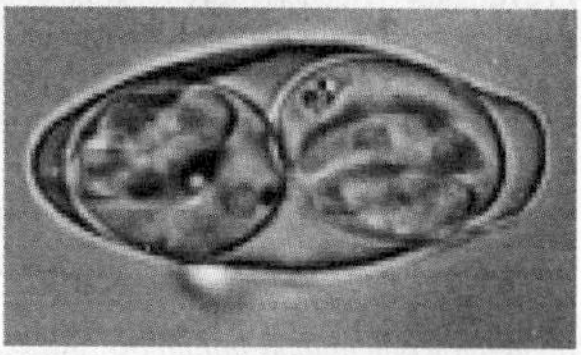

Fig 2. Sporulated (infective) oocyst of the protozoan *I. belli*; oocysts[76] are passed unsporulated, but can sporulate in 1-3 days, depending on T°, and the presence of O_2.

Figs 1 & 2 ©Prof D Duszynski

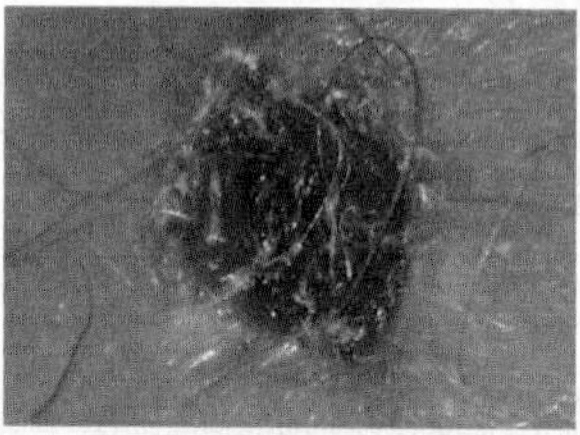

Fig 3. Dr Watson was treating this dentist's presumed septicaemia until Holmes went over his hindquarters with a hand-lens, revealing this ¼in lesion. "I see you have been hunting bushbuck in the Eastern Cape again, Mr S–. This eschar is the tell-tale *tache noire* of typhus." Prompt doxycycline averted disaster. Elementary? We are all uneasy amalgams of dullness and brilliancy, jackal and hind, haunted and hunted, as well as hunting. After AC Doyle; Courtesy of M Seare.

Gastroenteritis

Ingesting certain bacteria, viruses, and toxins is a common cause of D&V (p56 & p246). Contaminated food and water are common sources, but often no specific cause is found. Ask about details of food and water taken, cooking method, time until onset of symptoms, and whether fellow-diners were affected. Ask about swimming, canoeing, etc. **NB:** food poisoning is a notifiable disease (p373) in the UK.

Organism/Source	Incubation	Clinical features	Notes/sources of infection
Staph. aureus	1-6h	D&V, P, hypotension	Meat
Bacillus cereus	1-5h	D&V	Rice
Red beans	1-3h	D&V	
Heavy metals, eg zinc	5min-2h	V, P (?work exposure)	(delayed fever ± flu-like features)
Scrombotoxin	10-60min	D, flushing, sweating	Fish (NB may report hot mouth)
Mushrooms	15min-24h	D&V, P, fits, coma (LFT↑↑)	Image: p251 (hepatic & renal failure)
Salmonella	12-48h	D&V, P, fever, septicaemia	Meat, eggs, poultry
C. perfringens	8-24h	D, P afebrile	Meat
C. botulinum	12-36h	V, paralysis	Processed food
C. difficile	1-7d	Bloody D, P, GI perforation; toxic megacolon; hospital-acquired (1000 deaths/yr^UK^)	Antibiotic-associated; getting more virulent (eg strain BI/NAP1 with 20-fold ↑ in toxin A & B production).[77]
Vibrio cholerae	2h-5d	See p426	Water*
Vib. parahaemolyticus	12-24h	Profuse D; P, V	Seafood
Campylobacter	2-5d	Bloody D, P, T°↑, peritonism	Milk, poultry, water*
Listeria		Meningoencephalitis; "I've got flu"; miscarriages	Cheese, pâtés
E. coli type O157	12-72h	Cholera/typhoid-like;*	Haemolytic-uraemic sy., p308
Y. enterocolitica	24-36h	D, P, fever	Milk*
Cryptosporidium (**fig 1**)	4-12d	D in HIV	Cow→water→man
Giardia lamblia	1-4wks	p436 (D, malabsorption)	*Nappies, cats,[78] dogs, crows[79]
Entamoeba histolytica	1-4wks	See p436	*
Noroviruses, eg Norwalk SRVS (small round structured virus)	12-48h[80] mean≈34h	Fever, P, D & projectile V[81] 'winter vomiting illness'. Δ: no leucocytes in faeces; PCR	*Fecal-oral (vomit is infectious); very contagious, and common. Infectious for≤48h after symptoms resolve.[82]
Rotavirus	1-7d	D&V, fever, malaise	*(RotaTeq vaccine ?available for infants aged from 6 weeks)
Shigella	2-3d	Bloody D, P, fever	Any food

V=vomiting; **D** = diarrhoea; **P** = abdominal pain. *May be food- or water-borne.

Tests *Stool microscopy/ culture* if from abroad, an institution, or in day care, or an outbreak is suspected. In these circumstances culture of the food source may help.

Prevention Hygiene; if abroad, avoid unboiled/unbottled water, ice cubes, salads, and peel own fruit. Eat only freshly prepared hot food (or *thoroughly* rewarmed). Household water treatment and safe storage technologies can ↑ water quality and ↓ rates of diarrhoea, eg: chlorine or solar disinfection, and ceramic or biosand filtration.[1][83]

Management Usually symptomatic. Maintain ***oral fluid*** intake (±oral rehydration sachets). For severe symptoms (but not in dysentery), give ***anti-emetics***, eg ***prochlorperazine*** 12.5mg/6h IM + *antidiarrhoeals* (***codeine phosphate*** 30mg PO/IM or ***loperamide*** 4mg stat, then 2mg after each loose stool). *Antibiotics are only indicated if systemically unwell, immunosuppressed or elderly*; resistance is common.
Cholera: ***tetracycline*** reduces transmission.
Salmonella: ***ciprofloxacin*** 500mg/12h PO, 200–400mg/12h IVI over 60min (remember that antibiotic therapy in salmonella enteritis may ↑ number of chronic carriers).
Shigella & *Campylobacter*: ***ciprofloxacin*** as above.

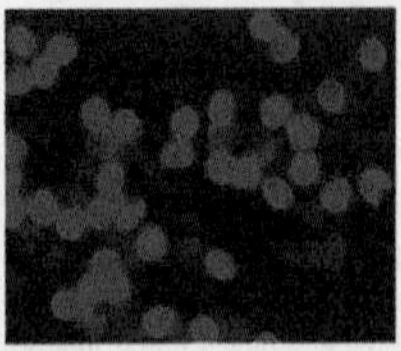

Fig 1. Cryptosporidium: indirect immunofluorescence (BF4 antibody).[84] It is a tiny protozoan (5μm) causing diarrhoea & cramps—life threatening if HIV+ve; self-limiting if CD4 ≥100; if <100, 14L of diarrhoea can be lost/d (bad news). It is a UK crime to sell water with >1 oocyst/10L. Spread: unboiled water; cattle. If found in stool, quantify excretion. If ℞ needed, ask a microbiologist (℞ often fails); optimize anti-HIV ℞. Consider: **nitazoxanide** 0.5g/12h PO for 3d (if >12yrs).

Courtesy of Prof S Upton; Kansas University.

1 The top few cm of sand traps most organisms, which develop into a highly active food chain (the *biological layer,* which must remain partially wet). Further filtration occurs in the lower layers of sand.

Immunization

www.immunisation.nhs.uk

Active immunization stimulates the immune system (humoral+cellular immunity). *Passive immunization* uses pre-formed antibody (nonspecific or antigen-specific).

Age	Immunization (L=live vaccine) (DoH[UK] 2009)
2 months	**Pediacel®**, ie 5-in-1 diphtheria + tetanus + acellular pertussis + inactivated polio + haemophilus B (Hib); if prem, still give at 2 mths; can give if ≤10 yrs if missed vacs + **Prevenar®** (7-valent pneumococcal)
3 months	**Pediacel® + Neisvac C® or Meningitec®** (Meningitis C vaccine)
4 months	**Pediacel® + Prevenar® + Neisvav C or Meningitec®**
12 mths	**Menitorix®** (*H. influenzae* with meningitis C)
13 mths	**MMR II vax pro®L** or **Priorix®L** (measles, mumps & rubella) + **Prevenar®**
3¼-5yrs	**Repevax®** or **Infanrix-IPV®** (diphtheria, tetanus, pertussis & polio) + **Priorix®L** or **MMR vax pro®L**
12-13yrs	**Gardasil®** 3 doses for girls at 0, 1 and 6mo (cervical ca., *OHCS* p272)
13-18+yrs	**Revaxis®** (low-dose diphtheria, tetanus, inactivated polio; can also be used for primary vaccination if >10yrs).
Any age	**BCG**L (not for everyone, since 2004 in UK) If at ↑risk of TB, eg for all in high-risk areas (eg London), or in groups at ↑risk, eg TB contact, or (grand) parents or from high-prevalence country, ie >40/100,000/yr—or a visitor to such a country for >1 month. May start at 3 days old. ***Hepatitis B:*** p271; universal (WHO advice) or if at ↑risk. ***MMR***L may be given at any age if the above is missed. One-off ***pneumococcal vaccine*** with 23-valent Pneumovax II® (**Prevenar®** × 2, as above, if <2yrs old); yearly ***flu vaccine*** if caring for a vulnerable person or if chronic heart, chest, liver, or renal disease; DM; immunosuppression (eg HIV +ve, cirrhosis, on chemotherapy, or spleen function↓, eg ∵ coeliac or sickle-cell disease). Consider 2nd pneumococcal vaccine if at ↑risk after >5yrs. [85]
Adults	Tetanus and diphtheria boosters (**Revaxis®**, as above). Travellers: p377.

►*An acute febrile illness is a contraindication to any vaccine.* Give live vaccines either together, or separated by ≥3wks. Caution with live vaccines in patients who are immune-deficient (transplants, cancer chemotherapy, steroids, HIV infection)—seek expert advice. ►*Contraindications to vaccines*: see *OHCS* p151.

►Bacille Calmette–Guérin (BCG) Live attenuated anti-TB vaccine (works in up to 80% of cases for ~10yrs). Make a 7mm blanched weal between the top and middle ⅓ of arm (deltoid's insertion) or, for cosmetic reasons, the upper, outer thigh. Expect to feel marked resistance as the injection is given. If, during injection, propagation of the weal stops, you are going too deep: re-insert the needle. A swelling appears after 2–6 wks, developing into a papule or small ulcer. Avoid air-occluding dressings. SE: pain, local abscess, regional lymphadenitis (the most common SE. The risk is ↑ in infants aged <30d, so give a reduced dose of vaccine). **CI:** immunosuppression, pregnancy, pyrexia, or eczema at vaccination site. [86] **T-spot-TB®/Mantoux test** (p398) Offer to those at risk of TB (see BCG, above). It is now not routinely needed for those <6yrs being referred for BCG on the above criteria. **Travel** p377. Get expert advice.[1] ►*Advice to travellers is more important than vaccination*: eg simple hygiene, malaria prophylaxis, and protective measures (mosquito nets, safe sex advice, etc).

Immunization in special situations If *splenectomized/hyposplenic (eg sickle cell):* meningitis vaccine; polyvalent pneumococcal; Hib (above); annual flu vaccine. *Chronic lung, heart, liver or kidney disease, diabetes:* pneumococcal; annual flu vaccine.

Further details Rotavirus vaccination for all infants (WHO 2009). Hepatitis B (p271); flu; pneumococcal (p160); meningococcal (Mengivac® = group A & C), for short-term use, eg travel abroad. Leave ≥2wks after routine MCC before giving Mengivac®.

1 *Schools of tropical medicine*: London: 020 7636 8636; Liverpool: 0151 708 9393); National Travel Health Network and Centre, **www.nathnac.org**

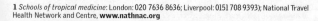

Nosocomial means hospital-acquired. Fever is common in hospitalized patients of all ages. Nosocomial fever usually results from exposure to pyrogens in the hospital environment or from a medical intervention. Nosocomial fever occurs in 2-30% of inpatients: most are bacterial infections.

Definition Two of the many commonly used definitions are as follows:

1 Oral temperature of 38.1°C that develops ≥24h after admission and is recorded on ≥2 consecutive occasions in patients with no history of fever in the preceding week.

2 Oral temperature >38.0°C that occurs at least 48h after admission and is recorded on at least two occasions during any 48-hour period.

Risk factors Alcoholism, cerebrovascular disease, CCF, 'Do-not-resuscitate' status, faecal incontinence, foot ulcers, indwelling bladder catheter, indwelling IV catheter, malignancy, number of procedures before febrile illness, pressure ulcers.

Causes can be grouped into five clinical entities:

1 ***Infections*** (the most common cause): UTI, pneumonia (eg post-op), bacteraemia, skin and soft tissue infections, CNS infection, catheter-related, GI infection, peritonitis, sinusitis, upper respiratory or other self-limiting viral infection, diverticulitis, cholangitis, vascular infections, device-related colitis, tuberculosis, AIDS.

2 ***Inflammation:*** Aspiration, ARDS, arthritis, autoimmune conditions, adrenal insufficiency, connective-tissue disorder, drug-induced fever, acalculous cholecystitis, phlebitis, procedure-related pancreatitis, haematoma, thrombosis, sickle-cell crisis, GI bleeding, graft-versus-host disease, IV contrast reaction.

3 ***Ischaemia:*** Stroke, MI, pulmonary embolism, bowel ischaemia.

4 ***Malignancy:*** Leukaemia, lymphoma, non-haematological cancer.

5 ***Drug-induced fever*** is another important cause.

Approach Nosocomial UTI is the most common cause in those on general medicine wards, whereas nosocomial pneumonia is the most common cause of nosocomial fever in ITU patients. The cause of nosocomial fever is often not apparent, especially when symptoms or obvious physical findings suggestive of a specific illness are absent. In such cases, follow these steps:

1 Get a detailed history and do a careful physical examination covering all systems including the skin. Elucidate the surgical history and procedures performed during hospitalization. Study the patient's medication list carefully (is it a drug fever?).

2 Initial lab and imaging studies should be noninvasive, inexpensive, and based on the findings of patient's history and physical examination: FBC, LFT, ESR, urinalysis, basic cultures (eg MSU, blood, swabs of suspect areas), CXR, ESR.

3 If the initial evaluation does not reveal the cause of nosocomial fever, more expensive and invasive studies may be needed. These studies should be based on clinical suspicion and the results of the initial studies. They include: US, CT scan, MRI, nuclear medicine scanning, and serology. These modalities, including directed biopsies where indicated, reduce the need for more invasive procedures. The use of radionuclide scanning, such as technetium ^{99m}Tc, gallium-67, or indium-labelled leukocytes, is warranted for obscure inflammatory or neoplastic conditions that are not diagnosed by conventional imaging studies.

Prevention Nosocomial infections result in a 4-fold ↑ in mortality, highlighting the importance of preventive measures—see BOX.

►Each country has its own risk profile, so get to know, and follow, local guidelines.

Preventing nosocomial infections [90,91]

Reducing person-to -person transmission *Hand decontamination:* The importance of hands in the transmission of hospital infections has been well demonstrated. There must be written policies and procedures for hand washing. Jewellery must be removed before washing. *Personal hygiene:* Nails must be clean and kept short. False nails should not be worn. Hair must be worn short or pinned up. Beard and moustaches must be kept trimmed short and clean.

Clothing *Working clothes:* In the UK there is a bare-below-the-elbows policy—and no white coats owing to the theoretical risk of cross-infection for cuffs and wrist-watches. In areas such as burn units or ITU (and on many ordinary UK wards), uniform trousers and a short-sleeved gown are required for men and women. In other units, women may wear a short-sleeved dress. *Shoes:* In aseptic units and in theatre, staff must wear dedicated shoes, which must be easy to clean. *Caps:* In aseptic units, theatre, or performing selected invasive procedures, staff must wear caps or hoods which completely cover the hair. *Masks:* Masks of cotton wool, gauze, or paper are ineffective. Paper masks with synthetic material for filtration are an effective barrier against microorganisms. Staff should wear masks to work in theatre, to care for immunocompromised patients or to puncture body cavities in order to protect the patient. In other situations, staff must wear masks to protect themselves (eg when caring for patients with airborne infections, or when performing bronchoscopy etc). Patients with infections which may be transmitted by air route must use surgical masks when outside their isolation room. *Gloves:* Staff should wear sterile gloves for surgery, care for immunocompromised patients, and invasive procedures which enter body cavities. Non-sterile gloves should be worn for all patient contacts where hands are likely to be contaminated, or for any mucous membrane contact. Staff should wear non-sterile gloves to protect themselves while caring for patients with communicable disease transmitted by contact, or performing bronchoscopy etc. Hands must be washed when gloves are removed or changed. Disposable gloves should not be reused.

Safe injection practices To prevent transmission of infections between patients with injections: • Eliminate unnecessary injections • Use sterile needle and syringe • Use disposable needle and syringes, if possible • Prevent contamination of medications • Follow safe sharps disposal practices.

Preventing transmission from the environment Adequate methods for cleaning, disinfecting and sterilizing must be in place. Written policies and procedures which are updated on a regular basis must be developed for each facility. *Cleaning of the hospital environment:* Routine cleaning is necessary to ensure that the hospital is visibly clean and free from dust and soil. 90% of microorganisms are present within 'visible dirt', and the purpose of routine cleaning is to eliminate this dirt. Neither soap nor detergents have antimicrobial activity, and the cleaning process depends essentially on mechanical action. There are 4 hospital zones:
Zone A: no patient contact (eg administration, library): Normal domestic cleaning.
Zone B: care of patients who are not infected, and not highly susceptible: clean by a procedure that does not raise dust. Dry sweeping or vacuum cleaners are not recommended. Using detergent solution improves the quality of cleaning. Disinfect any areas with visible contamination with blood or body fluids prior to cleaning.
Zone C: infected patients (isolation wards): Clean with a detergent/disinfectant solution, with separate cleaning equipment for each room.
Zone D: highly-susceptible patients (protective isolation) or protected areas, eg operating suites, delivery rooms, ITU, A&E and haemodialysis units: Clean using a detergent/disinfectant solution and separate cleaning equipment.

All horizontal surfaces in B, C and D, and all toilet areas should be cleaned daily.

►A child dies of malaria every 30 seconds; most are African children (WHO).[92] Check for it in any sick patient from an endemic area (>3 billion are at risk). *Species:*[93] *P. vivax:* incubation 10–17d, *'benign tertian malaria'*, fever spikes every 48h. *P. ovale:* similar to *P. vivax*; except untreated infection lasts less long. Both may produce true relapses by new invasion of the blood from latent hypnozoites in the liver, up to a few years after complete clearance of parasites from the blood.[94] *P. malariae:* incubation 18–40d, recurs 72hrly ('quartan'$^{1,4,7\ldots}$); may 'lie low' in the blood to recrudesce after 1–52yrs. It is rarely fatal but may cause glomerulonephritis. *P. falciparum:* incubation 7–10 days, symptoms recur 36–48hrly; fulminating disease. *P. knowlesi* is an emergent species (still rare in humans; common in monkeys).[95] See also **figs 1-5**.

Biology Plasmodium protozoa, injected by female *Anopheles* mosquitoes (~120 sporozoites/bite), multiply in RBCs (>10^8–10^{12} trophozoites per infection) causing haemolysis, RBC sequestration and cytokine release. *Fever periodicity* reflects synchronous rupture of mature schizonts (RBCs in which a ring trophozoite has multiplied into 6–24 merozoites, **fig 1**). NB: don't *rely* on periodicity to rule out any type of malaria!

Malaria paroxysms: **1** Shivering for ≤1h: "I feel so cold." **2** Hot stage for 2-6h: T≈41°C, flushed, dry skin ± headache, nausea, vomiting. **3** Sweating for 2-4h as T° falls.[96]

Protective factors: Sickle-cell trait, melanesian ovalocytosis, G6PD deficiency, some HLA B53 alleles enable T cells to kill parasite-infected hepatocytes in non-Europeans.

Falciparum malaria 90% of patients present within 1 month with flu-like prodrome: headache, malaise, myalgia, and anorexia followed by fever paroxysms (above) ± faints. Classic tertian fever and rigors are unusual initially. *Signs:* Anaemia, jaundice, and hepatosplenomegaly. No rash or lymphadenopathy. *Complications: Cerebral malaria* (p397): confusion; coma ± fits. Focal signs unusual. May have variable tone, extensor posturing; upgoing plantars, dysconjugate gaze; teeth-grinding. In children, seizures are common. Mortality: ~20%. *Metabolic (lactic) acidosis* giving laboured deep (Kussmaul) breathing is also a major cause of death. *Anaemia* is common due to haemolysis of parasitized and unparasitized RBCs, and may be particularly severe in young children. *Hyperparasitaemia* (>5% of RBCs parasitized). *Hypoglycaemia* occurs in severe malaria (25% of children, 8% of adults), pregnancy, or with quinine therapy. *Acute renal failure* from acute tubular necrosis, sometimes with haemoglobinuria (*'blackwater fever'*), and *pulmonary oedema* (ARDS, p178) are important causes of death in adults. Shock may develop in severe malaria (*algid malaria*) from supervening bacterial septicaemia, dehydration or, rarely, splenic rupture. In pregnancy, the risk of death (mother or fetus) is high (*OHCS* p27). Use chemoprophylaxis in pregnant women in endemic areas of transmission.

Diagnosis Serial thin & thick blood films (needs much skill, don't always believe -ve reports, or reports based on thin film examination alone); if *P. falciparum*, you must know the level of parasitaemia. Rapid stick tests are available if microscopy cannot be performed or previously treated seriously ill patient: see p383 for *Para*Sight F®. Serology is not useful. Other tests: FBC (anaemia, thrombocytopenia), clotting (DIC, p346), glucose (hypoglycaemia), ABG/lactate (lactic acidosis), U&E (renal failure), urinalysis (haemoglobinuria, proteinuria, casts), blood culture to rule out septicaemia.

Poor prognosis (in falciparum malaria) Age <3yrs, pregnancy, fits, coma, no corneal reflex, papilloedema, pulmonary oedema/ARDS (p178), HCO_3^- <15mmol/L, plasma or CSF lactate >5mmol/L, glucose <2.2mmol/L, hyperparasitaemia (>5% RBCs or 250,000/μL), Hb <5g/dL, DIC, creatinine >265μmol/L.[97] If ≥20% (or >10^4/μL) of parasites are mature trophozoites or schizonts, the prognosis is poor, even if few parasites seen (reflects critical mass of sequestered RBCs[98]); malaria pigment in >5% of neutrophils.

Preventing malaria deaths

Public health measures entail political will + money for indoor antimosquito spraying, insecticide treated bednets, good antenatal and paediatric care, and reliable distribution of malaria drugs (no wars, no corruption). The US leads here in terms of finance (>$1bn over 5yrs) and will.[99] PMI: US President's malaria initiative

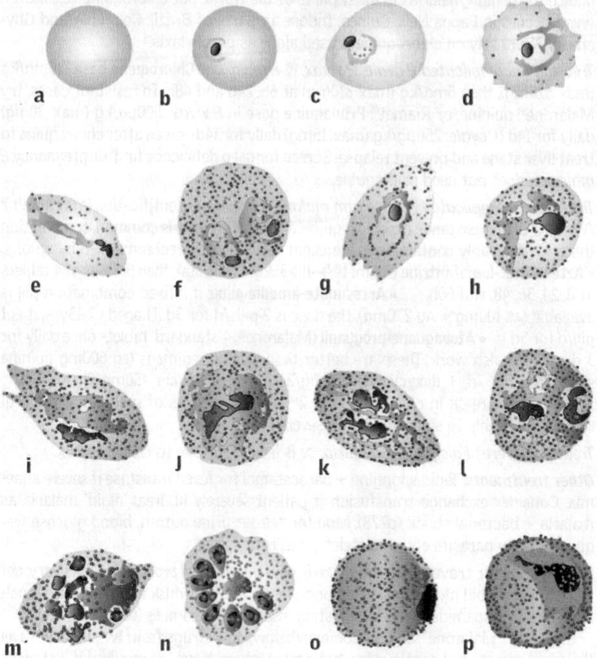

Fig 1 *P. ovale*. Plasmodia live inside erythrocytes: what a fantastic niche!—full of food and protected from prowling immunocytes. **a** is an RBC; **b–i** show trophozoites; **g**'s RBC is fimbriated and oval, giving the species its name; **k–n** are schizonts containing segmenting merozoites; **o–q** are ♀ & ♂ gametocytes. Having this marvellous knack of sexual reproduction (in the mosquito's gut) ensures the infinite variety of plasmodia and their co-evolution with man.[100]
After the Nicholson paintings[101] in Oatney's *Primate Malarias*.

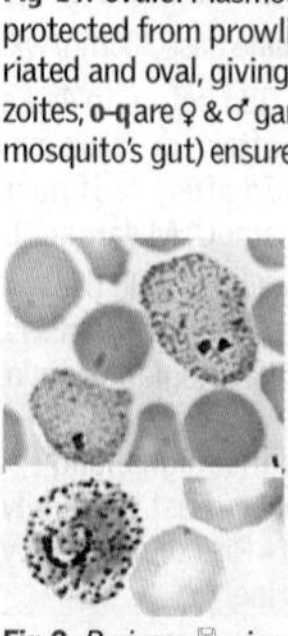

Fig 2. *P. vivax*[102] ring forms partly hidden by Schuffner's dots.[103]

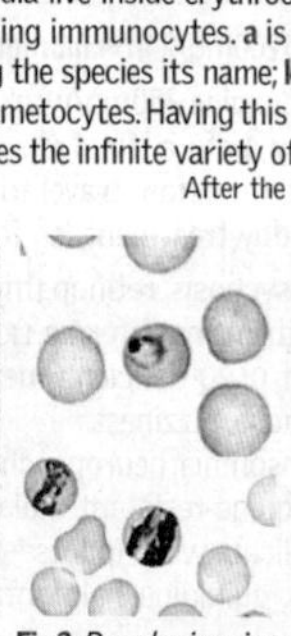

Fig 3. *P. malariae* ring & band forms from two specimens.[104]

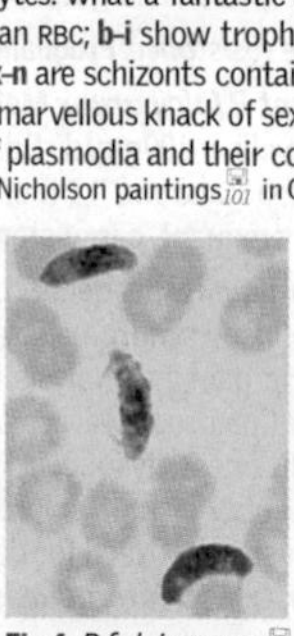

Fig 4. *P. falciparum*[105] sausage-shaped gametocytes in RBC ghosts.

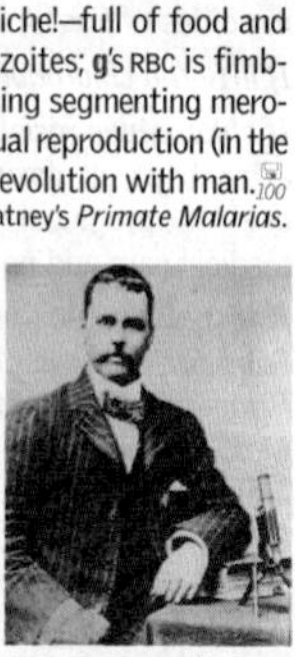

Fig 5. Ronald Ross who first described the malaria lifecycle.[106]

Fig 2 was stained and examined in the field (p383) by JML; figs 3–5 courtesy of Prof S Upton, Kansas Univ.

Treatment ►If the patient has taken prophylaxis, do not use the same drug for treatment. If species unknown or mixed infection, treat as *P. falciparum*. Nearly all *P. falciparum* is resistant to chloroquine and in many areas also to Fansidar® (*pyrimethamine + sulfadoxine*). If in doubt, consider as resistant. *Chloroquine*[108] is 1st choice for benign malarias in most parts of the world, but chloroquine-resistant *P. vivax* occurs in Papua New Guinea, Indonesia, parts of Brazil, Colombia, and Guyana.[109] Never rely on chloroquine if used alone as prophylaxis.

Treating uncomplicated P. ovale, P. vivax, & P. malariae: **Chloroquine base**:[1] 10mg/kg (max 620mg), then 5mg/kg (max 310mg) at 6h, 24h and 48h. In resistant cases, try Malarone®, quinine, or Riamet®. **Primaquine** dose in *P. vivax:* 500µg/kg (max. 30mg) daily for 14d (*P. ovale:* 250µg/kg (max. 15mg) daily for 14d—given after chloroquine to treat liver stage and prevent relapse. Screen for G6PD deficiency first. CI: pregnancy. *P. malariae* does not need primaquine.

Treating uncomplicated Falciparum malaria (or species identification is uncertain): As multi-drug resistance (to chloroquine, amodiaquine etc) is common, combination therapy, preferably containing artemisinin derivatives, is recommended by WHO.[110] • **Artemether-lumefantrine** (Riamet®[2])—if >35kg: 4 tabs stat, then 5 doses of 4 tablets at 8, 24, 36, 48, and 60h.[MET 111] • **Artesunate-amodiaquine**; if a fixed combination pill is available (AS 100mg + AQ 270mg), the dose is 2 pills/d for 3d. If aged ~7–13yrs, it is 1 pill/d for 3d.[112] • **Atovaquone-proguanil** (Malarone®; 4 'standard' tablets once daily for 3 days) may also work. These are better than **quinine** regimens (eg 600mg quinine salt/8h PO for 7d, + **doxycycline** 200mg/24h or **clindamycin** 450mg/8h for 7d).[113] Artemisinins are OK in children and in 2nd & 3rd trimesters of pregnancy. The oral route is OK if able to swallow and no severe signs.

Treating severe[3] Falciparum malaria: IV ℞ is needed. Take to ITU. ►►see BOX.

Other treatments: Tepid sponging + paracetamol for fever. Transfuse if severe anaemia. Consider exchange transfusion if patient severely ill. Treat 'algid' malaria as malaria + bacterial shock (p778). Monitor TPR, BP, urine output, blood glucose frequently. Daily parasite count, platelets, U&E, LFT.

Prophylaxis for travellers ►*Prophylaxis does not give full protection.* Risks vary; get local advice. Avoid mosquitos: wear long-sleeves between dusk and dawn, use repellents (diethyltoluamide/DEET), long-lasting insecticidal bed-nets (US$5; last ~5yrs).

Except for Malarone® and mefloquine (below), take drugs from 1wk before travel (to reveal any SE) and continue for 4wks after return. None are required if just visiting cities of East Asia. There is no good protection for parts of South East Asia.[114]

If little/no chloroquine resistance: **Proguanil** 200mg/24h + **chloroquine** base 300mg/wk.

If chloroquine resistant P. falciparum: **Mefloquine** 250mg/week (18d before to 4wks after trip) or **doxycycline** 100mg/d (1day before to 4wks after) or **atovaquone**^{250mg} + **proguanil**^{100mg} (Malarone®) 1 tab/d (1d before travel to 7d after).[115] If poor medical care and not pregnant, carry standby treatment (eg Riamet®, Malarone®).

Antimalarial SE *Chloroquine:* headache, psychosis, retinopathy (in chronic use).
Fansidar®: Stevens-Johnson syndrome, erythema multiforme, LFT↑, blood dyscrasias.
Primaquine: Epigastric pain, haemolysis if G6PD-deficient, methaemoglobinaemia.
Malarone®: Abdominal pain, nausea, headache, dizziness.
Mefloquine: Nausea, dizziness, dysphoria, insomnia, neuropsychiatric signs, long $t_{1/2}$. Avoid mefloquine if: • Low risk of chloroquine-resistant malaria • Past or family history of epilepsy, psychosis • Need for delicate work (pilots etc) • Risk of pregnancy within 3 months of last dose. ***Interactions:*** quinidine, halofantrine.

1 150mg chloroquine base ≈ 250mg chloroquine phosphate (PO) ≈ 200mg chloroquine sulfate IV.
2 Dispersable formulation example for children with uncomplicated malaria: Coartem® (20mg artemether + 120mg lumefantrine: 1 tab per dose if 5–14kg; 3 tabs/dose if 25–34kg; repeat if vomits within 1h.
3 Prostration, consciousness↓, fits, respiratory distress, unable to drink, uncontrolled vomiting, macroscopic haemoglobinuria, jaundice, systolic BP ≤70mmHg, bleeding/DIC, inability to sit or stand.

Severe *P. falciparum* malaria

Falciparum malaria is one of the great killers (mortality is ~100% in untreated severe malaria, 15–20% with treatment), so get expert help in anyone who could have travelled abroad particularly in the last few months, who is feverish with ↓consciousness. But fever is not *always* a feature of malaria, and signs may be unusual if prophylaxis has been given, and is partly effective. The central event in severe Falciparum malaria is sequestration of parasitized erythrocytes in the microvasculature of vital organs. Death rate: ~1 million deaths/yr, worldwide. 116

Key questions What is the parasite count, the plasma bicarbonate and the creatinine? Are there complications: shock (algid malaria), metabolic acidosis, hypoglycaemia, renal failure, or acute respiratory distress syndrome (ARDS, p178).

℞: (on ITU) Take advice. The main goal is to prevent death. Check FBC, daily parasite count, platelets, U&E, LFT, plasma glucose. Degree of acidosis is an important determinant of outcome. Assess fluid balance meticulously. ►► ***Start antimalarials in full dose as soon as possible.*** Parenteral drugs: quinine, quinidine, and artemisinin derivatives (artesunate, artemether, artemotil). Give **artesunate** (if *immediately* available[1]) or **quinine** (dihydrochloride) 20mg salt /kg IVI (max 1.4g) over 4h, then after 8h give 10mg/kg (max 700mg) over 4h every 8h.[2] Give IV until the patient can swallow; complete the course orally. Monitor for hypoglycaemia. Alternative: **artemether** (3.2mg/kg followed by 1.6mg/kg daily); in the UK, artemether is not always available: get local advice. Don't wait for an ideal drug if a good alternative is to hand: delay is fatal. 117

If swallowing OK and no complications (shock; ARDS, renal failure) give either:

a) Artemether-lumefantrine Riamet®, see p396.

b) Malarone® (atovaquone + proguanil; 4 tabs once daily for 3d with food).

c) Quinine (600mg salt/8h PO for 7d), with either **doxycyline** 200mg daily or **clindamycin** 450mg/8h for 7d PO.

ITU monitoring in cerebral malaria

- ►►Fluid requirements vary widely; careful fluid management is critical. Haemofilter early if renal failure. Ventilate early if pulmonary oedema.
- ►►Consider exchange transfusion in very seriously ill patients if feasible.
- ►►Monitor blood lactate (or bicarbonate) and glucose: quinine may cause hypoglycaemia. Do LFT and clotting studies and cross-match blood if haematocrit <20%.
- ►►Repeated U&E (and arterial blood gases if ARDS).
- ►►Arrange repeated skilled microscopy to monitor the parasite counts. 118

Expect a >75% decrease in the parasite count by 48h of treatment.

Pitfalls

- Failure to take a full travel history (including stop-overs) and failure to check if the patient has already received treatment (can make the blood smear negative).
- Delay in treatment while seeking lab confirmation.
- Failure to examine enough blood films before excluding the diagnosis.
- Belief that drugs will work, when the parasite is often one step ahead.
- Not having IV quinine available immediately. (Quinidine is an alternative.)
- Not observing falciparum patients closely for the first few days.
- Forgetting that malaria is an important cause of coma, deep jaundice, severe anaemia, and renal failure in the tropics.

1 **Artesunate** dose 2.4mg/kg as a bolus at 0, 12 & 24h, then daily. It is not universally available, but works better than quinine (15% mortality *vs* 22%), and has fewer SEs, White N 2005 *Lancet* 366 717 RTC

2 Do not give **quinine** loading doses if the patient has already definitely had quinine, quinidine or mefloquine in last 24h. Warn about tinnitus. In some countries, IV quinine is not available; **quinidine gluconate** is an alternative, eg a loading dose of 10mg/kg over 1–4h then 0.02mg/kg/min IVI by pump for 72h or until can swallow. ECG monitoring is essential when quinidine is given (not needed for quinine). Stop or ↓infusion if BP↓ or QTc prolonged by >25% (p90). Further details: A Omari 2004 *BMJ* **328** 154

TB kills 2 million people/yr; it is the cause of death of most people with HIV. TB is one reason why the poor stay poor—and then die. If HIV+ve, risk↑ if: CD4↓; ESR↑; many coinfections; poor nutrition; high viraemia. [119] **UK incidence** ~8200/yr; 350 deaths/yr.

Diagnosis *Latent TB:* Do a Mantoux test. If +ve, (or non-reliable) consider interferon-gamma testing (eg *Quantiferon TB Gold®* or *T-spot-TB®*, see below). ***Active TB:*** If CXR is suggestive of TB, take sputum samples (at least 3, with one early morning sample, before starting treatment if possible) and send for MC+S for AFB (acid-fast bacilli). If spontaneously produced sputum cannot be obtained, induction of sputum or bronchoscopy and lavage should be used. ***Active non-respiratory TB:*** try hard to get the relevant clinical samples: sputum, pleura & pleural fluid, urine, pus, ascites, peritoneum, bone marrow or CSF. Send surgical samples for culture. Microbiology staff should routinely perform TB culture on the above samples (even if it is not requested). [120] All patients with non-respiratory TB should have a CXR to exclude coexisting respiratory TB. AFB resist acid-alcohol decolourization under Ziehl–Neelsen (ZN) staining. Cultures undergo prolonged incubation (up to 12 weeks) on Lowenstein–Jensen medium. *PCR* allows rapid identification of rifampicin (and likely multidrug) resistance. Occasionally useful for diagnosis in sterile specimens. ***Histology:*** The hallmark is the presence of *caseating granulomata*. ***CXR signs:*** Consolidation, cavitation, fibrosis, and calcification. ***Immunological*** evidence of TB may be helpful: *Tuberculin skin test:* TB antigen is injected intradermally and the cell-mediated response at 48–72h is recorded. A +ve test indicates immunity. It may also indicate previous exposure or BCG. A strong +ve test probably means active infection. *False-negative tests* occur in immunosuppression (eg miliary TB, sarcoid, AIDS, lymphoma).

Quantiferon TB Gold® and the *T-spot-TB®* tests measure the delayed hypersensitivity reaction developed after contact with *M. tuberculosis*; they use specific, complex *M. tuberculosis* antigens and are better than older Mantoux tests, which rely on reactions to serial dilutions of TB antigen. [121]

Treatment of pulmonary TB (BOX 1 & 2) ►If the histology & clinical picture are consistent with TB, start treatment without waiting for culture results, and continue even if subsequent culture results are negative. [122] ***Before treatment:*** Stress importance of compliance/concordance (helps the patient and prevents spread of resistance). Check FBC, liver, and renal function. Test colour vision (Ishihara chart) and acuity before and during treatment as ethambutol may cause (reversible) ocular toxicity. ►Patients often forget to take pills, so consider *Directly Supervised Therapy* (DOT) as follows:

- ***Initial phase:*** 8wks on 4 drugs (depending on susceptibilities):
  1. *Rifampicin* 600–900mg (child 15mg/kg) PO 3 times/wk.
  2. *Isoniazid* 15mg/kg PO 3 times/wk max 900mg + pyridoxine 10mg/24h (if diabetic, malnourished, chronic renal failure, HIV +ve or alcoholic).
  3. *Pyrazinamide* 2.5g PO (2g if <50kg) 3 times/wk (child 50mg/kg).
  4. *Ethambutol* 30mg/kg PO 3 times a week for 2 months, or streptomycin 0.75–1g/24h IM (see BNF; child 15mg/kg/24h).
- ***Continuation phase*** (16wks on 2 drugs) rifampicin and isoniazid at same doses. Rifinah 300®=rifampicin 300mg + isoniazid 150mg; get advice about resistance.
- Give pyridoxine throughout treatment.
- Steroids are indicated in meningeal and pericardial disease.

Main side effects ►Seek help in renal or hepatic failure, or pregnancy.

Rifampicin: Hepatitis (a small rise of AST is acceptable, stop if bilirubin rises), orange discolouration of urine and tears (contact lens staining), inactivation of the Pill, flu-like syndrome with intermittent use. **Isoniazid:** Hepatitis, neuropathy, pyridoxine deficit, agranulocytosis. **Ethambutol:** Optic neuritis (colour vision is the first to deteriorate). **Pyrazinamide:** Hepatitis, arthralgia (CI: acute gout; porphyria).

WHO's/G8 'Stop TB' plan Sputum smear microscopy*et al* for all as needed; directly observed therapy (**DOT**) in front of a health worker for 6 months; aiming to treat 50 million people over 10yrs, and to reduce therapy duration to 8 weeks. [123]

Chemoprophylaxis for asymptomatic tuberculous infection

Immigrant or contact screening may identify patients with TB without symptoms or radiographic changes. In such patients, chemoprophylaxis may prevent disease progression. Prophylaxis entails one or two anti-TB drugs for shorter periods than for symptomatic disease (eg rifampicin and isoniazid for 3 months, or isoniazid alone for 6 months). Suitable patients for chemoprophylaxis include adults with documented recent tuberculin conversion, and some young immigrants (16–34yrs) who are T-spot-TB/Mantoux +ve, without prior BCG vaccination.[124] ►Seek expert advice, or consult the latest British Thoracic Society guidelines. brit-thoracic.org.uk ►Start standard anti-TB ℞ once any clinical or CXR evidence active TB is found.

Some clinical features of TB ►Ask about recent contact with TB

- *Pulmonary TB:* This may be silent or present with cough, sputum, malaise, weight loss, night sweats, pleurisy, haemoptysis (may be massive), pleural effusion, or superimposed pulmonary infection. Investigation and treatment: see p398. An aspergilloma/mycetoma (p 168) may form in the cavities.
- ***Miliary TB:*** Occurs following haematogenous dissemination. Signs may be non-specific. CXR shows characteristic reticulonodular shadowing. Look for retinal TB. Biopsy of lung, liver, lymph nodes, or marrow may yield AFB or granulomata.
- ***Genitourinary TB:*** May cause frequency, dysuria, loin/back pain, haematuria, sterile pyuria (p292; do 3 EMUs ± renal ultrasound). Renal TB may spread to bladder, seminal vesicles, epididymis, or fallopian tubes. Endometrial TB: see *OHCS* p274.
- ***Bone TB:*** (*OHCS* p696) Look for vertebral collapse & Pott's vertebra, p722.
- ***Skin TB (lupus vulgaris):*** Look for jelly-like nodules, eg on face or neck.
- ***Peritoneal TB:*** This causes abdominal pain and GI upset. Look for AFB in ascites (send a large volume to lab); laparotomy may be needed.
- ***Acute TB pericarditis:*** Think of this as a primary exudative allergic lesion. ***Chronic pericardial effusion and constrictive pericarditis:*** Fibrosis/calcification may be prominent with spread to myocardium. (Giving steroids to these patients for 11wks with their anti-TB drugs reduces need for pericardiectomy.) ***TB meningitis:*** *Prodrome:* Fever, headache, vomiting, drowsiness, meningism, and delirium often worsening over 1–3 weeks (rarely many months) ± seizures. *CNS signs:* Tremor, papilloedema; cranial nerve palsies. *Diagnosis:* LP (p782—the 1st few LPs may be normal); TB PCR; look for immunosuppression (HIV) and TB elsewhere (CXR etc). CT (obstructive hydrocephalus and basal enhancement). There may also be CNS tuberculomas.[125] *℞:* **Isoniazid + rifampicin** for 12 months, with **pyrazinamide** and **streptomycin** during the 1st 2 months is often used (*OTM*). *Ethambutol* or *ethionamide* are alternatives to streptomycin. Add *pyridoxine* 10–20mg/24h PO to regimens using isoniazid to prevent neuropathies.[126] In adults, daily single doses of 300mg of isoniazid, 600mg of rifampicin, and 1500mg of pyrazinamide are adequate. Higher doses are unnecessary and can cause hepatotoxicity. Always check sensitivities of the causative organism, and discuss the chances of multi-drug resistant TB with a microbiologist. TBM with resistance to isoniazid and rifampicin is likely to be fatal.[127] There is a role for **dexamethasone** (eg for 1st month),[128] but tuberculomas may start to appear.[129][130] **Mannitol** for ICP↑ (p840).[131] *Complications:* Hydrocephalus (may need surgery).[132] Cognition↓.

Anti-TB drug use in liver and renal failure[133]

►Monitor U&E + LFT before and after starting. In liver failure, get expert help.

If creatine clearance=10–50mL/min: **Rifampicin**: ↓dose by 50%. **Ethambutol**: monitor U&E; avoid if possible. No dose change for **ethionamide** or **isoniazid**.

Herpes simplex virus (HSV) Manifestations of primary infection:

1 *Genital herpes* is a chronic, life-long infection. Majority of cases (esp recurrent) are caused by HSV-2 (HSV-1 is taking over).[134] *Signs:* Flu-like prodrome, then grouped vesicles/papules develop around genitals, anus, or throat. These burst forming shallow ulcers (heal in ~3wks). Also: urethral discharge ± dysuria (esp if ♀); urinary retention. *OHCS* p268. *Tests:* PCR. ℞: Give analgesia. *Aciclovir* 400mg/8h PO, *famciclovir* 250mg/8h PO (500mg if immunocompromised[135]), or *valaciclovir* 500mg/12h for 5d (extend the treatment if healing is incomplete). If frequent (≥6/yr) or severe recurrences, continuous *aciclovir* 400mg/12h PO, *famciclovir* 250mg/12h PO or *valaciclovir* 500mg/12h.[136] *Prevention:* Condoms, even for oral sex.

2 *Gingivostomatitis:* Ulcers filled with yellow slough appear in the mouth.

3 *Herpetic whitlow:* Abrasions allow virus to enter the finger, causing a vesicle.

4 *Herpes gladiatorum:* Vesicles wherever HSV is ground into the skin by force.

5 *Eczema herpeticum:* HSV infection of eczematous skin; usually children.

6 *Herpes simplex meningitis:* This is uncommon and usually self-limiting (typically HSV II in women during a primary attack).

7 *HSV keratitis:* Corneal dendritic ulcers. *Avoid steroids*. See *OHCS* p416.

8 *Systemic infection* eg fever, sore throat, and lymphadenopathy may pass unnoticed. If immunocompromised, it may be life-threatening with fever, lymphadenopathy, pneumonitis, and hepatitis.

9 *Herpes simplex encephalitis:* Usually HSV-I. Spreads centripetally, eg from cranial nerve ganglia, to frontal and temporal lobes. ►*Suspect if* fever, fits, headaches, odd behaviour, dysphasia, hemiparesis, or coma or brainstem encephalitis, meningitis, or myelitis. Δ: Urgent PCR on CSF (it remains +ve ~5d after initiating treatment). CT/MRI or EEG may show nonspecific temporal lobe changes; brain biopsy rarely required. Seek expert help: careful fluid balance to minimize cerebral oedema, p840; ►►*prompt* aciclovir, eg 10mg/kg/8h IV for ≥10d, saves lives (p834). Mortality: 19%.

Tests: Rising antibody titres in 1° infection; culture; PCR for fast diagnosis.

Recurrent HSV: Dormant HSV in ganglion cells may be reactivated by illness, immunosuppression, menstruation, or sunlight. Cold sores (perioral vesicles) are one manifestation. Aciclovir cream may be disappointing.

Varicella zoster Varicella (chickenpox; fig 1) is a contagious febrile illness with crops of blisters of different ages starting on the back. Complications, eg purpura fulminans/DIC (get help; ►►may need heparin[137]), pneumonitis, and ataxia are commoner in pregnancy and adults than in children.[138] *Incubation:* 11–21d. *Infectivity:* 4d before the rash until all lesions are scabbed (~1 week). *OHCS* p144. After infection, virus is dormant in dorsal root ganglia. Reactivation causes **shingles** (affects 20% at some time; eg if old or immunosuppressed). Pain in dermatomal distribution precedes malaise and fever by some days; p458.

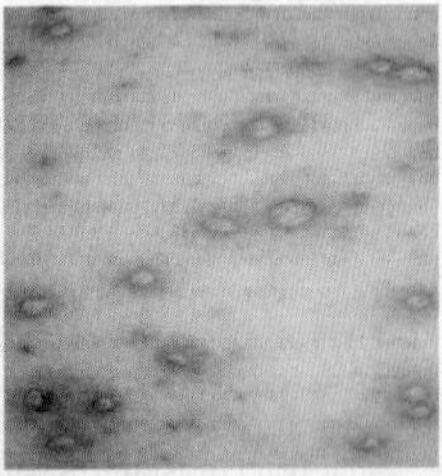

Fig 1. Chickenpox. ©Dr C Leung

Shingles ℞: Treating acute herpes zoster infection with oral aciclovir (eg 800mg 5 times/d PO for 5–7d if eGFR <25. If immunocompromised, give 10mg/kg/8h slowly IVI for 10d); famciclovir or valaciclovir can reduce the risk of progression to post-herpetic neuralgia (controversial).[139] Paracetamol ± amitriptyline (start with 10mg at night) for pain. If the conjunctiva is affected, apply 3% aciclovir ointment 5 times/d. Beware iritis. Measure acuity often. Say to report *any* visual loss at once. SE of aciclovir: renal impairment (check U&E) vomiting, urticaria, encephalopathy. *Post-herpetic neuralgia* in affected dermatomes can last years; it is hard to treat and intolerable.[140] Try topical lidocaine patches, amitriptyline or gabapentin (±carbamazepine, phenytoin, topical capsaicin counter-irritant). The role of opioids is controversial. Last resort: ablation of the ganglion; refer to a pain clinic. A live attenuated vaccine against herpes zoster given at the age of 65–70 yrs has shown promising results.[141]

Infectious mononucleosis (glandular fever)

This is a common disease in the young which may be unnoticed or cause acute illness. Spread: saliva or droplet (presumed). Incubation 4–5wks. Cause: Epstein-Barr virus (EBV, a DNA herpesvirus) infection of B-lymphocytes, causing proliferation of T cells ('atypical' mononuclear cells) which are cytotoxic to EBV-infected cells. The latter are 'immortalized' by EBV infection and can, very rarely, proliferate in a way indistinguishable from immunoblastic lymphoma in immunodeficient individuals (whose suppressor T cells fail to check multiplication of these B-cells).

Symptoms: Sore throat, T°↑, anorexia, malaise, lymphadenopathy, palatal petechiae, splenomegaly, hepatitis, haemolysis. ***Complications—CNS:*** • Meningitis • Encephalitis • Ataxia[142] • Cranial nerve lesions (eg VII, bilateral in 40%[143]) ± Guillain–Barré syndrome • Neuropathy • Depression • Chronic fatigue syndrome (the risk is ~5–6 times that of other common upper respiratory tract infections,[144] depending in part on features present at onset eg less fit premorbidly, no delay in Monospot® becoming +ve, and need for bed rest).[145] Fatigue is also part of 'severe chronic active EBV infection', eg with anaemia, platelets↓ and severe hepatosplenomegaly.[146] ***Others:*** Thrombocytopenia (±pancytopenia with a megaloblastic marrow),[147] ruptured spleen, splenic haemorrhage, upper airways obstruction (may need ITU admission), hepatitis (± fulminant hepatic failure[148]), secondary infection, myo- or pericarditis, pneumonitis/fibrosis,[149] renal failure, autoimmune haemolysis, and erythema multiforme. All are very rare.

Blood film shows a lymphocytosis (~20% of WBC) and atypical lymphocytes (large, irregular nuclei, **fig 1**). These may occur in viral infections (CMV, HIV, parvovirus, dengue), toxoplasmosis, typhus, leukaemia, lymphoma, drug hypersensitivity, and lead poisoning.

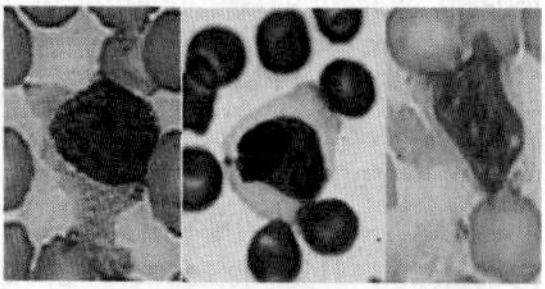

Fig 1. Atypical lymphocytes flowing around RBCs; dark cytoplasm at contact points. Courtesy of JML and Axel Schneider.

Heterophil antibody tests (Monospot®; Paul-Bunnell): Heterophil antibodies develop in 90% of patients by week 3, disappearing after ~3 months (≤1yr).[150] They agglutinate sheep RBCs and can be absorbed (and thus agglutination is prevented) by ox RBCs, but not guinea-pig kidney cells. This pattern distinguishes them from other heterophil antibodies. These antibodies don't react with EBV or its antigens. *False +ve* Monospot® tests may occur in hepatitis, parvovirus infection, lymphoma, leukaemia, rubella, malaria, carcinoma of pancreas, and SLE.[151] *Other false trails:* Older patients may have little pharyngitis or adenopathy, but fever & LFT↑ are more prolonged, often with no telltale lymphocytosis or atypical lymphocytes.[152] So, if Monospot –ve, they may be subjected to dangerous over-investigation unless you request EBV-specific IgM—implies current infection (IgG reflects past infection). PCR may reveal ↑↑serum EBV DNA levels and warn of fulminant infection.[153] **ΔΔ** Strep sore throat (may coexist), CMV, viral hepatitis, HIV seroconversion, toxoplasmosis, leukaemia, diphtheria. **℞:** Avoiding alcohol 'to protect the liver' is controversial. Steroids are sometimes used to treat complications, eg severe thrombocytopenia or severe lymphadenopathy obstructing the airway (uncomplicated cases don't need steroids).[154] *Never give ampicillin or amoxicillin for sore throats as they often cause a severe rash in those with acute EBV infection.*

EBV oncogenicity Lymphoma[155] (eg post-transplant);[156] **nasopharyngeal cancer** (esp. in Asia), **leiomyosarcoma**[157] and **oral hairy leucoplakia** (p238; aciclovir-responsive). A vaccine to prevent the disease has shown promising results.[158]

Other EBV-associated diseases Crescentic glomerulonephritis;[159] **haemophagocytic syndrome** (EBV over-activates T cells & macrophages, with overproduction of cytokines, eg causing fatal coagulopathy[160] ± central pontine myelinolysis).[161] The EBV **Gianotti–Crosti rash** (self-limiting papular acrodermatitis of childhood) consists of pale or red monomorphous 1–10mm papules and plaques placed symmetrically over extensor surfaces of limbs, buttocks, and face (also caused by streps, hep B, HIV, echo, Coxsackie, and respiratory syncitial viruses). forlag.fadl.dk/sample/derma/images/447.htm

Influenza

This (see **fig 1**) is the most important viral respiratory infection owing to its ubiquity, unpredictability, and complications (esp. if elderly). In a pandemic (see BOX) millions may die (1918 pandemic) or it may be global but milder (eg 1957). ***Spread:*** Droplets (to stop this, masks for medics must be well-fitted). ***Incubation:*** 1–4d. ***Infectivity:*** 1d before to 7d after symptoms start. ***Immunity*** is only to a strain that has already attacked you. ***Symptoms:*** T°↑, headache, malaise/mood↓, myalgia, prostration, nausea, vomiting, conjunctivitis/eye pain (± photophobia). **Δ:** ***Serology*** (paired sera; takes >2wks). ***Culture*** (1wk, from nasopharyngeal swabs). ***PCR:*** (eg 36h; sensitivity 94.2%; specificity ~100%).[162] ***Complications:*** Bronchitis (20%[163], pneumonia (esp. staph), sinusitis, otitis media, encephalitis, pericarditis, Reye's syndrome (coma, LFT↑).

Treatment ►Follow national guidelines. Bed rest ± paracetamol; if severe pneumonia, take to ITU to prevent shock/hypoxia (cover *strep pneumoniae* and resistant staphs, eg **ciprofloxacin** & **co-amoxiclav**).[164] **Oseltamivir** (*Tamiflu®*) is a neuraminidase inhibitor that is active against influenza A & B. It may be indicated in people >1yr old who present with recent (<48h) symptoms typical of flu, when flu virus is circulating in the community. Dosage (>13yrs old and eGFR >30): 75mg/12h PO for 5d. For children 1–12yrs old, adjust dose according to body weight.[165] **SE**: D&V, dyspepsia, headache, insomnia, dizziness, conjunctivitis, epistaxis, rash; rarely hepatitis, Stevens-Johnson, p724 ± ?flawed reports of hallucinations in children.[166] **Zanamivir** (**Relenza®**) is an inhaled neuraminidase inhibitor active against influenza A & B. It prevents viral release from infected cells and infection of adjacent cells. It is used to ↓symptoms in those >5yrs old with typical flu symptoms starting <48h ago (36h if a child)—when flu is circulating in the community.[167] Dose: 2 blisters (2×5mg)/12h for 5d (before any other inhalers). **NB:** inhalation is not an ideal route, eg if elderly. SE: bronchospasm; oropharyngeal oedema.[168] *Ensure he knows how to use the Diskhaler.*

Prevention • Hygeine: see BOX. • Use whole ***trivalent vaccine*** (from inactivated virus), reserving split vaccine (fragmented virus) for those <13yrs old. It is made from current serotypes and takes <2wks to work. Vaccination is indicated if at ↑risk: DM; COPD; asthma (not if mild), heart, renal or liver failure; immunosuppression (eg splenectomy; steroid use); haemoglobinopathy, medical staff/carers; ≥65yrs old (esp. in institutions).[169] [170] Vaccinating all at ↑risk poses logistic challenges in aging populations. **NB:** *routine* vaccination of children may be worthwhile (might save ~100 deaths/yr). *Dose:* 0.5mL SC (once). In children repeat after 6wks (½ dose if <3yrs old). *SE:* pain/swelling (17%). T°↑, headaches, and malaise. Guillain-Barré and pericarditis are rare. *Vaccine efficacy* is 'modest' (eg relative risk of pneumonia falls from 1 to 0.88 after vaccination for the elderly; all cause mortality *is* slightly reduced).[171] • ***Oseltamivir:*** Only use as **prophylaxis** after formal notice that flu A or B is circulating ***and*** >1yr old ***and*** <48h since exposure ***and*** in at-risk group. It is ***not*** needed if vaccinated >2wks ago with a well-matched vaccine ***unless*** living in a rest- or nursing-home*et al* when it can be used ***whatever*** the vaccination status.[172] Dose: 75mg/d (if 24–40kg, 60mg/d; 16–23kg, 45mg/d) all for ≥10d. Resistance to oseltamivir is now common (in some A/H1N1; B & A/H5N1).[173]

The common cold (coryza)

Rhinoviruses are the main culprits (>80 strains), and cause a self-limiting nasal discharge (becoming mucopurulent over a few days). ***Incubation:*** 1–4d. ***Complications:*** (6% in children) Otitis media, pneumonia, febrile convulsions. **℞:** None is usually needed. *Echinacea* (herbal extract, *OHCS* p161) is used by some as a preventive and to shorten symptoms.[174] Zinc gluconate yields conflicting results in trials.[175] [176] If nasal obstruction in infants hampers feeding, try 0.9% saline nose drops.

The ART of making and delaying new pandemics

When an animal source of virus couples with human virus (reassortment[1]) to form a novel hybrid with efficient replication and person-to-person transmission, a pandemic is born. Millions of deaths only occur if no previous immunological exposure *and* the new strain is highly pathogenic. What can we do? Early clusters may be containable, but once transmission is established, quarantine is probably futile and the pandemic will become global.[1] But strategic planning can help:

- Simulated exercises before the event to enhance preparedness.
- Stockpile vaccine (if it can be made in time), antivirals, and vital supplies. Masks (must be well-fitting) are recommended by WHO when health workers are within 1 metre of a probable case (eg on entering a room with such patients).[177]
- Seamless international co-operation with WHO and bodies such as the European Centre for Disease Prevention, eg to cancel mass events and give information.
- Buy time in spreading epidemics by moving hosts (eg free range hens) indoors.
- Quarantine restrictions around clusters of animal infections, eg a 3km zone where entry and exit are banned, with movements restricted in a further 10km monitoring zone with checking of residents, and their hosts destroyed.[178]
- Social distancing: less travel; no mass events (discos, theatre, cinema, schools).[179]
- Self-isolation at 1st sign of illness. Personal hygiene: wash hands, don't sneeze into your hand (your elbow may be better); carry, use, and bin tissues; use only once.

Prevention, containment, health systems response, and communications
This 4-part response to highly pathogenic flu pandemics depends on how far we have progressed down the pandemic path. Preceding a pandemic there is an *inter-pandemic period—phase 1:* no new subtypes. *Phase 2:* new circulating animal virus arrives; and then a *pandemic alert period. Phase 3:* 'human infections with a new subtype, [with] rare instances of spread to a close contact'. *Phase 4:* 'small clusters of highly localized spread' (virus isn't well adapted to us). In *phase 5* there are large clusters of human-to-human spread. A *pandemic* is declared when efficient human transmission is happening in ≥3 WHO regions.

How does pandemic influenza differ from seasonal influenza?

- Those with no immunity (eg the young) are at risk and prone to complications.
- Death rates are higher, depending on: **1** Numbers getting infected **2** Virulence factors (**fig 1**) **3** Host vulnerability **4** Preventive and treatment measures.
- Transmission is more efficient, occurring not only in autumn and winter.
- 2-3 waves of infection may occur; later waves may be more severe. Increased death rates are observed even in milder pandemics, over the next 3 winters.

Is the 2009–2010 H1N1 'swine flu' pandemic behaving as expected? Yes, so far. As predicted, containment was only briefly effective. It is not known if swine virus (S-OIV) will replace human H1 virus as the seasonal virus, and evolve antigenic variants each year—or whether S-OIV antigen in vaccine will cause side-effects.

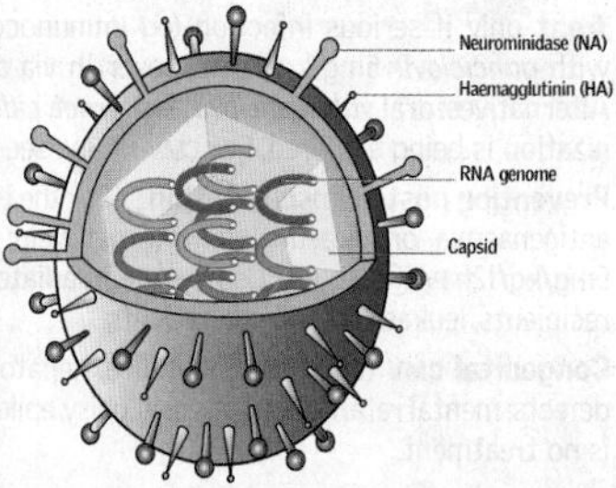

Fig 1. Influenza A. Orthomyxoviridae (RNA) have 2 genera: influenza A and B viruses—and influenza C, distinguishable by antigenic differences between their nucleoproteins (NP) and matrix (M) proteins. Influenza B & C are almost exclusively isolated from man (rarely pigs & seals). Influenza A infects many birds and mammals; they are subtyped by surface glycoproteins (haem-agglutinin, HA) and neuraminidase (NA). So far, 15 different HAs (H1 to 15) and 9 NAs (N1 to 9) have been described. Pathogenicity is partly determined by HA glycosylation patterns and amino acids at HA cleavage sites.

1 In genetic reassortment, 2 viral sources shuffle genetic material in someone with a dual infection. Also, simple stepwise single mutations can accumulate to produce new strains. Coulombier D, *BMJ* 2005 414

Toxoplasmosis

The protozoan *Toxoplasma gondii* infects via the gut (poorly cooked meat), lung, or broken skin. Life-cycle: **fig 2**. In humans, the oocysts release trophozoites, which migrate widely, with a predeliction for eye, brain, and muscle. Toxoplasmosis occurs worldwide, but is common in the tropics. Infection is lifelong. HIV may reactivate it.

The patient ►*In any granulomatous uveitis or necrotizing retinitis, think of toxoplasmosis, especially in the immunosuppressed.* See **figs 3, 4 & 5**. Most infections are asymptomatic: in the UK 50% have been infected by 70yrs. Symptomatic acquired toxoplasmosis resembles infectious mononucleosis, and is usually self-limiting. Eye infection, usually congenital, presents with posterior uveitis, often in the 2nd decade of life, and may cause cataract. In the immunocompromised (eg AIDS), myocarditis, encephalitis, focal neurological signs, stroke or fits may occur.

Tests Acute infection is confirmed by a 4-fold rise in antibody titre over 4wks or specific IgM (unreliable if HIV+ve). Reactivation of latent toxoplasmosis in HIV presents problems (you may need to look for toxoplasma antigen and IgG).[180] PCR may be rewarding.[181] Parasite isolation is difficult; lymph node or CNS biopsy may be diagnostic. CT: characteristic multiple ring-shaped contrast-enhancing CNS lesions.

Treatment Often not needed (get help).[182] If the eye is involved, or if immunocompromised, ***pyrimethamine*** + ***sulfadiazine***. ►If pregnant, get help. Sampling of fetal cord blood, at ~21wks for IgM indicates severe infection. For HIV, see p410.

Prevention: Cook food to safe temperatures (eg beef, lamb, and steak >145°F). Peel or wash fruits and vegetables before eating. Freezing meat can ↓chance of infection. Wash hands after contact with soil. ***Pregnancy or immunosuppression:*** Don't change cat litter. Don't adopt or handle stray cats, esp kittens.[183]

Congenital toxoplasmosis (*OHCS* p34) abortion, seizures, choroidoretinitis (**fig 2**), hydrocephalus, microcephaly, cerebral calcification. Worse prognosis if early infection.

Cytomegalovirus (CMV)

CMV (**fig 1**) is acquired by direct contact (doctors are at ↑risk),[184] blood transfusion, or organ transplantation. After acute infection, CMV becomes latent but the infection may reactivate at times of stress or immunocompromise. If immunocompetent, primary infection is usually asymptomatic, but acute hepatitis may occur. In transplant recipients or post marrow transplantation: fever > pneumonitis > colitis > hepatitis > retinitis. In AIDS: retinitis > colitis > CNS disease. (here, '>' means 'is commoner than').

Diagnosis of acute CMV infection is difficult; virus growth is slow and there may be prolonged CMV excretion from past infection. Serology helps; specific IgM indicates acute infection (unreliable if HIV +ve). CMV PCR (including quantitative tests) of blood, CSF & bronchoalveolar lavage is available.

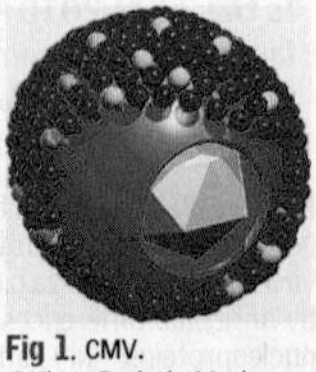

Fig 1. CMV.
©Klaus Radsak; Marburg

Treat only if serious infection (eg immunocompromised), with ***ganciclovir*** 5mg/kg/12h IVI over 1h via a central line. Alternatives: oral ***valganciclovir, foscarnet, cidofovir***. Immunization is being explored. For CMV in HIV, see p410.

Prevention post-transplantation[185] For the 1st 100 days do weekly PCR to detect CMV antigenaemia or viraemia; if +ve, get help; ganciclovir starting dose example: 5mg/kg/12h IV if eGFR OK). Use CMV-ve, irradiated blood when transfusing transplant recipients, leukaemics, or HIV patients.

Congenital CMV (*OHCS* p34) Jaundice, hepatosplenomegaly, and purpura. Chronic defects: mental retardation, cerebral palsy, epilepsy, deafness, and eye problems. There is no treatment.

Toxoplasma gondii: a subtle parasite

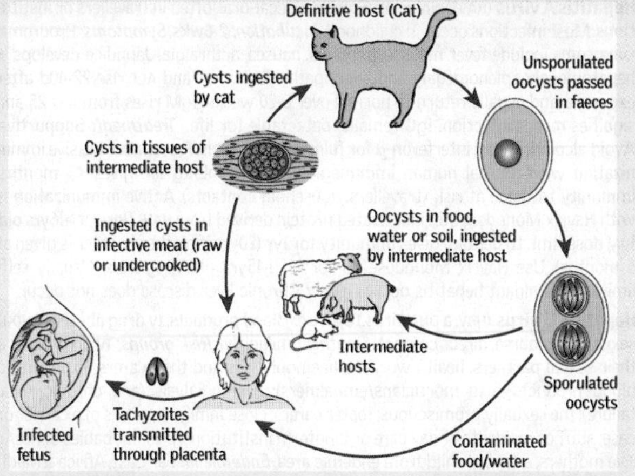

Fig 2. Oocysts in cat faeces can stay in the soil for months, where animals such as rats eat them. They get infected, and, under the direction of *Toxoplasma* in the amygdala, these rats lose their innate fear of cats, and so tend to get eaten. So parasites ensure their success by facilitating their jump from the intermediate to the definitive host.[186]
Data from Fernando Monroy; http://www2.nau.edu/~fpm/research/res.html

Humans with toxoplasmosis may show these features

- Confusion, seizures, and signs of brainstem or spinal cord injury.
- *A latent* phase of toxoplasmosis is recognized, as is subtle personality change. Loss of fear of cats is *not* reported in us, but there are changes in willingness to accept group moral standards, in proportion to the latent period's length.[187]
- Meningoencephalitis + localizing signs (fever+headache→drowsiness→coma→death, eg over a days or weeks). CSF: mild lymphocytic pleocytosis & protein↑.
- Multifocal myelin loss, and microglial nodules.
- *Pseudotumour cerebri* syndrome: transient intracranial hypertension.
- Space-occupying mass with ICP↑ mimicking a tumour or a brain abscess.
- Multiple mass lesions that can be the cause of hemisensory abnormalities, hemiparesis, cranial nerve palsy, aphasia, and tremors.
- In some areas, eg India, toxoplasmosis is the major HIV-associated CNS infection.[188]

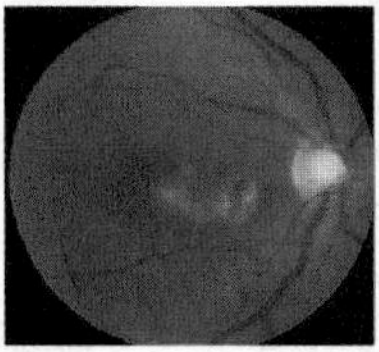

Fig 3. Retinal toxoplasmosis.

Figures 3–5 ©Prof. J Trobe.[189]

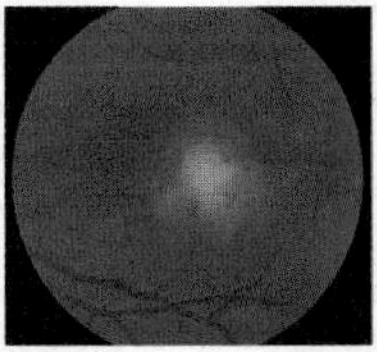

Fig 4. Ill-defined yellow infiltrates. ΔΔ: toxoplasmosis; herpes simplex/zoster; syphilis; sarcoidosis; leukaemia.[190]

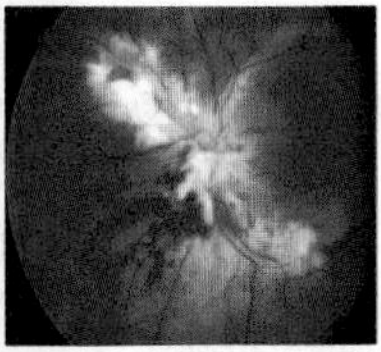

Fig 5. In HIV this 'pizza-pie' fundus means CMV retinitis. If CD4↓↓, re-examine in 2 days; ►is it progressing?[191]

Hepatitis A virus (HAV) RNA virus. *Spread:* Faecal–oral, often in travellers or institutions. Most infections occur in childhood. *Incubation:* 2–6wks. *Symptoms:* Prodromal symptoms include fever, malaise, anorexia, nausea, arthralgia. Jaundice develops ± hepatomegaly, splenomegaly, and adenopathy. *Tests:* AST and ALT rise 22–40d after exposure, and usually return to normal over 5–20 weeks. IgM rises from day 25 and signifies recent infection. IgG remains detectable for life. *Treatment:* Supportive. Avoid alcohol. Rarely, interferon-α for fulminant hepatitis. *Prevention:* Passive immunization with normal human immunoglobulin (0.02mL/kg IM) gives <3 months' immunity to those at risk (travellers, household contacts). Active immunization is with Havrix Monodose®, an inactivated protein derived from HAV. *Dose:* if >16yrs old, 1 IM dose (1mL to deltoid) gives immunity for 1yr (20yrs if further booster is given at 6 months). Use Havrix Monodose Junior® if 1–15yrs old. *Prognosis:* Usually self-limiting. Fulminant hepatitis occurs rarely. Chronic liver disease does not occur.

Hepatitis B virus (HBV, a DNA virus.) *Spread:* Blood products, IV drug abusers (IVDU), sexual intercourse, direct contact. *Deaths:* 1 million/yr. *Risk groups:* IV drug users & their sexual partners; health workers; haemophiliacs and their carers (exposure to blood products—also morticians/embalmers); haemodialysis (and chronic renal failure); the sexually promiscuous; foster carers; close family members of a carrier or case; staff or residents of day care or longterm institutions/prisons; babies of HBsAg +ve mothers; adopted child from endemic area. *Endemic in:* Far East, Africa & Mediterranean. *Incubation:* 1–6 months. *Signs:* Resemble hepatitis A but extrahepatic features are more common, eg arthralgia, urticaria. *Tests:* HBsAg (surface antigen) is present from 1 to 6 months after exposure. HBeAg (e antigen) is present for 1½–3 months after the acute illness and implies high infectivity. The persistence of HBsAg for >6 months defines carrier status and occurs in 5–10% of infections (chronic infection). Antibodies to HBcAg (anti-HBc) imply past infection; antibodies to HBsAg (anti-HBs) alone imply vaccination. HBV PCR allows monitoring of response to therapy. See **fig 1**. *Vaccination* (►p271) may be universal in childhood or just for high-risk groups. Passive immunization (specific anti-HBV immunoglobulin) may be given to non-immune contacts after high-risk exposure. *℞:* Supportive. Avoid alcohol. Chronic HBV may respond to PEGinterferon alfa-2a or other antivirals, eg lamivudine, entecavir[192], adefovir dipivoxil.[193] Telbivudine is no longer used for chronic hepatitis B.[194] Immunize sexual contacts. *Complications:* Fulminant hepatic failure (rare); relapse; prolonged cholestasis; chronic hepatitis (5–10%); cirrhosis; hepatocellular carcinoma (HCC: 10-fold ↑risk if HBsAg +ve, 60-fold ↑risk if both HBsAg and HBeAg +ve; preventable by interferon esp. in HBeAg-positive Asians);[195] glomerulonephritis; cryoglobulinaemia.

Hepatitis C virus (HCV) RNA flavivirus. *Spread:* Blood: transfusion (thousands of UK cases; compensation available via the Skipton Fund), IV drug abuse, sexual, acupuncture.[1] UK prevalence: 200,000–466,000.[196] Early infection is often mild/asymptomatic. ~85% develop chronic infection; 20–30% get cirrhosis within 20yrs; a few get hepatocellular cancer (HCC). *Tests:* LFT (AST:ALT <1:1 until cirrhosis develops, p282), anti-HCV antibodies, recombinant immunoblot assay, HCV-PCR; liver biopsy if HCV-PCR +ve to assess liver damage and need for treatment. Do HCV genotype (BOX 1). *Treatment:* see BOX 2.

Hepatitis D virus (HDV) Incomplete RNA virus, exists only with HBV. *Spread:* With HBV. *Signs:* Increased risk of acute hepatic failure and cirrhosis. *Tests:* Anti-HDV antibody. *Treatment:* Interferon-α has limited success in treatment of HDV infection.

Hepatitis E virus (HEV) RNA virus. Similar to HAV; common in Indochina. High mortality in pregnancy. **Δ**: Serology. *℞:* Nil specific. *Vaccine:* One is becoming available.[197]

Hepatitis GB Parenterally transmitted. Causes asymptomatic post-transfusion hepatitis. One type (HGB-C) can cause fulminant liver failure.

ΔΔ Alcohol; drugs; toxins; EBV/CMV; leptospirosis; malaria; Q fever; syphilis; yellow fever, chronic hepatitis (eg alcohol; drugs; autoimmune hepatitis, p268; Wilson's, p269).

1 In elderly, HCV is a more important cause of hepatocellular cancer than HBV. Shin 2006 *Intervir* 49 18

Serological markers of HBV infection

	Incubation	Acute	Carrier	Recovery	Vaccinated
LFT		↑↑↑	↑	Normal	Normal
HBsAg	+	+	+		
HBeAg	+	+	+/−		
Anti-HBs				+	+
Anti-HBe			+/−		
Anti-HBC IgM		+	+/−		
Anti-HBC IgG		+	+	+	

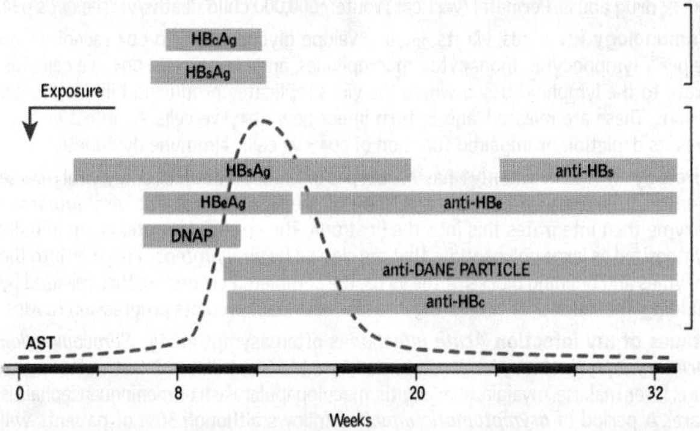

Fig 1. Virological events in acute hepatitis B in relation to serum amino-transferase (AST) peak. IF=immunofluorescence; Ag=antigen; HBS=hepatitis B surface; HBC=hepatitis B core; HBE=hepatitis B e antigen; DNAP=DNA polymerase.

Using ribavirin with PEGinterferon-α in HCV: *NICE advice*

In mild chronic disease the decision between immediate treatment and 'watchful waiting' until the disease has reached a moderate stage, should be made on individual basis.[198,199] Combination therapy, comprising PEGinterferon alfa-2a and ribavirin or PEGinterferon alfa-2b and ribavirin, is recommended for the treatment of chronic hepatitis C. For people who are unable to tolerate ribavirin, monotherapy with PEGinterferon alfa-2a or PEGinterferon alfa-2b is recommended.[200] Efficacy is less if: • HCV genotype G1, 4, 5, or 6 is involved[1] • ↑Viral load • Older patients • Excessive delay before ℞ starts • Blacks (*vs* Caucasians) • Males • HIV+ve.

NB: PEGylated interferon has an inert tail retarding its elimination (hence it is given SC once weekly). Giving these drugs is a specialist role, so the main thing for non-specialists is to know contraindications, to prevent inappropriate referral. **CI:** • Allergy to or past use of interferon • Autoimmune hepatitis • Severe liver dysfunction/decompensated cirrhosis • Age <3yrs • Severe, unstable or uncontrolled heart disease in past 6 months • Past severe psychiatric conditions (esp. depression) • Pregnancy/lactation • Haemoglobinopathies (a contraindication to ribavirin).

HIV and hepatitis C HCV prevalence is ~7% for sexually transmitted HIV and >90% for IV drug abuse transmission. Untreated HIV seems to accelerate the progression of HCV-induced liver fibrosis. Given the safety and efficacy of co-therapy with PEGinterferon + ribavirin and the bad effects of chronic hepatitis C, all HIV/HCV co-infected patients should be evaluated for therapy.[201]

1 Interferon-α ℞ is either for 24wks (genotype 2 & 3) or 48wks for G1 (commonest in UK) & G4-6, if, after 12 weeks, viral load is <1% of pre-treatment levels.

HIV1, a retrovirus (p376), is responsible for most cases. HIV2 causes a similar illness (?longer latent period). Over 30 million people are HIV +ve (2.5 million/yr; 2 million deaths/yr; most are in Africa (Africa has 25% of the world's *total* disease burden, 3% of total health workforce, and just 1% of wealth).[202] There is increasing HIV transmission in east Europe. *UK incidence:* 9100/yr; more heterosexually acquired than homosexually. ♂:♀ ≈3:1.[203] *UK prevalence:* ~73,000.

Transmission Sexual (75%, oral sex in 3–7%[204,205]), infected blood (>1200 cases in the UK), IV drug abuse. Perinatal (vertical) route: ~600,000 child deaths/yr: see *OHCS* p34.

Immunology HIV binds, via its gp120 envelope glycoprotein, to CD4 receptors on helper T lymphocytes, monocytes, macrophages, and neural cells. CD4 +ve cells migrate to the lymphoid tissue where the virus replicates producing billions of new virions. These are released, and in turn infect new CD4 +ve cells. As infection progresses depletion or impaired function of CD4 +ve cells ↓immune dysfunction.

Virology RNA retrovirus; HIV1 has 9 subtypes or 'clades'. After cell entry, viral reverse *transcriptase* enzyme makes a DNA copy of the RNA genome. The viral *integrase* enzyme then integrates this into the host DNA. The core viral proteins are initially synthesized as large polypeptides that are cleaved by viral *protease* enzymes into the enzymes and building blocks of the virus. The completed virions are then released by budding. The number of circulating viruses (viral load) predicts progression to AIDS.

Stages of HIV infection *Acute infection* is often asymptomatic. ***Seroconversion (primary infection)*** may be accompanied by a transient illness 2–6wks after exposure: fever, malaise, myalgia, pharyngitis, maculopapular rash or meningoencephalitis (rare). A period of ***asymptomatic infection*** follows although 30% of patients will have ***persistent generalized lymphadenopathy (PGL)***, defined as nodes >1cm diameter at ≥2 extra-inguinal sites, persisting for 3 months or longer. Later, constitutional symptoms develop: T°↑, night sweats, diarrhoea, weight↓, ± minor opportunistic infections, eg oral candida, oral hairy leucoplakia, herpes zoster, recurrent herpes simplex, seborrhoeic dermatitis, tinea infections. This collection of symptoms and signs is referred to as the ***AIDS-related complex (ARC)*** and is regarded as a prodrome to AIDS. ***AIDS*** is a stage in HIV infection characterized by the presence of an indicator disease (p410). CD4 count is usually ≤200 × 10^6/L (prognosis ~2yrs if untreated).

Diagnosis Serum (or salivary) HIV-Ab by ELISA, usually confirmed by Western blot. In case of recent infection, HIV-Ab might be negative (window period, usually 1–3wks after exposure). In this case, checking HIV RNA (PCR) or core p24 antigen in plasma, or repeating ELISA tests at 6 wks and 3 months can confirm the diagnosis. 4th generation kits can test for HIV-Ab and p24-Ag. Rapid test kits are available and give the result in 30min; however, positive results must be confirmed by Western blot.[206] OraQuick® uses oral fluid, and may be bought over the counter (false +ves are a problem, reducible if 2 tests done in parallel).[207] ***HIV subtypes*** A & B predominate in the UK; type D (commoner in Africa)[208] & hybrid/recombinant strains carry a worse prognosis as they bind to immune cells more readily.

Prevention Blood screening; disposable equipment; perinatal antiretrovirals for HIV+ve mothers ± Caesarean birth ± bottle-feeding (may ↑mortality if hygiene poor).

►*A stop-HIV sexual manifesto:* **Good HIV information** (TV, wind-up radios, eg in Africa; HIV issues in soap operas are most influential);[209] accessible **HIV tests** (with opt-out not opt-in when done in clinics;[210] expensive counselling reserved for those proving +ve). **Well-rehearsed sexual negotiation skills. Condoms** for *all* sexual contact, or **abstinence** (*very* unreliable![211]—also "I'd rather be dead than abstain"[212]). **Reframing of our bodies as a route to intimacy** rather than as instruments of gratification always entailing penetration. **Fewer sexual partners**. NB: 3 *simultaneous* partners is *much* riskier than 6 *serial* partners. **↓Alcohol use** (to avoid risky behaviour). Good trials find that **circumcision** prevents ~65% of HIV (and herpes[213]) infections over 1½yrs.[214] It is not a reliable preventive: circumcised men must not behave as if they are safe.

HIV, TB, poverty, and multi-drug resistance (MDR-TB)

TB is a common, serious complication of HIV. ~40% of those with AIDS in the developing world have TB. Morbidity due to HIV/AIDS/TB leads to a vicious circle: loss in productivity→failing economies→unbalanced health budgets→incomplete courses of TB drugs→selection of drug-resistant organisms→more TB deaths→ruin.[215] New cases of MDR-TB run at ~500000/yr; mortality >20%.[216] *Other HIV–TB interactions:*

- Mantoux tests may be negative and the presentation of TB may be atypical.
- Increased reactivation of latent TB infection (LTBI).[1]
- Previous BCG vaccination does not prevent development of TB.[217]
- Smears may be -ve for AFB. Smears that are +ve often have few AFB. This makes culture very important (and vital to characterize drug resistance).
- Atypical CXR, eg lobar or bibasal pneumonia, hilar lymphadenopathy.
- Extrapulmonary and disseminated disease is much more common.
- TB ℞ in poor countries entails a 4-drug initial phase (2 months of rifampicin, isoniazid, pyrazinamide & ethambutol) and a 2-drug continuation phase (4 months of rifampicin & isoniazid, or 6 months of isoniazid & ethambutol). HIV is known to increases case fatality and rates recurrent TB after this regimen.[218]
- There is ↑toxicity (D&V, hepatitis, rash neuropathy) from combining anti-TB and anti-HIV drugs (eg stavudine, lamivudine & nevirapine as twice-daily generic tablet, often used in resource-poor/WHO HAART, p414). NB: it may be best to delay HAART until 1–2 months after TB ℞ is started (unless CD4 <100×10⁶/L).[219]
- As HAART reconstitutes CD4 counts, paradoxical worsening of TB symptoms may occur (the 'immune reconstitution inflammatory response', IRIS).[220]
- HIV may or may not necessitate lifelong prophylaxis with isoniazid (may prevent TB deaths in children),[221][222] but either way, regular clinical monitoring is vital.

►Directly observed treatment strategy (DOTS) prevents MDR-TB.[223] In areas where MDR-TB is common, DOTS-plus (use of 2nd-line drugs) may be a solution.[224]

►Respiratory isolation is vital if TB patients are near HIV +ve people. Nosocomial (hospital-acquired) and MDR-TB are major problems worldwide, affecting HIV +ve and HIV -ve people. Mortality is ~80% in patient-to-patient spread. Test TB cultures against 1st and 2nd line agents; 5+ drugs may be needed in MDR-TB:[225]

First-line antitubercular agents:		Second-line antitubercular agents:	
Isoniazid	Streptomycin	Ofloxacin	Aminosalicylic acid
Rifampicin	Amikacin	Moxifloxacin	Clarithromycin
Pyrazinamide	Kanamycin	Cycloserine	Azithromycin
Ethambutol	Capreomycin	Ethionamide	

Reducing MDR-TB: chief goals Early identification; full treatment; isolation.[226] Early isolation of suspected TB. A suspicious CXR or past MDR-TB is enough.

- The ability to obtain Ziehl–Nielsen (ZN)/auramine stains 24h a day.
- Directly observing and confirming that patients take all prescribed drugs.
- Wearing of special masks by staff and patient if s/he leaves the isolation room.
- Sputum induction/expectoration being confined to isolation rooms.
- Doors to isolation rooms having automatic closing devices.
- Providing negative air pressure in isolation rooms.
- Only stop isolation after ≥3 sputum samples are AFB -ve on culture for MDR-TB.
- Frequent tuberculin skin surveillance tests for workers and contacts.

Extensively drug-resistant tuberculosis (XDR-TB) This most worrying strain (there may be almost no treatment options) is occurring in 45 countries. Most cases are in former Soviet Union, but cases are accelerating in Africa.[227] It is associated with the cumulative duration of past treatment with 2nd-line TB drugs.[228] Compulsory confinement of such patients is suggested, but the practicalities and ethics of this are highly problematic.[229][230]

1 LTBI implies no X-ray or clinical sign of active TB. 30% of the worlds population has LTBI. Targeted testing and treatment of LTBI in high-risk groups (eg born in endemic area or immunosuppressed) is advised in well-off countries. New tests for LTBI (QuantiFERON-TB; T-SPOT.TB) are better than tuberculin skin tests (too many false +ves and false -ves if immunosuppressed; a reaction >15mm *is* significant even if no risk factors). ℞: 9 months of daily isoniazid in rich low-prevalence countries.

►All patients with a new diagnosis of HIV should have a tuberculin test and be tested for toxoplasma, CMV, hepatitis B/C, and syphilis serology, to identify past or current infections that may develop as immunosuppression progresses.

TB p398. **Kaposi's sarcoma** p716. **Leishmaniasis** p439.

Pulmonary *Pneumocystis jiroveci* (*P. Carinii* is now known to be a rat strain) pneumonia (see **fig 1**): this fungus is the chief life-threatening opportunistic infection in AIDS (p162). ℞: high-dose co-trimoxazole IV (60mg/kg/12h for 14d PO or IV; special monitoring must be available); precede each dose by prednisolone 40mg (reduce after 5d, and tail off). *Primary prophylaxis:* If CD4 count <200×10^6/L: *co-trimoxazole* 960mg/24h PO—reducible to 480mg to improve tolerance or 960mg on alternate days (3 times a week), or 960mg/12h on alternate days (3 times a week). Secondary prophylaxis is essential after 1st attack until CD4 count >200×10^6/L.[231] Other pathogens: *pyogenic bacteria* (atypical presentation); *M. tuberculosis* (p398); *M. avium intracellulare* (MAI); *fungi* (*Aspergillus*, cryptococcus, histoplasma); *CMV*. Also: *Kaposi's sarcoma*, lymphoma, lymphoid interstitial pneumonitis, and non-specific pneumonitis.

Gut Oral pain may be caused by *candidiasis*, HSV or aphthous ulcers, or tumours. *Oral Candida* is treated with *nystatin* suspension 100,000U (1mL swill & swallow/6h)-or amphotericin lozenges/6h PO. *Oesophageal* involvement causes dysphagia ± retrosternal discomfort. ℞: fluconazole, ketoconazole, or itraconazole PO for 1–2 weeks. Relapse is common. *HSV* and *CMV* also cause oesophageal ulceration which may be difficult to differentiate from *Candida* by barium studies. *Anorexia and weight loss* are common in HIV infection. *LFT ↑ and hepatomegaly* are common; causes include drugs, viral hepatitis, AIDS sclerosing cholangitis, or MAI. *MAI* causes fever, night sweats, malaise, anorexia, weight↓, abdominal pain, diarrhoea, hepatomegaly, and anaemia. *Diagnosis:* blood cultures, biopsies (lymph node, liver, colon, bone marrow). ℞: *ethambutol + clarithromycin + rifabutin* (BOX). *Chronic diarrhoea* may be caused by bacteria (*Salmonella, Shigella, Campylobacter, atypical mycobacteria, C. difficile*), protozoa (*Cryptosporidium* p390, *Microsporidium, Isospora belli* **fig 1** p389, *cyclospora*), or viruses (*CMV, adenovirus*). *Perianal disease* may be from recurrent HSV ulceration, perianal warts, squamous cell cancer (rare). Kaposi's sarcoma (p716) and lymphomas can also affect the gut.

Eye *CMV retinitis* (acuity↓ ± blindness) may affect 45% of those with AIDS. Fundoscopy shows characteristic 'mozzarella pizza' signs, **fig 5** p405. *Treatment:* see BOX. *Ganciclovir*-containing intraocular implants are available (**NB:** risk of post-op retinal detachment, one implant does not prevent disease in the other eye). The need for maintenance therapy may be reviewed if CD4 ≥100×10^6/L—eg after immune restoration by HAART (p414), if retinitis is inactive.[232]

CNS *Acute HIV* is associated with transient meningoencephalitis, myelopathy, and neuropathy. *Chronic HIV* is associated with several CNS syndromes: AIDS-related dementia, HIV-related meningitis, CMV encephalitis, progressive multifocal leucoencephalopathy (PML, p376), and vacuolar myelopathy. *Toxoplasma gondii* (p404) is the main CNS pathogen in AIDS, presenting with focal signs. CT/MRI shows ring-shaped contrast enhancing lesions. Treat with *pyrimethamine* (+*folinic acid*) + *sulfadiazine* or *clindamycin* for 6 months. Lifelong secondary prophylaxis is needed. Pneumocystis prophylaxis also protects against toxoplasmosis.[233] *Cryptococcus neoformans* (**fig 2**; and p440) causes a chronic meningitis, eg with no neck stiffness. ℞: See BOX. *Tumours* affecting the CNS include primary cerebral lymphoma, B-cell non-Hodgkin's lymphoma. CSF JC virus PCR is useful in distinguishing PML from lymphoma.

Psychology HIV is *the* paradigm of a *biopsychosocial illness*. HIV is treatable, 100% preventable, yet very prevalent. Asking *why* tells us more about ourselves than about HIV-1.[234] Shame, sexual imperatives, pride and prejudice keep HIV underground and multiplying. ►Imagine you are pregnant and HIV+ve, perhaps as a result of rape, and you will appreciate some of the many many psychological problems of HIV (p414).

Managing opportunistic infections in HIV

Infection	Treatment/side effects/prophylaxis
Tuberculosis	The most lethal opportunistic infection; ►p398. Active pulmonary TB may develop when CD4 <200/mm^3, which usually responds to standard anti-TB therapy. If no active infection, prophylaxis may be needed if significant exposure, or tuberculin skin test >5mm induration (*isoniazid* 300mg/day + *pyridoxine* 10–20mg/day PO; get expert local help, eg on how long to continue prophylaxis).[235]
Pneumocystis jiroveci (=P. carinii)  **Fig 1.** *P. Jiroveci* (fluorescent stain × 1000).[236] © Subhash K Mohan	*Co-trimoxazole* (=trimethoprim 1 part + 5 parts sulfamethoxazole) 120mg/kg/d IVI in 2–4 divided doses for 14d. (SE: nausea, vomiting, fever, rash, myelosuppression) **or** *pentamidine isetionate* 4mg/kg/d by slow IVI for 14–21d (SE: BP↓, hyper- or hypoglycaemia, renal failure, hepatitis, myelosuppression, arrhythmias). *Prednisolone* 40–60mg PO daily (reducing dose) if severe hypoxia. *2nd line agents: Primaquine + clindamycin, pentamidine isetionate, atovaquone. Secondary prophylaxis,* eg *co-trimoxazole* 480mg/24h PO; same dose as 1° prophylaxis, essential after 1st attack.
Candidiasis (See figures on p441)	*Local ℞: Nystatin* suspension 100,000U swill & swallow/6h or *amphotericin* lozenges/6h. *Systemic ℞ if mucosal: Fluconazole* 50–100mg/d PO for 7–30d; *if invasive:* 400mg/d (continue according to response; SE: nausea, hepatitis, platelets↓) or *itraconazole* (SE: CCF, nausea, hepatitis). *Amphotericin B* (p168) is for *severe* systemic infection. Relapse is common.
Toxoplasmosis (fig 3, p405)	*Indications:* typical CNS signs & symptoms + lab data (CD4 <200 cells/μL, +ve toxoplasma IgG and ring-enhancing lesions on CT/MRI). *Acute phase: pyrimethamine* 200mg PO once, then 75mg/d + *sulfadiazine* 1.5g/6h PO + leucovorin (folinic acid) 5–20mg 3 times a week, continued for 1 week after stopping pyrimethamine (stop the latter 1 wk after 'cure').
Cryptococcal meningitis 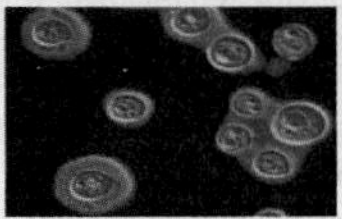 **Fig 2.** Cryptococcus[237]	*Amphotericin B* IV (p168) for 14d, then fluconazole 400mg/24h PO until CSF is sterile, eg 8 weeks. 20% mortality. Normalizing ICP (repeated LPs ± shunts) may help. Give secondary prophylaxis (fluconazole) until CD4 >150×10^6/L and cryptococcal antigen -ve.[238] Diagnosis: India ink stain (**fig 2**); CSF culture; cryptococcal antigen in blood & CSF. Note that the capsule is an essential virulence factor for this yeast. Fig 2 © Dr M McGinnis)
CMV retinitis (fig 4 on p405)	Induction: *ganciclovir* eye implant. *Valganciclovir* 900mg /12h PO for 3wks, then 900mg/24h PO *or cidofovir:* start with 5mg/kg IV once weekly for 2wks (with probenecid & IV fluids), then reduce to alternate weekly doses.
MAI Mycobacterium avium intracellulare (=MAC, *M. avium* complex, p410).	*Clarithromycin* 500mg/12h + *ethambutol* 15mg/kg/d + *rifabutin*[12] 300mg/d, all PO. Prophylaxis if CDC <50/mm^3: *azithromycin* 1.2g/wk PO.
Strep. pneumoniae	Prophylaxis: 23-valent pneumococcal vaccine, p391.[239]

►Get comfortable talking about sex and sexuality, and requesting HIV tests. It's vital that you do—literally. If you find this difficult, get help (*OHCS* p328). Keep practising! NB: asking "are you gay?" is not very helpful. If speaking to a man, ask about sex with other men, as many don't identify themselves as gay (esp. in repressive countries). Globally, men who have sex with men are 19-fold more likely to get HIV than others.[240]

Preventing HIV depends on us all promoting *lifelong* safer sex, condom use, and reduction in partner numbers and regular testing (for example in all new patients in areas where diagnosed rates of HIV are high. Videos, followed by interactive discussions, is one way to double condom use, and *100% condom programs* also help.

- Warn everyone about dangers of sexual tourism/promiscuity. Teach skills in sexual negotiation. Explain how alcohol can undermine safe sex messages.
- Promote human rights so groups driving HIV epidemics aren't driven underground.
- Introduce drug users to needle exchange schemes ("Don't share needles").
- Good control of other STDs ↓HIV incidence by 40%. Promote the work of STI clinics.
- Encourage HIV testing, eg in pregnancy (±Caesarean sections if +ve, *OHCS* p34).[1]
- Diagnose HIV *early*: have a high index of suspicion in all with TB, pneumonia, diarrhoea, meningitis, weight↓, lymphoma, severe fungal infections, or candida.[241]

Post-exposure prophylaxis (PEP)

Seroconversion rate post-needle-stick: ~0.4% (HIV); 30% for hep B if HBeAg +ve.

- Wash well. If needle-stick, encourage bleeding; do not suck or immerse in bleach.
- Note name, address, and clinical details of donor.
- Report incident to Occupational Health and fill in an accident form.
- Store blood from both parties (HIV, HBV & HCV tests).
- Immunize (active & passive) against hepatitis B at once, if needed (p271).
- Counsel and test recipient at 3 and 6 months.
- Weigh risks by questioning donor; if HIV+ve, what is the CD4 & viral load count?
- Before prophylaxis, do a pregnancy test. Was the inoculum big? Was injury deep?

Start PEP in case of a significant exposure to blood or other high-risk body fluid from a HIV +ve source, or any source which is at high risk of HIV infection. PEP is not indicated after low risk exposures (eg urine, vomit, saliva, faeces, unless they are visibly bloodstained) or the source is HIV –ve (proven by tests). Start PEP as soon as possible (certainly within 48–72h), and continue for at least 28d. PEP is not needed beyond 72h post-exposure. Do *follow-up testing* at 12 and 24wks post-exposure (or 24 wks after cessation of PEP) and continue for at least 12wks after the HIV exposure event (or for at least 12wks from when PEP was stopped). ***Starter regimen:*** One *Truvada* tab (245mg ***tenofovir*** and 200mg ***emtricitabine***) once a day plus two *Kaletra*® film-coated tabs (200mg ***lopinavir*** and 50mg ***ritonavir***) twice a day. *Truvada*® + *Kaletra*® is the preferred regimen, but *Combivir*® + *Kaletra*® may be considered as an option if there are difficulties sourcing starter packs containing *Truvada*®.[242]

Acute seroconversion. Early identification matters! Signs are like infectious mononucleosis (eg lymphadenopathy, myalgia, rash, headache; rarely meningitis); do tests if there are unusual signs, eg oral candidiasis, recurrent shingles, leucopenia, or CNS signs (antibody tests may be negative but viral p24 antigen and HIV RNA levels are ↑ in early infection). As ever, the first best 'test' is to take a thorough history. If you *do* identify acute seroconversion illness, get expert help—and advise unambiguously on preventing transmission. It is not known if early therapy is worthwhile.[243]

Other direct effects of HIV Osteoporosis; dementia (the brain is a sanctuary for HIV—and HAART may not prevent dementia from developing).[244]

When seeing HIV+ve people, ask... • Have you been to an STD clinic? (STDs promote spread of HIV). • Using condoms? • Sharing needles? • Have you told your partner(s)? • What is your CD4 cell count/HIV-1 RNA level? Viral load helps plan start of antiretrovirals; CD4 <200, <100, and <50/mm³ prompt prophylaxis for *pneumocystis*, *toxoplasma*, and *MAC* (p410), respectively • What is your CMV & toxoplasma titre? (if -ve, counsel to avoid infection, eg no uncooked meat; avoid cats etc) • Recent CXR? (eg TB; pneumocystosis) • Last cervical smear? (risk of neoplasia↑)[245] • Are you depressed?

HIV tests and counselling

Pre-test counselling does not need to be exhaustive (it is routine/'opt-out'[246] in antenatal & STI clinics, new patient medicals, etc).[247] [248] If in doubt, get help from STI clinic.

- Determine level of risk (eg unprotected sex; sex overseas; male-male sex; rape).
- Discuss test benefits: partner protection; avoiding vertical transmission; getting treatment.
- What are the difficulties? Will you tell family and friends? Explain possible effects on: job, mortgage, insurance (we have no obligation to disclose HIV status).
- Do post-test counselling (eg to re-emphasize ways to ↓risk exposure).

Rapid point-of-care HIV testing: This has great benefits—eg on labour ward. 2 rapid tests done in parallel improves accuracy (blood is better than saliva).[249]

Counselling throughout HIV illness: A key issue when a person is dying from HIV is making a will. Legal help may be needed on housing, next-of-kin, employment, and guardianship of children. Making advance directives needs special skill. Domiciliary genitourinary teams, GP, and hospices help with terminal care all have a role.

Aims of HAART & other strategies

- HAART (Highly Active Antiretroviral Therapy) aims to suppress plasma HIV RNA concentrations below the limit of detection and restore immune function. This is not a cure as latent replication-competent provirus exists in resting CD4+ T lymphocytes and persistent (but cryptic) viral replication remains intact.[250] Lifelong suppression of plasma HIV RNA is problematic—hence the need for strategies to *eradicate* HIV.
- In theory, these effects can be helped by any therapy which blocks histone deacetylase 1 (HDAC1 mediates virion production). This is the rationale behind studies of HDAC1 blockers such as valproic acid—which has been shown to ↓frequency of resting cell infection (mean reduction 75%).[251]

►HAART should be part of a holistic, integrated, individualized care plan proceeding with management of comorbidities, eg malnutrition, malaria etc.[252]

Monitoring HIV infection

Routine tests

- CD4 T cell count (every 3–6 months). CD4 counts are expensive. A reasonable alternative is the TLC—the total lymphocyte count: a TLC of 1400/μL ≈ a CD4 count of 200/μL as far as risk of mortality from HIV goes.[254]
- HIV RNA (every 3–6 months).
- Serum U&E, HCO_3, Cl, creatinine, bilirubin (total + direct)/LFT (every 6–12 months)
- FBC differential (every 3–6 months)
- Fasting lipid profile and glucose (annually)

Other tests

- Pregnancy test
- Drug resistance testing

Indications for initiating antiretroviral therapy[255]

- History of an AIDS-defining illness or with a CD4 count ≲350 cells/μL.[256]
- Antiretroviral therapy should also be initiated in the following groups of patients regardless of CD4 count: Pregnant women; patients with HIV-associated nephropathy; and patients coinfected with HBV when treatment is indicated for hepatitis B.
- Antiretroviral therapy may be considered in some patients with CD4 counts >350 cells/mm³ (high viral load, or when CD4 count is falling rapidly).

Useful web link: British HIV Association: www.bhiv.org.

1 Without interventions, rate of vertical transmission is 15–20%; prolonged breastfeeding doubles this, falling to <2% with antiretroviral prophylaxis, elective Caesars and bottle feeding.

►Seek expert help early. If no prior anti-retroviral therapy, aim to start with a combination of 1 NNRTI + 2 NRTIs or PI (preferably boosted with ritonavir) + 2 NRTIs.[257]

Nucleoside reverse transcriptase inhibitors (NRTI)

Zidovudine (AZT) was the 1st anti-HIV drug. Dose: 250–300mg/12h PO or 1–2mg/kg/4h IV. SE: anaemia, WCC↓, GI disturbance, fever, rash, myalgia. Stop treatment if ↑LFT, hepatomegaly, lactic acidosis. CI: anaemia, neutropenia, breast-feeding.

Didanosine (DDI; Videx EC®) 250mg/24h PO if > eGFR 80 and wt <60kg; 400mg/24h if ≥60kg. SE: pancreatitis, neuropathy, urate↑, GI disturbance, retinal and optic nerve changes, liver failure. Stop if significant rise in LFT or amylase. CI: breast-feeding.

Lamivudine (3TC)[258] is well-tolerated. Dose: 150mg/12h PO, take without food. SE: see zidovudine, but less common. Stop if: ↑LFT; big liver; lactic acidosis; pancreatitis.

Emtricitabine (FTC) It is like lamivudine, but is also active against hepatitis B.[259]

Stavudine (D4T) 40mg/12h PO if ≥60kg; 30mg/12h if <60kg; stop if neuropathy or LFT↑.

Tenofovir 245mg/24h PO. SE: see lamivudine.

Abacavir 300mg/12h PO. SE: hepatitis, lactic acidosis, hypersensitivity syndrome (3–5%)—rash, fever, vomiting; may be fatal if rechallenged.

Protease inhibitors (PI) slow cell-to-cell spread, and lengthen the time to the first clinical event. PIs are often given with low-dose ritonavir (100mg/12hr PO), which appears to enhance drug levels. All PIs are metabolized by the cytochrome p450 enzyme system. They may therefore increase the concentrations of certain drugs by competitive inhibition of their metabolism, if administered concomitantly.[260] PIs can cause metabolic syndrome (dyslipidaemia, hyperglycaemia, insulin resistance).

Indinavir 800mg/8h PO, 1h before or 2h after a meal. SE: dry mouth, taste disturbance, rash, pruritus, hyperpigmentation, alopecia, nephrolithiasis, anaemia, neutropenia, myalgia, paraesthesiae, ↑LFT.

Ritonavir Start with 300mg then ↑ by 100mg every 12h to 600mg/12h PO. SE: see indinavir.

Saquinavir 1g/12h PO within 2h of a meal. SE: oral ulcers, paraesthesiae, myalgia, headache, dizziness, pruritus, rash, pancreatitis.

Lopinavir/ritonavir (Kaletra®) 400mg (+100mg ritonavir)/12h PO. SE: see saquinavir.

• Others: *Fosamprenavir*. SE: see saquinavir; *atazanavir*; *tipranavir*, *darunavir*.

Non-nucleoside reverse transcriptase inhibitors (NNRTI) These may interact with drugs metabolized by the cytochrome p450 enzyme system, which they either induce or inhibit depending on the concomitantly administered drug.[261]

Nevirapine 200mg/24h for 2wks, then 200mg/12h PO. Resistance emerges readily. SE: Stevens–Johnson syndrome, toxic epidermal necrolysis, hepatitis.

Efavirenz Dose: 600mg/24h PO. SE: rash, insomnia, dizziness. Avoid in pregnancy.

Integrase inhibitors (Integrase is essential for HIV-1 replication) *Raltegravir*.[262] May be combined with tenofovir 245mg/d + lamivudine 300mg/d.[263]

CCR5 antagonists (CC-chemokine receptor 5) *Maraviroc* 300mg/12h PO.

Once-a-day tablets Atripla® contains tenofovir^{245mg}, emtricitabine^{200mg} + efavirenz^{600mg}; take on an empty stomach at bedtime (may cause strange dreams).[264]

Beyond pharmacology It's not all about drugs! There is little point in prolonging life if the negatives outweigh the positives. And there are many negatives: difficult regimens; repeat hospital appointments; low/suicidal mood; poor body image; low self-esteem; guilt; discrimination; stigma; safe-sex conundrums; intercurrent infections; financial and insurance difficulties; family conflicts; difficulties with about-to-be-orphaned children and bereavements. ►*Enable patients to become people in charge of their own destiny.* Treat low mood. Make symptoms less intrusive. Randomized trials show that even a single session of art therapy can achieve these ends.[265] Phone-delivered support[266] and conflict resolution workers can be *very* helpful. HIV+ve people can be involved in caring for other HIV people to mutual advantage.[267]

Golden rules in HAART (Highly Active Antiretroviral Therapy)

- Start HAART early, ideally before CD4 count <200 x 10^6/L.
- Explain to patients that regimens can be complex: negotiate strict adherence. Take time to harmonize pills with the patient's expectations and lifestyle.
- Is the patient suitable to include in an ongoing research trial?
- Aim for no more than twice-daily dosing, if possible.
- Use ≥3 drugs (minimizes replication and cross-resistance). No dual therapies.
- Monitor plasma viral load & CD4 count; *what seems like elimination of HIV often turns into reactivation when treatment stops.* Aim for undetectable viral loads 4 months after starting HAART. Suspect poor adherence if viral load rebounds.
- If viral loads remains high despite good adherence, if there is a consistent fall in CD4 count, or if new symptoms occur, change to a new combination of anti-HIV drugs and request resistance tests, eg genotyping for HIV reverse transcriptase/protease mutations (if available).
- Stay informed about new drugs, and emerging classes of drugs.

Examples and problems with HAART regimens

- Typical regimen for HIV-1: efavirenz 600mg/24h PO with 2 NRTIs (eg lamivudine 300mg/24h PO + tenofovir disoproxil fumarate 245mg/24h PO). Monitor U&E, eg tenofovir 245mg/2d if eGFR 30-50; 245mg/3-4d if eGFR 10-30.
- To avoid NRTI SE (eg lipoatrophy) non-NRTI regimens have been tried, eg efavirenz + lopinavir + ritonavir (efficacy is similar but drug resistance is more likely). NICE 268
- Other comparisons: efavirenz + tenofovir + emtricitabine is better than efavirenz + zidovudine + lamivudine. 269 270
- If other illnesses are present: no ddI if **pancreatitis**. If **polyneuropathy**, avoid using d-drugs (ddI, ddC/dideoxycitidine, d4T). **Non-insulin-dependent diabetes** may need insulin with PIs. Hepatotoxicity risk is ↑ for nevirapine or ritonavir if there are **liver problems**.
- Common initial regimens consist of two nucleoside analogues, combined with either a protease inhibitor, an NNRTI or a third nucleoside analogue. 271
- Managing highly antiviral-experienced HIV-infected patients is complicated by drug resistance, patient intolerabilities, drug interactions and quality-of-life issues. So potent regimens need expert input to maximize activity against resistant virus, eg enfuvirtide and tipranavir/ritonavir, have shown promising results in HAART regimens in those with extensive treatment histories and resistance profiles, if used in combination with other active agents. 272
- A few studies on simplification have been completed: for example, switching from complex regimes to didanosine-tenofovir-efavirenz provides a virological suppression rate at 12 months similar to that seen in patients who do not change from more complex therapy (and may obviate dyslipidaemias). 273
- Combination tablet examples: Trizivir® is abacavir 300mg, lamivudine 150mg, and zidovudine 300mg. Combivir® is zidovudine with lamivudine.

The UK top 10 STIs: genital warts, chlamydia, genital herpes, gonorrhoea, HIV, hepatitis B & C, pubic lice, syphilis, trichomonas. ►Refer early to genitourinary medicine clinic (GUM) for microbiology tests, contact tracing and notification. Some clinics offer walk-in services and on-call services. Avoid antibiotics until seen in GUM clinic.

UK incidence is rising alarmingly, by >10%/yr as 'safer sex' practices are being ignored. Prevalence of chlamydia is ~11%[UK] (>104,000 new cases of genital *Chlamydia*); 22,320 cases of gonorrhoea[UK], and >2250 cases of syphilis.[274]

History Ask about timing of last intercourse; contraceptive method; sexual contacts; duration of relationship; sexual practices and orientation; past sexual infections; menstrual and medical history; antimicrobial therapy.

Examination Detailed examination of genitalia including inguinal nodes and pubic hair. Scrotum, subpreputial space, and male urethra. PR examination and proctoscopy (if indicated); PV and speculum examination.

Signs Vaginal/urethral discharge (p418), genital lesions: herpes (p400); syphilis (p431); *Chlamydia* (BOX). Genital warts (*OHCS* p599). Salpingitis (*OHCS* p286). Lice (*OHCS* p608).

Tests Refer to GUM clinic. Urine: dipstick and MSU for MC+S. Ulcers: take swabs for HSV culture (viral transport medium) and dark ground microscopy for syphilis (*T. pallidum*). Urethral smear for Gram stain/culture for ***N. gonorrhoeae*** (send quickly to lab in Stuart's medium); urethral swab for ***Chlamydia*** (free tests also available from UK chemists, see BOX). High vaginal or swab in Stuart's medium for microscopy/culture (***Candida, Gardnerella vaginalis,*** anaerobes, ***Trichomonas vaginalis***); endocervical swab for ***Chlamydia trachomatis. Chlamydia*** (an obligate intracellular bacteria) is the trickiest STD to diagnose as it is asymptomatic, difficult to culture, and serology may be unhelpful as it cross-reacts with *C. pneumoniae*. Nucleic acid amplification assays (eg urine ligase chain reaction, PCR) are quite good screening tests, with sensitivity >90%. Other tests: include Chlamydia antigen and nucleic acid probe assays.[275] ***Blood tests:*** Syphilis, hepatitis, and HIV serology after counselling.

Follow-up At 1wk & 3 months, with repeat smears, cultures, and syphilis serology.

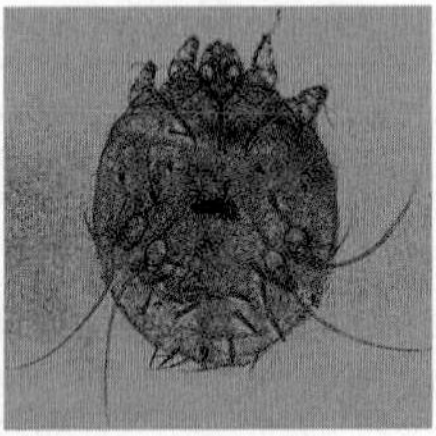

Fig 1. *Sarcoptes scabei*[276] ©Prof S. Upton; Kansas Univ.

Scabies *(Sarcoptes scabei*, an arachnid) Spread is common in families. ***The patient:*** Papular rash (on abdomen or medial thigh; itchy at night) + burrows (in digital web spaces and flexor wrist skin). ***Incubation:*** ~6wks (during which time sensitization to the mite's faeces and/or saliva occurs). Penile lesions produce red nodules. **Δ**: Tease a mite out of its burrow with a needle for microscopy (dropping oil and scraping with a scalpel may provide faeces or eggs). ***℞***: ►Bedding, clothing, etc of the patient and his close contacts should be decontaminated (eg washing in hot water and drying in a hot dryer). Give written advice (*OHCS* p608). Apply 5% ***permethrin*** over whole body including scalp, face (avoid eyes), neck and ears (*BNF*). Do not forget the soles. Wash off after 8–12h; repeat after 7d; use 5% cream on hands if washed before the 8h elapses.[277]

Lymphogranuloma *Signs:* Inguinal lymphadenopathy + ulceration ***Causes:*** *Lymphogranuloma venereum* (*Chlamydia trachomatis;* serovar L2 causes proctitis too, eg in HIV +ve European men),[278] chancroid (*Haemophilus ducreyi*),[1] or granuloma inguinale (*Klebsiella (Calymmatobacterium) granulomatis*, ie donovanosis). The latter causes extensive, painless, red genital ulcers and pseudobuboes (inguinal nodes abscess), with possible elephantiasis ± malignant change. ***Diagnosis:*** 'Closed safety-pin' inclusion bodies in cytoplasm of histiocytes. ***℞***: *Doxycycline* 100mg/12h PO until all lesions epithelialized—or ***azithromycin***, ***erythromycin***, or ***tetracycline***.

1 In the Tropics, chancroid is a common cause of sexually acquired genital ulcers, typically with a granular, yellow base, and ragged edges (± inguinal buboes, which may need draining via a wide-bore needle); the cause is *Haemophilus ducreyi*. WHO recommends erythromycin 500mg/6h PO for 7d, ceftriaxone 250mg IM (1 dose), or azithromycin 1g PO (1 dose). Chancroid facilitates spread of HIV.

Chlamydia screening to prevent pelvic inflammatory disease

Genital *Chlamydia trachomatis* is the commonest STI in the UK (>104,000 diagnoses in GUM clinics/yr). Highest rates are in men and women <24yrs old—implying longterm morbidity, as salpingitis, infertility, or ectopic pregnancy will occur in 2-4%.[279] These 2006 data (n=43,751) are at odds with older NICE data, casting doubt on some of NICE's strategies (below).

Shame, embarrassment about discussing STIs with partners, lack of appointments, and having to go out of one's way to be sensible are the main obstacles. Dialogue is the key; you can help by talking frankly with your patients about sex: see *OHCS* p328. As part of implementing the UK **National Chlamydia Screening Programme**, UK high street pharmacies (Boots) offer **free chlamydia tests** (NHS funded) to those aged 16-24yrs (eg in London, and if +ve, to their partners, of *any* age). Uptake of this service is patchy and it may be hard to sustain. Colleges, prisons, and armed forces are also targeted.[280] NB: only 0.5% of young adults respond to **mass media campaigns** inviting them in for screening.

Free home-based urine test kits may be distributed to garages, hairdressers, and supermarkets with results texted to **mobile phones**—removing the need to provide embarrassing samples at the doctor's surgery.

Walk-in STI clinics and **late-opening GP clinics** allow *prompt* treatment of uncomplicated genital chlamydial infection: **azithromycin** 1g PO as a single dose.

NICE advocates **opportunistic screening** of young adults (eg with nucleic acid amplification tests on urine) *wherever* they present to primary care, irrespective of presenting symptoms.[281] This might halve the incidence of pelvic inflammatory disease. Issues about efficient contact tracing are unresolved. NB: there is no good evidence to support using screening to halt transmission, of to reduce rates of orchitis,♂ ectopic pregnancy or infertility.

First-void (early morning) urine may be the single best diagnostic specimen (for *C. trachomatis* & *M. genitalium*—another common STI) detection by PCR. An additional endocervical specimen may also be needed.[282]

For genital chlamydial infection give **azithromycin** 1g PO as a single dose.

Leaping over barriers which perpetuate STD

A holistic approach to sexual health

A simple reading of this chapter supports the fallacy that the pathogen is everything—that we are simply the unvarying terrain on which pathogens wreak their havoc. Claude Bernard was one of the first to point out that **the terrain is more important than the pathogen**—get the terrain right, and the pathogen loses its grip. Louis Pasteur embodied the pathogen theory of disease; nevertheless, his deathbed words were: "Bernard is right; the pathogen is nothing; the terrain is everything." Bernard had drunk a glassful of cholera to prove his point (no one quite knows why he survived but French physiologists are a tough lot).

So when we look at sexual infections we must look at the terrain and the pathogen—and ask questions such as how does this couple stay healthy (the science of '**salutogenesis**'[283]) whereas another couple or triad keeps getting illnesses? Take thrush for example: always a commensal, but in some patients also a recurring problem. For the terrain to be optimum, nutrition and the immune system must be optimum too. If the subject has HIV, candida may become invasive—not because it changes but because the terrain changes—in this case probably HIV-related downregulation of anti-β-1,2-oligomannosidic epitopes (an epitope is a surface portion of an antigen capable of eliciting an immune response and of combining with the antibody produced to counter that response).[284]

Understand terrain (above) in its widest sense: it has local, individual, and social connotations. Each of these merit interventions in our efforts to reduce sexual infections. Also note that one pathogen often alters the terrain for another—for example one sexual infection makes further infections more likely as inflamed surfaces offer juicy portals of entry. ►So our job in infectious diseases is to get the terrain right. *If we simply focus on killing pathogens we will always fail.*

Non-offensive vaginal discharge may be physiological. Most which are smelly or itchy are due to infection. Foul discharge may be due to a foreign body (eg forgotten tampons, or beads in children). ►Discharges rarely resemble their classical descriptions. ►Untreated GU inflammation ↑viral shedding of HIV-1 in semen 3-fold.

Thrush ***(Candida albicans)*** Thrush is the commonest cause of discharge and is classically described as white curds. The vulva and vagina may be red, fissured, and sore. The partner may be asymptomatic. ***Risk factors:*** Pregnancy, immunodeficiencies, diabetes, the Pill, antibiotics. ***Diagnosis:*** Microscopy: strings of mycelium or oval spores. Culture on Sabouraud's medium. ***Treatment:*** A single imidazole vaginal pessary, eg **clotrimazole** 500mg, + cream for the vulva (and partner) is convenient. Alternative: 1 dose of **fluconazole** 150mg PO. Reassure that thrush is not necessarily sexually transmitted. Recurrent thrush: see *OHCS* p284.

Trichomonas vaginalis (TV) Produces vaginitis and a thin, bubbly, fishy smelling discharge. It is sexually transmitted. Exclude gonorrhoea (which may coexist). The motile flagellate may be seen on wet film microscopy, or cultured (**fig 1**). ℞: **Metronidazole** 400mg/12h PO for 5 days or 2g PO stat. Treat the partner. If pregnant, use the 5-day regimen.

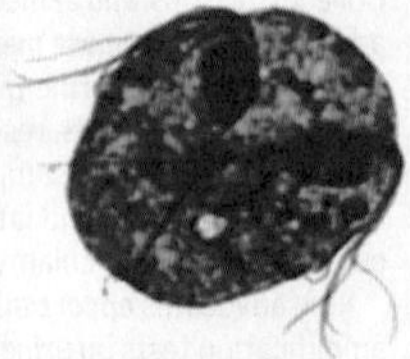

Fig 1. *T. vaginalis*.[285] ©Prof S Upton, Kansas Univ.

Bacterial vaginosis causes a fishy smelling discharge. The vagina is not inflamed. Itch is rare. Vaginal pH: >5.5, hence alteration of bacterial flora ± overgrowth, eg of *Gardnerella vaginalis*, *Mycoplasma hominis*, peptostreptococci, *Mobiluncus* & anaerobes, eg *Bacteroides* species with too few lactobacilli. There is ↑risk of pre-term labour ± amniotic infection. Δ: Stippled vaginal epithelial 'clue cells' on wet microscopy. Culture. ℞: **metronidazole** 400mg/12h PO for 5d (probiotic *Lactobacillus* GR-1 & RC-14 for 28d↑cure rates),[286] or **clindamycin** cream.

Gonorrhoea *Neisseria gonorrhoea* (gonococcus, GC; **fig 2**) can infect any columnar epithelium, eg urethra, cervix, rectum, pharynx, conjunctiva. Incubation: 2–10d. ♂: Urethral pus ± dysuria; tenesmus; proctitis ± discharge PR if gay. ♀: Often asymptomatic, but may have vaginal discharge, dysuria, proctitis. Pharyngeal disease is often asymptomatic. ***Complications— Local:*** Prostatitis, cystitis, salpingitis, epididymitis, Bartholinitis. ***Systemic:*** Septicaemia, eg with petechiae, hand or foot pustules, arthritis; Reiter's syndrome; SBE/IE. ***Obstetric:*** Ophthalmia neonatorum[ND] (*OHCS* p36). ***Long-term:*** Urethral stricture, infertility. ℞: ***Uncomplicated infection of cervix, urethra, and rectum:*** **ceftriaxone** 250mg IM single dose, or **cefixime** 400mg PO stat, plus treatment for Chlamydia (eg **doxycyline** 100mg/12h PO for 7d, or a stat dose of **azithromycin** 1g PO). *Also:* **spectinomycin** 2g IM stat, or single-dose cephalosporin regimens.[288]

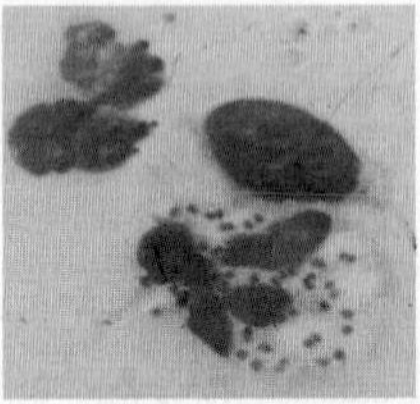

Fig 2. Gonococci in neutrophils; pairs of diplococci (long axes parallel), stained at the bedside by JML (Field's stain, p383).[287]

Non-gonococcal urethritis (NGU) is commoner than GC. Discharge is thinner and signs less acute (may not help diagnosis). Women (typically asymptomatic) may have cervicitis, urethritis, or salpingitis (pain, fever, infertility). Rectum and pharynx are not infected. ***Organisms:*** *C. trachomatis* (►special swabs are needed, *OHCS* p286); *Ureaplasma urealyticum*; *Mycoplasma genitalium*; *Trichomonas vaginalis*; *Gardnerella*; Gram –ve and anaerobic bacteria; *Candida*. ***Complications:*** Similar to local complications of GC. *Chlamydia* may cause Reiter's syndrome and neonatal conjunctivitis. ℞: **Azithromycin** 1g PO stat, or **doxycycline** 100mg/12h PO for 7d. *Also:* **Erythromycin** 500mg/6h PO for 7d, **ofloxacin** 300mg/12h for 7d, or **levofloxacin** 500mg/d PO for 7d. Trace contacts. Avoid intercourse during treatment and alcohol for 4wks.[289]

Non-infective urethritis Traumatic; chemicals; cancer; foreign body.

When do antibiotic guidelines become outdated?

The emergence of antibiotic resistance amongst pathogens represents one of the main obstacles in the fight against infectious diseases. Antibiotic guidelines, which exist on local, regional, and national levels, help ensure optimal therapy, but must be continually updated in the vain task of trying to keep up with pathogens. To monitor resistance patterns, sample infective isolates from different UK regions are collected centrally and tested against a variety of antibiotics to determine their sensitivities to the different drugs (as measured by the minimal inhibitory concentration (MIC) of drug required to prevent organism growth in culture). Such results can highlight the need to revise antibiotic guidelines.

One example is the emergence of ciprofloxacin resistance in *Neisseria gonorrhoea* isolates in England and Canada.[290] Resistance was found in 42% of isolates from southeast England in 2006[291]—a big rise from 10% of isolates in 2002, 3% in 2001, and 2% in 2000. National guidelines aim for chosen drugs to eliminate gonococcal infection in >95% of patients. Ciprofloxacin, previously 1st-line, now has to be replaced by cephalosporins (eg cefixime) in new guidelines.[292] Avoiding use of broad-spectrum antibiotics (eg cephalosporins, co-amoxiclav) may help reduce overall antibiotic resistance, but ill patients often need such drugs: a big dilemma.

Staphylococci When pathogenic, these are usually *Staph. aureus*. Often they infect skin, lids, or wounds. Severe *Staph. aureus* infections are: pneumonia, osteomyelitis; septic arthritis; endocarditis; septicaemia. Production of β-lactamase which destroys many antibiotics (p378–70) is the main problem. *Staph. aureus* toxins cause food poisoning (p390) and toxic shock syndrome toxin (TSST-1): shock, confusion, fever, a rash with desquamation, diarrhoea, myalgia, CPK↑, platelets↓ (associated with the use of hyperabsorbent tampons). *Staph. epidermidis* (*albus*) is recognized as a pathogen in the immunocompromised, particularly in connection with IV lines or any prosthesis. When isolated from a culture, *Staph. epidermidis* can usually be assumed to be a contaminant. It is often enough to remove infected lines. Deep *Staph.* infections need ≥4wks of ***flucloxacillin*** 500mg/6h IV ± removal of foreign bodies, eg prostheses.

Methicillin-resistant Staph. aureus (MRSA) is a high-profile hospital-acquired infection, causing pneumonia, septicaemia, wound infections, and death (risk ↑5-fold),[293] but MRSA only accounts for ~6% of total hospital-acquired infection (~40 cases of septicaemia/yr in England). ≥17 sub-types. NB: glycopeptide-resistant enterococci and *C. difficile* are worse (6500 deaths/yr, p247). In the UK it is mandatory to record all infections; despite stringent efforts rates are rising in 40% of UK hospitals—eg related to overcrowding, the inability to close affected wards, poor barrier-nursing facilities, and faulty hygiene (eg not washing hands between patients). Carriage rates (nasal): 1–10%. Risk factors: HIV, dialysis, being on ITU. MRSA is community-acquired in up to 40%. ℞: Discuss with a microbiologist. ***Vancomycin*** or ***teicoplanin*** are used, but strains with reduced sensitivity (vancomycin-intermediate *Staph. aureus* (VISA)—↓sensitivity to *both* drugs) have emerged. Here, ***linezolid*** (may be used 1st-line too)[294] or ***quinupristin/dalfopristin*** (Synercid®) may be tried. Preventive measures:

- Isolate recently admitted patients with suspected MRSA. Group MRSA cases on one ward (impractical if hospital has to run at 100% capacity).
- Wash your hands and your stethoscope! (also TV remote controls, etc).
- Ask about the need for eradication (with *mupirocin*).
- Be meticulous in looking after intravascular catheters.
- Surveillance swabs of patients and staff during outbreaks.
- Use gowns/gloves when dealing with infected or colonized patients. Masks may be needed during contact with MRSA pneumonia.

Streptococci Group A streps (eg *Strep. pyogenes*) are common pathogens, causing wound and skin infections (eg impetigo, erysipelas, *OHCS* p598), tonsillitis, scarlet fever[ND], necrotizing fasciitis (p662), toxic shock, or septicaemia (**fig 1**). Late complications are rheumatic fever and post-streptococcal glomerulonephritis. *Strep. pneumoniae* (pneumococcus, Gram +ve diplococcus) causes pneumonia, otitis media, meningitis, septicaemia, peritonitis (rare). Resistance to penicillin is a problem. *Strep. sanguis, Strep. mutans,* and *Strep. mitior* (of the 'viridans' group), *Strep. bovis*, and *Enterococcus faecalis* all cause endocarditis. *Enterococcus faecalis* also causes UTI, wound infections, and septicaemia. *Strep. mutans* is a very common cause of dental caries. *Strep. milleri* forms abscesses, eg in CNS, lungs, and liver. Most streps are sensitive to the penicillins, but *Enterococcus faecalis* and *Enterococcus faecium* may present some difficulties. They usually respond to a combination of ***ampicillin*** and an aminoglycoside, eg ***gentamicin*** (p381 & p767). Vancomycin-resistant enterococci (VRE) have been reported. Some strains of VRE are sensitive to either ***teicoplanin*** or ***Synercid***®; all appear sensitive to ***linezolid*** (p380).[1]

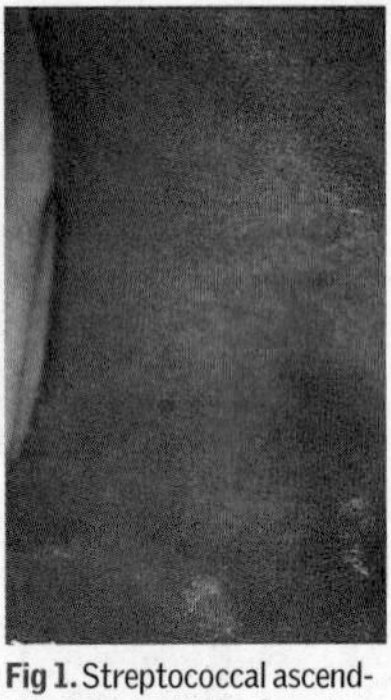

Fig 1. Streptococcal ascending lymphangitis from an infected (diabetic) ankle ulcer.[295] ©Prof Arthur Huntley

1 See reports of vancomycin-resistant *S. aureus* (VRSA), containing a *vanA* resistance gene

Anthrax[ND] *(Bacillus anthracis)* Occurs in Africa, Asia, China, Eastern Europe, and Haiti. Spread is by handling infected carcasses; well-cooked meat poses *no* risk. Terrorists have used long-lasting anthrax spores as a biological weapon.[296] *Signs:* Common form: local cutaneous black pustule. Oedema may be a striking sign ± fever and hepatosplenomegaly—or lung or GI anthrax with dyspnoea ± big GI bleeds or meningoencephalitis. *Tests:* CXR (wide mediastinum). Gram stain is sometimes diagnostic (Gram +ve rod). ℞: (for inhalational anthrax) **Ciprofloxacin** 400 mg/12h IVI or **doxycycline** (100mg/12h PO/IV) + **clindamycin** 7.5mg/kg/6h for 1-2 wks. Continue postexposure prophylaxis using **doxycycline** or any **quinolone** (eg **ciprofloxacin**, **levofloxacin**) for postexposure prophylaxis for 60d. If unable to take **penicillin** or **doxycycline**, use any **quinolone**. *Prevention:* Immunize animals at risk; enforce sound food-handling and carcass hygiene.[297]

Diphtheria[ND] is caused by *Corynebacterium diphtheriae* toxin. *Signs:* Tonsillitis ± a pseudomembrane over the fauces and lymphadenopathy ('bull neck'). ENT details: *OHCS* p158. ℞: *Erythromycin* 10-12mg/kg/6h IVI. Antitoxin, *OHCS* p158. *Prevention:* p391. Give non-immune contacts erythromycin 500mg/6h PO for 10d *before* swab results known.

Listeriosis is caused by *Listeria monocytogenes*, a Gram +ve bacillus with an odd ability to multiply at low temperatures. Possible sources of infection include pâtés, raw vegetables, unpasteurized milk, and soft cheeses (brie, camembert, and blue vein types). It may cause a non-specific flu-like illness, pneumonia, meningoencephalitis, ataxia, rash, or PUO, especially in the immunocompromised, in pregnancy, where it may cause miscarriage or stillbirth, and in neonates.[298] Δ: Culture blood, placenta, amniotic fluid, CSF, and any expelled products of conception. ►*Take blood cultures in any pregnant patient with unexplained fever for ≥48h.* Serology, vaginal, and rectal swabs don't help (it may be a commensal here). ℞: *Ampicillin* IV (*erythromycin* if allergic) + *gentamicin*; p378 & p381 for doses. *Prevention in pregnancy:* • Avoid soft cheeses, pâtés, and under-cooked meat. • Observe 'use by' dates and standing times if using microwaves. • Ensure reheated food is piping hot; throw away any left-overs.

***Nocardia* species** cause subcutaneous infection (eg Madura foot) in warm climes, and, if immunocompromised, abscesses (lung, liver, cerebral). Microscopy: branching chains of cocci. ℞: *Trimethoprim* 5mg/kg/8h IVI + *sulfamethoxazole* 25mg/kg/8h IVI for 3wks (do serum levels) then reduce + cefriaxone 1g/12h IV.

Clostridia Tetanus p424. *C. perfringens* causes wound infections and gas gangrene ± shock or renal failure after surgery or trauma (p592). ℞: Debridement is vital; benzylpenicillin 1.2-2.4g/6h IV + clindamycin 900mg/8h IVI, antitoxin and hyperbaric O_2 may also be used. Amputation may be necessary. *Clostridia* food poisoning (p390). *C. difficile:* Diarrhoea (the cause of pseudomembranous colitis following antibiotic therapy, p247). *C. botulinum:* (Botulism) *C. botulinum* toxin blocks release of acetylcholine causing flaccid paralysis. Botulism does not spread from one person to another. There are 2 adult forms of botulism: food-borne and wound botulism. ►*Risk is high in IV drug abusers* if heroin is contaminated with *C. botulinum*. *Signs:* Afebrile, flaccid paralysis ('descending', eg dysarthria, dysphagia, diplopia, ptosis, then difficulty in holding the head up, then dropping things—and *no* sensory signs).[299] Respiratory failure may supervene. Autonomic signs: dry mouth, fixed or dilated pupils. *Tests:* Find toxin in blood samples or, in wound botulism, identify *C. botulinum* in wound specimens by prompt referral to a reference lab. Samples include: serum, wound pus, swabs in anaerobic transport media (in the UK, phone 020 8200 6868).[300] ℞: Get help (on ITU). *Botulinum antitoxin* works if given early. Also give to those who have ingested toxin but are as yet asymptomatic. *C. botulinum* is sensitive to *benzylpenicillin* and *metronidazole*. In the UK, if out of hours, antitoxin is sourced via CDSC doctors (UK tel. 020 7210 300).[301]

Actinomycosis is caused by *Actinomyces israelii*. Usually causes subcutaneous infections, forming sinuses with pus which contains sulfur granules—eg on the jaw (or IUCDs, *OHCS* p298). It may cause abdominal masses (may mimic appendix mass). ℞: *Ampicillin* 12.5mg/kg/6h for 30d then penicillin V for 100d. Liaise with surgeons.

Enterobacteria Some are normal gut commensals, others environmental organisms. They are a big cause of UTI and intra-abdominal sepsis (eg post-op and in the acute abdomen), and a common cause of septicaemia. Unusually, they may cause pneumonia (especially *Klebsiella*), meningitis, or endocarditis. They may be sensitive to ampicillin and trimethoprim but resistance is growing. Resistance of *K. pneumoniae* to amikacin is seen in 50% (in some places), ceftazidime (90%) and tobramycin (90%)[302] so imipenem may be needed. ***Salmonella*** & ***Shigella*** are discussed on p426.

Pseudomonas aeruginosa is a serious pathogen (esp. if immunocompromised and in cystic fibrosis). It causes pneumonia, septicaemia (risk ↑ if: immunosuppressed, >90yrs old, recent antibiotic use, central venous or urinary catheter[303]), UTI, wound infection, osteomyelitis, and cutaneous infections. The main problem is its increasing antibiotic resistance. ℞: Piperacillin (p378) or mezlocillin + an aminoglycoside (p766). Ciprofloxacin, ceftazidime, and imipenem (p381) are useful against *Pseudomonas*.

Haemophilus influenzae typically affects unvaccinated children usually <4yrs old. It causes otitis media, acute epiglottitis, pneumonia, meningitis, osteomyelitis, and septicaemia. In adults it may cause exacerbations of chronic bronchitis. ℞: Unreliably sensitive to ampicillin; cefotaxime is more reliable. Capsulated types tend to be much more pathogenic than non-capsulated types. ***Prevention:*** Immunization (p391) has resulted in a dramatic fall in incidence.

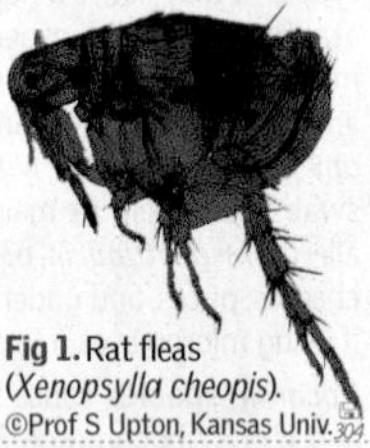

Fig 1. Rat fleas (*Xenopsylla cheopis*). ©Prof S Upton, Kansas Univ.[304]

Yersinia Plague[ND], caused by ***Yersinia pestis***, is a disease of small animals and their fleas (see **fig 1**), which can also infect humans. ***Transmission***: Flea bites, direct contact and via droplet inhalation. ***Incubation:*** 1–7d. *Signs:* Flu-like symptoms, sudden onset of fever, chills, head and body-aches and weakness, nausea and vomiting. ***Bubonic plague*** is the most common form. *Yersinia pestis* enters the skin from the site of the bite and travels through the lymphatic system to the nearest node. The swollen node, called a 'bubo', is very painful and can suppurate. ***Septicaemic plague*** occurs when infection spreads directly through the bloodstream without evidence of a bubo. More commonly advanced stages of bubonic plague will result in the presence of *Y. pestis* in the blood. ***Pneumonic plague*** is the most virulent and least common form. Typically, it is due to a secondary spread from an initial bubonic form. Primary form results from inhalation of aerosolized infective droplets and can be transmitted from human to human without involvement of fleas or animals. Untreated pneumonic plague has a ↑↑ high mortality rate. **Δ**: Phage typing of bacterial culture, or 4-fold ↑ in antibodies to F antigen. ℞: Isolate suspects; ***streptomycin*** up to 15mg/kg/12h IM for 10d. If in 1st ⅓ of pregnancy, ***amoxicillin*** 250–500mg/8h PO; if later, ***co-trimoxazole*** 480mg/12h PO children: co-trimoxazole.[305] Staying at home, quarantine (inspect daily for 1wk), insect sprays to legs/bedding, and avoiding dead animals helps stop spread. ***Vaccination:*** does not offer instant protection, so is not recommended for immediate protection in outbreaks. It is only recommended for high-risk groups (eg lab personnel).[306] [307]

Yersinia enterocolitica In Scandinavia this is a common cause of a reactive, asymmetrical polyarthritis of weight-bearing joints; in America, a common cause of enteritis. It also causes uveitis, appendicitis, mesenteric lymphadenitis, myositis, glomerulonephritis, thyroiditis, colonic dilatation, terminal ileitis and perforation, and septicaemia. *Diagnosis:* Serology is often more helpful than culture, as there may be quite a time-lag between infection and the clinical manifestations. Agglutination titres >1:160 mean recent infection. ***Treatment:*** None may be needed or ciprofloxacin 500mg/12h PO for 3–5d.

Pasteurella multocida causes skin infections (via cat or dog bites), septicaemia, pneumonia, UTI, or meningitis. ℞: Co-amoxiclav, p378, eg 1g/6–8h IV over 4min (dose expressed as amoxicillin).

Moraxella catarrhalis (Gram -ve diplococcus) is a cause of pneumonia, exacerbations of COPD, otitis media, sinusitis, and septicaemia. ℞: Clarithromycin 500mg/12h PO.

Brucellosis This zoonosis (p446) is spread via direct contact with animals, their droplet exhalations, or other products, eg unpasteurized goat (or human) milk. It is common in the Middle & Far East and Bosnia, eg in vets or farmers. ***Cause:*** *B. melitensis* (most virulent); *B. abortus*; *B. suis*; *B. canis*. ***Symptoms*** may be indolent and last for years, eg PUO, sweats, malaise, anorexia, weight↓, hepatosplenomegaly, rash, constipation, D&V, myalgia, backache, arthritis, spondylodiscitis (**fig 2**),[309] sacroiliitis, psoas abscess,[310] bursitis, orchitis, TIAs,[311] cranial nerve lesions (II, VI),[312] depression. ***Complications:*** Osteomyelitis, SBE/IE (culture -ve; a big cause of brucella deaths),[313] abscesses (liver, spleen, lung, breast), meningoencephalitis. **Δ**: Blood culture (≥6wks but rapid culture systems exist, contact lab); serology: if titres equivocal (eg >1:40 in non-endemic zones) do ELISA ± immunoradiometric assays; pancytopenia. **℞**: ~6wks ***doxycycline*** 100mg/12h PO + ***rifampicin + gentamicin*** (for 7d).[314] Oral regimens (doxycycline + rifampicin) might engender more relapses, a ***big*** problem, but not, ironically, if IM route leads to ↑defaulting: either way, the best doctors somehow negotiate to achieve ~100% concordance. In children, get expert help. ***Surgery:*** For abscesses or IE.

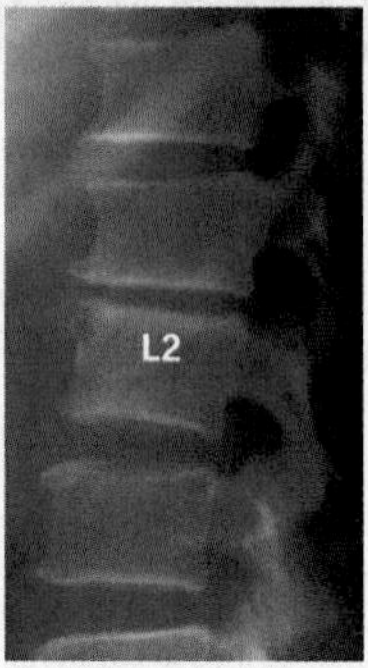

Fig 2. Loss of joint space between L1 & L2 + destruction of L2's anterior body.[308]
Courtesy of Prof Maurice Reeder & Dr. Frank McGuinness

Tularaemia is caused by *Francisella tularensis* (Gram -ve bacillus), which may be acquired by handling infected animal carcasses. It causes rash, fever, malaise, tonsillitis, headache, hepatosplenomegaly, and lymphadenopathy. There may be papules at sites of inoculation (eg fingers). ***Complications:*** Meningitis, osteomyelitis, SBE/IE, pericarditis, septicaemia. ***Diagnosis:*** Contact local microbiologist for advice. Only use laboratories with safety cabinets suitable for dangerous pathogens. Swabs and aspirates must be transported in approved containers. ***Treatment:*** Gentamicin or tobramycin. Oral tetracycline may be suitable for chemoprophylaxis. ***Prevention:*** Find the animal vector; reduce human contact with it as far as possible. Vaccination may be possible for high-risk groups.

Whooping cough[ND] is caused by *Bordetella pertussis*. After 7d of prodromal catarrhal, fever, and cough, the child develops the characteristic paroxysms of coughing and inspiratory whoops. Most children recover well, although the illness may last months. Some (esp the very young) may develop pneumonia (±bronchiectasis), convulsions or brain damage. **℞**: Hospitalise severe cases. Treat all household and close contacts with **erythromycin** (400mg/6h PO).[315] *Also:* **azithromycin** 500mg PO on day 1, then 250mg/d for the next 4d, **clarithromycin** 500mg/12h PO for 7-10d. *Immunization* (p391) has not controlled the disease in Europe: incidence in adults doubled over a recent 5yr period.[316]

Acinetobacter infections This Gram-ve coccobacillus (eg *A. baumannii*) causes pneumonia ± septicaemia in debilitated people. Risk↑ if vascular catheter *in situ*, ventilator use/tracheostomy, enteral feeding, or recent use of 3rd-generation cefalosporins or carbapenem. We carry it on our hands, and it inhabits ventilator equipment. ITU outbreaks occur in summer. **℞**: Imipenem ± aminoglycosides. Multidrug-resistance may require use of nephrotoxic polymyxins or tigecycline. ***Infection control:*** Clean the source; sterilize the reservoir, characterize transmission—and interrupt.[317] NEJM 2008

Cat-scratch disease Mostly due to *Bartonella henselae* (a small, curved, pleomorphic, Gram -ve rod) or *Afepilis felis*. Think of this when any three of the following coexist: an inoculating cat scratch; regional lymphadenopathy (with negative lab tests for other causes of lymphadenopathy, p29); positive cat scratch skin test antigen response; or microabscesses in lymph nodes. In HIV-infected patients, the skin lesions may resemble Kaposi's sarcoma. ***Treatment:*** Usually resolves spontaneously within 1-2 months. One trial found that azithromycin ↑speed of resolution of lymph nodes.[318] Other drugs that have been used include ciprofloxacin, rifampicin and co-trimoxazole. Usually unresponsive *in vivo* despite susceptibility *in vitro*.

See also **Spirochetes** p430; *Neisseria* p375, and *Legionella* p162.

Essence Tetanospasmin, *Clostridium tetani's* exotoxin, causes muscle spasms and rigidity, cardinal features of tetanus (='to stretch').

Incidence ~50 people/yr in the UK. Mortality: 40% (80% in neonates).

Pathogenesis Spores of *C. tetani* live in faeces, soil, dust, and on instruments. A tiny breach in skin or mucosa, eg cuts, burns, ear piercing, banding of piles, may admit the spores. Diabetics are at ↑risk. Spores then germinate and make the exotoxin. This travels up peripheral nerves and interferes with inhibitory synapses.

The Patient *20% have no evidence of recent wounds.*[319] Signs appear from 1d to several months from the (often forgotten) injury. There is a prodrome of fever, malaise, and headache before classical features develop: *trismus* (=lockjaw; Greek trismos = grinding, hence difficulty in opening the mouth); *risus sardonicus* (a grin-like posture of hypertonic facial muscles); *opisthotonus* (**fig 1**); *spasms* (which at first may be induced by movement, injections, noise, etc, but later are spontaneous; they may cause dysphagia & respiratory arrest); autonomic dysfunction (arrhythmias ± wide fluctuations in BP).

Differential diagnosis is dental abscess (both cause trismus), rabies, phenothiazine toxicity, and strychnine poisoning. Phenothiazine toxicity usually only affects facial and tongue muscles (see p855).

Poorer prognosis Incubation <1wk;[320] trismus leads to spasms in <48h; neonates; elderly; postinfective; postpartum (a big cause of maternal mortality worldwide).

Treatment ▸▸Get help on ITU. **ABC** (may need tracheostomy & ventilation). Monitor ECG + BP + SpO_2 (keep >92%, eg with O_2 mask + reservoir); careful fluid balance.

- **Human tetanus immunoglobulin** (HTIG) 5000–10,000U IVI to neutralize toxin.
- Aim to keep the patient asleep but rousable to obey simple commands. **Diazepam** 5–20mg/8h PO (mild disease) or, to control spasms, 0.05–0.2mg/kg/h IVI (≤140mg/d) **or phenobarbital** 1.0mg/kg/h IM or IV + **chlorpromazine** 0.5mg/kg/6h IM (IV bolus is dangerous) starting 3h after the phenobarbital. If this fails to control the spasms, paralyse and ventilate (get anaesthetist's help). Dose example (*OTM*): **pancuronium** 2–4mg IV/½–2h (or by continuous IVI).
- Antimicrobials: **metronidazole** (preferred to penicillin) eg 500mg/6h PO for 7–10d, **benzylpenicillin** 1.2g/4h IV.

Prevention See BOX. Active immunization with tetanus toxoid is part of the 3-stage vaccine during the 1st year of life (eg Pediacel®, p391). Boosters are given on starting school and in early adulthood. Once 5 injections have been given, revaccinate only at the time of significant injury, and consider a final one-off booster at ~65yrs.[321]

Primary immunization of adults: 0.5mL tetanus toxoid IM repeated twice at monthly intervals. In the UK, the formulation is Revaxis®, p391.

Secondary prevention: see BOX.

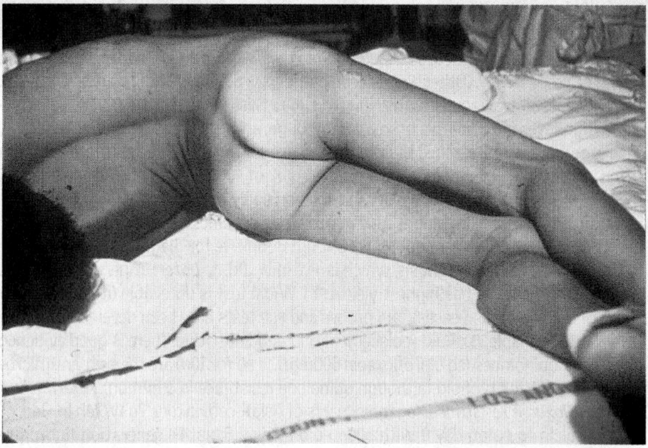

Fig 1. Spasm causing opisthotonus (arching of body with neck hyperextension).[322]
Courtesy of Centres for Disease Control & Prevention

Tetanus prophylaxis in wound management [323]

Clean, minor wounds

Uncertain history of previous vaccination or fewer than 3 doses: Give vaccine.
3 or more previous doses: No need to vaccinate unless ≥10 years since last dose.

All other wounds (wounds contaminated with dirt, faeces, soil, and saliva, puncture wounds, avulsions, and wounds caused by missiles, crushing, burns, and frostbite.

Uncertain history of previous vaccination or fewer than 3 doses: Give vaccine and Tetanus Immunoglobulin (TIG). The recommended dose of TIG for recent (<24h) wounds of average severity is 250 units IM (500 units if wound >24h old, and in burns or heavy contamination). When both tetanus vaccine and TIG are administered, use separate syringes and separate injection sites.

3 or more previous doses: Give vaccine if ≥5 years since last dose.

►If immune status is unknown, assume that the patient is nonimmune. Routine infant immunization started in 1961, so many adults are at risk.

►Hygiene education and wound debridement are of vital importance.

Enteric fever[ND] (200,000 deaths per year)

Typhoid & paratyphoid are caused by *Salmonella typhi* and *S. paratyphi* (types A, B, and C), respectively. (Other *Salmonella* cause D&V: p390 & p246.) *Incubation:* 3–21d. *Spread:* Faecal-oral (acid suppression from PPIs ↑risk). *Presentation:* Malaise, headache, high fever with relative bradycardia, cough, and constipation. CNS signs (coma, delirium, meningism, cerebellar signs, fits)[324] are serious. Diarrhoea is more common after the 1st week. Rose spots occur on the trunk of 40%, but may be difficult to see. Epistaxis, bruising, abdominal pain, and splenomegaly may occur. **Δ:** Can be made by isolation of *S. typhi* from blood, bone marrow or a specific anatomical lesion. Clinical symptoms or serology are suggestive but not definitive for diagnosis. Blood culture is the mainstay of the diagnosis, which is +ve in 1st 10d.[325] *Later:* urine/stool cultures. Bone marrow culture has highest yield. LFT↑. Widal test is unreliable (it can be -ve in ~30% of culture-proven cases). DNA probes and PCR tests have been developed, but are not widely available. *℞:* Fluid replacement and good nutrition. There is good evidence that fluoroquinolones (eg ciprofloxacin 500mg/12h PO for 10d) are the best antimicrobial treatment for typhoid (although quinolone resistance is common). ***Alternatives for ciprofloxacin resistance:*** (eg many parts of Asia)—ceftriaxone 2g IV/24h for 14d; or azithromycin 1g PO on day 0 with 500g PO on days 1-5. NB: 4th generation fluoroquinolones may not work in India. ***In severe disease***, give IV ciprofloxacin or IV cefotaxime for 10-14d. In encephalopathy ± shock, give dexamethasone 3mg/kg IV stat just before antibiotics, then 1mg/kg/6h for 48h. ***Complications:*** Osteomyelitis (eg in sickle-cell disease); GI bleed or perforation; cholecystitis; myocarditis; pyelonephritis; meningitis; abscess; DVT. Infection is cleared when 6 consecutive cultures of urine and faeces are -ve. 1% become chronic carriers; treat if at risk of spreading disease (eg food handlers). Ciprofloxacin 500mg/12h PO for 6wks ±cholecystectomy. ***Prognosis:*** If untreated, 10% die; if treated, 0.1% die. ***Vaccine:*** p377.

Bacillary dysentery[ND]

Shigella causes abdominal pain and bloody diarrhoea ± sudden fever, headache, and occasionally neck stiffness. CSF is sterile. UK school epidemics are often mild (often *S. sonnei*), but imported dysentery may be severe (often *S. flexneri* or *S. dysenteriae*). ***Incubation:*** 1–7d. ***Spread:*** Faecal-oral. ***Diagnosis:*** Stool culture. ***Treatment:*** Fluids PO. Avoid anti-diarrhoeal drugs. Drugs: ciprofloxacin 500mg/12h PO for 3-5d. Imported shigellosis is often resistant to several antimicrobials: sensitivity testing is important for all enteric fevers. There may be associated spondyloarthritis (p553).

Cholera[ND]

►***Cholera loves filth.*** Anything soiled, polluted or corrupt, where politics and tainted water mix, gives cholera life—and spells death to the poor and undernourished. Where there is no corruption there is no cholera. Clean water with clean politics abolishes it.[326] ***Cause:*** *Vibrio cholerae* (Gram -ve comma-shaped rod; **fig 1** on p364). Pandemics or epidemics may occur, eg outbreaks in Zimbabwe & Angola. ***Incubation:*** few hours to 5d. ***Spread:*** Faecal-oral. ***Signs:*** Profuse (eg 1L/h) watery ('rice water') stools, fever, vomiting, and rapid dehydration (the cause of death, with associated metabolic acidosis). **Δ:** Stool microscopy (eg dark ground) & culture. ***℞:*** Strict barrier nursing. ►►Prompt oral rehydration with pre-prepared sachets drunk in large amounts. (0.9% saline IVI if shocked; add 20mmol/L K^+ until U&E known; avoid plain Ringer's lactate: it may cause fatal K^+↓). Oral rehydration with WHO formula (20g glucose/L) is not as good as cooked rice powder solution (50-80g/L) in reducing stool volume.[327] Its high osmolarity (310mmol/L *vs* 200mmol/L) is also unfavourable to water absorption. Oral ***erythromycin*** or 1 dose of ***ciprofloxacin*** 1g PO may ↓fluid loss.[328] Zinc supplements shorten the illness (15mg elemental Zn/12h, as acetate). ***Mortality:*** 1%; up to 50% if the district is unprepared (war, ecological disaster). ***Prevention:*** Only drink boiled or treated water. Cook all food well; eat it hot. Avoid shellfish. Peel all vegetables. Heat-killed vaccine (serovar O1) gives limited protection, and is no longer needed for international travel; newer vaccines are non-standard.[329]

Whose deaths really matter?

In 2006, DNA analysis of pulp in the teeth of Athenians dying in the great plague of 430BC revealed that the cause was typhoid fever.330 30% of Athenians died, including Pericles, their leader. He gave us the Parthenon, juries, free theatre, and, in his own immortal oratory, the notion that it is better to die resisting than to live in submission.331 This is definitely *not* the right approach to infectious diseases: Pericles should have promulgated a third way: neither victory nor submission, but, more subtly, *accommodation*, or something even more symbiotic.

For the next 23 centuries, typhoid fever carried on killing, teaching us nothing much, until noon on 23 April 1851, when a little-known girl was quietly expiring in Malvern. Her name was Annie Darwin, her father's, Charles. Annie was his favourite fun-loving daughter, and with her lingering enteric death Darwin gave up all belief in a just and moral universe. Thus unimpeded, his mind was able to frame and compellingly justify the most devastating answer to the oldest question: that we are here by accident, thanks to natural selection, the survival of the fittest, and the 'wasteful, blundering, low & horridly cruel works of nature'.[1]

The next significant enteric death was 3 summers later at 40 Broad Street (**fig 1**, p664), in the Parish of St James, London, where a child became ill with diarrhoea in August 1854, dying on September 2. Her mother rinsed the soiled nappies into the house drains. These led within feet of the supply to the Broad Street pump. Both the drain and the pump's well had faulty brickwork allowing the waters to mix. From this confluence sprung the discipline of Public Health, for many of the 500 or so ensuing late summer deaths from cholera clustered around this Broad Street pump, as diagrammed by the local doctor, Dr John Snow. He used his now famous diagrams locating each death to motivate the Board of Guardians of St James's parish at its meeting of Sept. 7th 'In consequence of what I said, the handle of the pump was removed the following day'[2]—so inaugurating the control of cholera. If Snow were alive today, he might be busy unplugging all our carbon-emitting power-stations (as killing as cholera), but note that Snow worked through committees to save his countless lives, not by direct action.

These events illustrate two counter-intuitive truths: knowledge of the microscopic cause of a disease is not required for public health measures to succeed (*Vibrio cholerae* was as yet undiscovered)—and even the most parochial Church Council is capable of prompt and decisive action affecting the lives of millions, when informed by an intelligent doctor in command of the facts.

There is one metaphysical truth revealed by these enteric deaths, which would not have escaped Pericles had he only taken the trouble to become a medical student for long enough to realise that his overvalued ideal of heroism is often pointless.[3] Pericles never gave his condolences to parents who lost their sons in battle, because, he said, a hero's death was the finest thing that could befall a man. We meet many heroic deaths on our wards, but they seem oddly pointless in retrospect. This is why we award the palm to Annie, whose unheroic death so transforms the inner landscapes of the mind. And with her in mind, we can confidently relieve our patients of the notion that they must die fighting.

1 A remark of Darwin's in 1856, before starting his *Origin of Species*, quoted in *Darwin* (Desmond & Moore, Penguin). This reminds us of Thomas Hobbes' (1588-1679) dictum: owing to scarcity of natural resources, there is constant war of all against all (*'bellum omnium contra omnes'*). Life in the state of nature is 'solitary, poor, nasty, brutish & short'. It was Thomas Hobbes who first brought Pericles to our attention through his great translations of Thucydides, the biographer of Pericles.

2 J Snow 1854 *Med Times Gaz* **9** 321. Snow (a teetotaller, a vegetarian, and a virgin) is unfairly portrayed as secular saviour; he was really just the man on the spot who took logical decisions.

3 If you doubt that heroism is often pointless, visit the Somme where lies buried the old lie '*dulce et decorum est pro patria mori*'. Wilfred Owen (1893-1918) wrote in a letter to his mother: 'The famous Latin tag [Horace] means *It is sweet and meet to die for one's country*. Sweet! and decorous!...'

►In an endemic area, any individual should be regarded as having leprosy if they show **one** of the following signs: **1** skin lesion consistent with leprosy (**fig 1**) and with definite sensory loss, with or without thickened nerves. **2** positive skin smears. Leprosy is a chronic disease caused by *Mycobacterium leprae*. It affects millions of people in the tropics and subtropics. Since the widespread use of dapsone, and WHO elimination campaigns, prevalence has fallen (from 0.5% to 0.4/10,000 in Uganda; from 11% to 4/10,000 in parts of India).[332] Incidence remains stable, however, at about 800,000 new cases/yr worldwide, many of whom are children. It mainly affects the skin, peripheral nerves, mucosa of the upper respiratory tract and the eyes. ~1–2 million people are disabled, visibly and irreversibly, from leprosy, and need care in the community in which they live. **Diagnosis** is based on the clinical signs and symptoms, and laboratory and other investigations are rarely needed.[333] Skin lesions can be single or multiple, and usually manifests as hypopigmented anaesthetic macules, papules, or annular lesions (with raised erythematous rims). Erythema nodosum (**fig 1**, p564) occurs in 'lepromatous' disease, especially during the 1st year of treatment. Sensory loss is a typical feature of leprosy. The skin lesion may show loss of sensation to pin-prick and/or light touch. A thickened nerve is another feature of leprosy, and is often accompanied by other signs as a result of damage to the nerve (eg loss of sensation in the skin and weakness of muscles supplied by the affected nerve). Sometimes a thickened sensory nerve may be felt running into the skin lesion (eg ulnar nerve above the elbow, median nerve at the wrist, or the great auricular nerve running up behind the ear). In the absence of these signs, nerve thickening by itself, without sensory loss and/or muscle weakness is often not a reliable sign of leprosy. In a few cases, rod-shaped, red-stained leprosy bacilli, which are diagnostic of the disease, may be seen in the smears taken from the affected skin. *Eye lesions:* ►*Refer promptly to an ophthalmologist.* The lower temperature of the anterior chamber favours corneal invasion (so secondary infection and cataract). Inflammatory signs: chronic iritis, scleritis, episcleritis. There may be reduced corneal sensation (V nerve palsy), and reduced blinking (VII nerve palsy) and lagophthalmos (difficulty in closing the eyes), ± ingrowing eyelashes (trichiasis).

Classification[334] ***Paucibacillary ('tuberculoid') leprosy:*** there is a vigorous immune response, with granulomata containing epithelioid cells and lymphocytes, but few or no demonstrable bacilli. Patients show negative smears at all sites. ***Multibacillary ('lepromatous') leprosy:*** immune response is ↓. There are foamy histiocytes full of bacilli, but few lymphocytes. Patients show +ve smears at any site. ***Borderline:*** Between these two poles. ***Method of transmission:*** the exact method is not known,[335] however, it seems to be transmitted by contact between cases of leprosy and healthy persons. More recently, the possibility of transmission by the respiratory route has been gaining ground. There are also other possibilities, such as transmission through insects, which cannot be completely ruled out.

Treatment for adults (WHO):[336] Ask a local expert about: • Resistance patterns, eg to dapsone, when ethionamide may (rarely) be needed • Using prednisolone for severe complications • Is surgery ± physiotherapy needed as well as drug therapy? In the UK, seek advice from the panel of Leprosy Opinion. ***Paucibacillary leprosy:*** Rifampicin 600mg once a month, dapsone: 100mg/d. Duration: 6 months. ***Multibacillary leprosy:*** Rifampicin: 600mg once a month, dapsone: 100mg/d, clofazimine 300mg once a month (supervised) and 50mg/d. Duration: 12 months. ***Single skin lesion paucibacillary leprosy:*** a single dose of rifampicin 600mg, ofloxacin 400mg, minocycline 100mg.

►Beware sudden permanent *paralysis* from nerve inflammation caused by dying bacilli (± *orchitis*, *prostration*, or *death*); this 'lepra reaction' may be mollified by thalidomide (*NOT* if pregnant). Liaise urgently with a leprologist. Supervised therapy may be problematic as many patients find it hard to attend (nomads, jungle-dwellers). WHO has proposed 'accompanied' multi-drug therapy, where someone close to the patient takes responsibility for ensuring treatment compliance. This strategy is controversial.[337]

What is more communicable than leprosy?

This page is dedicated to Joseph deVeuster (Father Damien) of Kalawao, Molokai, in Hawaii, who befriended sufferers of leprosy in a remote Pacific colony. Here the leprosy victims, arriving by ship, were sometimes told to jump overboard and swim for their lives, so frightened were the sailors of this island of contagion. But when they arrived they found a friend who was both doctor and priest to them, whose self-imposed duty was to build their homes, their churches—and their coffins. Without any distinction of race or religion, he gave a voice to the voiceless, building a unique community where the joy of being together gave people new reasons for living.

It is said that after spilling hot water painlessly on his foot, he diagnosed his own leprosy. After that, his sermons beginning "We lepers..." had added veracity.

He gave everything to leprosy—and leprosy took all it could from him, including, on April 15th 1889, his life.

We may look upon that water flowing over his foot not so much as a death sentence, but as one of those initiation ceremonies devised by ancient shamans who realized that it was by these close encounters with death that we augment our spirituality, and so are able to heal.

Joseph deVeuster also invalidates all our definitions of health, and, more importantly, he demonstrates that optimism works and is more communicable than leprosy, proving that there is nothing that cannot be transcended.

►Why are doctors and lepers similar? Both will eventually stop feeling unless cherished.

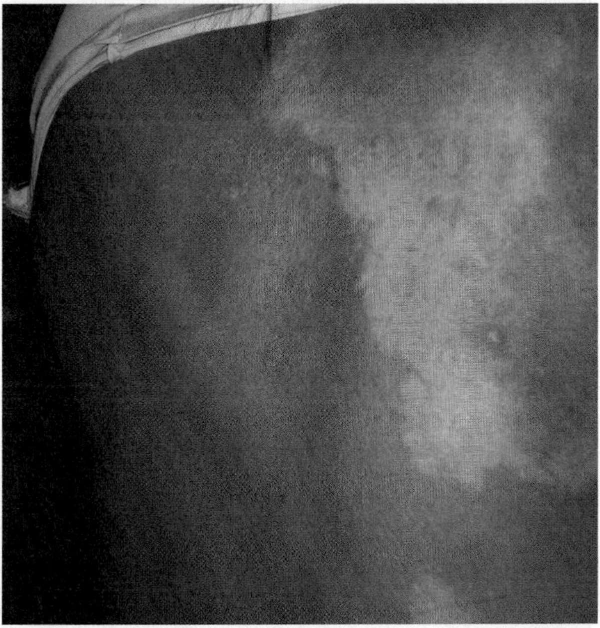

Fig 1. Think of leprosy in everyone with anaesthetic hypopigmented macules or plaques. Could this be vitiligo? No: vitiligo is more demarcated and **de**pigmented (chalk white).[338]
See **fig 4** on p565. Courtesy of Prof Jayakar Thomas

Lyme disease[339] is a tick-borne (eg **fig 1**) infection caused by *Borrelia burgdorferi*. *Signs:* ►≤75% remember the tick bite. The 1st sign is usually **erythema migrans**; a circular rash occurring in ~80%, which begins at the site of a tick bite after 3-30d (p564). It gradually expands, reaching up to 30cm across. Its centre may clear as it enlarges (bull's-eye appearance). *Also:* fatigue, chills, fever, headache, muscle and joint pain, lymphadenopathy, myocarditis; heart block; meningitis; ataxia; amnesia; cranial nerve palsies; neuropathy; lymphocytic meningoradiculitis (Bannwarth's syndrome). *Diagnosis* is based on symptoms, physical findings, and a history of exposure to infected ticks. Lab tests are not needed in presence of erythema migrans.[340] ℞: Skin rash: doxycycline 100mg/12h PO (amoxicillin or penicillin V if <8yrs or pregnant) for 14-21d. Later complications: high-dose IV benzylpenicillin, ceftriaxone. *Prevention:* Keep limbs covered; use insect repellent; tick collars for pets; check skin often when in risky areas. Vaccination is available eg if living in high-risk areas. Advice differs on prophylaxis after a tick bites. A single dose of doxycycline 200mg PO given within 72h of a bite is effective prophylaxis; in highly endemic areas, this may be worthwhile (eg if risk >1%). *Removing ticks:* Use fine (tick-removing) tweezers to grasp the tick very close to your skin. With a steady motion, pull the tick's body away; clean with soap & water. Don't worry if the tick's mouthparts remain in the skin—they won't transmit Lyme disease.[341] Skin complications: **acrodermatitis chronica atrophicans** (ACA; skin is as 'thin as cigarette paper'); **borrelia lymphocytoma** manifests eg as a blue/red discolouration of the earlobe.

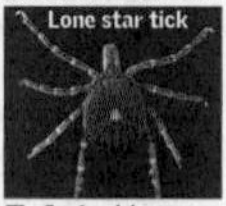

Fig 1. *Amblyomma americanum.* ©Prof S Upton; Kansas Univ.

Endemic treponematoses *Yaws* is caused by *T. pertenue* (serologically indistinguishable from *T. pallidum*). It is a chronic granulomatous disease common in children in the rural Tropics. Spread: direct contact, via skin abrasions, and is promoted by poor hygiene. The primary lesion (an ulcerating papule) appears ~4wks after exposure. Scattered 2nd lesions then appear, eg in moist skin, but can be anywhere. These may become exuberant. Tertiary lesions are subcutaneous gummatous ulcerating granulomata, affecting skin and bone. CVS and CNS complications do not occur. *Pinta* (*T. carateum*) affects only skin; seen in Central and S America. ***Endemic non-venereal syphilis*** (*bejel; T. pallidum*) is seen in Third World children, when it resembles yaws. In the developed world, *T. pallidum* causes ***syphilis*** (see BOX). **Δ**: Clinical. ℞: Procaine penicillin (p378).

Weil's diseaseND is caused by ***Leptospira interrogans*** (eg serogroup *L. icterohaemorrhagiae*). Spread is typically by contact with infected rat urine, eg in slums or while swimming, canoeing or cycling through puddles. After an incubation of 2-20d there is abrupt fever, myalgia/myositis, cough, chest pain ± haemoptysis—then recovery, or jaundice, meningitis, uveitis, and renal failure. **Δ**: Blood culture +ve only up to day 4 of illness; serology. **℞**: *Mild:* doxycycline, ampicillin, or amoxicillin. *Severe:* IV penicillin G. ***Alternatives:*** ampicillin, amoxicillin, erythromycin. Prophylaxis: doxycycline 200mg/wk *may* have a role—eg for water sports in dangerous places.

Canicola fever is an aseptic meningitis caused by *Leptospira canicola*.

Relapsing feverND This is caused by ***Borrelia recurrentis*** (louse-borne) or ***B. duttoni*** (tick-borne). It typically occurs in pandemics following war or disaster, and may kill millions. ***Incubation:*** 4-18d. ***Presentation:*** Abrupt onset fever, rigors, and headache. A petechial rash (which may be faint or absent), jaundice, and tender hepatosplenomegaly may develop. Serious signs: myocarditis, hepatic failure, and DIC. Crises of very high fever and tachycardia occur; on abating, fatal hypotension from vasodilatation may occur. Relapses occur, but are milder. *Tests:* Organisms are seen on Leishman-stained thin or thick films. ℞: Doxycyline 100mg/12h PO. The Jarisch-Herxheimer reaction (p431) is fatal in 5%: meptazinol 100mg IV slowly is given as prophylaxis with the tetracycline, repeated ½h later (with the chill phase) and during the flush phase (if systolic BP <75mmHg). Delouse the patient and their clothes.[342] Doxycycline (p380) is useful prophylaxis in high-risk groups.

Syphilis: the archetypal spirochete

►*Any anogenital ulcer or sore is syphilis until proven otherwise.*

UK incidence: >2250 infections/yr.[344] 1995–2007 saw a 1665% ↑ in UK incidence, with serious outbreaks in London, Manchester, and Brighton[345] [346] as safe-sex messages are forgotten, ignored, or trounced (some clubs ban condoms on 'raw nights').[347] ~75% of patients are in men who have sex with men. Female prevalence (screening in London antenatal clinics): 0.44% (*vs* 0.34% for HIV and 1.1% for hepatitis B).[348]

Treponema pallidum (**fig 1**) enters via a graze, during sex. All signs are due to an endarteritis obliterans. *Incubation:* 9–90d. 4 stages:

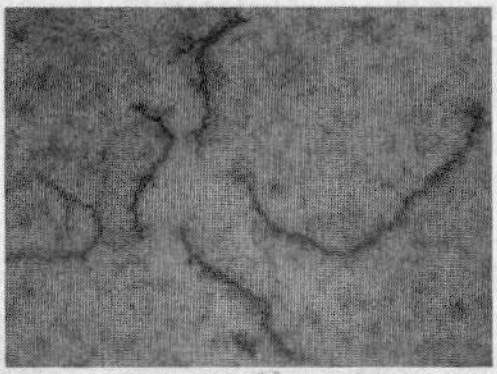

Fig 1. *T. pallidum.*[343] ©Prof S Spilatro.

Primary syphilis: Macule at site of sexual contact forms a painless hard ulcer (*primary chancre;* it is very infectious).

Secondary syphilis: Occurs 6 weeks to 6 months after infection: rash (trunk, face, palms, soles; may be scaly), malaise, lymphadenopathy, T°↑, tonsillitis, alopecia, condylomata lata (flat papules around or beyond genitals),[349] palatal or buccal snail-track ulcers, hepatitis (in up to ⅓, esp. if HIV +ve too[350]), hepatosplenomegaly, uveitis, optic neuritis, meningism, nephrosis, glomerulonephritis, and periosteitis.

Tertiary syphilis follows ≥2yrs latency (when patients are non-infectious): there are *gummas* (granulomas in skin, mucosa, bone, joints, viscera, eg lung, testis).

Quaternary *Vascular:* Ascending aortic aneurysm/aortic regurgitation. *Neurosyphilis* (Δ: CSF analysis; worth considering if RPR titre ≥1:32) *(a) Meningovascular:* Cranial nerve palsies (optic nerve, vision↓), stroke *(b) General paresis of insane (GPI):* Dementia, psychoses (fatal untreated; treatment *may* reverse it) *(c) Tabes dorsalis:* Ataxia, numb legs, chest, and bridge of nose, lightning pains ('like a bolt from the blue'), gastric crises, reflex loss, plantars↑↑, Charcot's joints (p520). *Argyll Robertson pupil* (p79). Classifications may subsume *quaternary* under *tertiary*.[351]

Cardiolipin antibody: Not treponeme-specific. Detectable in primary disease but wanes in late syphilis. Indicates active disease and becomes –ve after treatment. *False +ves* (with –ve treponemal antibody): pregnancy, immunization, pneumonia, malaria, SLE, TB, leprosy. Examples: **Venereal Disease Research Laboratory slide test (VDRL), rapid plasma reagin (RPR), Wassermann reaction (WR).**

Treponeme-specific antibody: Positive in 1° disease, remains so despite treatment. Examples: *T. pallidum* **haemagglutination assay (TPHA), fluorescent treponemal antibody (FTA)**, *T. pallidum* **immobilization test (TPI)**. Non-specific, also +ve in non-venereal yaws, bejel, or pinta. *ELISA:* Syphilis ELISA IgG and ELISA IgM.

Other tests In 1° syphilis, treponemes may be seen by *dark ground microscopy* of chancre fluid; serology at this stage is often –ve. In 2° syphilis, treponemes are seen in the lesions and both types of antibody tests are positive. In late syphilis, organisms may no longer be seen, but both types of antibody test usually remain +ve (cardiolipin antibody tests may wane). In neurosyphilis, CSF antibody tests (particularly FTA and TPHA) are +ve. ►*Look for other STIs.* If HIV+ve, serology may be negative during syphilis reactivation. PCR may help. Do contact tracing.

℞: Simplest regimen: 2–3 doses (one week apart) of **benzathine penicillin** G 1.8g.[352] As this is only available in the UK on a named-patient basis (see *BNF*) an alternative is **procaine penicillin** (=procaine benzylpenicillin) 0.6g–1.2/24h IM for ~28d (17d in early syphilis) + probenecid, eg 500mg/6h (to prevent penicillin loss in urine).[353] Or **doxycycline:** early syphilis, 100mg/12h for 14d; late latent syphilis, 100mg/12h for 28d. Neurosyphilis, **ceftriaxone** (unlicensed) 2g/d IM for 14d. ***If pregnant:*** **erythromycin** 500mg/6h PO (*OTM* dose).

Beware ***Jarisch–Herxheimer reaction:*** T°, pulse↑, and vasodilatation hours after the 1st dose of antibiotic (? from sudden release of endotoxin). Commonest in 2° disease; most dangerous in 3°. Consider steroids. If HIV+ve, penicillin may not stop neurosyphilis; consult microbiologist. ***Congenital syphilis:*** *OHCS* p35.

Viral haemorrhagic (and related) fevers[ND]

Yellow fever: An epidemic arbovirus disease spread by *Aedes* mosquitoes (Brazil, Bolivia, Peru, Central and West Africa). ***Immunization:*** p391. ***Incubation:*** 2–14d. ***The patient:*** In mild forms, fever, headache, nausea, albuminuria, myalgia, and relative bradycardia. If severe: 3 days of headache, myalgia, anorexia ± nausea, then abrupt fever, a brief remission, then prostration, jaundice (± fatty liver), haematemesis, other bleeding, oliguria. ***Mortality:*** <10% (day 5–10). Δ: ELISA. ℞: Symptomatic.

Lassa fever[ND], ***Ebola virus***[ND], ***Marburg virus***[ND], & ***dengue haemorrhagic fever*** (**DHF**—this 'unofficial' haemorrhagic fever is the commonest arbovirus disease).[354] They start with sudden headache, pleuritic pain, backache, myalgia, conjunctivitis, prostration, dehydration, facial flushing (dengue), and T°↑. Bleeding soon supervenes. There may be resolution, or renal failure, encephalitis, coma, and death. ℞: Primarily symptomatic; ribavirin is useful in Lassa fever if given early in disease. ►*Use special infection control measures (Lassa, Ebola, Marburg); get expert help at once.*

Poliomyelitis[ND]

Polio is a highly contagious picornavirus (**fig 1**), though only a few patients develop any illness from the infection. ***Spread:*** Droplet or faeco-oral. ***Incubation:*** 7 days. ***Signs:*** ***Flu prodrome*** for 48h then a ***pre-paralytic stage***: T°↑, pulse↑, headache, vomiting, neck stiffness, and unilateral tremor. In <50% this progresses to a ***paralytic stage:*** myalgia, LMN signs ± respiratory failure. No sensory signs. ***Tests:*** CSF: WCC↑, polymorphs then lymphocytes, otherwise normal; paired sera (14 days apart); throat swab & stool culture identify virus. **ΔΔ**: *Non-viral causes of flaccid paralysis:* Borrelia; mycoplasma; diphtheria; botulism; heavy metals; transverse myelitis; polymyositis. ***Natural history:*** <10% of those with paralysis die. There may be *delayed progression* of paralysis (***post-polio syndrome***, PPS). *Risk of severe paralysis* ↑ *if:* Adulthood; pregnancy; post-tonsillectomy; muscle fatigue/trauma during incubation period. *PPS* causes fatigue, weakness, myalgia, and worsening function, not necessarily at sites originally affected (advise enough exercise to prevent wasting but no so much as to ↑weakness in already damaged muscles). No drug works.[355] ***Vaccine:*** p391.

Rabies[ND]

Rabies is a rhabdovirus spread by bites from an infected mammal, eg bats, dogs, cats, foxes, or raccoons (bites may go unnoticed)[356]. There is slight risk from scratches, or licks to cuts, mouth or eyes. ***The patient:*** ~9–90 days' incubation, so give prophylaxis even several months after exposure. Prodrome: headache, malaise, odd behaviour, agitation, fever, and itch around the bite. Progresses to 'furious rabies', eg with water-provoked muscle spasms often accompanied by terror (hydrophobia). In 20%, 'dumb rabies' starts with flaccid paralysis in the bitten limb. ***Deaths/yr:*** 50,000

Advice in countries not declared rabies-free: Avoid animal contact; get help if bitten. Wash all bites meticulously with soapy water (takes 20min and ↓incidence by ~65%). ***Pre-exposure prophylaxis*** (vets, zoo-keepers, customs workers, bat handlers, travellers in rabies area for >1 month or at especial risk, or if access to post-exposure treatment is problematic): give human diploid cell strain vaccine (1mL IM, deltoid) on days 0, 7, & 28, and again at 2–3yrs if still at risk. ***Treatment if bitten where rabies is endemic*** (if unvaccinated): wash as above. ►Seek help (*Health Protection Agency, tel.:* UK020 8200 6868). Watch the biting animal to see if it dies (but it is possible that it may not die of rabies before the patient does).[357] ***If previously immunized:*** give vaccine (1mL IM) on days 0 & 3. ***If previously unimmunized:*** give vaccine on days 0, 3, 7, 14, and 30 and rabies immunoglobulin (RIG, 20U/kg on day 0; ½ given IM and ½ infiltrated around wounds). HRIG is probably unnecessary > a week after vaccination has started, as an active antibody response has already begun. ►Never mix vaccine and antiserum or inject in the same limb.[358] Rabies is 'always' fatal once symptoms start (survival has occurred, with optimal CNS/cardiorespiratory support). Vaccinate attending staff. ***Public health:*** Wherever rabies is a problem, put it on the national curriculum, along with dog-handling.[359] Philippines success story Make houses bat-proof.

Dengue fever (DF) and dengue haemorrhagic fever (DHF)

There is a global pandemic of this RNA flavivirus, related to poor vector control (*Aedes* mosquitoes), urbanization,[1] poor waste disposal, and rapid migrations bringing new strains (DEN-2) which become more virulent in those who have had mild dengue. Global warming is also important: a temperature rise of 1-3° increases transmission, leading to an extra 25,000 cases/yr. [WHO data] Incidence: 50-100×10⁶/yr; 250,000-500,000/yr get DHF.[2]

Infants typically have a simple febrile illness with a rash. Older children/adults have flushes (face, neck, chest) ± centrifugal maculopapular rash from day 3, or late confluent petechiae with round pale areas of normal skin ± headache, arthralgia, jaundice; hepatosplenomegaly; anuria. ***Haemorrhagic signs:*** (Unlikely if AST normal).[360] Petechiae, GI, gum or nose bleeds, haematuria; menorrhagia.

Monitor: BP; urine flow; WCC↓; platelets↓; PCV; +ve tourniquet test (>20 petechiae/inch^2) + PCV↑ by 20% are telling signs (rapid endothelial plasma leak is the key pathophysiology of DHF). **ΔΔ:** Chikungunya,[2] measles, leptospirosis, typhoid, malaria. ***Exclusion:*** If symptoms start >2wks after leaving a dengue area, or if fever lasts >2wks, dengue can be 'ruled out'. **℞:** Supportive. Prompt IV resuscitation, eg Ringer's lactate. ➡If shocked (mortality 40%), give a bolus of 15mL/kg; repeat every ½h until BP rises, and urine flow at >30mL/h.[361]

Polio: a tantalising exercise in prevention and (near) eradication

Eradication makes economic and humanitarian sense, even if it costs US$billions.[362]

- Pre-1950s, polio distribution was worldwide. In 1952, during an epidemic in Copenhagen, the cause of death was established as CO_2 retention. Mechanical ventilation began in special centres—the birth of intensive care units.[363]
- 12 April 1955: vaccination starts with Salk's inactivated vaccine.
- 1958: Sabin donated his 3 attenuated strains to Chumakov in Moscow, who produced the 3 vaccines, giving them to 15 million people in 1 year.
- 1960s: the 3 vaccines were mixed, to produce a single oral polio vaccine (OPV).
- 1988: Estimated 350,000 cases worldwide, occurring in 125 countries. The Global Polio Eradication Initiative, aiming to protect children worldwide through vaccination, is launched; the aim was eradication by the year 2000.
- 1991: Transmission interrupted in the West.
- 1993: China starts national immunization days; >80,000,000 vaccinated in 2 days; in 1994 only 5 cases of virus-confirmed wild polio.
- 1994: WHO declares the Americas polio-free.
- 1997: 1 case of wild polio in all of Europe.
- 1999: Only 7090 cases worldwide.
- 2000: WHO declares Western Pacific polio-free.
- 2001: 483 cases in 10 endemic countries.
- 2002: WHO declares Europe polio-free.
- 2004: 6 polio-endemic countries remain.[364]

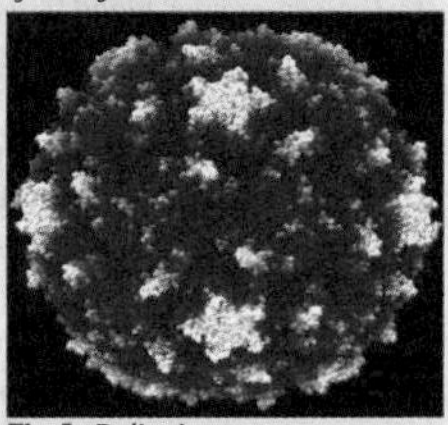

Fig 1. Poliovirus ©D Belnap (Utah Univ.) & J Hogle (Harvard Univ.)

- 2006: Transmission re-established in: Nigeria, Sudan, Egypt, Central African Republic, Mali, Côte D'Ivoire, Somalia, Burkina Faso, Uttar Pradesh.[365] [366]
- 2008: 1655 cases in 17 countries, 1491 in the 4 endemic countries (Nigeria, Afghanistan, India, and Pakistan).[367] OPV proves insufficient to ensure eradication.

Before 2005 most cases in the West were adult contacts of child vaccinees; these cases have stopped as live vaccine has been replaced by inactivated vaccine.

NB: Sabin viruses and their genetic revertants can cause chronic infection in immunodeficient people, who may shed neurovirulent virus in faeces for years. So programmes of oral vaccination should not continue one day longer than necessary to eliminate disease caused by wild virus.

1 Cities high in the Andes are free of dengue, as *Aedes* mosquitos cannot survive high altitudes.
2 Haemorrhagic features in Chikungunya virus infections are rare; arthralgia, fever, myalgia and a rash are more common, eg in Indian Ocean Islands.

Q fever is caused by *Coxiella burnetii* (100 cases/yr in the UK). It is so named because it was first labelled 'query' fever in workers in an Australian abattoir.

Epidemiology: Occurs worldwide, and is usually rural, with reservoirs in cattle and sheep. The organism is resistant to drying and is usually inhaled from infected dust. It can be contracted from unpasteurized milk, directly from carcasses in abattoirs, sometimes by droplet spread, and rarely from tick bites.

Clinical features Suspect Q fever in anyone with a PUO or atypical pneumonia. It may present with fever, myalgia, sweats, headache, cough, and hepatitis (± splenomegaly).[368] If the disease becomes chronic, suspect endocarditis (typically 'culture-negative'). This usually affects the aortic valve, but clinical signs may be absent. It also causes miscarriages and CNS infection.

Tests: CXR may show consolidation, eg multilobar or slowly resolving. Liver function tests may be hepatitic and biopsy may show granulomata. Diagnosis is serological: indirect immunofluorescence assay (IFA) is the most dependable and widely used method. Increased IgG and IgA antibodies to phase I are often indicative of Q fever endocarditis.[369] Phase I antigens suggest chronic infection; phase II antigens suggest acute infection. PCR may be used on tissue samples. CSF tests may be needed.

Treatment: Get expert microbiological help. *Acute:* Doxycycline 100mg/12h PO for 2–3wks. Minocycline, clarithromycin, ciprofloxacin (in pregnancy) and co-trimoxazole are used. *Q fever endocarditis:* Treatment is difficult, eg doxycycline plus hydroxychloroquine, eg 600mg/d PO for at least 18 months ± valve replacement.[370]

Prevention: Vaccination for those whose occupation places them at high risk.

Bartonellosis is caused by *Bartonella bacilliformis*, a Gram -ve, motile, bacillus-like organism which parasitizes RBCs. Spread is by sandflies in the Andes, Peru, Ecuador, Colombia, Thailand, and Niger. Transient immunosuppression leads to other infections (eg Salmonella). *Incubation:* 10–210 days (mean=60d).

Signs: Fever, rashes, lymphadenopathy, hepatosplenomegaly, jaundice, cerebellar syndromes, dermal nodules (verrucas), retinal haemorrhages, myocarditis, pericardial effusion, oedema, and rarely, meningo-encephalomyelitis.

Tests: Giemsa-stained blood films. Blood culture (prolonged). Coombs' -ve haemolytic anaemia, and hypochromic, macrocytic red cells with a megaloblastic marrow. CSF pleocytosis. Serological tests are not widely available.

Treatment: Responds to penicillin, but ciprofloxacin (500mg/12h PO for 10d) is often used because of frequent association with salmonelloses. Steroids may be indicated if there is severe neurological involvement.

Trench fever is caused by *Bartonella quintana* inoculated from infected louse faeces, not only in soldiers, but also in the homeless, and in alcoholics.

Clinical features: Fever, headache, myalgia, dizziness, back pain, macular rash, eye pain, leg pain, splenomegaly, endocarditis (rare). In HIV-infected patients, the sk

in lesions may resemble Kaposi's sarcoma. It is not fatal; it may relapse.

Tests: Blood culture, serology, PCR. ℞: Doxycycline 100mg/12h PO for 15 days.

Ehrlichiosis is caused by *Ehrlichia chaffeensis*, an obligate intracytoplasmic Gram -ve organism, related to Rickettsia. It is spread by ticks. It causes fever, headache, anorexia, malaise, abdominal pain, epigastric pain, conjunctivitis, lymphadenopathy, jaundice, rash, confusion, and cervical lymphadenopathy.

Tests: Leucopenia, thrombocytopenia, AST↑.[371] Serology/PCR are diagnostic.

Treatment: May respond to doxycycline 100mg/12h PO for 7–14d.

Typhus: the archetypal rickettsial disease

Rickettsiae are parasitic bacteria that are obligate intracellular parasites; they are bigger than viruses but smaller than classical bacteria. They are carried by host arthropods (**figs 1-3**) and invade human mononuclear cells, neutrophils, or blood vessel endothelium ('vasculotropic'). All the cataclysmic events of the last century (war, revolution, flood, famine, genocide, and overcrowding) have favoured lice infestation. As a result, Rickettsiae (especially typhus) have killed untold millions.

Pathology Widespread vasculitis and endothelial proliferation may affect any organ and thrombotic occlusion may lead to gangrene.

Signs ►*Think of typhus in all travellers or inhabitants of endemic areas who seem to have septicaemia, but have –ve blood cultures.*[372] Incubation: 2–23d. Infection may be mild/asymptomatic or severe/systemic, with sudden fever, frontal headache, confusion, and jaundice. With some species, an *eschar* (dark crusty ulcer at the site of a bite) is found. A rickettsial rash may be macular, papular, petechial, or haemorrhagic. Tests: haemolysis, neutrophilia, thrombocytopenia, clotting↓, hepatitis, renal impairment. Patients die of shock, renal failure, DIC (p346), or stroke.
Epidemic typhus (*R. prowazeki*): *Spread:* human lice *Pediculus humanus* (**fig 1**; faeces are inhaled or pass through skin). It may recrudesce decades later (Brill-Zinsser disease). The rash is truncal, then peripheral (opposite to *R. rickettsii*).
Rocky Mountain spotted fever (*R. rickettsii*) is tick-borne (**fig 2**). Endemic in Rocky Mountains & south-eastern USA. The rash (seen in 90%) begins as macules on hands/feet, spreading and becoming petechial or haemorrhagic in 50%.
Tick typhus (*R. conorii*; Mediterranean spotted fever/boutonneuse; African tick bite fever, Marseilles fever, Indian/Israeli tick typhus) is the chief imported rickettsial disease in the UK (endemic in Africa, the Mediterranean area, eg Croatia, and parts of Asia; sporadic in Laos, Korea, etc). Vector example: **fig 3**. The rash starts in the axillae, becoming purpuric as it spreads. *Other signs*: Conjunctival suffusion; jaundice; deranged clotting; meningoencephalitis; cerebritis;[373] renal failure.
Scrub typhus (*Orienta tsutsugamushi*) Most common in SE Asia. Signs: Eschar from chigger bite (75%); hepatomegaly (65%); cough (60%); lymphadenopathy (46%);[374] tachypnoea (35%); constipation (25%); abdominal pain (20%); oedema (20%); splenomegaly (15%); vomiting (15%); rash (15%); petechiae (5%); sudden deafness.[375] CXR: bilateral infiltrations (85%).[376] Blood: LFT↑ (90%); platelets↓ (80%); neutrophilia (60%); lymphocytosis ± atypical lymphocytosis (5%). Complications: pneumonia ± pulmonary oedema, meningitis, and shock.
Murine (endemic) typhus (*R. typhi*) is spread by fleas from rats to humans. It is more prevalent in warm, coastal ports (eg Dalmatia, Laos).[377]
Rickettsialpox (*R. akari*) Variegate rash: macular, papular, or vesicular.
Mediterranean spotted fever (*R. conorii*): meningoencephalitis; cerebellitis.[378]

Diagnosis This is difficult as often the picture is non-specific, the organisms are difficult to grow, and traditional heterophil antibody Weil–Felix tests are insensitive and nonspecific. A rise in antibody titre in paired sera is diagnostic. Latex agglutination, indirect immunofluorescence, ELISAs and PCR are available (may be done on the eschar).[379] An accurate, rapid dotblot immunoassay is available for scrub typhus. Skin biopsy may be diagnostic in Rocky Mountain spotted fever.

Treatment Doxycycline 100mg/12h PO/IV for 7d (or 48h after T° normal) **or** chloramphenicol 500mg/6h PO for 10–14d. Resistance has been reported in Thailand. Azithromycin 500mg (1 dose) may work in tick and scrub typhus.[380]

Poor prognostic factors Older age, male, Black, G6PD deficiency.

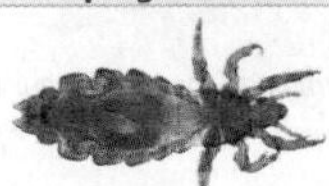

Fig 1. *Pediculus humanus*: endemic typhus vector.

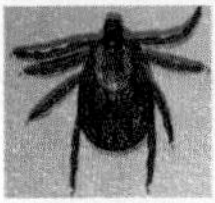

Fig 2. *Dermacentor variabilis* is a vector for Rocky Mountain spotted fever.

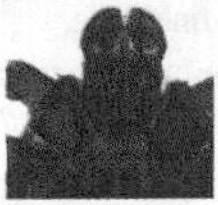

Fig 3. Dog tick
Figs 1-3 courtesy of Prof S Upton, Kansas Univ.

Some gastrointestinal protozoa

Giardia lamblia (**fig 1**) is a flagellate protozoon, which lives in the duodenum and jejunum. Spread: faecal–oral (↑ risk if eg immunosuppression, travel, anal sex, achlorhydria, playgroups,[382] and swimming)—or from pets or birds. Drinking water may be contaminated.

The patient: Giardiasis is often asymptomatic. Lassitude, bloating, flatulence, abdominal pain, loose stools ± explosive diarrhoea are typical. Malabsorption, weight loss, and lactose intolerance may occur.

Diagnosis: Direct fluorescent antibody (DFA) assay is considered the gold standard by many labs.[383] Repeated stool microscopy for cysts and trophozoites may be -ve. Duodenal fluid analysis (aspiration or absorption on to a piece of swallowed string, eg Enterotest®) may be tried, or ELISA/PCR or therapeutic trial. **ΔΔ:** Any cause of diarrhoea (p388, p390, p410), tropical sprue (p280), coeliac (p280). **℞:** Scrupulous hygiene. Tinidazole 2g PO stat (avoid alcohol); if pregnant, paromomycin 500mg/6h PO for 7d. If treatment fails, check for compliance and consider treating *all* the family. If diarrhoea persists, avoid milk as lactose intolerance may persist for 6wks.

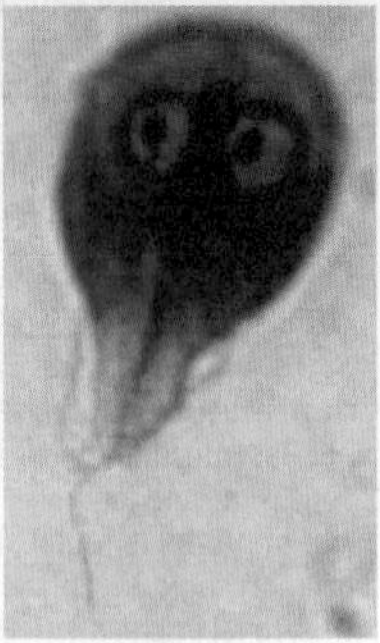

Fig 1. Giardia: the only diplomonadid to trouble us.[381]

Entamoeba histolytica (amoebiasis; see **figs 2-5**) occurs worldwide. Spread: faecal–oral. Boil water and infected food to destroy cysts. Trophozoites may remain in the bowel or invade extra-intestinal tissues, leaving 'flask-shaped' GI ulcers. Presentation may be asymptomatic, with mild diarrhoea or with severe amoebic dysentery.

Amoebic dysentery[ND] may occur some time after initial infection. Diarrhoea begins slowly, becoming profuse & bloody. An acute febrile prostrating illness can occur but high fever, colic, and tenesmus are rare. May remit and relapse. ***Diagnosis:*** stool microscopy shows trophozoites, blood, and pus cells. Faecal antigen detection may also be useful. Serology indicates previous or current infection and may be unhelpful in acute infection. **ΔΔ:** *Non-pathogenic amoebae* (eg *Entamoeba dispar*) are common in the tropics (cysts are indistinguishable). *Bacillary dysentery* often starts suddenly; it may cause dehydration. Stools are more watery. *Acute ulcerative colitis* has a more gradual onset and the stools are very bloody. For other causes of bloody diarrhoea, see p426 & p246.

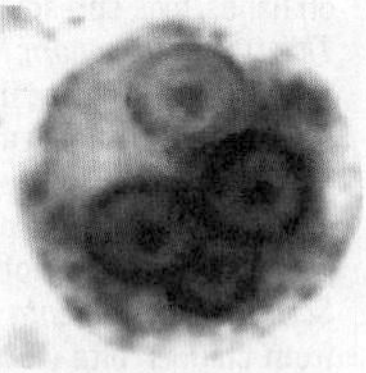

Fig 2. *E. histolytica* cyst with an endosome inside each of its 4 nuclei.[384]

Amoebic colonic abscess may perforate causing peritonitis.

Amoebomas are inflammatory masses, eg in the caecum (a cause of RIF masses).

Amoebic liver abscess is usually a single mass in the right lobe, and contains 'anchovy-sauce' pus. There is usually a high swinging fever, sweats, RUQ pain, and tenderness. WCC↑. LFT normal or ↑ (cholestatic). 50% have no history of amoebic dysentery. ***Diagnosis:*** ultrasound/CT ± aspiration; positive serology.

℞: Metronidazole 800mg/8h PO for 5d for acute amoebic dysentery (active against vegetative amoebae), then diloxanide furoate 500mg/8h PO for 10d to destroy gut cysts (SEs rare). Diloxanide is also best for chronic disease when *Entamoeba* cysts, not vegetative forms, are in stools. Amoebic liver abscess or severe infections: tinidazole 2g/24h for 5d; aspirate if no improvement within a few days; give diloxanide post-tinidazole.

Other GI protozoa *Cryptosporidium* (p390), *Microsporidium* and *Isospora* (occur in AIDS, p410), *Balantidium coli*, and *Sarcocyscocystis*.

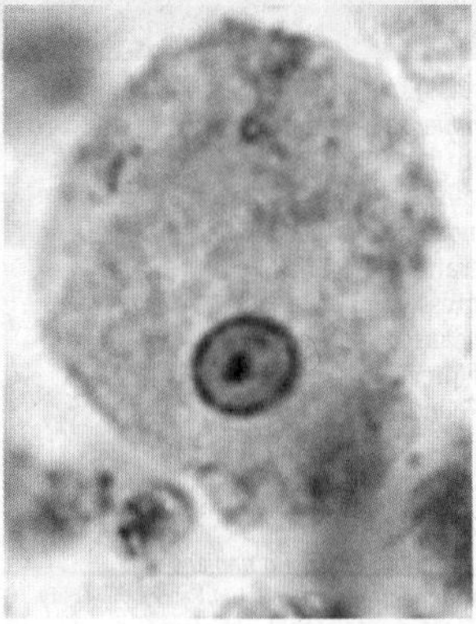

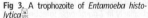

Fig 3. A trophozoite of *Entamoeba histolytica*.[385]

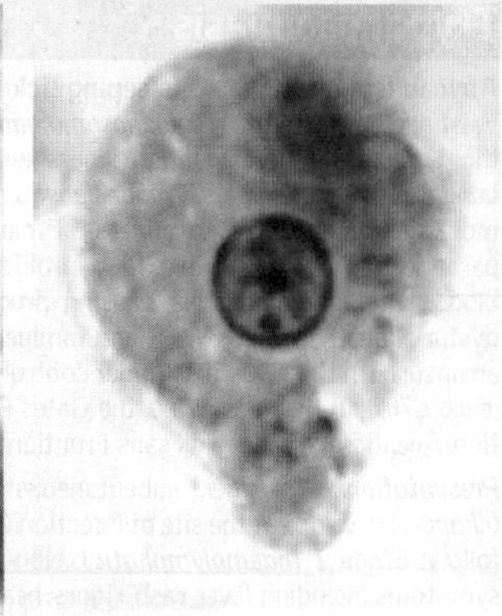

Fig 4. Another trophozoite of *Entamoeba histolytica*.[386]

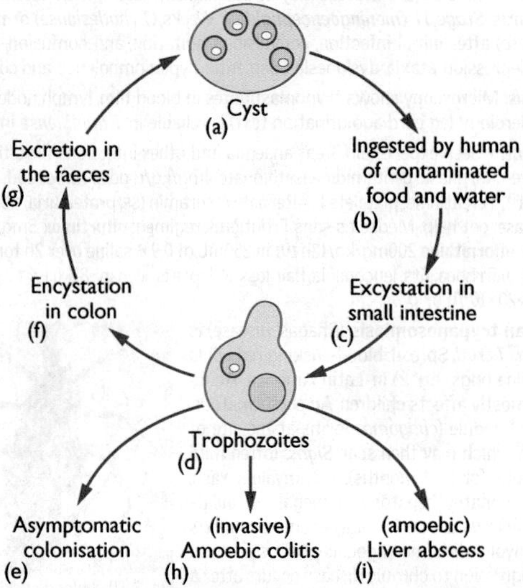

Fig 5. The life cycle of *Entamoeba histolytica* is in 2 stages: cysts and trophozoites. Cysts (10–15μm across) typically contain 4 nuclei; they are spread by ingesting faecally contaminated food or water. During excystation in the gut lumen, nuclear division is followed by cytoplasmic division, giving rise to 8 trophozoites. Trophozoites (10–50μm across) contain one nucleus with a central karyosome; they live in the caecum and colon. ~90% of individuals infected with *E. histolytica* are asymptomatic. Re-encystation of the trophozoites occurs in the colon, and excretion of cysts in faeces perpetuates the life cycle. Alternatively, trophozoites invade colonic epithelium, causing amoebic colitis (in ~10%).

E. histolytica can spread haematogenously after breaching colon epithelium and can establish persistent extra-intestinal infection (eg amoebic liver abscess).[387]

Figs 1–4 courtesy of Prof S Upton, Kansas University. Fig 5 is adapted with permission from *Expert Reviews in Molecular Medicine*, CUP, 1999; www-ermm.cbcu.cam.ac.uk/99000617h.htm.

African trypanosomiasis (sleeping sickness) In West and Central Africa, ***Trypanosoma gambiense*** **(fig 1)** causes a slow, wasting illness with long latency. In East Africa, ***T. rhodesiense*** causes a more rapidly progressive illness. Trypanosome parasites, spread by tsetse flies, proliferate in blood, lymphatics, and CNS, causing progressive dysfunction, then death. Wars and famine caused an upsurge in the 1990s, now under control (prevalence ≤70,000) thanks to WHO, the Gates Foundation, Aventis, and Médecins sans Frontières.[389]

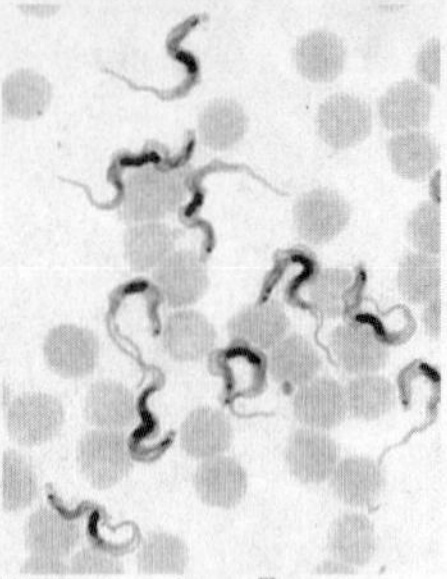

Fig 1. *T. gambiense*[388]
©Prof. S Upton, Kansas University

Presentation: A tender, subcutaneous nodule (*chancre*) develops at the site of infection. 2 stages follow: ***Stage I (haemolymphatic):*** Non-specific symptoms including fever, rash, rigors, headaches, hepatosplenomegaly, lymphadenopathy, and joint pains. Winterbottom's sign (posterior cervical nodes↑) is a reliable sign, particularly in *T. gambiense* infections. In *T. rhodesiense* infections, this stage may be particularly severe, with potentially fatal myocarditis. ***Stage II (meningoencephalitic):*** Weeks (*T. rhodesiense*) or months (*T. gambiense*) after initial infection, convulsions, agitation, and confusion—and then apathy, depression, ataxia, dyskinesias, dementia, hypersomnolence, and coma occur.

Diagnosis: Microscopy shows trypomastigotes in blood film, lymph node aspirate, or CSF. Serology (eg card agglutination text) is reliable in *T. gambiense* infections.

Treatment: ►Seek expert help. Treat anaemia and other infections first; then: Early (pre-CNS) phase: pentamidine isethionate 4mg/kg/d deep IM for 10d. SE: WCC↓, ↓BP, ↓Ca^{2+}, ↑creatinine, platelets↓. Alternative: suramin (SE: proteinuria, ↑creatinine). CNS disease: get help. Médecins sans Frontières regimen: **nifurtimox** 5mg/kg/8h PO for 10d + **eflornithine** 200mg/kg/12h IVI in 250mL of 0.9% saline over 2h for 7d.[390] SE: anaemia, diarrhoea, fits, leucopenia, hair loss. Relapse is seen in ~8% (risk↑ if CSF leucocytosis $>20\times10^9$/L or ♂).[391]

American trypanosomiasis (Chagas' disease) is caused by ***T. cruzi***. Spread: blood-sucking reduviids (triatomine bugs, **fig 2**) in Latin America. Acute disease mostly affects children. An erythematous, indurated nodule (*chagoma*) forms at the site of infection which may then scar. ***Signs:*** (often mild or insidious for 1st 2 months): T°↑, myalgia, rash, lymphadenopathy, hepatosplenomegaly ± unilateral conjunctivitis ± periorbital oedema (*Romaña's sign*) ± myocarditis/meningoencephalitis. In up to 30%, progression to chronic disease occurs after a latency of eg 20yrs. Multiorgan invasion causes megaoesophagus (dysphagia, aspiration), megacolon (abdominal distension, constipation) ± dilated cardiomyopathy (p146); CNS lesions, eg if immunosuppressed (HIV, lymphoma). **Δ:** (no gold standard): *Acute disease:* trypomastigotes seen in or grown from blood, CSF, or lymph node aspirate. *Chronic disease:* serology (Chagas' IgG ELISA).

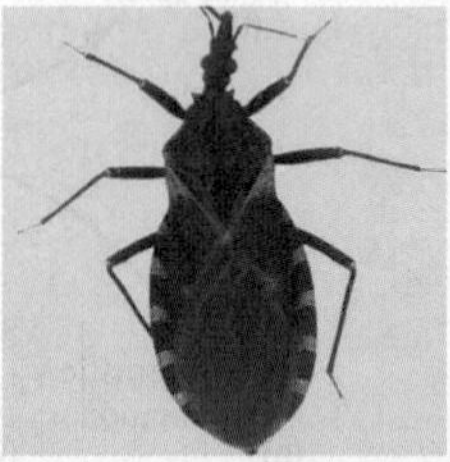

Fig 2. The blood-sucking vector (*Triatoma*) hides in thatch or cracks in walls (rural & urban). Transmission occurs when its faeces are rubbed into a wound or mucous membrane (or via infected blood). Vector control: spray buildings.[392]
©Prof. S Upton, Kansas University

Treatment: Unsatisfactory. **Nifurtimox** 2mg/kg/6h PO pc for 120d or **benznidazole** (2.5–3.5mg/kg/12h PO for 60d) in acute disease (toxic, and eliminate parasites in ≤50%). Chronic disease can only be treated symptomatically. Surgery may be tried. ***Prevention:*** Better housing, spraying houses with insecticides.

Leishmaniasis

Leishmania are protozoa (**fig 1**, inset, with 2 RBCs, from a spleen aspirate) that cause granulomata. They are spread by sandflies and occur in Africa, India, Latin America, the Middle East, and Mediterranean. Clinical effects reflect: **1** The ability of each species to induce or suppress the immune response, to metastasize, and to invade cartilage, and **2** the efficiency of our own immune response. *L. major*, is the most immunogenic and allergenic of cutaneous Old World *Leishmania*, and causes most necrosis. *L. tropica* is less immunogenic and causes less inflamed, slow-healing sores with relapsing lesions and a tuberculoid histology.

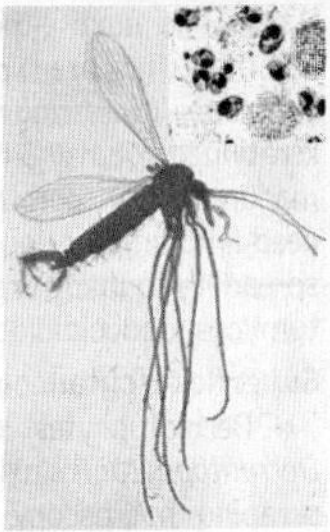

Fig 1. Sandfly.[393]
©Prof S Upton, Kasas Uni.

Cutaneous leishmaniasis (oriental sore) affects >300,000 people eg in Africa, India, and S. America; caused by *L. mexicana*, *L. major*, *L. tropica* or *L. amazonensis*.[394] Lesions develop at the bite site, beginning as an itchy papule; crusts fall off to leave an ulcer (*Chiclero's ulcer*). Most heal in ~2 (Old World disease) to 15 months, with scarring (disfiguring if extensive). *L. mexicana* may cause pinna destruction (*Chiclero's ear*). **Δ:** Microscopy and culture of aspiration from the base of the ulcer.[395] **℞:** May only be needed if unhealed by 6 months or lesion >4cm across (or multiple). Get help. Pentavalent antimony eg **meglumine antimoniate** (Glucantime) or **sodium stibogluconate** (Pentostam); 20mg/kg/d for 10d. **Pentamidine isethionate** 2mg/kg IM every other day for 7d. **Amphotericin B** (if antimony fails); 1mg/kg/day IV for 20 days.[396]

Mucocutaneous leishmaniasis (*L. brasiliensis*) occurs in S America. Primary skin lesions may spread to the mucosa of the nose, pharynx, palate, larynx, and upper lip and cause severe scarring. Nasopharyngeal lesions are called *espundia*. **Δ:** As parasites may be scanty, a Leishmanin skin test may be needed to distinguish the condition from leprosy, TB, syphilis, yaws, and cancer. Indirect fluorescent antibody tests and PCR tests are available. **℞:** Sodium stibogluconate (below). Treatment is unsatisfactory once mucosae are involved, so treat all cutaneous lesions early.

Visceral leishmaniasis (VL) (kala-azar, means black sickness) is the 2nd most deadly parasitic disease in the world following malaria (50000 deaths/year).[397] It occurs in Asia, Africa, S America, and the Mediterranean. Cause: *L. donovani*, *L. chagasi*, or *L. infantum* (or rarely, 'visceralizing' of *L. tropica*).[398] Incubation: months to years. Protozoa spread via lymphatics from minor skin lesions and multiply in macrophages of the reticuloendothelial system (Leishman-Donovan bodies). There are 30 subclinical cases for every overt case. ♀:♂>3:1. It can be HIV-associated. ***Signs:*** Dry, warty, hyperpigmented skin lesions; T°↑; sweats; burning feet; arthralgia; cough; epistaxis; abdo pain; splenomegaly (96%); hepatomegaly (63%); lymphadenopathy; emaciation; pancytopenia, hypergammaglobulinemia. **Δ:**[399] ***Microscopic exam*** of lymph nodes, bone marrow or spleen are confirmatory. ***Ab-detection:*** Indirect fluorescence antibody (IFA), ELISA, western blot, direct agglutination test (DAT) and rK39-based immunochromatographic test (ICT). Serology has 2 limitations: **1** Ab levels remain detectable for several years after cure. Therefore, VL relapse cannot be diagnosed by serology. **2** Tests are +ve in a significant number of healthy individuals in endemic areas with no history of VL. Serology may be –ve if HIV+ve. ***Ag-detection:*** detects a heat-stable Ag by latex agglutination. **℞:**[400] **Sodium stibogluconate**: 20mg/kg/24h IV/IM, up to 850mg/d, for 28d or **meglumine antimoniate** or **liposomal amphoterin B** (1st-line drug in Europe and USA), **miltefosine** (1st effective oral drug for VL; 0.75–1.2mg/kg/12h PO for 28d). There are increasing cases of antimony-resistant strains of *L. donovani* in some endemic regions (esp India).[401] **Amphotericin B** has shown promising results in this group.[402] Combination therapy (eg **sodium stibogluconate + paromomycin**) results in ↑ efficacy, ↓drug resistance, and ↓treatment duration. SE: arrhythmias and acute pancreatitis. ***Post kala-azar dermal leishmaniasis*** may occur months or years following successful treatment; lesions resemble leprosy.

Pathogenic fungi either produce toxins or allergic reactions. They are *superficial* (pityriasis versicolor), *cutaneous* (tinea/ringworm; intertrigo; restricted to keratinized skin, hair & nails), *subcutaneous* (mycetoma; madura foot or sporotrichosis; ℞ is complex and may need limb amputation)—or *systemic* (from the lung, spreading to many organs (eg histoplasmosis; blastomycosis; coccidioidomycosis; fungal meningitis).

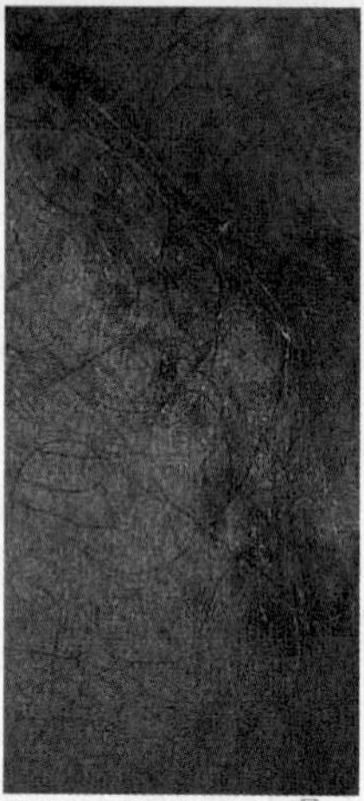

Fig 1. Candida intertrigo.[403]

Superficial/cutaneous mycoses ***Candida*** **(figs 1** & 3). Dermatophytes (*Trichophyton, Microsporum, Dermatophyton)* cause tinea (ringworm). **Δ**: Skin scraping microscopy. ℞: Topical clotrimazole 1%. Continue for 14d after healing. If intractable, try itraconazole (100–200mg/24h PO for 7d if eGFR >80; SE: D&V; CCF), terbinafine (250mg/24h PO for 4wks) or griseofulvin 0.5–1g/24h (SE: agranulocytosis↓; SLE). *Malassezia furfur* causes pityriasis versicolor: a macular rash which appears brown on pale skin and pale on tanned skin. **Δ**: Microscopy of skin scrapings under Wood's light. ℞: Ketoconazole cream (2%) or selenium shampoo used as a lotion; leave on for 30min (alternate days for 14d).

Systemic mycoses *Aspergillus fumigatus* may precipitate asthma, allergic bronchopulmonary aspergillosis (ABPA), or cause aspergilloma (p160). Pneumonia and invasive aspergillosis occur if immunosuppressed. There is evidence that **voriconazole** is better than **amphotericin B** in invasive aspergillosis,[404] especially in cerebral aspergillosis.[405] Systemic candidiasis also occurs in the immunocompromised: consider this *whenever* they get a PUO, eg *Candida* UTI in DM or as a rare cause of prosthetic valve endocarditis. Do repeated blood cultures. If infection does not resolve when the predisposing factor (eg IV line) is removed, the treatment is **amphotericin B** IV (p168) or, if not neutropenic, **fluconazole** 400mg stat then 200mg/d PO, halved if eGFR <50. **Caspofungin** (70mg/d IVI if >80kg on day 1, then 50mg/d) is an alternative.[406]
Cryptococcus neoformans causes meningitis or pneumonia. It is commonest in the immunocompromised, eg AIDS, sarcoid, Hodgkin's, or steroid ℞. The history may be long. Look for signs of ICP↑, eg confusion, papilloedema, cranial nerve lesions. **Δ**: Indian ink CSF stain; blood culture. Cryptococcal antigen is detected in CSF and blood by latex tests. ℞: It may be necessary to ↓CSF pressure by ~50% by removing CSF. *Non-AIDS meningitis:* Amphotericin B 0.7mg/kg/d IV + flucytosine 25mg/kg/6h PO for 2wks then fluconazole 200mg/d PO for 8wks. *AIDS meningitis:* As above, but continue fluconazole 400mg/d PO for 10wks, then 200mg/d PO until CD4 >200 for >6 months (or life-long). *Non-CNS infections* (AIDS or non-AIDS): do LP to rule out meningitis, then treat with fluconazole, itraconazole or flucytosine.[407] Prophylaxis with fluconazole 200mg/d PO is needed until CD4 >150 × 10^6/L and cryptococcal antigen –ve (p410).

New World and Africa fungi causing deep infection: Histoplasma, *Coccidioides immitis, Paracoccidioides brasiliensis* & *Blastomyces dermatitidis* may be asymptomatic or cause acute/chronic lung disease, or disseminated infection. Histoplasma pneumonitis: arthralgia, erythema nodosum (**fig 1**, p565), and multiforme (p565). Chronic disease causes upper-zone fibrosis ± CXR coin lesions. **Δ**: CXR, serology, culture, biopsy. ℞: *Histoplasmosis:* 1 week's methylprednisolone (0.5 mg/kg/d) + **amphotericin B** 0.7mg/kg/d IV, eg if HIV+ve & severe; liposomal form may be better (+less renal failure), then **itraconazole** 200mg/8–12h PO for 12wks. *Paracoccidioides:* **Itraconazole** 200mg/d PO for >26wks. *Blastomycosis:* **Itraconazole**.

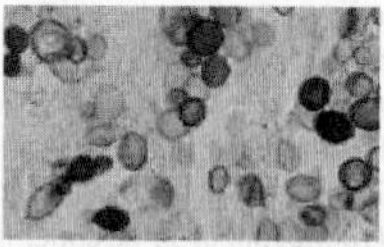

Fig 2. Histoplasma ×1000.[408]

Candida on ITU: colonization→invasion→dissemination

Not everyone with +ve yeast cultures needs treating: *Candida* is a common commensal on skin, pharynx, or vagina (p238; p418) but in some contexts (see MINIBOX) or if many sites are colonized (surgical drains, urine ± sputum), risk of invasion is high.[409] *Invasion* implies fungus in normally sterile tissues. *Dissemination* involves infection of remote organs via the blood (eg endophthalmitis + fungi in lung or kidney). Consider IV amphotericin (p440) or fluconazole (alternative: caspofungin) in at-risk circumstances (see MINIBOX—especially if your patient is deteriorating):[410]

Risk of dissemination↑ if:
- Prolonged ventilation
- Broad-spectrum antibiotics
- Urinary catheters
- Immunosuppression
- Intravascular lines
- IV nutrition

- A single well-taken +ve blood culture—if risk factors present (above).
- Isolation of *Candida* from any sterile site except urine.
- Yeasts on microscopy on a sterile-site specimen, before cultures are known.
- Positive histology from normally sterile tissues in those at risk (above).
- Removal/change of IV lines is essential in patients with candidaemia.

►Consult an ID physician/microbiologist before starting systemic antifungals.

Preventing fungal infections if immunocompromised Fluconazole 50–400mg/24h after cytotoxics or radiotherapy, preferably started before onset of neutropenia, and continued for 1 week after WCC returns to normal.

Facts of life for budding mycologists (figs 1–8)[1]

To the uninitiated, fungi are like bacteria, but their chitin cell walls and their knack of mitosis puts them in their own kingdom. They are larger than bacteria (eg 8μm across), and mostly reproduce by budding of germ tubes (**fig 4**), not by fission.

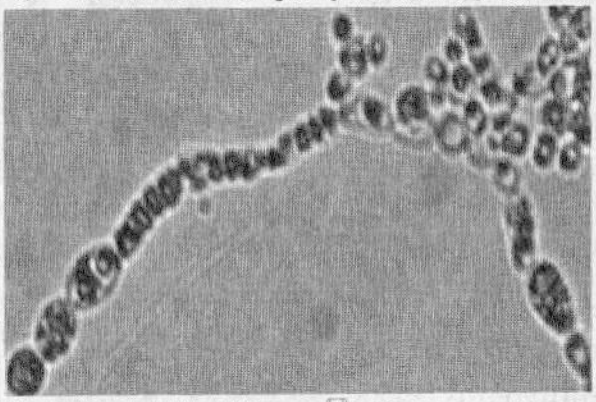

Fig 3. *Candida albicans.*[411] Some yeasts can be dimorphic: single cells at 37°C but forming structures called mycelia, containing fruiting bodies (hyphae), at room temperature.

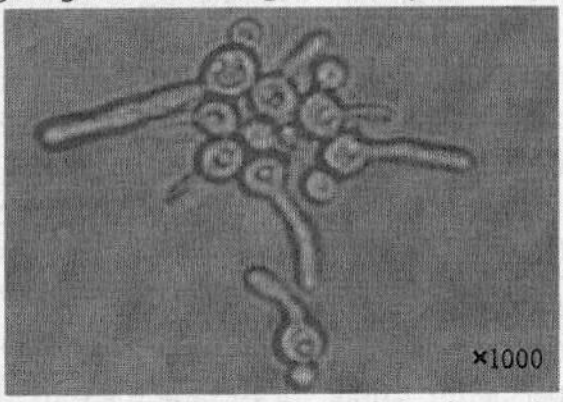

Fig 4. Germ tubes emerging from dimorphic *Candida albicans* blastospores.[412]

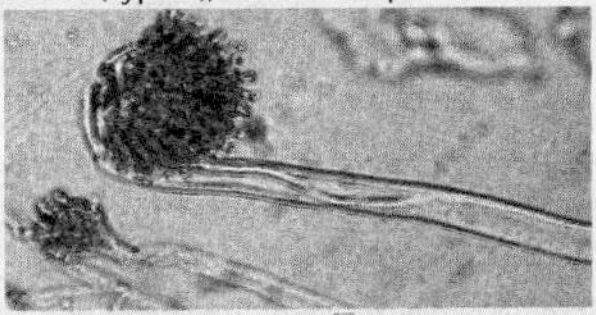

Fig 5. *Aspergillus niger.*[413] If spores are inhaled, aspergillosis can occur (rare, p169).[414] If HIV +ve, bone or eye infection may occur.

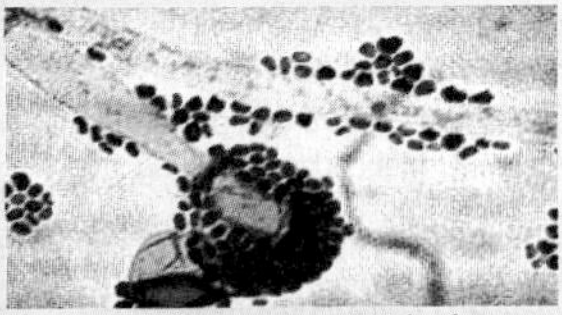

Fig 6. Mucor blastospores. Think of mucormycosis in diabetics with black pus in the nose ± proptosis/sinusitis or pneumonia. ℞: amphotericin B; posaconazole.[415]

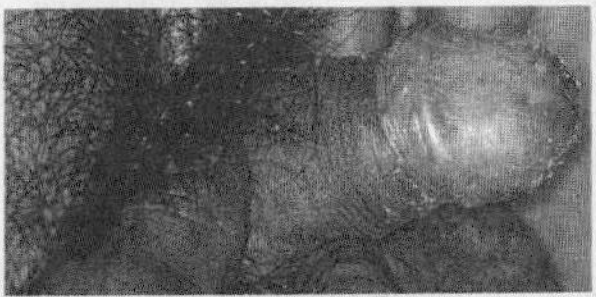

Fig 7. Candida of the glans.[416]

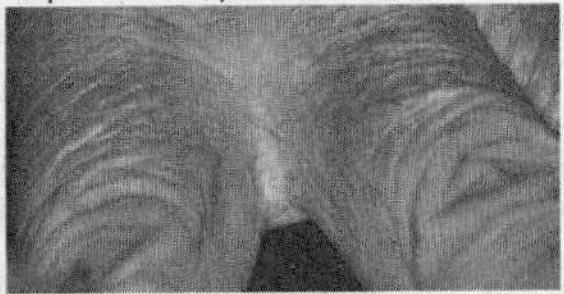

Fig 8. Web-space candida.[417]

1 Images courtesy of A Huntley (figs 1, 5 & 8), Subhash Mohan (fig 2) & P-Y Guillaume (figs 3, 4, 6 & 7).

1 billion people are hosts to nematodes (give or take a few hundred million[418]). Many live with us quite peacefully (even helpfully); but ascariasis can cause GI obstruction, hookworms can stunt growth, necatoriasis can cause anaemia, and trichuriasis causes dysentery/rectal prolapse. Mass use of albendazole 400mg/24h PO for 3d to school children or immigrants from endemic areas may be beneficial.

***Necator americanus* & *Ankylostoma duodenale* (hookworms)** occur in the Indian subcontinent, SE Asia, central/N Africa, and parts of Europe. Necator is also found in the Americas & sub-Saharan Africa. Many small worms attach to upper GI mucosa, causing bleeding (iron-deficiency anaemia). Eggs are excreted in faeces and hatch in soil. Larvae penetrate feet, so starting new infections. Oral transmission of *Ankylostoma* occurs. Δ: Stool microscopy (**fig 1**). ℞: Mebendazole 500mg PO stat (1 dose) ± iron.

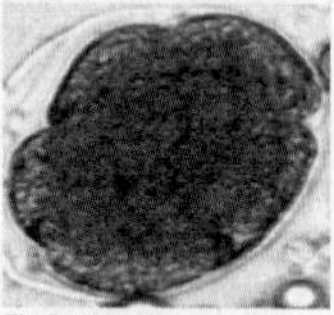

Fig 1. *Necator americanus* eggs. ~70×38µm.

Strongyloides stercoralis is endemic in the sub-tropics. Transmitted via skin, it causes migrating urticaria on legs & trunk (*cutaneous larva migrans*) ± pneumonitis, enteritis/malabsorption (chronic diarrhoea/abdominal; pain). Worms may take bacteria into the blood, causing septicaemia ± meningitis. Δ: Stool microscopy, serology, or duodenal aspiration. ℞: Ivermectin 0.2mg/kg/24h PO for 48h. Hyperinfestation occurs in AIDS; consider albendazole 400mg/12h PO for 7–10d)

Ascaris lumbricoides looks like a garden worm (*Lumbricus*). It has 3 finely toothed lips. Transmission: faecal-oral. It migrates through liver & lungs, settling in small bowel. Often asymptomatic; GI obstruction/perforation is rare. If in bile ducts, cholangitis or pancreatitis can result. Worms may be >25cm long with a hooked end if ♂, **fig 2**). Δ: Stool microscopy (ova stain orange in bile); worms on barium X-rays; eosinophilia. ℞: Albendazole (400mg PO once), mebendazole (100mg/12h PO for 3d), ivermectin (150–200µg/kg PO once).[419]

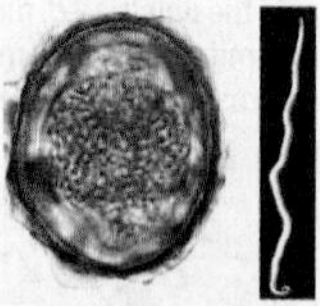

Fig 2. Ascaris eggs (45×40µm) & ♂ worm (20cm).

Enterobius vermicularis (threadworm; ~9mm long; **fig 3**) causes anal itch as it leaves the bowel to lay eggs on the perineum. Apply sticky tape there to identify eggs (~55 × 25µm) microscopically. ℞: Mebendazole 100mg PO stat. Repeat at 2wks if ≥2yrs. If aged <2yrs, try piperazine (see BNF). Treat the whole family. *Hygiene is more important than drugs* as adult worms die after 6wks. Continued symptoms means *reinfection*.

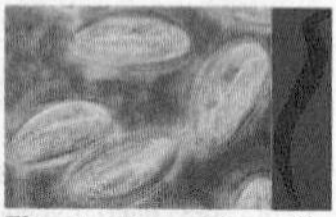

Fig 3. Enterobius: the folded worm is seen squirming in its egg. On the right is a ♀ worm.[420]

Trichuris trichiura (whipworm) causes non-specific abdominal pain. Δ: Stool microscopy. ℞: Mebendazole 500mg stat. ***Trichinella spiralis*** (worldwide) Transmitted by uncooked pork, it migrates to muscle/CNS,[421] causing myalgia, myocarditis, eyelid oedema ± T°↑. ℞: Albendazole 400mg/24h PO for 3d.

Toxocara canis is the main cause of visceral[1] & ocular larval migrans (eye granulomas, retinal detachment, ophthalmitis, uveitis, squint, blindness). Δ: Fundoscopy, serology, histology. ℞: Albendazole 400mg/12h PO for 5d. Severe lung, heart, or CNS disease may warrant steroids. In eye disease, visible larvae can be lasered. *Toxocara* is contracted by ingesting dirt, so de-worm pets often (exclude from play areas).

Dracunculus medinensis Guinea worm is the longest nematode (up to 70cm; in Ghana & Sudan); transmitted by water containing tiny crustaceans (copepods).[422] ℞: Slow extraction of pre-emerging worms as they exit through the skin helped by metronidazole (±steroids). WHO eradication date is set for 2009.[423]

1 Visceral larval migrans occurs when larvae migrate through a host's internal organs. We get it by ingesting parasite eggs, or by eating tissues from intermediate hosts containing larvae, eg Ascaris in raw beef. Signs vary with location, eg ↓appetite, T°↑, myalgia, big liver, asthma, cough, myeloradiculitis.

Figs 1&2 courtesy of Prof S Upton, Kansas Univ. Fig 3 (worm) courtesy of Prof S Upton &(eggs) JML.

Filarial infection

This is common—prevalence of lymphatic filariasis: 120 million worldwide.

1 **Onchocerciasis** (caused by *Onchocerca volvulus*, transmitted by the black fly) is the world's second leading infectious cause of blindness.[424] It causes **river blindness** in 72% of some communities in Africa and S America (17 million worldwide). A nodule forms at the site of the bite, shedding microfilariae to distant skin sites which develop altered pigmentation, lichenification, loss of elasticity, and poor healing. Signs are mainly from the localized host response to moribund microfilariae. Eye signs: keratitis, uveitis, cataract, fixed pupil, fundal degeneration, or optic neuritis/atrophy. Lymphadenopathy and elephantiasis also occur. *Diagnosis:* Visualization of microfilaria in eye or skin snips. Remove a fine shaving of clean, unanaesthetized skin with a scalpel. Put on slide with a drop of 0.9% saline and look for swimming larvae after 30min. ℞: ***Ivermectin*** 150-200μg/kg stat, repeat eg 6-monthly to suppress dermal and ocular microfilariae. If the eye is involved start ***prednisolone*** 1mg/kg/24h PO a few days before starting ivermectin (probably OK in pregnancy). Worm survival requires symbiosis with Wolbachia bacteria (susceptible to doxycycline 100mg/d PO for 6 weeks; give *before* ivermectin). Ivermectin resistance may be evolving.[425]

2 **Lymphatic filaria** occurs in Asia, Africa, & S. America and is transmitted by 5 genera of mosquito. Acute infection causes fever, lymphadenitis & chyluria.[1] *Wuchereria bancrofti* causes leg lymphoedema (elephantiasis) and hydroceles (may be huge). *Brugia malaya* causes elephantiasis below the elbow/knee. *Wuchereria* life cycle: a mosquito bites an infected human→ingested microfilariae develop into larvae→larvae migrate to mosquito's mouth→biting of another human→access to bloodstream→adult filariae lodge in the lymphatic system. Δ: Blood film (**fig 4**) and serology. A rapid immuno-chromatographic fingerprick test can be used in the field (as lymphedema may develop many years after infection, lab tests may be -ve). *Complications:* Immune hyperreactivity may cause tropical pulmonary eosinophilia (cough, wheeze, lung fibrosis, high eosinophil counts, IgE↑ and IgG↑). It is a major public health problem and is a WHO target for elimination by the year 2020 (starting with Nigeria, Samoa & Egypt). The current elimination strategy involves mass treatment with one yearly dose of 2 drugs for 5yrs: ***albendazole*** (400mg) + *either* ***ivermectin*** (200μg/kg) *or* ***diethylcarbamazine*** (6mg/kg).[427] Giving ***diethylcarbamazine***-fortified salt to families for 1yr is also effective. *Prevention:* Avoiding mosquito bites, annual mass treatment of the entire community.[428]

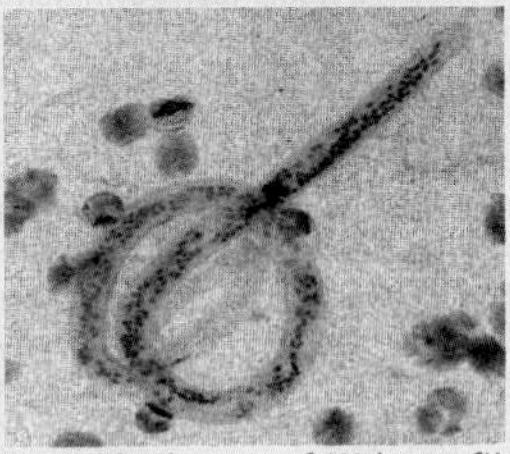

Fig 4. Blood smear of *W. bancrofti*; 290×8.5μm.[426] ©Prof S Upton, Kansas Univ.

3 **Loiasis (eye-worm)** is caused by *Loa loa*. It occurs in Africa/S. Europe[429] (transmitted by the *Chrysops* fly). It causes pruritus, urticaria, myalgia arthralgia, and mysterious wandering Calabar swellings.[2] The worm may migrate over the surface of the eye ("Something's wiggling in my eye, doctor"). This eerie voyage across the globe causes intense conjunctivitis, which luckily heals OK if left alone (don't treat until the transmigration is over: on detecting your therapy the worm tends to panic).[430] Check for glomerulonephritis, eosinophilia, and encephalitis. Δ: Blood smears (often -ve, or show squirming microfilariae),[431 video link] serology, or PCR. ℞: ***Diethylcarbamazine***.

1 **Chyluria** entails fistulae (eg pyelo-lymphatic) between lymphatic and urinary systems: hence milky lymph in urine (ΔΔ: filariasis, TB, trauma, neoplasia, congenital; it is also associated with nephrosis).

2 **Calabar swellings** occur anywhere (face, arms, legs, eg induced by local trauma). Oedema is preceded by local pain or itching lasting 1-2h. There then develops a 10-20 cm non-erythematous, non-pitting swelling, resolving after 2 days to several weeks. Severe swellings can cause paraesthesiae or entrapment neuropathy. Recurrences are common at the same site (or elsewhere). Cause: unknown (?allergic responses to antigens released in the tracks of adult migrating parasites).

Taenia solium (pork tapeworm; fig 1) infection occurs by eating uncooked pork, or from drinking contaminated water.[1] *T. saginata* is contracted from uncooked beef. Both cause vague abdominal symptoms and malabsorption. Contaminated food and water contain cysticerci which adhere to the gut and develop into adult worms. On swallowing the eggs of *T. solium* they may enter the circulation and disseminate throughout the body, becoming cysticerci within the human host (*cysticercosis*). This tapeworm encysts in muscle, skin, heart, eye, and CNS, causing focal signs. ***Subcutaneous cysticercosis*** causes subcutaneous nodules (arms, legs, chest). ***Ocular cysticercosis*** causes conjunctivitis; uveitis; retinitis; choroidal atrophy; blindness.

Neurocysticercosis is the chief cause of seizures in some places, eg Mexico. Other features: focal CNS signs, eg hemiplegia, odd behavioural, dementia—or no symptoms. Cysticerci may cluster like bunches of grapes ('racemose' form) in the ventricles (causing hydrocephalus) and basal cisterns (causing basal meningitis, cranial nerve lesions, and ↑ICP). Spinal cysticerci may cause radicular or compressive symptoms (p470). *Diagnosis:* • Stool microscopy and examination of perianal swabs.

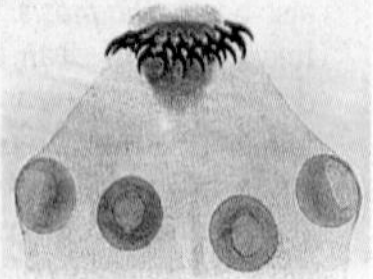

Fig 1. *Tinea solium* (note the two rows of hooks).[432]

• Serology: indirect haemagglutination test. • CSF: may show eosinophils in neurocysticercosis, and a CSF antigen test is available. • CT or MRI scan may locate cysts. • SXR and x-rays of soft tissues may show calcified cysts. • Detecting *T. solium* DNA in brain biopsy tissue.[433] ℞: Get help (*tel:* 0151 708 9393[UK]). Neurocysticercosis: albendazole, eg 7.5mg/kg/12h PO for 8–30d, or praziquantel. Allergic responses to dying larvae should be covered by dexamethasone 0.1mg/kg/d for 29d. The role of steroids in the routine treatment of neurocysticercosis is controversial. **NB:** if CSF ventricles are involved, you may need to shunt before starting drugs. Drugs may worsen the acute phase of cysticercotic encephalitis.[434]

Hymenolepis nana; H. diminuta (dwarf tapeworm; rarely symptomatic). ℞: Praziquantel 25mg/kg PO (1 dose; adults & children) or niclosamide 500mg/day for 3d.

Diphyllobothrium latum (**fig 2**) is a fish tapeworm (via uncooked fish) causing similar symptoms to *T. solium*. It is a cause of vitamin B_{12}↓. ℞: Praziquantel 5–10mg/kg stat PO.

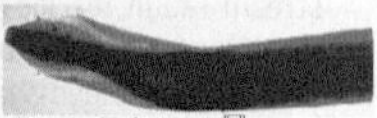

Fig 2. *D. latum*.[435]

Hydatid disease Cystic hydatid disease is a zoonosis caused by eating eggs of the dog parasite *Echinococcus granulosus* (**fig 3**) eg in rural sheep-farming regions. Hydatid is a worldwide public health problem (not confined to traditional rural areas in China, Russia, Alaska, Wales, Italy, India, Pakistan, and Japan). ***Signs:*** Most cysts are asymptomatic, but liver cysts may present with hepatomegaly, obstructive jaundice, cholangitis, or PUO. Lung cysts present with dyspnoea, chest pain, haemoptysis, or anaphylaxis. Parasites migrate almost anywhere, eg CNS; or it turns up incidentally on CXR. Other sites involved: breast, bone, kidney, adrenals, bladder, heart, psoas.[437] *Diagnosis:* Plain x-ray, ultrasound, CT/MRI. Appearances may look like a tumour.[438] A good serological test has replaced the variably sensitive Casoni intradermal test. ℞: Get help (including surgical). 1st-choice: albendazole before & after drainage (if >60kg, 400mg/12h; if <60kg, 7.5mg/kg/12h with food). Excise/drain symptomatic cysts. Beware spilling cyst contents (causes anaphylaxis; give praziquantel here). The **PAIR** approach is often used: puncture→aspirate cyst→inject hypertonic saline→re-aspirate after 25min—and continue albendazole for 28 days to prevent recurrence.[439] (NB: alveolar hydatid is caused by *E. multilocularis*.)

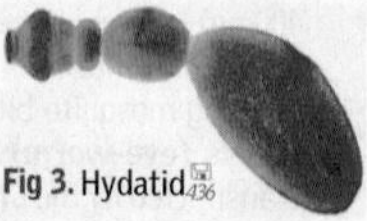

Fig 3. Hydatid.[436]

1 While eating undercooked pork is the only way to acquire intestinal *T. solium*, any food contaminated by faeces from hosts infected with cysticerci can carry the eggs that may lead to development of cysticercosis. Even vegetarians are at risk. The lack of public awareness of this poses big problems.

Figs 1, 2 & 3 courtesy of Professor Steve Upton, Kansas University.

Trematodes (flukes)

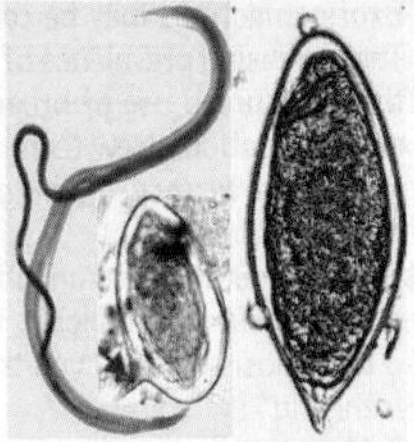

Fig 1. *S. mansoni* ♂/♀ mating; right: egg with sublateral spine (red arrow) **Fig 2.** (enlarged) *S. haematobium*; terminal spine. Figs 1-3 ©Prof S Upton Kansas University.[440]

Schistosomiasis (bilharzia) is the most prevalent disease caused by flukes (~200 million people in Africa; now also introduced to S America/Caribbean). Snail vectors release cercariae that penetrate skin, eg during paddling, causing itchy papular rashes ('swimmer's itch'). The cercariae shed their tails to become schistosomules and migrate via lungs to liver where they grow. ~2wks later, there may be fever, urticaria, diarrhoea, cough, wheeze, and hepatosplenomegaly ('Katayama fever'). In ~8wks, flukes are mature (14♂–20♀mm long), mate (**fig 1**), and migrate to resting habitats, ie bladder and vulval veins (*haematobium*) or mesenteric veins (*mansoni* & *japonicum*). Eggs released from these sites cause granulomata and scarring and are important sites of HIV entry. Clinical signs reflect our immune response to eggs (type IV hypersensitivity, eg for *S. mansoni*).

Signs: S. mansoni: abdominal pain; D&V; later, hepatic fibrosis, granulomatous inflammation, anaemia, and portal hypertension (variceal bleeding is common, but transformation into true cirrhosis has not been well-documented). *S. japonicum*, often the most serious, occurs in SE Asia, tends to affect the bowel and liver, and may migrate to lung and CNS ('travellers' myelitis'). Urinary schistosomiasis (*S. haematobium*) occurs in Africa, the Middle East, and the Indian Ocean. Signs: frequency, dysuria, haematuria (± haematospermia), incontinence. It may progress to hydronephrosis and renal failure. There is an ↑risk of squamous cell carcinoma of the bladder. **Δ:** Eggs in urine (*S. haematobium;* **fig 2**, with 3 RBCs for scale) or faeces (*S. mansoni* & *japonicum*) or rectal biopsy (all types). AXR may show bladder calcification in chronic *S. haematobium* infection. Ultrasound (renal obstruction, hydronephrosis ± thickened bladder wall). Detecting Ab to *S. mansoni*, *S. haematobium*, and *S. japonicum* adult worm microsomal Ag are specific for all 3 species (ELISA and immunoblot assays).[441] **℞:** Praziquantel: 40mg/kg PO with food divided into 2 doses separated by 4-6h for *S. mansoni* & *S. haematobium*, or 20mg/kg/8h for 1d in *S. japonicum*. Sudden transitory abdominal pain ± bloody diarrhoea may occur shortly after. Oxamniquine is an alternative for *S. mansoni* infection.

Fasciola hepatica (liver fluke) is spread by sheep, water, and snails. It causes T°↑, abdominal pain, diarrhoea, weight↓, jaundice, hepatomegaly, liver fibrosis and eosinophilia. *Tests:* Stool microscopy, serology. **℞:** Get help. Triclabendazole 10mg/kg PO, 1 dose, or bithionol 30mg/kg alternate days for 10–15 doses, max 2g/day IM.

Opisthorchis & ***Clonorchis*** are liver flukes common in SE Asia, where they cause cholangitis, cholecystitis & cholangiocarcinoma. ***Risk factor:*** Raw fish. *Tests:*[443] Stool microscopy; PCR. **℞:** Praziquantel 25mg/kg/8h PO for 2d.

Fasciolopsis buski is a big intestinal fluke ~7cm long causing ulcers or abscesses at the site of attachment. **℞:** Praziquantel 25mg/kg/8h PO for 1d.

Paragonimus westermani (lung fluke) is got by eating raw freshwater crabs and crayfish. Parasites migrate through gut and diaphragm to invade lungs (hence cough, dyspnoea, haemoptysis, ± lung abscess/bronchiectasis). It occurs in the Far East, S America, and Congo; often mistaken for TB (similar signs & CXR). *Tests:* Sputum in ova. 
Do MRI OR CT for CNS/lung lesions. **℞:** Praziquantel (25mg/kg/8h PO for 2d).

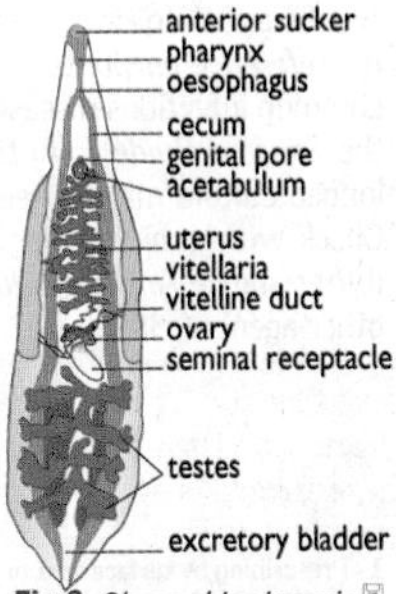

Fig 3. *Clonorchis sinensis*[442]

Exotic infections may be *community-acquired* or *nosocomial*, ie acquired in hospital. The increasing prevalence of immunosuppression, both drug induced and innate, and the widespread use of broad-spectrum antibiotics have resulted in an increase in exotic infections. New techniques such as PCR have identified more putative infective agents. *The history—and a good gossip:* Don't expect to find the pertinent question in any textbook—eg:

1 "Have you delivered any infected babies in the last year?" You can more than impress your obstetrician friends who don't know about baby-to-obstetrician brucellosis who tell you that "I'm so depressed about not being able to shake off this flu".[444]
2 "Are your carp well at present?" (*Mycobacterium marinum* skin infection).[445]
3 "Who has been licking your face recently?" (*Pasteurella multocida*).[446]
4 "Has your dog been on holiday this year?" (monkeypox from prairie dogs).
5 "Has your pet hedgehog lost weight?" (salmonella).[447]
6 "I expect you have a pet magpie causing your headache" (zoonotic transmission of *Cryptococcus neoformans* causing meningitis in an immunocompetent adult).[448]
7 "Did you have a stray pig living under your house when the monsoon started?" (pigs + standing water + mosquitoes ≈ Japanese encephalitis).
8 "Any contact with invasive snails?" Angiostrongyliasis→eosinophilic meningitis.[449]
9 "Do you sometimes wonder if your goat miscarried last year?" (brucellosis).[450]

When you suspect infection (T°↑, sweats, inflammation, D&V, WCC↑, or *any* unexplained symptom), ask about: • Foreign travel (recent and past) • Foreign bodies (hip prosthesis, heart valve) • Work or hobby or family exposure to infectious agents • Any bites/stings • Sexual exploits • Any necrotic tissue? • HIV risk or reason for immunosuppression (eg pregnancy; steroids) • Any pets, exotic or otherwise?

Diagnosis Take appropriate cultures (blood, urine, stool, CSF) or swabs as clinically indicated. Liaise early with an infectious diseases physician or microbiologist. Consider CXR, ultrasound, or CT as clinically indicated. If the infection appears to be localized, consider surgical debridement ± drainage. Do not give up if you cannot culture an organism; tests may need to be repeated. Perhaps the organism is 'fastidious' in its nutritional requirement or requires prolonged incubation? Even if culture *is* achieved, it may be that the organism is pathogenic, or it could be a commensal (ie part of the normal flora for that patient). If culture is not possible, look for antibodies or antigen in the serum or other body fluids. It is generally agreed that a 4-fold increase in antibody titres in convalescence (compared with the acute sera) is indicative of recent infection, although not diagnostic. PCR is increasingly being used to make identifications; however, it is far from infallible, and contamination with DNA from the lab or elsewhere is a frequent problem.

Treatment Empirical therapy (p382) may be needed if the patient is ill. *The TABLE is for reference purposes only:* no one can remember *all* the details about even the common infectious diseases, let alone rare ones. The principle source for the BOX is the *Sanford Guide to Antimicrobial Therapy 2009* (ISBN 978-1-930808-54-6). Prolonged culture may be needed. The draining of pus is as important as antibiotics. Check with a microbiologist for local patterns of disease and antibiotic sensitivity/resistance. *Antibiotic doses:* Penicillins (p378); cephalosporins (p379); gentamicin;[1] other agents (p380).

1 Prescribing by **surface area**, or **lean** body weight (LBW), eg for gentamicin, or **ideal** body weight (IBW):
Body surface area = $0.20247 \times \text{Height (metres)}^{0.725} \times \text{Weight(kg)}^{0.425}$
Lean body weight (♂) = $(1.10 \times \text{Weight in kg}) - 128 (\text{Weight}^2/(100 \times \text{Height in metres})^2)$
Lean body weight (♀) = $(1.07 \times \text{Weight in kg}) - 148 (\text{Weight}^2/(100 \times \text{Height in metres})^2)$
Ideal body weight (♂) = 50 + 2.3 for every inch over 5ft tall
Ideal body weight (♀) = 49 + 1.7 for every inch over 5ft tall. halls.md/ideal-weight/devine.htm

Organism	*Site or type of infection* *IE=infective endocarditis*	*Treatment example*
Acanthamoeba	Corneal ulcers	Propamidine + neomycin
Acinetobacter calcoaceticus	UTI; CSF; lung; bone; conjunctiva.	p423 ?Imepenem ± gentamicin
Actinobacillus lignieresii	CSF; IE; wounds; bone; lymph nodes	Ampicillin ± gentamicin
Actinobacillus ureae	Bronchus; CSF post-trauma; hepatitis	Ampicillin ± gentamicin
Aerococcus viridans	Empyema; UTI; CSF; bone; IE	Penicillin ± gentamicin
Aeromonas hydrophila	IE; CSF; cornea; bone; D&V; liver abscess	Ciprofloxacin
Afipia broomeae	Marrow; synovium	Imipenem or ceftriaxone
Aggregatibacter actinomycetemcomitans	IE; CNS; UTI; bone; thyroid; lung; periodontitis; abscesses	Penicillin ± gentamicin
Alcaligenes species	Dialysis peritonitis; ear; lung	co-amoxiclav or cetazidime
Arachnia propionica	Actinomycosis; tear ducts; CNS	Penicillin
Arcanobacterium	Throat; cellulitis; leg ulcer	Penicillin
Babesia microti (protozoa)	PUO ± haemolysis if old/splenectomy	Atovoquone + azithromycin
Bacillus cereus	Wounds; eye; ear; lung; UTI; IE	Vancomycin
Bifidobacterium	Vagina; UTI; IE; peritonitis; lung	Penicillin
Bordetella bronchiseptica	URTI; CSF (after animal contact)	Co-amoxiclav
Burkholderia cepacia, etc (formerly *pseudomonas*)	Wounds; feet; lungs; IE; CAPD; UTI ecthyma gangrenosa; peritonitis	Ciprofloxacin or meropenem
Burkholderia pickettii	CSF (formerly a pseudomonas)	Cefalosporin
Burkholderia pseudomallei (formerly *Pseudomonas pseudomallei*)	Melioidosis: self-reactivating septicaemia + multiorgan, protean signs eg in rice-farmers, via water/soil in Papua, Thailand, Vietnam, Torres Straits	Ceftazidime (14d) + co-trimoxazole for 3 months
Capnocytophaga	Oral ulcer; stomatitis; arthritis Blood; cervical abscess; joints	Ertapenem
Cardiobacterium hominis	IE (=infective endocarditis)	Ceftrixone for 4wks
Chromobacterium violaceum	Nodes; eye; bone; liver; pustules	Gentamicin, chloramphenicol
Citrobacter koseri/diversus	CSF; UTI; blood; cholecystitis	Imipenem
Corynebacterium jeikeium	IE; CSF; otitis; leg ulcer; lung	Vancomycin
Corynebacterium pseudoTB	Lymphadenitis	Ciprofloxacin
Corynebacterium ulcerans	Diphtheria-like ± CNS signs	Rifampicin+diphtheria antitoxin
Cyclospora cayetanensis	Diarrhoea (via raspberries)	Co-trimoxazole
Edwardsiella tarda	Cellulitis; abscesses; BP↓; dysentery via penetrating fish injuries	Cefuroxime + gentamicin
Eikenella corrodens	Sinus; ears; PE post-jugular vein phlebitis (postanginal sepsis) via bites	Penicillin ± gentamicin
Erysipelothrix rhusiopathiae	Erysipelas-like (*OHCS* p598); IE	Penicillin
Eubacterium	Wounds; gynaecologic sepsis; IE	Penicillin + cefoxitin
Flavobacterium meningosepticum	Lungs; epidemic neonatal meningitis; post-op bacteraemia; contact lens keratitis	Piperacillin
Flavobacterium multivorum	Peritonitis (spontaneous); pneumonia in HIV patients	Ciprofloxacin
Gemella haemolysans	IE; meningitis after neurosurgery	Linezolid + chloramphenicol
Helicobacter cinaedi	Proctitis in homosexual men	Ciprofloxacin + rifampicin
Kingella kingae	Throat; larynx; eyelid; joint; skin	Penicillin ± cephalosporin
Lactobacillus	Teeth; chorioamnionitis; pyelitis	Penicillin or ampicillin
Mobiluncus curtisii/mulieris	Vagina	Clindamycin (topical)
Moraxella osloensis and ***M. nonliquefaciens***	Conjunctiva; wound; vagina; UTI; CSF CNS; bone; haemorrhagic stomatitis	Co-amoxiclav
Pasteurella multocida[451] [452] (Gram-ve rod)	Skin; bone; lung; CSF; UTI; pericarditis epiglottitis. From cat or dog bites	β-lactam antibiotics
Pasteurella pneumotrophica	Wounds; joints; bone; CSF	Penicillin; cipro-/moxifloxacin
Peptostreptococcus	Bone/joint/discitis; wound; teeth; face	Clindamycin or metronidazole
Plesiomonas shigelloides	D&V; eye; sepsis post fishbone injury	Ciprofloxacin
Propionibacterium acnes (see *OHCS* p600)	Face; wounds; CSF shunts; bone; IE; liver granuloma (botyromycosis)	Tetracycline or ceftriaxone
Prototheca wickerhamii[453] & ***zopfii=achlorophyllous algae***	Subcutaneous granuloma; plaques; bursitis; adenitis; nodules	Amphotericin or ketoconazole
Providencia stuartii	UTI; purple urine bag syndrome	Ceftriaxone
Pseudomonas maltophilia	stenotrophomonas Wounds; ear; eye; lung; UTI; IE [454]	Co-trimoxazole or cefepine
Pseudomonas putrefaciens	CSF post CNS surgery/head trauma	Cefotaxime
Rothia dentocariosa[455]	Appendix abscess; infective emboli	Penicillin + gentamicin
Serratia marcescens (may be non-pathogenic)[456]	Wound; burns; lung; UTI; liver; CSF; bone; IE; red diaper/nappy syndrome	Imipenem, ceftazidime, ciprofloxacin
Sphingomonas paucimobilis	Superficial leg ulcer; CSF; UTI	Ceftazidime
Streptococcus bovis	IE if colon cancer; do colonoscopy	Penicillin + gentamicin
Vibrio vulnificus	Wounds; muscle; uterus; fasciitis	Tetracycline + cephalosporin

Contents

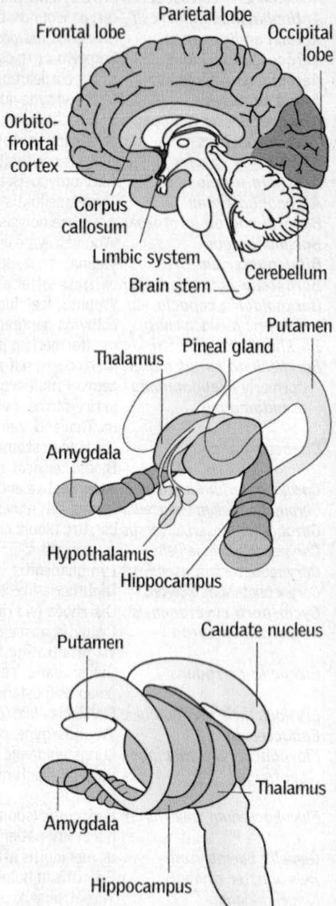

Fig 1. *Conflicting systems:* cerebral hemispheres & limbic system (last 2 images) 'We know... about how there isn't a unitary ego—how we're made up of conflicting, interacting systems.' A.S.Byatt *Possession* Our bodies are not a bicycle with a single rider—more like a tandem with various processes in various saddles. The front(al) drivers may decide to bear right, but if the rear drivers now lean left we go awry, and our will seems mysteriously subverted. Those few doctors whose processes are in perpetual harmony are at a disadvantage here as they never understand what makes their patients good and bad.

Pages elsewhere Neurological examination (p72-p80); mental state (p82); LP (p782); headache emergencies (p794); coma (p800); GCS (p802); meningitis (p832); encephalitis (p832); cerebral abscess (p835); status epilepticus (p836); head injury (p838); ↑ICP (p840).

We dedicate this page to those carers who find themselves responsible for a friend or relative who has a chronic neurological illness, such as stroke, Parkinson's disease, Alzheimer's disease, or motor neuron disease. As a thought experiment, try spending a morning imagining that you are such a carer, trying to expunge the smell of soiled sheets from your clothes, while awaiting a visit from a neighbour, who said he would 'sit with him' so you can catch the bus into town, and, like a guilty hedonist, play truant from your role as nurse for a few sanity-giving hours of normal life. You wait. No one comes. You stop bothering about the smell on your clothes, and turn towards your husband, about to say something, but when your eyes meet his, you realize he does not recognize you—and you keep your thoughts to yourself. Knuckles whiten as you grasp his collar to lift him forward on the commode, and you seem to hear a mocking voice over your shoulder saying: "... so I see we're getting angry with him today, are we?" The ceaseless round from mouth to anus, from bed to chair, from twilight to twilight, continues, *ad infinitum*.

It is all we can do to spend *2 minutes* on this thought experiment, let alone a morning—or the rest of our lives. We need to be aware of the strategies we adopt to avoid involvement with the naked truth of the shattered lives, which, like a tragic subplot, stand behind the farce of morning surgery or outpatients in which we hear ourselves for ever saying in plummy complacency: "And how are *you* today Mrs Salt—your husband, I know... marvellous how you manage. You are a real support to each other. Let me know if I can do anything." We pretend to be busy, we ensure that we *are* busy, we surround ourselves with students, with white coats, and a miasma of technical expertise—we surround ourselves with *anything* to ensure that there is no chink through which Mrs Salt can shine her rays of darkness. Poor Mrs Salt. Poor us—to be frightened of the darkness, panicking at the thought that we might not have anything to offer, or that we might be called to offer up our equanimity as a sacrifice to Mrs Salt. How dare one little grain upset our carefully contrived universe?

Respite care, medical charities, meals on wheels, laundry services, physiotherapy, occupational therapy (OT), transport, day care centres, clubs for carers, visits from the doctor (which may cure the plummy complacency), district nurses or from a nurse-matron specializing in chronic diseases will go some way to mitigate Mrs Salt's problems. As ever, the way forward is by taking time to listen. Carers' needs evolve. First there is uncertainty, and the need for help in handling this. Next comes the moment of diagnosis with the numbness, denial, and anger that may follow. Then there may be an adjustment to reality, with frenzied searching for information and advice, or a careful titration by the carer of how much information he or she can handle.

Issues of driving, mobility, finance, sex, and employment are likely to occur throughout the illness, and advice will need to be constantly tailored to suit individual circumstances. But the best thing you can ever offer is the unwritten contract that, come what may, you will be there, available, often ineffectual, but incapable of being alienated by whatever the carer may disclose to you.

Revising for exams? Skip this page? Not really...what if the question is "What's the most important issue in neurology?" Answer: caring for the carers.

We thank Dr Thomas Hughes who is our Specialist Reader for this chapter.

Is there a **focal lesion** (illness of all cells in one part of the brain, eg a stroke)?—or:
- A **general insult**, eg trauma, encephalitis, anoxia, poisoning, or post-ictal states.
- **Widespread neurodegeneration** (may have specific local effects, eg amnesia).
- Loss of **a specific type of nerve cell**, eg motor neuron disease; subacute combined degeneration of the cord (B_{12}↓, p328); loss of pre-Bötzinger neurons in the medulla causes central sleep apnoea (and death during sleep in the elderly).[2]
- A **disorder of function** (migraine; epilepsy) or **connectivity** (in autism, face processing areas do not connect well to fronto-parietal areas directing attention).[3]
- **Medically unexplained symptoms**, eg associated with psychological problems.

A key feature in determining if a focal lesion is present is lack of symmetry—eg one pupil dilated, or one upgoing plantar response.

Where is the lesion? Localizing the lesion depends on recognizing characteristic patterns of cognitive, cranial nerve, motor, and sensory deficits that occur with lesions at different sites in the nervous system.

Patterns of motor deficits Weakness can arise from lesions of the cortex, corona radiata, internal capsule, brainstem, spinal cord, roots, plexi, peripheral nerves, neuromuscular junction, or muscle. Is the pattern upper or lower motor neuron (UMN or LMN; see BOXES)? *Cortical lesions* may cause an unexpected pattern of weakness of all movements of a hand or foot, with normal or even ↓tone—but ↑reflexes more proximally in the arm or leg will suggest an UMN rather than LMN lesion. *Internal capsule* and *corticospinal pathway* brainstem lesions cause contralateral hemiparesis with a pyramidal distribution of weakness (BOX 1). If the hemiplegia occurs with epilepsy, ↓cognition, or homonymous hemianopia (p453), the lesion is in a cerebral hemisphere. A cranial nerve palsy (III–XII) contralateral to a hemiplegia implicates the brainstem on the side of the cranial nerve palsy. *Cord lesions* causing paraparesis (both legs) or quadriparesis/tetraplegia (all limbs) are suggested by finding a motor and reflex level (ie power is unaffected above the lesion, with LMN signs *at* the level of the lesion, and UMN signs *below* the lesion). *Peripheral neuropathies:* (p506) Most cause a distal weakness (foot-drop; weak hand), but in Guillain-Barré syndrome weakness is often *proximal* (due to root involvement). Involvement of a single nerve (mononeuropathy) occurs with trauma or entrapment (carpal tunnel, p507); involvement of several nerves (mononeuritis multiplex) is seen eg in DM or vasculitis.

Sensory deficits The distribution of sensory loss and the range of modalities involved (pain, temperature, touch, vibration, and joint-position sense) can add information about the site of a lesion. Pain and T° sensations travel along small fibres in peripheral nerves and the *anterolateral (spinothalamic) tracts* in the cord and brainstem (p520), whereas joint-position and vibration sense travel in large fibres in peripheral nerves and the large *dorsal columns* of the cord. *Distal sensory loss* suggests a neuropathy and may involve all sensory modalities or be more selective, depending on the nerve fibre size involved in the peripheral nerve. Individual nerve lesions are identified by their anatomical territories, which are usually more sharply defined than those of root lesions (dermatomes, p458), which often show considerable overlap. A *sensory level* is the hallmark (albeit a rather unreliable one) of a cord lesion—ie decreased sensation below the lesion (eg the legs) with normal sensation above this level (eg in abdomen, trunk, and arms). Hemi-cord lesions cause Brown-Séquard syndrome (p710) with dorsal column loss on the side of the lesion and contralateral spinothalamic loss. *Dissociated sensory loss* may occur with cervical cord lesions—selective loss of pain and temperature sensation with sparing of joint position sense and vibration (eg syringomyelia, p520; or cord tumours). Lateral brainstem lesions show both dissociated and crossed sensory loss with pain and T° loss on the side of the face ipsilateral to the lesion, and contralateral arm and leg sensory loss. Lesions above the brainstem give a contralateral pattern of generalized sensory loss. In *cortical lesions*, sensory loss is confined to more subtle and discriminating sensory functions (2-point discrimination and stereognosis; p503).

UMN lesions (upper motor neuron)

These are caused by damage to motor pathways anywhere from motor nerve cells in the precentral gyrus of the frontal cortex, through the internal capsule, brainstem, and cord, to the anterior horn cells in the cord. UMN weakness affects ***muscle groups***, not individual muscles. Weakness is typically 'pyramidal'[1] in distribution, ie weakness involving physiological extensors of the arm (shoulder abduction; elbow, wrist, and finger extension; and the small muscles of the hand) and the flexors of the lower limb (hip flexion, knee flexion, and ankle dorsiflexion and everters). There is no muscle wasting and ***loss of skilled fine finger movements*** may be greater than expected from the overall grade of weakness (BOX 3). ***Spasticity*** develops in stronger muscles (eg arm flexors and leg extensors). It is manifest increased tone that is *velocity-dependent and non-uniform*,[2] ie as resistance to passive movement that can suddenly be overcome (clasp-knife feel). There is ***hyperreflexia:*** reflexes are brisk; ***plantars are upgoing*** (+ve Babinski sign) ± ***clonus*** (elicited by rapidly dorsiflexing the foot; ≤3 rhythmic, downward beats of the foot are normal; more suggest an UMN lesion) ± a positive ***Hoffman's reflex***: brief flexion of thumb and index finger in a pincer movement following a flick to the pulp of the middle finger (it is a stretch reflex so the often-used way of flicking the finger *towards* the palm isn't ideal).[4] Neck extension is said to increase sensitivity of this test.[5] **NB:** UMN lesions can mimic LMN lesions in the first few hours before the spasticity and hyperreflexia develop.

LMN lesions (lower motor neuron)

These are caused by damage anywhere from anterior horn cells in the cord, nerve roots, plexi, or peripheral nerves. The distribution of weakness corresponds to those muscles supplied by the involved cord segment, nerve root, part of plexus, or peripheral nerve. See p456. A combination of anatomical knowledge, good muscle testing technique, and experience is needed to distinguish, eg a radial nerve palsy from a C7 root lesion, or a common peroneal nerve palsy from an L5 root lesion (p456).[3] Affected muscles show ***wasting*** ± ***fasciculation*** (spontaneous involuntary twitching), and the limb feels soft and floppy, providing little resistance to passive stretch (***hypotonia/flaccidity***). ***Reflexes are reduced*** or absent, the ***plantars remain flexor***. The chief differential is weakness from primary muscle disease—here there is symmetrical loss, reflexes are lost later than in neuropathies, and there is no sensory loss. Myasthenia gravis (p516) causes weakness worsening with use (fatiguability); there is little wasting, normal reflexes, and no sensory loss.

Reflexes and spinal cord level: p73. ***Spinal roots for each muscle:*** p456.
For *mixed LMN and UMN signs*, see p471 (MND, ↓ B_{12}, taboparesis, etc).

Muscle weakness grading (MRC classification)

Grade 0	No muscle contraction	**Grade 3**	Active movement against gravity
Grade 1	Flicker of contraction	**Grade 4**	Active movement against resistance
Grade 2	Some active movement	**Grade 5**	Normal power (allowing for age)

Grade 4 covers a big range: **4–**, **4**, and **4+** denote movement against slight, moderate, and stronger resistance; avoid fudging descriptions—'strength 4/5 throughout' suggests a mild quadriparesis or myopathy. It is better to document 'poor effort' and the maximum grade for each muscle tested.

1 ***Pyramidal neurons*** have basal dendrites and an apical dendrite pointing towards the dorsal cortical border. They are a distinctive cortical feature and are specialized in their dendritic morphology, projection patterns, and localization in the 6 cortical layers. ***'Extrapyramidal'*** denotes CNS motor phenomena relating to the basal ganglia. Pyramidal lesions result in paresis and spasticity, but extrapyramidal lesions cause abnormality in initiation and maintenance of movement—negative symptoms include bradykinesia/akinesia (slow/absent movement) and loss of postural reflexes; positive symptoms are tremor, rigidity, and involuntary movements (p472, eg chorea, athetosis, ballismus, and dystonia).
2 Whereas with ***rigidity***, ↑ tone is not velocity-dependent but constant throughout passive movement.
3 The booklet *Aids to the Examination of the Peripheral Nervous System* is invaluable here. ISBN 0-7020-2512-7

Cerebral artery territories

Knowledge of the anatomy of the blood supply of the brain helps in diagnosing and managing cerebrovascular disease (p474–p482). Always try to identify the area of brain that correlates with a patient's symptoms and identify the affected artery.

Cerebral blood supply The brain is supplied by the two internal carotid arteries (anteriorly) and the basilar artery (posteriorly—formed by the joining of the two vertebral arteries). These 3 vessels feed into an anastomotic ring at the base of the brain called the circle of Willis (below). This arrangement may lessen the effects of occlusion of a feeder vessel proximal to the anastomosis by allowing supply from unaffected vessels. The anatomy of the circle of Willis is, however, highly variable and in many people it does not provide much protection from ischaemia due to carotid, vertebral, or basilar artery occlusion. Anastomotic supply from other vessels in the neck may mitigate occlusions of feeder vessels—occlusion of the internal carotid in the neck, for example, may not cause infarction if flow from the external carotid artery enters the circle of Willis via its anastomosis with the ophthalmic artery.

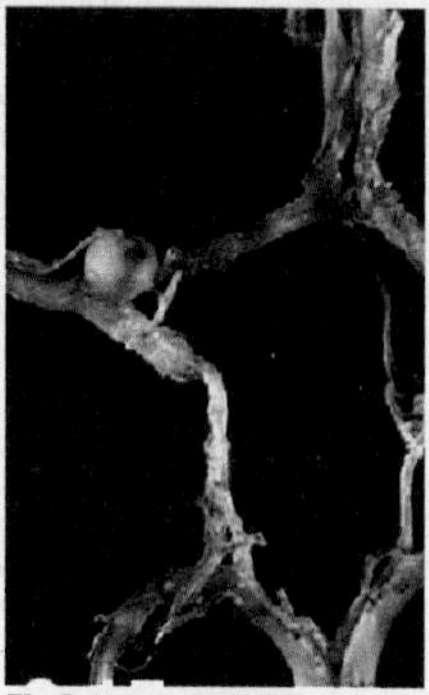

Fig 1. Where (and what) is the lesion? Answer: p482. 6

Courtesy of Dr D Hamoundi

The circle of Willis at the base of the brain

(see also CT on p483)

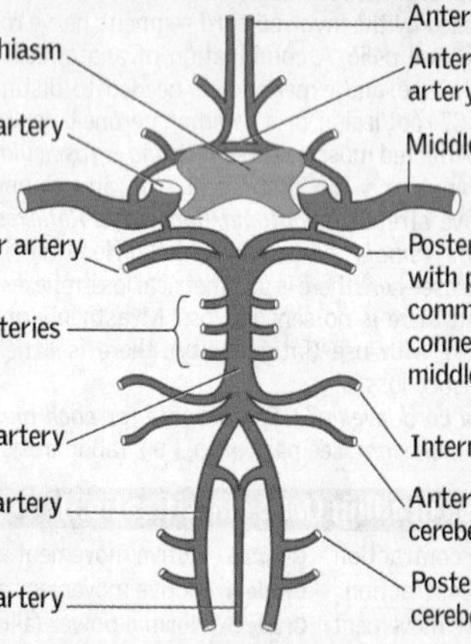

Footnotes in history: Willis

Thomas Willis (1621–75) is one of those happy Oxford heroes who hold a bogus DM degree—awarded in 1646 for his Royalist sympathies while at Christ Church, the most staunchly Royalist college in the University at that time. He had a busy life inventing terms such as 'neurology' and 'reflex'. Not only has his name been given to his famous circle, but he was the first to describe myasthenia gravis, whooping cough, and the sweet taste of diabetic urine. He was the first person (few have followed him) who knew the course of the spinal accessory nerve. He is unusual among Oxford neurologists in that, at various times, he developed the practice of giving his lunch away to the poor. He also developed the practice of iatrochemistry: a theory of medicine according to which all morbid conditions of the body can be explained by disturbances in the fermentations and effervescences of its humours.

Occlusion of the cerebral arteries

(see also figs 3 & 4, p761)

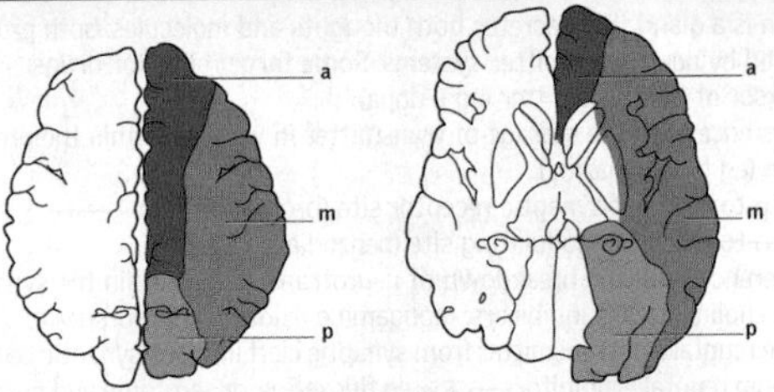

Fig 2. See text.

Carotid artery Internal carotid artery occlusion may, at worst, cause total (and usually fatal) infarction of the anterior two-thirds of the ipsilateral hemisphere and basal ganglia (lenticulostriate arteries). More often, the picture is similar to a middle cerebral artery occlusion (below).

Cerebral arteries 3 pairs of arteries leave the circle of Willis to supply the cerebral hemispheres: the anterior, middle, and posterior cerebral arteries. The anterior and middle cerebrals are branches of the carotid arteries; the basilar artery divides into the 2 posterior cerebral arteries. Ischaemia due to occlusion of any one of them may be reduced, if not prevented, by retrograde supply from meningeal vessels.

Anterior cerebral artery: (a in **Fig 2**) Supplies the frontal and medial part of the cerebrum. Occlusion may cause a weak, numb contralateral leg ± similar, if milder, arm symptoms. The face is spared. Bilateral infarction can cause akinetic mutism from damage to the cingulate gyri (also a rare cause of paraplegia).

Middle cerebral artery: (m in **Fig 2**) Supplies the lateral (external) part of each hemisphere. Occlusion may cause contralateral hemiparesis, hemisensory loss (esp. face and arm), contralateral homonymous hemianopia due to involvement of the optic radiation, cognitive change including dysphasia with dominant hemisphere lesions, and visuo-spatial disturbance (eg cannot dress; gets lost) with non-dominant lesions.

Posterior cerebral artery: (p in **fig 2**; also **fig 3**) Supplies the occipital lobe. Occlusion gives contralateral homonymous hemianopia (often with macula sparing).

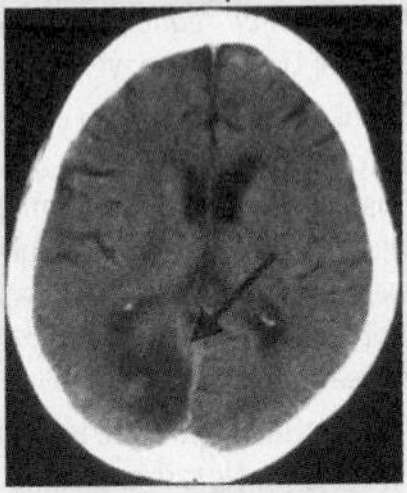

Fig 3. CT of stroke (arrow) in the distribution of the posterior cerebral artery.

Image courtesy of Prof. J Trobe.

Vertebrobasilar circulation Supplies the cerebellum, brainstem, occipital lobes, and occlusion may cause a combination of symptoms relating to any or all three: hemianopia; cortical blindness; diplopia; vertigo; nystagmus; ataxia; dysarthria; dysphasia; hemi- or quadriplegia; unilateral or bilateral sensory symptoms; hiccups; coma. Infarctions of the brainstem can produce various syndromes, eg *lateral medullary syndrome*, in which occlusion of one vertebral artery or the posterior inferior cerebellar artery causes infarction of the lateral medulla and the inferior cerebellar surface producing vertigo, vomiting, dysphagia, nystagmus, ipsilateral ataxia, soft palate paralysis, ipsilateral Horner's syndrome, and a crossed pattern sensory loss (analgesia to pin-prick on ipsilateral face and contralateral trunk & limbs). *Locked-in syndrome* is caused by damage to the ventral pons due to pontine artery occlusion. Patients are unable to move, but retain full awareness and cognitive function. They may be able to communicate by blinking.

Subclavian steal syndrome: Subclavian artery stenosis proximal to the origin of the vertebral artery may cause blood to be *stolen* by retrograde flow down this vertebral artery down into the arm, causing brainstem ischaemia typically after use of the arm. Suspect if the BP in each arm differs by >20mmHg.

Drugs and the nervous system

The brain is a gland that secretes both thoughts and molecules: both products are modulated by neurotransmitter systems. Some target sites for drugs:

1 Precursor of the transmitter (eg L-dopa).
2 Interference with the storage of transmitter in vesicles within the pre-synaptic neuron (eg tetrabenazine).
3 Binding to the post-synaptic receptor site (bromocriptine).
4 Binding to receptor-modulating site (benzodiazepines).
5 Interference with the breakdown of neurotransmitter within the synaptic cleft (acetylcholinesterase inhibitors; monoamine oxidase inhibitors—MAOIs).
6 Reduce reuptake of transmitter from synaptic cleft into pre-synaptic cell (selective serotonin reuptake inhibitors—SSRIs, eg fluoxetine, or serotonin and noradrenaline reuptake inhibitors—SNRIs, eg mirtazapine).[1]
7 Binding to presynaptic autoreceptors. There are 3 kinds of autoreceptors: neurotransmitter release modulators, synthesis modulators, and impulse modulators. These offer sites for intervention.[8] Augmenting antidepressant therapy with 5HT autoreceptor antagonists such as pindolol is possible.[9]

The proven neurotransmitters include:

Amino acids Glutamate & aspartate act as excitatory transmitters on NMDA & non-NMDA receptors (BOX)—relevant in epilepsy and CNS ischaemia. γ-aminobutyric acid (GABA) is mostly inhibitory. ***Drugs enhancing GABA activity:*** Used in epilepsy and neuropathic pain (gabapentin, valproate); spasticity (baclofen, benzodiazepines).

Peptides Opioids and substance P.

Histamine and **Purines** (such as ATP) Clinical relevance is not clear.

Dopamine (DA) ***Drugs enhancing DA activity:*** Used in Parkinson's; hyperprolactinaemia; acromegaly. SE: vomiting; BP↓; chorea; dystonia; hallucinations/psychosis. ***Drugs which reduce DA activity:*** Used in schizophrenia (*OHCS* p360, D_2 antagonists); chorea; tics; nausea; vertigo. SE: parkinsonism; dystonias; akathisia.

Serotonin (5-hydroxytryptamine; 5HT) There are many types of receptor, eg $5HT_{1-4}$. $5HT_1$ has 5 subtypes ($5HT_{1A-E}$). ***Agonists:*** Lithium_{1A}; sumatriptan_{1D}. ***Partial agonists:*** Buspirone_{1A}; LSD_2. ***Antagonists:*** Ondansetron_3, $\text{pizotifen}_{1\&2}$, $\text{methysergide}_{1\&2}$, clozapine_{2C}—known as low D_2–high $5HT_2$, while risperidone is high D_2–high $5HT_2$ (low D_2 means <60% D_2 occupancy at conventional doses; traditional antipsychotics are just high D_2, ie 60–80%). ***Reuptake inhibitors:*** Fluoxetine, sertraline, venlafaxine. Ecstasy increases nerve-terminal 5HT release.[10]

Adrenaline (epinephrine) and noradrenaline (norepinephrine) 4 receptor types: α_1, α_2, β_1, β_2. Noradrenaline is more specific for α-receptors but both transmitters affect all receptors. In the periphery, α-receptor stimulation leads to arteriolar vasoconstriction and pupillary dilatation, β_1 stimulation leads to increase in pulse and myocardial contractility, and β_2 stimulation leads to bronchodilatation, uterine relaxation, and arteriolar vasodilatation.

Drugs enhancing adrenergic activity: Used in asthma (β_2); anaphylaxis (adrenaline); heart failure (dobutamine); depression (MAOIs and tricyclics; the latter may act by increasing synaptic norepinephrine in the CNS).[1]

Drugs reducing adrenergic activity: Used in angina, ↑BP, arrhythmias (β_1); anxiety, thyrotoxicosis (β); ↑BP from phaeochromocytoma, prostatism (α).

Acetylcholine (Muscarinic and nicotinic receptors)

Centrally acting anticholinergics: Used in parkinsonism, dystonias, motion sickness. Central toxic effects (especially in the elderly): confusion, delusions.

Peripherally acting antimuscarinics: Used in asthma (ipratropium); incontinence; to dry secretions pre-op; to dilate pupils; to ↑ heart rate (atropine).

Peripherally acting cholinergic agonists: Used in glaucoma (pilocarpine); myasthenia (anticholinesterases). SE: sweating, hypersalivation, colic.

1 Noradrenaline may be more involved in the symptoms of anergia, fatigue and loss of drive in depression, and 5-HT may be more involved in the alteration in subjective mood and anxiety.

Neurotransmitters and CNS drugs

Here we list drugs used to modify CNS transmitters. When prescribing bear in mind that: • The drug (or a metabolite) must be able to pass through the blood-brain barrier to have an effect. • The consequences of any sedative effects may be severe. • There will be short- and long-term side effects (eg tardive dyskinesia with neuroleptic drugs). • Drugs may affect many neurotransmitters, increasing therapeutic scope (and uncertainty). • One neurotransmitter may have many effects, eg dopaminergic neurons go awry in Parkinson's disease, schizophrenia, and addiction to drugs and gambling, by affecting motor control, motivation, effort, reward, analgesia, stress, learning, attention, and cognition.

Drugs increasing activity (≈agonists)	Drugs decreasing activity (≈antagonists)
Dopamine	
Pergolide; apomorphine; amantadine Bromocriptine (D_2) Pramipexole (D_3) to do with mood behaviour & rewards Selegiline (MAOI-B inhibitor)	Benzisoxazoles (D_2) eg risperidone Haloperidol, chlorpromazine Metoclopramide (D_2)
Non-adrenaline & adrenaline (=norepinephrine & epinephrine)	
Salbutamol (β_2); adrenaline ?Tricyclic antidepressants MAOIs	Propranolol (β); bisoprolol, metoprolol (β_1) Clonidine (α_2-agonist) Phentolamine (α)
Serotonin (5HT)	
LSD and other hallucinogens Sumatriptan ($5HT_{1B\,\&\,1D}$) Some tricyclic antidepressants, eg trazodone Buspirone, lithium Fluoxetine	Pizotifen Benzisoxazoles ($5HT_2$), eg risperidone Olanzapine, clozapine ($5HT_{2A}$) Mirtazapine, ondansetron ($5HT_3$)
Acetylcholine	
Carbachol Pilocarpine anticholinesterases, eg donepezil, rivastigmine, pyridostigmine	Atropine; scopolamine Ipratropium Benzhexol (=trihexyphenidyl) Orphenadrine; procyclidine
GABA (=gamma aminobutyric acid—an inhibitory neurotransmitter)	
Benzodiazepines ($GABA_A$) Valproate Gabapentin, pregabalin Barbiturates Acamprosate (used in alcohol addiction; taurine & GABA analogue)	Baclofen ($GABA_B$) Alcohol abuse:[1] *acute effects* block *N*-methyl-D-aspartate (NMDA) receptors; *with chronic use*, numbers of NMDA receptors rise, mediating alcohol craving
Glutamate[1] (an excitatory amino acid)	
None	Lamotrigine (used in epilepsy) Topiramate (used in epilepsy)[1] Acamprosate (↓craving in alcoholics) Memantine (Alzheimer's, p492) Zonisamide (+ carbonic anhydrase activity, and modulates T-TYPE Ca^{2+} channels)

New drugs are often aimed at multiple neurotransmitters, eg *risperidone* (blocks D_2, $5HT_2$, α_1 and α_2 adrenoceptors, *OHCS* p360). The smoking-cessation drug *bupropion* (=*amfebutamone*) is said to act by increasing dopamine in the mesolimbic system (mediates dependence) *and* via noradrenergic effects in the locus ceruleus (mediates symptoms of nicotine withdrawal).

1 Alcoholics have more glutamate binding sites, facilitating midbrain dopamine neurotransmission (pathways, which, in the ventral tegmental area, mediate alcohol's rewarding effects). Topiramate and baclofen facilitate GABA function, antagonizing glutamate at kainate receptors, and ↓craving in alcoholism.

Upper limb		
Nerve root	**Muscle**	**Test by asking the patient to:**
C3, 4	Trapezius	Shrug shoulder (via accessory nerve)
C5, 6, 7	Serratus anterior	Push arm forward against resistance; look for winging of scapula (p515) if weak
C5, 6	Pectoralis major (P major) clavicular head	Adduct arm from above horizontal, and push it forward
C6, 7, 8	P major sternocostal head	Adduct arm below horizontal
C5, 6	Supraspinatus	Abduct arm the first 15°
C5, 6	Infraspinatus	Externally rotate semi-flexed arm, elbow at side
C6, 7, 8	Latissimus dorsi	Adduct arm from horizontal position
C5, 6	Biceps	Flex supinated forearm
C5, 6	Deltoid	Abduct arm between 15° and 90°
Radial nerve (p506)		
C6, 7, 8	Triceps	Extend elbow against resistance
C5, 6	Brachioradialis	Flex elbow with forearm half way between pronation and supination
C5, 6	Extensor carpi radialis longus	Extend wrist to radial side
C6, 7	Supinator	Arm by side, resist hand pronation
C7, 8	Extensor digitorum	Keep fingers extended at MCP joint
C7, 8	Extensor carpi ulnaris	Extend wrist to ulnar side
C7, 8	Abductor pollicis longus	Abduct thumb at 90° to palm
C7, 8	Extensor pollicis brevis	Extend thumb at MCP joint
C7, 8	Extensor pollicis longus	Resist thumb flexion at IP joint
Median nerve (p506)		
C6, 7	Pronator teres	Keep arm pronated against resistance
C6, 7	Flexor carpi radialis	Flex wrist towards radial side
C7, 8, T1	Flexor digitorum superficialis	Resist extension at PIP joint (with proximal phalanx fixed by the examiner)
C7, 8	Flexor digitorum profundus I & II	Resist extension at index DIP joint of index finger
C7, 8, T1	Flexor pollicis longus	Resist thumb extension at interphalangeal joint (fix proximal phalanx)
C8, T1	Abductor pollicis brevis	Abduct thumb (nail at 90° to palm)
C8, T1	Opponens pollicis	Thumb touches base of 5th finger-tip (nail parallel to palm)
C8, T1	1st lumbrical/interosseus (median & ulnar nerves)	Extend PIP joint against resistance with MCP joint held hyperextended
Ulnar nerve (p506)		
C7, 8, T1	Flexor carpi ulnaris	Flex wrist to ulnar side; observe tendon
C7, C8	Flexor digitorum profundus III and IV	Resist extension of distal phalanx of 5th finger while you fix its middle phalanx
C8, T1	Dorsal interossei	Finger abduction: cannot cross the middle over the index finger (tests index finger adduction too)[14]
C8, T1	Palmar interossei	Finger adduction: pull apart a sheet of paper held between middle and ring finger DIP joints of both hands; the paper moves on the weaker side[1] [15]
C8, T1	Adductor pollicis	Adduct thumb (nail at 90° to palm)
C8, T1	Abductor digiti minimi	Abduct little finger
C8, T1	Flexor digiti minimi	Flex little finger at MCP joint

1 Also, metacarpophalangeal joint flexion may be more on the affected side as flexor tendons are recruited—the basis of Froment's paper sign. Wartenberg's sign is persistent little finger abduction.

Lower limb

Femoral nerve		
L1, 2, 3	Iliopsoas (also supplied via L1, 2, & 3 spinal nerves)	Flex hip against resistance with knee flexed and lower leg supported: patient lies on back
L2, 3, 4	Quadriceps femoris	Extend at knee against resistance Start with knee flexed
Obturator nerve		
L2, 3, 4	Hip adductors	Adduct leg against resistance
Inferior gluteal nerve		
L5, S1, S2	Gluteus maximus	Hip extension ('bury heel into the couch')—with knee in extension
Superior gluteal nerve		
L4, 5, S1	Gluteus medius & minimus	Abduction and internal hip rotation with leg flexed at hip and knee
Sciatic (and common peroneal*) and sciatic (and tibial) nerves**		
*L4, 5	Tibialis anterior	Dorsiflex ankle
*L5, S1	Extensor digitorum longus	Dorsiflex toes against resistance
*L5, S1	Extensor hallucis longus	Dorsiflex hallux against resistance
*L5, S1	Peroneus longus & brevis	Evert foot against resistance
*L5, S1	Extensor digitorum brevis	Dorsiflex proximal phalanges of toes
**L5, S1, 2	Hamstrings	Flex knee against resistance
**L4, 5	Tibialis posterior	Invert plantarflexed foot
**S1, 2	Gastrocnemius	Plantarflex ankle or stand on tiptoe
**L5, S1, 2	Flexor digitorum longus	Flex terminal joints of toes
**S1, 2	Small muscles of foot	Make the sole of the foot into a cup

Quick screening test for muscle power

Shoulder	Abduction	C5	**Hip**	Flexion	L1–L2
	Adduction	C5–C7		Adduction	L2-3
Elbow	Flexion	C5–C6		Extension	L5–S1
	Extension	C7	**Knee**	Flexion	L5–S1
Wrist	Flexion	C7-8		Extension	L3–L4
	Extension	C7	**Ankle**	Dorsiflexion	L4
Fingers	Flexion	C8		Eversion	L5–S1
	Extension	C7		Plantarflexion	S1–S2
	Abduction	T1	**Toe**	Big toe extension	L5

Remember to test proximal muscle power: ask the patient to sit from lying, to pull you towards himself, and to rise from squatting (if reasonably fit).

►Observe walking—easy to forget, even if the complaint is of difficulty walking!

►Sources vary in ascribing particular nerve roots to muscles, and there is some biological variation in individuals. The above is a reasonable compromise, based on MRC/*Brain* 2001 guidelines: ISBN 0-7020-2512-7.
►We don't react to nerve damage according to simple anatomy; eg ulnar neuropathy may initiate dystonic flexion or tremor of 4th & 5th digits by inducing a central motor disorder.

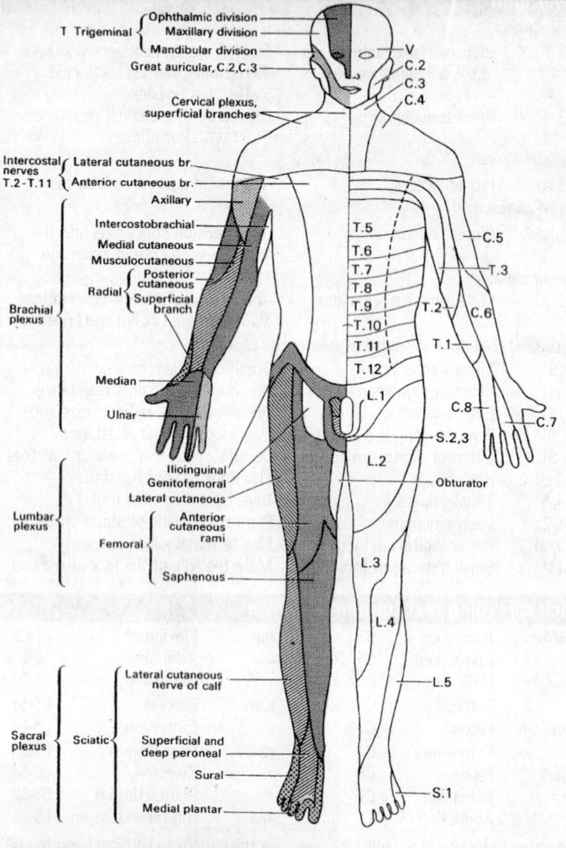

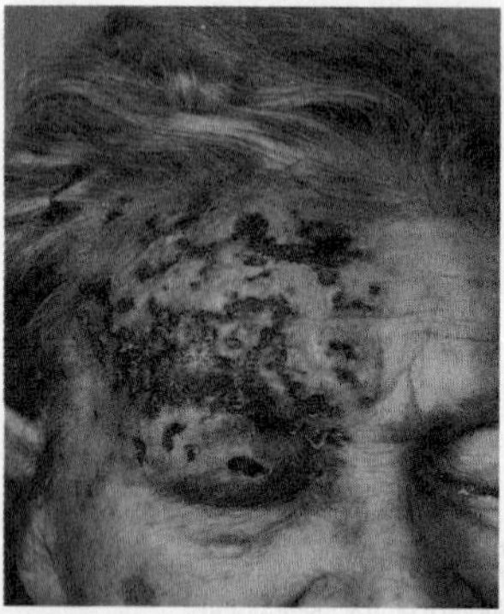

Pain in a dermatomal distribution suggests a problem with a cranial nerve or dorsal root ganglion (radiculopathy)—where the cell bodies of sensory fibres live.[17] What is the dermatome? What is the lesion? See p400.

Dermatomes

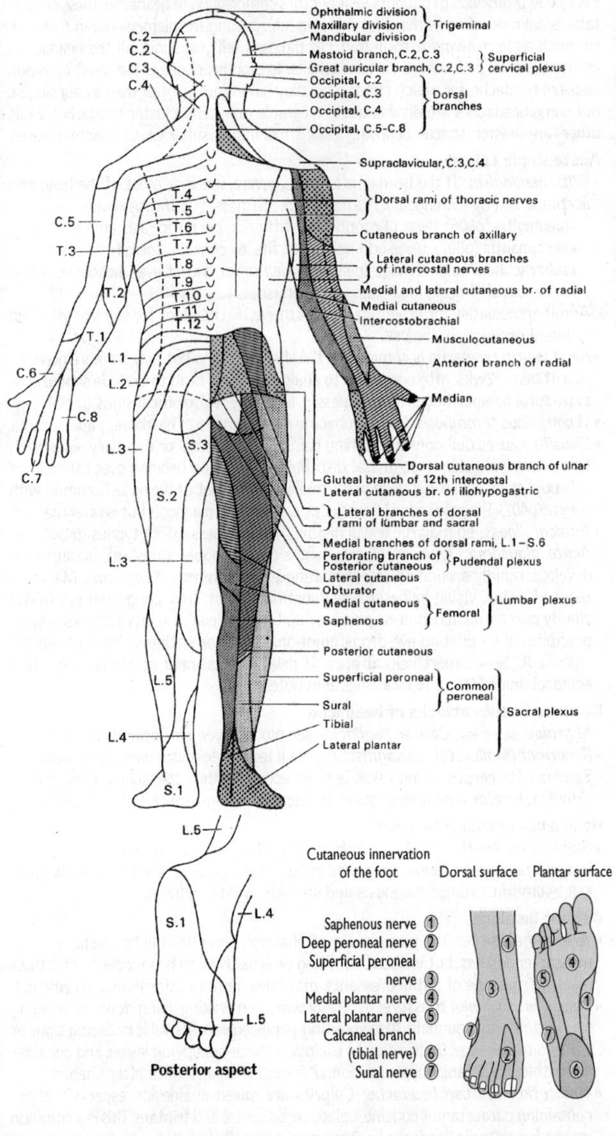

Ophthalmic division
Maxillary division
Mandibular division
Trigeminal
Mastoid branch, C.2, C.3
Great auricular branch, C.2, C.3
Superficial cervical plexus
Occipital, C.2
Occipital, C.3
Occipital, C.4
Occipital, C.5–C.8
Dorsal branches
Supraclavicular, C.3, C.4
Dorsal rami of thoracic nerves
Cutaneous branch of axillary
Lateral cutaneous branches of intercostal nerves
Medial and lateral cutaneous br. of radial
Medial cutaneous
Intercostobrachial
Musculocutaneous
Anterior branch of radial
Median
Dorsal cutaneous branch of ulnar
Gluteal branch of 12th intercostal
Lateral cutaneous br. of iliohypogastric
Lateral branches of dorsal rami of lumbar and sacral
Medial branches of dorsal rami, L.1 – S.6
Perforating branch of
Posterior cutaneous
Pudendal plexus
Lateral cutaneous
Obturator
Medial cutaneous
Saphenous
Femoral
Lumbar plexus
Posterior cutaneous
Superficial peroneal
Common peroneal
Sural
Tibial
Lateral plantar
Sacral plexus
C.2
C.2
C.3
C.4
C.5
T.3
T.2
T.1
C.6
C.8
C.7
T.4
T.5
T.6
T.7
T.8
T.9
T.10
T.11
T.12
L.1
L.2
L.3
S.3
S.2
L.3
L.5
L.4
S.1
L.5
S.1
L.4
L.5
Posterior aspect
Cutaneous innervation of the foot
Dorsal surface
Plantar surface
Saphenous nerve 1
Deep peroneal nerve 2
Superficial peroneal nerve 3
Medial plantar nerve 4
Lateral plantar nerve 5
Calcaneal branch (tibial nerve) 6
Sural nerve 7

Headache

Every day, *thousands* of patients visit doctors complaining of headache. These consultations are rewarding as the chief skill is in interpreting the history—not in *taking* it, so much as in *allowing* it to unfold. Let patients tell you about all the headache's associations, or even *who* their headache is. Tension headache is the most common cause of headache, for which stress relief may have more to offer than a neurologist, but some headaches are disabling and treatable (migraine, cluster headache), while others are sinister (space-occupying lesions, meningitis, subarachnoid haemorrhage).

Acute single episode

- *With meningism:* If the headache is acute, severe, felt over most of the head and accompanied by meningeal irritation (neck stiffness) you must exclude:
  - **meningitis** (p806): fever, photophobia, stiff neck, purpuric rash, coma
  - **encephalitis** (p807): fever, odd behaviour, fits, or consciousness↓
  - **subarachnoid haemorrhage** (p482): *sudden*-onset, 'worst ever' headache, often occipital, stiff neck, focal signs, consciousness↓.

  Admit immediately for urgent CT head. If CT -ve, do LP to look for signs of infection or blood products in the CSF.
- *Head injury:* Headache is common at the site of trauma but may be more generalized. It lasts ~2wks; often resistant to analgesia. Do CT head to exclude **subdural** or **extradural haemorrhage** if drowsiness ± lucid interval, or focal signs (p486).
- *Venous sinus thrombosis:* (p484) Subacute or sudden-onset headache, papilloedema.
- *Sinusitis* causes dull, constant, aching pain over the frontal or maxillary sinus, with tender overlying skin ± postnasal drip. Pain is worse on bending over. Ethmoid or sphenoid sinus pain is felt deep in the midline at the root of the nose. Common with coryza (p402). The pain lasts ~1-2 weeks. CT can confirm diagnosis but is rarely needed.
- *Tropical illness:* eg malaria: travel history, flu-like illness (p388); typhus (p435).
- *Acute glaucoma:* Typically elderly, long-sighted people. Constant, aching pain develops rapidly around one eye, radiating to the forehead. *Symptoms:* Markedly reduced vision, visual haloes, nausea/vomiting. *Signs:* Red, congested eye (p563); cloudy cornea; dilated, non-responsive pupil, may be oval; ↓acuity. Attacks may be precipitated by dilating eye-drops, emotional upset or sitting in the dark, eg the cinema. *℞:* Seek expert help at once. If delay in treatment of >1h is likely, start acetazolamide 500mg IV over several minutes.

Recurrent acute attacks of headache

Migraine: see p462. *Cluster headache:* see BOX 1. *Trigeminal neuralgia:* see BOX 2.

- *Recurrent (Mollaret's) meningitis:* Suspect if fever/meningism with every headache. Send CSF for herpes simplex PCR. Is there access to the subarachnoid space via a skull fracture, or a recurring cause of aseptic meningitis (SLE, Behçet's, sarcoid)?

Headaches of subacute onset

- *Giant cell arteritis:* (p558). *Exclude in all >50yrs old with a headache that has lasted a few weeks.* Tender, thickened, pulseless temporal arteries; jaw claudication; ESR >40mm/h. Prompt diagnosis and steroids avoid blindness.

Chronic headache

- *Tension headache:* The usual cause of bilateral, non-pulsatile headache ± scalp muscle tenderness, but without vomiting or sensitivity to head movement. Stress relief, eg massage or antidepressants, may have more to offer than a neurologist.
- *Raised intracranial pressure:* Typically worse on waking, lying down or bending forward, or with coughing. Also vomiting, papilloedema, fits, false localizing signs or behavioural change. Do imaging to exclude a space-occupying lesion, and consider idiopathic intracranial hypertension. *LP is contraindicated* until after imaging.
- *Medication overuse headache:* Culprits are mixed analgesics, especially those containing paracetamol, codeine, opiates, ergotamine and triptans. This is a common reason for episodic headache becoming chronic daily headache. Analgesia must be withdrawn—aspirin or naproxen may mollify the rebound headache. A preventive may help once other drugs withdrawn (eg tricyclics, valproate, gabapentin; p508). Advise patients to use over-the-counter analgesia no more than 6 days per month.

Cluster headache (AKA migrainous neuralgia)

One theory (among many) is that this is caused by superficial temporal artery smooth muscle hyperreactivity to 5HT. There are related hypothalamic grey matter abnormalities. An autosomal dominant gene also has a role. ♂:♀ ≥5:1; onset at any age; commoner in smokers.

Symptoms
Rapid onset severe pain around one eye which may become watery and bloodshot with lid swelling, lacrimation, facial flushing, rhinorrhoea, miosis ± ptosis (20% of attacks; permanent in 5%). Pain is strictly unilateral and almost always affects the same side. It lasts 15-160min, occurs once or twice a day, and is often nocturnal. Clusters last 4-12wks and are followed by pain-free periods of months or even 1-2yrs before the next cluster. Sometimes it is chronic rather than episodic.

Management
Acute attack: 100% O_2 for ~15min via non-rebreathable mask (CI in COPD);[18] **sumatriptan** SC 6mg at the attack's onset. *Preventives:* 1st line are **verapamil** or **topiramate**. Also lithium, steroids, methysergide (highly effective but SE of retroperitoneal fibrosis ∴ take a 1 month 'drug holiday' every 6 months).

The father in extremis
'...I am careful not to wake the children as I make my way down the stairs. If they were to witness my nightly cluster ritual, they would never see me the same way again. Their father, fearless protector, diligent provider, crawling about in tears, beating his head on the hard wood floor. The pain is so intense I want to scream, but I never do. I go down 3 flights of stairs where I can't be heard, and drop to my knees. I place my hands on the back of my neck, and lock my fingers together. I bind my head between my arms and squeeze as hard as I can in an attempt to crush my skull. I begin to roll around, banging my head on the floor, pressing my left eye with full force of my palm. I search for the phone that has always been my weapon of choice for creating a diversion, and I beat my left temple with the hand piece. I create a rhythm as I strike my skull, cursing the demon with each blow...'[19]

Trigeminal neuralgia

Symptoms: Paroxysms of intense, stabbing pain, lasting seconds, in the trigeminal nerve distribution. It is unilateral, typically affecting mandibular or maxillary divisions. The face screws up with pain (hence *tic doloureux*). *Triggers:* Washing affected area, shaving, eating, talking, dental prostheses. *Typical patient:* ♂ >50yrs old; in Asians ♀:♂ ≈2:1. *Secondary causes:* compression of the trigeminal root by anomalous or aneurysmal intracranial vessels or a tumour, chronic meningeal inflammation, MS, zoster, skull base malformation (eg Chiari). *MRI* is necessary to exclude secondary causes (~14% of cases).[20] *R̷x:* **Carbamazepine** (start at 100mg/12h PO; max 400mg/6h; **lamotrigine**; **phenytoin** 200-400mg/24h PO; or **gabapentin** (p508). If drugs fail, surgery may be necessary. This may be directed at the peripheral nerve, the trigeminal ganglion or the nerve root. *Microvascular decompression:* Anomalous vessels are separated from the trigeminal root. Stereotactic gamma knife surgery can work, but length of pain relief and the time to treatment response are limiting factors. *Facial pain ΔΔ:* p71.

Migraine

Migraine causes much misery and costs the UK economy >£200 million a year in lost production. Its prevalence is 8%. ♀:♂≈2:1.

Symptoms *Classically:* • Visual or other aura (see below) lasting 15-30min followed within 1h by unilateral, throbbing headache. *Or:* • Isolated aura with no headache; • Episodic severe headaches without aura, often premenstrual, usually unilateral, with nausea, vomiting ± photophobia/phonophobia (*'common migraine'*). There may be allodynia—all stimuli produce pain: "I can't brush my hair, wear earrings or glasses, or shave, it's so painful". *Signs:* None. *Associations:* Obesity (weight loss may ↓ excess oestrogen/estradiol production in adipose tissue—but benefit is unproven);[21] patent foramen ovale (some say catheter closure may help).[22] *Tests:* None if typical history.

Prodrome: Yawning, food cravings, or changes in sleep, appetite or mood may precede the headache by hours or days.

Aura: Precedes the headache by minutes and may persist during it. • *Visual:* chaotic cascading, distorting, 'melting' and jumbling of lines, dots, or zigzags, scotomata or hemianopia; • *Somatosensory:* paraesthesiae spreading from fingers to face; • *Motor:* dysarthria and ataxia (basilar migraine), ophthalmoplegia, or hemiparesis; • *Speech:* (8% of auras) dysphasia or paraphasia, eg phoneme substitution.

Diagnostic criteria if no aura ≥5 headaches lasting 4-72h with either nausea/vomiting or photo/phonophobia, *and* ≥2 of: • Unilateral; • Pulsating; • Interferes with normal life; • Worsened by routine activity, eg climbing stairs.

Triggers CHOCOLATE *or:* Cheese, oral contraceptives, caffeine (or its withdrawal), alcohol, anxiety, travel, or exercise. In ~50%, no trigger is found, and in only a few does avoiding triggers prevent *all* attacks.

Differential Cluster or tension headache, cervical spondylosis, ↑BP, intracranial pathology, sinusitis/otitis media, caries. TIAs may mimic migraine aura. Migraine is rarely a sign of other pathology: don't look *too* hard for antiphospholipid syndrome, arteriovenous malformations, or microemboli (but in some they may be important).

Treatment NSAIDs (eg **ketoprofen** 100mg, dispersible **aspirin** 900mg/6h) are preferred as there is less chance of developing medication misuse headache (p460), and they have similar efficacy to oral 5HT agonists (triptans and ergot alkaloids).[23] Triptans are generally better tolerated than ergots: in one QALY-based study, **rizatriptan** was better/cheaper than **sumatriptan**[1], which was better/cheaper than **Cafergot**® (below).[24] Triptans are CI if IHD, coronary spasm, uncontrolled ↑BP, recent lithium, SSRIs, or ergot use. Rare SEs: arrhythmias or angina ± MI, even if no pre-existing risk. **Ergotamine** 1mg PO as headache starts, repeated at ½h, up to 3mg in a day, and 6mg in a week; or better, as a *Cafergot® suppository* (2mg ergotamine + 100mg caffeine up to 2 in 24h; then ≥4 days without). Emphasize dangers of ergotamine (gangrene, vascular damage). CI: the Pill (*OHCS* p300); peripheral vascular disease, IHD; pregnancy; breast-feeding; hemiplegic migraine; Raynaud's; liver or renal impairment; BP↑.

Prophylaxis (eg if frequency > twice a month). *1st line:* **Propranolol** 40-120mg/12h, **topiramate** 25-50mg/12h (SE: memory impairment),[25] or **amitriptyline** 25-75mg nocte (SE: drowsiness, dry mouth, blurred vision). *2nd-line agents:* **Valproate**, **pizotifen** (effective, but unacceptable weight gain in some), **gabapentin**, **pregabalin** or NSAIDs.[26] There is less evidence for levetiracetam, tiagabine and lamotrigine.[27] If one drug does not work after 3 months, try another—be guided by patient choice and SEs. Most (>65%) achieve ~50% ↓ in attack frequency.

Non-pharmacological therapies: Warm or cold packs to the head, or rebreathing into paper bag (↑P_aCO_2) may help abort attacks.[28] Spinal manipulation,[29] riboflavin[30] and magnesium may have a role. ►Migraine often co-exists with other chronic conditions—and the combined negative impact is immense. Don't treat each disease in isolation. Rather, attempt to restore a good relationship with the self—and the recovery of the purpose of life. This is the hardest and the most rewarding task. Can these structured holistic dialogues help? Yes, definitely,[31] so don't be daunted.

What is going on in migraine?

The old theory was vascular: constriction during aura, with dilatation causing pain. But MRIs during attacks show episodic cerebral oedema, dilatation of intracerebral vessels, and ↓water diffusion not respecting vascular territories, so the primary event may be neurological.[32] PET (p752) implicates ↑hypothalamic activity; this matches food cravings and neuroendocrine data.[33]

Is migraine due to a hyperexcitable brain? Magneto-encephalographic (MEG) studies have shown resting (interictal) hyperexcitability at least in the visual cortex, suggesting a failure of inhibitory circuits.[34] Cortical hyperexcitability may relate to imbalance between neuronal inhibition (mediated by GABA, p455) and excitation (via excitatory amino acids). Putative causes: ↓cerebral Mg^{2+} levels, mitochondrial abnormalities, dysfunctions related to ↑nitric oxide, and Ca^{2+} channelopathy.[35]

How do triptans work? Triptans are $5HT_{1B/1D}$ agonists, constricting cranial arteries. They also inhibit the release of a number of neurotransmitters involved in pain pathways, such as substance P, and of pro-inflammatory neuropeptides. They appear to be especially effective at blocking transmission from the trigeminal nerve to 2nd-order neurons in the trigeminal nucleus caudalis,[36] hence use in any process that activates trigeminal fibres, including migraine, cluster headache & subarachnoid haemorrhage.

Migraine considerations in women

Migraine, stroke, and the Pill *(combined oral contraception, COC)* Incidence of migraine + Pill-related ischaemic stroke is 8/100,000 if aged 20; and 80/100,000 in those aged 40yrs. Low-dose COCs only should be used. Those with migraine with aura are known to be at especial risk, precluding use of the combined Pill (but no problem with progesterone-only or non-hormonal contraception). Risk is further augmented by: • Smoking; • Age >35yrs; • BP↑; • Obesity (body mass index >30); • Diabetes mellitus; • Hyperlipidaemia; • Family history of arteriopathy when aged <45yrs. Warn women with migraine to stop Pills at once if they develop aura or worsening migraine—see *OHCS* p301.

If the problem is migraine without aura in the pill-free interval consider: • Alternative contraception method or a pill with a lower dose of the same progestogen or lowest available dose of a different progestogen. • Tri-cycling: take the pill continuously for 3 packets (9 weeks) followed by a 7 day pill-free interval, so that the number of menstrual bleeds is reduced. • Oestrogen supplements (below) from 3 days before menses, continuing for 7 days.

Peri-menstrual migraine *Prophylaxis:* If no asthma, CCF, peptic ulcer etc, NSAID (eg mefenamic acid) at onset of menses to last day of bleeding ± transdermal estradiol 50-100μg patches 3 days before menses, continue for 7 days.

Pregnancy Be optimistic: migraine often improves; if not, get help—evidence suggests that worsening migraine in pregnancy is associated with a greater risk of pre-eclampsia and cardiovascular complications.[37] *Prophylaxis:* stop, or use **amitriptyline** (most, especially the anti-convulsants, are teratogenic). *Anti-emetic:* **cyclizine** or **promethazine**. *Analgesia:* **ibuprofen** or **aspirin** may be used up to 30 weeks' gestation. If attacks persist in the 2nd and 3rd trimesters (uncommon) and **paracetamol** is insufficient, try partial agonist opioids.[38] Don't use aspirin if breastfeeding.

1 Of the oral triptans, **rizatriptan** is said to have quick efficacy; **rizatriptan** & **zolmitriptan** are available as rapid-dissolving wafers. **Imigran Recover®** may be bought 'over the counter'. **Almotriptan** is similar to oral sumatriptan, but ?fewer SEs; 12.5mg is an effective, well-tolerated alternative if there is a poor response to sumatriptan 50mg. A poor response to one triptan doesn't predict a poor response to all. Rizatriptan interacts with propranolol (halve rizatriptan dose).

History It is vital to establish exactly what patients mean by 'blackout'. Do they mean loss of consciousness (LOC)? A fall to the ground without loss of consciousness? A clouding of vision, diplopia, or vertigo? Take a detailed history from the patient *and* a witness (see BOX).

Vasovagal (neurocardiogenic) syncope Due to reflex bradycardia ± peripheral vasodilatation provoked by emotion, pain, fear or standing too long. Onset is over seconds (*not* instantaneous), and is often preceded by nausea, pallor, sweating and closing in of visual fields (pre-syncope). *It cannot occur if lying down.* The patient falls to the ground, being unconscious for ~2min. Brief clonic jerking of the limbs may occur (reflex anoxic convulsion due to cerebral hypoperfusion), but there is no stiffening or tonic→clonic sequence. Urinary incontinence is uncommon (but can occur), and there is no tongue-biting. Post-ictal recovery is rapid.

Situation syncope Syncopal symptoms are as described for vasovagal syncope.
- *Cough syncope:* Syncope after a paroxysm of coughing.
- *Effort syncope:* Syncope on exercise; cardiac origin, eg aortic stenosis, HOCM.
- *Micturition syncope:* Syncope during or after micturition. Mostly men, at night.

Carotid sinus syncope Hypersensitive baroreceptors cause excessive reflex bradycardia ± vasodilatation on minimal stimulation (eg head-turning, shaving).

Epilepsy Attacks vary with the type of seizure (p494), but certain features are more suggestive of epilepsy: attacks when asleep or lying down; aura; identifiable triggers, eg TV; altered breathing; cyanosis; typical tonic-clonic movements; incontinence of urine; tongue-biting (ask about a sore tongue after the fit); prolonged post-ictal drowsiness, confusion, amnesia and transient focal paralysis (Todd's palsy).

Stokes–Adams attacks Transient arrhythmias (eg bradycardia due to complete heart block) causing ↓cardiac output and LOC. The patient falls to the ground (often with *no* warning except palpitations), pale, with a slow or absent pulse. Recovery is in seconds, the patient flushes, the pulse speeds up, and consciousness is regained. Injury is typical of these intermittent arrhythmias. As with vasovagal syncope, a few clonic jerks may occur if an attack is prolonged, due to cerebral hypoperfusion (reflex anoxic convulsion). Attacks may happen several times a day and in any posture.

Drop attacks Sudden weakness of the legs causes the patient, usually an older woman, to fall to the ground. There is no warning, no LOC and no confusion afterwards. The condition is benign, resolving spontaneously after a number of attacks. *Other causes:* hydrocephalus (these patients, however, may not be able to get up for hours); cataplexy—triggered by emotion (associated with narcolepsy, p714).

Other causes ***Hypoglycaemia:*** Tremor, hunger, and perspiration herald light-headedness or LOC; rare in non-diabetics but see p206. ***Orthostatic hypotension:*** Unsteadiness or LOC on standing from lying in those with inadequate vasomotor reflexes: the elderly; autonomic neuropathy (p509); antihypertensive medication; overdiuresis; multi-system atrophy (MSA; p499). ***Anxiety:*** Hyperventilation, tremor, sweating, tachycardia, paraesthesiae, light-headedness, and no LOC suggest a panic attack. ***Factitious blackouts:*** pseudoseizures, Münchausen's (p720). ***Choking:*** If a large piece of food blocks the larynx, the patient may collapse, become cyanotic, and be unable to speak. Do the Heimlich manoeuvre immediately to eject the food.

Examination Cardiovascular, neurological. BP lying and standing.

Investigation ECG ± 24h ECG (arrhythmia, long QT, eg Romano–Ward, p90);[1] U&E, FBC, glucose; tilt-table tests; EEG, sleep EEG; echocardiogram; CT/MRI brain; HUT.[2] P_aCO_2↓ in attacks suggests hyperventilation as the cause.

►*While the cause is being elucidated, advise against driving.*

1 Consider elevating V1–V3 leads from 4th to the 2nd intercostal space to reveal saddle-shaped ST elevation, a telltale sign of **Brugada syndrome** (p709)—a SCN5A channelopathy predisposing to VT.

2 **Head-up tilt (HUT) tests** distinguish vasodepressor from cardio-inhibitory syncope. HUT is +ve if symptoms are associated with a BP drop >30mmHg (vasodepressor; consider β-blockers to counter ↑sympathetic activity)—or bradycardia (cardio-inhibitory; consider pacing).

Taking a history of blackouts

Ask a witness:

- Does the patient lose awareness?
- Does the patient injure himself?
- Does the patient move? Are they stiff or floppy? (Not everything that twitches is epilepsy—a few clonic jerks may occur with syncope or arrhythmias, but are not preceded by a tonic phase. Ask for exact details of movements.)
- Is there incontinence? (More common in epilepsy, but can occur with syncope.)
- Is the complexion changed? (Cyanosis suggests epilepsy; white or red suggests arrhythmia, but may also occur in temporal lobe seizures.)
- Does the patient bite the side of his tongue? (Suggests epilepsy.)
- What is the patient's pulse like? (Abnormalities suggest a cardiological cause.)
- Any associated symptoms (palpitations, sweats, pallor, chest pain, dyspnoea)?
- How long does the attack last?
- If a 'drop attack', is the patient always sleepy? (Narcolepsy, p714.)

Before the attack:

- Is there any warning?—eg typical epileptic aura or cardiac pre-syncope.
- In what circumstances do attacks occur? (If watching TV, presume epilepsy).
- Can the patient prevent attacks?

After the attack:

- How much does the patient remember about the attack afterwards?
- Muscle ache afterwards suggests a tonic-clonic seizure.
- Is the patient confused or sleepy? (Suggests epilepsy).

Background to attacks:

- When did they start?
- Are they getting more frequent?
- Is anyone else in the family getting them? Sudden arrhythmic death syndrome (SADS)[1] may leave no cardiac trace at post mortem, or there may be hereditary cardiomyopathy.

►Witnesses often give conflicting accounts: the most reliable may not be the one with the most medical knowledge. He or she may know what you expect to hear, and furnish you with extra (imagined) material.

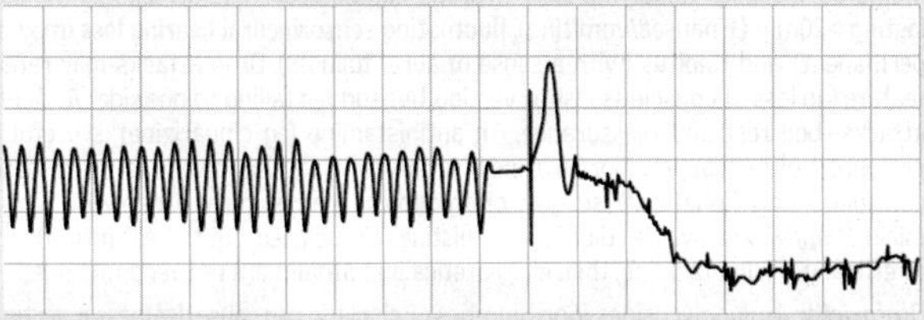

Fig 1. What is the cause of this patient's blackouts (also illustrated on p126)? Try to work out how they have been treated before reading footnote 1 opposite. What is the event illustrated here, and what happens just afterwards? Clue: DDDMS (p126). ►All with recurrent syncope (or falls) need cardiac assessment—urgently if associated with palpitations, arrhythmias, 3rd-degree AV block, or prolonged QT interval (p725).[39] Also refer those with a relative who has had a sudden unexplained death (<40yrs old)—genetic counselling is vital: bshg.org.uk/genetic_centres/uk_genetic_centres.htm

Vertigo and dizziness

Complaints of 'dizzy spells' are very common and are used by patients to describe many different sensations. The key to diagnosis is to find out exactly what the patient means by 'dizzy' and then decide whether or not this represents vertigo.

Is this vertigo? *Definition:* An illusion of movement, often rotatory, of the patient or his surroundings. In practice, simple 'spinning' is rare—the floor may tilt, sink, or rise, or "I veer sideways on walking as if pulled by a magnet". Vertigo is always[1] worsened by movement. *Associated symptoms:* Difficulty walking or standing (may even fall suddenly to the ground), relief on lying or sitting still; nausea, vomiting, pallor, sweating. Associated hearing loss or tinnitus implies labyrinth or VIIIth nerve involvement. ***What is not vertigo:*** *Faintness* may be due to anxiety with associated palpitations, tremor, and sweating. *Light-headedness* may be due to anaemia, orthostatic hypotension, or effort in an emphysematous patient. But in all of these there is no illusion of movement or typical associated symptoms. *Lost awareness* during attacks should prompt thoughts of epilepsy or syncope rather than vertigo.

Causes The labyrinth, vestibular nerve, vestibular nuclei, or their central connections are responsible for almost all vertigo. Only rarely are other structures involved (BOX).

Causes of vertigo

Labyrinth & VIIIth nerve
- Ménière's disease
- Vestibular neuronitis (ie acute labyrinthitis)
- Benign positional vertigo (*OHCS* p554)
- Motion sickness
- Trauma
- Ototoxic drugs
- Zoster (ie Ramsay Hunt syndrome, p505)

Brainstem, cerebellum, cerebello-pontine angle
(Look for nystagmus and cranial nerve lesions)
- MS
- Stroke/TIA
- Haemorrhage
- Migraine
- Acoustic neuroma

Cerebral cortex
- Vertiginous epilepsy

Alcohol intoxication

Benign positional vertigo is due to canalolithiasis—debris in the semicircular canal, disturbed by head movement, resettles causing vertigo that lasts a few seconds after the movement (often turning over in bed). Nystagmus on performing the Hallpike manoeuvre is diagnostic. The Epley manoeuvre clears the debris from the semicircular canals (*OHCS* p554).

Acute labyrinthitis (vestibular neuronitis): Abrupt onset of severe vertigo, nausea, vomiting ± prostration. No deafness or tinnitus. *Causes:* virus; vascular lesion. Severe vertigo subsides in days, complete recovery takes 3–4wks. *℞:* Reassure. Sedate.

Ménière's disease: Endolymphatic hydrops causes recurrent attacks of **vertigo** lasting >20min (± nausea/vomiting), fluctuating sensorineural **hearing loss** (may be permanent), and **tinnitus** (with a sense of aural fullness). Drop attacks may rarely feature (no loss of consciousness or vertigo, but sudden falling to one side). *℞:* Acute attacks—bed rest and reassurance. An antihistamine (eg cinnarizine) is useful if prolonged, or buccal prochlorperazine if severe, for up to 7d. In very severe disease, consider endolymphatic sac surgery or ablation of the vestibular organ with gentamicin. *Prophylaxis:* low-Na^+ diets or betahistine may be tried, but there is no evidence of efficacy.[40] Trimetazidine, thiazide diuretics and lithium are not recommended.

Ototoxicity: Aminoglycosides, loop diuretics or cisplatin can cause deafness ± vertigo.

Acoustic neuroma (**figs 1 & 2**) is doubly misnamed: it is a Schwannoma (not neuroma) arising from the vestibular (not auditory) nerve. It often presents with unilateral hearing loss, with vertigo occurring later. With progression, ipsilateral V[th], VIth, IXth, & X[th] nerves may be affected (also ipsilateral cerebellar signs). Paradoxically, the VIIth nerve is rarely involved pre-operatively. Signs of ↑ICP occur late, indicating a large tumour. They account for 80% of cerebello-pontine angle tumours (ΔΔ meningioma).[41] Commoner in ♀; also in neurofibromatosis (esp. NF2, p518). Not all need removing.

Traumatic damage involving the petrous temporal bone or the cerebello-pontine angle often affects the auditory nerve, causing vertigo, deafness and/or tinnitus.

Herpes zoster: Herpetic eruption of the external auditory meatus; facial palsy ± deafness, tinnitus, and vertigo (Ramsay Hunt syndrome, see p505).

1 The single exception is *mal de debarquement*, in which vertiginous motion sickness persists long after alighting from, for example, the ship or train that triggered the motion sickness.

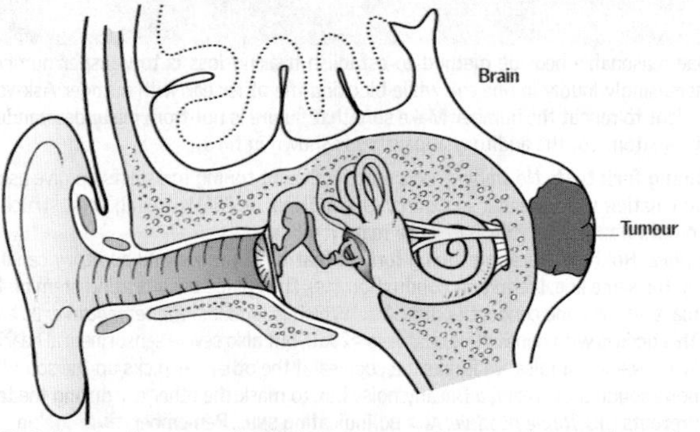

Fig 1. An acoustic neuroma (vestibular Schwannoma) growing dangerously near the facial nerve. It is helpful to understand their natural history, since you may be able to save patients a difficult and dangerous operation. For each patient growth rate is constant and predictable after a few years of serial MRIs: ~30% do not progress; ~50% grow slowly (1-2mm/yr); and ~20% grow >2mm/yr per year. Malignancy is rare but not negligible, and every so often we all get tricked by these tumours. ***Microsurgical removal*** has ~1% operative mortality. Near-normal post-op facial movement, sensation and perhaps hearing is the aim, but damage to VIIth nerve is common. Likelihood of surgical cure is >95%.[42]

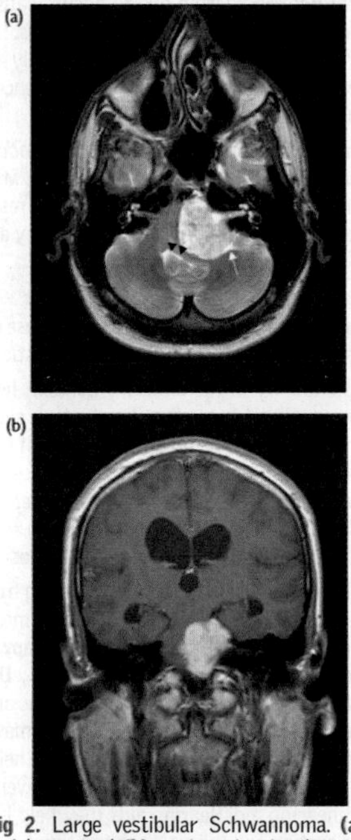

Fig 2. Large vestibular Schwannoma. **(a)** Axial T2W and **(b)** post-contrast enhanced coronal MRI.[43]

 ►See *OHCS* p550 for management

Hearing loss

One reasonable bedside method to establish hearing loss is to whisper numbers increasingly loudly in one ear while blocking the other ear with a finger. Ask your patient to repeat the number. Make sure that failure is not from misunderstanding. The anatomy of the auditory apparatus is shown in **fig 1**.

Tuning fork tests No single test is diagnostic, but tuning fork tests do give useful information (also popular in exams). Use a 512Hz or 256Hz tuning fork, struck ⅓ from its free end on your patella to make it vibrate.

- *Rinne:* Hold the vibrating tuning fork so that the 2 prongs and auditory canal lie on the same line, testing air conduction (AC). Then place the vibrating stem on the mastoid for bone conduction (BC). Ask "Which is louder?" ***Rinne negative:*** BC > AC. This occurs with conductive deafness >20dB, but also severe sensorineural hearing loss (SNHL)—ie a false -ve Rinne: the cochlea of the other ear picks up the sound by bone conduction. Using a Barany noise box to mask the other ear during the test, prevents this. ***Rinne positive:*** AC > BC, indicating SNHL. Remember '**SNAC–RIP**': in sensorineural loss & normal ears, air conduction is better—Rinne is positive.
- *Weber:* With the vibrating tuning fork on the vertex, forehead or upper incisors(!), ask the patient which ear the sound is heard in. Sound localizes to the affected ear with conductive loss (>10dB loss), to the contralateral ear in SNHL, and to the midline if both ears are normal (or if bilateral sensorineural loss).

Conductive deafness *Causes:* wax (remove eg by syringing with warm water after softening with olive oil drops), otosclerosis, otitis media, or glue ear (*OHCS* p546).

Chronic sensorineural deafness Often due to accumulated environmental noise toxicity, presbyacusis or inherited disorders. ***Presbyacusis:*** Loss of acuity for high-frequency sounds starts before 30yrs old. We do not usually notice it until hearing of speech is affected. Hearing is most affected in the presence of background noise. Hearing aids are the usual treatment.

Sudden sensorineural deafness ►Get an ENT opinion *today*! *Causes:* noise exposure; gentamicin/other toxin; mumps; acoustic neuroma; MS; stroke; vasculitis; TB. *Tests:* ESR, FBC, LFTs, pANCA, viral titres & TB Elispot; evoked response audiometry; CXR; MRI; lymph node & nasopharyngeal biopsy for malignancy and TB culture.

Tinnitus

(See also *OHCS* p552)

This ringing or buzzing in the ears is common, and may cause depression or insomnia. ►Investigate unilateral tinnitus fully to exclude an acoustic neuroma (p466).

Causes Focal hyper-excitability in the auditory cortex,[1] hearing loss (20%), wax, viral, presbyacusis, excess noise (eg gunfire), head injury, septic otitis media, post-stapedectomy, Ménière's, anaemia, ↑BP (in up to 16%, but it may not be causative).[44] *Drugs:* Aspirin (reversible), loop diuretics, aminoglycosides. ***Psychological associations:*** Redundancy, divorce, retirement. ***Mean age at onset:*** 40–50yrs. ♂≈♀. ***Causes of pulsatile tinnitus:*** Carotid artery stenosis or dissection,[45] AV fistulae, and glomus jugulare tumours (*OHCS* p552). May be audible with stethoscope. Do an MRI.

Management Psychological support is very important (eg from a hearing therapist). Exclude serious causes; reassure that tinnitus does not mean madness or serious disease and that it often improves in time. **Cognitive therapy** helps, as does 'tinnitus coping training'. Patient support groups can help greatly.[46] **Drugs** are disappointing. Avoid tranquillizers, particularly if depressed (use tricyclic antidepressants here, eg amitriptyline[47] or nortriptyline).[48] Hypnotics at night may help. Carbamazepine rarely helps. If Ménière's disease is the cause, betahistine helps only a few. **Masking** may give relief. White noise (like an off-tuned radio) is given via a noise generator worn like a post-aural hearing aid. **Hearing aids** may help by amplifying desirable sounds. **Cochlear nerve section** can relieve disabling tinnitus in 25% (at the expense of deafness). Repetitive **transcranial magnetic stimulation** of the auditory cortex can help (a novel and non-standard therapy).[49]

1 Postulated to be the cause of common tinnitus

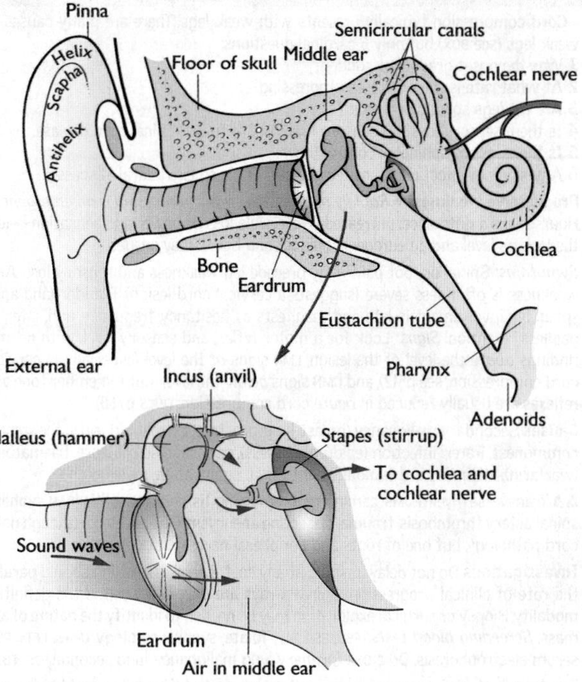

Fig 1. The anatomy of the auditory apparatus

►Cord compression typically presents with weak legs. There are many causes of weak legs (see BOX) but only 6 cardinal questions:

1 Was the onset gradual or sudden?
2 At what rate is the weakness progressing?
3 Are the legs spastic or flaccid?
4 Is there sensory loss?[1] A sensory level usually means spinal cord disease.
5 Is there loss of sphincter control (bowels, bladder)?
6 Any signs of infection (spine tenderness, WCC↑; eg extradural abscess)?

Progressive weakness ►*Rapidly progressing cord compression is an emergency.*[1] Hours make a difference: untreated, irreversible loss of power and sensation below the lesion's level and a neurogenic bladder and bowel may ensue.

Symptoms: Spinal or root pain[2] may precede leg weakness and sensory loss. Arm weakness is often less severe (suggests a cervical cord lesion). Bladder (and anal) sphincter involvement is late and manifests as hesitancy, frequency, and, later, as painless retention. *Signs:* Look for a motor, reflex, and sensory level, with normal findings *above* the level of the lesion, LMN signs *at* the level (especially in cervical cord compression, see p512), and UMN signs *below* the level (but remember tone and reflexes are usually reduced in *acute* cord compression; *OHCS* p768).

Causes Secondary malignancy (breast, lung, prostate, thyroid, kidney) in the spine is commonest. Rarer: infection (epidural abscess), cervical disc prolapse, haematoma (warfarin), intrinsic cord tumour, atlanto-axial subluxation, myeloma.

ΔΔ Transverse myelitis, MS, carcinomatous meningitis, cord vasculitis (PAN, syphilis), spinal artery thrombosis, trauma, dissecting aneurysm, Guillain-Barré (though not a cord pathology, but one of roots and peripheral nerves ∴ LMN; p716).

Investigations Do not delay imaging at any cost. Speed of imaging should parallel the rate of clinical progression. Spinal x-rays are unreliable; MRI is the definitive modality. Biopsy or surgical exploration may be needed to identify the nature of any mass. *Screening blood tests:* FBC, ESR, B_{12}, folate, syphilis serology, U&Es, LFTs, PSA, serum electrophoresis. Do a CXR (primary lung malignancy, lung secondaries, TB).

Treatment If malignancy, give dexamethasone IV 4mg/6h while considering more specific therapy, eg radiotherapy or chemotherapy ± decompressive laminectomy; which is most appropriate depends on tumour type, quality of life, and likely prognosis. Epidural abscesses must be surgically decompressed and antibiotics given.

Cauda equina and conus medullaris lesions The big difference between these lesions and those high up in the cord is that leg weakness is flaccid and areflexic, not spastic and hyperreflexic. *Causes:* As above, plus congenital lumbar disc disease and lumbosacral nerve lesions. *Clinical features:* **Conus medullaris lesions** feature a mixed UMN/LMN leg weakness; early urinary retention and constipation; back pain; sacral sensory disturbance; and erectile dysfunction. **Cauda equina lesions** feature back pain and radicular pain down the legs; asymmetrical, atrophic, areflexic paralysis of the legs; sensory loss in a root distribution; and ↓sphincter tone; do PR.

Paralysed patients need especial care Avoid pressure sores by turning. Review weight-bearing areas often. Avoid thrombosis in paralysed limbs by frequent passive movement and pressure stockings ± low molecular weight heparin (p344). Bladder care is vital; catheterization is only one option. Do not control incontinence by decreasing fluid intake (*OHCS* p774). Bowel evacuation may be manual or aided by suppositories. Increasing dietary fibre intake may help. Exercise of unaffected or partially paralysed limbs is important to avoid unnecessary loss of function.

1 Get help *today* from a neurosurgeon or your spinal cord compression co-ordinator. Prevent DVTs and pressure sores. See p526.

2 *Nerve root sensations* may be sharp or dull (like angina if T3–T4 affected) or 'warm glows', or 'as if icy bandages were wrapped round my leg' or rubbed with sandpaper, or sprayed with hot water. *Dorsal column damage* may cause hypersensitivity or vibratory feelings, as if on the deck of a ship under full power, or the limbs may feel twice their normal size. *Spinothalamic symptoms* may be 'as if my bones burned, and the flesh was torn away'.

Other causes of leg weakness

Unilateral foot drop: DM, common peroneal nerve palsy, stroke, prolapsed disc, MS.
Weak legs with no sensory loss: MND, poliomyelitis and parasagittal meningioma (a rare exception to the 'rule' that weak legs mean cord or more distal problems).
Chronic spastic paraparesis: MS, intrinsic cord tumours (astrocytomas, ependymomas, haemangioblastomas),[51] cord metastases (melanoma, lung),[52] MND, syringomyelia, subacute combined degeneration of the cord (vit B_{12} deficiency; **fig 1**), hereditary spastic paraparesis, taboparesis,[1] rare non-neoplastic lesions—eg histiocytosis X, schistosomiasis, other parasites (look for eosinophilia).[53]
Chronic flaccid paraparesis: Peripheral neuropathies, myopathies (rare; arms also involved).
Absent knee jerks and extensor plantars: Combined cervical and lumbar disc disease, conus medullaris lesions, or a '**MAST**': **M**ND (or **m**yeloradiculitis[2]), Friedreich's **a**taxia, **s**ubacute combined degeneration of the cord (vit B_{12} deficiency; **fig 1**), **t**aboparesis.[1]

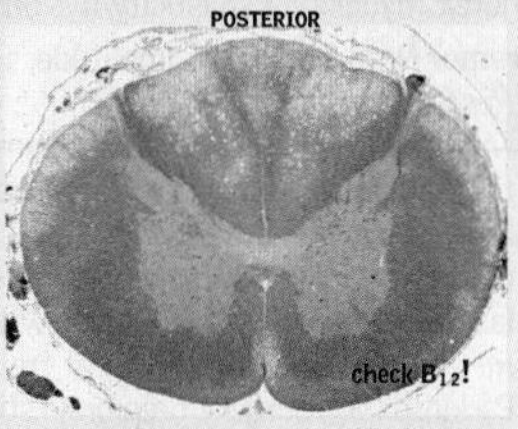

Fig 1. Subacute combined degeneration of the cord, due to vitamin B_{12} deficiency. Why 'combined'? Both lateral (motor) *and* dorsal (sensory) columns lose myelin (at ~C5–T3 level), then axons. Eventually *all* the cord's rim will be affected, if vit B_{12} injections are delayed (p328).

Image courtesy of Prof Dimitri Agamanolis.[50]

Gait disorders

(Even the best professionals have to employ extraordinary tactics just to *describe* gaits accurately,[3] never mind *diagnose* them accurately.)
Spastic: Stiff, circumduction of legs ± scuffing of the foot.
Extrapyramidal: Flexed posture, shuffling feet, slow to start, postural instability. *Example*: Parkinson's disease.
Apraxic: Pathognomonic '**gluing-to-the-floor**' on attempting walking or a wide-based unsteady gait with a tendency to fall, like a novice on an ice-rink. *Causes:* normal pressure hydrocephalus, multi-infarct states.
Ataxic: Wide-based; falls; cannot walk heel-to-toe. *Causes:* cerebellar lesions (eg MS, posterior fossa tumours, alcohol, phenytoin toxicity); proprioceptive sensory loss (eg sensory neuropathies, ↓B_{12}). Often worse in the dark, or with eyes closed.
Myopathic: Waddle (hip girdle weakness). Cannot climb steps or stand from sitting.
Psychogenic: Often a bizarre gait not conforming to any pattern of organic gait disturbance. Suspect if there is profound gait disturbance with inability even to stand, without any signs when examined on the couch ('astasia abasia')—but this may occur with midline cerebellar lesions, normal pressure hydrocephalus, and other rare tumours.[54] Video analysis reveals 6 signs of psychogenicity, seen in 97% of patients in one study:[55]

- Fluctuations in response to suggestion or distraction.
- Excessive hesitation of locomotion incompatible with CNS disease.
- 'Psychogenic' building-up of sway amplitudes on Romberg test.
- Uneconomic postures wasting muscular energy.
- 'Walking on ice' gait, ie small cautious steps, with ankle joints fixed.
- Sudden buckling of the knees, usually without falls.

Tests Spinal X-rays, MRI; FBC, ESR, syphilis serology, serum B_{12}, U&Es, LFTs, PSA, serum electrophoresis; CXR; LP; EMG; muscle ± sural nerve biopsy.

1 Tertiary syphilis (p431): in **tabes dorsalis** the afferent pathways from muscle spindles are lost, with reduced tone and tendon reflexes (without weakness). Later, additional involvement of the pyramidal tracts causes **taboparesis**—a spastic paraparesis with the peculiar combination of extensor plantars (from the taboparesis) and absent tendon reflexes (from the tabes dorsalis).
2 Infections can inflame roots *and* cord (eg visceral larva migrans); hence the mixed picture.
3 Unda her brella mid piddle med puddle she ninnygoes nannygoes nancing by. James Joyce *Finnegans Wake*

Movement disorders are clinically and pathologically heterogeneous, and are characterized by impairment of the planning, control or execution of movement.[56] [57] They may manifest with symptoms of ataxia, dystonia, gait problems (p471), parkinsonism, chorea, myoclonus, spasticity, dyskinesia, tics and tremor.

Tremor Note frequency, amplitude, and exacerbating factors (stress; fatigue).
- *Rest tremor:* abolished on voluntary movement. *Cause:* parkinsonism (p498).
- *Intention tremor:* irregular, large-amplitude, worse at the end of purposeful acts, eg finger-pointing or using a remote control. *Cause:* cerebellar damage (eg MS, stroke).
- *Postural tremor:* absent at rest, present on maintained posture (arms outstretched) and may persist (but is not worse) on movement. *Causes:* Benign essential tremor (autosomal dominant; improves with alcohol), thyrotoxicosis, anxiety, β-agonists.
- *Re-emergent tremor:* postural tremor developing after a delay of ~10sec (eg in Parkinson's).[58] Surgery/deep brain stimulation (DBS) helps some tremors.[59]

Chorea, athetosis, and hemiballismus *Chorea:*[1] Non-rhythmic, jerky, purposeless movements flitting from one place to another—eg facial grimacing, raising the shoulders, flexing/extending the fingers. *Causes:* Huntington's disease, Sydenham's chorea (choreoathetoid movements as a rare complication of strep infection). The anatomical basis of chorea is uncertain but it may be the pharmacological mirror image of Parkinson's disease (L-dopa worsens chorea). *Hemiballismus:* Large-amplitude, flinging hemichorea (affects proximal muscles) contralateral to a vascular lesion of the subthalamic nucleus (often elderly diabetics). Recovers spontaneously over months. *Athetosis:* Slow, sinuous, confluent, purposeless movements (esp. digits, hands, face, tongue), often difficult to distinguish from chorea. *Causes:* commonest is cerebral palsy (*OHCS* p214). Most other 'athetoid' patterns may now be better classed as dystonias. *Pseudoathetosis* is caused by severe proprioceptive loss.

Tics Brief, repeated, stereotyped movements which patients may suppress for a while. Tics are common in children (and usually resolve). In *Tourette's syndrome* (p714), motor and vocal tics occur. Consider psychological support, clonazepam or clonidine if tics are severe (haloperidol may help but risks tardive dyskinesia).

Myoclonus Sudden involuntary focal or general jerks arising from cord, brainstem, or cerebral cortex, seen in metabolic problems (below), neurodegenerative disease (eg lysosomal storage enzyme defects), CJD (p710), and myoclonic epilepsies (infantile spasms). *Benign essential myoclonus:* childhood onset with frequent generalized myoclonus, without progression. Often autosomal dominant. It may respond to valproate, clonazepam or piracetam. *Asterixis ('metabolic flap'):* Jerking (~1-2 jerks/sec) of outstretched hands, worse with wrists extended, from loss of extensor tone—ie incoordination between flexors and extensors (='negative myoclonus'). *Causes:* liver or kidney failure, ↓Na^+, ↑CO_2, gabapentin, thalamic stroke (consider if unilateral).[60]

Tardive syndromes Tardive means 'delayed onset', in this case after chronic exposure to dopamine antagonists (eg antipsychotics, antiemetics). Tardive syndromes are a source of much distress and disability, and may be permanent, despite discontinuing all drugs. *Classification:*[61] • *Tardive dyskinesia* (orobuccolingual, truncal, or choreiform movements, eg vacuous chewing and grimacing movements); • *Tardive dystonia* (sustained, stereotyped muscle spasms of a twisting or turning character, eg retrocollis and back arching/opisthotonic posturing); • *Tardive akathisia* (unpleasant inner sense of restlessness or unease ± repetitive, purposeless movements (stereotypies, eg pacing); • *Tardive myoclonus;* • *Tardive tourettism* (p714); • *Tardive tremor* (may respond to donepezil).[62] *Treating tardive dyskinesia:* Get help. Gradually withdraw neuroleptics and wait 3–6 months. If still a problem, consider **tetrabenazine** 12.5–50mg/8h PO.[63] Quetiapine, olanzapine and clozapine are examples of atypical antipsychotics that are less likely to cause tardive syndromes.

1 Paracelsus used the term *chorea* to describe the jerking movements of medieval pilgrims travelling to the healing shrine of St Vitus—reflecting the ancient Greek round dance accompanied by singing (hence chorus; choreography). He recognized 3 types: chorea arising from the imagination (chorea imaginativa), or from sexual desire (chorea lasciva)—and chorea arising from corporeal causes (chorea naturalis).

Dystonia

Dystonia describes prolonged muscle contractions causing abnormal posture or repetitive movements. Verbatim example of dystonic symptoms (writer's cramp, in this example): "I cannot, for example, draw the instrument [pen, pencil] toward me in a circular motion, eg the left arc of a circle, or the letter O. If I force the move, the movements become jerky and I lose all smoothness in the character. The same thing will happen when eating and trying to use a fork...I end up moving my mouth to the fork...instead of moving my hand to my mouth—awkward."[64]

Classification can be by *age of onset*—childhood (<12yrs old), adolescent (13-20yrs) or adult (>20yrs); by *part of the body affected*; or by *cause* (there are many).

Idiopathic generalized dystonia is suggested by onset in childhood and often starts with dystonia in one leg, spreading to that side of the body over 5-10yrs. Autosomal dominant inheritance is common (genetics often show a deletion in DYT1). Treatment is challenging; exclude Wilson's disease and dopa-responsive dystonia (often better after sleep; needs an L-dopa trial). High-dose **trihexyphenidyl** (=benzhexol, an anticholinergic) and **deep-brain stimulation** may help.[65]

Focal dystonias are confined to one part of the body, eg *spasmodic torticollis* (head pulled to one side), *blepharospasm* (involuntary contraction of orbicularis oculi, *OHCS* p460), *writer's cramp*. Focal dystonias in adults are typically idiopathic, and rarely generalize. They are worsened by stress. Patients may develop a *geste antagonistique* to try to resist the dystonic posturing (eg a touch of the finger to the jaw in spasmodic torticollis).[66] Injection of **botulinum toxin** into the overactive muscles (*OHCS* p460) is usually effective, but there may be SEs.

Writer's cramp (scrivener's palsy; graphospasm) When trying to write, the pen is driven into the paper and flow of movement is poor. "I would look at [my fingers] and tell them to do one thing, and they'd do jagged things instead, I'd have full muscle control for everything, except putting a pen to a piece of paper."[67] Look for hand and forearm spasm, dystonic arm posture, focal tremor, myoclonus, and dominant-hand muscle hypertrophy.[68] *Association:* obsessive-compulsive disorder.[69] *EMG:* May correlate with physiological events: ↓reciprocal inhibition of wrist flexor motor neurons at rest, and ↑co-contraction of antagonist muscles of the forearm during voluntary activity.[70] *EEG:* Abnormal motor command (sensorimotor region β rhythm).[71] ℞: β-blockers and valproate often fail. Breath-holding or arm-cooling may work, as may botulinum toxin and EMG biofeedback.[72]

Acute dystonia (**fig 1**) may occur on starting many drugs, including neuroleptics and some antiemetics (eg metoclopramide, cyclizine). There is torticollis (head pulled back), trismus (oromandibular spasm), and/or oculogyric crisis (eyes drawn up). You may mistake this for tetanus or meningitis, but such reactions rapidly disappear after a dose of an anticholinergic, see p855.

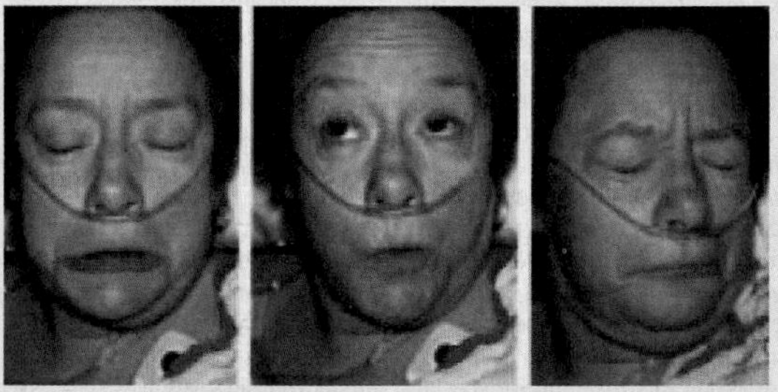

Fig 1. Oromandibular/oculogyric crisis in acute dystonia.

From *Mayo Clinic Proc* 2003; 78:1150-2. Used with permission.[73]

Strokes result from ischaemic infarction or bleeding into part of the brain, manifest by rapid onset (eg seconds–minutes) of focal CNS signs and symptoms. It is the major neurological disease of our times (1.5/1000/yr, rising with age to 10/1000/yr at 75yrs).

Causes • Small vessel occlusion (thrombosis *in situ*)
• Cardiac emboli (AF; endocarditis; MI—see BOX on p476)
• Atherothromboembolism (eg from carotids)
• CNS bleeds (BP↑, trauma, aneurysm rupture, anticoagulation, thrombolysis)

Other causes: (less common in the elderly, but important to consider in younger patients) sudden BP drop by ≥40mmHg ('watershed' stroke, eg in sepsis), carotid artery dissection (spontaneous, or from neck trauma or fibromuscular dysplasia), vasculitis, subarachnoid haemorrhage, venous sinus thrombosis (acute venous infarct, p484), antiphospholipid syndrome, thrombophilia, Fabry's disease (p712), CADASIL.[1]
►Do not hesitate to get a neurology, cardiology, or haematology opinion.

Risk factors BP↑, smoking, DM, heart disease (valvular, ischaemic, AF), peripheral vascular disease, past TIA/stroke, ↑PCV, carotid bruit, the Pill, lipids↑, alcoholism, clotting↑ (eg ↑plasma fibrinogen, ↓antithrombin III, p368), ↑homocysteine, syphilis.

Signs Sudden onset, occasionally with further progression over hours (rarely days). In theory, focal signs relate to distribution of the affected artery (p452), but collateral supplies cloud the issue. ►Ischaemic and haemorrhagic stroke are *not* reliably distinguishable clinically but pointers to haemorrhage are: meningism, severe headache, and coma within hours. Ischaemic pointers: carotid bruit, AF, past TIA, IHD.

- *Cerebral hemisphere infarcts:* (50%) depending on site there may be contralateral hemiplegia—initially flaccid (floppy limb, falls like a dead weight when lifted), then becomes spastic (UMN), contralateral sensory loss, dysphasia, homonymous hemianopia, visuo-spatial deficit.
- *Brainstem infarcts:* (25%) wide range of effects, which include quadriplegia, disturbances of gaze and vision, locked-in syndrome (aware, but unable to respond).
- *Lacunar infarcts:* (25%) small infarcts around basal ganglia, internal capsule, thalamus, and pons. Five lacunar syndromes are classically described: pure motor, ataxic hemiparesis, pure sensory, mixed sensorimotor, and dysarthria/clumsy hand. Cognition and consciousness remain intact (except thalamic lacunes).

Acute management (First hours; see p476–7 for further management)

1 *Ensure patent airway* to avoid hypoxia or aspiration.
2 *Monitor blood glucose:* keep BM 4–11 mmol/L. Use insulin sliding scale if diabetic or BM not controlled.
3 *Monitor BP*, but treating even very high levels may harm (unless there is encephalopathy, or aortic dissection): even a 20% fall may compromise cerebral perfusion, as autoregulation is impaired. If on HRT, stop it.
4 *Urgent CT/MRI if:* thrombolysis considered, cerebellar stroke (cerebellar haematomas may need urgent referral for evacuation),[74] unusual presentation (ie if alternative diagnosis likely; see BOX 2), or high risk of haemorrhage (↓GCS, signs of ↑ICP, severe headache, meningism, progressive symptoms, known bleeding tendency or anticoagulation). Otherwise imaging can wait (aim <24hrs). Diffusion-weighted MRI is most sensitive for an acute infarct, but CT will rule out primary haemorrhage.
5 *Thrombolysis:* consider if aged 18–80yrs and onset of symptoms <4.5h ago; BOX 1.
6 '*Nil by mouth*' until swallowing is assessed.
7 *Keep hydrated*, but don't overhydrate (risk of cerebral oedema).
8 *Explain what has happened.* ►Communicate fully with patient, relatives and carers over difficult decisions, eg deciding on the kindest level of intervention taking into account quality of life, coexisting conditions, and prognosis.
9 *Antiplatelet agents:* once haemorrhagic stroke is excluded, give aspirin 300mg.
10 *Admission to stroke unit* for specialist nursing/physio saves lives,[75] and is a great motivator (see p478).

1 cerebral Autosomal Dominant Arteriopathy with Subcortical Infarcts and Leucoencephalopathy (CADASIL) presents with TIA/stroke from 4th decade ± migraine. Due to a mutation on the notch 3 gene.

▸▸Thrombolysis in acute non-haemorrhagic stroke

If an expert team (neuroimaging and clinicians) is in place, *and* the patient is seen within 4.5h[1] of the onset of symptoms, *and* no contraindication exists (see below), refer with *utmost urgency* for consideration of reperfusion with IV recombinant tissue plasminogen activator (tPA: alteplase—eg 0.9mg/kg over 1h). This reduces death and dependency (odds ratio 0.64) despite a small increase in intracranial haemorrhage (but these are usually small and asymptomatic).[76] Recent use of antiplatelet agents does not appear to increase this risk of haemorrhage.[77] All patients who are thrombolysed should have a CT head 24h post-thrombolysis to identify haemorrhage. Consider registering each case with the *Safe Implementation of Thrombolysis in Stroke* (SITS) database at www.acutestroke.org.

CI: • Major infarct or haemorrhage on CT; • Mild (non-disabling) deficits; • Recent surgery, trauma or obstetric delivery; • Past CNS haemorrhage; • AVM or aneurysm; • Severe liver disease, varices or portal hypertension; • Seizures at presentation; • Recent arterial or venous puncture at a non-compressible site; • Anticoagulants or PTT >15s; • Platelets <100 × 10^9/L; • BP >220/130.

Differential diagnosis of stroke

- Head injury
- Subdural haemorrhage
- Hypoglycaemia
- Hyperglycaemia
- Intracranial tumours
- Hemiplegic migraine
- Epilepsy (Todd's palsy)
- CNS lymphoma
- Pneumocephalus (air entry via: otitis, mastoid air cells, trauma)
- Wernicke's encephalopathy
- Drug overdose (if coma)
- Hepatic encephalopathy
- Mitochondrial cytopathies[2]
- Herpes encephalitis
- HIV; HTLV-1
- Toxoplasmosis (AIDS)[78]
- Abscesses (eg typhoid)
- Mycotic aneurysm[79]
- Coccidioides immitis[80]
- Acanthamoeba/naegleria[82]

NB: status epilepticus *can* cause CNS infarcts.[81]

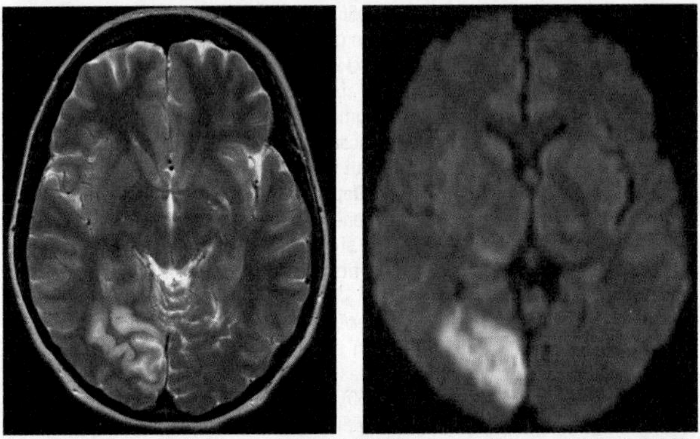

Fig 1. The image on the left is T2-weighted (p760); the more water present, the more white the appearance. In the right occipital lobe, the cerebral cortex is abnormal with high signal, most likely from oedema. If so, it is cytotoxic oedema from cell ischaemia and death, rather than vasogenic oedema from leaky capillaries that involves more of the white matter. The diagnosis could be an infarct (distribution is the right PCA territory), inflammation, or tumour. The diffusion-weighted image on the right shows limited (abnormal) diffusion in the region, indicating this is an infarct. Courtesy of Prof Peter Scally.

1 Alteplase is licensed for use within 3h of onset of focal neurological symptoms. However, the ECASS 3 and SITS studies have demonstrated efficacy up to 4.5h, and the IST 3 trial is currently investigating efficacy at 4.5–6h. ▸▸In any case, maximum efficacy is within the first 90min, so don't dawdle!

2 Mitochondrial Encephalopathy with Lactic Acidosis and Stroke-like episodes (MELAS). Episodes triggered by metabolic stress, with lactic acidosis ± seizures. Due to a point mutation in mitochondrial DNA.

Primary prevention (ie before a stroke) Control risk factors (p474): Look for and treat hypertension, DM, ↑lipids (p704; statins ↓risk by ~17%),[83] and cardiac disease (see BOX). Exercise helps (↑HDL, ↑glucose tolerance). Folate supplements[1] may also help (↓ serum homocysteine).[84] *Help quit smoking:* ►p87. In middle-aged men (especially if ↑BP), quitting ↓risk of stroke, with benefits seen in ≤5yrs (switching to pipes or cigars achieves little; former heavy smokers retain some excess risk). Use *lifelong anticoagulation* if rheumatic or prosthetic heart valves on left side, and consider in chronic non-rheumatic atrial fibrillation (AF), especially if there are other vascular risk factors (see BOX). For prevention post-TIA see p480.

Secondary prevention (ie preventing further strokes) Control risk factors (as *Primary prevention* above). Several large studies suggest considerable advantages from lowering blood pressure and cholesterol (even if not particularly raised). *Antiplatelet agents after stroke:* Unless imaging shows primary haemorrhage, give **aspirin** 300mg/24h for 2wks, then 75mg/day.[85] **Dipyridamole MR** (200mg/12h) in combination with aspirin improves outcomes.[86] Clopidogrel is at least as good as aspirin as monotherapy,[87] and may be as good as aspirin plus dipyridamole MR.[88] If aspirin-intolerant, add PPI, p242; if aspirin-hypersensitive, substitute **clopidogrel** (p480). Dipyridamole-associated headache can be reduced by slow titration to the above dose. *Anticoagulation after stroke:* **Warfarin** should be used instead of antiplatelet agents only for embolic stroke (see BOX) or chronic AF (p124), and only from 2 weeks after the stroke (if clinically and radiologically a small stroke, consider from 7-10 days). Use antiplatelet therapy until anticoagulated; if anticoagulated already, hold anticoagulant and replace with antiplatelet for 1 week. Use antiplatelet therapy if risk of falls etc. Warfarin plus aspirin ↑ risk of haemorrhage without added benefit.

Tests (see p464 for imaging) Investigate promptly to identify risk factors for further strokes, but consider whether results will affect management. Look for:

- *Hypertension:* Look for retinopathy (p562), nephropathy, and a big heart on **CXR**. Raised BP is common in early stroke. In general, don't treat acutely.
- *Cardiac source of emboli:* (see also BOX) **24° tape ECG** to look for atrial fibrillation (p124). **CXR** may show an enlarged left atrium. **Echocardiogram** may reveal mural thrombus due to AF or a hypokinetic segment of cardiac muscle post-MI. It may also show valvular lesions in infective endocarditis or rheumatic heart disease. Trans-oesophageal echo is more sensitive than transthoracic.
- *Carotid artery stenosis:* Do **carotid Doppler ultrasound** ± **CT/MRI angiography**. Carotid endarterectomy shows clear benefit for fit patients with ≥70% stenosis on Doppler.[89] Endovascular carotid artery stenting is an alternative if not suitable for surgery, but safety and long-term benefits (in-stent re-stenosis is common) remain under investigation.[90]
- *Hypoglycaemia, hyperglycaemia, hyperlipidaemia* and *hyperhomocysteinaemia.*
- *Vasculitis:* ↑ESR, ANA +ve, etc (p558). VDRL to look for active, untreated syphilis (p431).
- *Prothrombotic states:* eg thrombophilia (p368), antiphospholipid syndrome (p556).
- *Hyperviscosity:* eg polycythaemia (p360), sickle-cell disease (p334).
- *Thrombocytopenia* and other bleeding disorders.
- *Genetic tests* for Fabry's disease and CADASIL (p474).

Prognosis Good nursing (eg to prevent pressure sores—see **fig 1**) on a stroke unit, antiplatelet agents, and prompt intervention (eg after carotid Doppler imaging) are the key. For those with a minor ischaemic stroke/TIA, urgent assessment and treatment saves lives (p480). *Overall mortality:* 60,000/yr;[UK] 20% at 1 month, then ≤10%/yr. *Full recovery:* ≤40%. Drowsiness≈poor prognosis. *Complications:* Aspiration pneumonia (keep 'nil by mouth' until assessed, p478); pressure sores (**fig 1**; turn regularly and keep dry—consider catheter); contractures; constipation; depression; "I'm a prisoner in my body"; stress in spouse (eg alcoholism), p449.

1 Folate ('good') and homocysteine ('bad') have a complex link with risk of haemorrhagic stroke.

Cardiac causes of stroke

Cardioembolic causes are the source of stroke in >30% of patients in population studies. These may recur, unless you prevent them.

►So examine the heart with as much attention as you examine the brain.

- *Non-valvular atrial fibrillation* is associated with an overall risk of stroke of 4.5% per year. Advancing age, prior stroke/TIA, diabetes and hypertension are additive risks. Ischaemic strokes in AF are often worse than ischaemic stroke with sinus rhythm. Warfarin is effective for primary and secondary prevention of ischaemic stroke, reducing ↓risk by 68%. Aspirin alone is adequate when there are few or no additional risk factors. It is safer and needs no monitoring.[91] Explain risks and benefits of warfarin, and let the patient decide, giving an evidence-based steer towards warfarin if there are additional risk factors—provided there are no contraindications (falls, poor compliance/concordance). If warfarin is chosen, aim for an INR of 2.5-3.5 (stroke risk is twice as much for those with an INR of 1.7 as opposed to 2). Adding aspirin to warfarin does not confer additional protection.
- *External cardioversion* is complicated in 1-3% by peripheral emboli: pharmacological cardioversion may carry similar risks.
- *Prosthetic valves* risk major emboli; anticoagulate (INR 3.5-4.5, p345).
- *Acute myocardial infarct* with large left ventricular wall motion abnormalities on echocardiography predispose to left ventricular thrombus. Emboli arise in 10% of these patients in the next 6-12 months; risk is reduced by two-thirds by warfarin anticoagulation. Mural thrombus is best seen by echocardiography.
- *Paradoxical systemic emboli* via the venous circulation in those with patent foramen ovale, atrial and ventricular septal defects.
- *Cardiac surgery*, eg bypass graft, carries particular risk (0.9-5.2%).
- *Valve vegetations from SBE/IE* may embolize (p144). 20% of those with endocarditis present with CNS signs due to septic emboli from valves. ►Is there fever or a murmur? Treat as endocarditis; ask a cardiologist's opinion.

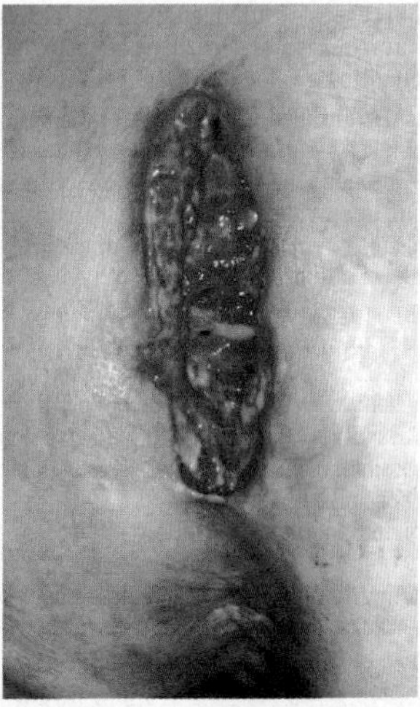

Fig 1. Sacral pressure sore after a stroke. Easy to prevent, given good nurses; so hard to treat, and so often a prelude to death.[92]

Rehabilitation is about improving quality of life for people with any chronic disorder. It uses multidisciplinary teamwork, dialogue and programs tailored for individual needs.[93] *Points in the early management of stroke which bear on later rehab plans:*

- Watch the patient swallow a small volume of water; if signs of aspiration (a cough or voice change) make *nil by mouth* until formal assessment by a speech therapist. Use IV fluids, then semi-solids (eg jelly; avoid soups and crumbly food). Avoid early NG tube feeds (needed only in the few with established chronic swallowing problems). Speech therapists skilled in assessing swallowing difficulties are invaluable here.
- Avoid falls and damaging patients' shoulders through careless lifting.
- Ensure good bladder and bowel care through frequent toileting. Avoid early catheterization which may prevent return to continence.
- Position the patient to minimize spasticity (occurs in ~40%). Get prompt physiotherapy. Botulinum toxin injections are helpful for focal spasticity.[94]
- Measure time taken to sit up, and to transfer from lying to sitting in a chair; this is a good way to monitor progress with physio/occupational therapy.[95]
- In pseudo-emotionalism/emotional lability (sobbing unprovoked by sorrow, from failure of cortical inhibition of the limbic system), tricyclics or fluoxetine may help.

►Involve the carer/spouse with all aspects of care-giving. Good rehab saves lives.

Screen for depression[1] 33% are depressed, and, untreated, this worsens motor function and ↑mortality (↑vascular disease).[96] Depression may lift with specific therapy (p11), exercise, diet, and a 'can-do' mentality, which builds on small successes.

Tests Asking to point to a named part of the body tests perceptual function. Copying matchstick patterns tests spatial ability. Dressing or copying a clock face tests for *apraxia* (p80). Picking out and naming easy objects from a pile tests for agnosia (acuity OK, but cannot mime use; guesses are way-out, semantically, and phonetically).

Neurorehabilitation takes a functional approach building on what patients can do—with speech- and physio-therapy (most importantly in restoring balance and gait). Making physio fun aids motivation, eg swimming (a hemiplegic arm may be supported on a special float), music and video games (↑recovery by aiding coordination).[97] The aim is to promote cerebral reorganization. To this end, constraint of the good arm has been found to be helpful (*constraint-induced movement therapy*).[98]

End-of-life decisions '...And thus the native hue of resolution is sicklied o'er with the pale cast of thought' *Hamlet* Act III:i —the more we think on these issues, the more we tie ourselves in knots. We intended these precepts to bisect these snares, not to reveal deep, hidden truths, but to provide a workable framework at the bedside.

- If the patient's views are known, comply with them, except perhaps where doing so entails an illegal act, or one that clearly harms others.
- No person has authority to impose views on end-of-life decisions. You cannot tell a nurse to stop feeding someone, and expect her to obey you. Consensus is the only practical way. Try to get the opinion of more than one relative, and more than one shift of nurses (eg at changeover time). Let everyone have their say. You may learn new and important facts about your patient, which make decisions easier—or harder.
- If consensus is impossible, recourse to the Courts is one option: but remember that judges have no special skill in this area.
- Beware guidelines giving doctors special powers (such as the BMA guidelines).[99] Doctors may be the worst decision-makers as closeness to life and death may make them tolerant of ending life—eg if the bed could be used for 'something better'. Even if *not* the case, if society thinks this, then doctors are in an untenable position. We *do* have a role, though, in facilitating consensus, and documenting it.

Success is often impossible (there are too many grey areas), but if you can stumble from one ambiguity to another without being disheartened, then that is good enough. Your patients will respect your honesty.

1 Have you been bothered by **little interest or pleasure** in doing things? Have you been **feeling down, depressed**, or **hopeless** in the last month? If 'yes' ask about sleep disturbance, appetite change, low self-esteem, and anhedonia, and whether their feelings have caused distress or impaired ability to function.

Assessing handicap, disability, and independence in daily life

Handicap entails inability to carry out social functions. 'A disadvantage for a given individual, resulting from an impairment or disability, that limits or prevents the fulfilment of a role.' Two people with the same *impairment* (eg paralysed arm) may have different *disabilities* (one can dress, the other cannot). Disabilities are likely to determine quality of future life. Treatment is often best aimed at reducing disability, not curing disease. For example, Velcro® fasteners in place of buttons may enable a person to dress.

A person with a severe hearing impairment may seem to you to have no disability if they can lip-read. But ask yourself (and your patients, when you get to know them) about the price they pay for rising above their disabilities. Lip-reading, for example, is exhausting, requiring 100% vigilance to make sense of transitory and incomplete visual clues.

Barthel's index of activities of daily living

Bowels	0	Incontinent (or needs to be given enemas)
	1	Occasional accidents (once a week)
	2	Continent
Bladder	0	Incontinent, or catheter inserted but unable to manage it
	1	Occasional accidents (up to once per 24h)
	2	Continent (for more than seven days)
Grooming	0	Needs help with personal care: face, hair, teeth, shaving
	1	Independent (implements provided)
Toilet use	0	Dependent
	1	Needs some help but can do some things alone
	2	Independent (on and off, wiping, dressing)
Feeding	0	Unable
	1	Needs help in cutting, spreading butter, etc.
	2	Independent (food provided within reach)
Transfer	0	Unable to get from bed to commode: the vital transfer to prevent the need for 24-hour nursing care
	1	Major help needed (physical, 1-2 people), can sit
	2	Minor help needed (verbal or physical)
	3	Independent
Mobility	0	Immobile
	1	Wheelchair-independent, including corners, etc.
	2	Walks with help of one person (verbal or physical)
	3	Independent
Dressing	0	Dependent
	1	Needs help but can do about half unaided
	2	Independent (including buttons, zips, laces, etc.)
Stairs	0	Unable
	1	Needs help (verbal, physical, carrying aid)
	2	Independent up and down
Bath/shower	0	Dependent
	1	Independent (must get in and out unaided and wash self)

The aim is to establish the degree of independence from any help.

Mahoney FI, Barthel DW: Functional evaluation: the Barthel Index. Maryland State Medical Journal. 1965; 14:61-65. Used with permission.

Barthel's paradox The more we contemplate Barthel's eulogy of independence, the more we see it as a mirage reflecting a greater truth about human affairs: ►there is no such thing as independence[1]—only **inter-dependence,** and in fostering this interdependence lies our true vocation.

1 **No man is an Island,** *intire of it selfe; every man is a peece of the Continent, a part of the maine; if a Clod bee washed away by the Sea, Europe is the lesse, as well as if a promontorie were, as well as if a Mannor of thy friends or of thine owne were. Any man's death diminishes me, because I am involved in mankinde; And therefore never send to know for whom the bell tolls: It tolls for thee*. **John Donne** 1572-1631; Meditation XVII. What happens when we take up John Donne's offer of meditation? Some very interesting CNS events: brain activity slows, and blood is relocated to the anterior cingulate and dorsolateral prefrontal areas.

Transient ischaemic attack (TIA)

The sudden onset of focal CNS phenomena due to temporary occlusion of part of the cerebral circulation, usually by emboli, is termed a TIA if symptoms last <24h (often much shorter). Incidence: 0.4/1000/yr. ⏩15% of 1st strokes are preceded by TIAs; they are also harbingers of MI, so...*good management may avert disaster.*

Signs of TIA Attacks are single or many. Features of a TIA should always mimic those of a stroke in the same arterial territory (p453), and may be the same or different for each TIA. *Global* events (eg syncope, dizziness) are **not** typical of TIAs. Multiple highly stereotyped attacks suggest a critical intracranial stenosis (commonly the superior division of the MCA, p452). Emboli may also pass to the retinal artery, causing **amaurosis fugax** (one eye's vision is progressively lost "like a curtain descending over my field of view"). Limb-shaking TIAs may be mistaken for a focal motor seizure.

Signs of causes Carotid bruit (p72), but absence does not rule out a carotid source of emboli: tight stenoses often have *no* bruit;[100] BP↑; heart murmur from valve disease; atrial fibrillation. Fundoscopy during TIAs may show retinal artery emboli.

Causes (see also p474) *Atherothromboembolism* from the carotid is the chief cause. *Cardioembolism:* mural thrombus post-MI or in AF, valve disease, prosthetic valve. *Hyperviscosity:* (p366), eg polycythaemia, sickle-cell anaemia, WCC↑↑ (leukostasis; may need urgent chemotherapy), myeloma.[101] *Vasculitis* (eg cranial arteritis, PAN, SLE, syphilis, etc) is a rare cause, and perhaps shouldn't be classified as TIA.

Differential Hypoglycaemia, migraine aura (symptoms spread and intensify over minutes, often with visual scintillations), focal epilepsy (symptoms spread over seconds and often include twitching and jerking), hyperventilation, retinal bleeds. *Rare mimics of TIA:* Malignant hypertension, MS (paroxysmal dysarthria), intracranial tumours, peripheral neuropathy, phaeochromocytoma, somatization.

Tests Aim to find the cause and define vascular risk: FBC, ESR, U&Es, glucose, lipids, CXR, ECG, carotid Doppler ± angiography, CT or diffusion-weighted MRI (any existing infarcts? If bilateral, it suggests cardioembolism), echocardiogram (rarely shows cardiac cause if no suggestive signs).

Treatment ⏩Time to intervention is crucial. Risk of stroke within 90 days of TIA is 2% in those treated within 72h of TIA, compared to 10% in those treated by 3 wks.[102]

- *Control cardiovascular risk factors:* ↑BP (cautiously lower; aim for <140/85mmHg, p134); hyperlipidaemia (p704); DM (p198); help to stop smoking (p87 & *OHCS* p512).
- *Antiplatelet drugs:* **Aspirin** 300mg/d if no peptic ulcer (then after 2 weeks 75mg/d *for life*; probably reduces non-fatal strokes and MI by 25%, and vascular death by 15%), and, for the next 2 years, **dipyridamole MR** (200mg/12h). Dipyridamole ↑cAMP and ↓thromboxane A2. If aspirin-intolerant use **clopidogrel** (75mg/d), a thienopyridine that inhibits platelet aggregation by modifying platelet ADP receptors.
- *Warfarin indications:* Cardiac emboli (eg AF, mitral stenosis, recent big septal MI).
- *Carotid endarterectomy* If ≥70% stenosis at the origin of the internal carotid artery and operative risk is good.[1][103][104] Surgery should be performed within 2 weeks of first presentation.[105] Operating on 50–70% stenoses may be valuable if the team's peri-operative stroke and mortality rate <3%.[106] Intra-operative transcranial Doppler can monitor middle cerebral artery flow. Using patches may reduce chance of restenosis. Do not stop aspirin beforehand. Endovascular carotid artery stenting is an alternative if not suitable for surgery, but safety and long-term benefits (in-stent restenosis is common) remain under investigation.[107]

Driving Avoid for 1 month; patients in the UK should inform the DVLA only if multiple attacks in short period or residual deficit.

Prognosis The combined risk of stroke and MI is ~9%/yr; if carotid stenosis is ≥70% risk of stroke ↑ to 12% in 1st year and up to 10% subsequently. More frequent TIAs ↑ risk yet further. Mortality is ~3-fold that of a TIA-free matched population. In one Dutch study in 2005, 60% of patients were dead within 10 years of a TIA.[108]

1 *Who risks death/CVA from endarterectomy?* ♀ sex, >75yrs old, systolic BP↑, contralateral artery occluded; stenosis of ipsilateral carotid syphon/external carotid; wide-territory TIAs (against just amaurosis fugax).

▸▸When should TIA lead to prompt or emergency referral?

An ABCD2 score[109] of ≥6 (see TABLE) strongly predicts a stroke (8.1% within 2 days, 35.5% in the next week). Patients with a score ≥4 should be assessed by a specialist within 24hrs, and all patients with a suspected TIA should be seen within 7 days.

Age ≥60 yrs old	1 point
Blood pressure ≥140/90	1 point
Clinical features	
Unilateral weakness	2 points
Speech disturbance without weakness	1 point
Duration of symptoms	
Symptoms lasting ≥1h	2 points
Symptoms lasting 10-59 mins	1 point
Diabetes	1 point

In assessing urgency, bear in mind Warlow's 2005 data: in stroke patients who had a preceding TIA, 17% occurred on the day of the stroke, 9% on the previous day, and 43% at some point during the 7 days before the stroke.[110] These sobering figures should remind us to rehearse routes for referral for emergency endarterectomy—at present this is typically performed >90 days post-TIA.[111]

ABCD2 score reproduced from *The Lancet*, 366, Rothwell *et al*, A simple score (ABCD) to identify individuals at early risk of stroke after transient ischaemic attack. pp29-36.

Subarachnoid haemorrhage (SAH)

Spontaneous bleeding into the subarachnoid space is often catastrophic. Annual incidence: 9/100,000; typical age: 35–65. *Causes:* Rupture of saccular aneurysms (80%); arterio-venous malformations (AVM; 15%). No cause is found in <15%. *Risk factors:* Smoking, alcohol misuse, BP↑,[1] bleeding disorders, mycotic aneurysm (SBE), perhaps post-menopausal ↓ oestrogen (♀:♂=3:2 once >45 yrs old).[113] Close relatives of those with SAH have 3–5× risk of SAH.[114]

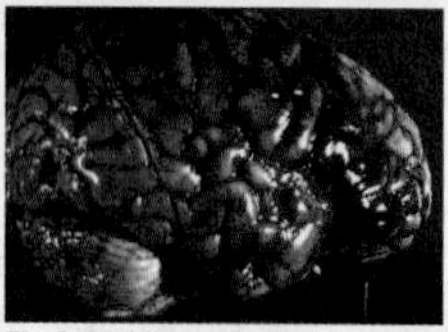

Fig 1. Middle cerebral artery SAH at the Sylvian fissure.[112] ©Dr D Hamoudi

Berry aneurysms Common sites: junction of posterior communicating with the internal carotid or of the anterior communicating with the anterior cerebral artery or bifurcation of the middle cerebral artery (**figs 1,3**; and **fig 1**, p452). 15% are multiple. Some are hereditary. *Associations:* Polycystic kidneys, coarctation of the aorta, Ehlers-Danlos syndrome (hypermobile joints with ↑skin elasticity, *OHCS* p642).

Symptoms Sudden (usually, but not always, within seconds)[115] devastating typically occipital headache—"I thought I'd been kicked in the head". Vomiting, collapse, seizures & coma often follow. Coma/drowsiness may last for days. **Signs** Neck stiffness, Kernig's sign (takes 6hrs to develop), retinal or subhyaloid haemorrhage. Focal neurology *at presentation* may suggest site of aneurysm (eg pupil changes indicating a IIIrd nerve palsy with a posterior communicating artery aneurysm) or intracerebral haematoma. Later deficits suggest complications (see below).[116]

Differential In primary care, only 25% of those with severe, sudden 'thunderclap' headache have SAH. In 50–60%, no cause is found; the remainder have meningitis, migraine, intracerebral bleeds, or cortical vein thrombosis (p484).

Sentinel headache SAH patients may earlier have experienced a sentinel headache, perhaps due to a small warning leak from the offending aneurysm (~6%), but recall-bias clouds the picture.[117] As surgery is more successful in the least symptomatic, be suspicious of any *sudden* headache especially with neck or back pain.[118]

Investigations **CT** detects >90% of SAH within the 1st 48hrs (**fig 2**).[119] **LP** if CT –ve and no contraindication >12h after headache onset. **CSF** in SAH is uniformly bloody early on, and becomes xanthochromic (yellow) after several hours due to breakdown products of Hb (bilirubin). Finding xanthochromia confirms SAH, showing that the LP was not a 'bloody tap' (don't rely on finding fewer CSF RBCs in each successive bottle).

Management ►Refer all proven SAH to neurosurgery immediately.
- **Re-examine** CNS often; chart BP, pupils and GCS (p802). Repeat CT if deteriorating.
- **Maintain cerebral perfusion** by keep well hydrated, and aim for SBP ≥160mmHg. Treat ↑BP only if very severe.
- **Nimodipine** (60mg/4h PO for 3wks, or 1mg/h IVI) is a Ca^{2+} antagonist that reduces vasospasm and consequent morbidity from cerebral ischaemia.
- **Endovascular coiling** is preferable to **surgical clipping** where possible (7% ↑ in independent survival over 7yrs follow-up, although ↑ risk of rebleeding).[120] Do **catheter** or **CT angiography** to identify single *vs* multiple aneurysms prior to intervention. **Intracranial stents** and **balloon remodelling** make possible the treatment of wide-necked aneurysms. Microcatheters can now traverse tortuous vessels to treat previously unreachable lesions.[121] AV malformations and fistulae may also benefit from this procedure.

Complications *Rebleeding* is the commonest cause of death, and occurs in 20%, often in the 1st few days. *Cerebral ischaemia* due to vasospasm may cause a permanent CNS deficit, and is the commonest cause of morbidity. If this happens, surgery is not helpful at the time but may be so later. *Hydrocephalus*, due to blockage of arachnoid granulations, requires a ventricular or lumbar drain. *Hyponatraemia* is common but should not be managed with fluid restriction. Seek expert help.

1 For each 20mmHg rise in systolic BP, relative risks of ischaemic stroke, intracerebral haemorrhage, and subarachnoid haemorrhage are 1.8, 2.5, and 1.6 in ♂, and 1.6, 3.1, and 2.3 in ♀, respectively.

Mortality in subarachnoid haemorrhage

Grade	Signs	Mortality: %
I	None	0
II	Neck stiffness and cranial nerve palsies	11
III	Drowsiness	37
IV	Drowsy with hemiplegia	71
V	Prolonged coma	100

Almost all the mortality occurs in the 1st month. Of those who survive the 1st month, 90% survive a year or more.

Unruptured aneurysms: 'the time-bomb in my head'

Bear in mind the old adage: 'if it ain't broke; don't fix it'—usually, risks of *preventive* intervention outweigh any benefits, except perhaps in young patients (more years at risk, and surgery is twice as hazardous if >45yrs old)[122] who have aneurysms >7mm in diameter, especially if located at the junction of the internal carotid and the posterior communicating cerebral artery, or at the rostral basilar artery bifurcation, and especially if there is uncontrolled hypertension or a past history of bleeds.[123] Data from the 2003 International Study of Unruptured Intracranial Aneurysms (ISUIA) show that relative risk of rupture for an aneurysm 7-12mm across is 3.3 compared with aneurysms <7mm across; if the diameter is >12mm, the relative risk is 17.[124]

Patients with a *previous SAH* have a raised risk for new aneurysm formation and enlargement of untreated aneurysms. Screening these patients might be beneficial, eg if multiple aneurysms, hypertension, or a history of smoking.[125]

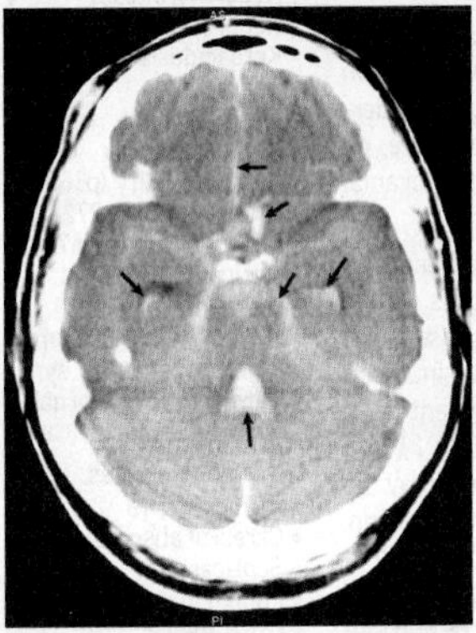

Fig 2. Blood from a ruptured aneurysm occupies the interhemispheric fissure (top arrow), a crescentic intracerebral area presumably near the aneurysm (2nd arrow), the basal cisterns, the lateral ventricles (temporal horns), and the 4th ventricle (bottom arrow).

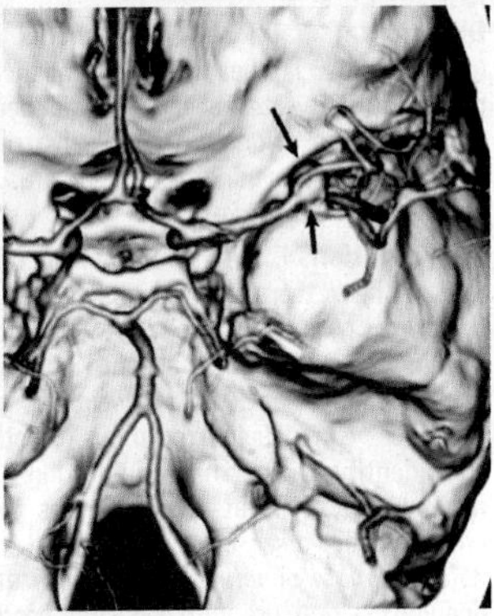

Fig 3. CT images can be manipulated to show only high-density structures such as bones and arteries containing contrast. Here is a middle cerebral artery aneurysm.

We thank Prof. Peter Scally for these CT images and the commentaries on them.

Dural venous sinus thrombosis Most commonly sagittal sinus thrombosis (**figs 1 & 2**; 47% of all IVT) or transverse sinus thrombosis (35%). Sagittal sinus thrombosis often coexists if other sinuses are thrombosed. Symptoms come on gradually over days or weeks. Thrombosis within a dural venous sinus may extend into the cortical veins and cause infarction within a venous territory (**fig 3**; see under *Cortical vein thrombosis* below for symptoms & signs).

- *Sagittal sinus:* Headache, vomiting, seizures, ↓vision, papilloedema.
- *Transverse sinus:* Headache ± mastoid pain, focal CNS signs, seizures, papilloedema.
- *Sigmoid sinus:* Cerebellar signs, lower cranial nerve palsies.
- *Inferior petrosal sinus:* V^{th} & VIth cranial nerve palsies, ie Gradenigo's syndrome.
- *Cavernous sinus* (**fig 1** on p83): Often due to spread from facial pustules or folliculitis, causing headache, chemosis, oedematous eyelids, proptosis, painful ophthalmoplegia, fever.[129]

Cortical vein thrombosis (CVT) Often causes venous infarcts, with stroke-like focal symptoms that develop over days. However, the associated headache may come on suddenly (thunderclap headache).[130] Seizures are common, unlike in arterial stroke, and focal (p494). It usually occurs with sinus thromboses.[131] Galen vein thrombosis is a rare cause of CVT and is usually associated with vascular malformation.[132] *Signs:* encephalopathy, focal seizures, headache (including thunderclap headache), slowly evolving focal deficits (paresis, speech disorders, cognition↓, vision↓).

Differential diagnosis Subarachnoid haemorrhage (p482; thunderclap headaches also occur in dissection of a carotid or vertebral artery, and in benign thunderclap headache, triggered by Valsalva manoeuvre, eg cough, coitus); meningitis, encephalitis, intracranial abscess, arterial stroke.

Investigations Exclude SAH if thunderclap headache (p482). Check there are no signs of meningitis (p832). *Imaging:* CT/MRI venography may show the absence of a sinus (**fig 1**), though an absent transverse sinus can be a normal variant. MRI T2*-weighted gradient echo sequences can visualize thrombus directly (**fig 2**), and also identify haemorrhagic infarction.[133] CT may be normal early; then at ~1wk develops the delta sign, where a transversely cut sinus shows a contrast filling defect. *Lumbar puncture* (unless CI by MRI/CT): if raised opening CSF pressure, with persistent headache and SAH excluded, suspect cerebral vein thrombosis. CSF may be normal, or show RBCs and xanthochromia.

Management Seek expert help. Heparin improves outcome,[134] possibly even in those with haemorrhagic venous infarction. Fibrinolytics (eg streptokinase) have been used via selective catheterization.[135][136] Thrombophilia screen and ENT review to help identify the cause.

Common causes
- Pregnancy/puerperium
- Oral contraceptives
- Head injury
- Dehydration
- Blood dyscrasias
- Intracranial malignancy (local invasion/pressure)
- Extracranial malignancy (hypercoagulability)
- Recent LP

Systemic causes
- Hyperthyroidism
- Nephrosis
- Ketoacidosis[126]
- Heart failure
- SLE
- Homocystinuria
- Hyperviscosity (p366)
- Crohn's or UC (p272-4)
- Behçet's disease (p708)
- Activated protein C resistance (p368)
- Antiphospholipid syn
- Klippel-Trénaunay syn
- Paroxysmal nocturnal haemoglobinuria

Infectious causes
- Meningitis; TB
- Cerebral abscess
- Septicaemia
- Fungal infections
- Otitis media
- Cerebral malaria
- HIV with nephrosis

Drug causes
- Androgens, eg oxymetholone[127]
- Antifibrinolytics, eg tranexamic acid
- Infliximab[128]

Prognosis Variable. Death is mainly due to transtentorial herniation from unilateral focal mass effects or diffuse oedema, and multiple parenchymal lesions. Independent predictors of death in one study were coma (odds ratio OR≈8.8), deep cortical vein thrombosis (OR≈8.5), posterior fossa lesion (OR≈6.5) right intracerebral haemorrhage (OR≈3.4), and mental disturbance (OR≈2.5). Evolving focal deficits are also associated with ↑ mortality.[137]

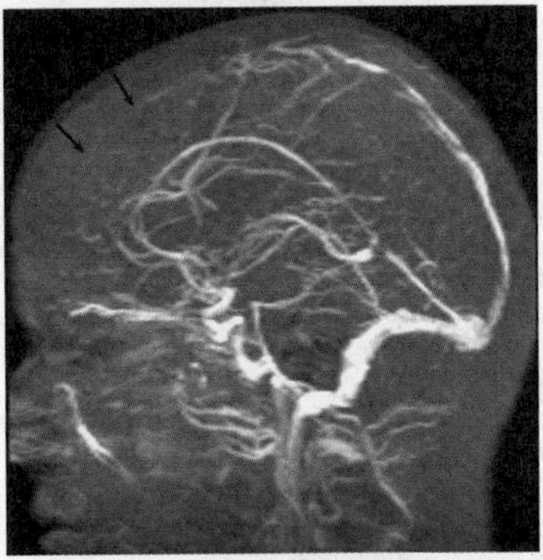

Fig 1. This magnetic resonance venogram (MRV) could look normal at first glance: the hardest thing to see in imaging is often that which is not there. Much of the superior sagittal sinus is not seen because it is filled with clot—a superior sagittal sinus thrombosis. The arrows point to where it should be seen. Posteriorly, the irregularity of the vessel indicates non-occlusive clot.

Image and commentary courtesy of Prof. Peter Scally

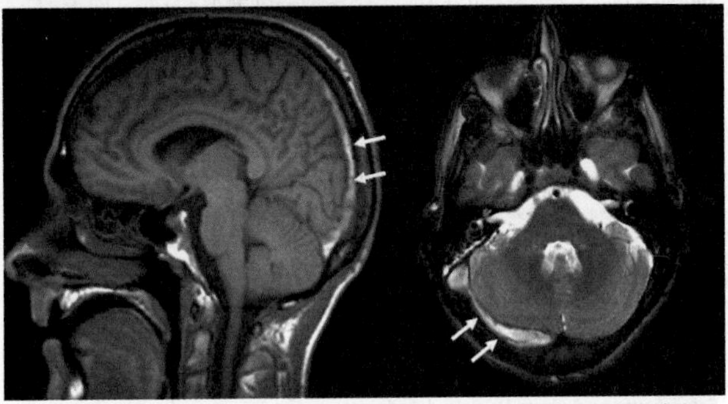

Fig 2. MRI showing thrombus (arrows) in the sagittal sinus (sagittal T1-weighted image, LEFT), and in the right transverse sinus (axial T2-weighted image, RIGHT). Often more than one sinus is involved.

Image courtesy of Dr David Werring

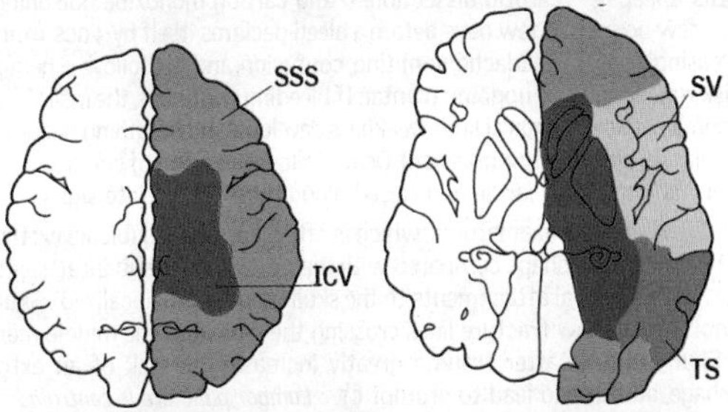

Fig 3. Venous territories (compare with arterial territories on p453). SSS—superior saggital sinus; TS—transverse sinus; SV—Sylvian veins; ICV—internal cortical veins.

There is much greater variation in venous anatomy between individuals than there is in arterial anatomy, so this diagram is only a rough guide. The key point is to realize that infarction that crosses boundaries between arterial territories may be venous in origin.

Subdural haemorrhage

►Consider this very treatable condition in all whose conscious level fluctuates, and also in those having an 'evolving stroke', especially if on anticoagulants. Bleeding is from bridging veins between cortex and venous sinuses (vulnerable to deceleration injury), resulting in accumulating haematoma between dura and arachnoid. This gradually raises ICP, shifting midline structures away from the side of the clot and, if untreated, eventual tentorial herniation and coning. Most subdurals are from trauma but the trauma is *often forgotten as it was so minor or so long ago* (up to 9 months).[138] It can also occur without trauma (eg ↓ICP;[1] dural metastases).[139] The elderly are most susceptible, as brain atrophy makes bridging veins vulnerable. *Other risk factors:* falls (epileptics, alcoholics); anticoagulation.

Symptoms Fluctuating level of consciousness (seen in 35%) ± insidious physical or intellectual slowing, sleepiness, headache, personality change, and unsteadiness.

Signs ↑ICP (p840); seizures. Localizing neurological symptoms (eg unequal pupils, hemiparesis) occur late and often long after the injury (mean=63 days).

Imaging (figs 1 & 2) CT/MRI shows clot ± midline shift (but beware bilateral isodense clots). Look for crescent-shaped collection of blood over 1 hemisphere. The sickle-shape differentiates subdural blood from extradural haemorrhage.

ΔΔ Stroke, dementia, CNS masses (eg tumours, abscess, neurocysticercosis).[140]

Treatment Irrigation/evacuation, eg via burr twist drill and burr hole craniostomy, can be considered 1st-line; craniotomy is 2nd-line,[141] if the clot has organized.[142] Address causes of the trauma (eg falls due cataract or arrhythmia; abuse).

Extradural (epidural) haemorrhage

►*Suspect this if, after head injury, conscious level falls or is slow to improve, or there is a lucid interval.* Extradural bleeds are often due to a fractured temporal or parietal bone causing laceration of the middle meningeal artery and vein, typically after trauma to a temple just lateral to the eye. Any tear in a dural venous sinus will also result in an extradural bleed. Blood accumulates between bone and dura.

Symptoms and signs Beware deteriorating consciousness after any head injury that initially produced no loss of consciousness or after initial drowsiness post-injury seems to have resolved. This **lucid interval** pattern is typical of extradural bleeds (ΔΔ: epilepsy,[143] carotid dissection,[144] and carbon monoxide poisoning).[145] It may last a few hours to a few days before a bleed declares itself by ↓GCS from rising ICP. Increasingly severe headache, vomiting, confusion, and fits follow, ± hemiparesis with brisk reflexes and an upgoing plantar. If bleeding continues, the ipsilateral pupil dilates, coma deepens, bilateral limb weakness develops, and breathing becomes deep and irregular (brainstem compression). Death follows a period of coma and is due to respiratory arrest. Bradycardia and raised blood pressure are late signs.

Tests CT **(fig 3)** shows a haematoma, which is often lens-shaped (biconvex; the blood forms a more rounded shape compared with the sickle-shaped subdural haematoma because the tough dural attachments to the skull keep it more localized). Skull x-ray may be normal or show fracture lines crossing the course of the middle meningeal vessels. Skull fracture after trauma greatly increases the risk of an extradural haemorrhage, and should lead to prompt CT. ►*Lumbar puncture is contraindicated.*

Management ►►Stabilize and transfer urgently (with skilled medical and nursing escorts) to a neurosurgical unit for clot evacuation ± ligation of the bleeding vessel. Care of the airway in an unconscious patient, and measures to ↓ICP often mandate intubation and ventilation (+ mannitol IVI, p840).

Prognosis Excellent if diagnosis and operation early. Poor if coma, pupil abnormalities, or decerebrate rigidity are present pre-op.

1 *Intracranial hypotension* (↓ICP) is due to CSF leaks, amenable to epidural blood patches over the leak. Suspect if headaches are worse on standing. *Causes:* meningeal diverticula; after lumbar puncture or epidural anaesthesia; dehydration; hyperpnoea (↑tidal volume). *MRI:* engorged venous sinuses, meningeal enhancement, and subdural fluid.

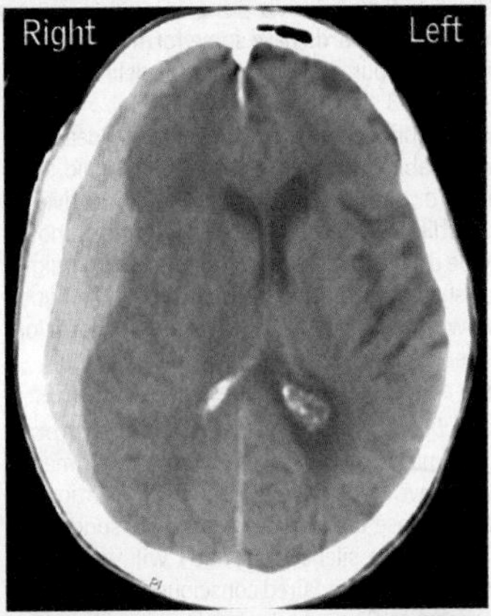

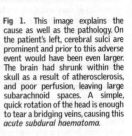

Fig 1. This image explains the cause as well as the pathology. On the patient's left, cerebral sulci are prominent and prior to this adverse event would have been even larger. The brain had shrunk within the skull as a result of atherosclerosis, and poor perfusion, leaving large subarachnoid spaces. A simple, quick rotation of the head is enough to tear a bridging veins, causing this *acute subdural haematoma*.

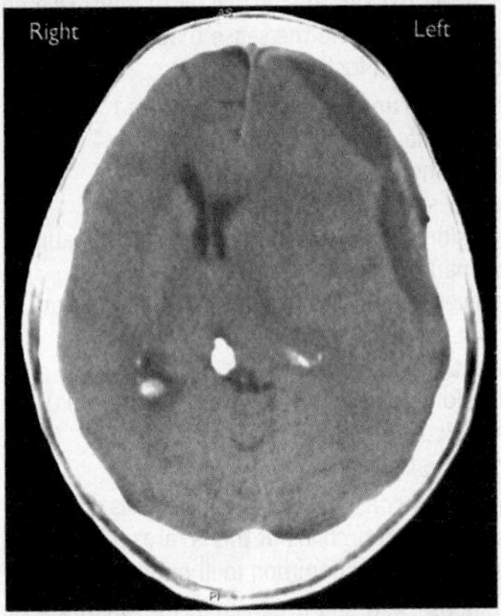

Fig 2. This fluid collection is of low attenuation compared to the brain, except for a small area of increased attenuation. It is an *acute on chronic subdural haematoma*. But there is more! Look at the shift of midline structures across under the falx cerebri—subfalcine herniation. It is not just caused by the subdural. The left hemisphere is swollen as a result of the compression of the bridging veins in the subdural space, shifting the ventricles and calcified pineal across to the right.

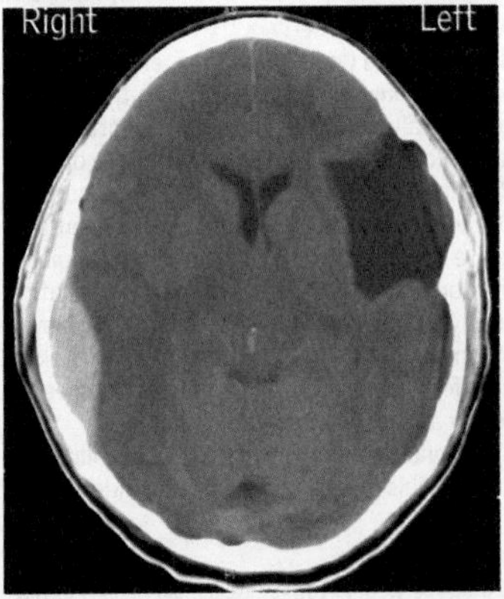

Fig 3. The blood (high attenuation, fusiform or biconvex collection) on the right side is limited anteriorly by the coronal suture and posteriorly by the lambdoid suture. This is therefore an *extradural haematoma*. The low attenuation CSF density collection on the left is causing scalloping of the overlying bone. It is in the typical location of an arachnoid cyst; an incidental finding of a congenital abnormality.

We thank Professor Peter Scally for the images and commentary.

Delirium (acute confusional state)

20% of elderly patients on medical and surgical wards have some form of delirium:[1] consider *any* acute fluctuating baffling behaviour change as possible delirium. Look for organic causes (UTI, pneumonia, MI). The 8 signs of **DELIRIUM** are:

Disordered thinking: slow, irrational, rambling, jumbled up, incoherent ideas.
Euphoric, fearful, depressed or angry: Labile mood, eg anxious then torpid.
Language impaired: Speech is reduced or gabbling, repetitive, and disruptive.
Illusions/delusions/hallucinations: Tactile or visual (auditory suggests psychosis)
Reversal of sleep-awake cycle: May be drowsy by day, and hypervigilant at night.
Inattention: Focusing, sustaining, or shifting attention is poor; no real dialogue.
Unaware/disorientated: Doesn't know it's evening, or his own name, or location.
Memory deficits: Often marked. (Later he may be amnesic for the episode.)

Summary: Globally impaired cognition and impaired awareness/consciousness.

Illustration from Conrad's ***Heart of Darkness*** 'The wastes of his weary brain were haunted by shadowy images now—images of wealth and fame...Sometimes he was contemptibly childish. He desired to have kings meet him at railway-stations on his return from some ghastly Nowhere..."Close the shutter", said Kurtz suddenly "I can't bear to look at this." I did so. There was a silence. "Oh, but I will wring your heart yet!" he cried at the invisible wilderness.' 146 Impaired consciousness is difficult to describe (which is why we have to resort to Conrad—the master of multi-layered descriptions). When you talk to the patient you have the sense that he is not with you, but away with the fairies—inaccessible and lost.

Causes (Pain and other psychological states are important co-factors.)

- Systemic infection: pneumonia, UTI, malaria, wounds, IV lines.
- Intracranial infection: encephalitis, meningitis.
- Drugs: opiates, anticonvulsants, L-dopa, sedatives, recreational, post-GA.
- Alcohol withdrawal (2-5d post-admission; ↑LFTs, ↑MCV; history of alcohol abuse). Also drug withdrawal. See p282 for management of alcohol withdrawal.
- Metabolic: hypoglycaemia, uraemia, liver failure, Na^+↑↓, anaemia, malnutrition.
- Hypoxia: respiratory or cardiac failure.
- Vascular: stroke, myocardial infarction.
- Head injury, ↑ICP, space-occupying lesions (eg tumour, subdural haematoma).
- Epilepsy: non-convulsive status epilepticus (see BOX), post-ictal states.
- Nutritional: thiamine, nicotinic acid, or B_{12} deficiency.

Differential If agitated, is it **anxiety**? Check conscious level. If delusions or hallucinations, is it a **primary mental illness** (eg schizophrenia) but this is rare on the wards (especially if no past history) and delirium is very common in ill patients.

Tests Consider FBC, U&E, LFTs, blood glucose, ABG, septic screen (urine dipstick, CXR, blood cultures); also ECG, malaria films, LP, EEG, CT/MRI.

Management After identifying and treating the underlying cause, aim to:

- Reduce distress and prevent accidents; encourage family to sit with the patient.
- Nurse in a *moderately lit*, quiet room, ideally with the *same* staff in attendance (minimizes confusion) where the patient can be watched closely. Improve orientation to time and place—**hunt down hearing aids/glasses**, give repeated reassurance.
- Do not use physical restraints—and remove catheters and other impedimenta.
- Augment self-care. Discourage passive dependency and inappropriate napping.
- Use the 3M non-drug cures for agitation: **m**usic, **m**assage, and **m**uscle relaxation.
- Minimize medication (especially sedatives); but if disruptive, some sedation may be needed, eg haloperidol 0.5-2mg, or chlorpromazine 50-100mg, PO if they will take it, IM if not (p11). Wait 20min to judge effect—further doses can be given if needed. **NB:** Avoid chlorpromazine in the elderly and in alcohol withdrawal (p282).

►Be aware that delirium may persist beyond the duration of the original illness by several weeks in the elderly. Do not assume this must be dementia—provide support and reassess 1-2 months later.

1 Delirium, from the latin *de* (from) and *lira* (ridge between furrows), meaning 'out of one's furrow'.

Tests of consciousness, and an explanation of dissociative states

Consciousness results wherever four entities co-exist: perception, memory, emotion, and orientation in space and time. Remorse, for example, is a blend of these constructs. If a black box exhibited remorse no further test would be needed to establish its consciousness. Patients are often black boxes to us: we are never *sure* what is going on inside. How do we find out? Dialogue is the first method. Patients with clouding of consciousness often engage in dialogue, but we get the feeling that they are not quite with us. A conversation may suggest clouding of consciousness—until the moment when the patient makes an ironic remark, banishing the need for formal tests of consciousness.

If a patient knows where he is, the time of day, and his memory is OK, we think there is no problem with consciousness—and move on to more mundane issues. This is a pity because changes in consciousness are often subtle—and we need to ask others who know the patient well if there has been any change. So elucidating changes in consciousness depends on triangulation between 3 interacting centres of consciousness—our own, the patient's, and a third party. These issues are exemplified in the next boxes, where we illustrate the concept of derealization. Here, it is enough to say that ***depersonalization*** and ***derealization*** are part of the ***dissociative states*** (one example of a disorder of consciousness). Dissociation is a mechanism that separates streams of memories or thoughts from 'now' consciousness. These fragments may resurface and persue a life of their own. *Causes:* migraine, epilepsy, head injury, stress, and prolonged sleeplessness (which is why all doctors instinctively understand this odd syndrome).

Non-convulsive status epilepticus as a cause of confusion

Non-convulsive status epilepticus is under-diagnosed, and may manifest itself as confusion, impaired cognition/memory, odd behaviour, and dreamy derealization[147] (the external world appears unfamiliar and unreal—its objects, anchored neither in space nor time, float as in a more or less lucid dream). Other features: aggression, psychosis ± abnormalities of eye movement, eyelid myoclonus, and odd postures. It may occur in the context of classic convulsive seizures (eg prolonged 'post-ictal' state) or ischaemic brain injury (especially haemorrhagic).[148] Other causes and associations: drugs (eg antidepressants), infections (eg arboviruses; HIV; syphilis), neoplasia, dementia, sudden ↑↓Ca^{2+},[149] renal failure (eg with cephalosporin therapy or peritoneal dialysis). ***Diagnosis:*** EEG evidence of rhythmical discharges (eg prolonged 3-per-second spike-wave complexes). Subsequent MRI may show focal oedema (eg in the hippocampus). ℞: lorazepam 2mg IV as first line. Valproate IV may be indicated (this requires specialist evaluation).

Ganser syndrome—an example of dissociative symptoms

There are absurd or approximate answers to questions (*paralogias*)—wrong but suggesting that the answers are unconsciously known but have been passed by or half-ignored by the current (dissociated) stream of consciousness. There are also: clouding of consciousness (or hypervigilance); somatic conversion symptoms (eg inexplicable paralysis—formerly known as hysterical symptoms); hallucinations; and amnesia, regarding the episode. ***Causes/associations:*** head injury, Munchausen's syndrome, solitary confinement, very stressful events.[150]

When asked to spell WORLD backwards, one Ganser patient replied 'EBOLG'. When asked to recall the words 'honesty', 'window', and 'lace', he replied 'modesty', 'house', and 'shoes'.[151] *NB:* ►ictal and post-ictal states may present with similarly impaired consciousness, perceptual abnormalities, and odd behaviour.

Can you ganser? A common experience is to be perusing a patient's results while he is talking at you: suddenly he asks "Is my PSA OK?" and you say "Yes". "What was it?" he insists. You say "5" off the top of your head. You think you had better check. It turns out that the PSA was 5.09. Unconsciously you had taken in the data, and rounded it down, instinctively giving the patient the benefit of the doubt. Ganser would be proud of you. Ganser is the essence of multitasking.

Dementia

Dementia is a syndrome encompassing progressive deficits in several cognitive domains. The initial presentation is usually of memory loss over months or years (►if over days think infection or stroke; if over weeks think depression). In later stages, non-cognitive symptoms such as agitation, aggression or apathy may complicate care, which becomes increasingly difficult requiring specialist input.

Prevalence Rare <55yrs of age, 5–10% in those >65yrs, 20% >80yrs and 70% >100yrs.

Diagnosis The key is a good history both from the patient and someone who knows them well (eg spouse, relatives, or friends). Ask about the *timeline* of the progression of their impaired cognition/memory, what was noticed first and what particular aspects of it they have most difficulty with (autobiographical,[1] political, etc). Ask also about how it affects their *activities of daily living*, and their ability to cope with tasks such as *financial affairs* and *medications*—some may cope well with significant impairment, others may be disproportionately affected. Examples from the spouse or relative will be helpful. There may also be agitation, aggression, wandering, hallucinations, slow repetitious speech, apathy, mood disturbance (NB: depression is common in dementia, but can also *cause* cognitive impairment). *Cognitive testing:* use a validated dementia screen such as the AMTS (p70), TYM (p85), or similar, plus short tests of verbal recall (eg HVLT, which is more sensitive in mild impairment)[152] and executive function (eg CLOX).[153] *Mental state examination* may reveal anxiety, depression or hallucinations. *Physical examination* may identify a physical cause of the cognitive impairment, risk factors (esp. for vascular dementia), or parkinsonism.

Investigations FBC, ESR, U&E, Ca^{2+}, LFTs, TSH, autoantibodies, B_{12}/folate (treat low-normals).[154] CT/MRI (for vascular damage, haemorrhage or structural pathology). Consider also syphilis serology, EEG, CSF, functional imaging (FDG, PET, SPECT).[155] Metabolic, genetic or HIV tests if indicated, after appropriate counselling.

Commonest causes *Alzheimer's disease (AD)* See p492.

Vascular dementia: ~25% of all dementias. It represents the cumulative effects of many small strokes, thus sudden onset and stepwise deterioration is characteristic (but often difficult to recognise). Look for evidence of vascular pathology (BP↑, past strokes, focal CNS signs).

Lewy body dementia: the 3rd commonest cause (15–25%) after Alzheimer's and vascular causes, typically with *fluctuating* cognitive impairment, detailed visual hallucinations (eg small animals or children) and later, parkinsonism (p498). Histology is characterized by Lewy bodies[3] in brainstem *and* neocortex.

Ameliorable causes
• T4↓; B_{12}/folate↓; thiamine↓ (eg alcohol)
• Depression
• Syphilis
• Tumours (meningioma)
• Subdural haematoma
• Parkinson's (p498)
• CNS cysticercosis (p444)
• HIV (± cryptococcosis)
• Normal pressure hydrocephalus[2]
• Pellagra (p278)
• Whipple's disease (p730)

Fronto-temporal dementia: (Frontal and temporal atrophy without Alzheimer histology, p493). *Signs:* Executive impairment; behavioural/personality change; early preservation of episodic memory and spatial orientation; disinhibition; hyperorality, stereotyped behaviour, and emotional unconcern. The disinhibition is not *always* bad.[4]

Rarer causes: Alcohol/drug abuse; repeated head trauma; pellagra (p278), Whipple's disease (p730); Huntington's (p716); CJD (p710); Parkinson's (p498); Pick's disease; HIV; cryptococcosis (p440); familial autosomal dominant Alzheimer's; CADASIL (p474).

1 Autobiographical and political memory are held in different areas: S Black 2004 *Neuropsychologia* **42** 25

2 Normal pressure hydrocephalus gives dilated ventricles *without* enlarged cerebral sulci (?from obstructed CSF outflow from the subarachnoid space). *Signs:* gait apraxia, incontinence, dementia. CSF shunts help.

3 Lewy bodies are eosinophilic intracytoplasmic neuronal inclusion bodies; there is overlap between Lewy body dementia, Alzheimer's and Parkinson's (PD), making treatment hard as L-dopa can precipitate delusions, and antipsychotic drugs worsen PD. Rivastigmine may help all 3.

4 An artist who had been constrained by over-adherence to one school of art had a fascinating blossoming of creativity and emotional insight with the arrival of fronto-temporal dementia. Similarly, the unique writing style of 19th century critic and author John Ruskin is thought to be a consequence of CADASIL. This poses the question of what counts as a disease. If you can answer this question unequivocally perhaps you are over-endowed, fronto-temporally? Let some ambiguity in!

The positive features of dementia (Auntie Kathleen's syndrome)

Positive features include **wandering**, **aggression**, **flight of ideas**, and **logorrhoea**: "Not for her a listless, dull-eyed wordless decline; with her it is all rush, gabble, celerity. She had always been a talker, but now her dementia unleashes torrents of speech...one train of thought switching to another without signal or pause, rattling across points and through junctions at a rate no listener can follow... Following the sense is like trying to track a particular ripple in a pelting torrent of talk." **Alan Bennett** *Untold Stories*, **87**

Practical issues in managing dementia

Patients with dementia become increasingly dependent and develop increasing complex needs as the disease progresses. Most will at some stage experience behavioural or psychological symptoms, which can be particularly distressing for the carer. ►See *Living with neurological disease*, p449. Issues to consider are:

- ***A care coordinator*** (via Social Services or the local Old Age Community Mental Healthcare Team) is vital to coordinate the various teams and services that may at various times become necessary, and to arrange the *special help* that is available for those caring for demented relatives at home, eg in the UK:
  - Laundry services for soiled linen
  - Car badge giving priority parking
  - Carers' groups for mutual support
  - Help from occupational therapist, district nurses, and community psychiatric nurses
  - Attendance allowance
  - Respite care in hospital
  - Day care/lunch clubs
  - Council tax rebate (forms from local council office)
- ***Capacity:*** can the patient make decisions regarding medical or financial affairs? Wherever possible, allow the patient to guide decisions. If currently capacitous suggest making an advanced directive or appointing a Lasting Power of Attorney.
- ***Develop routines:*** routines learned early on are retained till late in the disease, helping patients to maintain their independence for longer. Habitually keeping house keys in the same place, for example, will help to avoid losing them by forgetting their whereabouts later on.
- ***Plan ahead:*** relocation to a new house or to a care home can be very disruptive for a patient with dementia. Discuss this with the patient and their family. If the family are keen to help but live far away, consider moving earlier rather than later, when a new environment will be harder to become accustomed to. Equally, regular respite visits to the same care home may make a final move there easier at a later date.
- ***Day services*** can be invaluable for stimulating patients and providing regular, much-needed breaks for carers. Multisensory stimulation, massage, music,[156] animal therapy and aromatherapy[157] can help mood, aggression, anxiety, and speech.[158] Structured conversation and exercise also help.[159]
- ***Who will care for the carers?*** Carer stress is inevitable, causing ↑morbidity *and* mortality. Support groups, telephone helplines, respite care and your unswerving loyalty can all ease the burden; eg UK Alzheimer's Disease Society: **0845 300 0336**.
- ***Challenging behaviour:*** First rule out pain and infection as the cause of the worsening behaviour. Then, if non-pharmacological therapies fail, consider trazodone (50-300mg ON) or lorazepam (0.5mg OD to 2mg BD). If the agitation is severe, get help: antipsychotics such as quetiapine, risperidone and olanzapine may improve positive symptoms (ABOVE), but cognition, verbal fluency, and longevity may be worsened.[160] Haloperidol (0.5–4mg) can be useful in the short term.

►Avoid using antipsychotics for agitation in Lewy body dementia (↑↑risk of SE). There is some evidence that acetylcholinesterase inhibitors may help (see p493).

- ***Depression*** is common. Try an SSRI (eg citalopram 10–20mg OD) or, if severe, mirtazapine (15–45mg at night if eGFR >40). Cognitive behavioural therapy can help with social withdrawal and catastrophic thinking.
- ***Avoid drugs that impair cognition*** (eg neuroleptics, sedatives, tricyclics, p11).

This leading cause of dementia is *the* big neuropsychiatric disorder of our times, dominating not just old age psychiatry wards, but the lives of countless children and spouses who have given up work, friends, and all accustomed ways of life to support relatives through their long final years. Their lives can be tormented—"*I am chained to a corpse*" (p449)—or transformed, depending on how gently patients exit into their "*worlds of preoccupied emptiness*".[161] ***Onset*** may be from 40yrs (earlier in Down's syndrome, in which AD is inevitable). ***Mean survival:*** 7 years from onset.

Presentation See p490 for a general approach to diagnosing dementias. Suspect Alzheimer's in adults with enduring,[1] progressive and global cognitive impairment (unlike other dementias which may affect certain domains but not others): **visuo-spatial skill** (gets lost), **memory**, **verbal abilities** and **executive function** (planning) are all affected (use neuropsychometric testing to identify affected domains; see p490), and there is **anosognosia**[2]—a lack of insight into the problems engendered by the disease, eg missed appointments, misunderstood conversations or plots of films, and mishandling of money and clerical work.[162] Later there may be irritability; mood disturbance (depression or euphoria); behavioural change (eg aggression, wandering, disinhibition); psychosis (hallucinations or delusions); agnosia (may not recognize self in the mirror). There is no standard natural history. Cognitive impairment is progressive, but non-cognitive symptoms may come and go over months. Towards the end, often but not invariably, patients become sedentary, taking little interest in anything.

Cause Modest concordance between monozygotic and dizygotic twins, suggests that environmental and genetic factors both play a role. Accumulation of β-amyloid peptide, a degradation product of amyloid precursor protein, results in progressive neuronal damage, neurofibrillary tangles, ↑numbers of amyloid plaques, and loss of the neurotransmitter *acetylcholine* (**fig 1**). Defective clearance of β-amyloid plaques by macrophages appears to relate to altered macrophage gene expression.[3] Neuronal loss is selective—the hippocampus, amygdala, temporal neocortex and some subcortical nuclei, eg the nucleus basalis of Meynert, are especially vulnerable (p448).[163] Vascular effects are also important—95% of AD patients show evidence of vascular dementia.

Risk factors First-degree relative with AD; Down's syndrome; homozygosity for the apolipoprotein E (ApoE) e4 allele; PICALM, CLI and CLU gene mutations;[164] [165] vascular risk factors such as ↑BP, diabetes, hyperlipidaemia, ↑homocysteine, and atrial fibrillation; low physical and cognitive activity; depression; evidence on alcohol and smoking is not consistent: ↑EtOH ≥2 drinks/day accelerated onset of AD by 4.8yrs in one study (but others report that red wine may be protective); ≥20 cigarettes/day≈2.3yrs; ApoE e4 genotype≈3yrs. Delaying onset by 5yrs would ↓ prevalence by ~50%.[166] 2008 data. n=938

Management ►See p491 for a general approach to management in dementia. • Refer to a specialist memory service. • Acetylcholinesterase inhibitors (BOX). • Meticulous BP control helps[167] due to the complex interaction between vasculopathy and AD.[4] • There is little evidence that HRT, statins, or NSAIDs confer any benefit.[168] Vitamin E and ginkgo biloba get some support from one trial each;[169] data on other antioxidants is mixed. The limited data on huperzine A looks promising.[170]

Prevention Many theories are being tested, but good replicated randomized trials are lacking.[171] Interventions are likely to be most effective if started early, and MRI/PET can predict decline/dementia in the cognitively normal,[172] but even if we could count neurofibrillary tangles with post-mortem accuracy we could not say 'this brain is becoming demented' as there is no simple relationship between structure and function.[173]

1 'Enduring' doesn't mean unfluctuating: cognition comes and goes, allowing poetic insights, as in Iris Murdoch's poignant self-diagnosis: 'I am sailing into the dark'.

2 Anosognosia, from the Greek *nosos* (disease) and *gnosis* (knowledge)

3 This is partly correctable by bisdemethoxycurcumin, found in the turmeric component of curries; just one reason why AD may be less prevalent in India: 0.5% *vs* 1.7% in USA.

4 In heart failure there is a ~2-fold ↑risk of AD; excess risk halves if antihypertensives are used. In a 2006 study of **transcranial Doppler** middle cerebral artery monitoring for 1 hour, **small emboli** occurred in 40% of those with Alzheimer's compared with ~15% for controls.

Pharmacological treatment of cognitive decline

Is it better to be useless or cruel?

Acetylcholinesterase inhibitors: Evidence that acetylcholinesterase inhibitors are modestly effective in treating Alzheimer's is good.[174] There is also limited evidence for their efficacy in the dementia of Parkinson's disease,[175] and rivastigmine may improve behavioural symptoms in Lewy body dementia.[176] They appear to help the laying down of new memories more than accessing old ones,[177] and delay the need for institutional care, but not necessarily its duration.[178] They are currently available in the UK only through specialist memory services, for patients whose MMSE lies between 10 and 20. However, one cannot say "Stop these drugs as he has only scored x on the MMSE" (notoriously variable from day to day) if the wife says "but he's brighter, more motivated".[179] ►Be aware that using QALYs (p10) relentlessly can make us cruel; sentiment (the alternative to QALYs) may make us useless, but it is better to be useless than cruel. The Scottish Intercollegiate Guidelines Network (SIGN) states that all AD patients could benefit from acetylcholinesterase inhibitors, although this did not take into account a cost-benefit analysis.

- **Donepezil:**[1] 5mg ON initially, ↑ to 10mg ON at 1 month.
- **Rivastigmine:**[2] 1.5mg bd initially, ↑ to 3–6mg bd. Patches are also available.
- **Galantamine**: initially 4mg bd, ↑ to 8–12mg bd. Originally isolated from daffodils.

SE: D&V, cramps, incontinence, headache, dizziness, insomnia, LFTs↑; rarely, but importantly, heart block and cardiac arrhythmias, hallucinations, peptic ulcers. ►The cholinergic effects of acetylcholinesterase inhibitors may exacerbate peptic ulcer disease and heart block. Always ask about dyspepsia and cardiac symptoms, and do an ECG before starting treatment.

Antiglutamatergic treatment: Randomized trials show that **memantine** (an NMDA antagonist, see p455) is reasonably effective in late stage disease, although its use in the UK is currently restricted to clinical trials. *Dose:* 5mg/24h initially, ↑by 5mg/d weekly to 10mg/12h. *SE:* hallucinations, confusion, hypertonia, hypersexuality.

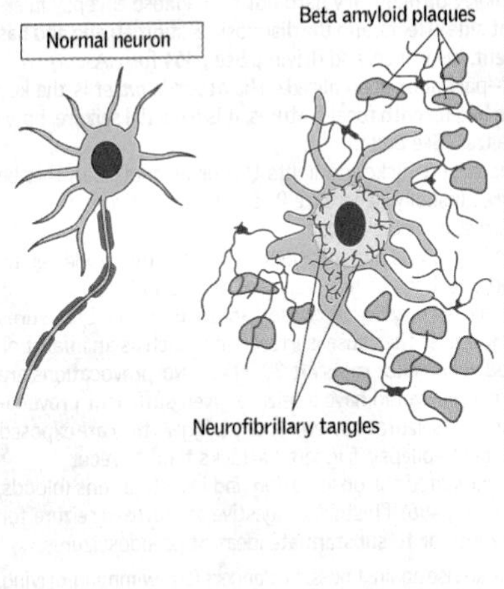

Fig 1. Alzheimer's has 2 hallmarks: senile plaques and neurofibrillary tangles. A quarter of a century ago their proteins were identified, precipitating an avalanche of molecular research and promises of new drugs. So why have we failed to make any landmark progress? Perhaps we need a paradigm shift from the reductionism that defines amyloid-beta and tau hypotheses—to recognition that AD pathology is a manifestation of cellular adaptation, eg a defence against oxidative injury. If AD pathology is a host response rather than a manifestation of protein injury, it is unlikely to be a fruitful target for therapeutic intervention

1 Pre-treatment orbitofrontal signs (agitation, disinhibition, odd motor activity) may predict good response to donepezil.

2 Pre-treatment hallucinations predict a response to rivastigmine.

Epilepsy is a recurrent tendency to spontaneous, intermittent, abnormal electrical activity in part of the brain, manifest as *seizures*.[1] These may take many forms, but for each individual patient they tend to be stereotyped. *Convulsions* are the motor signs of electrical discharges. Many of us would have seizures in abnormal metabolic circumstances—eg Na^+↓, hypoxia (eg reflex anoxic seizures in faints): we would not normally be said to have epilepsy. The prevalence of active epilepsy is ~1%.

Elements of a seizure A *prodrome* lasting hours or days may rarely precede the seizure. It is not part of the seizure itself: the patient or others notice a change in mood or behaviour. An *aura* is part of the seizure of which the patient is aware, and may precede its other manifestations. The aura may be a strange feeling in the gut, or an experience such as *déjà vu* (disturbing sense of familiarity), or strange smells or flashing lights. It implies a partial (focal) seizure, often, but not necessarily, from the temporal lobe. *Post-ictally* there may be headache, confusion, myalgia, and a sore tongue; or temporary weakness after a focal seizure in motor cortex (Todd's palsy, p726), or dysphasia following a focal seizure in the temporal lobe.

Causes ⅔ are idiopathic (often familial). ***Structural:*** Cortical scarring (eg head injury years before onset), developmental (eg dysembryoplastic neuroepithelial tumour or cortical dysgenesis), space-occupying lesion, stroke, hippocampal sclerosis (eg after a febrile convulsion), vascular malformations. ***Others:*** Tuberous sclerosis, sarcoid, SLE, PAN. ***Non-epileptic causes of seizures:*** Trauma, stroke, haemorrhage, ↑ICP; alcohol or benzodiazepine withdrawal; metabolic disturbance (hypoxia, Na^+↑↓, Ca^{2+}↓, glucose↑↓, uraemia); liver disease; infection (eg meningitis, encephalitis, syphilis, cysticercosis, HIV); T°↑; drugs (tricyclics, cocaine, tramadol, theophylline); pseudoseizures (p496).

Diagnosis There are three key questions to consider:

1 *Are these really seizures?* A detailed description from a witness of 'the fit' is vital (but ask yourself: "Are they reliable?" In the heat of the moment many witnesses report twitching when none took place). Tongue-biting and a slow recovery are very suggestive. Not everything that twitches is epilepsy—reflex anoxic convulsions due to syncope are particularly difficult. Try hard not to diagnose epilepsy in error—therapy has significant side effects, and the diagnosis is stigmatizing and has implications for employment, insurance, and driving. See p464 for ΔΔ.

2 *What type of seizure is it*—partial or generalized? The attack's *onset* is the key concern here. If the seizure begins with focal features, it is a partial seizure, however rapidly it then generalizes. See BOX 1.

3 *What, if anything, triggers it?* Eg flickering lights (TV) or alcohol? Can this be avoided? TV-induced seizures (usually generalized) rarely require drugs.

In assessing a first-ever seizure, consider also:

- *Is it really the first?* Ask the family and patient about past funny turns/odd behaviour. Déjà vu and odd episodic feelings of fear may well be relevant.
- *Was the seizure provoked?* (see *'Non-epileptic causes'* above) Provoked 1st seizures are less likely to recur (3–10%, unless the cause is irreversible, such as an infarct or glioma); if it was unprovoked, recurrence rates are 30–50%.[180] **NB:** provocations are different to triggers: most people would have a seizure given sufficient provocation, but most people do not have seizures however many triggers they are exposed to, so triggered seizures suggest epilepsy. Triggered attacks tend to recur.
- Admission for ~24h may be indicated for observation and investigations (bloods, drugs screen, CT/MRI, LP, EEG—see p496) if history suggestive of provoked seizure, for intractable or recurrent seizures, or to substantiate ideas of pseudoseizures.

Counselling After any seizure, advise against possible dangers (eg swimming, driving, heights) until a diagnosis is established. After diagnosis, *individualized* counselling is needed regarding issues such as employment, insurance and conception. Driving is a difficult area—advise them that they cannot drive until seizure-free for >1yr and must (in the UK) contact DVLA themselves (p153).[181] Document your discussion carefully.

1 ↑Membrane excitation (epileptogenicity) may be related to disorders of synaptic transmission, K^+ channelopathies, or α-subunit mutations (eg SCN2A; SCN1A) of voltage-gated Na^+ channel. *Lancet* 2003 1238

Seizure classification

Partial seizures Focal onset, with features referable to a part of one hemisphere (see BOX 2). Often seen with underlying structural disease.

- *Simple partial seizure:* Awareness is unimpaired, with focal motor, sensory (olfactory, visual, etc), autonomic or psychic symptoms. No post-ictal symptoms.
- *Complex partial seizures:* Awareness is impaired. May have a simple partial onset (=aura), or impaired awareness at onset. Most commonly arise from the temporal lobe. Post-ictal confusion is common with seizures arising from the temporal lobe, whereas recovery is rapid after seizures in the frontal lobe.
- *Partial seizure with secondary generalization:* In ⅔ of patients with partial seizures, the electrical disturbance, which starts focally (either as a simple or complex partial seizure), spreads widely causing a secondary generalized seizure, which is typically convulsive.

Primary generalized seizures Simultaneous onset of electrical discharge throughout cortex, with no localizing features referable to only one hemisphere.

- *Absence seizures:* Brief (≤10s) pauses, eg suddenly stops talking in mid-sentence, then carries on where left off. Presents in childhood.
- *Tonic–clonic seizures:* Loss of consciousness. Limbs stiffen (tonic), then jerk (clonic). May have one without the other. Post-ictal confusion and drowsiness.
- *Myoclonic seizures:* Sudden jerk of a limb, face or trunk. The patient may be thrown suddenly to ground, or have a violently disobedient limb: one patient described it as *'my flying-saucer epilepsy'*, as crockery which happened to be in the hand would take off.
- *Atonic (akinetic) seizures:* Sudden loss of muscle tone causing a fall, no LOC.
- *Infantile spasms* (OHCS p206) Commonly associated with tuberous sclerosis.

NB: the classification of *epileptic syndromes* is separate to the classification of seizures, and is based on seizure type, age of onset, EEG findings and other features such as family history. Seizure classifications based on semiology also exist.[183]

Localizing features of partial (focal) seizures

Temporal lobe • Automatisms—complex motor phenomena, but with impaired awareness and no recollection afterwards, varying from primitive oral (lip smacking, chewing, swallowing) or manual (fumbling, fiddling, grabbing) movements, to complex actions (singing, kissing, driving a car and violent acts);[184] • Abdominal rising sensation or pain (± ictal vomiting; or rarely episodic fevers[185] or D&V[186]); • Dysphasia (ictal or post-ictal); • Memory phenomena—*déjà vu* (when everything seems strangely familiar), or *jamais vu* (everything seems strangely unfamiliar); • Hippocampal involvement may cause emotional disturbance, eg sudden terror, panic, anger or elation, and derealization (out-of-body experiences)[187], which in combination may manifest as excessive religiosity;[1][188] • Uncal involvement may cause hallucinations of smell or taste and a dreamlike state[189] & seizures in auditory cortex may cause complex auditory hallucinations, eg music or conversations, or palinacousis[190]; • Delusional behaviour; • Finally, you may find yourself not believing your patient's bizarre story—eg "Canned music at Tesco's always makes me cry and then pass out, unless I wear an earplug in one ear"[191] or "I get orgasms when I brush my teeth" (right temporal lobe hyper- and hypo-perfusion, respectively).[192]

Frontal lobe • Motor features such as posturing, versive movements of the head and eyes,[193] or peddling movements of the legs • Jacksonian march (a spreading focal motor seizure with retained awareness, often starting with the face or a thumb) • Motor arrest • Subtle behavioural disturbances (often diagnosed as psychogenic) • Dysphasia or speech arrest • Post-ictal Todd's palsy (p726).

Parietal lobe • Sensory disturbances—tingling, numbness, pain (rare) • Motor symptoms (due to spread to the pre-central gyrus).

Occipital lobe • Visual phenomena such as spots, lines, flashes.

1 The temporolimbic system tags certain stimuli as derealized, crucially important, harmonious, and/or joyous or ecstatic, making us prone to describe these experiences within religious frameworks.

Children: OHCS p206

General principles ►*Involve patients in all decisions.* Compliance depends on communication and doctor-patient concordance (p3). Living with *active* epilepsy creates many problems (eg inability to drive or operate machinery, drug side effects) and fears (eg of sudden death). Neurologists may have little time to explore these issues, while GPs may have no special interest in epilepsy. Enlist the help of an **epilepsy nurse specialist**, who can provide telephone advice and annual reviews to monitor drug efficacy and side-effects, to address employment, leisure, and reproductive issues, and, after a few seizure-free years, to consider drug withdrawal.

Drug therapy Most specialists would not recommend treatment after one fit, unless the risk of recurrence is high (eg structural brain lesion, focal neurological deficit, or unequivocal epileptiform EEG) but would start treatment after a second. ►Discuss options with the patient. If your patient has only 1 fit every 2yrs, he or she may accept the risk (particularly if there is no need to drive or operate machinery) rather than have to take drugs every day. Drug choice depends on seizure type and epilepsy syndrome, other medications and co-morbidities, and patient preference:

- ***Generalized tonic-clonic seizures:*** **Sodium valproate** or **lamotrigine** (often better tolerated,[194] and less teratogenic) are 1st line, then carbamazepine or topiramate. Others: levetiracetam, oxcarbazepine, clobazam.
- ***Absence seizures:*** **sodium valproate**, **lamotrigine** or **ethosuximide**.[195]
- ***Tonic, atonic*** and ***myoclonic seizures:*** As for generalized tonic-clonic seizures, but avoiding carbamazepine and oxcarbazepine, which may worsen seizures.
- ***Partial seizures ± secondary generalization:*** **Carbamazepine** is 1st-line, then sodium valproate, lamotrigine, oxcarbazepine or topiramate. Others: levetiracetam, gabapentin, tiagabine, phenytoin, clobazam.

Treat with *one* drug and with *one* doctor in charge only. Slowly build up doses over 2-3 months (see BOX) until seizures are controlled, side effects are intolerable, or maximum dosage is reached. If ineffective or not tolerated, switch to the next most appropriate drug. To switch drugs, introduce the new drug (see BOX), and only withdraw the first drug once established on the second. Newer drugs are often costly (eg £100/month *vs* £12), but cost-effective.[196] Dual therapy is necessary in <10% of patients—consider if all appropriate drugs have been tried singly at their top dose.

The role of electroencephalography (EEG) EEG cannot *of itself* exclude or refute epilepsy; it forms part of the context for diagnosis, so don't do one if the likely diagnosis is simple syncope (often false +ve). It helps classification and prognosis: in 1st unprovoked seizures, unequivocal epileptiform activity on EEG helps assess risk of recurrence.[197] Only do *emergency* EEGs if non-convulsive status is the problem (p489). Other tests: MRI (structural lesions, p494). Serum drug levels (is he taking the tablets?). Magnetoencephalography (MEG), PET, cognitive assessment, and ictal SPECT (p761) may help localize the epileptogenic focus when evaluating for epilepsy surgery.

Non-epileptic attack disorder ***(pseudo- or psychogenic seizures)*** These are not infrequent: suspect this if there are uncontrollable symptoms, no learning disabilities, and CNS exam, CT, MRI, and EEG are normal.[198] It may coexist with true epilepsy.

Further therapeutic options Occasionally, despite multiple medications, a patient's epilepsy will be refractory to medication. If a single epileptogenic focus can be identified (see above) such as hippocampal sclerosis or a small low-grade tumour, **neurosurgical resection** offers up to 70% chance of seizure freedom, depending on the location of the focus, with the risk of causing focal neurological deficits such as memory impairment, dysphasia or hemianopia.[199] An alternative is **vagal nerve stimulation**, which can reduce seizure frequency and severity in ~33%.

When it all goes wrong *Sudden unexpected death in epilepsy* ***(SUDEP)*** is more common in uncontrolled epilepsy, and may be related to nocturnal seizure-associated apnoea or asystole.[200] Those with epilepsy have a mortality rate 3-fold that of controls. >700 epilepsy-related deaths are recorded/yr in the UK; up to 17% are SUDEPs. For help with families of those with SUDEP, contact *Epilepsy Bereaved*[UK] 01235 772852.

Antiepileptic drugs (AED): doses & side-effects (see formulary for details)

Carbamazepine: (as slow-release) Initially 100mg/12h, increase by 200mg/d every 2wks up to max 1000mg/12h. SE: *leucopenia*, diplopia, blurred vision, impaired balance, drowsiness, mild generalized erythematous rash, SIADH (rare; see p687).

Lamotrigine: As monotherapy, initially 25mg/d, ↑ by 50mg/d every 2wks up to 100mg/12hr (max 250mg/12h). ►Halve monotherapy dose if on valproate; double if on carbamazepine or phenytoin (max 350mg/12h). SE: maculopapular rash—occurs in 10% (but 1/1000 develop *Stevens-Johnson syndrome* or *toxic epidermal necrolysis*) typically in 1st 8wks, esp if on valproate; warn patients to see a doctor at once if rash or flu symptoms develop; also associated with hypersensitivity (fever, ↑LFTs & disseminated intravascular coagulopathy). Other SEs: diplopia, blurred vision, photosensitivity (SLE-like), tremor, agitation, vomiting, aplastic anaemia.

Levetiracetam: If >16yrs, initially 250mg/12h, increase by 250mg/12h every 2wks up to max 1.5g/12h (if eGFR >80). Psychiatric side effects are common, eg depression, agitation. Other SEs: D&V, dyspepsia, drowsiness, diplopia, blood dyscrasias.

Phenytoin: Effective and well-tried, but no longer 1st line for generalized or partial epilepsy due to toxicity (nystagmus, diplopia, tremor, dysarthria, ataxia) and SEs (↓intellect, depression, coarse facial features, acne, gum hypertrophy, polyneuropathy, blood dyscrasias). Dosage is difficult—do blood levels (p766).

Sodium valproate: Initially 300mg/12h, increase by 100mg/12h every 3 days up to max 30mg/kg (or 2.5g) daily. Nausea is very common (take with food).

Vigabatrin: Only used in infantile spasms (due to a high incidence of visual field defects).

Valproate side effects

- Appetite↑, weight gain.
- Liver failure (watch LFTs during 1st 6 months).
- Pancreatitis.
- Reversible hair loss (grows back curly).
- Oedema.
- Ataxia.
- Teratogenicity, tremor, thrombocytopaenia.
- Encephalopathy (due to hyperammonaemia).

►Carbamazepine, phenytoin and barbiturates are liver enzyme inducing.

Women with epilepsy

- *Teratogenicity of AEDs:* Women of child-bearing age should take *folic acid* 5mg/d. Valproate in particular should be avoided (use lamotrigine).
- *Pre-conception counselling* is vital due to 5% risk of fetal abnormality (*OHCS* p29).
- *Breastfeeding:* most AEDs except carbamazepine and valproate are present in breast milk. Lamotrigine is not thought to be harmful to infants.
- *Contraception:* Non-enzyme-inducing AEDs have no effect on the Pill. With other AEDs ≥50μg of oestrogen may be needed (Norinyl-1®; ↓pill-free days from 7 to 4; use condoms too) or Depo-Provera® (10-weekly IM). The progesterone-only pill is also affected. The coil is suitable for emergency contraception, or levonorgestrel 3mg PO stat.

Stopping anticonvulsants

►*Discuss risks and benefits with patients. Informed choices are vital.* Most patients are seizure-free within a few years of starting drugs. More than 50% remain so when drugs are withdrawn. After assessing risks and benefits for the individual patient (eg the need to drive), withdrawal may be tried, if the patient meets these criteria: normal CNS examination, normal IQ, normal EEG prior to withdrawal, seizure-free for >2yrs, and no juvenile myoclonic epilepsy. In one study (*N* =459), over 5yrs 52% remained seizure-free, compared with 67% who continued their medication.[201] However, in another study, resuming medication did not return the patient to his/her status quo, and not all seizures could be controlled (risk factors: cognitive deficits and partial epilepsy).[202] One way to withdraw drugs in adults is to decrease the dose by 10% every 2-4wks (for carbamazepine, lamotrigine, phenytoin, valproate, and vigabatrin) and by 10% every 4-8wks for phenobarbital, benzodiazepines, and ethosuximide.[203]

Parkinsonism

Classical triad of signs: **tremor**, **rigidity**, **bradykinesia/hypokinesia**.

- *Tremor:* Worse at rest. Characteristic 'pill-rolling' action of thumb over fingers. 4-6 cycles/sec (slower than cerebellar tremor). Distinguish from essential tremor, which is a symptomatic postural ± action tremor of the upper limbs and head.
- *Rigidity:* ↑Tone. Superimposed tremor causes 'cogwheel rigidity'.
- *Bradykinesia/hypokinesia:* Slowness of movement initiation with progressive reduction in speed and amplitude of repetitive actions. Paucity of movement, eg expressionless face, ↓blink rate, monotonous hypophonic speech, micrographia. *Gait:* reduced arm-swing, festinance (short shuffling steps with flexed trunk as if forever a step behind one's centre of gravity), freezing at obstacles & doors.

Causes of parkinsonism

- Idiopathic Parkinson's disease
- Multiple cerebral infarcts
- Parkinson's-plus syndromes: PSP, MSA, CBD, & Lewy body dementia (see BOX)
- Post-encephalopathy
- Drug-induced, eg neuroleptics, prochlorperazine, metoclopramide
- Toxin-induced, eg MPTP, manganese, copper (Wilson's disease)
- Trauma (pugilistic encephalopathy)

Parkinson's disease (PD)

Presentation Syndrome of bradykinesia/hypokinesia plus at least one of rest tremor, postural instability without other cause (late sign), or muscular rigidity. Usually asymmetric onset, with persistent asymmetry affecting side of onset worst. Reconsider diagnosis if red flag features are present (see BOX).

Non-motor features of idiopathic Parkinson's disease:

- Anosmia
- Depression
- Dementia
- Visual hallucinations
- Dribbling saliva
- Postural instability
- REM behavioural sleep disorder
- Mild urinary frequency & urgency
- L-dopa SEs (see BOX)

Pathophysiology Degeneration of dopaminergic neurons in the substantia nigra pars compacta, associated with Lewy bodies, causes ↓ striatal dopamine levels. Degeneration is thought to be related to mitochondrial DNA dysfunction.[204]

Epidemiology Mean age of onset 65 years old; prevalence is 1.6% in Europe, rising from 0.6% at age 60-64 to 3.5% at age 85-89.

Management ►Get help. Parkinson's disease is progressive and incurable. As the disease progresses from the early, stable stage, through more complex stages with increasing motor and non-motor complications, and finally becomes palliative, priorities and goals will change. A multidisciplinary approach is vital to improve the patient's quality of life throughout the course of the disease. Involve a neurologist, PD nurse, physiotherapist, occupational therapist, social worker, GP and carers.[205]

- **Assess disability** and cognition regularly and objectively (eg UPDRS—Unified Parkinson's Disease Rating Scale). Postural exercises, eg Chinese qigong, may help both.[206]
- **Medical therapy** (see BOX). The key decision is when to start L-dopa, and patients should be involved in this. L-dopa remains the gold standard, but end-of-dose wearing off and dopamine-induced dyskinesias develop over time (~5-10yrs). Start in the elderly (>70yrs) or when PD seriously interferes with life. NICE now recommends referring patients unmedicated to a neurologist. Dopamine agonists and MAO-B inhibitors may be useful to delay starting L-dopa, and in conjunction with L-dopa allow lower doses of L-dopa to be used.
- **Neuropsychiatric complications**, such as depression, dementia and psychosis, are common and may reflect disease progression or drug SEs. Use SSRIs for depression. Distinguish drug-induced psychosis (consider reducing DA-agonist doses) from disease progression (use atypical antipsychotics, eg quetiapine, olanzapine).
- **Respite care** is much valued by carers in advanced disease.
- **Surgery** to interrupt overactive basal ganglia circuits (eg subthalamic nuclei) by surgical lesions or deep brain stimulation are available in specialist centres for those who are dopamine-responsive but remain poorly controlled.

Medical therapy in Parkinson's disease

►No neuroprotective effect has yet been proven for any PD therapy.

Levodopa is used combined with a dopa-decarboxylase inhibitor as **Madopar** (co-beneldopa) or **Sinemet** (co-careldopa). Modified-release preparations have little benefit over normal preparations. Dispersible preparations have rapid bio-availability and may be useful to 'jump-start' patients in the morning, or for rescue during sudden 'off' freezing. Initial side effects of nausea and vomiting can be treated with domperidone. Efficacy reduces with time, requiring larger and more frequent dosing, with worsening side effects. In the long term, dyskinesias, painful dystonias, and response fluctuations such as unpredictable 'off' freezing and pronounced end-of-dose reduced response are common side effects (~50% at 6 yrs). Non-motor side effects include psychosis and visual hallucinations.

Dopamine agonists **Ropinirole** and **pramipexole** are used as monotherapy to delay starting L-dopa in the early stages of PD, and as an adjunct to allow lower doses of L-dopa as the PD symptoms progress. **Rotigotine** transdermal patches are also available as mono- or adjunctive therapy. SEs include drowsiness, nausea, hallucinations and compulsive behaviour. Ergot-derived DA-agonists such as **bromocriptine**, **pergolide** and **cabergoline** may cause cardiac valvulopathy and serosal fibrosis, and are no longer favoured.[207] **Amantadine** is a weak DA-agonist useful for drug-induced dyskinesias in advanced PD.

Apomorphine is a potent DA agonist used subcutaneously as a continuous infusion to even out end-of-dose effects, or as a rescue-pen for sudden 'off' freezing. Injection-site reactions and ulceration can be severe.

Anticholinergics (eg **benzhexol**, **orphenadrine**) help tremor, but cause confusion in the elderly. SEs include dry mouth, dizziness, vision↓, urinary retention, pulse↑, anxiety, confusion, excitement, hallucinations, insomnia, memory↓.

MAO-B inhibitors (eg **rasagiline**, **selegiline**) are an alternative to dopamine agonists in early PD. SEs include postural hypotension and atrial fibrillation.[208]

COMT inhibitors (eg **entacapone**, **tolcapone**) may lessen the 'off' time in those with end-of-dose wearing off. Tolcapone has better efficacy, but may cause severe hepatic complications and requires close monitoring of LFTs.[209]

Future therapies: Non-dopaminergic receptors within the basal ganglia are providing new therapeutic avenues: **istradefylline**, an adenosine A_{2A} receptor blocker, potentiates responses to low-dose L-dopa and reduces 'off' time,[210] and *endocannabinoid receptors* have been successfully targeted in PD mouse models.[211] Animal studies also hint at a possible neuroprotective and neuroregenerative role for glial cell line-derived neurotrophic factor (GDNF), by using **gene therapy** to increase local GDNF levels.[212] **Neural stem cell transplantation** remains unproven.[213]

Parkinson's-plus syndromes

The following are *red flag features* to look for in a patient presenting with parkinsonism that might indicate a (rare) alternative cause to idiopathic PD.

Progressive supranuclear palsy: (PSP, Steele-Richardson-Olszewski syndrome) Early postural instability and falls; vertical gaze palsy; rigidity of trunk > limbs; symmetrical onset; speech and swallowing problems; tremor is unusual.

Multiple system atrophy: (MSA, Shy-Drager syndrome) Early autonomic features (postural ↓BP, bladder dysfunction); cerebellar and pyramidal signs; rigidity>tremor.

Cortico-basal degeneration: (CBD) Akinetic rigidity involving one limb; cortical sensory loss (eg astereognosis); apraxia (in the extreme there may be autonomous interfering activity of affected limb—the 'alien limb' phenomenon).

Lewy body dementia: (p490) Early dementia with fluctuating cognition and visual hallucinations.

Vascular parkinsonism: Parkinsonism is worse in legs than arms; pyramidal signs; prominent gait abnormality.

Cause Discrete plaques of demyelination occur at sites throughout the CNS, caused by a T-cell-mediated immune response. The trigger is unknown. Demyelination heals incompletely causing *relapsing and remitting* symptoms. Prolonged demyelination causes axonal loss, and clinically *progressive* symptoms. ***Prevalence:*** commoner in temperate areas (England ≥42:100,000; SE Scotland 200:100,000;[214] rarer in Black Africa/Asia). Lifetime UK risk 1:1000. Adult migrants take their risk with them; children acquire the risk of where they settle. ***Mean age of onset:*** 30yrs. ♀:♂ ≥3:1.[215]

Early exposure to sunlight/vitamin D seems to be important, and circulating vit D status relates to improved symptoms and prevention of MS.[216] Vitamin D also directly interacts with the major locus determining genetic susceptibility (HLA-DRB1*15).[217]

Presentation Usually monosymptomatic: unilateral optic neuritis (pain on eye movement & rapid ↓ central vision); numbness or tingling in the limbs; leg weakness; brainstem or cerebellar symptoms (eg diplopia, ataxia). Other signs: see BOX. Symptoms may worsen with heat (eg hot bath) or exercise. Rarely polysymptomatic. *Progression:* Early on, relapses (which can be stress induced)[218] may be followed by remission and full recovery. With time, remissions are incomplete, so disability accumulates. Steady progression of disability from the outset also occurs, while some patients experience no progressive disablement at all. ***Poor prognostic signs:*** Older ♂; motor signs at onset; many relapses early on; many MRI lesions; axonal loss.

Diagnosis This is clinical, as no test is pathognomonic. It requires demonstration of *lesions disseminated in time and space*, unattributable to other causes; thus after a first episode further evidence is needed. ►Early diagnosis and treatment reduce relapse rates and disability. A careful history may reveal previous episodes, eg unexplained blindness for a week, and careful examination may reveal deficits other than the presenting problem. *MRI* is sensitive but not specific for plaque detection, but can provide evidence of lesions disseminated in time (see BOX for the *McDonald criteria*). ~90% presenting with an MS-like first episode and consistent MRI lesions go on to develop MS.[219] MRI may also exclude other causes, eg cord compression. *CSF:* oligoclonal bands of IgG on electrophoresis that are not present in serum suggest CNS inflammation. Delayed visual, auditory, and somatosensory ***evoked potentials***. NMO-IgG antibodies are highly specific for Devic's syndrome.[1] MOG and MBP antibodies in those with a single MS-like clinical lesion can predict time to conversion to definite MS.[220]

Treatment Methylprednisolone 1g/24h IV/PO for 3d shortens relapses; use sparingly (max twice/yr, due to steroid SEs—see p371). It does not alter the overall prognosis. *Interferon (IFN-1β & IFN-1α):* ↓ relapses by ~30% in active relapsing-remitting MS;[221] they also ↓lesion accumulation on MRI.[222] Their power to ↓disability is modest, as is their role in primary and secondary progressive MS. SE: flu-like symptoms, depression, abortion. **Glatiramer** is an alternative with similar efficacy. ***Monoclonal antibodies:*** **Natalizumab** (*Tysabri*) acts against the VLA-4 receptor that allows immune cells to adhere to and cross the blood-brain barrier. It ↓ relapses in relapsing-remitting MS by ⅔, and reduces MRI lesions by ~90%.[223] There are few SEs, but antibody-mediated resistance may develop against natalizumab, and a number of cases of progressive multifocal leucoencephalopathy have been reported. **Alemtuzumab** (*Campath*-1H®) acts against T cells, and is a 2nd-line agent in relapsing-remitting MS.

Other drugs: **Azathioprine** may be as effective as interferons for relapsing-remitting MS and is 20× cheaper.[224] **Mitoxantrone** (doxorubicin analogue) helps in secondary progressive MS; safety is an issue. There is no effective ℞ for primary progressive MS.[225]

Palliation: ►Help to live well with disability. ***Spasticity:*** Start all drugs at a low dose, and build up at weekly intervals. **Baclofen** 5-25mg/8h PO; **diazepam** 5mg/8-24h PO (addictive); **dantrolene** 25mg/24h (max 100mg/6h); **tizanidine** 2mg/24h PO, ↑ at intervals of >3d in steps of 1mg/12h (max 9mg/6h). Intrathecal baclofen, phenol nerve block, botulinum toxin, and cannabis are less evidence-based. ***Urgency/frequency:*** If post-micturition residual urine >100mL teach intermittent self-catheterization; if <100mL, try **oxybutynin** 2.5mg/8h or **tolterodine**.

Clinical features (and some personal/social consequences) of MS

Sensory:	• Dysaesthesia[2] • Pins and needles • Vibration sense ↓ • Trigeminal neuralgia	*GI:* Swallowing disorders; constipation. ***Eye:*** Diplopia; hemianopia; optic neuritis;[3] visual phenomena (eg on exercise);[3] bilateral internuclear ophthalmoplegia (p78); pupillary defects.[4]
Motor:	• Spastic weakness • Transverse myelitis[1]	***Cerebellum:*** Trunk and limb ataxia; intention tremor; scanning (ie monotonous) speech; falls.
Sexual/ GU: *(don't be too shy to ask!)*	• Erectile dysfunction • Anorgasmia; urine retention; incontinence	***Cognitive/visuospatial decline*** ►a *big* cause of unemployment, accidents/isolation;[226] amnesia; mood ↑ or ↓ (avoid ECT); ↓executive functioning.

NB: T° ↑, malaise, nausea, vomiting, positional vertigo, seizures, aphasia, meningism, bilateral optic neuritis, CSF leucocytosis and ↑ CSF protein are rare in MS, and may suggest non-MS recurrent demyelinating disease, eg vasculitis or sarcoidosis.[227]

McDonald criteria for diagnosing MS[228]

►MS remains a clinical diagnosis! These criteria may accord too much weight to MRI.[229]

Clinical presentation	**Additional data needed**
2 or more attacks (relapses) with 2 or more objective clinical lesions	None; clinical evidence will do; imaging evidence desirable; must conform to MS
2 or more attacks with 1 objective clinical lesion	Typical disseminated lesions on MRI *or* +ve CSF *and* ≥2 MRI lesions consistent with MS *or* 2nd attack at a new site
1 attack with 2 or more objective clinical lesions	Dissemination in ***time:*** • MRI *or* 2nd clinical attack
1 attack with 1 objective clinical lesion (monosymptomatic presentation)	Dissemination in ***space:*** • MRI *or* +ve CSF if ≥2 MRI lesions consistent with MS • *and* dissemination in time shown by MRI *or* 2nd clinical attack[3]
Insidious neurological progression suggestive of MS (primary progressive MS)	+ve CSF *and* dissemination in space, ie: • MRI evidence of ≥9 T2 brain lesions; *or* 2 or more cord lesions; *or* 4-8 brain and 1 cord lesion; *or* +ve visual evoked potential (VEP) with 4-8 MRI lesions; *or* +ve VEP + <4 brain lesions + 1 cord lesion *and* dissemination in time seen on MRI; *or* continued progression for ≥1yr

Attacks must last >1h, eg weakness etc (see above), with >30d between attacks.

MRI abnormality: 3 out of 4:
- Gadolinium-enhancing *or* ≥9 T2 hyperintense lesions if no Gd-enhancing lesion
- 1 or more infratentorial lesions • 1 or more juxtacortical lesions
- ≥3 periventricular lesions (1 spinal cord lesion = 1 brain lesion)

CSF: Oligoclonal IgG bands in CSF (and not serum) or ↑IgG index.

Evoked potentials: (EP) This counts if delayed but well-preserved waveform.

What provides MRI evidence of dissemination in time? A Gd-enhancing lesion demonstrated in a scan done at least 3 months following onset of clinical attack at a site different from attack, *or* if no Gd-enhancing lesions at a 3-month scan, follow-up scan after another 3 months showing Gd-lesion or new T2 lesion.[230]

"I'm not worried about losing my life; but I am worried about losing my demeanour, my mind, my interaction with life..." **J Hinkleton**

1 Loss of motor, sensory, autonomic, reflex, and sphincter function below the level of a lesion indicates transverse myelitis. **Devic's syndrome** (neuromyelitis optica—NMO) is an MS variant with transverse myelitis and optic atrophy, distinguishable from MS by the presence of NMO-IgG antibodies (p712).

2 In **Lhermitte's sign,** neck flexion causes 'electric shocks' in trunk/limbs. Also +ve in cervical spondylosis, cord tumours & subacute combined degeneration of the cord (B_{12}↓).

3 Optic neuritis symptoms: • Acuity↓; • **Uhthoff's phenomenon** (vision worsens on exercise, eating a hot meal, or in hot baths); • Phosphenes (flashes) on eye movement; • The **Pulfrich effect** (latencies between the eyes are unequal, causing disorientation, eg in moving traffic as straight trajectories seem curved).

4 Efferent, afferent or relative afferent pupillary defect (see p79). An **Argyle Robertson**-type pupil is rarer (p79; ΔΔ: syphilis, DM, MS or sarcoidosis—lesion in or near the **Edinger-Westphal** nucleus).

Signs • ↑*ICP* (see p840): Headache worse on waking, lying down, bending forward, or with coughing (p460); vomiting; papilloedema (only in 50% of tumours); ↓GCS.
• *Seizures:* Seen in ≤50%. Exclude SOL in all adult-onset seizures, especially if focal, or with a localizing aura or post-ictal weakness (Todd's palsy, p726).
• *Evolving focal neurology:* See BOX for localizing signs. ↑ICP causes *false localizing signs:* VIth nerve palsy is commonest (p76) due to its long intracranial course.
• *Subtle personality change:* Irritability, lack of application to tasks, lack of initiative, socially inappropriate behaviour.

Causes Tumour (primary or metastatic, below), aneurysm, abscess (25% multiple); chronic subdural haematoma, granuloma (p187, eg tuberculoma), cyst (eg cysticercosis). *Tumours:* 30% are metastatic (eg breast, lung, melanoma). *Primaries:* astrocytoma, glioblastoma multiforme (opinion remains divided over association with mobile phone use),[231] [232] oligodendroglioma, ependymoma. Also meningioma (♀:♂≈2:1), primary CNS lymphoma (eg as non-infectious manifestation of HIV), and cerebellar haemangioblastoma.

Differential diagnosis Stroke, head injury, venous sinus thrombosis, vasculitis (p558; eg SLE, syphilis, PAN, giant cell arteritis), MS, encephalitis, post-ictal (Todd's palsy, p726), metabolic, or U&E disturbance. Also colloid cyst of the 3rd ventricle and idiopathic intracranial hypertension (see BELOW).

Tests CT ± MRI (good for posterior fossa masses). Consider biopsy. Avoid LP before imaging (risks *coning*, ie cerebellar tonsils herniate through the foramen magnum).

Tumour management *Benign:* Removal if possible but some may be inaccessible. *Malignant:* **Excision** of gliomas is hard as resection margins are rarely clear, but surgery does give a tissue diagnosis, it debulks pre-radiotherapy, and makes a cavity for inserting **carmustine wafers**[233] (may cause serious cerebral oedema).[234] If a tumour is inaccessible but causing hydrocephalus, a **ventriculo-peritoneal shunt** can help. **Chemo-radiotherapy** is used post-op for gliomas or metastases, and as sole therapy if surgery is impossible. Oligodendroglioma with 1p/19q deletions is especially sensitive. In glioblastoma, **temozolomide** (a new alkylating agent) ↑survival[235] (benefit is mainly if tumours have methylated methylguanine methyltransferase gene promoters and are thus unable to repair chemotherapy-induced DNA damage).[236] **Seizure prophylaxis** (eg phenytoin) is important, but often fails. **Treat headache** (eg **codeine** 60mg/4h PO). *Cerebral oedema:* **dexamethasone** 4mg/8h PO; **mannitol** if ↑ICP acutely (p841). Plan meticulous palliative treatment (p532).

Prognosis Poor but improving (<50% survival at 5yrs) for CNS primaries; 40% 20yr survival for cerebellar haemangioblastoma; benign tumours are curable by excision.

Third ventricle colloid cysts These congenital cysts declare themselves in adult life with amnesia, headache (often positional), obtundation (blunted consciousness), incontinence, dim vision, bilateral paraesthesiae, weak legs, and drop attacks. ℞: Excision or ventriculo-peritoneal shunting.

Idiopathic intracranial hypertension

AKA *pseudotumor cerebri.* Think of this in those presenting as if with a mass (headache, ↑ICP and papilloedema)—*when none is found.* Typical patients are obese women with blurred vision ± diplopia, VIth nerve palsy, and an enlarged blind spot, if papilloedema is present (it usually is). Consciousness and cognition are preserved.

Cause: Often unknown, or secondary to venous sinus thrombosis, or drugs, eg tetracycline, minocycline, nitrofurantoin, vitamin A, isotretinoin, danazol, and somatropin.

℞: Weight loss, acetazolamide, loop diuretics, and prednisolone (start at ~40mg/24h PO; more SE than diuretics) *may* reverse papilloedema.[237] Consider optic nerve sheath fenestration or lumbar-peritoneal shunt if drugs fail and visual loss worsens.[238]

Prognosis: Often self-limiting. Permanent significant visual loss in 10% (ie not so benign). CSF shunting or optic nerve sheath fenestration can help vision.[239]

Localizing features

(see p448 for cerebral and limbic anatomy)

►Ask first *where* the mass is then *what it is.* Localizing features of SOLs can be thought of as dividing into *negative symptoms* (deficits caused by direct pressure or tumour invasion), and *positive symptoms* (due to localized seizure activity caused by irritation of the brain parenchyma). Both depend on the function of the area of the brain affected. Negative symptoms are listed below. See p495 for positive (seizure) symptoms. Frontal lobe, midline, and non-dominant temporal lobe masses present late.

Temporal lobe • Dysphasia (p80); • Contralateral homonymous hemianopia (or upper quadrantanopia if only Meyer's loop affected); • Amnesia; • Many odd or seemingly inexplicable phenomena, p495.

Frontal lobe • Hemiparesis; • Personality change (indecent, indolent, indiscreet, facetious, tendency to pun; see also orbitofrontal syndrome below); • Release phenomena such as the grasp reflex (fingers drawn across palm are grasped), significant only if unilateral; • Broca's dysphasia (p80), or more subtle difficulty with initiating and planning speech with intact repetition and no anomia—but loss of coherence; • Unilateral anosmia (loss of smell); • General lack of drive or initiative; • Concrete thinking; • Perseveration (unable to switch from one line of thinking to another); • Executive dysfunction (unable to plan tasks); • ↓verbal fluency, eg unable to list words beginning with the letter 'A' or 'F' (normal is ~15 words in 1 min). 240

Orbitofrontal[1] *syndrome* (**fig 1**, p448): Lack of empathy; over-eating; disinhibition; impulsive behaviour; ↓social skills; over-familiar; unconscious imitation of postures (eg when you put your feet on the desk, or sit on the floor); 'utilization behaviour' (whatever is provided is used, eg hand the patient spectacles, and he puts them on, hand him another pair, and this goes on his nose too, ditto for a 3rd pair).

Parietal lobe • Hemisensory loss; • ↓2-point discrimination; • Astereognosis (unable to recognize an object by touch alone); • Sensory inattention; • Dysphasia (p80); • Gerstmann's syndrome (p714).

Occipital lobe • Contralateral visual field defects; • Palinopsia;[2] • Polyopia (seeing multiple images).

Cerebellum Remember DASHING: **d**ysdiadochokinesis (impaired *rapidly alternating* movements, p80) & **d**ysmetria (past-pointing); **a**taxia (limb/truncal);[3] **s**lurred speech (dysarthria); **h**ypotonia; **i**ntention tremor; **n**ystagmus; **g**ait abnormality.

Cerebellopontine angle (eg acoustic neuroma/vestibular Schwannoma; p468) Causes ipsilateral deafness, nystagmus, ↓corneal reflex, facial weakness (rare), ipsilateral cerebellar signs (above), papilloedema, VIth nerve palsy (p77).

Corpus callosum (a rare site for lesions) Severe rapid intellectual deterioration with focal signs of adjacent lobes and signs of loss of communication between lobes (eg left hand unable to carry out verbal commands).

Midbrain (eg pineal tumours or midbrain infarction) Failure of up or down gaze; light/near dissociated pupil responses (p79), with convergence globe-retracting nystagmus 241 from co-contraction of opposing horizontal muscles, on attempted up-gaze. 242 Elicited by looking at a down-moving target. 243 video link

1 The orbitofrontal cortex (**fig 1**, p448) and right amygdala appreciate beauty (and sexual allure). The poets were nearly right that ***Beauty is in the eye of the beholder***: it is ~1cm *above* the orbit.

2 Palinopsia: persisting or recurring images, once the stimulus has left the field of view, from the Greek word *palin* meaning 'again'.

3 If truncal ataxia is worse on eye closure, blame the dorsal columns, not the cerebellum.

Bell's palsy (idiopathic facial nerve palsy)

Bell's palsy is partly a diagnosis of exclusion, but features distinguishing it from other causes of facial palsy (BOX) are: abrupt onset (typically overnight or after a nap) with complete unilateral facial weakness at 24 to 72h; ipsilateral numbness or pain around the ear; ↓taste (ageusia); hypersensitivity to sounds (ie hyperacusis from stapedius palsy).[247] Other pathologies may be indicated by bilateral symptoms,[1] UMN signs, other cranial neuropathies (eg V or XII, but also seen in 8% of idiopathic cases),[248] limb weakness, and rashes.

Causes of VIIth nerve palsy
Bell's palsy (75% of cases)
Ramsay Hunt syn. (BOX)
Lyme disease (*Borrelia* sp.)
Meningitis (eg fungal)
TB; viruses (HIV, polio)
Mycoplasma (rare)
Brainstem lesions
Stroke, tumour, MS
Cerebello-pontine angle
Acoustic neuroma (p466)
Meningioma
Systemic disease
Diabetes mellitus
Sarcoidosis[244]
Guillain-Barré syndrome (usually bilateral palsy)
ENT and other causes
Orofacial granulomatosis
Parotid tumours
Cholesteatoma
Otitis media
Trauma to skull base
Diving (barotrauma+temporal bone pneumocoele)[245]
Intracranial hypotension[246]

Incidence 15–40/100,000/yr (~1 patient/2yrs/GP).[249] ♂≈♀. Risk ↑ in pregnancy (×3) and in diabetes (×5).

Other symptoms of VIIth palsy (from any cause)
• Unilateral sagging of the mouth, which is drawn upwards on the normal side on smiling, producing a grimace; • drooling of saliva; • food trapped between gum and cheek; • speech difficulty; • failure of eye closure may cause a watery or dry eye, ectropion (sagging and turning-out of the lower lid), injury from foreign bodies, or conjunctivitis.

Signs Ask the patient to wrinkle up the forehead and close the eyes forcefully (bilaterally innervated and thus spared in a LMN lesion). Whistling/blowing out the cheeks tests buccinator (*buccina* is Latin for trumpet).

Investigations Explore other diagnoses in atypical presentations (although Lyme disease may be indistinguishable clinically):[250] ***MRI*** may show space-occupying lesions, stroke or MS; ***CSF*** may suggest infection. ***Serology:*** ↑ *Borrelia* antibodies in Lyme disease, or ↑VZV antibodies in Ramsay Hunt syndrome (BOX).[251] ***Nerve conduction studies*** at 2 weeks predict delayed recovery by showing axonal degeneration but do not influence treatment (and is therefore not routinely done).

Prognosis ***Incomplete paralysis*** without axonal degeneration usually recovers completely within a few weeks. Of those with ***complete paralysis*** ~80% make a full spontaneous recovery, but ~15% have axonal degeneration (~50% in pregnancy) in which case recovery is delayed, starting after ~3 months, and may be complicated by aberrant reconnections: ***synkinesis***, eg eye blinking causes synchronous upturning of the mouth; misconnection of parasympathetic fibres (red in **fig 1**) can produce ***crocodile tears*** (gusto-lacrimal reflex) when eating stimulates unilateral lacrimation, not salivation (intra-lacrimal gland botulinum toxin may help).[252]

Management If given within 72hrs of onset, **prednisolone** (eg 60mg/d PO for 5 days, tailing by 10mg/d) improved recovery time in two large recent RCTs, (with 95% making a full recovery; NNT=8),[253] [254] supposedly by reducing axonal oedema and thus damage. Neither study found benefit from antivirals (eg aciclovir), and although some 'Bell's cases' are thought to be associated with HSV-1, no-one has shown actively replicating virus (which may be why results are equivocal).[255] There is little data to guide treatment if presenting after 72hrs of onset, although corticosteroids are widely used, and no advice on the use of steroids is universally agreed in pregnancy.[256] **Protect the eye:** • dark glasses and artificial tears (eg hypromellose) if evidence of drying; • encourage regular eyelid closure by pulling down the lid by hand; • use tape to close the eyes at night. **Surgery:** if the ectropion is severe, lateral tarsorrhaphy (partial lid-to-lid suturing) can help; if no recovery in 1yr, plastic surgery to help lid closure and to straighten the drooping face can be tried. Botulinum toxin can augment facial symmetry,[257] and hence self-esteem (beauty *is* symmetry according to Greek ideals—and *Vogue*).[258] There is no evidence that physiotherapy or electrical stimulation therapy improve recovery.[259]

1 Common causes for bilateral facial palsy include Lyme disease, Guillain-Barré syndrome, leukaemia, sarcoidosis, EBV, and trauma. Myasthenia gravis may also mimic a bilateral facial nerve palsy.

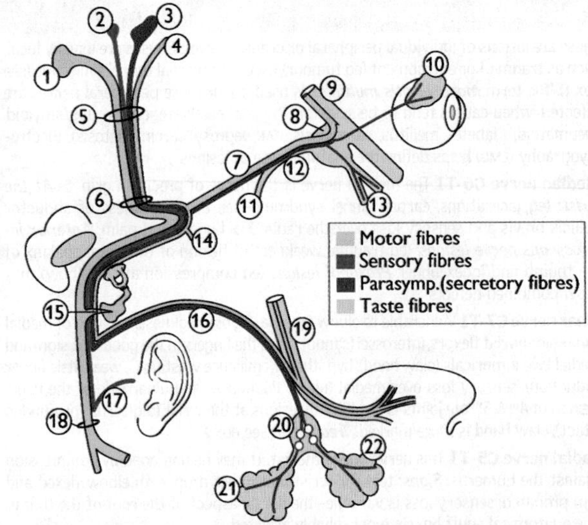

1 Facial nerve (VIIth) nucleus, deep in the reticular formation of lower pons
2 Spinal nucleus of V
3 Superior salivary nucleus
4 Solitary tract
5 Porus acusticus internus
6 Meatal foramen
7 Large petrosal nerve
8 Sphenopalatine ganglion
9 Superior maxillary nerve
10 Lacrimal gland
11 Large deep petrosal nerve
12 Vidian nerve
13 Nose & palate gland nerves
14 Small petrosal nerve at geniculate ganglion[260]
15 Stapedial nerve
16 Chorda tympani
17 Auricular branch
18 Stylomastoid foramen
19 Lingual nerve—visceral motor^VII & taste^VII & general sensory to tongue (V^3)[261]
20 Submandibular ganglion
21 Submandibular gland
22 Sublingual gland

Fig 1. Facial nerve branches. The motor part supplies moves the muscles of the face, scalp, and ears—also buccinator (puffs out the cheeks), platysma, stapedius, and the posterior belly of the digastric. It also contains the sympathetic motor fibres (vasodilator) of the submaxillary and sublingual glands (via the chorda tympani nerve). The sensory part contains the fibres of taste for the anterior ⅔ of the tongue and a few somatic sensory fibres from the middle ear region.

After Baylor College of Medicine www.bcm.edu/oto/studs/face.html

Ramsay Hunt syndrome

First described by the American neurologist James Ramsay Hunt in 1907,[262] the syndrome occurs when latent varicella zoster virus (see also p400) reactivates within the geniculate ganglion of the VIIth cranial nerve, causing ***symptoms*** of a painful vesicular rash in the auditory canal (*herpes zoster oticus*), ± ear-drum, pinna, tongue or hard palate. There is associated ipsilateral facial weakness, loss of taste, dry mouth or eyes, vertigo, tinnitus or deafness. However, the rash may be subtle or absent (*herpes sine herpete*). It is rare: ***incidence*** is ~5/100,000 and it is more common in those > 60yrs old. The ***diagnosis*** is clinical, as antiviral treatment is thought to be most effective within the first 72hrs, while the virus is replicating. ***Treatment*** is with antivirals (eg **aciclovir** 800mg PO five times daily for 5-7d; if eGFR low, see p834) and corticosteroids (eg **prednisolone**, as for Bell's palsy, p504), supported by a few small retrospective analyses,[263] although there are no definitive RCTs. ***Prognosis:*** treated within 72hrs, rates up to 75% full recovery are reported; otherwise approximately ⅓ make a good recovery, ⅓ a reasonable recovery, and ⅓ a poor recovery.

These are lesions of individual peripheral or cranial nerves. Causes are usually local, such as trauma,[1] or entrapment (eg tumour), except for carpal tunnel syndrome (see BOX 1). The term ***mononeuritis multiplex*** is used if 2 or more peripheral nerves are affected, when causes tend to be systemic ('**WARDS PLC**'): **W**egener's, **A**IDS/amyloid, **r**heumatoid, **d**iabetes mellitus, **s**arcoidosis, **P**AN, **l**eprosy, **c**arcinomatosis). Electromyography (EMG) helps define the anatomic site of lesions.

Median nerve C6–T1 The median nerve is the nerve of precision grip. 264 ***At the wrist:*** (eg lacerations, carpal tunnel syndrome—see BOX) weakness of abductor pollicis brevis and sensory loss over the radial 3½ fingers and palm. ***Anterior interosseous nerve lesions:*** (eg trauma) weakness of flexion of the distal phalanx of the thumb and index finger. ***Proximal lesions*** (eg compression at the elbow) may show combined defects.

Ulnar nerve C7–T1 Vulnerable to elbow trauma. ***Signs:*** weakness/wasting of medial (ulnar side) wrist flexors, interossei (cannot cross the fingers in the good luck sign) and medial two lumbricals (claw hand); hypothenar eminence wasting (∴ weak little finger abduction); sensory loss over medial (ulnar) 1½ fingers and ulnar side of the hand. Flexion of 4th & 5th DIP joints is weak. With lesions at the wrist (digitorum profundus intact), claw hand is more marked. ***Treatment:*** see BOX 2.

Radial nerve C5–T1 This nerve opens the fist. It may be damaged by compression against the humerus. ***Signs:*** test for wrist and finger drop with elbow flexed and arm pronated; sensory loss is variable—the dorsal aspect of the root of the thumb (the anatomical snuff box) is most reliably affected.

Brachial plexus Pain/paraesthesiae and weakness in the affected arm in a variable distribution. *Causes:* trauma, radiotherapy (eg for breast carcinoma), prolonged wearing of a heavy rucksack, cervical rib, neuralgic amyotrophy,[2] thoracic outlet compression (also affects vasculature).

Phrenic nerve C3–5 C3, 4, 5 keeps the diaphragm alive Consider phrenic nerve palsy if orthopnoea with raised hemidiaphragm on CXR. ***Causes:*** Lung cancer, myeloma, thymoma, cervical spondylosis/trauma, thoracic surgery, C3-5 zoster, HIV, Lyme disease, TB, paraneoplastic syndromes, muscular dystrophy, big left atrium, phrenic nucleus lesion (eg MS, rare).

Lateral cutaneous nerve of the thigh L2–L3 *Meralgia paraesthetica* is anterolateral burning thigh pain from entrapment under the inguinal ligament.

Sciatic nerve L4–S3 Damaged by pelvic tumours or fractures to pelvis or femur. Lesions affect the hamstrings and all muscles below the knee (foot drop), with loss of sensation below the knee laterally.

Common peroneal nerve L4–S1 Originates from sciatic nerve just above knee. Often damaged as it winds round the fibular head (trauma, sitting cross-legged). ***Signs:*** foot drop, weak ankle dorsiflexion/eversion, and sensory loss over dorsum of foot.

Tibial nerve L4–S3 Originates from the sciatic nerve just above the knee. Lesions lead to an inability to stand on tiptoe (plantarflexion), invert the foot, or flex the toes, with sensory loss over the sole.

1 **Hereditary neuropathy with liability to pressure palsies** is an autosomal dominant hereditary neuropathy presenting as recurrent isolated or multiple neuropathies. Onset is during teenage years.
2 **Neuralgic amyotrophy** (Parsonage-Turner syndrome) is a poorly understood inflammatory condition affecting the brachial plexus on one side only. Sudden onset severe pain, followed over hours by profound weakness, resolving completely over several days. It may rarely involve the phrenic or lower cranial nerves.

Carpal tunnel syndrome: the commonest mononeuropathy

The median nerve and 9 tendons compete for space within the wrist. Compression is common, especially in women who have narrower wrists but similar-sized tendons to men. For similar reasons, the tibial nerve may be compressed: the tarsal tunnel syndrome, causing unilateral burning sole pain, eg on walking or standing.

The patient: Aching pain in the hand and arm (especially at night), and paraesthesiae in thumb, index, and middle fingers, all relieved by dangling the hand over the edge of the bed and shaking it (remember 'wake and shake'). There may be sensory loss and weakness of abductor pollicis brevis ± wasting of the thenar eminence. Light touch, 2-point discrimination, and sweating may be impaired.

Associations: Pregnancy, diabetes mellitus, rheumatoid, hypothyroidism, renal dialysis, trauma, acromegaly.[265]

Tests: Neurophysiology helps by confirming the lesion's site and severity (and likelihood of improvement after surgery). Maximal wrist flexion for 1 min (*Phalen's test*) may elicit symptoms (unreliable!). Tapping over the nerve at the wrist induces tingling (*Tinel's test*; also rather non-specific).

Treatment: Splinting, local steroid injection (*OHCS* p710) ± decompression surgery; many alternative therapies are tried: meta-analyses are doubtful.[1]

Managing ulnar mononeuropathies from entrapments

The ulnar nerve asks for trouble in at least 5 places at the elbow, starting proximally at the *arcade of Struthers* (a musculofascial band ~8cm proximal to the medial epicondyle), and ending distally where it exits the flexor carpi ulnaris muscle in the forearm.[266] Most often, compression occurs at the *epicondylar groove* or at the point where the nerve passes between the 2 heads of flexor carpi ulnaris (true *cubital tunnel syndrome*). Trauma can easily damage the nerve against its bony confines (the medial condyle of the humerus—the 'funny bone'). Normally, stretch and compression forces on the ulnar nerve at the elbow are moderated by its ability to glide in its groove. When normal excursion is restricted, irritation ensues. This may cause a vicious cycle of perineural scarring, consequent loss of excursion, and progressive symptoms—without antecedent trauma. Compressive ulnar neuropathies at the wrist (*Guyon's canal*—between the pisiform and hamate bones) are less common, but they can also result in disability.

Treatment centres on rest and avoiding pressure on the nerve, but if symptoms continue, night-time soft elbow splinting (to prevent flexion to >60°)[267] is warranted, eg for 6 months.[268] A splint for the hand may help prevent permanent clawing of the fingers. For chronic neuropathy associated with weakness, or if splinting fails, a variety of *surgical procedures* have been tried. For moderately severe neuropathies, decompressions *in situ* may help, but often fail. Medial *epicondylectomies* are effective in ≲50% (but many will recur). Subcutaneous *nerve re-routing* (transposition) may be tried. Intramuscular and submuscular transpositions are more complicated, but the latter may be preferable.[269]

1 *Cochrane meta-analysis of 21 carpal tunnel trials:* 7 (but not 2) weeks' ultrasound can help. Compared to placebo, diuretics & NSAIDs gave no benefit. Vit B_6 did not help (N = 50). Those adopting the namaste (prayer) posture in yoga may obviate need for surgery: the forced wrist extension helps (N = 53). Trials of ergonomic keyboards give equivocal results for pain and function. Trials of magnet therapy, laser acupuncture, and exercise showed no benefit. Chiropractic care can increase distress.

Polyneuropathies

Polyneuropathies are generalized disorders of peripheral or cranial nerves, whose distribution is usually symmetrical and widespread, often with distal weakness and sensory loss ('glove & stocking'). They are classified by time course (*acute or chronic*), by affected functions (*motor, sensory, autonomic, or mixed*), or by underlying pathology (*demyelination, axonal degeneration, + both*). For example, Guillain-Barré syndrome (p716) is an acute, predominantly motor, demyelinating neuropathy, whereas chronic alcohol abuse leads to a chronic, initially sensory then mixed, axonal neuropathy.

Mostly motor	**Mostly sensory**
Guillain-Barré syndrome (p716)	Diabetes mellitus
Lead poisoning	Renal failure
Charcot-Marie-Tooth syndrome[1]	Leprosy

Diagnosis The history is vital: be clear about the time course, the precise nature of the symptoms, and any preceding or associated events (eg D&V before Guillain-Barré syndrome; weight↓ in cancer; arthralgia from a connective tissue disease). Ask about travel, alcohol and drug use, sexual infections, and family history. If there is palpable nerve thickening think of leprosy or Charcot-Marie-Tooth. Examine other systems for clues to the cause, eg alcoholic liver disease.

Sensory neuropathy: Numbness, pins & needles, 'feels funny' or burning sensations, affecting the extremities first ('glove & stocking' distribution—map out each modality, p450). There may be difficulty handling small objects such as buttons. Signs of trauma (eg finger burns) or joint deformation may indicate sensory loss. Diabetic and alcoholic neuropathies are typically painful.

Motor neuropathy: Often progressive (may be rapid) weakness or clumsiness of the hands; difficulty walking (falls, stumbling); respiratory difficulty. Signs are of LMN lesion: wasting and weakness most marked in the distal muscles of hands and feet (foot or wrist drop). Reflexes are reduced or absent. Involvement of the respiratory muscles may be shown by a falling vital capacity.

Cranial nerves: Swallowing/speaking difficulty; diplopia.

Autonomic neuropathy: See BOX.

Tests FBC, ESR, glucose, U&Es, LFTs, TSH, B_{12}, electrophoresis, ANA & ANCA (p555), CXR, urinalysis, and consider an LP ± specific genetic tests for inherited neuropathies (eg for PMP22 in Charcot-Marie-Tooth),[270] lead levels, and antiganglioside antibodies. Nerve conduction studies help distinguish demyelinating from axonal neuropathies.

Management Treat the cause. Involve **physio & OT** (p449). **Foot care** and **shoe choice** are important in sensory neuropathies to minimize trauma. Splinting of joints can help prevent contractures in prolonged paralysis. In Guillain-Barré and CIDP[2] **IV immunoglobulin** helps.[271] For vasculitic causes, **steroids** or immunosuppressants may help. Treat neuropathic pain with **amitriptyline** or **nortriptyline** (10–25mg at night; may not work in HIV neuropathy).[272] If this fails, try **gabapentin**[3] or **pregabalin**.[273]

Causes of polyneuropathy

Metabolic
Diabetes mellitus, Renal failure, Hypothyroidism, Hypoglycaemia, Mitochondrial disorders

Vasculitides (p558)
Polyarteritis nodosa, Rheumatoid arthritis, Wegener's granulomatosis

Malignancy
Paraneoplastic syndromes
Polycythaemia rubra vera

Inflammatory
Guillain-Barré syndrome
Sarcoidosis; CIDP[2]

Infections
Leprosy, HIV, syphilis
Lyme disease (p430),

Nutritional
↓ vit B_1, B_{12}, (eg EtOH abuse)
↓ vit E, folate
↑ vit B_6 (if >100mg/d)

Inherited syndromes
Charcot-Marie-Tooth (p710)
Refsum's syndrome (p724)
Porphyria (p706)
Leucodystrophy

Toxins Lead, arsenic

Drugs Vincristine
Alcohol, Cisplatin
Isoniazid, Nitrofurantoin
Phenytoin, Metronidazole

Others
Paraproteinaemias
Amyloidosis (p364)

1 The *presentation* of Charcot-Marie-Tooth is typically motor, although the sensory deficit is present on examination, because the sensory loss is so gradual & long-standing that it feels 'normal' to the patient.
2 Chronic inflammatory demyelinating polyradiculoneuropathy (CIDP) is an autoimmune demyelinating disease of peripheral nerves causing distal onset of weakness & sensory loss in limbs, with peripheral nerve enlargement and ↑ CSF protein.
3 300mg on day 1, 300mg/12h on day 2, 300mg/8h on day 3, then ↑ according to response in steps of 100mg/8h; max 600mg/8h if eGFR >80. SE: diarrhoea, dry mouth, dyspepsia, vomiting, oedema, dizziness.

Autonomic neuropathy

Sympathetic and Parasympathetic neuropathies may be isolated or part of a generalized sensorimotor peripheral neuropathy.

Causes DM, amyloid, Guillain-Barré syndrome, HIV, paraneoplastic syndromes (eg LEMS, p516), leprosy, SLE,[274] toxic, genetic.

Signs Postural hypotension[s] (faints on standing, eating, or hot bath), erectile dysfunction[p]/ejaculatory failure[s] (remember 'point & shoot'), sweating↓[s], constipation/nocturnal diarrhoea, urine retention[p], Horner's[s] (p716), Holmes–Adie pupil[p] (p79).[275]

Autonomic function tests • *Postural drop* of ≥20/10mmHg is abnormal. ℞: p68.
- *ECG:* A variation of <10bpm with respiration is abnormal.
- *Cystometry:* bladder pressure studies.
- *Pupils:* Instil 0.1% epinephrine (dilates if post-ganglionic sympathetic denervation, not if normal); 2.5% cocaine (dilates if normal; not if sympathetic denervation); 2.5% methacholine (constricts if parasympathetic lesion). These are rarely used.
- *Antibodies:* anti-HU & anti-nicotinic acetylcholine receptor antibodies may be +ve.

Primary autonomic failure Occurs alone, as part of multisystem atrophy (MSA, p498), or with Parkinson's disease. Typically a middle-aged or elderly man. Insidious onset (symptoms as above).

Motor neuron disease (MND)

MND is a cluster of major degenerative diseases characterized by selective loss of neurons in motor cortex, cranial nerve nuclei, and anterior horn cells. Upper and lower motor neurons are affected but there is *no* sensory loss or sphincter disturbance, thus distinguishing MND from MS and polyneuropathies. MND never affects eye movements, distinguishing it from myasthenia (p516). The cause is unknown, but as MND, like polio, affects anterior horn cells, viruses are suggested. ≤10% of MND is familial, of whom ~20% show Cu/Zn superoxide dismutase mutations (SOD1).

There are 4 clinical patterns: **1** *Amyotrophic lateral sclerosis* (ALS, the archetypal MND—50%) Loss of motor neurons in both motor cortex and the anterior horn of spinal cord, thus weakness with UMN signs *and* LMN wasting (p451). Worse prognosis if bulbar onset, ↑age or ↓FVC; risk ↑ in Gulf War veterans. **2** *Progressive bulbar palsy* (10%) Only affects cranial nerves IX–XII. Symptoms as BOX 1. Often progresses to ALS. **3** *Progressive muscular atrophy* (10%) Anterior horn cell lesion only, thus no UMN signs. Affects distal muscle groups before proximal. Better prognosis than ALS. **4** *Primary lateral sclerosis* Loss of Betz cells in motor cortex, thus mainly UMN signs, with marked spastic leg weakness and pseudobulbar palsy. No cognitive decline.

►Think of MND in those >40yrs with stumbling spastic gait, foot-drop ± proximal myopathy, weak grip (door-handles are hard) and shoulder abduction (hair-washing is hard), or aspiration pneumonia. Look for UMN signs: spasticity, brisk reflexes, ↑plantars; and LMN signs: wasting, fasciculation of tongue, abdomen, back, thigh. Is speech or swallowing affected? Fasciculations are not enough to diagnose an LMN lesion: look for weakness too. Fronto-temporal dementia is seen in 10–35%.

Diagnostic criteria: See BOX 2. There is no diagnostic test. Brain/cord MRI helps exclude structural causes, LP helps exclude inflammatory ones, and neurophysiology can detect subclinical denervation and help exclude mimicking motor neuropathies.[1]

Prevalence 6/100,000. ♂:♀≈3:2. Median UK age at onset: 60yrs. Often fatal in 2–4yrs.

Treatment Due to MND's implacable course, its rarity, and its frightening nature, a multidisciplinary approach is best:[276] neurologist, palliative nurse,[277] hospice, physio, OT, speech therapist, dietician, social services—all orchestrated by the GP. Death by choking is rare, so warmly reassure that a dignified end is the rule. MNDassociation.org tel.UK 08457 626262

Antiglutamatergic drugs: **Riluzole** (see BOX 3) prolongs life by ~3 months; it is costly. *Cautions:* LFTs↑. Do regular LFTs every month for 3 months. SE: vomiting, weakness, pulse↑, somnolence, headache, dizziness, vertigo, pain, LFTs↑.

Drooling: **Propantheline** 15–30mg/8h PO; **amitriptyline** 25–50mg/8h PO.

Dysphagia: Blend food; would he or she like a nasogastric tube, or percutaneous catheter gastrostomy?—or would this prolong death? *Spasticity:* See MS (p500).

Joint pains and distress: Analgesic ladder—NSAIDs etc, then opioids (p534).

Respiratory failure (± aspiration pneumonia and sleep apnoea): Non-invasive ventilation at home in selected patients may give valuable palliation.

Ethical problems: beyond autonomy Patients with MND may be ventilated, for example, and then decide that they want this intervention withdrawn.[278] In some patients, this is likely to be fatal, making these decisions difficult for everyone. Ethicists tend to speak in black-and-white prose: "Do whatever promotes autonomy", and this is the *raison d'être* of assisted-suicide organizations such as Dignitas (increasingly popular, worldwide, even where illegal). But sometimes nature contrives something more ambiguous and poetic, in which rationality and rage,[279] uncertainty and the forked emotions of hope and despair produce a heady internal world which the ethicist can never quite catch or tame. If this internal world is one of perpetual change and oscillating will, ideas of autonomy become incoherent. Rather than aiming to apply Kantian universal rules (p15), our role may be more to offer a well-placed hug to signal metaphysical complicity, and to stand beside our patients, come what may.

1 If no UMN signs and distal arm muscles are affected in the distribution of individual nerves, suspect **multifocal motor neuropathy with conduction block** (diagnose on nerve conduction studies; ℞: IV Ig). Gynaecomastia, atrophic testes ± infertility suggests **Kennedy syndrome** (bulbospinal muscular atrophy).

Bulbar and pseudobulbar palsy

Bulbar palsy is a term most commonly used for diseases of the nuclei of cranial nerves IX–XII in the medulla. ***Signs*** are of a *LMN lesion* of the tongue and muscles of talking and swallowing: flaccid, fasciculating tongue (p76, like a sack of worms); jaw jerk is normal or absent, speech is quiet, hoarse, or nasal. ***Causes:*** MND, Guillain–Barré, polio, myasthenia gravis, syringobulbia (p520), brainstem tumours, central pontine myelinolysis (p686).

Corticobulbar (pseudobulbar) palsy *UMN lesion* of muscles of swallowing and talking due to bilateral lesions above the mid-pons, eg corticobulbar tracts (MS, MND, stroke, central pontine myelinolysis). It is commoner than bulbar palsy. ***Signs:*** Slow tongue movements, with slow deliberate speech; ↑jaw jerk; ↑pharangeal and palatal reflexes; weeping unprovoked by sorrow or mood-incongruent giggling (emotional incontinence *without* mood change is also seen in MS, dementia and head injury).[280]

Revised El Escorial diagnostic criteria for ALS

Definite Lower + upper motor neuron signs in 3 regions.
Probable Lower + upper motor neuron signs in 2 regions.
Probably with lab support Lower + upper motor neuron signs in 1 region, or upper motor neuron signs in ≥1 region + EMG shows acute denervation in ≥2 limbs.
Possible Lower + upper motor neuron signs in one region.
Suspected Upper *or* lower motor neuron signs only—in 1 or more regions.

Following in the footprints of free radicals

Post-mortem studies show that changes to proteins and DNA that are signs or 'footprints' of free-radical damage are more pronounced in MND brains than in controls.[281] Also, cultured fibroblasts from MND brains show high sensitivity to oxidative insults. But these findings don't explain two key MND phenomena:

Why is there a predilection for motor neurons? One answer may be the sheer length and complex cytoarchitecture of motor cells, with their 1 metre axons and high levels of neurofilament proteins, and low levels of Ca^{2+}-buffering proteins (thought to be protective). We note that motor cells with the shortest axons (to the extraocular muscles) are unaffected in MND; this is not true of the tongue, which only requires slightly longer axons. Another answer is that it is *not* only motor neurons which are affected: changes are seen in other areas, and we note that specific aphasia-dementia syndromes occur in MND.[282]

Why do some mnd brains have excess levels of glutamate? (Glutamate is the chief excitatory neurotransmitter.) This is thought to be from ↓ activity of the excitatory amino acid transporter (EAAT2), which mops up glutamate—hence the notion that MND is an 'excitotoxic' phenomenon. Motor cells have high levels of Cu/Zn superoxide dismutase (thought to protect normal motor cells from glutamate toxicity/oxidative stress). But a high level may itself be damaging, given certain genetic or acquired vulnerabilities.[283] Transgenic mice exhibiting high levels of superoxide dismutase do indeed develop an MND phenotype.

These ideas are speculative,[284] but help understanding and criticism of future therapies. **Riluzole** is an Na^+-channel blocker inhibiting glutamate release. Neurotrophic factors can protect motor neurons in animal studies, but clinical trials have proved disappointing. CI: hepatic and renal impairment. Effects of free-radical manipulation can be unpredictable. The antioxidant **vitamin E** protects transgenic mice from developing an MND-like picture, and in at least one human trial high intake of polyunsaturated fatty acids and vitamin E was associated with a 50% decreased risk of developing ALS (these nutrients appear to act synergistically).[285]

Apoptosis is a hallmark of MND,[286] and overexpression of proteins inhibiting cell death via apoptosis (Bcl-2) in transgenic mice can slow MND degeneration.

Cervical spondylosis

Cervical spondylosis with compression of the cord (myelopathy) and nerve roots is the leading cause of progressive spastic quadriparesis with sensory loss below the neck.[287] Most people with cervical spondylosis have no impairment, however—just degeneration of the annulus fibrosus of cervical intervertebral discs ± osteophytes, which narrow the spinal canal and intervertebral foramina. As the neck flexes and extends, the cord is damaged as it is dragged over these protruding bony spurs anteriorly and indented by a thickened ligamentum flavum posteriorly.

Signs Limited, painful neck movement ± crepitus—be careful! Neck flexion may produce tingling down the spine—a positive Lhermitte's symptom. This does not help decide if cord or roots (or both) are involved.

Root compression (radiculopathy): Pain in arms or fingers at the level of the compression (see TABLE), with dull reflexes, dermatomal sensory disturbance (numbness, tingling, ↓pain & T°), LMN weakness and eventual wasting of muscles innervated by the affected root. Below the level of the affected root (examine the legs) there may be UMN signs suggestive of a cord compression: spasticity, weakness, brisk reflexes, and upgoing plantars. Position & vibration sense may be lost. Examine for a sensory level.

Complaints may be of:
- Neck stiffness (but common in anyone >50yrs old)
- Crepitus on moving neck
- Stabbing or dull arm pain (brachialgia)
- Forearm/wrist pain

Signs of cord compression:
- Spastic leg weakness (often 1 leg > than other)
- Weak, clumsy hands
- Numbness in hands
- 'Heavy' legs
- Foot-drop/poor walking
- Incontinence, hesitancy & urgency are often late[288]

►*Worrying symptoms:* nocturnal pain, weight loss, fever, immunosuppression.

Typical motor and sensory deficits from individual root involvement

Nerve root (disc)		
C5	(C4/C5)	Weak deltoid & supraspinatus; ↓supinator jerks; numb elbow.
C6	(C5/C6)	Weak biceps & brachioradialis; ↓biceps jerks; numb thumb & index finger.
C7	(C6/C7)	Weak triceps & finger extension; ↓triceps jerks; numb middle finger.
C8	(C7/T1)	Weak finger flexors & small muscles of the hand; numb 5th & ring finger.

Investigations MRI to localize the lesion (**fig 1**). An AP compression ratio ≥30% usually induces histopathological changes in the cord (cadaver studies). Time to walk 30m helps monitor progress (valid & cheap).[289]

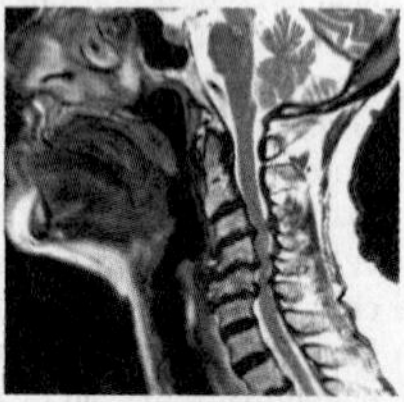

Fig 1. A T2-weighted MRI (∴ CSF looks bright). The spinal cord is compressed between the osteophytes anteriorly and the ligamentum flavum posteriorly.

Image courtesy of Prof. P Scally

Differential diagnosis MS, nerve root neurofibroma, subacute combined degeneration of the cord (↓B_{12}), compression by vertebral (bony) or cord tumours.

Management A firm neck collar restricts anterior-posterior movement of the neck so may relieve pain, but patients dislike them. Don't dismiss those with chronic root pain in the arm as suffering simply from 'wear and tear' spondylosis. Be optimistic: they may improve over months; if not, they *may* benefit greatly from surgical root decompression (**laminectomy, fig 2** or **laminoplasty, fig 3**) if there is significant MRI abnormality,[290] and especially if the history is short and the neurological deficit is progressing. As a rule of thumb, opt for conservative treatment if the spinal transverse area is >70mm², the patient is elderly, and motor conduction time is normal.[291] If surgery *is* done, progression is usually halted and leg weakness may improve. Operative risk is less than with **anterior spinal fusion** (requires bone grafts with additional complications with no extra benefit).[292] **Transforaminal steroid injection** is gaining popularity on the rationale that nerve root inflammation causes radicular pain. Pain reduction is reported (but no RCTs yet).

Rare complications Diaphragm paralysis;[293] spinal artery syndrome mimicking angina (due to spinal artery compression; pain & T° are lost before vibration sense).[294]

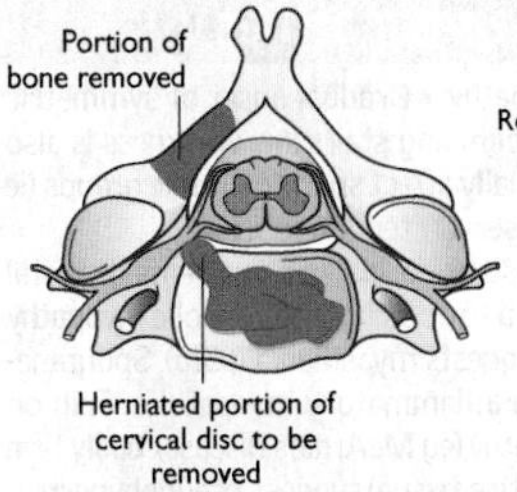

Fig 2. Laminectomy 295

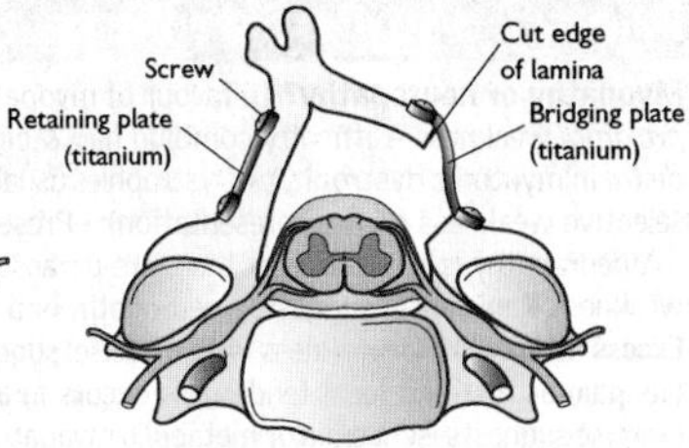

Fig 3. Laminoplasty (screws & plates) 296

Laminectomy or laminoplasty? **Laminectomy and laminoplasty improve gait, strength, sensation, pain, and degree of myelopathy. To a roughly equal extent, but in one study of 44 consecutive patients, laminoplasty was associated with more pain reduction and fewer late complications (but there was more neck stiffness). 297 At appropriate level, the ligamentum flavum (overlies the dura) is incised and cut away with part of adjacent laminae, as necessary to expose the extradural space. 298**

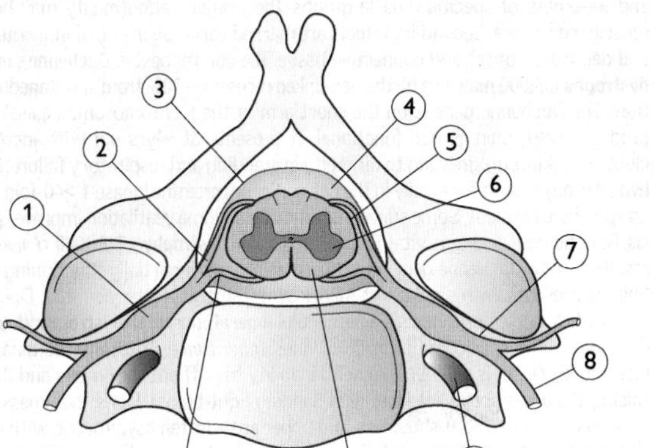

Fig 4. Cervical vertebra. 299

1 Dorsal root ganglion
2 Dorsal root
3 Dura mater
4 Subarachnoid space
5 Pia mater
6 Grey matter
7 Spinal nerve
8 Ventral ramus
9 Vertebral artery in the transverse foramen
10 White matter
11 Ventral spinal nerve

Image after Dr Carey Carpenter.

Primary disorders of muscle (myopathies)

Myopathy or neuropathy? In favour of myopathy: • Gradual onset of symmetric *proximal* weakness—difficulty combing hair & climbing stairs (NB: weakness is also *distal* in myotonic dystrophy); • Dystrophies usually affect specific muscle groups (ie selective weakness on first presentation); • Preserved tendon reflexes.

A neuropathy is more likely if there are paraesthesiae, bladder problems or distal weakness. **Rapid onset** suggests a neuropathy or a toxic, drug, or metabolic myopathy. **Excess fatigability** (↑weakness with exercise) suggests myasthenia (p516). Spontaneous **pain** at rest and local tenderness occurs in inflammatory myopathies. Pain on exercise suggests ischaemia or metabolic myopathy (eg McArdle's disease). **Oddly firm** muscles (due to infiltrations with fat or connective tissue) suggest pseudohypertrophic muscular dystrophies (eg Duchenne's). **Lumps** are commonly caused by haematoma, herniation of muscle through fascia, and tendon rupture. Muscle tumours are rare. **Fasciculation** suggests anterior horn cell or root disease. Look for evidence of systemic disease. ***Tests:*** ESR, CK, AST & LDH may be raised. Do EMG and tests relevant to systemic causes (eg TSH↑↓, p208). Many genetic disorders of muscle are detectable by DNA analysis: use muscle biopsy only if genetic tests are non-diagnostic.

Muscular dystrophies are a group of genetic diseases with progressive degeneration and weakness of specific muscle groups. The primary abnormality may be in the muscle membrane. Secondary effects are marked variation in size of individual fibres and deposition of fat and connective tissue. The commonest is **Duchenne's muscular dystrophy** (3/1000 male live births; sex-linked recessive—30% from spontaneous mutation). The Duchenne gene is on the short arm of the X chromosome (Xp665), and its product, dystrophin, is non-functional. It presents at ~4yrs old with increasingly clumsy walking, progressing to difficulty in standing and respiratory failure. Pseudohypertrophy is seen, especially in the calves. Serum creatine kinase ↑ >40-fold. There is no specific treatment. Some survive beyond 20yrs. Home ventilation improves prognosis. Genetic counselling is vital. **Becker's muscular dystrophy** (~0.3/1000 ♂ live births) results from a Duchenne gene mutation that produces partially functioning dystrophin. It presents with similar but milder symptoms, at a later age than Duchenne's, and with a better prognosis. **Facioscapulohumeral muscular dystrophy (Landouzy-Dejerine)** is almost as common as Duchenne's. *Inheritance:* Autosomal dominant (gene locus 4q35). *Onset* is ~12-14yrs old, with inability to puff out the cheeks and difficulty raising the arms above the head (eg changing light-bulbs). *Signs:* Weakness of face ('ironed out' expression), shoulders, and upper arms (often asymmetric with deltoids spared), foot-drop, winging of the scapulae (**fig 1**),[300] scoliosis, anterior axillary folds,[301] and horizontal clavicles.[302] ≤20% need a wheelchair by 40yrs old.

Myotonic disorders cause tonic muscle spasm (myotonia). *Histology:* long chains of central nuclei within muscle fibres. The chief one is **dystrophia myotonica** (DM1), an autosomal dominant **Cl^- channelopathy**.[303] *Typical onset:* 25yrs old with distal-onset weakness (hand/foot drop), weak sternomastoids, and myotonia. Facial weakness and muscle wasting give a long, haggard appearance. *Also:* cataracts, male frontal baldness, diabetes mellitus, testis/ovary atrophy, cardiomyopathy, and mental impairment. Most patients die in middle age of intercurrent illness. Mexiletine, phenytoin and acetazolamide may help. Genetic counselling is important. Myotonia caused by **Na^+ channelopathy**: paramyotonia congenita, adynamia episodica hereditaria.

Acquired myopathies of late onset are often part of systemic disease—eg hyperthyroidism, malignancy, Cushing's, hypo- and hypercalcaemia.

Inflammatory myopathies Inclusion body myositis is the chief example if aged >50yrs. Aggregates of Alzheimer tau proteins suggest a 'peripheral tauopathy'.[304] ***Signs:*** weakness starts with quads, finger flexors or pharyngeal muscles. Ventral extremity muscle groups are more affected than dorsal or girdle groups. Wheelchair dependency is <3%. ***Histology:*** ringed vacuoles + intranuclear inclusions. ℞: nothing is consistently effective. For **polymyositis** and **dermatomyositis,** see p554.

Drug causes Alcohol; statins; steroids; chloroquine; zidovudine; vincristine; cocaine.

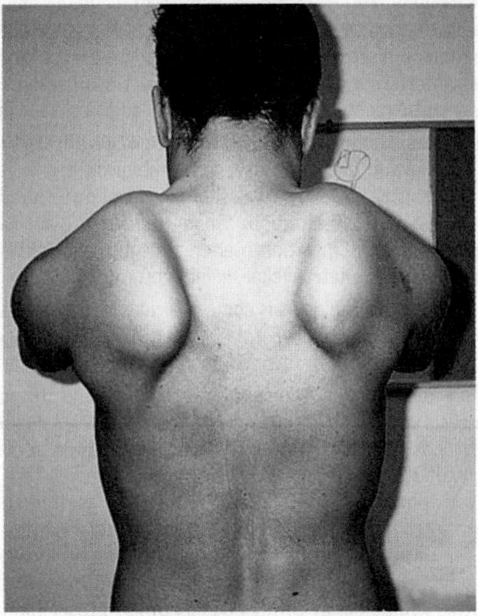

Fig 1. Winging of both scapulae in facioscapulohumeral muscular dystrophy. Winging is due to weakness of thoracoscapular muscles.

Myasthenia gravis (MG)

MG is an autoimmune disease mediated by antibodies to nicotinic acetylcholine receptors (AChR), interfering with the neuromuscular transmission via depletion of working post-synaptic receptor sites (**fig 1**). Both B and T cells are implicated.[305,306]

Presentation Increasing muscular fatigue. Muscle groups affected, in order: extra-ocular; bulbar (swallowing, chewing); face; neck; limb girdle; trunk. Look for: ptosis, diplopia, myasthenic snarl on smiling, 'peek sign'.[1] On counting to 50, the voice deteriorates (dysphonia is a rare presentation). *Tendon reflexes* are normal. Weakness is worsened by: pregnancy, K^+↓, infection, over-treatment, change of climate, emotion, exercise, gentamicin, opiates, tetracycline, quinine, procainamide, β-blockers.

Associations If under 50yrs old, MG is commoner in women, associated with other autoimmune diseases and thymic hyperplasia. Over 50, it is commoner in men, and associated with thymic atrophy or thymic tumour. Also rheumatoid arthritis and SLE.

Investigations • *Tensilon® test:* If resuscitation facilities and atropine are to hand, prepare 2 syringes, 1 with 10mg edrophonium and 1 with 0.9% saline. Give 1st 20% of each separately IV as test dose. Ask an independent observer to comment on the effect of each; wait 30s before giving rest of each syringe. The test is +ve if edrophonium improves power in ~1min. The test may not be as dramatic as is stated. • *Antibodies:* Anti-AChR antibodies ↑ in 90% (70% in ocular-confined MG); if sero-negative look for MuSK antibodies (muscle specific tyrosine kinase; ♀:♂≈15:2).[307] • *Neurophysiology:* Decremental muscle response to repetitive nerve stimulation ± ↑single-fibre jitter. • *Imaging:* CT of thymus.[308] • *Other:* ptosis improves by >2mm after ice application to the (shut) affected lid for >2min—a neat, non-invasive test.[309]

Treatment ***Symptom control*** Anticholinesterase, eg **pyridostigmine** (60–120mg PO up to 6×daily; max 1.2g/d). Cholinergic SE: salivation↑, lacrimation, sweats, vomiting, miosis. Other SE: diarrhoea, colic (controllable with propantheline 15mg/8h PO).
Immunosuppression: Treat relapses with **prednisolone**—start at 5mg on alternate days, ↑by 5mg/wk up to 1mg/kg on each treatment day. ↓dose on remission (may take months). Give osteoporosis prophylaxis. SE: weakness (hence low starting dose). Steroids may be combined with **azathioprine** 2.5mg/kg/day (do FBC & LFT weekly for 8wks, then 12-weekly) or weekly **methotrexate**.[310] IV methylprednisolone has a role.
Thymectomy: Consider if onset before 50yrs old and disease is not easily controlled by anticholinesterases. Expect remission in 25% and worthwhile benefit in a further 50%. Thymectomy is also necessary for thymomas to prevent local invasion (but MG symptoms are often unaffected). Some give **IV immunoglobulin** (**IV Ig**) 0.4g/kg daily for 5 days pre-op.[311]

Myasthenic crisis Weakness of the respiratory muscles during a relapse can be life-threatening. ►Monitor forced vital capacity. **Ventilatory support** is unlikely to be needed if vital capacity >20mL/kg.[312] Treat with **plasmapheresis** or **IV Ig**[313] and identify and treat the trigger for the relapse (eg infection, medications).

Prognosis Relapsing or slow progression. If thymoma, 5yr survival is 68%.[314]

Other causes of muscle fatigability Polymyositis; SLE; Takayasu's arteritis (fatigability of the extremities); botulism (see BOX). For other myopathies, see p514.

Lambert-Eaton myasthenic syndrome (LEMS, *ALSO* ELMS)

LEMS can be paraneoplastic (from small-cell lung cancer) or autoimmune.[2] Unlike true MG there is: • Gait difficulty before eye signs; • Autonomic involvement (dry mouth, constipation, impotence); • Hyporeflexia & weakness, which improve after exercise; • Less response to edrophonium; • Antibody to the pre-synaptic membrane's voltage-gated Ca^{2+} channels (see **fig 2**; anti-P/Q type VGCC antibodies are +ve in 85%).[315] • Electrical post-tetanic potentiation with >60% ↑ in post-exercise facilitation of abductor digiti quinti.[316] ℞: 3,4-diaminopyridine or IV immunoglobulin (get specialist help).[317] ►Do regular CXRs/HRCTs as symptoms may precede the cancer by >4 years.

1 After brief opposition to gentle sustained lid closure, the lids separate ('peek') to show white sclerae.
2 64% of those with non-tumour LEMS have a family member with autoimmune thyroid disease or DM.

How synapses work—the neuromuscular junction

1 Before transmission can occur, neurotransmitter must be packed into synaptic vesicles. At the neuromuscular junction (NMJ) this is acetylcholine (ACh). Each vesicle contains ~8000 ACh molecules.

2 When an action potential arrives at the pre-synaptic terminal, depolarization opens voltage-gated Ca^{2+} channels (VGCC). In **Lambert-Eaton** syndrome anti-P/Q type VGCC antibodies disrupt this stage of synaptic transmission.

3 Influx of Ca^{2+} through the VGCCs triggers fusion of synaptic vesicles with the pre-synaptic membrane (a process that **botulinum toxin** interferes with), and neurotransmitter is released from the vesicles into the synaptic cleft.

4 Transmitter molecules cross the synaptic cleft by diffusion and bind to receptors on the post-synaptic membrane, causing depolarization of the post-synaptic membrane (the end-plate potential). This change in the post-synaptic membrane triggers muscle contraction at the NMJ, or onward transmission of the action potential in neurons. In **myasthenia gravis**, antibodies block the post-synaptic ACh receptors, preventing the end-plate potential from becoming large enough to trigger muscle contraction—and muscle weakness ensues.

5 Transmitter action is terminated by enzyme-induced degradation of transmitter (eg acetylcholinesterase), uptake into the pre-synaptic terminal or glial cells, or by diffusion away from synapse.318 Anticholinesterase treatments for myasthenia gravis, such as **pyridostigmine**, reduce the rate of degradation of ACh, increasing the chance that it will trigger an end-plate potential.

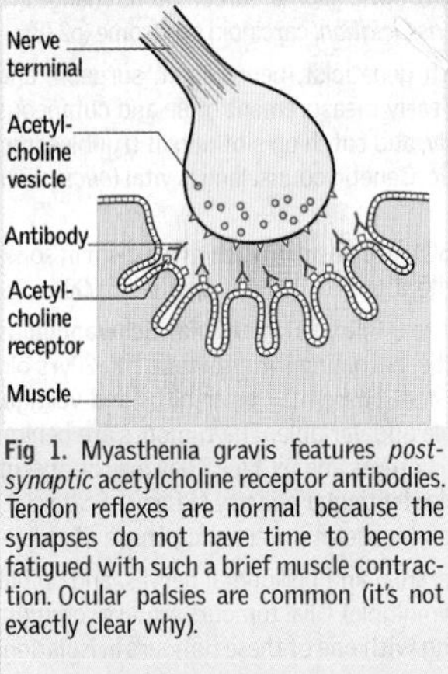

Fig 1. Myasthenia gravis features *post-synaptic* acetylcholine receptor antibodies. Tendon reflexes are normal because the synapses do not have time to become fatigued with such a brief muscle contraction. Ocular palsies are common (it's not exactly clear why).

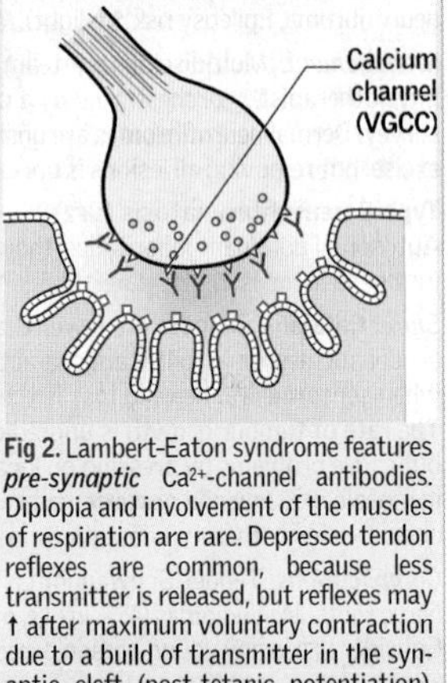

Fig 2. Lambert-Eaton syndrome features *pre-synaptic* Ca^{2+}-channel antibodies. Diplopia and involvement of the muscles of respiration are rare. Depressed tendon reflexes are common, because less transmitter is released, but reflexes may ↑ after maximum voluntary contraction due to a build of transmitter in the synaptic cleft (post-tetanic potentiation). Dysfunction of the autonomic nervous system is also common.

Type 1 neurofibromatosis (NF1, von Recklinghausen's disease)

Autosomal dominant inheritance (gene locus 17q11.2). Expression of NF1 is variable, even within a family. *Prevalence:* 1 in 2500, ♀:♂≈1:1; no racial predilection.

Signs: **Café-au-lait spots:** flat, coffee-coloured patches of skin seen in 1st year of life (clearest in UV light), increasing in size and number with age. Adults have ≥6, >15mm across. They do *not* predispose to skin cancer. **Freckling:** typically in skin-folds (axillae, groin, neck base, and submammary area♀), and usually present by age 10. **Dermal neurofibromas:** small, violaceous nodules, gelatinous in texture, which appear at puberty, and may become papillomatous. They are not painful but may itch. Numbers increase with age. **Nodular neurofibromas** arise from nerve trunks. Firm and clearly demarcated, they can give rise to paraesthesiae if pressed. **Lisch nodules (fig 1)** are tiny harmless regular brown/translucent mounds (hamartomas) on the iris (use a slit lamp) ≤2mm in diameter. They develop by 6yrs old in 90%. Also short stature and macrocephaly.

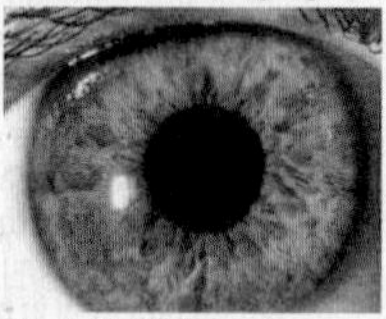

Fig 1. Multiple brown Lisch nodules on the iris.[319]
Courtesy of Jon Miles

Complications: Occur in 30%. Mild learning disability is common. *Local effects of neurofibromas:* Nerve root compression (weakness, pain, paraesthesiae);[320] GI—bleeds, obstruction; bone—cystic lesions, scoliosis, pseudarthrosis. BP↑ (6%) from renal artery stenosis or phaeochromocytoma. Plexiform neurofibromas (large, subcutaneous swellings). *Malignancy* (5% patients with NF1): optic glioma, sarcomatous change in a neurofibroma. Epilepsy risk ↑ (slight). *Rare association:* carcinoid syndrome (p278).[321]

Management: Multidisciplinary team with geneticist, neurologist, surgeon, and physiotherapist,[322] orchestrated by a GP. Yearly measurement of BP and cutaneous survey. Dermal neurofibromas are unsightly, and catch on clothing; if troublesome, excise, but removing all lesions is unrealistic. Genetic counselling is vital (*OHCS* p154).

Type 2 neurofibromatosis (NF2)

Autosomal dominant inheritance, though 50% are *de novo*, with mosaicism in some (NF2 gene locus is 22q11). Rarer than NF1 with a prevalence of only 1 in 35,000.

Signs: **Café-au-lait spots** are fewer than in NF1. **Bilateral vestibular Schwannomas** (= acoustic neuromas; p466) are characteristic, becoming symptomatic by ~20yrs old when sensorineural hearing loss is the 1st sign. There may be tinnitus and vertigo. The rate of tumour growth is unpredictable and variable. The tumours are benign but cause problems by pressing on local structures and by ↑ICP. They may be absent in mosaic NF2. **Juvenile posterior subcapsular lenticular opacity** (a form of cataract) occurs before other manifestations and can be useful in screening those at risk.

Complications: Tender Schwannomas of cranial and peripheral nerves, and spinal nerve roots. Meningiomas (45% in NF2, often multiple). Glial tumours are less common. Consider NF2 in any young person presenting with one of these tumours in isolation.

Management: Hearing tests yearly from puberty in affected families, with MRI brain if abnormality is detected. A normal MRI in the late teens is helpful in assessing risk to any offspring. A clear scan at 30yrs (unless a family history of late onset) indicates that the gene has not been inherited. Treatment of vestibular Schwannomas is neurosurgical and complicated by hearing loss/deterioration and facial palsy. Mean survival from diagnosis is reported at 15yrs,[323] but with best practice should be better.[324]

Schwannomatosis

A recently described syndrome of multiple tender cutaneous Schwannomas without the bilateral vestibular Schwannomas that are characteristic of NF2. Indistinguishable from mosaic NF2, where vestibular Schwannomas are also absent, except by genetic analysis of tumour biopsies.[325] There is typically a large tumour load, assessable only by whole-body MRI. INI1 gene mutations with autosomal dominant inheritance and spontaneous NF2 mutations have both been described.[326] Life expectancy is normal.

Diagnostic criteria for neurofibromatosis

NF1 (von Recklinghausen's disease)

Diagnosis is made if 2 of the following are found:

1 ≥6 *café-au-lait* macules >5mm (prepubertal) or >15mm (post-pubertal)
2 ≥2 neurofibromas of any type or 1 plexiform
3 Freckling in the axillary or inguinal regions
4 Optic glioma
5 ≥2 Lisch nodules
6 Distinctive osseous lesion typical of NF1, eg sphenoid dysplasia
7 First-degree relative with NF1 according to the above criteria

Differential: McCune–Albright syndrome (*OHCS* p649), multiple lentigenes,[1] urticaria pigmentosa (*OHCS* p610).

NF2

Diagnosis is made if either of the following are found:

1 Bilateral vestibular Schwannomas seen on MRI or CT
2 First-degree relative with NF2, and either:
  a) Unilateral vestibular Schwannoma; or
  b) One of the following:
  - Neurofibroma
  - Meningioma
  - Glioma
  - Schwannoma
  - Juvenile cataract (NF2 type)

Differential: NF1, Schwannomatosis.

1 May be part **LEOPARD** syndrome: autosomal dominant **L**entigines, **E**CG anomalies, **O**cular hypertelorism (eyes wide-spaced), **P**ulmonary stenosis, **A**nomalies of genital organs, **R**etarded growth, **D**eafness.

Syringomyelia

Syrinx was one of those versatile virgins of Arcadia who, on being pursued by Pan beside the river Ladon, turned herself into a reed, from which Pan made his pipes, so giving her name to various tubular structures, eg syringe, and syrinx, which is a tubular or slit-like cavity in or close to the central canal of the cervical cord. It may extend up or down. *Mean age of onset:* 30yrs. *Incidence:* 8/100,000/yr. Symptoms may be static for years, but then worsen fast—eg on coughing or sneezing, as ↑ pressure causes extension, eg into the brainstem (*syringobulbia*).[327]

Causes *Typically*, blocked CSF circulation (without 4th ventricular communication), with ↓flow from basal posterior fossa to caudal space, eg Arnold-Chiari malformation (cerebellum herniates through foramen magnum); basal arachnoiditis (after infection, irradiation, subarachnoid haemorrhage); basilar impression/invagination;[1] masses (cysts, rheumatoid pannus, encephalocoele, tumours). *Less commonly*, a syrinx may develop after myelitis, cord trauma or rupture of an AV malformation, or within spinal tumours (ependymoma or haemangioblastoma) due to fluid secreted from neoplastic cells or haemorrhage.

Cardinal signs: Dissociated sensory loss (absent pain & T° sensation, with preserved light touch, vibration, and joint-position sense) due to pressure from the syrinx on the decussating anterolateral pathway (**fig 1**) in a root distribution reflecting the location of the syrinx (eg for typical cervical syrinx then sensory loss is over trunk & arms); **wasting/weakness** of hands ± **claw-hand** (then arms→shoulders→respiratory muscles). Anterior horn cells are also vulnerable.

Other signs: Horner's syndrome; UMN leg signs; body asymmetry, limb hemi-hypertrophy, or unilateral odo- or chiromegaly (enlarged hand or foot), perhaps from release of trophic factors via anterior horn cells; *Syringobulbia* (brainstem involvement): nystagmus, tongue atrophy, dysphagia, pharyngeal/palatal weakness, Vth nerve sensory loss. ***Charcot's (neuropathic) joints:*** Increased range of movement (from lost joint proprioception), destroys the joint, which becomes swollen and mobile (see **fig 2**, p540).[329] *Causes:* tabes dorsalis (eg knee), diabetic neuropathy, paraplegia (eg hips),[330] syringomyelia (shoulder, wrist),[331] leprosy, spinal osteolysis/cord atrophy (systemic sclerosis).[332]

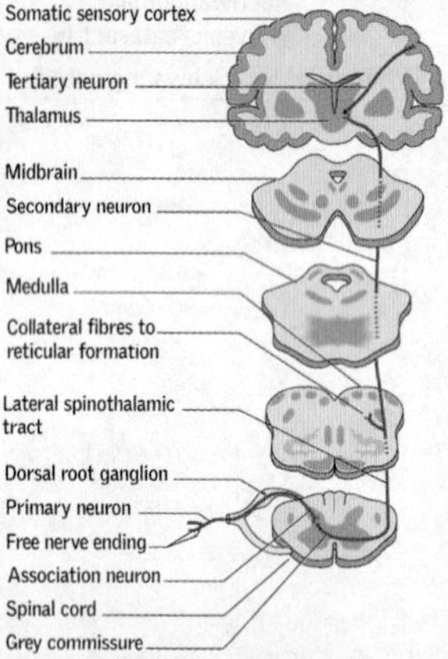

Fig 1. The anterolateral system.[328]

MRI imaging How big is the syrinx? Any base-of-brain (Chiari) malformation?

Surgery Don't wait for gross deterioration to occur. Decompression at the foramen magnum may be tried in Chiari malformations, to promote free flow of CSF, and so prevent syrinx dilatation. Surgery may relieve pain, and slow progression.[333]

Retroviruses and neurology

HIV/AIDS is part of the differential diagnosis of meningitis (eg fungal/TB), intracranial mass lesions (toxoplasmosis), dementia, encephalomyelitis, cord problems,[334] and peripheral nerve problems, eg mononeuritis multiplex & Guillain-Barré syndrome.

Tropical spastic paraplegia/HTLV-1 myelopathy is a slowly progressing spastic paraplegia, with paraesthesiae, sensory loss, and disorders of micturition.

1 The top of the odontoid process (part of C2) migrates upwards (congenitally, or in rheumatoid arthritis or osteogenesis imperfecta) causing foramen magnum stenosis ± medulla oblongata compression. Consider basilar invagination if the odontoid tip is ≥4mm above McGregor's line (drawn from the upper surface of the posterior edge of the hard palate to the most caudal point of the occipital curve).

Models of brain functioning

A superficial reading of the foregoing pages might lead one to the conclusion that the structure of the adult brain is fixed, and that a circumscribed lesion will cause reproducible, predictable results (if we remember our neuroanatomy correctly). Furthermore, if a certain phenomenon appears when part of the brain (say area A) is stimulated, and is lost when the same part of the brain is injured, we happily conclude that area A is the centre for laughter, fear, or whatever the phenomenon is. A lesion here, and you will stop laughing for ever, we might think. An area on the hard disk of our mind has been scratched. The grey cells do not regenerate themselves, so the brain carries on as before with this one defect. The more we look at the brain, the more wrong this model becomes.

If our brains were like a computer, the more tasks we did at the same time, the slower we would do any one task. In fact, our performance can *improve*, the more simultaneous tasks we take on. This is why music helps some of us concentrate. Experiments using functional MRI show that listening to polyphonic music recruits memory circuits, promotes attention, and aids semantic processing, target detection, and some forms of imagery.[335]

Another way in which our brains are not like a computer is that we are born with certain predispositions and expectations. Our hard disk was never blank. Just as the skin on the feet of new-born babies is thicker than other areas, as if feet were made with a prior knowledge of walking or somehow expecting walking, so our brains are made expecting a world of stimuli, which need making sense of by reframing sequential events in terms of cause and effect. We cannot help unconsciously imposing cause and effect relationships on events which are purely sequential. This unconscious reframing no doubt has survival value.

The model we have of brain function is important because it influences our attitude to our patients. If we are stuck with a neuroanatomical model, we will be rather pessimistic and guarded in our assessment of how patients may recover after neurological events. If we use a model which is more holistic and reality-based, such as the Piaget-type model in which the brain is seen as intrinsically unstable and continually re-creating itself, we will grant our patients more possibilities.[336] Our model of the brain must encompass its ability to set goals for itself, and to be self-actuating.[337] Unstructured optimism is unwarranted, but structured optimism is to some extent a self-fulfilling prognosis. For many medical conditions, the more optimistic we are, and the more we involve our patients in their own care and its planning, the faster and better they will recover.[338] If we combine this with the observed fact that those with an optimistic turn of mind are less likely to suffer stroke,[339] we can reach the conclusion that emotional wellbeing predicts subsequent functional independence and survival. When this hypothesis is tested directly in a prospective way, the effect of emotional wellbeing is found to be direct and strong and independent of other factors such as functional status, sociodemographic variables, chronic conditions, body mass index, etc.[340]

So the conclusion is that the brain has an unknown amount of inherent plasticity, and an unknown potential for healing after injury—uninjured areas may take on new functions, and injured parts may function in new ways.[1] The great challenge of neurology is to work to maximize this potential for recovery and re-creation. This demands knowledge of your patient, as well as knowledge of neuroanatomy and neurophysiology. The point is that there is no predefined limit to what is possible.

1 In early frontotemporal dementia, artistic creativity may blossom—suggesting that language is not required for, and may even inhibit, certain types of visual creativity. See p490.

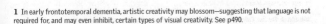

Contents

Relevant pages in other chapters: Active management of death (p7); leukaemias/lymphomas (p346–p356); myeloma (p362); immunosuppressive drugs (p370); pain (p 576); dying at home (*OHCS* p498). For specific cancers, see relevant chapters, eg *Surgery*, p566.

Communication

This forms the first step in understanding, treating, or coming to terms with cancer. A range of overwhelming feelings can surface on receiving this diagnosis, including shock, numbness, denial, panic, anger and resignation ("I knew all along..."). Some doctors instinctively turn away from 'undisciplined squads of emotions' and try to stop them taking over consultations. A more positive approach is to try to use these to benefit and motivate your patient, through listening to and addressing their worst fears. ►*Include your patient in all decision-making processes.* Many patients (not just the young and well informed) will appreciate this, and the giving of information and the sharing of decisions is known to reduce treatment morbidity. So, even when this is physically exhausting (the same ground may need covering many times) it is definitely worth spending this time. A huge amount is forgotten or fails to register initially, so videos and written information are important. Be sure to question, in an open way, about use of alternative therapies, which can indicate psychosocial distress and is frequently a sign of undisclosed worry of recurrence. Ask about this and through good communication and the promotion of autonomy, your patient's fear-driven wish to try dangerous or untried therapies may be trumped by a spirit of rational optimism.

We thank Dr Ian Cairns, who is our Specialist Reader for this chapter.

Looking after people with cancer

No rules guarantee success, but getting to know your patient, making an agreed management plan, and seeking out the right expert for each stage of treatment *all* need to be central activities in oncology. The patient will bring worries from all aspects of their family, work and social life. Communication is central to resolving these issues and the personal attributes of the doctor as a physician are key. Remember, it is never too early to start palliative care (*with* other treatments) and that *quality of life* is of the utmost importance.

Psychological support Meta-analyses have suggested that psychological support can improve outcome measures such as survival.[2] Examples include:

- *Allowing negative feelings*, eg fear or anger (anger can anaesthetize pain).
- *Counselling*, eg with a breast cancer nurse in preparation for mastectomy.
- *Biofeedback and relaxation therapy* can ↓ side effects of chemotherapy.[3]
- *Cognitive behavioural therapy* reduces psychological morbidity associated with cancer treatments. See OHCS p370.
- *Group therapy* (OHCS p376) reduces pain, mood disturbance and the frequency of maladaptive coping strategies.

Streamlining care pathways Care pathways map journeys in a health system: symptoms felt→unknown psychic processes[1]→GP appointment→referral→hospital appointment→consultant clinic→imaging→initial treatment (surgery, etc). Each arrow represents a possibly fatal delay. 48h access to GPs, GP referral under a '2-week rule' (hospital must see within 2wks, inevitably making other equally or more deserving patients wait longer) and *e*-booking (like on-line airline reservations) are unreliable ways of speeding up the crucial arrow pointing to initial treatment.[4] The only way to do this is to increase capacity (beds, nurses, doctors, equipment, theatres).

Hints for breaking bad news[5,6]

1. Set the environment up carefully. Choose a quiet place where you will not be disturbed. Make sure family are present if wanted. Be sure of your facts.
2. Find out what the patient already knows or surmises (often a great deal). This may change rapidly, and different perceptions may all be relevant.
3. Ascertain how much the person wants to know. You can be surprisingly direct. "If anything were amiss, would you want to know all the details?"
4. Give some warning—"There is some bad news for us to address". Offer small amounts of information at a time, as this can soften the impact.
5. Share information about diagnosis and treatments. Specifically list supporting people (eg nurses) and institutions (eg hospices). Ask "Is there anything else you want me to explain?" Don't hesitate to go over the same ground repeatedly. Allow denial: don't force the pace, give them time.
6. 'Cancer' has negative connotations for many people. Address this, and explain that ~50% of cancers are cured in the developed world.[7]
7. Listen to any concerns raised; encourage the airing of feelings and empathize.
8. Prognosis questions are often hardest to answer, doctors are usually too optimistic.[8] Encourage an appropriate level of hope, refer to an expert.
9. Summarize and make a plan. Offer availability.
10. Follow through. ►Leave the patient with the strong impression that come what may, you are with them, and that this unwritten contract will not be broken.

Don't imagine that a single blueprint will always work. Use whatever the patient gives you—closely observe both verbal and non-verbal cues.[9] Practise in low-key interactions with patients, so that when great difficulties arise you have a better chance of helping. Humans are very complex, and we all frequently fail—don't be put off: keep trying, and recap with colleagues afterwards, so you keep learning.

1 Why is there so much variation in European cancer 5-yr survival rates? In breast cancer, 5yr survival is 78% in England, 86% in Sweden, and 93% in Iceland. One reason is NHS inefficiency; another is cultural. If an English woman feels a lump she may say "I haven't got time to be ill," or "Let's see if it goes away," or "If this is how I'm going to die, so be it," but others may say "I'd better get this sorted *now*."

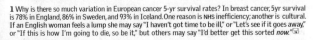

Some commoner cancer-predisposing gene mutations are given in the BOX.

Familial breast/ovarian cancer Most breast and ovarian cancer is sporadic, but ~5% is due to germline mutation in BRCA1 (17q) or BRCA2 (13q). Both genes function as tumour suppressors. Carrying a BRCA1 mutation confers a lifetime risk of developing breast cancer of 70–80%, and ovarian cancer of 30–40%. Mutations in BRCA2 are much less likely to cause ovarian cancer, but may cause male breast cancer. Incidence of mutations varies among populations. In families with ≥4 cases of breast cancer collected by the Breast Cancer Linkage Consortium, the disease was linked to BRCA1 in 52% of families and BRCA2 in 32%. Individuals from families in which a mutation has not been detected can be given risk estimation based on number of individuals affected and age of onset of cancer. There is no consensus on efficacy of mammographic and ovarian ultrasound screening or analysis of CA125 and CEA (carcionembryonic antigen) serum markers in individuals at moderate risk.

There is debate about cost-benefits of screening and risks of radiation exposure from regular mammography. MRI assists early detection.[10] Those at high risk of breast or ovarian cancer may opt for prophylactic mastectomy and oophorectomy both of which lower, but do not remove, the risk of developing cancer derived from those sites. No drug has been fully assessed for *prevention* in high-risk patients: tamoxifen is associated with unacceptable adverse side effects, aromatase inhibitors (eg anastrozole) are more promising but still under trial (eg MAP III).[11]

Familial prostate cancer ~5% of those with prostate cancer have a family history: the genetic basis is multifactorial. There is a modestly elevated lifetime risk of prostate cancer for male carriers of BRCA1 and BRCA2 mutations, although the molecular basis of this remains to be elucidated. Mutations in BRCA1/BRCA2 or in the genes on chromosomes 1 and X do not account for all family clusters of prostate cancer and so it is clear that other genes must be involved. In one twin study, 42% of the risk was found to be genetic.[12]

Familial colorectal cancer ~20% of those with colorectal cancer have a family history of the disease. An individual's relative risk (RR) of colorectal cancer is related to the degree of family history—refer to a genetic clinic if: • Two affected 1st-degree relatives aged <70 (RR×5); • One affected 1st degree relative aged <45yrs at diagnosis (RR×3); • three close relatives affected with average age at onset <60yrs (RR×2); • Familial adenomatous polyposis (below); • Potential family history of HNPCC (below).

Familial adenomatous polyposis is due to germline mutations in the APC gene. Offspring are at 50% of risk of being a gene carrier, and gene penetrance approaches 100% for colorectal cancer by 50yrs old.

Peutz–Jeghers syndrome has a 10–20% lifetime risk of colorectal cancer, and has been shown to be due to germline mutations in STK11, a serine threonine kinase (locus: 19p14).

Hereditary non-polyposis colorectal cancer (HNPCC) entails familial aggregation of colorectal cancer (HNPCC 1) ± cancer of uterus, ovary, stomach, renal pelvis, small gut, or pancreas (HNPCC 2) with mutations in 1 of 5 DNA mismatch repair genes. Suspect a family history if ≥3 affected relatives in an autosomal dominant pattern (incomplete penetrance), of whom one was affected <50 yrs old. Genetic testing and surveillance colonoscopy may be indicated. Lifetime risk of colorectal cancer for relatives who carry a mutation is 60%, and women with a mutation have a 40% lifetime risk of endometrial cancer. These mutations cause ~2% of all UK colorectal cancers.

Genetic tests can also tell if chemotherapy is likely to work: chemotherapy fails in 17% of colon cancer patients—ie those with certain mutations.[1]

1 Shown by the microsatellite instability status being 'high frequency'. Microsatellites are stretches of DNA in which a short section is repeated several times. 5-fluorouracil only improves survival in microsatellite stable or low-frequency microsatellite unstable tumours.

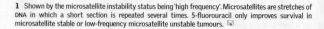

Examples of cancers with a familial predisposition

Cancer/syndrome	Gene	Chromosome	
Breast and ovarian cancers	BRCA1	17q	(p524)
	BRCA2	13q	
Hereditary non-polyposis colorectal cancer (HNPCC)	MSH2	2p	(p524)
	MLH1	3p	
	PMS2	7p	
Familial polyposis (colon/rectum)	APC	5q	(p524)
von Hippel-Lindau (kidney, CNS)	VHL	3p	(p726)
Carney complex	PRKAR1A	17q	(p215)
Multiple endocrine neoplasia type 1 (pituitary, pancreas, thyroid)	MEN1	11q	(p215)
Multiple endocrine neoplasia type 2	RET	10q	(p215)
Basal cell naevus syndrome (CNS, skin)	PTCH	9q	
Retinoblastoma (eye, bone)	Rb	13q	(*OHCS* p421)
Li-Fraumeni syndrome (multiple)	TP53	17p	(*OHCS* p648)
Neurofibromatosis type 1 (CNS; rare)	NF1	17q	(p518)
Neurofibromatosis type 2 (common—meningiomas, auditory neuromas)	NF2	22q	(p518)
Nijmegen breakage syndrome (melanoma, NHL, colon, prostate)	NBS1	8q	
Bloom syndrome (haematological malignancies, tongue, oesophagus, colon)	RECQL3	15q	
Hereditary paraganglioma	SDBH	1p	
	SDHC	1q	
	SDHD	11q	
Familial melanoma	INK4a	9p	

►A patient who becomes acutely unwell can often be made more comfortable with simple measures, but some problems require specific treatment.

Febrile neutropenic patients See p346.

Spinal cord compression (see also p470) Requires urgent and efficient treatment to preserve neurological function. A high index of suspicion is essential (BOX). ***Causes:*** Typically extradural metastases. *Other causes:* extension of tumour from a vertebral body, direct extension of the tumour, or crush fracture. ***Signs & symptoms:*** Back pain, weakness or sensory loss with a root distribution (or a sensory level), bowel and bladder dysfunction (more detail: p470). Have a low threshold for investigating patients with known cancer, who present with new or worsening back pain (especially thoracic or cervical) and *any* deterioration in mobility or sensation. ***Investigations:*** Urgent MRI of the whole spine. ***Management:*** **Dexamethasone** 8–16mg IV then 4mg/6h PO. Discuss with a neurosurgeon and clinical oncologist immediately.

Superior vena cava (SVC) obstruction with airway compromise SVC obstruction is not an emergency unless there is tracheal compression *with airway compromise:* otherwise there is usually time to plan optimal treatment, which is preferable to rushing into therapy that may not be beneficial.[13] ***Causes:*** Typically lung cancer. *Rare causes:* mediastinal enlargement (eg germ cell tumour), thymus malignancy, mediastinal lymphadenopathy (eg lymphoma), thrombotic disorders (eg Behçet's or nephrotic syndromes), thrombus around an IV central line, hamartoma, ovarian hyperstimulation (*OHCS* p311), and fibrotic bands (lung fibrosis after chemotherapy). ***Signs & symptoms:*** Dyspnoea, orthopnoea, plethora/cyanosis, swollen face & arm, cough, headache and engorged veins. ***Pemberton's test:*** Lifting the arms over the head for >1min causes facial plethora/cyanosis, JVP↑ (non-pulsatile), and inspiratory stridor. ***Investigations:*** CXR, CT, venography, sputum cytology. ***Management:*** Get a tissue diagnosis if possible, but bronchoscopy may be hazardous. Give oral **dexamethasone** 4mg/6h. Consider balloon **venoplasty** and SVC stenting,[14] eg prior to radical or palliative **chemo**- or **radiotherapy** (depending on tumour type).

Hypercalcaemia (see also p690) Affects 10–20% of patients with cancer, and 40% of those with myeloma. ***Causes:*** Lytic bone metastases, myeloma, production of osteoclast activating factor or PTH-like hormones by the tumour. ***Symptoms:*** Lethargy, anorexia, nausea, polydipsia, polyuria, constipation, dehydration, confusion, weakness. Most obvious with corrected serum Ca^{2+} >3mmol/L (but >2.6mmol/L may be enough in some patients). ***Management:*** The best treatment is control of underlying malignancy. Consider maintenance therapy with IV or PO **bisphosphonate**, or, if resistant, with **calcitonin**. See p690 for treatment of *acute hypercalcaemia*.

Raised intracranial pressure (see also p346). Due to either a primary CNS tumour or metastatic disease. ***Signs & symptoms:*** Headache (often worse in the morning, coughing or bending over), nausea, vomiting, papilloedema, fits, focal neurological signs. ***Investigations:*** Urgent CT/MRI is important to diagnose an expanding mass, cystic degeneration, haemorrhage within a tumour, cerebral oedema, or hydrocephalus due to tumour or blocked shunt since the management of these scenarios can be very different. ***Treatment:*** **Dexamethasone** 4mg/6h PO, radiotherapy, and surgery as appropriate depending on cause. **Mannitol** may be tried for symptom relief for cerebral oedema (not evidence-based).[15]

Tumour lysis syndrome Rapid cell death on starting chemotherapy for rapidly proliferating leukaemia, lymphoma, myeloma, and some germ cell tumours can result in a rise in serum urate, K^+, and phosphate, precipitating renal failure. Prevention is with good **hydration** and **allopurinol** started 24h before chemotherapy (300mg/12h PO if good renal function; if creatinine >100μmol/L give 100mg on alternate days).[16] Haemodialysis may be needed in renal failure. A more potent uricolytic agent is **rasburicase** (recombinant urate oxidase) 200μg/kg/d IVI for 5–7d. SE: fever, D&V, headache, rash, bronchospasm, and haemolysis.[17] It may interfere with uric acid tests.

Inappropriate ADH secretion p687.

When you suspect cord compression from metastases... NICE 2008

►Get advice today—eg from a neurosurgeon, or, where appointed, from your *metastatic spinal cord compression co-ordinator*. He or she will want to know:
- Why you think it is urgent—eg back pain disturbing sleep (p544), radicular pain, local spinal tenderness with weak legs, sphincter disturbance, or a sensory level.
- Has a tissue diagnosis of cancer been made?
- Is the patient too frail for specialist treatment?
- How is the compression progressing? If paraplegic for >24h, you may be too late.
- How long is the patient likely to live? Is it >3 months? ***Urgent radiotherapy*** may have a role. If longer, ***spinal reconstruction*** with a bone graft may be appropriate. ***Vertebral body reinforcement*** is one option for pain. ***Laminectomy*** alone should only be done for isolated epidural tumours or neural arch metastases.
- What is the fluid status (over-hydration is a danger)?
- Has DVT prophylaxis been considered (p568)?
- Have bisphosphonates (p696) been started? (Needed in all those with vertebral involvement from myeloma or breast cancer—they help pain and stability.)
- Has the option of palliative radiotherapy been considered?

Cancer affects 30% of the population; 20% die from it. Management requires a multidisciplinary team, and communication is vital (p522). Most patients wish to have some part in decision-making at the various stages of their treatment, and to be informed of their options. Patients are becoming better informed through self-help groups and access to the internet. Most patients undergo a variety of therapies during the treatment of their cancer and your job may be to orchestrate these.

Surgery In many cases a tissue diagnosis of cancer is made with either a biopsy or formal operation to remove the primary tumour. Although it is sometimes the only treatment required in early tumours of the GI tract, soft tissue sarcomas, and gynaecological tumours, it is often the case that best results follow the combination of surgery and chemotherapy. Surgery also has a role in palliating advanced disease.

Radiotherapy Uses ionizing radiation to kill tumour cells. See p530.

Chemotherapy Cytotoxics should be given under expert guidance by people trained in their administration. Drugs are given with a variety of intents, often in combination: *Neoadjuvant*—to shrink tumours to reduce the need for major surgery (eg mastectomy). There is also a rationale that considers early control of micro-metastasis. *Primary therapy*—as the sole treatment for haematological malignancies. *Adjuvant*—to reduce the chance of relapse, eg breast and bowel cancers. *Palliative*—to provide relief from symptomatic metastatic disease and possibly to prolong survival.

Important classes of drugs include:
- *Alkylating agents*, eg cyclophosphamide, chlorambucil, busulfan.
- *Antimetabolites*, eg methotrexate, 5-fluorouracil.
- *Vinca alkaloids*, eg vincristine, vinblastine.
- *Antitumour antibiotics*, eg actinomycin D, doxorubicin.
- *Monoclonal antibodies*, eg bevacizumab (for renal cell carcinoma), or antibodies against epidermal growth factor receptors such as panitumumab and cetuximab (over-expression of epidermal growth factor receptors correlates with poor prognosis in many cancers).
- *Others*, eg etoposide, taxanes, platinum compounds.

Side effects depend on the types of drugs used, and include:
- *Vomiting* is a source of much anxiety and should be prevented before the 1st dose, thus avoiding anticipatory vomiting: eg **dexamethasone** 4mg/12h, **metoclopramide** 10–20mg/8h and **ondansetron** 4–8mg/8h can be effective. See p241, BOX 3.
- *Alopecia* can also have a profound impact on quality of life.
- *Neutropenia* is most commonly seen 10–14d after chemotherapy (but can occur within 7d for taxanes). ►►Neutropenic sepsis requires immediate attention (p346).

Extravasation of a chemotherapeutic agent: Suspect if there is pain, burning or swelling at infusion site. ***Management:*** Stop the infusion, attempt to aspirate blood from the cannula, and then remove. Take advice. Administer steroids and consider antidotes.[1] [18] Elevate the arm and mark site affected. Review regularly and apply steroid cream. Apply cold pack (unless a vinca alkaloid, in which case a heat compress should be applied). Consider report to National Extravasation Scheme. Early liaison with plastic surgeon may be needed.

Communication ►*Include the patient in the decision-making process,* p522.

1 Some recommend (on scant evidence) topical dimethylsulfoxide (DMSO) and cooling after extravasation of anthracyclines or mitomycin, locally injected hyaluronidase if vinca alkaloids involved, and locally injected sodium thiosulfate (sodium hyposulfite) if chlormethine (mechlorethamine; mustine).

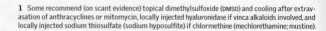

Avoiding pointless procedures in patients with cancer

Surgery is often performed with curative intent (eg for colorectal cancers), while other operations aim to restore function, deal with local recurrence, or reduce tumour bulk. But ambitious surgery is often pointless if the cancer has already spread beyond the organ in question. A key process in planning the right procedure is to interest a radiologist in your problem. This may require more than scrawling a brief request on an x-ray form. The range of imaging available is constantly changing, so discussing the request in person with a radiologist may help direct the use of the most appropriate modality to answer your question.[19]

CT: Extensive application in many cancers.

MRI: Used for precise staging in areas occult to CT (eg marrow, CNS). See p748.

Bone scan: Used for staging/follow-up of prostate, breast, and lung cancer.

Sestamibi scan: Used for localizing active disease in breast cancer and thyroid (eg if not iodine-avid). Like bone scans, it uses technetium (^{99m}Tc).

Thallium scan: Used to localize viable tissue, eg in brain tumours.

Gallium scan: Used for staging and follow-up in lymphoma.

Octreotide scan: Used to demonstrate cancers with somatostatin receptors (eg pancreas, medullary thyroid, neuroblastoma, and carcinoid tumours).

Monoclonal antibodies: ^{99m}Tc-labelled tumour antibodies are used in staging by detecting tumour antigen, eg in lung, colon, and prostate cancer.

FDG PET: 2-[^{18}F] fluoro-2-deoxy-D-glucose positron emission tomography detects high rates of aerobic metabolism, eg in lung, colon, breast, and testis.

MIBG scan (^{131}I): Used to localize noradrenaline production, eg phaeochromocytoma. MIBG = meta-iodobenzylguanidine.

Radiotherapy uses ionizing radiation to produce free radicals which damage DNA. Normal cells are better at repairing this damage than cancer cells, so are able to recover before the next dose (or fraction) of treatment.

Radical treatment is given with curative intent. The total doses given range from 40-70Gy (1Gy = 100cGy = 100rads) in 15-35 daily fractions. Some regimens involve giving several smaller fractions a day with a gap of 6-8h. Combined chemoradiation is used in some sites, eg anus and oesophagus, to increase response rates.

Palliation aims to relieve symptoms. Doses are 8-30Gy, given in 1, 2, 5, or 10 fractions. Bone pain, haemoptysis, cough, dyspnoea, and bleeding are helped in >50% of patients. "*Will this patient benefit from radiotherapy?*" is a frequently asked question.[20, 21] When in doubt, ask an expert (or two).

Early reactions occur during or soon after treatment.

- *Tiredness:* Common after radical treatments. It can last weeks to months.
- *Skin reactions:* These vary from erythema to dry desquamation to moist desquamation to ulceration. On completing treatment, use moisturizers.
- *Mucositis:* All patients receiving head and neck treatment should have a dental check-up before therapy. Avoid smoking, alcohol, and spicy foods. Antiseptic mouthwashes may help. Aspirin gargle and other soluble analgesics are helpful. Treat oral thrush, eg with **Nystatin** oral solution (1mL swill & swallow every 6h) ± fluconazole 50mg/24h PO.
- *Nausea and vomiting:* Occur when stomach, liver, or brain treated. Try **metoclopramide** (dopamine antagonist) 10-20mg/8h PO, or **domperidone** (blocks the central chemoreceptor trigger zone) 10-20mg/8h PO. If unsuccessful, try a serotonin ($5HT_3$) antagonist, eg **ondansetron** 4-8mg/8h PO/IV.
- *Diarrhoea:* Usually after abdominal or pelvic treatments. Maintain good hydration. Avoid high-fibre bulking agents; try **loperamide**.
- *Dysphagia:* Following thoracic treatments.
- *Cystitis:* After pelvic treatments. Drink plenty of fluids. Use NSAIDs, eg **diclofenac**.
- *Bone marrow suppression:* More likely after chemotherapy unless large areas are being irradiated. Usually reversible.

Late reactions occur months or years after the treatment.

- *CNS: Somnolence*, 6-12wks after brain radiotherapy. Treat with steroids. *Spinal cord myelopathy*—progressive weakness. MRI is needed to exclude cord compression. *Brachial plexopathy*—numb, weak, and painful arm after axillary radiotherapy. Reduced IQ can occur in children receiving brain irradiation if <6yrs old.
- *Lung: Pneumonitis* may occur 6-12wks after thoracic treatment, eg with dry cough ± dyspnoea. Treat with **prednisolone** 40mg OD reducing over 6wks.
- *GI: Xerostomia*—reduced saliva. Treat with **pilocarpine** 5mg/8h PO or artificial saliva with meals (*OHCS* p579). Care must be taken with all future dental care as healing is reduced. *Benign strictures*—of oesophagus or bowel. Treat with dilatation. *Fistulae* need surgery. *Radiation proctitis* may be a problem after prostate irradiation. *NB:* those having radiotherapy for rectal cancer seem to have a *lower* than expected incidence of prostate cancer in the next decade (risk ↓ by 72%).[22]
- *GU: Urinary frequency:* small fibrosed bladder after pelvic treatments. *Fertility:* pelvic radiotherapy (and cytotoxics) may ↓ fertility, so consider ova or sperm storage. This is a complex area: get expert help. See BOX. In premature female menopause or reduced testosterone, replace hormones. *Vaginal stenosis* and *dyspareunia*. *Erectile dysfunction* can occur several years after pelvic radiotherapy.
- *Others: Panhypopituitarism* following radical treatment involving pituitary fossa. Children need hormones checking regularly as growth hormone may be required. *Hypothyroidism*—neck treatments, eg for Hodgkin's lymphoma. *Secondary cancers*, eg sarcomas, usually wait 10 or more years before appearing. *Cataracts*.

Fertility issues in cancer patients

Plan with patients *before* treatment.

Chemotherapy and radiotherapy often damage germ cell spermatogonia (causing impaired spermatogenesis or male sterility), and may hasten oocyte depletion (premature menopause). GNRH agonists may offer some benefit to women if taken during chemotherapy.[23] As treatments become more effective and survival improves, there are more survivors in the reproductive years for whom parenting is a top priority.[24] There is nothing like the hope of creating new life to sustain patients through the difficult times of radio- and chemotherapy, so make sure this hope is well founded.[25]

Semen cryopreservation from men and older boys with cancer must be offered before therapy. With modern fertility treatment (*OHCS* p293), even poor quality samples can yield successful pregnancies.[26] Another option is use of sperm from cryopreserved testicular tissue followed up with intracytoplasmic sperm injection (ICSI). If your patient is a man some years after cancer therapy who is unable to have children, refer him to a specialist. ►*Do not write him off as infertile*—testicular sperm extraction (TESE) with ICSI can yield normal pregnancies.[27]

Cryopreservation of embryos and ***ovarian tissue banking*** are harder options in women.[28] Harvesting and storing ovarian cortical tissue from girls and young women before potentially gonadotoxic therapy is only available in some centres.[29] Success depends on the integrity of the uterus, and in some cancers this may have been badly affected by radiotherapy.

For ethical issues and the UK Human Embryology Authority, see *OHCS* p293.

Survival—European figures

Early diagnosis, a full range of treatment options, and the money spent by nations on health care have all had an impact on improved survival. On average, 47.3% of men and 55.8% of women in Europe survive >5yrs after a cancer diagnosis (44.8% and 52.7%, respectively, in England). These statistics are based on 5-yr survival rates for 2.7 million adults diagnosed between 2000 and 2002.[30] England's rates are improving, but remain behind most other European countries (and remain the second worst in Europe compared with the total national expediture on health—on a par with countries spending ⅓ of that spent on the NHS).[31]

Palliative care is the medicine of palliating symptoms. Though this most often applies in the later stages of a malignancy, it does not necessarily have to—something that doctors and patients all too often forget. Take time to find out exactly what is troubling a patient and approach problems holistically. Remember each person comes with a set of emotions, preconceptions and a family already attached. Most hospitals now have a dedicated palliative care team for help and advice.

Pain See p534.

Nausea and vomiting Causes include chemotherapy, constipation, GI obstruction, drugs, severe pain, cough, squashed stomach syndrome, oral thrush, infection and uraemia. *Management:* Aim to treat reversible causes, eg with laxatives, fluconazole, analgesia or antibiotics; consider stopping, reducing or changing drugs or route. Anti-emetic choice should be based on mechanism and site of drug action, and oral if possible, but remember alternative routes (IV/SC/IM/PR). Give anti-emetics regularly, not just PRN. A third of patients will need more than one medication.[32] *Oral agents:* **Cyclizine** 50mg/8h (antihistamine, central action, covers most causes); **domperidone** 10–20mg/8h (blocks the central chemoreceptor trigger zone, good for younger patients since no acute dystonic SEs); **metoclopramide** 10mg/8h (central antidopaminergic *and* peripheral prokinetic effects, good in gastric stasis); **haloperidol** 0.5-1.5mg/12h (dopamine antagonist, effective in drug or metabolic induced nausea); **ondansetron** 4-8mg/8h (serotonin antagonist, good second-line agent); **levomepromazine** 3-12.5mg/12h (useful for morphine-induced nausea, broad spectrum, but can sedate).[33]

Constipation Very common SE with opiates, and better prevented than treated. Use **bisacodyl** 5mg at night, or combine a stimulant with a softener (**co-danthramer** 5-10mL nocte). **Movicol®** sachets 2-4/12h are useful in resistance, and if oral therapy fails try **glycerol** suppositories or an arachis oil enema.

Breathlessness Consider fans, air supply, and **supplementary O_2. Morphine** reduces respiratory drive, and thus relieves the sensation of breathlessness. Use of relaxation techniques and benzodiazepines can be useful. Look for pleural or pericardial effusion. Consider thoracocentesis ± pleurodesis for a significant pleural effusion. If there is a malignant pericardial effusion, a number of options exist including pericardiocentesis (p786), pleuropericardial windows, & external beam radiotherapy.[34]

Coated/dry mouth Treat any candida infection (p530) or other underlying cause. Simple measures such as chewing ice chips, pineapple chunks (release proteolytic enzymes) or gum should be tried. Good oral hygiene with mouth washes, chorhexidine and saliva substitutes, such as Biotene Oralbalance® gel can help.

Pruritus (itching) See p26.

Venepuncture problems Repeated venepuncture with the attendant risk of painful extravasation and phlebitis may be avoided by insertion of a single or multilumen skin-tunnelled catheter (eg a Hickman line) into a major central vein (eg subclavian or internal jugular) using a strict aseptic technique. Patients can look after their own lines at home, and give their own drugs. Problems include: infection, blockage (flush with 0.9% saline or dilute heparin, eg every week), axillary, subclavian, or superior vena cava thrombosis/obstruction, and line slippage. Convenient portable delivery devices are available, allowing drugs to be given at a preset time, without the patient's intervention.

The last days and weeks of life (p7) Once a decision has been made that a patient is entering the very final weeks of their illness, comfort should be the main concern. Think about stopping observations, unnecessary blood tests and medications (such as those for long-term prophylaxis). Ensure that a decision regarding resuscitation status has been made and clearly documented; this should usually be done by a senior doctor. Consider with the family and patient whether transfer to an alternative location or hospice may be appropriate and if going home is a priority—this can be arranged at very short notice to enable comfort during final hours.

Other agents

Other agents and procedures to know about (alphabetically listed)

- **C(h)olestyramine** 4g/6h PO (1h after other drugs) helps itch in jaundice.
- **Dexamethasone** 8mg IV stat relieves symptoms of superior vena cava or bronchial obstruction, and lymphangitis carcinomatosa. 4mg/12-24h PO may stimulate appetite, reduce ↑ICP headache, or induce (in some patients) a satisfactory sense of euphoria.
- **Fluconazole** 50mg/24h PO for candida
- H_2-antagonists (eg **cimetidine** 400mg/12h PO) help relieve gastric irritation, eg associated with gastric carcinoma.
- **Haloperidol** 0.5-5mg/24h PO helps agitation, nightmares, hallucinations, and vomiting.
- **Hyoscine hydrobromide** 0.4-0.6mg/8h SC or 0.3mg sublingual: vomiting from upper GI obstruction or noisy bronchial rattles.
- **Low-residue diets** may be needed for post-radiotherapy diarrhoea.
- **Metronidazole** 400mg/8h PO mitigates anaerobic odours from tumours; so do **charcoal dressings** (Actisorb®).
- **Naproxen** 250mg/8h with food: fevers caused by malignancy or bone pain from metastases (consider splinting joints if this fails).
- **Nerve blocks** may lastingly relieve pleural or other resistant pains.
- **Sodium chloride nebulisers** 5mL as needed, can aid persistent cough
- **Spironolactone** 100mg/12h PO + **bumetanide** 1mg/24h PO for ascites.

Syringe drivers

Syringe drivers allow a continuous subcutaneous infusion of fluids and drugs, and are often helpful for avoiding repeated cannulation attempts. Several drugs can be administered subcutaneously to palliate a number of symptoms:

- *Terminal secretions:* **hyoscine hydrobromide**[1] 0.6-2.4mg/24h, or **glycopyrronium** 0.6-1.2mg/24h.
- *Pain:* **diamorphine** is preferred to morphine due to its greater solubility, reducing risk of precipitation at higher doses. See p535 for opiate equivalence dosing table, and p7 for dose increments.
- *Agitation:* **midazolam** 20-100mg/24h (also helpful for seizure control if no longer able to take anticonvulsants orally).
- *Nausea and vomiting:* **cyclizine** 150mg/24h, or **haloperidol** 2.5-10mg/24h.
- *Bowel colic:* **hyoscine butylbromide**[1] 20-60mg/24h.

1 Do not confuse the vastly different doses for hyoscine hydrobromide and hyoscine butylbromide!

(See also p7)

Pain is one of the most feared sequelae of a terminal diagnosis and yet is largely preventable. Studies show that cancer pain is particularly poorly managed in most settings,[35] especially in the elderly. No patient should live or die with unrelieved pain; aim to prevent or eliminate it.

Assessment Don't assume a cause—take a detailed history and examine to understand the aetiology. Evaluate severity, nature, functional deficit and psychological state—depression occurs in up to 25% of cancer patients.[36] Pain from nerve infiltration or local pressure damage may respond better to amitriptyline or gabapentin than to opioids.

Management Explain and plan rehabilitation goals. Aim to modify the pathological process when possible, eg radiotherapy, hormones, chemotherapy, surgery. Effective analgesia is possible in 70–90% of patients[37] by adhering to 5 simple guidelines:

1 *By the mouth* - give orally wherever possible.
2 *By the clock* - give at fixed intervals to give continuous relief.
3 *By the ladder* - following the WHO stepwise approach (BOX 1).
4 *For the individual* - there are no standard doses for opiates, needs vary.
5 *With attention to detail* - inform, set times carefully, warn of side effects.

Use the WHO ladder (BOX 1; **fig 1**) until pain is relieved. Monitor the response carefully—review of results and side effects is crucial to good care. Start regular laxatives and anti-emetics with strong opiates. **Paracetamol** PO/PR/IV at step 1 may have an opiate-sparing effect, and should be continued at steps 2 and 3.[38]

Morphine Start with **oral solution** 5–10mg/4h PO with an equal breakthrough dose as often as required. A double dose at bedtime can enable a good night's sleep. Patient needs will vary greatly and there is no maximum dose; aim to control symptoms with minimum side effects. Change to **modified release preparations** (MST 12h) once daily needs are known by totalling 24h use and dividing by 2. Give 1/6 of the total daily dose as breakthrough. Side effects (common) are drowsiness, nausea and vomiting, constipation, dry mouth. Hallucinations and myoclonic jerks are signs of toxicity and should prompt dose review. ►*If the oral route is unavailable* try **diamorphine** IV/SC (see BOX 2 for conversions). **Oxycodone** PO/IV/SC/PR is a newer more potent opioid as effective as morphine, which may have fewer side effects.[39] **Oxynorm** is the oral liquid form. There are also **fentanyl transdermal patches** which should usually be started under specialist supervision in those already opiate-exposed for easy titration. Remove after 72h, and place a new patch at a different site. 25, 50, 75, and 100μg/h patches are made. $t_{1/2} \approx$ 17h. *Suppositories* for pain: try oxycodone 30mg PR (eg 30mg/8h ≈ 30mg morphine). *Syringe drivers* See BOX on p533.

Unfounded fears: Patients often shrink from using morphine analgesia, usually as a result of common misconceptions—that it is addictive, for the dying, signifying 'The End'. It is important to address and allay these fears. Addiction is not a problem in the palliative care setting, neither is respiratory depression with correct titration—pain stimulates the respiratory centre. Reassure the patient that it is simply a good painkiller, used in many situations. There is evidence it has no effect on life expectancy.[40]

Prescribing morphine and other controlled drugs: include the total quantity in both words and figures, and include the formulation (tablets, capsules, oral liquid etc). On charts rewrite medications in full if doses change and always give the amount in milligrams, especially when using liquid preparations.

Morphine-resistant pain Consider methadone or ketamine, and **adjuvants** such as NSAIDs, steroids, muscle relaxants or anxiolytics. If *neuropathic pain* is suspected, try **amitriptyline** (10–25mg ON) or **gabapentin** (300mg/8h; p508). *Depression* is common, and can amplify pain, so consider starting an SSRI.

The analgesic ladder[41]

(See p576 for NNT)

Rung 1	*Non-opioid*	Aspirin; paracetamol; NSAID
Rung 2	*Weak opioid*	Codeine; dihydrocodeine; tramadol
Rung 3	*Strong opioid*	Morphine; diamorphine; hydromorphine; oxycodone; fentanyl (± adjuvant analgesics)

If one drug fails to relieve pain, move up the ladder—do not try other drugs at the same level. In new, severe pain, rung 2 may be omitted.[42]

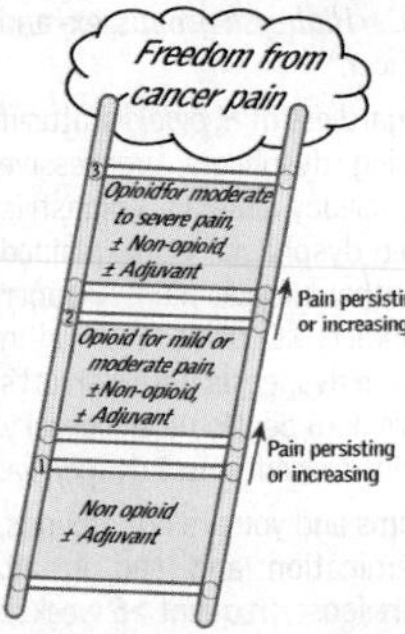

Fig 1. WHO's pain relief ladder.

Opiate dose equivalents

	Daily dose, mg	4h dose, mg	Relative potency to oral morphine
Morphine PO	30	5	1×
Morphine IV	15	2.5	2×
Diamorphine IV	10	2	3×
Oxycodone PO	15	2.5	2×
Oxycodone IV	10	2	3×
Fentanyl patch	0.2	—	150×

These conversions are not exact; the table is intended only as a rough guide. The potency figures particularly can vary widely. If in doubt, use a dose below your estimate when converting between opioids and titrate up according to response.

A variety of clinical scenarios and symptoms should alert you to the possible presence of malignancy and prompt urgent referral to the appropriate specialist. The list below is by no means exhaustive but covers the commonest presentations.[43]

Lung • Immediate referral if there are signs of superior vena caval obstruction or stridor; • Urgently with persistent haemoptysis (smokers or non-smokers over 40); • Suggestive CXR (pleural effusion, slowly resolving consolidation); • Normal CXR but high suspicion; • History of asbestos exposure and recent chest pain or dyspnoea; • Unexplained systemic symptoms with suspicious CXR. ►*High-risk groups:* ex- and current smokers, COPD, asbestos exposure, previous cancer.

Upper gastrointestinal • Urgent referral should be regardless of *H. pylori* status if there is *dyspepsia* plus any one of chronic GI bleeding, dysphagia, progressive unintentional weight loss, persistent vomiting, iron-deficiency anaemia, epigastric mass, or suspicious barium meal result. *Also:* • Isolated dysphagia; • Unexplained upper abdominal pain and weight loss, with or without back pain; • Upper abdominal mass without dyspepsia; • Obstructive jaundice; • Consider referral in vomiting or iron deficiency anaemia with weight loss, or in dyspepsia with Barrett's oesophagus, dysplasia, atrophic gastritis or old (>20yrs ago) peptic ulcer surgery. ►*For endoscopy:* those over 55 with persistent unexplained recent onset dyspepsia.

Lower gastrointestinal If there are equivocal symptoms and you are not anxious, it is reasonable to watch and wait. Do PR examination and FBC in all. • Over 40 with PR bleeding *and* bowel habit change (more loose/frequent >6 weeks); • Any age with a right lower abdominal mass likely to be bowel; • Palpable rectal mass; • Men or non-menstruating women with unexplained iron-deficiency anaemia and Hb less than 11 or 10 respectively. ►*High-risk groups:* Ulcerative colitis; it is unproven whether a family history of colon cancer assists decisions in symptomatic patients (p524).

Breast • Discrete, hard lump with fixation; • Over 30 with a discrete lump persisting after a period or presenting post-menopause; • Under 30 with an enlarging lump, fixed and hard lump, or family history; • Previous breast cancer with a new lump or suspicious symptoms; • Unilateral eczematous skin or nipple change unresponsive to topical treatment; • Recent nipple distortion; • Spontaneous bloody unilateral nipple discharge; • Men over 50 with a unilateral firm subareolar mass; • Consider referral if under 30 with a lump or persistent breast pain.

Gynaecology • Examination suggestive of cervical cancer (don't wait for a smear test); • Postmenopausal bleeding in non-HRT patients or those on HRT after 6 weeks cessation; • Vulval lump or bleeding; • Consider in persistent intermenstrual bleeding. ►*Ultrasound:* any abdominal or pelvic mass not GI or urological in origin. Do pelvic and abdominal examinations, with speculum as appropriate.

Urology • Hard irregular prostate (refer with PSA result); • Normal prostate but raised PSA (p538) and urinary symptoms; • Painless macroscopic haematuria at any age; • Over 40 with persistent or recurrent UTI and haematuria; • Over 50 with unexplained microscopic haematuria; • Any abdominal mass arising from the urinary tract; • Swelling or mass in the body of the testis; • Ulceration or mass in the penis.

Central nervous system • New onset cranial nerve palsy or unilateral sensorineural deafness (p467); • Recent-onset headaches with features of raised intracranial pressure (eg vomiting, drowsiness, posture-related headache, pulse-synchronous tinnitus; p460) or other CNS symptoms; • A new and different unexplained headache of progressive severity; • Recent-onset seizures; • Consider in rapid progression of subacute focal deficit, unexplained cognitive impairment, or personality change with features indicative of a tumour.

Haematological p346; ***Thyroid*** p602.

Is the energy we expend in speeding up referrals paying off?

Possibly not. There is evidence that reducing breast cancer waits from a few months to a few weeks is helpful—but there is little evidence that a few weeks here or there make any difference in colon and other cancers.[44] There are problems with the guidelines in that patients can meet national criteria and still be deemed 'inappropriate' by the consultant, while patients not meeting the criteria can present with suspicious signs—but they will not be seen soon because these possibly less serious cases are forced to jump the queue. This is just one example of the aphorism that *all targets distort clinical priorities.*

In one NHS trust ~66% of referrals for suspected cancer of breast, skin, and colon were deemed appropriate, and 80-100% of gynaecological, upper GI, lung, and urological cancer referrals were judged appropriate.[45]

Studies of how well dermatology cancer guidelines work conclude that the best way forward is by education regarding recognition of benign conditions.[46] It also seems likely that dialogue between local consultants and referring GPs is a key factor—and that this dialogue will become harder and less coherent as current moves for 'choose and book' and patient-choice agendas lead to referrals over ever wider geographical areas.

On the good side, establishing clear referral responsibilities forces everyone to look at what they are doing—and this has facilitated many care pathways.

▶Tumour markers are rarely sufficiently specific to be of diagnostic value. Their main value is in monitoring the course of an illness and the effectiveness of treatment.

Alpha-fetoprotein (AFP) ↑ in hepatocellular carcinoma (p270), germ cell tumours (not pure seminoma). *Also:* hepatitis, cirrhosis, pregnancy, open neural-tube defects.

CA 125 Raised in carcinoma of the ovary, uterus, breast, and hepatocellular carcinoma. *Also:* pregnancy, cirrhosis, and peritonitis.

CA 15-3 Raised in carcinoma of the breast and benign breast disease.

CA 19-9 Raised in colorectal and pancreatic carcinoma, and cholestasis.

CA 27-29 Raised in breast carcinoma, with better sensitivity and specificity than CA 15-3, being raised in ⅓ women with early breast cancer.

Carcino-embryonic antigen (CEA) Raised in gastrointestinal neoplasms, especially colorectal CA. Also cirrhosis, pancreatitis, and smoking.

Human epidermal growth factor receptor 2 (HER-2/NEU) Over-expression of the HER-2 gene in breast cancer carries a worse prognosis, but may be targeted with the monoclonal antibody trastuzumab (Herceptin). *Also:* ovarian, stomach & uterine ca.

Human chorionic gonadotrophin (β-HCG) Raised in pregnancy and germ cell tumours. For hydatidiform moles and choriocarcinoma, see *OHCS* p264.

Neuron-specific enolase (NSE) ↑ in small-cell lung cancer and neuroblastoma.

Monoclonal immunoglobulins Seen in multiple myeloma.

Placental alkaline phosphatase (PLAP) ↑ in pregnancy, seminoma, smoking.

Prostate specific antigen (PSA)

As well as being a marker of prostate cancer, PSA is (unfortunately) raised in benign prostatic hyperplasia. See p647 for advising men who ask for a PSA test. 25% of large benign prostates give PSA up to 10 µg/L. PSA may also be raised if: • BMI <25 (22% ↑ compared with BMI >35);[48] • Black Africans; • Taller men; • Recent ejaculation (avoid for 24h prior to measurement); • Recent rectal examination (usually insignificant); • Prostatitis; • UTI (PSA levels may not return to baseline for some months after a UTI).[49] Plasma reference interval is age specific; an example of the top end of the reference interval for total PSA is:

Healthy males, by age (yrs)	PSA µg/L
40-49	2.5
50-59	3.5
60-69	5.0
70-79	6.5
80-89	7.5

The above is a rough guide; reference ranges and populations vary. More specific assays, such as free PSA/total PSA index and PSA density, are also available, which may partly solve these problems. It is shown to illustrate the common problem of interpreting a PSA of ~8—and as a warning against casual requests for PSAs in the (vain) hope of simple answers. The following indicates the proportion of patients with a raised PSA and benign hypertrophy or carcinoma.

	PSA, µg/L	
Benign prostatic hyperplasia	<4 in 91%	PSA will be ~50% lower after 6 months on 5α reductase inhibitors (to ↓prostate size, see p644)
	4-10 in 8%	
	>10 in 1%	
Prostate carcinoma	<4 in 15%	
	4-10 in 20%	
	>10 in 65%	

Antineuronal antibody-associated paraneoplastic disorders

Paraneoplastic syndromes are rare, fascinating, non-metastatic manifestations of malignancy mediated by hormones, cytokines, or antibodies. Their importance is that they often pre-date symptoms associated with the cancer itself. Some antibody-mediated paraneoplastic syndromes are listed below.

Antibody	Neuronal reactivity	Protein antigens	Cloned genes	Tumour	Paraneoplastic symptoms
Anti-Hu	Nucleus > cytoplasm (all neurons)	35-40 kDa	HuD, HuC, Nel-N1	Small cell lung neuroblastoma, sarcoma, prostate	Encephalomyelitis sensory neuropathy, cerebellar degeneration
Anti-Yo	Cytoplasm Purkinje cells	34, 36 kDa	CDR34, CDR62	Ovary, breast, lung	Cerebellar degeneration
Anti-Ri	Nucleus > cytoplasm (CNS neurons)	55, 80 kDa	Nova	Breast, gynae, lung, bladder	Ataxia, opsoclonus[1]
Anti-Tr	Cytoplasm Purkinje cells	?	–	Hodgkin's disease	Cerebellar degeneration
Anti-VGCC[2]	Presynaptic neuromuscular junction	64 kDa	P/Q type MysB	small cell lung cancer	Lambert-Eaton myasthenic syn (p516)
Anti-retinal	Photoreceptor ganglion cells	23, 65, 145, 205 kDa	Recoverin	Small cell lung ca, melanoma, gynae cancers	Cancer- & myeloma-associated retinopathy
Anti-amphiphysin	Presynaptic	128 kDa	Amphiphysin	Breast, small cell lung ca	Stiff-person syn, encephalitis
Anti-CRMP5 (Anti-CV2)	Oligodendrocytes, neurons, cytoplasm	66 kDa	CRMP5 (POP66)	Small cell lung ca, thymoma	Encephalomyelitis, cerebellar degeneration, chorea, sensory neuropathy
Anti-PCA2	Purkinje cytoplasm and other neurons	280 kDa		Small cell lung cancer	Encephalomyelitis cerebellar degen, Lambert-Eaton
Anti-Ma1	Neurons (subnucleus)	40 kDa	Ma1	Lung, others	Brainstem
Anti-Ma2	Neurons (subnucleus)	41.5 kDa	Ma2	Testis	Limbic brainstem encephalitis
ANNA3	Nuclei, Purkinje cells	170 kDa		Lung cancer	Sensory neuropathy, encephalomyelitis

Data from the *OTM*

1 *Opsoclonus* entails continuous arrhythmic, multidirectional, involuntary, high-amplitude conjugate saccades ± synchronous blinking ± myoclonus of trunk, limbs, head ± ataxia.
2 Voltage-gated Ca^{2+} channels.

Contents

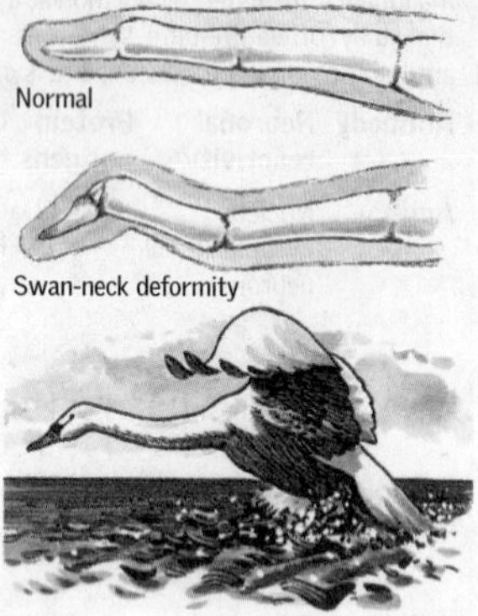

Fig 1. Swan-neck finger deformity.

We like to see our rheumatology patients before destructive changes take place. Rheumatic disease can present a baffling array of symptoms, however, and so the skill of the rheumatologist is to be able to stand back and see the whole from a different angle (**fig 2**). This greatest of clinical skills belongs not only in making a diagnosis, but also in understanding the relationship between patient and disease. The swan is famously mute, and serene, just as our most afflicted patients can appear so serene when we see them in our clinics, stoically bearing the arthritic agony of daily life. But when you see painted fingernails at the end of swan-neck fingers (**fig 1**), remember the great effort the swan must make to take flight:

"What time did you get up to get ready?"

"Who helped you get dressed?"

"And that nail-varnish! Surely you need help with that?"

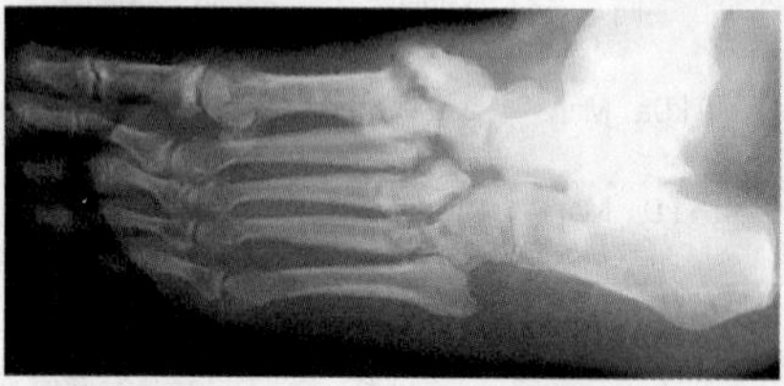

Fig 2. An oblique view of Charcot's foot (p520) with destroyed tarso-metatarsal joints, terminal osteolysis, and fracture & dislocation of fragments. Also loss of foot arch (pes planus).

Relevant pages elsewhere: Cervical spondylosis (p512); Charcot's joints (**fig 2** & p520); osteoporosis (p696); Behçet's disease (p708); Sjögren's syndrome (p724); Wegener's granulomatosis (p728). ***Orthopaedics:*** *OHCS* chapter 11.

We thank Dr Nigel Cox who is our Specialist Reader for this chapter.

Some points to note in a rheumatological history

In the assessment of an arthritic presentation, pay particular attention to the distribution of joint involvement (including spine) and the presence of symmetry. Also look for disruption of joint anatomy, limitation of movement (by pain or contracture), joint effusions and peri-articular involvement (see p542 for a fuller assessment). Ask about, and examine for, ***extra-articular features:*** skin and nail involvement (include scalp, hairline, umbilicus, genitalia, and natal cleft—psoriasis can easily be missed); eye signs (see p562); lungs (eg fibrosis); kidneys; heart; GI (eg mouth ulcers, diarrhoea); GU (eg urethritis, genital ulcers); and CNS.

3 screening questions for musculo-skeletal disease:

1 Are you free of any pain or stiffness?
2 Can you dress alright?
3 Can you manage stairs?

If *yes* to all 3, muscle/joint problems are unlikely.

Presenting symptoms:
- Pattern of involved joints
- Symmetry (or not)
- Morning stiffness >30min (eg RA)
- Pain, swelling, loss of function, erythema, warmth

Extra-articular features:
- Rashes, photosensitivity (eg SLE)
- Raynaud's (SLE; CREST; polymyositis and dermatomyositis)
- Dry eyes or mouth (Sjögren's)
- Red eyes, iritis (eg ank. spond.)
- Diarrhoea/urethritis (Reiter's)
- Nodules or nodes (eg RA; TB; gout)
- Mouth/genital ulcers (eg Behçet's)
- Weight loss (eg malignancy, any systemic inflammatory disease)

Related diseases:
- Crohn's/UC (in ankylosing spondylitis), gonorrhoea, psoriasis

Current & past drugs:
- NSAIDs, disease modifying drugs (p533)

Family history:
- Arthritis, psoriasis, autoimmune disease

Social history:
- Age
- Occupation
- Ethnicity (eg SLE is commoner in Afro-Caribbeans and Asians)
- Ability to function eg dressing, grooming, writing, walking
- Domestic situation, social support, home adaptations
- Smoking (may worsen RA)

Patterns of presentation of arthritis

Monoarthritis	Oligoarthritis (≤5 joints)	Polyarthritis (>5 joints involved)	
		Symmetrical:	*Asymmetrical:*
Septic arthritis	Crystal arthritis	Rheumatoid arthritis	Reactive arthritis
Crystal arthritis (gout, CPPD)	Psoriatic arthritis	Osteoarthritis	Psoriatic arthritis
Osteoarthritis	Reactive arthritis, eg *Yersinia, Salmonella, Campylobacter*	Viruses (eg hepatitis A, B & C; mumps)	
Trauma, eg haemarthrosis	Ankylosing spondylitis	Systemic conditions[1] (can be either)	
	Osteoarthritis		

▸▸Exclude septic arthritis in any acutely inflamed joint, as it can destroy a joint in under 24h (p546). Inflammation may be less overt if immunocompromised (eg steroids) or if there is underlying joint disease. Joint aspiration (p543) is the key investigation, and if you are unable to do it, find someone who can.

1 Connective tissue disease (eg SLE & relapsing polychondritis), sarcoidosis, malignancy (eg leukaemia), endocarditis, haemochromatosis, sickle-cell anaemia, familial Mediterranean fever, Behçet's.

Assessing the locomotor system

This aims to screen for most rheumatological conditions, and to assess motor disability. It is based on the GALS locomotor screen (Gait, Arms, Legs, Spine).

Essence 'Look, feel and move' (active and passive). If a joint *looks normal* to you, *feels normal* to the patient, and has *full range of movement*, it usually *is* normal. Make sure the patient is comfortable, and obtain their consent before examination. The GALS screening examination should be done in light underwear.

Spine: Observe from behind: Is muscle bulk normal (buttocks, shoulders)? Is the spine straight? Symmetrical paraspinal muscles? Swellings/deformities? *Observe from the side:* Normal cervical and lumbar lordosis? Kyphosis? *"Touch your toes, please":* Is lumbar spine flexion normal, eg Schober's test?[1] *Observe from in front* from now on. *"Tilt head towards shoulders"* (without moving the shoulders): is lateral neck flexion normal? Palpate for typical fibromyalgia tender points (see p560).

Arms: "Try putting your hands behind head"—tests functional shoulder movement. *"Arms straight"*—tests elbow extension and forearm supination/pronation. *Examine the hands*: See p32. Any deformity, wasting, or swellings? *Squeeze across 2nd–5th metacarpophalangeal joints. Repeat for metatarsophalangeal (MTP) joints.* Pain may denote joint or tendon synovitis. *"Put index finger on thumb"*—tests pincer grip. Assess dexterity.

Legs: Observe legs: Normal quadriceps bulk? Any swelling or deformity or length discrepancy? *Internally/externally rotate each hip in flexion.* Passively flex knee and hip to the full extent. Is movement limited? Any crepitus? *Find any knee effusion:* With patient supine, do the patella tap test. If there is fluid, consider aspirating and testing it for crystals or infection. *Observe feet:* Any deformity? Are arches high or flat? Any callosities? These may indicate an abnormal gait of some chronicity. *MTP squeeze:* see above. Also: although not in the GALS system, palpation of the heel and Achilles tendon is useful for identifying the plantar fasciitis and Achilles tendonitis often associated with seronegative rheumatological conditions.

Gait: "Walk over there please": Is the gait smooth? Good arm swing? Stride length OK? Normal heel strike and toe off? Can he turn quickly?

The GALS system for quickly recording your findings

G (Gait)	✓	
	Appearance:	*Movement:*
A (Arms)	✓	✓
L (Legs)	✓	✓
S (Spine)	✓	✓

✓ means normal. If not normal, then put a cross with a note to explain what the exact problem is.

Range of joint movement is noted in degrees, with anatomical position being the neutral position—eg elbow flexion 0°–150° normally, but with fixed flexion and limited movement, range may be reduced to 30°–90°. A valgus deformity deviates laterally (away from mid-line); a varus deformity points towards.

1 **Schober's test:** make a mark on the lumbar spine at the level of the posterior iliac spine. Measure out a line from 5cm below to 10cm above the mark. Ask the patient to bend forward as far as they can. If the line does not lengthen by at least 5cm, there is reduced lumbar flexion eg in ankylosing spondylitis.

Some important rheumatological investigations

Joint aspiration is the most important investigation in any monoarthritic presentation (see also OHCS p708). Send synovial fluid for urgent white cell count, Gram stain, polarized light microscopy (for crystals, p550) and culture. The risk of inducing septic arthritis, using sterile precautions, is <1:10,000. Look for blood, pus, and crystals (gout or CPPD crystal arthropathy; p550).

Synovial fluid in health and disease

	Appearance	*Viscosity*	*WBC/mm³*	*Neutrophils*
Normal	Clear, colourless	↔	≤200	None
Osteoarthritis	Clear, straw	↑	≤1000	≤50%
Haemorrhagic[1]	Bloody, xanthochromic	Varies	≤10,000	≤50%
Acutely inflamed:				
• *RA*	Turbid, yellow	↓	1-50,000	Varies
• *Crystal*	Turbid, yellow	↓	5-50,000	~80%
Septic	Turbid, yellow	↓	10-100,000	>90%

Blood tests FBC, ESR, urate, U&E, CRP. Blood culture for septic arthritis. Consider rheumatoid factor, antinuclear antibody, other autoantibodies (p555), and HLA B27 (p552) guided by presentation. Consider causes of reactive arthritis (p552), eg viral serology, urine chlamydia PCR, hepatitis and HIV serology if risk factors are present.

Radiology Look for erosions, calcification, widening or loss of joint space, changes in underlying bone of affected joints (eg periarticular osteopenia, sclerotic areas, osteophytes). Characteristic features for various arthritides are shown in **figs 1-3**. Irregularity of the lower half of the sacroiliac joints is seen in spondyloarthritis. Ultrasound and MRI are more sensitive in identifying effusions, synovitis, enthesitis and infection than plain radiographs—discuss further investigations with your radiologist. Do a CXR for RA, SLE, vasculitis, TB and sarcoid.

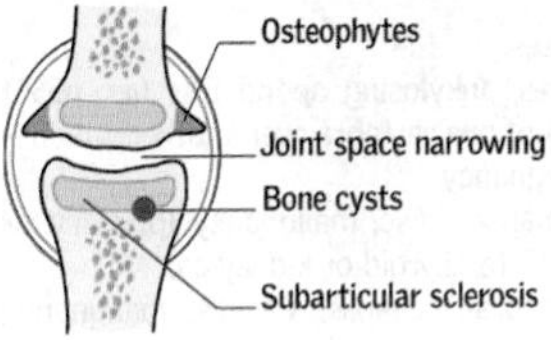

Fig 1. Imaging in osteoarthritis

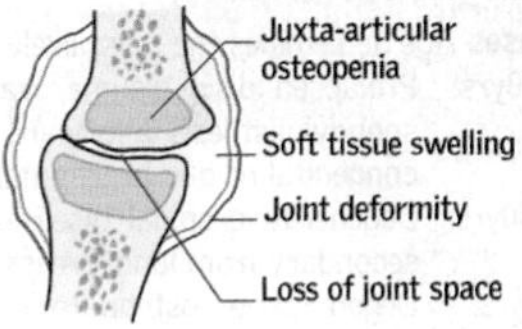

Fig 2. Imaging in rheumatoid arthritis

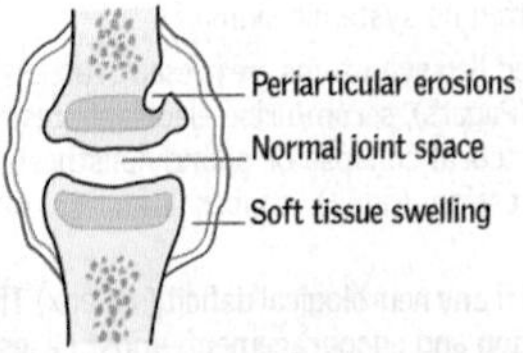

Fig 3. Imaging in gout

1 Eg trauma, tumour or haemophilia.

Back pain

Back pain is very common, and often self-limiting, but *be alert to sinister causes,* ie malignancy, infection or inflammatory causes. See below for red-flag symptoms, and BOX opposite for neurosurgical emergencies.

Red flags for sinister causes of back pain

- ►Aged <20yrs or >55yrs old
- ►Acute onset in elderly people
- ►Constant or progressive pain
- ►Nocturnal pain
- ►Worse pain on being supine
- ►Fever, night sweats, weight loss
- ►History of malignancy
- ►Abdominal mass
- ►Thoracic back pain
- ►Morning stiffness
- ►Bilateral or alternating leg pain
- ►Neurological disturbance (incl sciatica)
- ►Sphincter disturbance
- ►Current or recent infection
- ►Immunosuppression, eg steroids/HIV
- ►Leg claudication or exercise-related leg weakness/numbness (spinal stenosis)

Examination:

1 With the patient standing, gauge the extent and smoothness of lumbar forward/lateral flexion and extension (see p542).

2 Clinical tests for sacroiliitis: direct pressure, lateral compression, sacroiliac stretch test (pain on adduction of the hip, with the hip and knee flexed).

3 Neurological deficits (see BOX): test lower limb sensation, power, and deep tendon and plantar reflexes. Digital rectal examination for perianal tone and sensation.

4 Examine for nerve root pain: this is distributed in relevant dermatomes, and is worsened by coughing or bending forward. *Straight leg test* (L4, L5, S1): positive if raising the leg with the knee extended causes pain below the knee, which increases on foot dorsiflexion (Lasègue's sign). It suggests irritation to the sciatic nerve. The main cause is lumbar disc prolapse. Also *femoral stretch test* (L4 and above): pain in front of thigh on lifting the hip into extension with the patient lying face downwards and the knee flexed.

5 Signs of generalized disease—malignancy? Examine other systems (eg abdomen) as pain may be referred.

Causes Age determines the most likely causes:

15-30yrs: Prolapsed disc, trauma, fractures, ankylosing spondylitis (AS; p552), spondylolisthesis (a forward shift of one vertebra over another, which is congenital or due to trauma), pregnancy.

30-50yrs: Degenerative spinal disease, prolapsed disc, malignancy (primary or secondary from lung, breast, prostate, thyroid or kidney ca).

>50yrs: Degenerative, osteoporotic vertebral collapse, Paget's, malignancy, myeloma, spinal stenosis.

Rarer: Cauda equina tumours, spinal infection (eg discitis, usually staphylococcal but also *Proteus, E. coli, S. typhi* & TB—there are often no systemic signs).

Investigations are usually only necessary if red flag symptoms are present: FBC, ESR & CRP (myeloma, infection, tumour), U&E, ALP (Paget's), serum/urine electrophoresis (myeloma), PSA. *X-rays* may show Paget's, vertebral collapse or spondylolisthesis. *MRI* is best for disc prolapse, cord compression (**fig 1**), cancer, infection or inflammation (eg sacroiliitis).

Management: ►►Urgent neurosurgical referral if any neurological deficit (see BOX). If there is no serious pathology, focus on **education** and encouragement—most cases are self-limiting. Address **psychosocial issues**, which may predispose to developing chronic pain and disability (see p561). **Analgesia** (regular paracetamol ± NSAIDs ± codeine) and returning to normal activities as soon as possible is better than bed rest (which should not be advised).[5] Avoid precipitants and refer to **physiotherapy** if not improving. Local injections, eg facet joints, may help. Surgical options may be considered in selected patients with intractable symptoms who fail to respond to other measures. There is no evidence that antidepressants are of benefit.[6]

Neurosurgical emergencies

(see also p470)

- ►*Acute cauda equina compression:* Alternating or bilateral root pain in legs, saddle anaesthesia (perianal), loss of anal tone on PR, bladder ± bowel incontinence.
- ►*Acute cord compression:* Bilateral pain, LMN signs at level of compression, UMN and sensory loss below, sphincter disturbance.
- ►*Immediate urgent treatment* prevents irreversible loss, eg laminectomy for disc protrusions, radiotherapy for tumours, decompression for abscesses.
- ►*Causes* (same for both): bony metastasis (look for missing pedicle on X-ray), large disc protrusion, myeloma, cord or paraspinal tumour, TB (p398), abscess.

Nerve root lesions

Nerve root	Pain	Weakness	Reflex affected
L2	Across upper thigh	Hip flexion and adduction	Nil
L3	Across lower thigh	Hip adduction, knee extension	Knee jerk
L4	Across knee to medial malleolus	Knee extension, foot inversion and dorsiflexion	Knee jerk
L5	Lateral shin to dorsum of foot and great toe	Hip extension and abduction Knee flexion Foot and great toe dorsiflexion	Great toe jerk
S1	Posterior calf to lateral foot and little toe	Knee flexion Foot and toe plantar flexion Foot eversion	Ankle jerk

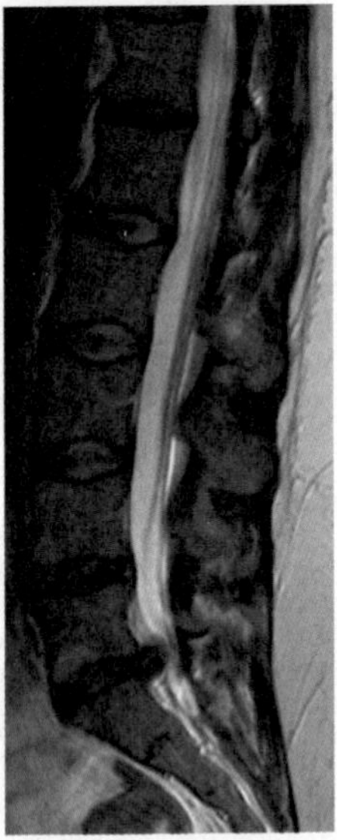

Fig 1. Sagittal T2 weighted MRI of the lumbar spine showing a herniated L5–S1 disc.

Courtesy of Norwich Radiology Department

Osteoarthritis (OA) is the commonest joint condition. ♀:♂≈3:1, onset typically >50yrs. It is usually primary (generalized), but may be secondary to joint disease or other conditions (eg haemochromatosis, obesity, occupational).

Signs & symptoms *Localised disease* (usually knee or hip): pain on movement and crepitus, worse at end of day; background pain at rest; joint gelling—stiffness after rest up to ~30mins; joint instability. *Generalised disease* (primary OA): with Heberden's nodes ('nodal OA', seen mainly in post-menopausal ♀), commonly affected joints are the DIP joints, thumb carpo-metacarpal joints and the knees. There may be joint tenderness, derangement and bony swelling (Heberden's nodes at DIP, Bouchard's nodes at PIP), ↓range of movement and mild synovitis.

Investigations Plain radiographs show loss of joint space, subchondral sclerosis and cysts, and marginal osteophytes (see **fig 1** on p543). CRP may be slightly elevated.[7]

Management Do exercises to improve muscle strength and joint stability (eg quadriceps exercises in knee OA, hydrotherapy in hip OA) and keep active. Regular paracetamol ± codeine for pain. Consider NSAIDs only if paracetamol ineffective (see BOX). Weight loss if BMI>28, walking aids, supportive footwear, physio, topical NSAIDs and capsaicin (derived from chillies) may help. Intra-articular steroid injections help severe symptoms temporarily. Joint replacement is the best way to deal with severe OA. The role of hyaluronic acid injections is unclear. Glucosamine & chondroitin sulfate 'failed' a 2006 *NEJM* trial.[8]

Septic arthritis

▸▸Consider septic arthritis in any acutely inflamed joint, as it can destroy a joint in under 24h. Inflammation may be less overt if immunocompromised (eg steroids) or if there is underlying joint disease.

Risk factors Pre-existing joint disease (especially rheumatoid arthritis); diabetes mellitus, immunosuppression, chronic renal failure, prosthetic joints (where infection is particularly difficult to treat).[9]

Investigations Urgent joint aspiration for synovial fluid microscopy and culture is the key investigation (p543), as plain radiographs and CRP may be normal. The main differential diagnoses are the crystal arthropathies (p550). Blood cultures may be helpful for guiding antibiotic choice later.

Ask yourself "How did the organism get there?" Is there immunosuppression, or another focus of infection (eg pneumonia is present in up to 50% of those with pneumococcal arthritis)?[10]

Treatment If in doubt, start empirical IV antibiotics until sensitivities are known. Common causative organisms are *Staph. aureus*, streps, *Neisseria gonococcus* and Gram -ve bacilli, thus: **flucloxacillin** 0.5-1g/6h IV (or vancomycin if MRSA); cefotaxime for Gram -ve organisms (p379). If HIV +ve, look for atypical mycobacteria and fungi. Ask a microbiologist how long to continue treatment (eg ≥2 weeks IV, then 4 weeks PO).[11] Ask for orthopaedic advice for consideration of arthrocentesis, lavage and debridement, especially if there is a prosthetic joint involved.[12] This may be done arthroscopically (eg for knee) or open under GA (eg for hip; this allows for biopsy—helpful in TB). Splint for ≤48h; then give physiotherapy.

Prescribing NSAIDs: dialogue with patients

NSAIDs cause ~1000 deaths/yr in the UK[13] so only use after risk-benefit analysis individualized for each patient, including indication, dose, proposed duration of use, and comorbidity. The main serious side effects are GI bleeding and renal impairment. NSAIDs are also contraindicated in severe heart failure.

Major risk factors for NSAID SEs ↑age, polypharmacy, history of peptic ulcers, renal impairment (review before *and after* starting therapy, as NSAIDs can cause renal impairment and exacerbate existing impairment), smoking, alcohol excess.

Inform your patients Many patients prescribed NSAIDs do not need them all the time, so say "Take the lowest possible dose for the shortest possible time". *Bleeding is more common in those who know less about their drugs.*[14] Explain:

- Drugs are to relieve symptoms: on good days, don't take any. In rheumatoid arthritis, cod liver oil (eg 10g/d) reduces reliance on NSAIDs by 30%.[15]
- Abdominal pain may be a sign of impending gut problems: stop the tablets, and come back for more advice if symptoms continue.
- Ulcers may occur with no warning: report black motions (± faints) at once.
- Don't supplement prescribed NSAIDs with ones bought over the counter (eg ibuprofen): mixing NSAIDs can increase risks 20-fold.
- Smoking and alcohol increase NSAID risk.

When should COX-2 selective NSAIDs be tried? Not often: perhaps *only* when an NSAID is essential *and* there is past peptic ulceration (but risk is not eliminated, and bleeds that do occur may be very serious) *if* an ordinary NSAID with PPI (eg omeprazole) is problematic *or* >65yrs old (not on aspirin) *or* needing high-dose NSAID over a long time. If at very high risk of GI bleed, combine a COX-2 (eg celecoxib 200mg/12h; avoid if eGFR <30) with a PPI.[16]

COX-2 (cyclo-oxygenase-2) selective NSAIDs are not as safe as we had hoped. There is ↑ risk of heart failure, MI & stroke.[17] This ↑ risk may also apply to conventional NSAIDs.[18] So avoid if known renal failure or vascular disease (past MI or stroke). There is insufficient experience with newer COX-2 selective inhibitors (etoricoxib, parecoxib) to recommend their use as 1st-line COX-2 agents.[19]

RA is a chronic systemic inflammatory disease, characterised by a symmetrical, deforming, peripheral polyarthritis. ***Epidemiology:*** Prevalence is ~1% (↑ in smokers). ♀:♂ >2:1. Peak onset: 5th–6th decade. HLA DR4/DR1 linked (associated with ↑ severity).

Presentation *Typically:* symmetrical swollen, painful, and stiff small joints of hands & feet, worse in the morning. This can fluctuate and larger joints may become involved. *Less common presentations:* • Sudden onset, widespread arthritis; • Recurring mono/polyarthritis of various joints (*palindromic RA*);[1] • Persistent monoarthritis (often knee, shoulder or hip); • Systemic illness with extra-articular symptoms, eg fatigue, fever, weight loss, pericarditis and pleurisy, but initially few joint problems (commoner in ♂); • Polymyalgic onset—vague limb girdle aches; • Recurrent soft tissue problems (eg frozen shoulder, carpal tunnel syndrome, de Quervain's tenosynovitis).

Signs *Early* (inflammation, no joint damage): swollen MCP, PIP, wrist, or MTP joints (often symmetrical). Look for tenosynovitis or bursitis. *Later* (joint damage, deformity): ulnar deviation of the fingers and dorsal wrist subluxation. Boutonnière and swan-neck deformities of fingers (**fig 1** on p540) or Z-deformity of thumbs occur (**fig 1**). Hand extensor tendons may rupture. Foot changes are similar. Larger joints can be involved. Atlanto-axial joint subluxation may threaten the spinal cord.

Extra-articular Nodules—elbows & lungs; lymphadenopathy; vasculitis; fibrosing alveolitis, obliterative bronchiolitis; pleural & pericardial effusion; Raynaud's; carpal tunnel syndrome; peripheral neuropathy; splenomegaly (seen in 5%; only 1% have Felty's syndrome: RA + splenomegaly + neutropenia, see p712); episcleritis, scleritis, scleromalacia, keratoconjunctivitis sicca (p562); osteoporosis; amyloidosis (p364).

Investigations Rheumatoid factor (RhF) is positive in ~70% (p555). A high titre is associated with severe disease, erosions and extra-articular disease. Anti-cyclic citrullinated peptide antibodies (anti-CCP) are highly specific (~98%) for RA. There is often anaemia of chronic disease. Inflammation causes ↑platelets, ↑ESR, ↑CRP. ***X-rays*** show soft tissue swelling, juxta-articular osteopenia and ↓joint space. Later there may be bony erosions, subluxation or complete carpal destruction (see **fig 2** on p543). Ultrasound and MRI can identify synovitis more accurately, and have greater sensitivity in detecting bone erosions than conventional X-rays.[20]

Diagnostic criteria 4 out of 7 of: Morning stiffness (>1 hour lasting >6 weeks), arthritis of ≥3 joints, arthritis of hand joints, symmetrical arthritis, rheumatoid nodules, +ve rheumatoid factor and radiographic changes.[21]

Management ►Refer early to a rheumatologist (before irreversible destruction).
- Disease activity is measured using the DAS28.[2] Aim to reduce score to <3.
- Early use of **DMARDs** and **biological agents** improves long-term outcomes (see BOX).
- **Steroids** rapidly reduce symptoms and inflammation, but avoid giving until seen by a rheumatologist as they mask symptoms and impede diagnosis. They are useful for treating acute exacerbations ('flares') of disease, eg with IM depot injections of methylprednisolone 80–120mg. Intra-articular steroids have a rapid but short-term effect (*OHCS* p708–711). Oral steroids (eg prednisolone 7.5mg/d) may control difficult symptoms, but side effects preclude routine long term use.
- **NSAIDs** are good for symptom relief, but have no effect on disease progression. Paracetamol and weak opiates are rarely effective. One cannot predict which NSAID a patient will respond to, so try several eg ibuprofen, diclofenac, etodolac (see p547).
- Encourage regular exercise; physio- and occupational therapy, eg for aids, splints.
- Surgery (eg ulna stylectomy, joint prosthesis) may relieve pain and improve function.
- There is ↑ risk of cardiovascular and cerebrovascular disease, as atherosclerosis is accelerated in RA. Manage risk factors (p87). Smoking also ↑ symptoms of RA.

1 *Palin dromo* is Greek for 'I run to and fro' or 'I recur'. In rheumatological palindromes, arthritis lasting hours or days runs to and fro, visiting and revisiting 3 or more sites, typically knees, wrists, & MCP joints. It may presage RA, SLE, Whipple's, or Behçet's disease. Remissions are (initially) complete, leaving no radiological mark.

2 28-joint Disease Activity Score—assesses tenderness & swelling at 28 joints (MCPs, PIPs, wrists, elbows, shoulders, knees), ESR and patient's self-reported symptom severity using a 100-point visual analogue score (VAS). DAS28 = $0.555\times\sqrt{(\text{tender joints})} + 0.284\times\sqrt{(\text{swollen joints})} + 0.7\times\log_n(\text{ESR}) + 0.0142\times\text{VAS}$.

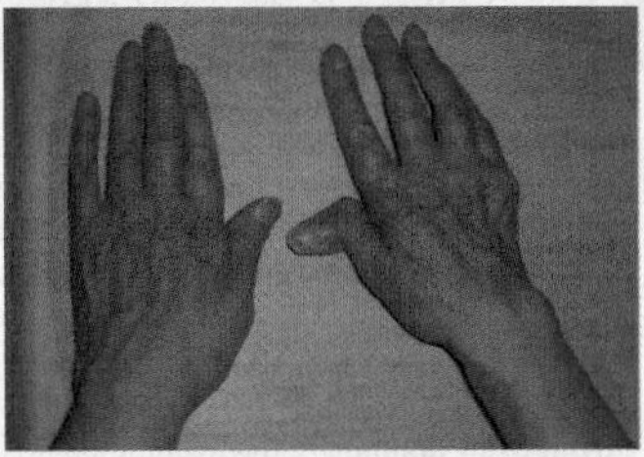

Fig 1. Z-deformity at the interphalangeal joint of the right thumb in RA. Note swelling of the right MCP joints and 'guttering' between the right extensor tendons over the metacarpals, denoting a little wasting of the small muscles of the hand (interossei and lumbricals).

Image courtesy of Thomas Jaconelli.

Influencing biological events in RA

The chief biological event is inflammation. Monocytes traffic into joints, cytokines are produced, fibroblasts and endothelial cells are activated, and tissue proliferates. Fluid is generated (effusion) and cytokines and cellular processes erode cartilage and bone. Tumour necrosis factor α (TNFα) and interleukins 1 & 6 (IL-1, IL-6) are cytokines over-produced in RA synovium, and are the site of action of the new generation of biological (monoclonal antibody) agents. Cytokines also produce the systemic effects seen in RA: fatigue, accelerated atherosclerosis, and accelerated bone turnover.

Disease-modifying anti-rheumatic drugs (DMARDs; non-biological agents) DMARDs are first-line for treating RA. Early DMARD therapy is associated with better long-term prognosis. They can take 6-12 weeks for symptomatic benefit. Best results are often achieved with a combination of **methotrexate**, **sulfasalazine** and **hydroxychloroquine**.[23] Other DMARDs that may be tried include **leflunomide** and IM **gold**. The role of penicillamine, azathioprine and ciclosporin is less clear.
►*Myelosuppression* (bone marrow suppression) is a potentially serious SE of DMARDs which can result in pancytopenia, with ↑susceptibility to infection and overwhelming neutropenic sepsis (p346). Regular FBC monitoring is required.[24]
Other SE: • methotrexate—pneumonitis (get urgent respiratory help), oral ulcers, hepatotoxicity (folic acid eg 5mg/48hr reduces SE); • sulfasalazine—rash, ↓sperm count, oral ulcers; • leflunomide—teratogenicity (male and female), oral ulcers, ↑BP, hepatotoxicity, diarrhoea; • hydroxychloroquine—irreversible retinopathy (check acuity annually, and refer to an ophthalmologist if deteriorating).[25]
TNFα inhibitors (AKA anti-cytokines; biological agents) **Infliximab** (chimeric murine/human anti-TNF antibody, IV every 8wks, p275), **etanercept** (TNFα receptor/IgFc fusion protein, SC twice weekly), and **adalimumab** (fully human anti-TNF monoclonal antibody, SC every 2wks) are approved by NICE for severe active RA after failure to respond to 2 DMARDs (DAS28 > 5.1).[26] Clinical response can be striking, with improved function and health outcomes. *CI:* pregnancy, breast feeding, active infection, severe heart failure (NYHA class III or IV), demyelinating disease, haematological malignancy, acute hepatitis B or C. *SE:* (Usually well tolerated) injection reaction, infections, reactivation of TB (∴ screen & consider prophylaxis), worsening of heart failure. Long-term safety is unknown (no clear evidence for ↑ risk of cancer). Neutralizing antibodies may ↓ efficacy with infliximab; ANA and reversible SLE-type illness may evolve.

Rituximab is an anti-CD20 chimeric monoclonal antibody that eliminates mature circulating B-cells. It is used in combination with methotrexate for severe active RA where TNFα blockers have failed, given as an IV infusion every 6-12 months. Due to its expense, its continuing use is recommended only where there is an improvement in DAS28 of at least 1.2.[27]

Other agents Anakinra, an IL-1 inhibitor, **toclizumab**, an anti IL-6 receptor monoclonal antibody, and **abatacept**, a selective T-cell co-stimulation modulator (cost/QALY≈£40,000, p10—so not favoured by NICE),[28] are currently being assessed (eg TOWARD, OPTION, RADIATE phase III trials). SE include ↑lipids, ↑LFTs, neutropenia, rash.

Gout typically presents with an acute monoarthropathy with severe joint inflammation (**fig 1**). ~60% occur at metatarsophalangeal joint of big toe (podagra). Other common joints are the ankle, foot, small joints of the hand, wrist, elbow or knee. It can be polyarticular. It is caused by deposition of monosodium urate crystals in and near joints, precipitated for example by trauma, surgery, starvation, infection or diuretics. It is associated with raised plasma urate. In the long-term, urate deposits (tophi, eg in pinna, tendons, joints; see **fig 2**) and renal disease (stones, interstitial nephritis) may occur. ***Prevalence:*** ~1%. ♂:♀≈5:1.

Differential diagnoses The main differentials for an acute monoarthropathy are septic arthritis (p532), haemarthrosis, pseudogout (below) and palindromic RA (p546).

Causes Hereditary, ↑dietary purines, alcohol excess, diuretics, leukaemia, cytotoxics (tumour lysis), renal impairment.

Associations Gout is often a marker for other conditions such as hypertension, ischaemic heart disease and metabolic syndrome. These should always be checked for and excluded.

Investigations Polarized light microscopy of synovial fluid shows *negatively bi-refringent* urate crystals (**fig 3**). Serum urate is usually raised but may be normal.[29] Radiographs show only soft-tissue swelling in the early stages. Later, well-defined 'punched out' erosions are seen in juxta-articular bone (see **fig 3** on p543). There is no sclerotic reaction, and joint spaces are preserved until late.

Treatment of acute gout Use a strong **NSAID** (eg diclofenac 50mg/8h PO or indometacin 50mg/8h PO—etoricoxib 120mg/d, for up to 8d, is as effective and may have fewer SEs).[30] If CI (eg peptic ulcer), use **colchicine** (0.5mg/6h PO if eGFR >50) until pain goes or D&V occurs or 6mg given. **NB:** in renal impairment, NSAIDs and colchicine are problematic. Steroids (oral, IM or intra-articular) may also be used.[31]

Prevention Lose weight. Avoid prolonged fasts, alcohol excess, purine-rich foods[1] and low-dose aspirin (↑serum urate). Use **allopurinol** (~200mg/24h; max 300mg/8h) if recurrent attacks, tophi, or renal stones. Introduction of allopurinol may trigger an attack so wait until 3 weeks after an acute episode, and cover with regular NSAID or colchicine (0.5mg/12h PO) for first 3 months. Adjust dose according to serum urate (aim <0.36mmol/L).[32] SE: rash, fever, WCC↓ (especially with azathioprine). Caution in renal impairment. Avoid stopping allopurinol in acute attacks once established on treatment. ***Uricosuric drugs*** (↑urate excretion) are rarely used (eg probenecid, available on a named-patient basis, for prevention of cidofovir nephropathy); they may precipitate urate in the kidney.

Calcium pyrophosphate dehydrate arthropathy

Acute CPPD (pseudogout) also presents as an acute monoarthropathy, similar to gout, and typically affects larger joints: knee, wrist or hip. It is usually spontaneous and self-limiting, but can be provoked by illness, surgery or trauma.

Chronic CPPD Destructive changes like OA, but more severe. It can present as a poly-arthritis (pseudo-rheumatoid).

Risk factors Old age, OA, diabetes mellitus, hypothyroidism, hyperparathyroidism, haemochromatosis, Wilson's disease, ↓PO_4^{3-}, ↓Mg^{2+}.

Investigations Polarized light microscopy of synovial fluid shows *weakly positively birefringent* crystals (**fig 4**). It is associated with chondrocalcinosis—soft tissue calcium deposition on X-ray, eg triangular ligament in wrist or in knee cartilage.

Management Analgesia, NSAIDs. If ineffective, try steroids (intra-articular, IM or PO) or hydroxychloroquine 200mg/d.[33]

1 There is a higher risk of gout with diets rich in meat (beef, pork or lamb) and seafood, but not with consumption of purine-rich vegetable protein. Low-fat dairy-rich diets give low risk. n=47150

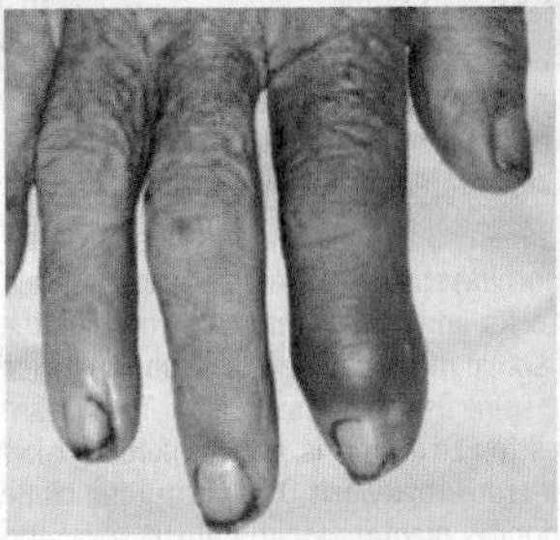

Fig 1. Acute monoarthritis in gout

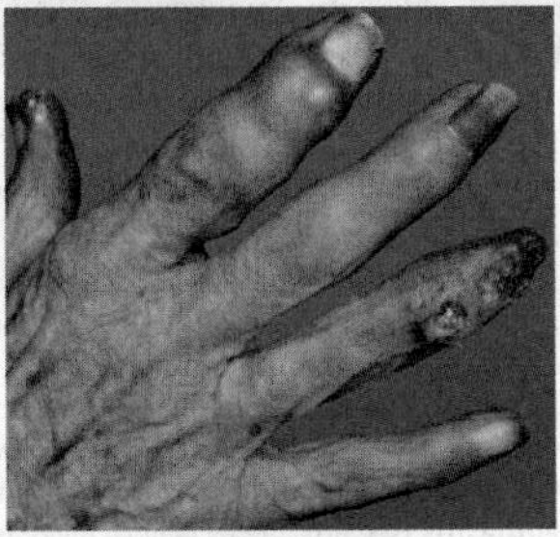

Fig 2. Ulcerated tophi in gout.

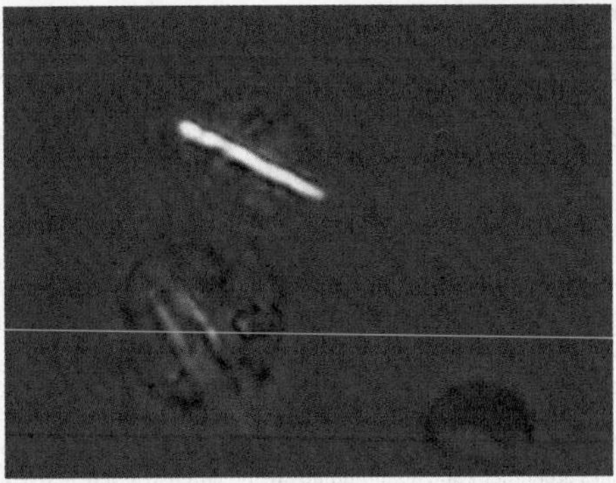

Fig 3. Needle-shaped monosodium urate crystals found in gout, displaying negative birefringence under polarised light.

Reproduced with permission from Oxford Textbook of Rheumatology. © OUP, 2004.

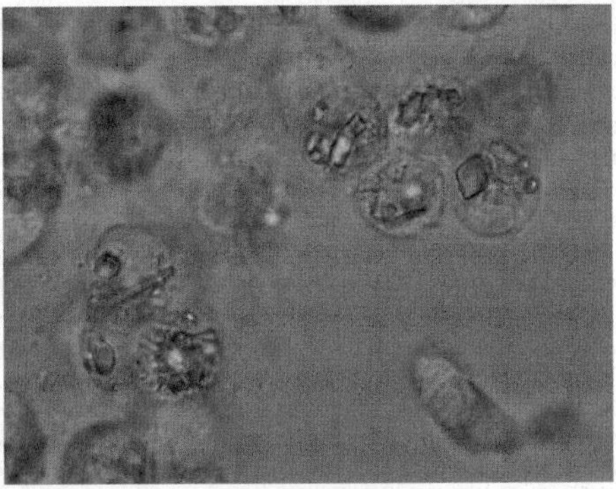

Fig 4. Rhomboid-shaped calcium pyrophosphate dihydrate crystals in pseudogout, showing positive birefringence in polarised light.

Image courtesy of Prof. Eliseo Pascual, Sección de Reumatología, Hospital General Universitario de Alicante.

1 Ankylosing spondylitis (AS) is a chronic inflammatory disease of the spine and sacroiliac joints, of unknown aetiology. *Prevalence:* 0.25–1%. *Men present earlier:* ♂:♀~6:1 at 16yrs old, and ~2:1 at 30yrs old. >95% are HLA B27 +ve.

Symptoms & signs: The typical patient is a man <30yrs old with gradual onset of low back pain, worse at night, with spinal morning stiffness relieved by exercise. Pain radiates from sacroiliac joints to hips/buttocks, and usually improves towards the end of the day. There is progressive loss of spinal movement (all directions)—hence ↓thoracic expansion. See p542–4 for tests of spine flexion and sacroiliitis. The disease course is variable. In a few, there is progression to kyphosis, neck hyperextension (question mark posture; see **fig 1**), and spino-cranial ankylosis. Other features include **enthesitis** (see BOX), especially Achilles tendonitis, plantar fasciitis, at the tibial and ischial tuberosities, and at the iliac crests. Anterior mechanical chest pain due to costochondritis and fatigue may feature. **Acute iritis** occurs in ~⅓ of patients, which may lead to blindness if untreated (but may also have occurred many years before, so enquire directly). AS is also associated with osteoporosis (common—up to 60%), aortic valve incompetence (<3%) and pulmonary apical fibrosis.

Investigations: Diagnosis is clinical, and radiological features appear late (MRI is most sensitive). Sacroiliitis is the earliest feature: look for irregularities, erosions, or sclerosis affecting the lower half of the sacroiliac joints, especially the iliac side. Vertebral *syndesmophytes* are characteristic (often T11–L1 initially): bony proliferations due to enthesitis between ligaments and vertebrae. These fuse with the vertebral body above, causing ankylosis. In later stages, calcification of ligaments with ankylosis lead to a 'bamboo spine' appearance. *Also:* FBC (normocytic anaemia), ↑ESR, ↑CRP, HLA B27.

Management: **Exercise**, not rest, for backache, eg badminton, swimming, or intense exercise regimens to maintain posture and mobility with a physiotherapist with a special interest in AS. **NSAIDs** (eg ibuprofen, diclofenac or naproxen, if no CI—see p547) usually relieve symptoms within 48h, and they may slow radiographic progression.[34] **TNFα blockers** etanercept and adalimumab are indicated in severe active AS if NSAIDs fail (p549).[35] Golimumab is currently undergoing phase III trials.[36] Local steroid injections provide temporary relief. Surgery includes hip replacement to improve pain and mobility if the hips are involved, and rarely spinal osteotomy. There is ↑risk of osteoporotic spinal fractures (bisphosphonates may prevent this).

Mortality: Higher than expected ×1.5–4 (eg secondary amyloidosis, heart disease).

2 Enteropathic spondyloarthropathies *Associations:* inflammatory bowel disease, GI bypass surgery, (possibly coeliac & Whipple's disease, p730). ~50% are HLA B27 +ve.

3 Psoriatic arthritis (*OHCS* p594) Occurs in 10–40% with psoriasis and can present before skin changes. Patterns are: • Symmetrical polyarthritis (like RA); • DIP joints; • Asymmetrical oligoarthritis; • Spinal (similar to AS); • Psoriatic arthritis mutilans (rare, ~3%, severe deformity). *Radiology:* Erosive changes, with 'pencil-in-cup' deformity in severe cases. Associated with nail changes in 80% (**fig 2**), synovitis (dactylitis—see BOX), acneiform rashes and palmo-plantar pustulosis. *Management:* NSAIDs, sulfasalazine, methotrexate and ciclosporin. Anti-TNF agents are also effective.

4 Reactive arthritis A *sterile* arthritis, typically affecting the lower limb ~1–4 weeks following urethritis (p416; *Chlamydia* or *Ureaplasma* sp.), or dysentery (*Campylobacter, Salmonella, Shigella,* or *Yersinia* sp.). It may be chronic or relapsing. Also there may be iritis, keratoderma blenorrhagica (brown, raised plaques on soles and palms), circinate balanitis (a painless serpiginous penile ulceration secondary to *Chlamydia trachomatis*), mouth ulcers, enthesitis (plantar fasciitis, Achilles tendonitis) and aortic incompetence (rare). *Reiter's syndrome* is a triad of urethritis, arthritis, and conjunctivitis. *Investigations:* ESR & CRP↑. Culture stool if diarrhoea. Infectious serology. Consider a sexual health review. X-ray (or ultrasound) may show enthesitis with periosteal reaction. *Management:* Rest; splint affected joints acutely; treat with NSAIDs or local steroid injections. Consider sulfasalazine or methotrexate. Treating the original infection may make little difference to the arthritis.

Shared features of the spondyloarthropathies

The spondyloarthropathies show much overlap, with several clinical features in common:

1 Seronegativity (rheumatoid factor -ve).
2 HLA B27 association (also in ~5% UK population, most do not have disease).
3 'Axial arthritis': pathology in spine (spondylo-) and sacroiliac joints.
4 Asymmetrical large-joint oligoarthritis (ie <5 joints) or monoarthritis.
5 Enthesitis: inflammation of the site of insertion of tendon or ligament into bone, eg plantar fasciitis, Achilles tendonitis, costochondritis.
6 Dactylitis: inflammation of an entire digit ('sausage digit'), due to soft tissue oedema, and tenosynovial and joint inflammation.
7 Extra-articular manifestations: eg iritis (anterior uveitis), psoriaform rashes, oral ulcers, aortic valve incompetence, inflammatory bowel disease.

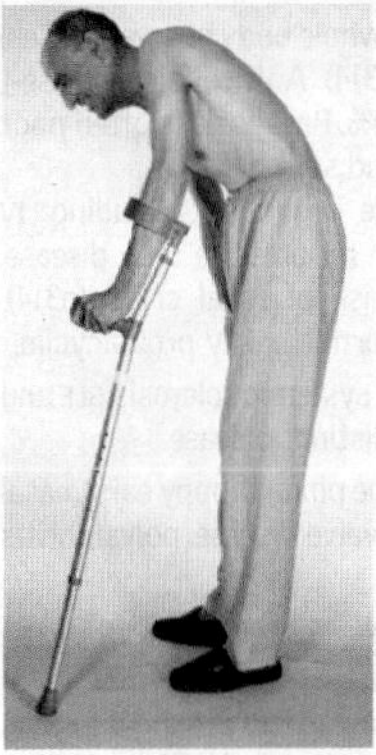

Fig 1. Question mark posture (ankylosing spondylitis).

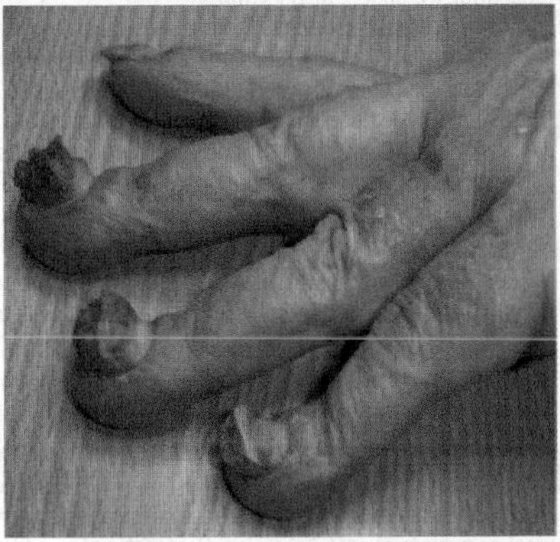

Fig 2. Nail changes in psoriasis: gross onycholysis is seen.

Essence Included under this heading are SLE (p556), diffuse and limited systemic sclerosis, primary Sjögren's syndrome (p724), idiopathic inflammatory myopathies (myositis—see below), mixed connective tissue disease, relapsing polychondritis, and Behçet's disease (p708). They overlap with each other, affect many organ systems, and often require immunosuppressive therapies (p370). Consider connective tissue disease in ill patients with multi-organ involvement, especially if there is no infection.

Systemic sclerosis features scleroderma (skin fibrosis) and vascular disease:
• *Limited systemic sclerosis:* (of which CREST syndrome is part) **C**alcinosis (subcutaneous tissues), **R**aynaud's, o**e**sophageal and gut dysmotility, **S**clerodactyly, and **T**elangiectasia. Skin involvement is limited to the face, hands and feet. It is associated with anti-centromere antibodies in 70–80%. Pulmonary hypertension is often present subclinically, and can become rapidly life-threatening, so should be looked for (℞: sildenafil, bosentan).
• *Diffuse systemic sclerosis:* 'Diffuse' skin involvement (whole body in severe cases) and organ fibrosis: lung, cardiac, and renal disease (p314). Anti-topoisomerase-1 [Scl70] antibodies in 40% and anti-RNA polymerase in 20%. Prognosis is often poor. Control BP meticulously, with annual echocardiogram and spirometry.
Management: Currently no cure. Immunosuppressive regimens, including IV cyclophosphamide, are used for organ involvement or progressive skin disease. Regular ACE-i or angiotensin-II receptor blockers ↓ risk of renal crisis (p314). *Raynaud's:* Hand warmers, Ca^{2+}-channel blockers, or intermittent IV prostacyclin.

Mixed connective tissue disease combines features of systemic sclerosis, SLE and polymyositis. Debate continues as to whether this is a distinct disease.[37,38]

Relapsing polychondritis attacks cartilage, affecting the pinna (floppy ears), nasal septum and larynx (hence stridor). *Associations:* aortic valve disease, polyarthritis and vasculitis. ℞: Steroids and immunosuppressives.

Polymyositis and dermatomyositis

Both typically feature insidious onset of progressive symmetrical proximal muscle weakness from *striated* muscle inflammation (myositis), associated with myalgia ± arthralgia. Muscle weakness may also cause dysphagia, dysphonia (ie poor phonation, *not* dysphasia), or respiratory weakness. The myositis (especially in dermatomyositis) may be a paraneoplastic phenomenon, commonly from an underlying lung, pancreatic, ovarian or bowel malignancy.

Dermatomyositis features myositis plus skin signs: • Macular rash (*shawl sign* is +ve if over back & shoulders); • Lilac-purple *(heliotrope)* rash on eyelids often with oedema; • Nailfold erythema *(dilated capillary loops);* • Roughened red papules over the knuckles, also seen on elbows, knees *(Gottron's papules*—pathognomonic if CK↑ + muscle weakness); • Subcutaneous calcifications; • *Mechanic's hands:* a painful rough skin cracking, affecting the tips and lateral aspects of the fingers.

Extra-muscular signs in both conditions include fever, arthralgia, Raynaud's, interstitial lung fibrosis and myocardial involvement (myocarditis, arrhythmias).

Investigations Muscle enzymes (ALT, AST, LDH & CK) ↑ in plasma; electromyography (EMG) shows fibrillation potentials; muscle biopsy confirms the diagnosis. *Autoantibody associations:* anti-Mi2, anti-Jo1—associated with a syndrome of acute onset, T°↑, interstitial lung fibrosis, Raynaud's, arthritis and mechanic's hands (above).

Differential diagnoses Carcinomatous myopathy, inclusion-body myositis, muscular dystrophy, endocrine/metabolic myopathy (including steroids), rhabdomyolysis, infection (eg HIV), drugs (penicillamine, colchicine, statins or chloroquine).

Management Screen thoroughly for malignancy. Start prednisolone (eg 1mg/kg/d PO). Immunosuppressives (p370) and cytotoxics are used early in resistant cases, eg azathioprine, methotrexate, cyclophosphamide or ciclosporin. Hydroxychloroquine, dapsone, thalidomide or topical tacrolimus may help with skin disease. A more aggressive form with prominent vasculitis and calcinosis occurs in children.

Plasma autoantibodies (Abs): disease associations

►Always interpret in the context of clinical findings:

Rheumatological **Rheumatoid factor (RhF)** positive in:

Sjögren's syndrome	≤100%	Mixed connective tissue disease	50%
Felty's syndrome	≤100%	SLE	≤40%
RA	70%	Systemic sclerosis	30%
Infection (SBE/IE; hepatitis)	≤50%	Normal	2-10%

Anti-cyclic citrullinated peptide Ab (anti-CCP): rheumatoid arthritis (~96% specificity)

Anti-nuclear antibody (ANA) positive by immunofluorescence in:

SLE	>95%	Systemic sclerosis	64%
Autoimmune hepatitis	75%	RA	30%
Sjögren's syndrome	68%	Normal	0-2%

ANA titres are expressed according to dilutions at which antibodies can be detected, ie 1:160 means antibodies can still be detected after the serum has been diluted 160 times. Titres of 1:40 or 1:80 may not be significant. The pattern of staining may indicate the disease (although these are not specific):

• *Homogeneous*	SLE	• *Nucleolar*	Systemic sclerosis
• *Speckled*	Mixed connective tissue disease	• *Centromere*	Limited systemic sclerosis

Anti-double-stranded DNA (dsDNA): SLE (60% sensitivity, but highly specific).

Anti-histone Ab: Drug-induced SLE (~100%).

Anti-phospholipid Ab (eg anti-cardiolipin Ab): antiphospholipid syndrome, SLE.

Anti-centromere Ab: limited systemic sclerosis.

Anti-extractable nuclear antigen (ENA) antibodies (usually with +ve ANA):

• **Anti-Ro (SSA)**	SLE, Sjögren's syndrome, systemic sclerosis. Associated with congenital heart block.
• **Anti-La (SSB)**	Sjögren's syndrome, SLE (15%).
• **Anti-Sm**	SLE (20-30%).
• **Anti-RNP**	SLE, mixed connective tissue disease.
• **Anti Jo-1; Anti-Mi-2**	Polymyositis, dermatomyositis.
• **Anti-Scl70**	Diffuse systemic sclerosis.

Gastrointestinal (for liver autoantibodies, see p268).

Anti-mitochondrial Ab (AMA): Primary biliary cirrhosis (>95%), autoimmune hepatitis (30%), idiopathic cirrhosis (25-30%).

Anti-smooth muscle Ab (SMA): Autoimmune hepatitis (70%), primary biliary cirrhosis (50%), idiopathic cirrhosis (25-30%).

Gastric parietal cell Ab: Pernicious anaemia (>90%), atrophic gastritis (40%), 'normal' (10%).

Intrinsic factor Ab: Pernicious anaemia (50%).

α-gliadin Ab, anti-tissue transglutaminase, anti-endomysial Ab: Coeliac disease.

Endocrine **Thyroid peroxidase Ab:** Hashimoto's thyroiditis (~87%), Graves' (>50%).

Islet cell Ab (ICA), glutamic acid decarboxylase (GAD) Ab: Type 1 diabetes mellitus (75%).

Renal **Glomerular basement membrane Ab (anti-GBM):** Goodpasture's disease (100%).

Anti-neutrophil cytoplasmic Ab (ANCA):

- **Cytoplasmic (c-ANCA)**, specific for **serine proteinase-3 (PR3 +ve).** Wegener's granulomatosis (90%); also microscopic polyangiitis (30%), polyarteritis nodosa (11%).
- **Perinuclear (p-ANCA)**, specific for **myeloperoxidase (MPO +ve)**. Microscopic polyangiitis (45%), Churg-Strauss, some pulmonary-renal vasculitides (Goodpasture's syndrome).

Unlike immune-complex vasculitis, in ANCA-associated vasculitis no complement consumption or immune complex deposition occurs (ie pauci-immune vasculitis). 39

ANCA may also be +ve in UC/Crohn's, sclerosing cholangitis, autoimmune hepatitis, Felty's, RA, SLE, or drugs (eg anti-thyroid, allopurinol, ciprofloxacin).

Neurological **Acetylcholine receptor Ab:** Myasthenia gravis (90%).

Anti-voltage-gated K^+-channel Ab: Limbic encephalitis.

Anti-voltage-gated Ca^{2+}-channel Ab: Lambert-Eaton syndrome.

Paraneoplastic anti-neuronal Ab: see p539.

Systemic lupus erythematosus (SLE)

SLE is a multisystemic autoimmune disease in which autoantibodies are made against a variety of autoantigens (eg ANA). Immunopathology results in polyclonal B-cell secretion of pathogenic autoantibodies and the formation of immune complexes that deposit in sites such as the kidneys. *Prevalence:* ~0.2%. ♀:♂ ≈9:1, typically women of child-bearing age. Commoner in Afro-Caribbeans, Asians, and if HLA B8, DR2 or DR3 +ve. ~10% of relatives may be affected. It may be triggered by EBV (p401).[40]

Clinical features It is a remitting and relapsing illness, typically presenting with non-specific constitutional symptoms of malaise, fatigue, myalgia and fever. See BOX opposite for specific features. Other features include lymphadenopathy, weight loss, alopecia, nail-fold infarcts, non-infective endocarditis (Libman-Sacks syndrome), Raynaud's (30%; see p722), migraine (40%), stroke, and retinal exudates.

Immunology >95% are ANA +ve. A high anti-double-stranded DNA (dsDNA) antibody titre is highly specific, but only +ve in ~60% of cases. ENA may be +ve in 20-30% (anti-Ro, anti-La, anti-Sm, anti-RNP), while 40% are RhF +ve (p555). Anticardiolipin antibodies may cause false +ve syphilis serology (below). SLE may be associated with other autoimmune conditions: Sjögren's (15-20%), autoimmune thyroid disease (5-10%).

Monitoring activity *3 best tests:* **1** Anti-dsDNA antibody titres. **2** Complement: C3↓, C4↓ (denotes consumption of complement, hence C3 and C4↓, and C3d and C4d↑, their degradation products). **3** ESR. *Also:* BP, urine for casts or protein (lupus nephritis, below), FBC, U&E, LFTs, CRP (usually normal) ►*think of SLE whenever someone has a multisystem disorder and ↑ESR but CRP normal.* If ↑CRP, think instead of infection, serositis or arthritis. Skin or renal biopsies may be diagnostic.

Drug-induced lupus Causes (>50 drugs) include isoniazid, hydralazine (if >50mg/24h in slow acetylators), procainamide, quinidine, chlorpromazine, minocycline, phenytoin. It is associated with antihistone antibodies in ~100%. Skin and lung signs prevail (renal and CNS are rarely affected). The disease remits if the drug is stopped. Sulfonamides or the oral contraceptive pill may worsen idiopathic SLE.

Antiphospholipid syndrome can be associated with SLE (20-30%). More often it occurs as a primary disease. Antiphospholipid antibodies (anti-cardiolipin & lupus anticoagulant) cause **CLOT**s: **C**oagulation defect, **L**ivedo reticularis (p559), **O**bstetric (recurrent miscarriage), **T**hrombocytopenia (↓platelets). There is a thrombotic tendency, affecting the cerebral, renal and other vessels. ℞: Low-dose aspirin, or warfarin if recurrent thromboses (aim INR of 2-3).[41] Seek advice in pregnancy.

Management should be through specialist SLE and lupus nephritis clinics.

- ►►*Severe flares:* Acute SLE (eg haemolytic anaemia, nephritis, severe pericarditis or CNS disease) requires urgent IV **cyclophosphamide** + **high-dose prednisolone.**
- *Cutaneous symptoms:* treat rashes with topical steroids. Prevent rashes with high-factor sunblock creams. Sun exposure may also trigger acute systemic flares.
- *Maintenance:* use **NSAIDs** and **hydroxychloroquine** (see p549 for SE) for joint and skin symptoms. Low-dose steroids may be of value in chronic disease. **Azathioprine**, **methotrexate** and **mycophenolate** are used as steroid-sparing agents.
- *Lupus nephritis:* (p314) May require more intensive immunosuppression with steroids and **cyclophosphamide** (monthly IV or daily PO). SE (p370): myelosuppression, nausea, alopecia, haemorrhagic cystitis, infertility (important in this patient group). NB: immunosuppressed patients are prone to infection (especially atypicals). BP control is vital: ACE-i, α-blockers (eg doxazosin) or Ca^{2+}-channel blockers (eg nifedipine). Renal replacement therapy (p304) may be needed if disease progresses; nephritis recurs in ~50% post-transplant, but is a rare cause of graft failure.[42]
- *B-cell depletion* with the chimeric anti-CD20 monoclonal antibody **rituximab** (p356) shows great promise in open clinical trials;[43] results of randomized-controlled trials are awaited. Phase II trials of humanized anti-CD20 and anti-CD22 monoclonal antibodies, ocrelizumab and epratuzumab, respectively, are under way.

Prognosis is ~80% survival at 15 years.[44] There is an increased long-term risk of cardiovascular disease and osteoporosis.

Revised criteria (serial or simultaneous) for diagnosing SLE

Diagnose SLE in an appropriate clinical setting if ≥4 out of 11 criteria are present:

1 *Malar rash (butterfly rash):* Fixed erythema, flat or raised, over the malar eminences, tending to spare the nasolabial folds (**fig 1**). Occurs in up to 30%.

2 *Discoid rash:* Erythematous raised patches with adherent keratotic scales & follicular plugging ± atrophic scarring (**fig 2**). Think of it as a 3-stage rash affecting ears, cheeks, scalp, forehead, and chest: erythema→pigmented hyperkeratotic oedematous papules→atrophic depressed lesions.

3 *Photosensitivity:* On exposed skin representing unusual reaction to light. Exposure to sun may also cause disease to flare, so sunblocks are advised.

4 *Oral ulcers:* Oral or nasopharyngeal ulceration, usually painless.

5 *Non-erosive arthritis:* Involving ≥2 peripheral joints (tenderness, swelling, or effusion). Joint involvement is seen in 90% of patients, and may present similarly to RA. A reversible deforming arthropathy may occur due to capsular laxity (Jaccoud's arthropathy). Aseptic bone necrosis may also occur.

6 *Serositis:* (a) **Pleuritis** (presents as pleuritic pain or dyspnoea due to pleural effusion—80% have lung function abnormalities) OR (b) **Pericarditis** (chest pain, ECG, pericardial rub or signs of pericardial effusion).

7 *Renal disorder:* (a) **Persistent proteinuria** >0.5g/d (or >3+ on urinalysis) OR (b) **Cellular casts**—may be red cell, granular, or mixed. See p314.

8 *CNS disorder:* (a) **Seizures**, in the absence of causative drugs or metabolic imbalance, eg uraemia or ketoacidosis, OR (b) **Psychosis** in the absence of causative drugs/metabolic derangements, as above.

9 *Haematological disorder:* (a) **Haemolytic anaemia** (p330), OR (b) **Leukopenia** $<4\times10^9$/L on ≥2 occasions, OR (c) **Lymphopenia** $<1.5\times10^9$/L on ≥2 occasions, OR (d) **Thrombocytopenia** $<100\times10^9$/L, in the absence of a drug effect.

10 *Immunological disorder:* (a) **Anti-dsDNA** antibody, (b) **Anti-Smooth muscle** antibody, OR (c) **Antiphospholipid** antibody +ve based on:
- An abnormal serum level of IgG or IgM anticardiolipin antibodies,
- Positive result for lupus anticoagulant using a standard method, or
- False +ve syphilis serology, +ve for >6 months and confirmed by -ve *Treponema pallidum* immobilization & fluorescent treponemal antibody absorption tests.[46]

11 *Antinuclear antibody (ANA):* +ve in >95%.

A useful mnemonic is 'A RASH POINTS AN MD'...to a possible diagnosis.[47] **A**rthritis, **R**enal disorder, **A**NA, **S**erositis, **H**aematological, **P**hotosensitivity, **O**ral ulcers, **I**mmunological disorder, **N**eurological disorder, **M**alar and **D**iscoid rash.

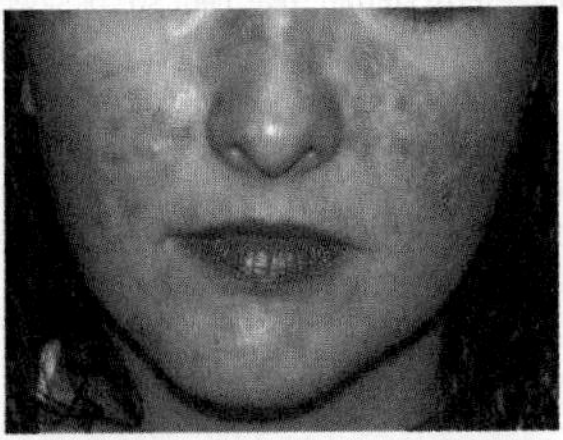

Fig 1. Malar rash, with sparing of the nasolabial folds.[48]

Courtesy of David F Fiorentino, MD, PhD; by kind permission of *Skin & Aging*.

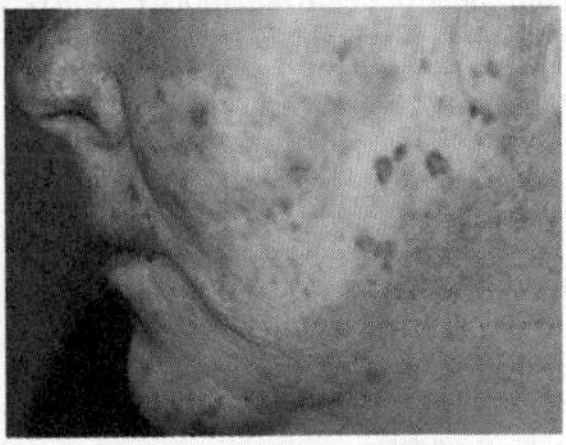

Fig 2. Discoid rash.[49]

Courtesy of Amy McMichael, MD; by kind permission of *Skin & Aging*.

Vasculitis is defined as an inflammatory disorder of blood vessel walls. It can affect the vessels of any organ, and the presentation will depend on which organs are involved. They are categorized according to the main size of blood vessel affected:

- *Large:* Giant cell arteritis, Takayasu's arteritis (p726).
- *Medium:* Polyarteritis nodosa, Kawasaki disease.
- *Small:*
  - **ANCA +ve:** (associated with glomerulonephritis): microscopic polyangiitis, Wegener's granulomatosis (p728), Churg-Strauss syndrome (p710).
  - **ANCA -ve:** Henoch-Schönlein purpura (p716), Goodpasture's syndrome (p714), cryoglobulinaemia.

Vasculitis may also be secondary to other diseases, eg SLE, RA, hepatitis B & C, HIV.

Symptoms: Different vasculitides preferentially affect different organs, causing different patterns of symptoms (see BOX 1), but the presentation may often be of only overwhelming fatigue with ↑ESR/CRP.

▸▸***Consider vasculitis in any unidentified multisystem disorder.*** Acute vasculitis is a medical emergency. If suspected, seek urgent help, as organ damage may occur rapidly (eg critical renal failure <24h).

Tests: ESR/CRP↑. ANCA may be +ve. ↑Creatinine if renal failure. Urine: proteinuria, haematuria, casts on microscopy. Angiography ± biopsy may be diagnostic.

Management: Large-vessel vasculitis: steroids in most cases. Medium/small: standard therapy is steroids and IV **cyclophosphamide** (15mg/kg).[50] **Azathioprine** may be useful as a steroid-sparing maintenance treatment.

Giant cell arteritis (GCA)

AKA cranial or temporal arteritis. It is common in the elderly, but rare in those under 55yrs. It is associated with polymyalgia rheumatica (see BOX 2) in 50%. *Symptoms:* Headache, temporal artery and scalp tenderness (eg when combing hair), jaw claudication, amaurosis fugax, or sudden blindness, typically in one eye. Extracranial symptoms may include dyspnoea, morning stiffness, and unequal or weak pulses.[51] ▸▸If you suspect GCA, do ESR and start **prednisolone** 40–60mg/d PO *immediately*. The risk is irreversible bilateral visual loss, which can occur suddenly if not treated (some advocate higher doses if visual symptoms—ask an ophthalmologist). *Investigations:* ESR & CRP↑↑, platelets↑, alk phos↑, Hb↓. Get a temporal artery biopsy within 3 days of starting steroids. Skip lesions occur, so don't be put off by a negative biopsy. *Prognosis:* Typically a 2-year course, then complete remission. Reduce prednisolone after 5–7d guided by symptoms and ESR; ↑dose if symptoms recur. The main cause of death and morbidity in GCA is long-term steroid treatment so consider risks and benefits! Give gastric and bone protection (PPI; alendronate, p696).

Polyarteritis nodosa (PAN)

PAN is a necrotizing vasculitis that causes aneurysms and thrombosis in medium-sized arteries, leading to infarction in affected organs, with severe systemic symptoms. ♂:♀≈2:1. It may be associated with hepatitis B, and is rare in the UK. *Symptoms:* Typically systemic features, plus predominantly skin (rash and 'punched out' ulcers), renal (main cause of death, though glomerulonephritis is *not* seen), cardiac, GI and GU involvement. See BOX 1. Coronary aneurysms occur in *Kawasaki disease* (childhood PAN variant, *OHCS* p646). *Investigations:* Often WCC↑, mild eosinophilia (in 30%), anaemia, ESR↑, CRP↑, ANCA -ve. Renal or mesenteric angiography, or renal biopsy can be diagnostic. *Treatment:* Control BP meticulously. Refer to experts. Most respond to corticosteroids and cyclophosphamide. Hepatitis B should be treated with an antiviral (lamivudine or interferon-α) after initial treatment with steroids.[52]

Microscopic polyangiitis

A necrotizing vasculitis affecting small and medium-sized vessels. *Symptoms:* Rapidly progressive glomerulonephritis usually features; pulmonary haemorrhage occurs in up to 30%; other features are rare. *Investigations:* pANCA (MPO) +ve (p555).

Features of vasculitis

The presentation of vasculitis will depend on the organs affected:

Systemic: fever, malaise, weight loss, arthralgia, myalgia.
Skin: purpura, ulcers, livedo reticularis (**fig 1**), nail-bed infarcts, digital gangrene.
Eyes: episcleritis, scleritis, visual loss.
ENT: epistaxis, nasal crusting, stridor, deafness.
Pulmonary: haemoptysis and dyspnoea (due to pulmonary haemorrhage).
Cardiac: Angina or MI (due to coronary arteritis), heart failure and pericarditis.
GI: Pain or perforation (infarcted viscus), malabsorption (chronic ischaemia).
Renal: Hypertension, haematuria, proteinuria, casts, and renal failure (renal cortical infarcts; glomerulonephritis in ANCA +ve vasculitis).
Neurological: Stroke, fits, chorea, psychosis, confusion, impaired cognition, altered mood. Arteritis of the vasa nervorum may cause mononeuritis multiplex or a sensorimotor polyneuropathy.[53]
GU: Orchitis—testicular pain or tenderness.

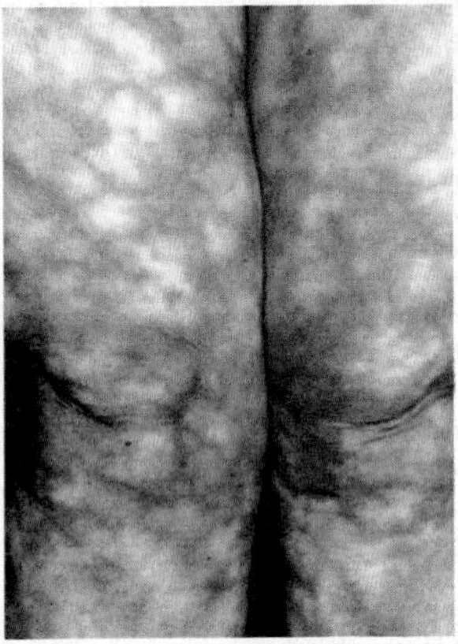

Fig 1. Livedo reticularis: pink-blue mottling caused by capillary dilatation and stasis in skin venules. Causes: physiological, eg cold weather, or vasculitis.[54]

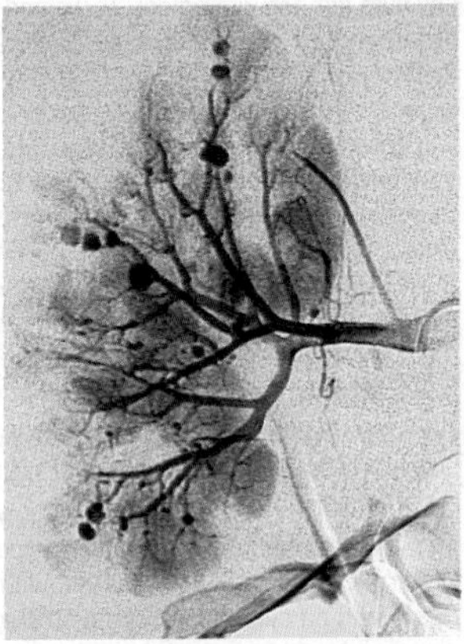

Fig 2. Renal angiogram showing multiple aneurysms in PAN.[55]

Courtesy of Dr William Herring.

Polymyalgia rheumatica (PMR)

PMR is not a true vasculitis, but shares the same demographic characteristics as GCA, and the two conditions often co-exist in the same patient.

Symptoms: Subacute onset (< 2 weeks) of symmetrical aching, tenderness and morning stiffness in shoulders and proximal limb muscles ± mild polyarthritis, tenosynovitis, and carpal tunnel syndrome (10%). Fatigue, fever, weight↓, anorexia and depression.

Investigations: CRP, plasma viscosity & ESR ↑; CK ↔; alk phos may be ↑.

Differential diagnoses: Recent onset RA, polymyositis, hypothyroidism, primary muscle disease, occult malignancy or infection, osteoarthritis (especially cervical spondylosis, shoulder OA), neck lesions, bilateral subacromial impingement (*OHCS* p664), spinal stenosis (*OHCS* p674).

Management: **Prednisolone** 10-15mg/d PO. Expect a dramatic response within 4 days. ↓dose slowly, eg by 1mg/month (according to symptoms & ESR). Most need steroids for ≥2yrs, so give gastric and bone protection (PPI; alendronate, p696).

Fibromyalgia and chronic fatigue syndrome are part of a diffuse group of overlapping syndromes, sharing similar demographic and clinical characteristics, in which chronic symptoms of fatigue and widespread pain feature prominently. Their existence as discrete entities is controversial, especially in the absence of clear pathology, and some find such dysfunctional diagnoses frustrating. However, a correct diagnosis enables the doctor to give appropriate counselling and advise appropriate therapies, and allows the patient to begin to accept and deal with their symptoms.

Fibromyalgia

Fibromyalgia comprises up to 10% of new referrals to the rheumatology clinic.[56] ***Prevalence:*** 0.5-4%. ♀:♂ ≈10:1. ***Risk factors:*** BOX 1. Also female sex, middle age, low household income, divorced, low educational status. ***Associations:*** Other somatic syndromes such as chronic fatigue syndrome, irritable bowel syndrome and chronic headaches syndromes. Also found in ~25% of patients with RA, AS and SLE.

Features: Diagnosis depends on pain that is *chronic* (>3months) and *widespread* (involves left and right sides, above and below the waist, and the axial skeleton) in the absence of inflammation; and the presence of pain on palpation of at least 11/18 '*tender points*'—left- and right-sided: • suboccipital muscle insertions; • anterior aspects of the inter-transverse spaces at C5–C7; • midpoint of the upper border of trapezius; • origin of supraspinatus near the medial border of the scapular spine; • costochondral junction of 2nd rib; • 2cm distal from lateral humeral epicondyle; • upper outer gluteal quadrant; • posterior to the greater trochanter; • knee, at medial fat pad proximal to joint line. Patients may have more tender points than those listed, but these are the most consistent and helpful diagnostically.[57] Healthy individuals may also have tender points, but it is their widespread and severe nature that indicates fibromyalgia. *Additional features:* morning stiffness (~80-90%), fatigue (~80-90%, often severe), poor concentration, low mood and sleep disturbance (~70%).

Investigations are all normal. Over-investigation can consolidate illness behaviour; however, other causes of pain and/or fatigue must be excluded (eg RA, PMR, vasculitis, hypothyroidism, myeloma).

Management: the manner in which management is discussed is almost as important as the management itself, which should focus on **education** of the patient *and their family* and on developing coping strategies. Such a diagnosis may be a relief or a disappointment to the patient. *Explain* that fibromyalgia is a relapsing and remitting condition, with no easy cures, and that they will continue to have good and bad days. *Reassure* them that there is no serious underlying pathology, that their joints are not being damaged, and that no further tests are necessary, but be sympathetic to the fact that they may have been seeking a physical cause for their symptoms. Discuss psychosocial issues (see BOX 1). **Cognitive-behavioural therapy** aims to help patients develop coping strategies and set achievable goals.[58] Pacing of activity is vital to avoid over-exertion and consequent pain and fatigue. Long-term **graded exercise programs** improve functional capacity.[59][60] ***Pharmacotherapy:*** Pain in fibromyalgia rarely responds to NSAIDs and steroids as there is no inflammation (if it does respond, reconsider your diagnosis!). Low-dose tricyclic antidepressants (eg **amitriptyline** 10–20mg at night) and **pregabalin** (150-300mg/12h PO) may improve pain (especially combined with tramadol), sleep and morning stiffness, but effects may not be apparent for up to a month.[61] High-dose **venlafaxine** may also be effective. SSRIs appear to be less useful.

Chronic fatigue syndrome (AKA myalgic encephalomyelitis)

Chronic fatigue syndrome is defined as persistent disabling fatigue lasting >6 months, affecting mental and physical function, present >50% of the time, plus ≥4 of: myalgia (~80%), polyarthralgia, ↓ memory, unrefreshing sleep, fatigue after exertion >24h, persistent sore throat, tender cervical/axillary lymph nodes. Management principles are similar to fibromyalgia above. No pharmacological agents have yet been proved effective for chronic fatigue syndrome (see also *OHCS* p528).

Yellow flags[62]

Psychosocial risk factors for developing persisting chronic pain and long-term disability have been termed 'yellow flags'. These include:

- ►Belief that pain and activity are harmful.
- ►Sickness behaviours such as extended rest.
- ►Social withdrawal.
- ►Emotional problems such as low mood, anxiety or stress.
- ►Problems or dissatisfaction at work.
- ►Problems with claims for compensation or time off work.
- ►Overprotective family or lack of support.
- ►Inappropriate expectations of treatment, eg low active participation in treatment.

An Existential approach to difficult symptoms

We all at some stage come across a patient with difficult symptoms and an exasperating lack of pathology to explain them. Investigations are all normal, and medications do not seem to work. It is tempting to dismiss such patients as malingerers, but often this conclusion comes from the clinician approaching the problem from the wrong angle. The patient has symptoms that are real and disabling to them, and that will not improve without help. Perhaps a more pragmatic approach is to take advice from the Danish philosopher Kierkegaard who wrote to a friend in 1835, '*What I really lack is to be clear in my mind what I am to do, not what I am to know ... The thing is to understand myself ... to find a truth which is true for me.*' Listen to the patient and accept their story. Then help them to focus on what they can *do* to improve their situation, and to move away from dwelling on finding a physical answer to their symptoms.

Is fibromyalgia a real disease?

The current hypothesis is that fibromyalgia is caused by aberrant peripheral and central pain processing. Two key features of the condition are *allodynia* (pain in response to a non-painful stimulus) and *hyperaesthesia* (exaggerated perception of pain in response to a mildly painful stimulus), examined for by palpation of tender points. Research is beginning to suggest that certain antidepressants can relieve pain and other symptoms, and especially those that have both serotonergic and noradrenergic activity (tricyclics and venlafaxine). Those acting on serotonergic receptors only are less effective. There is also some evidence to support the use of alternative therapies such as acupuncture and spa therapies, which have been postulated to act through similar spinal pain-modulatory pathways.[63] Thus far, trials have involved relatively small numbers of patients or short time periods, and lack the power to draw strong conclusions. However, it is interesting to note that the CSF of patients with fibromyalgia appears to have increased levels of substance P, while levels of noradrenaline and serotonin metabolites are decreased. All three are neurotransmitters involved in descending pain-modulatory pathways in the spinal cord.[64] [65] Evidence from PET imaging suggests that patients with fibromyalgia may have an abnormal central dopamine response to pain.[66] The critical question is: Is this cause or effect?

The eye is host to many diseases: the more you look, the more you'll see, and the more you'll enjoy, not least because the eye is as beautiful as its signs are legion.

Granulomatous disorders Syphilis, TB, sarcoidosis, leprosy, brucellosis, and toxoplasmosis may inflame either the front chamber (anterior uveitis/iritis) or back chamber (posterior uveitis/choroiditis). Refer to an ophthalmologist.

Systemic inflammatory diseases may manifest in any part of the eye: *iritis* in ankylosing spondylitis and Reiter's; *conjunctivitis* in Reiter's; *scleritis* or *episcleritis* in RA, vasculitis and SLE. Scleritis in RA and Wegener's may damage the eye. Refer urgently if eye pain. GCA causes optic nerve ischaemia presenting as sudden blindness.

Keratoconjunctivitis sicca is a reduction in tear formation, tested by the Schirmer filter paper test (<5mm in 5min). It causes a gritty feeling in the eyes, and a dry mouth (xerostomia from ↓ saliva production). It is found on its own (Sjögren's syndrome), or with other diseases, eg SLE, RA, sarcoidosis. ℞: artificial tears/saliva (eg tears naturale, hypromellose drops, Salivese® oral spray).

Hypertensive retinopathy ↑BP accelerates atherosclerosis in retinal vessels. Hardened arteries are shiny ('silver wiring'; **fig 1**) and nip veins where they cross (AV nipping; **fig 2**). Narrowed arterioles may become blocked, causing localized retinal infarction, seen as cotton-wool spots. Leaks from these in severe hypertension manifest as hard exudates or macular oedema. Papilloedema (**fig 3**) or flame haemorrhages suggest malignant hypertension (p132) requiring urgent treatment.

Vascular occlusion Emboli passing through the retinal vasculature may cause *retinal artery occlusion* (global or segmental retinal pallor) or *amaurosis fugax* (p480). *Roth spots* (small retinal infarcts, **fig 1** on p386) occur in infective endocarditis. In dermatomyositis, there is orbital oedema with retinopathy showing cotton-wool spots (micro-infarcts). ***Retinal vein occlusion*** is caused by ↑BP, age, or hyperviscosity (p366). Suspect in any acute fall in acuity. If it is the central vein, the fundus is like a stormy sunset (those angry red clouds are haemorrhages). In branch vein occlusion, changes are confined to a wedge of retina. Get expert help.

Haematological disorders *Retinal haemorrhages* occur in leukaemia; comma-shaped *conjunctival haemorrhages* and retinal *new vessel formation* may occur in sickle-cell disease. *Optic atrophy* is seen in pernicious anaemia (and also MS).

Metabolic disease Diabetes mellitus: p202. Hyperthyroid exophthalmos: p211. Lens opacities are seen in hypoparathyroidism. Conjunctival and corneal calcification can occur in hypercalcaemia. In gout, conjunctival urate deposits may cause sore eyes.

Systemic infections Septicaemia may seed to the vitreous causing endophthalmitis. Syphilis can cause iritis (+ pigmented retinopathy if congenital). Systemic fungal infections may affect the eye, eg in the immunocompromised or in IV drug abusers, requiring intra-vitreal antibiotics. **AIDS & HIV:** CMV retinitis (pizza-pie fundus, p405) may be asymptomatic but can cause sudden visual loss. If present, it implies full-blown AIDS (CD4 count <100 × 10^6/L; p410). Cotton-wool spots on their own indicate HIV retinopathy and may occur before the full HIV picture. Kaposi's sarcoma may affect the lids or conjunctiva.

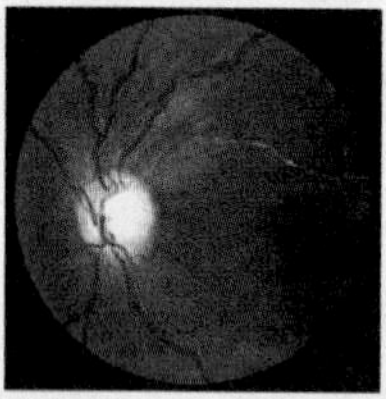

Fig 1. Silver wiring

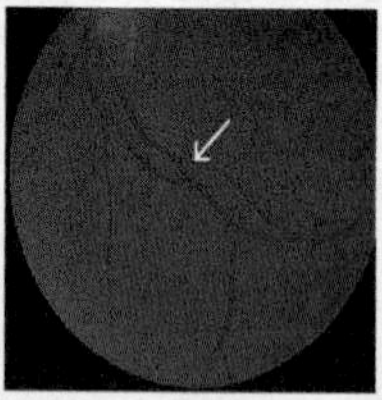

Fig 2. AV nipping

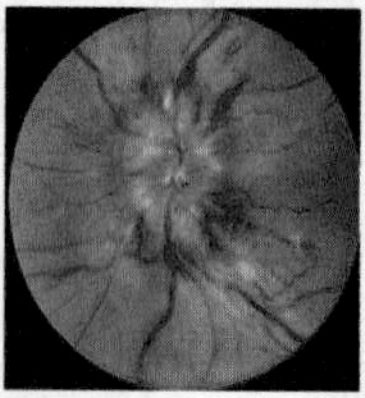

Fig 3. Papilloedema

Figs 1-3©Prof Jonathan Trobe

Differential diagnosis of a red eye

	Conjunctiva	Iris	Pupil	Cornea	Anterior chamber	Intraocular pressure	Appearance
Acute glaucoma	Both ciliary and conjunctival vessels injected. Entire eye is red See *OHCS* p430	Injected	Dilated, fixed, oval	Steamy, hazy	Very shallow	Very high	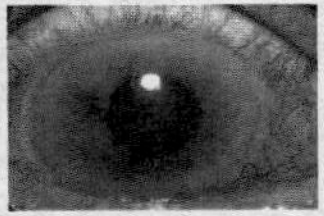
Anterior uveitis (Iritis)	Redness most marked around cornea, which doesn't blanch on pressure. Usually unilateral. *Causes:* ankylosing spondylitis, rheumatoid arthritis, Reiter's, sarcoidosis, herpes simplex, herpes zoster, and Behçet's disease *NB:* a similar scleral appearance but without papillary or anterior chamber involvement may be *scleritis* (eg RA, SLE, vasculitis)	Injected	Small, irregular due to adhesions between the anterior lens and the pupil margin	Normal	Turgid	Normal	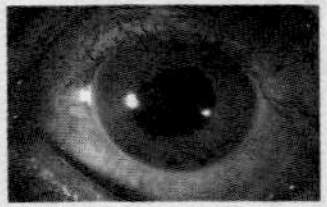
Conjunctivitis	Often bilateral. Conjunctival vessels injected, greatest toward fornices, but blanching on pressure Mobile over sclera Purulent discharge	Normal	Normal	Normal	Normal	Normal	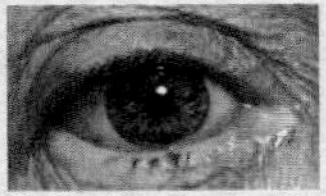
Subconjunctival haemorrhage	Bright red sclera with white rim around limbus *Causes:* BP↑; leptospirosis; bleeding disorders; trauma; snake venom; haemorrhagic fevers	Normal	Normal	Normal	Normal	Normal	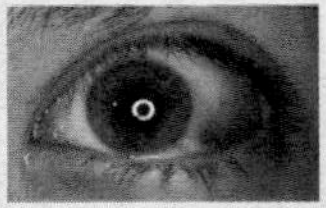

After RD Judge, GD Zuidema, FT Fitzgerald *Clinical diagnosis* 5/e, Little Brown, Boston. Images courtesy of Prof. Jonathan Trobe. 68

Erythema nodosum (fig 1) Painful, blue-red, raised lesions on shin fronts (± thighs/arms). *Causes:* sarcoidosis, drugs (sulfonamides, the Pill, dapsone), streptococcal infection. *Less common:* Crohn's/UC, BCG vaccination, leptospirosis, *Mycobacterium* (TB, leprosy), *Yersinia* or various viruses and fungi.

Erythema multiforme (fig 3) 'Target' lesions: symmetrical ± central blister, on palms/soles, limbs, and elsewhere. *Stevens-Johnson syndrome* (p724): a rare, severe variant with fever and mucosal involvement (mouth, genital, and eye ulcers), associated with a hypersensitivity reaction to drugs (NSAIDs, sulfonamides, anti-convulsants, allopurinol) or infections (herpes, *Mycoplasma*, orf—p376). Also seen in collagen disorders. 50% of cases are idiopathic. Get expert help in severe disease.

Erythema chronicum migrans Presents as a small papule which develops into a spreading large erythematous ring, with central fading. It lasts from 48h to 3 months. May be multiple. *Cause:* Lyme disease (p430).

Erythema marginatum Pink coalescent rings on trunk which come and go. It is seen in rheumatic fever (or rarely other causes, eg drugs).

Pyoderma gangrenosum (fig 2) Recurring nodulo-pustular ulcers, ~10cm wide, with tender red/blue overhanging necrotic edge, purulent surface, and healing with cribriform scars on leg, abdomen, or face. *Associations*: UC/Crohn's, autoimmune hepatitis, Wegener's, myeloma, neoplasia. ♀>♂. *Treatment*: Get help. Saline toilet, high-dose oral or topical steroids ± ciclosporin ± topical antibiotic.[69]

Vitiligo (fig 4) *Vitellus* is Latin for *spotted calf:* typically white patches ± hyper-pigmented borders. Sunlight makes them itch. *Associations:* autoimmune disorders; premature ovarian failure. Treat by camouflage cosmetics and sunscreens (± steroid creams ± dermabrasion). UK Vitiligo Society: 0800 018 2631.

Specific diseases and their skin manifestations

Crohn's Perianal/vulval ulcers; erythema nodosum; pyoderma gangrenosum.

Dermatomyositis Gottron's papules; shawl sign; heliotrope rash on eyelids. It may be associated with lung, bowel, ovarian or pancreatic malignancy (p554).

Diabetes mellitus Ulcers, *necrobiosis lipoidica* (shiny yellowish area on shin ± telangiectasia; **fig 5**), *granuloma annulare* (OHCS p586), *acanthosis nigricans* (pigmented, rough thickening of axillary, neck or groin skin with warty lesions; **fig 6**).

Gluten-sensitive enteropathy (coeliac disease) *Dermatitis herpetiformis*—itchy blisters, in groups on knees, elbows, and scalp. The itch (which can drive patients to suicide) responds to dapsone 25-200mg/24h PO within 48h—and this may be used as a diagnostic test. The maintenance dose may be as little as 50mg/wk. A gluten-free diet should be adhered to, but in 30% dapsone will need to be continued. SE (dose-related): haemolysis (CI: anaemia, G6PD-deficiency), hepatitis, agranulocytosis (monitor FBC and LFTs). There is an ↑ risk of small bowel lymphoma with coeliac disease *and* dermatitis herpetiformis—so surveillance is needed.

Hyperthyroidism *Pretibial myxoedema*—red oedematous swellings above lateral malleoli, progressing to thickened oedema of legs and feet, *thyroid acropachy*—clubbing + subperiosteal new bone in phalanges. ***Other endocrinopathies:*** p197.

Liver disease Palmar erythema; spider naevi; gynaecomastia; decrease in pubic hair; jaundice; bruising; scratch marks.

Malabsorption Dry pigmented skin, easy bruising, hair loss, leuconychia.

Neoplasia *Acanthosis nigricans:* (see above under diabetes & **fig 6**) associated with stomach cancer. *Dermatomyositis*—see above. *Thrombophlebitis migrans:* Successive crops of tender nodules affecting blood vessels throughout the body, associated with pancreatic cancer (especially body and tail). *Acquired ichthyosis:* Dry scaly skin associated with lymphoma. *Skin metastases:* Especially melanoma, and colonic, lung, breast, laryngeal/oral, or ovarian malignancy.

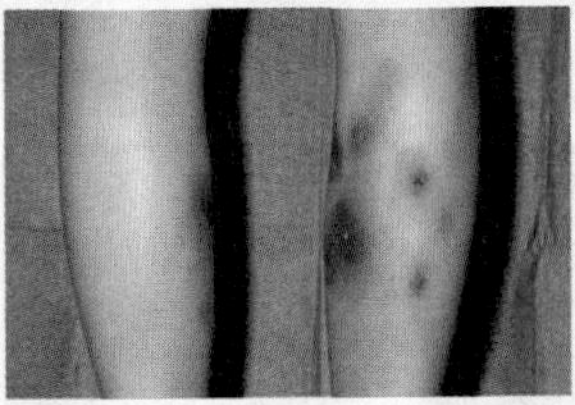

Fig 1. Erythema nodosum.

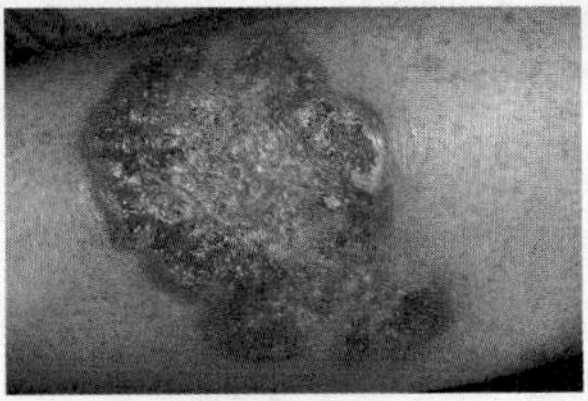

Fig 2. Pyoderma gangrenosum.[70]

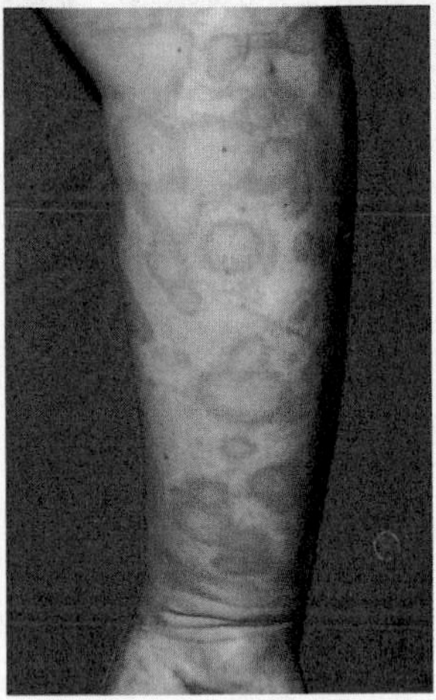

Fig 3. Erythema multiforme.

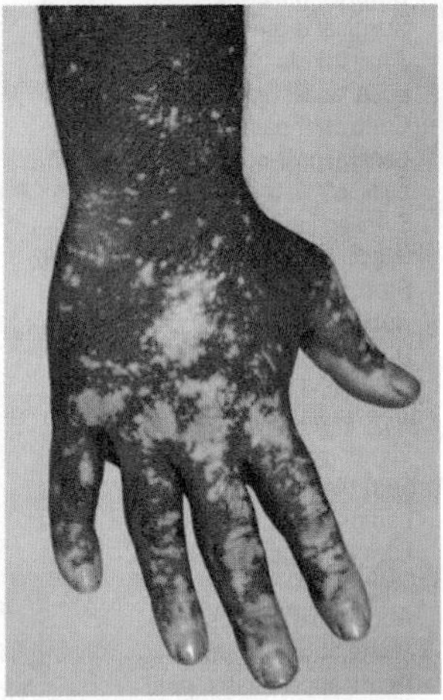

Fig 4. Vitiligo. Compare with fig 1, p429.

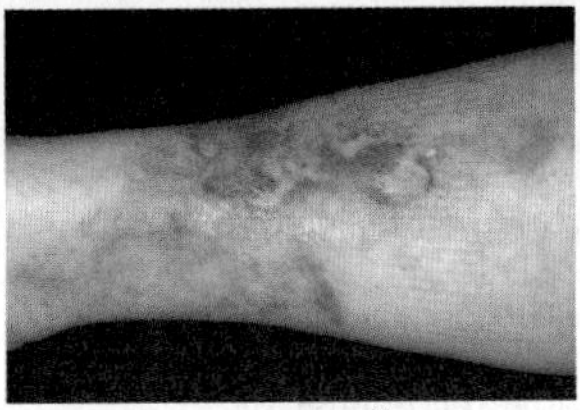

Fig 5. Necrobiosis lipoidica.[71]

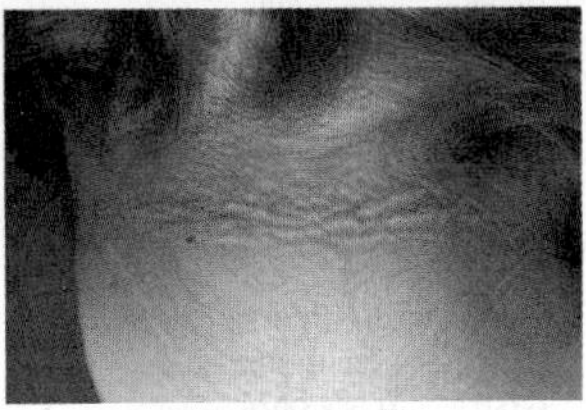

Fig 6. Acanthosis nigricans.[72]

Figures 2, 5 and 6 courtesy of Professor Thomas Habif

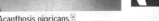

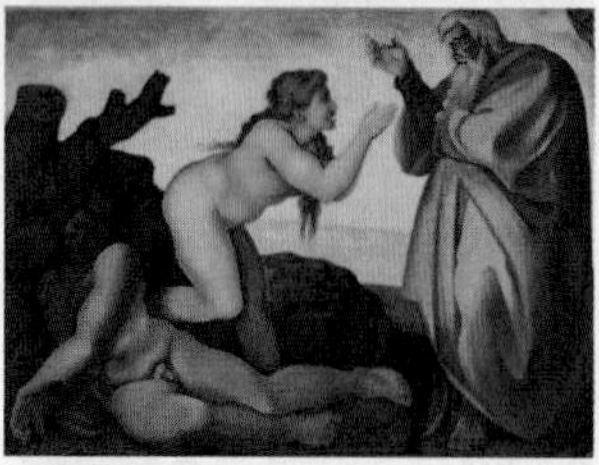

Fig 1. The *Creation of Eve*, from the rib of Adam...the first operation? Reproduced with permission from Gary Bevans (after Michelangelo).

Contents

See also in other chapters: **Gastroenterology** (p234), **Radiology** (p732), UTI (p286); haematuria (p286); prostatism (p65); gynaecological urology (*OHCS* p306); IV fluids (p680)

We thank Mr Barry Paraskeva FRCS who is our Specialist Reader for this chapter

The language of surgery

Abdominal areas:

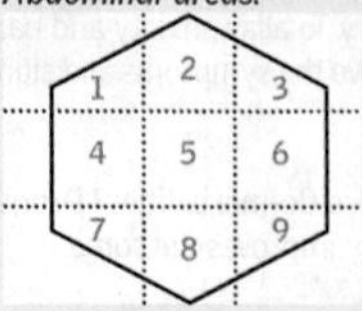

1 Right upper quadrant (RUQ) or hypochondrium
2 Epigastrium
3 Left upper quadrant (LUQ) or hypochondrium
4 Right flank (merges posteriorly with right loin, p57)
5 Peri-umbilical or central area
6 Left flank (merges posteriorly with left loin, p57)
7 Right iliac fossa (RIF)
8 Suprapubic area
9 Left iliac fossa (LIF)

Incisions:

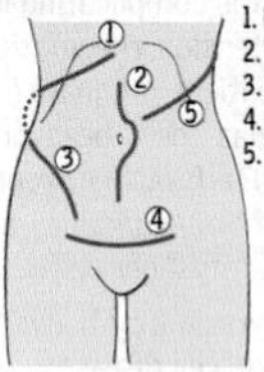

1. Kocher
2. Midline
3. Muscle splitting loin (ureter)
4. Pfannenstiel
5. Thoraco-abdominal (oesophagogastrectomy 9th or 10th ICS)

Paramedian 1.
McBurney 2.
Lanz 3.
Muscle-cutting transverse 4.
Roof-top 5.
McEvedy (femoral hernia) 6.
Inguinal hernia incision 7.

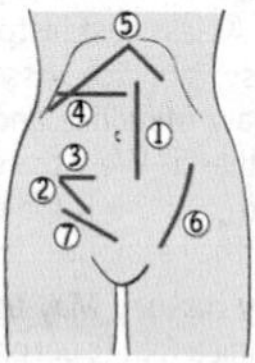

-ectomy	Cutting something out.
-gram	A radiological image.
-pexy	Anchoring of a structure to keep it in position.
-plasty	Surgical refashioning in order to regain good function.
-scopy	Procedure with instrumentation for looking into the body.
-stomy	An artificial union between a conduit and the outside or another conduit
-tomy	Cutting something open to the outside world.
-tripsy	Fragmentation of an object

angio-	Tube or vessel	**lith-**	Stone
appendic-	Appendix	**mast-**	Breast
chole-	Relating to gall/bile	**meso-**	Mesentery
colp-	Vagina	**nephr-**	Kidney
cyst-	Bladder	**orchid-**	Testicle
-doch-	Ducts	**oophor-**	Ovary
enter-	Small bowel	**phren-**	Diaphragm
eschar-	Dead tissue, eg from burn	**pyloro-**	Pyloric sphincter
gastr-	Stomach	**pyel-**	Renal pelvis
hepat-	Liver	**proct-**	Anal canal
hyster-	Uterus	**salping-**	Fallopian tube
lapar-	Abdomen	**splen-**	Spleen

abscess	A cavity containing pus. Remember: *if there is pus about, let it out.*
cyst	Fluid-filled cavity lined by epi/endothelium
fistula	An abnormal connection between two epithelial surfaces. Fistulae often close spontaneously, but will not in the presence of malignant tissue, distal obstruction, foreign bodies, chronic inflammation, and the formation of a muco-cutaneous junction (eg stoma).
hernia	The protrusion of a viscus/part of a viscus through a defect of the wall of its containing cavity into an abnormal position.
ileus	Used in this book as a term for adynamic bowel.
colic	Intermittent pain caused by obstruction of a hollow viscus
sinus	A blind-ending tract, typically lined by epithelial or granulation tissue, which opens to an epithelial surface.
stent	An artificial tube placed in a biological tube to keep it open.
stoma	(p584) An artificial union between conduits or a conduit and the outside.
ulcer	(p662) Interruption in the continuity of an epi/endothelial surface
volvulus	(p613) Twisting of a structure around itself. Common GI sites include the sigmoid colon and caecum, and more rarely the stomach.

epi-	Upon	**Pan-**	Whole	**peri-**	Around
end-	Inside	**para-**	Alongside	**sub-**	Beneath
mega-	Enlarged	**per-**	Going through	**trans-**	Across

Aims ►To provide diagnostic & prognostic information. To ensure the patient understands the nature, aims, and expected outcome of surgery. To allay anxiety and pain

- Ensure that the right patient gets the right surgery. Have the symptoms and signs changed? If so, inform the surgeon.
- Get informed consent (p570).
- Assess/balance risks of anaesthesia, and maximize fitness. Co-morbidities? Drugs? Smoker? Optimizing oxygenation **before** major surgery improves outcome.
- Check anaesthesia/analgesia type with anaesthetist.

Pre-op checks Assess cardiorespiratory system, exercise tolerance, existing illnesses, drugs, and allergies. Is the neck unstable (eg arthritis complicating intubation)? Assess past history of: MI,[1] diabetes, asthma, hypertension, rheumatic fever, epilepsy, jaundice. Assess any specific risks, eg is the patient pregnant? Is the neck/jaw immobile and teeth stable (intubation risk)? Has there been previous anaesthesia? Were there any complications (eg nausea, DVT)? ►Is DVT/PE prophylaxis needed (p580)? ►If for 'unilateral' surgery, mark the correct arm/leg/kidney, according to the recommendations of the UK National Patient Safety Agency.

Family history May be relevant, eg in malignant hyperpyrexia (p574); dystrophia myotonica (p514); porphyria; cholinesterase problems; sickle-cell disease.

Drugs Any drug/plaster/antiseptic allergies? ►Inform the anaesthetist about **all** drugs even if 'over-the-counter'. ►Steroids: see p592; diabetes, p590.

- ***Antibiotics:*** *Tetracycline* and *neomycin* may ↑neuromuscular blockade.
- ***Anticoagulants:*** ►**Tell the surgeon**. Avoid epidural, spinal, and regional blocks. *Aspirin* should probably be continued unless there is a major risk of bleeding. Discuss stopping *clopidogrel* therapy with the cardiologists/neurologists.
- ***Anticonvulsants:*** Give as usual pre-op. Post-op, give drugs IV (or by NGT) until able to take orally. *Valproate*: give usual dose IV. *Phenytoin*: give IV slowly (<50mg/min; monitor ECG). IM *phenytoin* absorption is unreliable.
- ***β-blockers:*** Continue up to and including the day of surgery as this precludes a labile cardiovascular response.
- ***Contraceptive steroids:*** See *BNF*. Stop 4wks before major/leg surgery; ensure alternative contraception is used. Restart 2wks after surgery, provided mobile.
- ***Digoxin:*** Continue up to and including morning of surgery. Check for toxicity (ECG; plasma level); do plasma K^+ and Ca^{2+} (*suxamethonium* can ↑K^+ and lead to ventricular arrhythmias in the fully digitalized).
- ***Diuretics:*** Beware hypokalaemia, dehydration. Do U&E (and bicarbonate).
- ***Eye-drops:*** β-blockers get absorbed; anticholinesterases ↑[*suxamethonium*].
- ***HRT:*** As with contraceptive steroids there may be an increased risk of DVT/PE.
- ***Levodopa:*** Possible arrhythmias when patient under GA.
- ***Lithium:*** Get expert help; it may potentiate neuromuscular blockade and cause arrhythmias. See *OHCS* p354.
- ***MAOIs:*** Get expert help as interactions may cause hypotensive/hypertensive crises.
- ***Thyroid medication:*** see p593.
- ***Tricyclics:*** These enhance *adrenaline* (epinephrine) and arrhythmias.

Preparation ►Fast patient; NBM ≥2h pre-op for clear fluids and ≥6h for solids.

- Is any bowel or skin preparation needed, or prophylactic antibiotics (p572)?
- Start DVT prophylaxis as indicated, eg graduated compression stockings (not if there is peripheral arterial disease) + *heparin* 5000U SC 2h pre-op, then every 8-12h SC for 7d or until ambulant. Low molecular weight heparin (LMWH, p344): eg *enoxaparin* 20mg/d SC, increased to 40mg/d in major-risk surgery.
- Write up the pre-meds (p574); book any pre-, intra-, or post-operative x-rays or frozen sections. Book post-operative physiotherapy.
- If needed, catheterize (p776) and insert a Ryle's tube (p773) before induction. These can reduce organ bulk, making it easier to operate in the abdomen.

1 If within the last 6 months, the peri-operative risk of reinfarction (up to 40%) makes most elective surgery too risky. ECHO & stress testing (+ exercise ECG or MUGA scan, p755) should be done.

Pre-operative examination and tests—see NICE guidelines[3]

►**Careful planning is the key to preventing peri-operative death.**[1] A good thought exercise is to imagine yourself at the next surgical *Mortality Meeting* and ask "If I were looking back at the pre-op period, knowing that this patient had died, would I still consider that surgery was indicated?" The UK National Confidential Enquiry into Perioperative Deaths (NCEPOD) found that 'too many' operations are performed on moribund patients.[5]

It is the anaesthetist's duty to assess suitability for anaesthesia. The ward doctor assists with a good history & examination, and can also reassure, inform, and get informed written consent (p570; ideally this should be from the surgeon).

Be alert to chronic lung disease, BP↑, arrhythmias, and murmurs.

Pre-op checklist
- Blood tests (inc. group & save or crossmatch)
- IV cannula
- ECG + CXR
- Drug chart:
  - regular medications
  - analgesia/antiemetic
  - antibiotics
  - LMWH/heparin
- Compression stockings
- Consent
- Marked site/side
- Anaesthetist informed
- Theatres informed
- Infection risk? (eg MRSA/HIV/HBV/HCV)
- NBM since when?

...not all will be required

WHO Surgical Safety checklists ensure pre-operative preparation, intraoperative monitoring and post-operative review[4]

Tests ►Be guided by the history and examination and local/NICE protocols.

- ***U&E, FBC, and ward tests for blood glucose in most patients.*** If Hb <10g/dL tell anaesthetist. Investigate/treat as appropriate. U&E are particularly important if the patient is starved, diabetic, on diuretics, a burns patient, has hepatic or renal disease, has an ileus, or is parenterally fed.
- ***Crossmatching:*** Examples: Group and save (G&S) for mastectomy or cholecystectomy. Crossmatch 2 units for Caesarean section; 4 units for a gastrectomy; 6 units for abdominal aortic aneurysm (AAA) surgery.
- ***Specific blood tests:*** LFT in jaundice, malignancy, or alcohol abuse. Amylase in acute abdominal pain. Blood glucose if diabetic (p590). Drug levels as appropriate (eg *digoxin, lithium*). Clotting studies in liver or renal disease, DIC (p346), massive blood loss, eg if on *valproate, warfarin,* or *heparin*. HIV, HBsAg in high-risk patients, after counselling. Sickle test in those from Africa, West Indies, or Mediterranean—and if origins are in malarial areas (including most of India). Thyroid function tests in those with thyroid disease.
- ***CXR*** if known cardiorespiratory disease, pathology or symptoms, possible lung metastases, or >65yrs old. Remember to check the film prior to surgery.
- ***ECG*** if >55yrs old or poor exercise tolerance, or history of myocardial ischaemia, hypertension, rheumatic fever, or other heart disease.
- ***Echocardiogram*** may be performed if there is a suspicion of poor LV function.
- ***Pulmonary function tests*** in known pulmonary disease/obesity
- ***Lateral cervical spine x-ray*** (flexion & extension views) if history of rheumatoid arthritis/ankylosing spondylitis/Down's syndrome, to warn of difficult intubations.
- ***MRSA screen:*** Rising above the frenzied media headlines, it is still important make every effort to reduce spread of MRSA. Colonisation is **not** a contra-indication to surgery, and if on balance surgery is appropriate, the case should be last on the list to minimize transmission to others (with appropriate theatre protocol). Cover with appropriate antibiotic prophylaxis, eg **vancomycin**.

American Society of Anesthesiologists (ASA) classification

Class I	Normally healthy
Class II	Mild systemic disease
Class III	Severe systemic disease that limits activity but is not incapacitating
Class IV	Incapacitating systemic disease which poses a constant threat to life.
Class V	Moribund: not expected to survive 24h even with operation

You will see a space for an ASA number on most anaesthetic charts. It is a health index at the time of surgery. The prefix E is used in emergencies.

1 Risk of mortality from elective surgery is currently about 1:100 000 to 1:150 000.

In which of the following situations would you seek 'informed written consent' from a patient? 1 Feeling for a pulse. 2 Taking some blood. 3 Inserting a central line. 4 Removing a section of small bowel during a laparotomy for division of adhesions. 5 Orchidectomy after a failed operation for testicular torsion.

English law states that **any** intervention or treatment needs consent—ie all of the above—yet, for different reasons, we know that, for some, informed formal consent is not regularly sought! In fact, **written** consent itself is not required by law, but it does constitute 'good medical practice' in the best interests of the patient and practitioner. Sometimes actions and words can imply valid consent, eg by simply entering into conversation or holding out an arm. In these situations your actions and their consequences are understood by the patient as a product of their knowledge, previous interactions with doctors and learning through experience.[1] However, if the consequences are not clear to the patient and they have the capacity to give consent (see below & BOX), you should seek informed written consent, as this serves as a record of your conversation together.[6]

For consent to be valid:

- It can be given any time before the intervention/treatment is initiated. Earlier is better as this will give the patient time to think about the risks, benefits and alternatives—he may even bring forward questions on issues that you had not considered relevant. Think of consent as an ongoing process throughout the patient's time with you, not just the moment of signing the form.
- The proposed treatment or test must be clearly understood by the patient, taking into account the benefits, risks (including complication rates if known), additional procedures, alternative courses of action and their consequences.
- It must be given **voluntarily.** This can be difficult to evaluate—eg when live organ donation is being considered—see BOX for other difficult situations.
- The doctor who is providing treatment or undertaking the test needs to ensure that the patient has given valid consent. The act of seeking consent is ultimately the responsibility of the doctor looking after the patient, though the task may be delegated to another health professional, as long as they are suitably trained and qualified. Sometimes you may have be certified to get consent.
- The patient must have the **capacity** (can understand, believe, retain, and weigh the necessary information) to give consent. Assessment of capacity must be time and decision-specific.

When taking consent:

- Think about whether you are the right person to be obtaining consent.
- Use words the patient understands and avoid jargon and abbreviations.
- Ensure that he believes your facts and can retain 'pros' and 'cons' long enough to inform his decision. Fact sheets/diagrams for individual operations help.
- Make sure his choice is free from pressure from others, and explain that after he has signed the form he is free to choose not to have the proposed treatment (ie withdraw consent) at any time. Some patients may view the consent form as a contract from which they cannot *renege*.
- If the patient is illiterate, a witnessed mark does endorse valid consent. Similarly, if the patient is willing but physically unable to sign the consent form, then an entry into the medical notes stating so is valid.
- Remember to discuss further procedures that may become necessary during the proposed treatment. This avoids waking up to a nasty surprise (eg a missing testicle as in scenario 5 above).
- If you suspect the patient is not capable of giving consent then a formal assessment needs to be documented in the medical notes.

Consent is complex, but remember that it exists for the benefit of the patient **and** the doctor, giving you an opportunity to revisit expectations and involve the patient in his own care.

Special circumstances for consent...and who to ask

There are some areas of treatment or investigation for which it may be advisable to seek specialist advice if it is not part of your regular practice:

- Photography of a patient.
- Innovative or novel treatment.
- Living organ donation.
- Storage, use, or removal of human tissue (for any length of time), as regulated under the Human Tissue Act 2004.
- The storage, loss, or use of gametes, as regulated under the Human Fertilisation and Embryology Act 1990.
- The use of patient records or tissue in research or teaching.
- In the presence of an advanced directive or living will expressly refusing a particular treatment, investigation or action.
- Consent if <16yrs—consent form 3 in NHS.[7] In the UK, those >16yrs can give valid consent. Those <16yrs can give consent for a medical decision provided they understand what it involves—the concept of *Gillick* competence.[8] It is still good practice to involve the parents in the decision, if the child is willing. If **<18yrs and refusing life-saving surgery**, talk to the parents and your senior; the law is unclear. You may need to contact the duty judge in the High Court.
- Consent in the incapacitated (NHS consent form 4).[9] No one (parents, relatives, or even members of a healthcare team) is able to give consent on behalf of an adult in England, and the High Court may be required to give a ruling on the matters of lawfulness of a proposed procedure. Proceeding in a patient's best interest is decided by the clinician overseeing their care, although it is always good practice to involve family in the proposed course of treatment.

Who to ask if you are unsure?
• Your team's senior/consultant
• Your employing organisation
• Legal defence organisation
• National medical association
• Local research ethics committee

The right to refuse treatment

Their's not to make reply,
Their's not to reason why,
Their's but to do and die. **Alfred, Lord Tennyson from *The Charge of the Light Brigade*, 1854**

The rights of a patient are something of an antithesis to this military macabre of Tennyson, and it is our responsibility to respect the legal and ethical rights of those we treat. We do this not only for the sake of the individual, but also for the sake of an enduring trust between the patient and doctor, remembering that is the patient's right to refuse treatment (if a fully competent adult) even when this may result in death of the patient, or even the death of an unborn child, whatever the stage of pregnancy. The only exception is in circumstances outlined by the Mental Health Act 2007 (amends Mental Health act 1983 and Mental Capacity Act 2005).

5 Principles of capacity:

1 Assumption of capacity unless it is established a person lacks capacity

2 A person is not to be treated as unable to make a decision unless all practicable steps to help him to do so have been taken without success

3 A person is not to be treated as unable to make a decision merely because he makes an unwise decision

4 An act done, or decision made for or on behalf of a person who lacks capacity must be done, or made, in his best interests

5 Before the act is done or the decision is made, regard must be paid as to whether the purpose for which it is needed can be effectively achieved in a way that is less restrictive of the person's rights and freedom of action.

1 In agreeing to a blood test, the patient understands that it may be an uncomfortable experience, perhaps with some bruising, but he also knows that the results of the test may help you in making a diagnosis and hopefully restore him to full health and vigour. But grey areas exist everywhere: when he extends his arm towards you, does he know that you could accidentally injure an artery or nerve, with all the complications that follow—does he need to know...?

Prophylactic antibiotics in surgery

Prophylactic antibiotics are given to counter the risk of wound infection (p582), which occurs in ~20% of elective GI surgery (up to 60% in emergency surgery); they are also given if infection elsewhere, although unlikely, would have severe consequences (eg when prostheses are involved). They are given 15-60min prior to the procedure so that the skin concentration is maximised[10] and may be given as a single dose, 3 doses, or more depending on local guidelines and contamination at the site of surgery (see TABLE). A single dose given before surgery has been shown to be just as beneficial as more prolonged regimens in biliary surgery and colorectal surgery.[11] [12] ►Wound infections are not necessarily trivial since sepsis may lead to haemorrhage, wound dehiscence, and initiate a fatal chain of events, so take measures to minimise the risk of wound infection:

- Time administration correctly.
- Use antibiotics which will kill anaerobes and coliforms.
- Consider use of perioperative supplemental oxygen. This is a practical method of reducing the incidence of surgical wound infections.[13]
- Practice strictly sterile surgical technique. (Ask for a hand with scrubbing up if you are not sure—Sister will be more than pleased to help!)

Antibiotic regimens Check for local or personal preferences. Examples:

- *Biliary surgery:* **Cefuroxime** 1.5g, for 1 dose IV + metronidazole (below).
- *Appendectomy:* If uncomplicated, a single dose **cefuroxime** 1.5g IV is effective.[14]
- *Colorectal surgery: Cefuroxime* 1.5g/8h + **metronidazole** 500mg/8h, 1-3 doses IV. *Tazocin*® 4.5g/8h, 1-3 doses IV can be used if there is heavy soiling.
- *Vascular surgery:* **Co-amoxiclav** 1.2g IV on induction; if penicillin-allergic, **cefuroxime** 1.5g IV/IM + **metronidazole** 500mg IV. Anaerobic cover is not always needed.
- MRSA is an increasing concern, and so may warrant vancomycin prophylaxis.[15]

Bowel preparation in colorectal surgery

The place of bowel preparation in colorectal surgery has recently come under much scrutiny.[16] Whereas there are clear benefits when visualisation of the lumen is required (eg colonoscopy), the intended benefit for elective open procedures of minimizing post-operative infection may well be outweighed by the complications:[17]

- Liquefying bowel contents which are spilled during surgery
- Perforation
- Electrolyte loss leading to hyponatraemia and seizures[18]
- Dehydration
- A higher rate of post-operative anastomotic leakage[19]

Usually no laxatives are needed for right-sided operations (eg right hemicolectomy); the patient is just put on a 'low-residue' diet for a few days pre-op, then clear fluids the day before. For left-sided operations and rectal operations (eg left hemicolectomy, anterior resection), laxatives and enemas may still be used. ►If in doubt, check with the surgeon as to what preparation he or she prefers.

Example: 1 sachet of Picolax® (10mg **sodium picosulfate + magnesium citrate**) at 8AM; another 6-8h later on the day before surgery.

Sutures

Sutures (stitches) are central to the art of surgery. The trainee may face several long evenings practising knots over a pint of beer before they are allowed back to tie at the table! In their broadest sense they are absorbable or non-absorbable, synthetic or natural, and their structure may be divided into monofilament, twisted, or braided. See TABLE (BOX 3) for some examples and their uses.

Monofilament sutures are quite slippery but minimize infection and produce less reaction (natural fibres of any type produce quite a vigorous reaction). Braided sutures have plaited strands and provide secure knots, but they may allow infection to occur between their strands. Twisted sutures have 2 twisted strands and similar qualities to braided sutures. 3-0 or 4-0 (smaller) are the best sizes for skin closure.

Classification of surgical procedures and wound infection risk

Category	Description	Infection risk
Clean	Incising uninfected skin without opening a viscus	<2%
Clean-contaminated	Intraoperative breach of a viscus (but not colon)	8-10%
Contaminated	Breach of a viscus + spillage or opening of the colon	12-20%
Dirty	The site is already contaminated with pus or faeces, or from exogenous contagion eg trauma	25%

Table after *MRCS Core Modules: Essential Revision Notes*, S. Andrews, Pastest, ISBN 1901198715

Surgical drains in the post-operative period

The decision when to insert and remove drains may seem to be one of the great surgical enigmas—but there are basically 3 types to get a grip on.

1 Most are inserted to drain the area of surgery and are often put under suction or -ve pressure (Redivac® uses a 'high vacuum'). These are removed when they stop draining. They protect against collection, haematoma and seroma formation (in breast surgery this can cause overlying skin necrosis).

2 The second type of drain is used to protect sites where leakage may occur in the post-operative period, such as bowel anastomoses. These form a tract and are removed after about 1 week.

3 The third type (eg Bellovac®) collects red blood cells from the site of the operation, which can then be autotransfused within 6h, protecting from the hazards of allotransfusion—it is used commonly in orthopaedics.

'Shortening a drain' means withdrawing it (eg by 2cm/day) to allow the tract to seal, bit by bit. Evidence suggests that certain types of drain are not effective and may even lead to more complications, such as when used to protect colorectal anastomoses.[20] ►Check the individual surgeon's wishes before altering a drain.

Some commonly encountered suture materials

The perfect suture material is monofilament, strong, easy to handle, holds knots well, has predictable absorption and causes minimal tissue reaction. Unfortunately no single suture fits the bill for every occasion, and so suture selection (including size) depends on a the job in hand:

Absorbable

Name	Material	Construction	Use
Monocryl®	Poliglecaprone	Monofilament	Subcuticular skin closure
PDS®	Polydioxanone	Monofilament	Closing abdominal wall
Vicryl®	Polyglactin	Braided multifilament	Tying pedicles; bowel anastomosis; subcutaneous closure
Dexon®	Polyglycolic acid	Braided multifilament	Very similar to vicryl®

Non-absorbable

Name	Material	Construction	Use
Ethilon®	Polyamide	Monofilament	Closing skin wounds
Prolene®	Polypropylene	Monofilament	Arterial anastomosis
Mersilk®N	Silk	Braided multifilament	Securing drains
Metal	Eg steel	Clips or monofilament	Skin wound/ sternotomy closure

N = natural; other natural materials (eg cotton and catgut) are rarely used these days.

Timing the removal of sutures

The timing of suture removal depends on site and the general health of the patient. Face and neck sutures may be removed after 5d (earlier in children), scalp and back of neck after 5d, abdominal incisions and proximal limbs (including clips) after ~10d and those on the distal extremities after 14d. In patients with poor wound healing, eg on steroids, with malignancy, infection, cachexia (p29), the elderly, or smokers, the sutures may need 14d or longer.

Before anaesthesia, explain to the patient what will happen and where he will wake up, otherwise the recovery room or ITU will be frightening. Explain that he may feel ill on waking. The premedication aims to allay anxiety and to make the anaesthesia itself easier to conduct (see BOX). Typical regimens might include:

- *Anxiolytics:* Benzodiazepines, eg ***temazepam*** 10–20mg PO. In children, ***midazolam*** 0.3–0.5mg/kg rectally 30min prior to procedure is effective.
- *Analgesics: See* p576. The patient should not be in pain prior to surgery. **Opioids, local anaesthetic blocks,** *paracetamol* and **NSAIDs** (beware bleeding risk) are all used. In children or anxious adults, local anaesthetic cream (eg **Emla®, Ametop®**) may be used on a few sites for the anaesthetist's IVI (►they may prefer to site the cannula themselves!)
- *Antiemetics:* 5HT3 antagonists (eg *ondansetron* 4mg IV/IM) are the most effective agents; others eg *metoclopramide* 10mg/8h IV/IM/PO are also used—see p241.
- *Antacids: Ranitidine* 50mg IV in patients at particular risk of aspiration.
- *Antisialogues: Glycopyrronium* (200–400µg in adults, 4–8µg/kg in children; given IV/IM 30–60min before induction) is sometimes used to decrease secretions that may cause respiratory obstruction in smaller airways.
- *Antibiotics: See* p572.

Give oral premedication 1–2h before surgery (1h if IM route used).

Side effects of anaesthetic agents

- *Hyoscine, atropine:* Anticholinergic ∴ tachycardia, urinary retention, glaucoma, sedation (especially in the elderly).
- *Opioids:* Respiratory depression, cough reflex↓, nausea & vomiting, constipation.
- *Thiopental:* (For rapid induction of anaesthesia) laryngospasm.
- *Propofol:* Respiratory depression, cardiac depression, pain on injection.
- *Volatile agents eg isoflurane:* Nausea & vomiting, cardiac depression, respiratory depression, vasodilatation, hepatotoxicity (see *BNF*).

The complications of anaesthesia are due to loss of:

- *Pain sensation:* Urinary retention, diathermy burns, pressure necrosis, local nerve injuries (eg radial nerve palsy from arm hanging over the table edge).
- *Consciousness:* Cannot communicate 'wrong leg/kidney'. **NB:** in some patients (eg 0.15%) *retained* consciousness is the problem.[21] Awareness under GA sounds like a contradiction of terms, but remember that anaesthesia is a process rather than an event. Such awareness can lead to ill-defined, delayed neuroses and post-traumatic stress disorder (*OHCS* p347).[22]
- *Muscle power:* Corneal abrasion (∴ tape the eyes closed), no respiration, no cough (leads to pneumonia and atelectasis—partial lung collapse causing shunting ± impaired gas exchange: it starts minutes after induction, and may be related to the use of 100% O_2, supine position, surgery and age as well as to loss of power). Cannot phonate (speak) and unable to impart vital information when paralysed—eg "I am in pain ...".

Local/regional anaesthesia If unfit/unwilling to undergo general anaesthesia, local nerve blocks (eg brachial plexus) or spinal blocks (contraindication: anticoagulation, local infection) using long-acting local anaesthetics such as *bupivacaine* may be indicated. See TABLE for doses and toxicity effects.

Drugs complicating anaesthesia ►Inform anaesthetist. See p568 for lists of specific drugs, and actions to take.

Malignant hyperpyrexia This is a rare complication, precipitated by eg *halothane* or *suxamethonium*, exhibiting autosomal dominant inheritance. There is a rapid rise in temperature (>1°C every 30min); masseter spasm may also be an early sign. Complications include hypoxaemia, hypercarbia, hyperkalaemia, metabolic acidosis, and arrhythmias. ►Get expert help immediately. Prompt treatment with *dantrolene*,[1] cooling and supportive care can reduce mortality significantly.

1 Give 1mg/kg every 5min IV—up to 10mg/kg in total (*OHCS* p628).

Surgery

Principles and practical conduct of anaesthesia

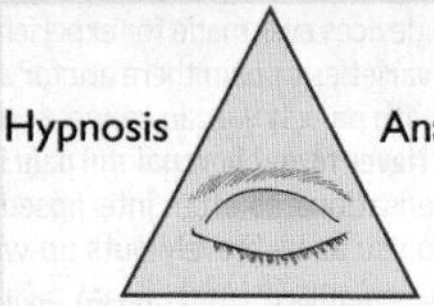

►The general principles of anaesthesia centre on the triad of hypnosis, analgesia, and muscle relaxation.

The conduct of anaesthesia typically involves:

- *Induction:* Either intravenous (eg *propofol* 1.5-2.5mg/kg IV at a rate of 20-40mg every 10s; *thiopental* is an alternative) or, if airway obstruction or difficult IV access, gaseous (eg *sevoflurane* or *nitrous oxide*, mixed in O_2).
- *Airway control:* Either using a face mask, an oropharyngeal (Guedel) airway or by intubation. The latter usually requires muscle relaxation with a depolarizing/non-depolarizing neuromuscular blocker (*OHCS* p622).
- *Maintenance of anaesthesia:* Either a volatile agent added to N_2O/O_2 mixture, or high-dose opiates with mechanical ventilation, or IV infusion anaesthesia (eg *propofol* 4-12mg/kg/h IVI).
- *End of anaesthesia:* Change inspired gases to 100% oxygen only, then discontinue any anaesthetic infusions and reverse muscle paralysis. Once spontaneously breathing, place patient in recovery position and give oxygen by face mask.
- For further details, see the *Anaesthesia* chapter in *OHCS* (p612)

Local anaesthetic toxicity and maximum doses

After a few minutes conversation with an anaesthetist at work, it becomes apparent that they are masters of the drug dose by weight! It is important to remember the maximum doses for local anaesthetics, not least because we use them so frequently, but because the effects of overdose can be lethal.

Local anaesthetic toxicity starts with perioral tingling and paraesthesiae, progressing to drowsiness, seizures, coma and cardiorespiratory arrest. If suspected (the patient feels 'funny' and develops early signs) then stop administration immediately and commence ABC resuscitation as required.

Handy to remember (though it can be worked out with a pen, paper and SI units) is that a 1% concentration is equivalent to 10mg/mL. Local anaesthetics are also basic, and so do not work well in acidic environments, eg abscesses.

%age	Lidocaine conc^n (mg/mL)	Approx. allowable volume (mL/kg)
0.25%	2.5	1.12
0.5%	5	0.56
1%	10	0.28
2%	20	0.14

Humans are the most exquisite devices ever made for experiencing of pain: the richer our inner lives, the greater the varieties of pain there are for us to feel, and the more resources we have for dealing with pain. If we can connect with patients' inner lives we may make a real difference. **Never forget how painful pain is,** nor how fear magnifies pain. Try not to let these sensations, so often interposed between your patient and his recovery, be invisible to you as he bravely puts up with them.

Guidelines for success (see also analgesic ladder, p535). Review and chart each pain carefully and individually.

- Identify and treat the underlying pathology wherever possible.
- Give **regular** doses rather than on an as-required basis.
- Choose the best route: PO, PR, IM, epidural, SC, inhalation, or IV.
- Explanation and reassurance contribute greatly to analgesia.
- Allow the patient to be in charge. This promotes wellbeing, and does not lead to overuse. Patient-controlled continuous IV morphine delivery systems are useful.
- Liaise with the Acute Pain Service, if possible.

Non-narcotic (simple) analgesia *Paracetamol* 0.5-1.0g/4h PO (up to 4g daily) [15mg/kg/4h IV over ¼h in children >10kg; up to 60mg/kg/d]. Caution in liver impairment. NSAIDs, eg *ibuprofen* 400mg/8h PO [10mg/kg/8h in children >5kg] or *diclofenac* 50mg/8h PO, or 100mg PR, or 75mg IM stat; these are good for musculoskeletal pain and renal or biliary colic. CI: peptic ulcer, clotting disorders, anticoagulants. Cautions: asthma, renal or hepatic impairment, pregnancy, and the elderly. *Aspirin* is contraindicated in children due to the risk of Reye's syndrome (*OHCS* p652).

Opioid drugs for severe pain *Morphine* (eg 10-15mg/2-4h IV/IM) or *diamorphine* (5-10mg/2-4h PO, SC, or slow IV, but you may need much more) are best. **NB:** these are 'controlled' drugs. For palliative care, see p534. ***Side effects of opioids:*** These include nausea (so give with an antiemetic, eg *prochlorperazine* 12.5mg stat IM), respiratory depression, constipation, cough suppression, urinary retention, BP↓, and sedation (do not use in hepatic failure or head injury). Dependency is rarely a problem. *Naloxone* (eg 100-200μg IV, followed by 100μg increments, eg every 2min until responsive) may be needed to reverse the effects of excess opioids (p854).

How effective are standard analgesics? Pain is subjective, but its measurement by patients is surprisingly consistent and reproducible. The table below gives 'number needed to treat' (NNT, p671), ie the number of patients who need to receive the drug for one to achieve at least 50% pain relief over 4-6h (the range is 95% confidence intervals).

Codeine^{60mg}	11-48	Paracetamol^{1000mg}	3-4
Tramadol^{50mg}	6-13	Paracetamol^{1000mg}/codeine^{60mg}	2-3
Aspirin^{650mg}/codeine^{60mg}	4-7	Diclofenac^{50mg} or ibuprofen^{400mg}	2-3

Epidural analgesia Opioids and anaesthetics are given into the epidural space by infusion or as boluses. Ask the advice of the Pain Service. SE: thought to be less as drug more localized: watch for respiratory depression; local anaesthetic-induced autonomic blockade (BP↓).

Adjuvant treatments Eg radiotherapy for bone cancer pain; anticonvulsants, antidepressants, *gabapentin* or steroids for neuropathic pain, antispasmodics, eg *hyoscine butylbromide*[1] (Buscopan® 10-20mg/8h PO/IM/IV) for intestinal, renal tract colic. If brief pain relief is needed (eg for changing dressings or exploring wounds), try inhaled *nitrous oxide* (with 50% O_2—as Entonox®) with an 'on-demand' valve. Transcutaneous electrical nerve stimulation (TENS), local heat, local or regional anaesthesia, and neurosurgical procedures (eg excision of neuroma) may be tried but can prove disappointing. Treat conditions that exacerbate pain (eg constipation, depression, anxiety).

1 Not to be confused with *hyoscine hydrobromide;* used for drying secretions and in motion sickness.

Why is controlling post-operative pain so important?

- **Psychological reasons:** Pain control is a humanitarian undertaking.
- **Social reasons:** Pain relief makes surgery less feared by society.
- **Biological reasons:** There is evidence for the following sequence: pain → autonomic activation → increased adrenergic activity → arteriolar vasoconstriction → reduced wound perfusion → decreased tissue oxygenation → delayed wound healing → serious or mortal consequences.

Looking for infection:
Check for signs of:
- Peritonism
- Chest infection
- UTI
- Wound infection
- Cannula site erythema
- Meningism
- Endocarditis

Pyrexia Mild pyrexia in the 1st 48h is often from atelectasis (needs prompt physio, not antibiotics), tissue damage/necrosis or even from blood transfusions, but still have a low threshold for infection screen. See MINIBOX for where to look for infection—also check the legs for DVT (causes ↑°T). Send blood for FBC, U&E, CRP, and cultures (±LFT). Dipstick the urine. Consider MSU, CXR, and abdominal ultrasound/CT depending on clinical findings.

Confusion may manifest as agitation, disorientation, and attempts to leave hospital, especially at night. Gently reassure the patient in well-lit surroundings. See p488 for a full work-up. The common causes are:
- Hypoxia (pneumonia, atelectasis, LVF, PE)
- Drugs (opiates, sedatives, and many others)
- Urinary retention
- MI or stroke
- Infection (see above)
- Alcohol withdrawal (p282)
- Liver/renal failure

Occasionally, sedation is necessary to examine the patient; consider *midazolam* (see p787; antidote: *flumazenil*) or *haloperidol* 0.5–2mg IM. Reassure relatives that post-op confusion is common (seen in up to 40%) and reversible.

Dyspnoea or hypoxia Any previous lung disease? Sit up and give O_2, monitoring peripheral O_2 sats by pulse oximetry (p156). Examine for evidence of: • Pneumonia, pulmonary collapse or aspiration • LVF (MI; fluid overload) • Pulmonary embolism (p182); • Pneumothorax (p182; due to CVP line, intercostal block or mechanical ventilation). *Tests* FBC; ABG; CXR; ECG. Manage according to findings.

BP↓ If severe, tilt bed head down and give O_2. Check pulse & BP yourself; compare it with pre-op values. Post-op ↓BP is often from hypovolaemia resulting from inadequate fluid input, so check fluid chart and replace losses. Monitor urine output (may need catheterization). A CVP line can help monitor fluid resuscitation (normal is 0–5cm H_2O relative to sternal angle). Hypovolaemia may also be caused by haemorrhage so review wounds and abdomen. If unstable, return to theatre for haemostasis. Beware cardiogenic and neurogenic causes and look for evidence of MI + PE. Consider sepsis and anaphylaxis. ***Management:*** p804.

BP↑ may be from pain, urinary retention, idiopathic hypertension (eg missed medication) or inotropic drugs. Oral cardiac medications (including anti-hypertensives) should be continued throughout the peri-operative period even if NBM. Treat the cause, consider increasing the regular medication, or if not absorbing orally try 50mg *labetalol* IV over 1 min (see p134).

Urine output↓ (oliguria) Aim for output of >30mL/h in adults (or >½mL/kg/h). **Anuria** often means a blocked or malsited catheter (see p777) rather than ARF and never, we hope, an impending lawsuit from both ureters tied. Flush or replace catheter. **Oliguria** is usually due to too little replacement of lost fluid. Treat by increasing fluid input. ►Acute renal failure may follow shock, drugs, transfusion, pancreatitis or trauma.
- Review fluid chart and examine for signs of volume depletion.
- Urinary retention is also common, so examine for a palpable bladder.
- Establish normovolaemia (a CVP line may help here); you may need 1L/h IVI for 2–3h. A 250–500mL bolus of colloid (eg Gelofusin®) over 30min may also help.
- Catheterize bladder (for accurate monitoring)—see p776; check U&E.
- If intrinsic renal failure is suspected, refer to a nephrologist early.

Nausea/vomiting Any mechanical obstruction, ileus, or emetic drugs (opiates, digoxin, anaesthetics)? Consider AXR, NGT, and an antiemetic (►**not** *metoclopramide* because of its prokinetic property). See p241 for choice of different anti-emetics.

↓Na^+ What was the pre-op level? SIADH (p687) can be precipitated by perioperative pain, nausea, and opioids as well as chest infection. Over-administration of IV fluids may exacerbate the situation. Correct slowly (p687).

Post-operative bleeding

Primary haemorrhage: Continuous bleeding, starting during surgery. Replace blood loss. If severe, return to theatre for adequate haemostasis. Treat shock vigorously (p804).

Reactive haemorrhage: Haemostasis appears secure until BP rises and bleeding starts. Replace blood and re-explore wound.

Secondary haemorrhage (caused by infection) occurs 1-2 weeks post-op.

Talking about post-op complications...

When asked to give your thoughts on the complications of an operation—may be with an examiner or a patient—a good starting point is to divide them up accordingly (and for each of the following stratify as immediate, early and late):

- *From the anaesthetic* (p574) eg respiratory depression from induction agents.
- *From surgery in general:* (see p578 and BOX 1) eg wound infection, haemorrhage, neurovascular damage, DVT/PE.
- *From the specific procedure:* eg saphenous nerve damage in stripping of the long varicose vein.

Tailor the discussion towards the individual who, eg if an arteriopath, may have a significant risk of cardiac ischaemia during hypotensive episodes whilst under the anaesthetic. For some other post-op complications, see:

- Pain (p576) • DVT (p580 & **figs 1-4**) • Pulmonary embolus (p182; massive, p828)
- Wound dehiscence (p582) • Complications in post-gastric surgery (p624)
- Other complications of specific operations (p582).

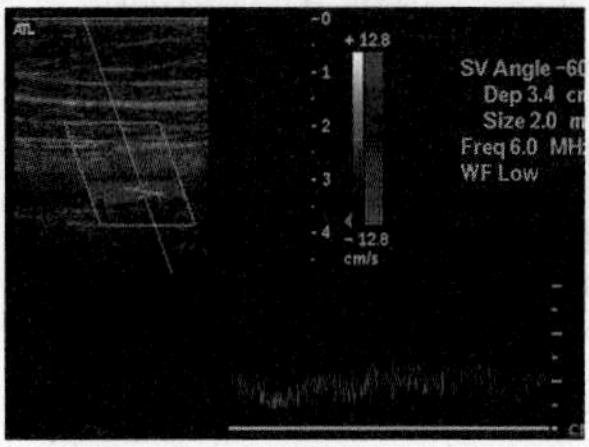

Fig 1. A normal duplex ultrasound (sagittal view) of the superficial femoral vein with a normal Doppler trace. Compression ultrasound (**fig 2**) is the best image in suspected DVT. Figs 1-4 courtesy of Norwich Radiology Dept.

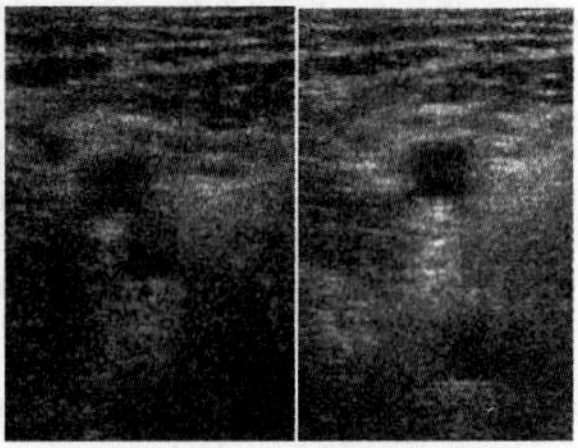

Fig 2. Transverse ultrasound of the superficial femoral vein and artery with (right) and without compression (left). Collapse of the vein (deeper to the artery) on compression means absence of thrombus.

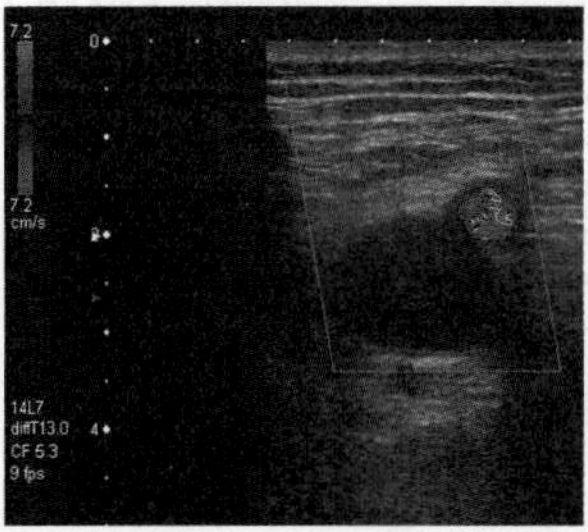

Fig 3. Ultrasound showing evidence of an acute thrombus within a dilated superficial femoral vein. This will not always show an intraluminal echo (compare with **fig 4**) and so confirm its presence by lack of compression of the vein with the ultrasound probe.

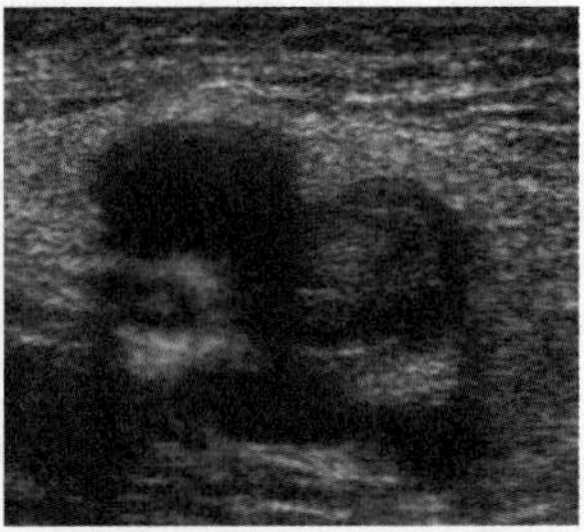

Fig 4. Ultrasound showing a transverse view of the femoral artery and vein. Here, the lumen of the femoral vein (deeper and medial to the artery) is occluded by thrombus, giving a hyperechoic signal compared to the arterial lumen.

Deep vein thrombosis (DVT)

See figs, p579

DVTs occur in 25–50% of surgical patients, and many non-surgical patients. 65% of below-knee DVTs are asymptomatic; these rarely embolize to the lung.

Risk factors Age↑, pregnancy, synthetic oestrogen, trauma, surgery (especially pelvic/ orthopaedic), past DVT, cancer, obesity, immobility, thrombophilia (p368).

Signs • Calf warmth/tenderness/swelling/erythema • Mild fever • Pitting oedema. Homans' sign (↑resistance/pain on forced foot dorsiflexion) should not be tested for as it may dislodge thrombus.

ΔΔ: Cellulitis; ruptured Baker's cyst. Both may coexist with a DVT.

Tests ***D-dimer blood tests*** are sensitive but not specific for DVT (also ↑ in infection, pregnancy, malignancy, and post-op).[23] A -ve result, combined with a low pretest clinical probability score (see BOX) is sufficient to exclude DVT.[24] If D-dimer↑, or the patient has a high/intermediate pretest clinical probability score, do ***compression US*** **(fig 3**, p579).[25] If this is -ve, a repeat US may be performed at 1wk to catch early but propagating DVTs. ***Venography*** is rarely necessary. Do ***thrombophilia tests*** (p368) **before** commencing anticoagulant therapy if there are no predisposing factors, in recurrent DVT, or if there is a family history of DVT.

Prevention • Stop the Pill 4wks pre-op. • Mobilize early. • ***Heparin*** 5000U/12h SC until mobile; low molecular weight heparin (LMWH, eg ***enoxaparin*** 20mg/24h SC, ↑ to 40mg for high-risk patients, starting 12h pre-op, or ***dalteparin***) may be better (less bleeding, no monitoring needed). • Support hosiery ('thromboembolic deterrent (TED) stockings') (CI: ischaemia). • Intermittent pneumatic pressure, until 16h post-op. • ***Fondaparinux*** (a factor Xa inhibitor, approved in the EU) may be better than LMWH.[26]

Treatment Meta-analyses have shown LMWH (eg ***enoxaparin*** 1.5mg/kg/24h SC) to be superior to ***unfractionated heparin***; APTT, p344, guides dosing, but extensive ileofemoral thrombi may still require unfractionated heparin as such patients were excluded from the trials. Start ***warfarin*** simultaneously with LMWH as it is prothrombotic for the first 48h, stopping heparin when INR is 2-3; treat for 3 months if post-op (6 months if no cause is found; lifelong in recurrent DVT or thrombophilia). ***Inferior vena caval filters*** may be used in active bleeding, or when anticoagulants fails, to minimize risk of pulmonary embolus. ***Post-phlebitic change*** can be seen in 10-30%. Prevention with thrombolytic therapy (to reduce damage to venous valves) and graduated compression stockings have both been tried, but neither has been conclusively shown to be beneficial.[27]

Swollen legs

see also p29; treatment—see BOX

Bilateral oedema implies systemic disease with ↑venous pressure (eg right heart failure) or ↓intravascular oncotic pressure (any cause of ↓albumin, so test the urine for protein). It is **dependent** (distributed by gravity), which is why legs are affected early, but severe oedema extends above the legs. In the bed-bound, fluid moves to the new dependent area, causing a sacral pad. The exception is the local increase in venous pressure occurring in IVC obstruction: the swelling neither extends above the legs nor redistributes. ***Causes:*** • Right heart failure (p128); • Albumin↓ (p700, eg renal or liver failure); • Venous insufficiency: acute, eg prolonged sitting, or chronic, with haemosiderin-pigmented, itchy, eczematous skin ± ulcers; • Vasodilators, eg ***nifedipine;*** • Pelvic mass (p57, p606); • Pregnancy—if BP↑ + proteinuria, diagnose pre-eclampsia (*OHCS* p48): find an obstetrician urgently. In all the above, both legs need not be affected to the same extent.

Unilateral oedema: Pain ± redness implies DVT or inflammation, eg cellulitis or insect bites (any blisters?). Bone or muscle may be to blame, eg tumours; necrotizing fasciitis (p662); trauma (check for sensation, pulses and severe pain esp. on passive movement: ►a **compartment syndrome** with ischaemic necrosis needs prompt fasciotomy). Impaired mobility suggests trauma, arthritis, or a Baker's cyst (p708). **Non-pitting oedema** is oedema you cannot indent: see p29.

Pretest clinical probability scoring for DVT: the Wells score[28]

In patients with symptoms in both legs, the more symptomatic leg is used.

Clinical features	Score
Active cancer (treatment within last 6 months or palliative)	1 point
Paralysis, paresis, or recent plaster immobilization of leg	1 point
Major surgery or recently bedridden for >3d in last 4wks	1 point
Local tenderness along distribution of deep venous system	1 point
Entire leg swollen	1 point
Calf swelling >3cm compared with asymptomatic leg (measured 10cm below tibial tuberosity)	1 point
Pitting oedema (greater in the symptomatic leg)	1 point
Collateral superficial veins (non-varicose)	1 point
Alternative diagnosis as likely or more likely than that of DVT	−2 points

Wells score: **≥*3 points:*** High pretest probability—treat as suspected DVT and perform compression US. ***1–2 points:*** Intermediate pretest probability—treat as suspected DVT and perform compression US. **≤*0 points:*** Low pretest probability of DVT—perform D-dimer test. If +ve then treat as suspected DVT and perform compression US. If -ve, DVT reliably excluded.

Air travel and DVT

In 1954, Homans first reported an association between air travel and venous thromboembolism. Recently, the supposed risk of DVT and subsequent pulmonary emboli associated with air travel (the so-called 'economy-class syndrome') has been the subject of much public scrutiny. Factors such as dehydration, immobilization, decreased oxygen tension, and prolonged pressure on the popliteal veins resulting from long periods in confined aircraft seats have all been suggested to be contributory factors. While the evidence linking air travel to an increased risk of DVT is still largely circumstantial, the following facts may help answer questions from your patients, family, and friends:

- The risk of developing a DVT from a long-distance flight has been estimated at 0.01–0.04% for the general population.
- The incidence of DVT in **high-risk** groups has been shown to be 4–6% for flights >10h. Prophylaxis with one dose of LMWH **may** be justified.[29]
- There is ↑risk of pulmonary embolus associated with long-distance air travel.[30]
- Compression stockings may decrease the risk of DVT, though they may also cause superficial thrombophlebitis.
- The role of prophylactic *aspirin* is still unclear and under investigation though at present not well supported
- Measures to minimize risk of DVT include leg exercises, increased water intake, and refraining from alcohol or caffeine during the flight.

9 questions to ask those with swollen legs

1 Is it **both** legs?	**2** Is she pregnant?	**3** Is she mobile?
4 Any trauma?	**5** Any pitting (p29)?	**6** Past diseases/on drugs?
7 Any pain?	**8** Any skin changes?	**9** Any oedema elsewhere?

Tests ►Look for proteinuria (+hypoalbuminaemia (≈nephrotic syndrome)). Is there CCF (echocardiogram)?

Treatment of leg oedema Treat the cause. Giving diuretics to everyone is not an answer. Ameliorate dependent oedema by elevating the legs (ankles higher than hips—do not just use footstools); raise the foot of the bed. Graduated support stockings may help (CI: ischaemia).[31]

Laparotomy In the elderly, or the malnourished, the wound may break down from a few days to a few weeks post-op, eg if infection or haematoma is present, or this is major surgery in a patient already compromised, eg by cancer, or this is a 2nd laparotomy. The warning sign of wound dehiscence (incidence ≈3.5%) is a pink serous discharge. Always assume that the defect involves the whole of the wound. Serious wound dehiscence may lead to a 'burst abdomen' with evisceration of bowel (mortality 15-30%). If you are on the ward when this happens, put the guts back into the abdomen, place a sterile dressing over the wound, give IV antibiotics (eg **cefuroxime** + **metronidazole**; see local guidelines) and call your senior. Allay anxiety, give parenteral pain control, set up an IVI, and return patient to theatre. ***Incisional hernia*** is a common problem (20%), repairable by mesh insertion.[32]

Biliary surgery After exploration of the common bile duct (CBD), a T-tube is usually left in the bile duct draining freely to the exterior. A T-tube cholangiogram is done at 8-10d and if there are no retained stones, the tube may be pulled out.
Retained stones may be removed by ERCP (p756), further surgery, or instillation of stone-dissolving agents (via T-tube). If there is distal obstruction in the CBD, fistula formation may occur with a chronic leakage of bile. Other complications of biliary surgery are CBD stricture; cholangitis; bleeding into the biliary tree (haemobilia) which may lead to biliary colic, jaundice, and haematemesis; pancreatitis; leak of bile causing biliary peritonitis. If jaundiced, it is important to maintain a good urine output as there is a danger of hepatorenal syndrome (p259). See TABLE for ***laparoscopic cholecystectomy***.

Thyroid surgery (also see p602) Recurrent (± superior) laryngeal nerve palsy (→hoarseness) can occur permanently in 0.5% and transiently in 1.5%[33]—warn the patient that **their voice will be different** for a few days post-op because of intubation and local oedema. **NB:** pre-operative fibreoptic laryngoscopy should be performed to exclude pre-existing vocal cord dysfunction); hypoparathyroidism (p214), causing hypocalcaemia (p692) that is permanent in 2.5%; hypothyroidism in the long term; thyroid storm (p844); tracheal obstruction due to haematoma in the wound may occur: ▸▸relieve by immediate removal of stitches or clips using the cutter/remover that should remain at the beside; may require urgent surgery.

Mastectomy Arm lymphoedema in up to 20% of those undergoing axillary node sampling or dissection—see BOX;[34] skin necrosis.

Arterial surgery Bleeding; thrombosis; embolism; graft infection; MI; AV fistula formation. ***Complications of aortic surgery:*** Gut ischaemia; renal failure; respiratory distress; aorto-enteric fistula; trauma to ureters or anterior spinal artery (leading to paraplegia); ischaemic events from distal trash from dislodged thrombus.

Colonic surgery Sepsis; ileus; fistulae; anastomotic leak (10% for anterior resection); obstruction from adhesions (BOX); haemorrhage; trauma to ureters or spleen.[35]

Small bowel surgery Short gut syndrome (best defined **functionally,** though anatomically ≤250cm in the adult) may result from substantial resections of small bowel. Diarrhoea and malabsorption (particularly of fats) lead to a number of metabolic abnormalities including deficiency in vitamins A, D, E, K, & B_{12}, hyperoxaluria (causing renal stones), and bile salt depletion (causing gallstones).[36]

Tracheostomy Stenosis; mediastinitis; surgical emphysema.

Splenectomy Acute gastric dilatation (a serious consequence of not using a NGT, or to check that the one in place is working); thrombocytosis; sepsis. ▶Lifetime sepsis risk is partly preventable with pre-op vaccines—ie *Haemophilus* type B, meningococcal, & pneumococcal (p391 & p160) and prophylactic penicillin (p367).

Genitourinary surgery Septicaemia (from instrumentation in the presence of infected urine)—consider a stat dose of ***gentamicin***; urinoma—rupture of a ureter or renal pelvis leading to a mass of extravasated urine.

Gastrectomy See p624. **Prostatectomy** p645. **Haemorrhoidectomy** p632.

Adhesions—legacy of the laparotomy, bane of the surgeon

When re-operating on the abdomen, the struggle against adhesions tests the farthest and darkest boundaries of patience of the abdominal surgeon and the assistant. The skill and persistence required to gently and atraumatically tease apart these fibrous bands that restrict access and vision makes any progression, no matter how slight, cause for subdued celebration. Perseverance is the name of this game—also known as ***adhesiolysis***.

Any surgical procedure that breaches the abdominal or pelvic cavities can predispose to the formation of adhesions, which are found in up to 90% of those with previous abdominal surgery; this is why we do not rush to operate on small bowel obstruction: the operation predisposes to yet more adhesions. Handling of the serosal surface of the bowel causes inflammation, which over weeks to years can lead to the formation of fibrous bands that tether the bowel to itself or adjacent structures—though adhesions can also form secondary to infection, radiation injury and inflammatory processes such as Crohn's disease. Their main sequelae are intestinal obstruction (the cause in ~60% of cases—see p612) and chronic abdominal or pelvic pain. Studies have shown that adhesiolysis may help relieve chronic pain, though for a small proportion of patients the pain never improves or even worsens after directed intervention.[37]

As far as prevention is concerned, the best approach is to avoid operating, though there is evidence to suggest that laparoscopy compared with laparotomy reduces the rate of local adhesions,[38] and that there may be a role for the insertion of synthetic films to prevent adhesions to the anterior abdominal wall.[39]

Lymphatic drainage of the breast

Risk of lymphoedema increases with the level of axillary dissection:

- **Level 1** dissection remains inferior to pectoralis minor
- **Level 2** goes behind pectoralis minor
- **Level 3** goes superior to pectoralis minor (rarely done).

The higher the dissection, the greater the risk of interference with lymphatic drainage of the arm and, therefore, of lymphoedema.

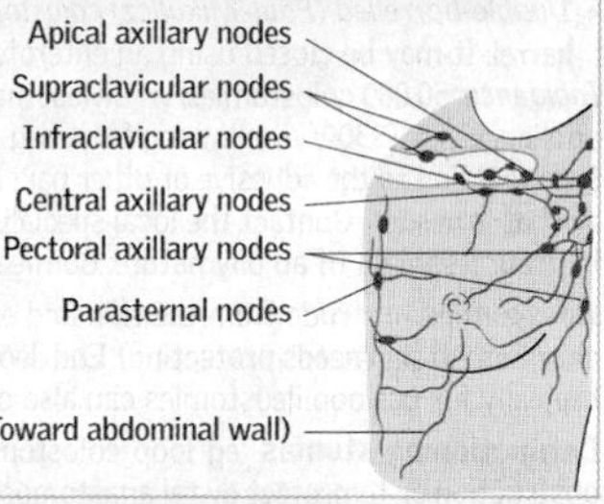

The complications of laparoscopic cholecystectomy

Complications that should be discussed include:	Risk
Conversion to open procedure	5%
CBD injury[1]	0.32%
Bile leak	0.2%
Post-operative haemorrhage	0.1%
Intra-abdominal abscess	0.07%
Mortality secondary to operative injury	0.04%

These complication rates are taken from one study that reviewed 39,238 cases.[40]

NB: total operative mortality may be nearer 0.1%

1 The nasty long-term sequela of this is permanent CBD stricture and a life of misery along with it. CBD damage rate during laparoscopic surgery is twice that of open surgery. However, the 'critical view of safety' method, in which the cystic duct and cystic artery are approached through a meticulous dissection of the upper border of the triangle of Calot along the underside of the gallbladder, can reduce rates of bile duct injury in comparison with the originally described infundibular technique of laparoscopic cholecystectomy.

Stoma care

A stoma (Greek στομα=mouth) is an artificial union made between 2 conduits (eg a choledochojejunostomy) or, more commonly, between a conduit and the outside—eg a colostomy, in which faeces are made to pass through a hole in the abdominal wall into an adherent plastic bag, ideally as 1-2 formed motions/day.

The physical and psychological aspects of stoma care must not be undervalued. Be alert to any vicious cycle in which a skin reaction leads to leakage → fear of going out into the world → fear of eating → poor skin nutrition → further skin reactions → further leakage → more depression. These cycles can be circumvented by the *stoma nurse*, who is **the** expert in fitting secure, odourless devices.[41] Ensure patients have his/her phone number for use before and after surgery. His/her visits are more useful than any doctor's in explaining what is going to happen, what the stoma will be like, and in troubleshooting post-op problems. ►**Early direct self-referral prevents problems.** Without him/her, a patient may reject his colostomy, never attend to it, or even become suicidal.

Colostomies Pre-op, confirm that he is unsuited to one of the newer colostomy avoiding operations (see below). Is he suitable for a laparoscopic operation?[42]

- *Loop colostomy:* A loop of colon is exteriorized, opened, and sewn to the skin. A rod under the loop prevents retraction and may be removed after 7d. This can be a defunctioning stoma (below), though faeces may pass beyond the loop. It is often temporary, and more prone to complications than end colostomies.
- *End colostomy:* The bowel is divided; the proximal end brought out as a stoma; the distal end may be: **1 resected**, eg abdominoperineal resection (inspect the perineum for absent anus when examining a stoma); **2 closed** & left in the abdomen (Hartman's procedure); **3 exteriorized**, forming a 'mucous fistula'.
- *Double-barrelled (Paul–Mikulicz) colostomy:* The colon is brought out as a double-barrel. It may be closed using an enterotome. See **figs 1** & **3**.

Incidence: 50,000 colostomies/yr[UK]. Most manage their colostomies well. The cost for appliances is ~£1300/yr (allowing for a bag-use rate of 1-3/d). If there is an allergic-type reaction to the adhesive or other part of the device, a change of device may be all that is needed. Contact the local specialist nurse. Avoid most creams, which can be troublesome if of an oily nature; Comfeel® is an exception.

Ileostomies protrude from the skin and emit fluid motions which contain active enzymes (so skin needs protecting). End ileostomy usually follows proctocolectomy, typically for UC; loop ileostomies can also be formed. See **fig 2**.

Defunctioning stomas (eg loop colostomy/ileostomy) are used to relieve distal obstruction or to protect distal anastomoses. Although they do not reduce leakage rates, they probably minimise the severity of leakage when it does occur.[43]

The alternatives to colostomy *Total anorectal reconstruction* uses gracilis muscle disconnected distally and wound around the anus and induced to contract by a pulse generator implanted in the abdomen, with bowel action triggered by a hand-held radiofrequency controller. It is still rather experimental, but patients will ask about it. Warn them that it is not without complications and that normal-quality continence will not be achieved because of lack of sensation of the arrival of stools.[44] *Posterior sagittal anorectoplasty (PSARP)* is also possible.

There is some evidence from non-randomized trials that sphincter-saving operations are not associated with poorer disease-free survival compared with abdominoperineal resection in those with rectal carcinoma near the anal verge.[45]

Urostomies are fashioned after total cystectomy, bringing urine from the ureters to the abdominal wall via an *ileal conduit* that is usually incontinent. Formation of a catheterizable valvular mechanism may retain continence. Advances in urological surgery have seen an increase in continence-saving procedures such as orthotopic neobladder reconstruction.[46]

Complications of stomas

►Liaise with the stoma nurse, starting pre-operatively.

Early:

- Haemorrhage at stoma site
- Stoma ischaemia—colour progresses from dusky grey to black
- High output (can lead to $K^+\downarrow$)—consider *loperamide* ± *codeine* to thicken output
- Obstruction secondary to adhesions (see p583)
- Stoma retraction

Delayed:

- Obstruction (failure at operation to close lateral space around stoma)
- Dermatitis around stoma site (worse with ileostomy)
- Stoma prolapse
- Stomal intussusception
- Stenosis
- Parastomal hernia (risk increases with time)[47]
- Fistulae (p567)
- Psychological problems

Choosing a stoma site[1]

When choosing the site for a stoma, avoid:

- Bony prominences (eg anterior superior iliac spine, costal margins)
- The umbilicus
- Old wounds/scars—there may be adhesions beneath
- Skin folds and creases
- The waistline
- The site should be assessed pre-operatively by the stoma nurse, with the patient both lying and standing

When placing the first bag at the end of the operation, think about whether the patient will be sitting up or mobile (direct bag towards feet) or whether they will be recumbent for a period (direct bag towards the flank).

Colostomies are most often placed in the left iliac fossa whereas a stoma in the right iliac fossa is more likely to be an ileostomy/ileal conduit.

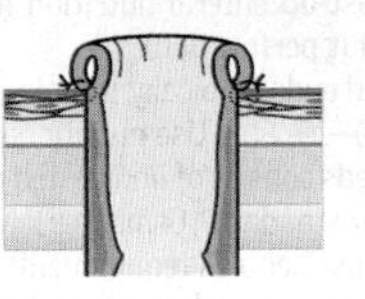

Fig 1. Colostomy

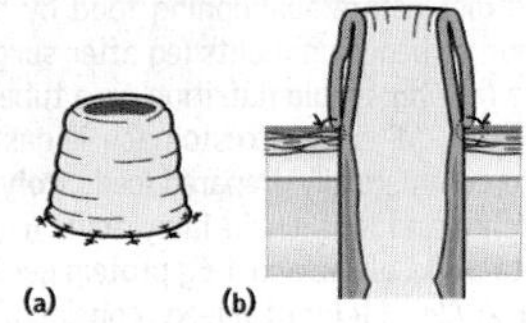

Fig 2. Ileostomy

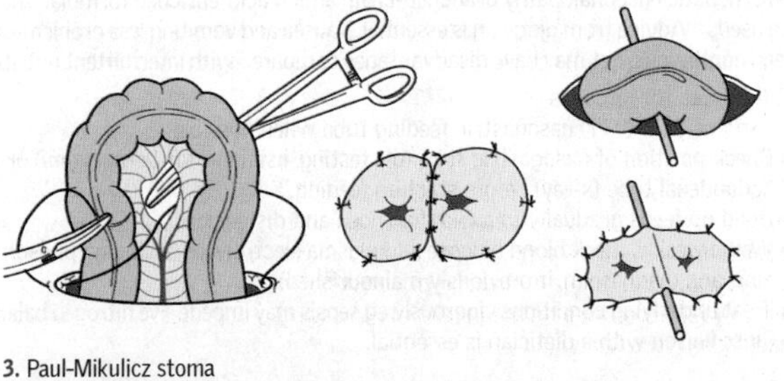

Fig 3. Paul-Mikulicz stoma

1 The same principles apply when choosing a drain site, though since they are usually only *in situ* for a few days, pre-operative assessment is rarely required—see p573.

Surgery

►Over 25% of hospital inpatients may be malnourished. Hospitals can become so focused on curing disease that they ignore the foundations of good health— malnourished patients recover more slowly and experience more complications.[1]

Why are so many hospital patients malnourished?

1 Increased nutritional requirements (eg sepsis, burns, surgery)
2 Increased nutritional losses (eg malabsorption, output from stoma)
3 Decreased intake (eg dysphagia, sedation, coma)
4 Effect of treatment (eg nausea, diarrhoea)
5 Enforced starvation (eg prolonged periods nil by mouth)
6 Missing meals through being whisked off, eg for investigations
7 Difficulty with feeding (eg lost dentures; no one available to give enough help)
8 Unappetizing food

Identifying the malnourished patient

- *History:* Recent weight↓ (>20%, accounting for fluid balance); recent reduced intake; diet change (eg recent change in consistency of food); nausea, vomiting, pain, diarrhoea which might have led to reduced intake.
- *Examination:* State of hydration (p688): dehydration can go hand-in-hand with malnutrition, and overhydration can mask the appearance of malnutrition. Evidence of malnutrition: skin hanging off muscles (eg over biceps); no fat between fold of skin; hair rough and wiry; pressure sores; sores at corner of mouth. Calculate body mass index (p236); BMI <20kg/m^2 suggests malnourishment. Anthropomorphic indices, eg mid arm circumference, skin fold measures and grip strength also used.
- *Investigations:* Generally unhelpful. Low albumin suggestive, but is affected by many things other than nutrition. ↑Albumin can be helpful in monitoring recovery.

Prevention of malnutrition Assess nutrition state and weight on admission, and eg weekly thereafter. Identify those at risk (see above). Ensure that meals are uninterrupted, when possible. Provide appetizing food to the patient when he wants to eat it. If patient requires nutritional support, seek help from dietician.

Enteral nutrition (ie nutrition given into gastrointestinal tract) If at all possible, give nutrition by mouth. An all-fluid diet can meet requirements (but get advice from dietician). If danger of choking or aspiration (eg after stroke), consider semi-solid diet before abandoning food by mouth. Post-op enteral nutrition has been shown to benefit patients (eg after surgery for gut perforation).[48]

Tube feeding: Liquid nutrition via a tube, eg placed endoscopically, radiologically, or surgically (directly into stomach, ie gastrostomy)—see BOX. Use nutritionally complete, commercially prepared feeds. **Polymeric** feeds consist of undigested proteins, starches and long chain fatty acids (eg Nutrison standard®, Osmolite®). Normally contain ~1kCal/mL and 4–6g protein per 100mL. Most people's requirements are met with 2L/24h. **Elemental** feeds consist of individual amino acids, oligo- and monosaccharides needing minimal digestion. Also **disease specific** feeds eg in liver cirrhosis with hepatic encephalopathy branched-chain amino acid-enriched formulae should be used.[49] Advice from dietician is essential. Nausea and vomiting less problematic if feed continuous, but may have disadvantages compared with intermittent nutrition.

Guidelines for success

- Use fine-bore (9 Fr) nasogastric feeding tube when possible.
- Check position of nasogastric tube (pH testing, listening for *borborygmi*) or nasoduodenal tube (X-ray) before starting feeding.
- Build up feeds gradually to avoid diarrhoea and distension.
- Weigh weekly, check blood glucose and plasma electrolytes (including phosphate, zinc, and magnesium, if previously malnourished).
- Treat underlying conditions vigorously, eg sepsis may impede +ve nitrogen balance.

►Close liaison with a dietician is essential.

1 For an in depth guide to nutrition see *Manual of Dietetic Practice, 4e*, Briony Thomas, Blackwell

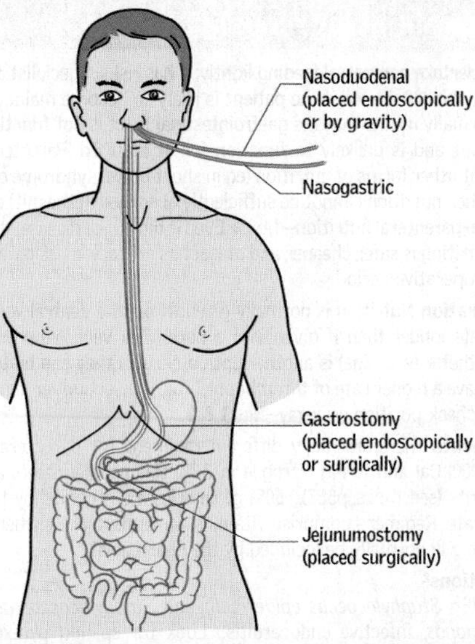

Fig 1. Enteral tube feeding

Daily energy and nutritional requirements

Substance	Requirement (/kg/d)	Notes
Energy	20-40kCal	Normal adult requirements will be 2000-2500kCal/d; even catabolic patients rarely require >2500kCal/d. Very high calorie diets (eg >4000kCal/d) can lead to a fatty liver.
	84-168kJ	Multiply kCal by a factor of 4.2.
Nitrogen	0.2-0.4g	6.25g of enteral protein gives 1g of nitrogen. Considering nitrogen balance is important because although catabolism is inevitable, replenishment is vital.
Protein	0.5g	Contains 5kCal/g.
Fat	3g	Contains 10kCal/g.
Carbohydrate	2g	Contains 4kCal/g.
Water	30-35ml	+500ml/d for each °C of pyrexia.
Na/K/Cl	1.0mmol each	Electrolytes need to be considered, even if not on IVI.

Nil by mouth (NBM) before theatre

If in doubt about what is acceptable oral intake prior to induction for general anaesthesia (eg GI surgery), it is best to liaise with the anaesthetist concerned. However, guidelines have been published by the Royal College of Nursing, the European Society for Clinical Nutrition and Metabolism, American Society of Anaesthesiologists, and The Association of Anaesthetists of Great Britain and Ireland to outline what is safe in the perioperative period. **In emergency surgery**, ≥6h NBM prior to theatre is best. For **adult elective surgery** in healthy patients without GI co-morbidity, water or clear fluids (eg black tea/coffee) are allowed up to 2h beforehand, with all other intake up to 6h beforehand. 50

Do not undertake parenteral feeding lightly: it has risks. Specialist advice is vital. It should only be considered if the patient is likely to become malnourished without it—this normally means that the gastrointestinal tract is not functioning (eg bowel obstruction), and is unlikely to function for at least 7d. Parenteral feeding may supplement other forms of nutrition (eg in short bowel syndrome or active Crohn's disease, when nutrition cannot be sufficiently absorbed in the gut) or it can be used alone (total parenteral nutrition—TPN). ►Even if there is GI disease, studies show that enteral nutrition is safer, cheaper, and at least as efficacious as parenteral nutrition in the perioperative period.[1] [51]

Administration Nutrition is normally given through a central venous line as this usually lasts longer than if given into a peripheral vein. A peripherally inserted central catheter (PICC line) is another option, though they can be trickier to insert and may have a higher rate of thrombophlebitis.[52] Insert under strict sterile conditions and check position on x-ray—**figs 1 & 2**.

Requirements There are many different regimens for parenteral feeding. Most provide 2000kCal and 10-14g nitrogen in 2-3L; this usually meets a patient's daily requirements (see TABLE, p587). ~50% of calories are provided by fat and ~50% by carbohydrate. Regimens comprise vitamins, minerals, trace elements, and electrolytes; these will normally be included by the pharmacist.

Complications[2]

- ***Sepsis:*** (Eg *Staphylococcus epidermidis* and *Staphylococcus aureus; Candida; Pseudomonas;* infective endocarditis.) Look for spiking pyrexia and examine wound at tube insertion point. Take line **and** peripheral cultures. If central venous line-related sepsis is suspected, the safest course of action is always to remove the line. Do not attempt to salvage a line when *S. aureus* or *Candida* infection has been identified. Antimicrobial-impregnated central lines decrease the incidence of line-related infections.[53]
- ***Thrombosis:*** Central vein thrombosis may occur, resulting in pulmonary embolus or superior vena caval obstruction (p526). ***Heparin*** in the nutrient solution may be useful for prophylaxis in high-risk patients, though there is little clear-cut evidence in adult studies.
- ***Metabolic imbalance*** Electrolyte abnormalities—see BOX; deranged plasma glucose; hyperlipidaemia; deficiency syndromes (TABLE, p281); acid-base disturbance (eg hypercapnia from excessive CO_2 production).
- ***Mechanical:*** Pneumothorax; embolism of IV line tip.

Guidelines for success

►Liaise closely with line insertion team, nutrition team and pharmacist.

- Meticulous sterility. Do not use central venous lines for uses other than nutrition. Remove the line if you suspect infection. Culture its tip.
- Review fluid balance at least twice daily, and requirements for energy and electrolytes daily.
- Check weight, fluid balance, and urine glucose daily throughout period of parenteral nutrition. Check plasma glucose, creatinine and electrolytes (including calcium and phosphate), and FBC daily until stable and then 3 times a week. Check LFT and lipid clearance three times a week until stable and then weekly. Check zinc and magnesium weekly throughout.
- Do not rush. Achieve the maintenance regimen in small steps.
- Treat underlying conditions vigorously—eg sepsis may impede +ve nitrogen balance.

1 Enteral feeding promotes integrity of the gut mucosal barrier, thus preventing bacterial and endotoxin translocation across the gut wall, which can lead to multiple organ dysfunction syndrome (MODS) and perpetuation of a systemic inflammatory response—even when the gut is not the primary source of pathology.

2 For children, see Brit. Assoc. Parenteral and Enteral Nutr. 2000 *Guidelines* ISBN 1899467408.

Refeeding syndrome

At risk with:
- Malignancy
- Anorexia nervosa
- Alcoholism
- GI surgery
- Starvation

►This is a life-threatening metabolic complication of refeeding *via* any route after a prolonged period of starvation.[54] As the body turns to fat and protein metabolism in the starved state, there is a drop in the level of circulating insulin (because of the paucity of dietary carbohydrates). The catabolic state also depletes intracellular stores of phosphate, although serum levels may remain normal (0.85-1.45mmol/L). When refeeding begins, the level of insulin rises in response to the carbohydrate load, and one of the consequences is to increase cellular uptake of phosphate.

A hypophosphataemic state (<0.50mmol/L) normally develops within 4d and is mostly responsible for the features of '**refeeding syndrome**', which include: rhabdomyolysis; red and white cell dysfunction; respiratory insufficiency; arrhythmias; cardiogenic shock; seizures; sudden death.

Prevention requires at-risk patients to be identified, assessed and monitored closely during refeeding (glucose, lipids, sodium, potassium, phosphate, calcium, magnesium, and zinc). Close involvement of a nutritionist is required.

Treatment is of the complicating features and includes parenteral phosphate administration (eg 18mmol/d) in addition to oral supplementation.[55]

The venous system at the thoracic outlet

When trying to judge the position of a central venous line tip on CXR (see **figs 1** & **2**) it helps to know the anatomical landmarks of the venous system. The subclavian veins join the internal jugular veins behind the sternoclavicular joints to form the brachiocephalic veins. These come together behind the right 1st sternocostal joint to form the superior vena cava (SVC), which runs from this point to the right 3rd sternocostal joint. The right atrium starts here.

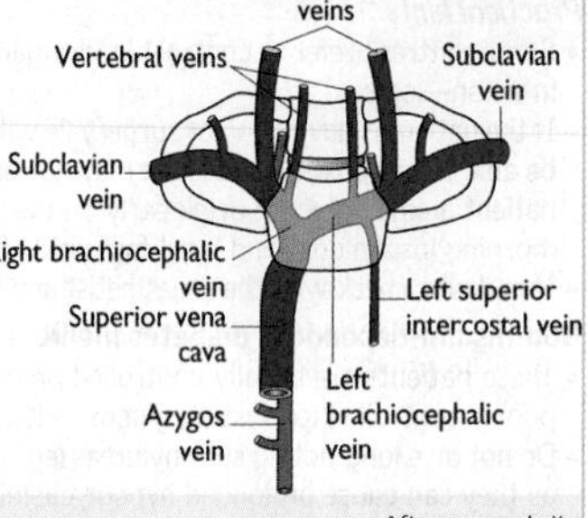

After RCSI website.

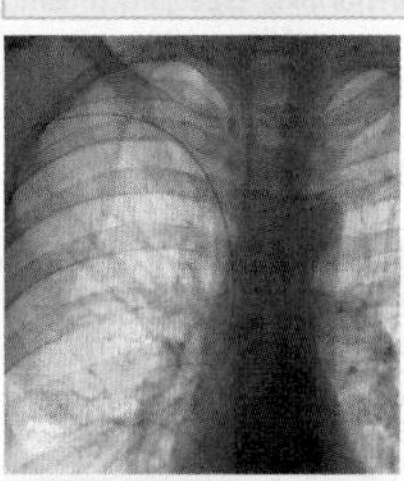

Fig 1. Right arm PICC (peripherally inserted central catheter) still with a wire in the lumen. This is a radiograph at the time of insertion to determine if placement is correct. The tip lies in the SVC—ie good positioning for long term antibiotic therapy. The tip of a Hickman line, for cytotoxic administration, is better in the right atrium, to avoid possible irritation of the SVC and consequent thrombosis or stenosis. Both images courtesy of Prof Peter Scally.

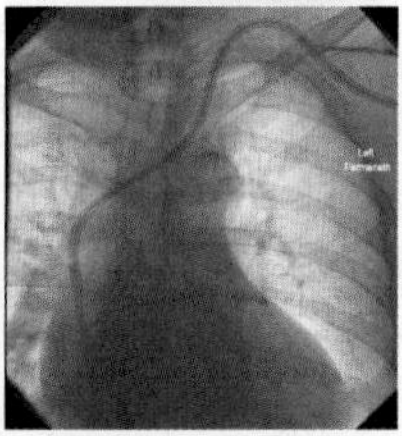

Fig 2. CXR showing placement of a dual lumen haemodialysis catheter. It is tunnelled through the subcutaneous tissues, enters the left internal jugular vein, and travels through the left brachiocephalic vein and SVC to enter the right atrium. The tip lies best in the SVC or right atrium, any further and it might damage the tricuspid valve.

Both images were acquired in the angiography room, where radio-opaque material appears black (it is easier to see contrast media against a white background).

Insulin-dependent diabetes mellitus (eg type 1 diabetes mellitus)

- Patients are often well informed about their diabetes; involve them fully when managing their diabetic care.
- Stress or intercurrent illness increases basal insulin needs (see p198).
- Always try to put the patient first on the list (surgery, endoscopy, bronchoscopy, etc). Inform the surgeon and anaesthetist early.
- Stop all long-acting insulin the night before. Get IV access before you need it urgently. If surgery is in the morning, stop all SC morning insulin. If surgery is in the afternoon, have the usual short-acting insulin in the morning at breakfast. No medium- or long-acting insulin. It may be feasible to continue *glargine* (p201) as baseline therapy throughout the peri-operative period though there have been no large studies into this.[56]
- Check blood glucose hourly. Aim for 7–11mmol/L during surgery.
- Check U&E pre-op. Start an IVI of 1L of 5% dextrose with 20mmol KCl/8h. Dextrose saline can be given if Na^+ low, but do not give only saline; dextrose may need constant infusion to maintain blood glucose.
- Start an infusion pump with 50U short-acting insulin (eg Actrapid®) in 50mL 0.9% saline. Give according to a sliding scale (see TABLE) adjusted in the light of blood glucose.
- Post-op, continue IV insulin + dextrose until patient tolerating food. Check finger-prick glucose every 2h. Switch to usual SC regimen around a meal.

Practical hints:

- Some centres prefer to control blood sugar with a glucose-potassium-insulin (GKI) infusion—see BOX.
- If the patient is having minor surgery (ie will not be NBM for >6h) and will definitely be able to eat post-op, IV insulin may not be necessary. Some advocate giving the patient a small glucose drink early on the morning of surgery, and delaying their morning insulin dose and breakfast until after the procedure.
- If in doubt, check with the anaesthetist and liaise with a diabetes specialist nurse.

Non-insulin-dependent diabetes mellitus (≈type 2 diabetes)

- These patients are usually controlled on oral hypoglycaemics (p200). If diabetes poorly controlled (eg fasting glucose >10mmol/L), treat as for type 1 diabetes.
- Do not give long-acting sulfonylureas (eg *glibenclamide*) on the morning of surgery, as they can cause prolonged hypoglycaemia on fasting.
- Beware lactic acidosis in patients on biguanides (eg *metformin*), especially if using IV contrast agents and/or renal function poor (creatinine >150μmol/L).
- If the patient can eat post-operatively, simply omit tablets on the morning of surgery and give post-op with a meal.
- If the patient is having major surgery with restrictions on eating post-op, check fasting glucose on the morning of surgery and start IV or SC insulin given according to sliding scale. Post-op, consult the diabetic team as the patient may need a phase of insulin to supplement their oral hypoglycaemics.

Diet-controlled diabetes Usually no problem, though patient may briefly be insulin dependent post-op. Monitor fingerprick glucose before meals and bedtime. Avoid giving 5% dextrose IVI as a fluid replacement as blood glucose will rise.

Peri-operative morbidity and mortality Diabetes mellitus is classed as in intermediate risk factor for increased perioperative cardiovascular risk by the American Heart Association, so screen for the presence of asymptomatic cardiac and renal disease (p569) and be aware of possible 'silent' myocardial ischaemia.[57]

One retrospective study on those undergoing major vascular surgery showed that although long-term survival was poorer for patients with diabetes, perioperative cardiovascular morbidity and mortality were only increased in the presence of congestive heart failure and haemodialysis—ie **not** diabetes alone.[58]

An example of an IV sliding scale

Fingerprick glucose	IV soluble insulin[1]	Alternative SC insulin[2]
<2 ⏩See p844	None–50% glucose IV + Glucogel® PO	
2–5	No insulin	No insulin
5–10	1U/h	2U/h (rough guide only)
10–15	2U/h	5U/h
15–20	3U/h	7U/h
>20	6U/h–get urgent diabetic review	

NB: this is a guide only: individual scales may vary between institutions

GKI infusions (glucose, K^+ & insulin)

►A problem when giving IV insulin and IV dextrose simultaneously through separate intravenous lines is that if one cannula becomes blocked, the patient may become hypo- or hyperglycaemic. If the glucose and insulin are given through the same cannula, however, and the 3-way converter becomes blocked, the syringe driver may retrogradely fill the infusion set with insulin. When the cannula is subsequently resited and the infusion restarted, the patient will receive this large accumulated dose of insulin. This has caused lethal hypoglycaemia, so some centres now use GKI infusions instead of sliding scales.

A 500mL bag of 5% or 10% dextrose ± KCl is given over 6h, with a short-acting insulin (eg Actrapid®) added according to blood glucose:59

Blood glucose (mmol/L)	Insulin dose (units/bag)	Serum K^+ (mmol/L)	KCl to be added (mmol/bag)
<4	None	<3	20
4–6	5	3–5	10
6–10	10	>5	None
10–20	15		
>20	20		

- Check blood glucose every 3h. If levels too high or low, start a new 500mL bag of 5% dextrose with the correct insulin dose.
- Check U&E daily.
- GKI infusions are useful when close monitoring of blood glucose is not possible, but are not suitable in poorly controlled diabetes. If the patient is under a fluid restriction then it is possible to halve the bag volume and double the dextrose concentration (eg 250 mL of 10–20% dextrose), dosing the insulin per bag just as before. If the patient is ***hyponatraemic*** then a concomitant infusion of 0.9% saline should be considered.
- **NB:** regimens vary and sometimes more insulin will be required; eg if shocked, severely ill, or if on steroids or sympathomimetics, 2–4 times as much insulin may be needed. See *BNF* section 6.1.

1 Check glucose hourly and adjust insulin accordingly.
2 ►Only use SC route if IV route is problematic as it is associated with much variability; check fingerprick glucose every 2–4h if NBM, or pre-meals if using SC insulin to supplement other hypoglycaemics.

Jaundiced patients undergoing surgery

Operating in jaundiced patients is best avoided, especially with the availability of ERCP. Patients with obstructive jaundice are prone to developing renal failure after surgery, perhaps from the toxic effect of bilirubin and any concomitant sepsis (see hepatorenal syndrome—p259). In practice this means that good urine output must be maintained in such patients around the time of surgery.

Pre-operative preparation Avoid *morphine* in the premedication.

- Give antibiotic prophylaxis (p572); treat sepsis to ↓ risk of endotoxaemia, p805.[60]
- Insert IV line and give 1L of 0.9% saline over ½–1h following pre-med (unless the patient has heart failure), to produce a moderate diuresis peri-operatively. A loop diuretic (eg *furosemide*) may be needed to ensure diuresis. Pre-op **mannitol** is no longer routine in jaundiced patients—it may even be deleterious.[61]
- Insert a urinary catheter.
- A 'renal' dose *dopamine* (2–5μg/kg/min) IVI **may** be indicated. See [62] but also [63]. Remember there may be side-effects from any central line used, and from the drug:
  - Sepsis (immune dysfunction)
  - Arrhythmias
  - Gut + myocardial perfusion↓
  - Diuresis when hypovolaemic
  - Catabolism↑
  - Gastric motility decreased
  - Pulmonary hypertension
  - Impaired hypoxic ventilatory responses[64]
- Check clotting and consider giving prophylactic *vitamin K* (p338), even if normal.

During surgery Measure urine output hourly, give 0.9% saline IV to match output

For 48h after surgery Measure urine output every 2h; measure U&E daily.

- Give 0.9% saline at rate to match urine output and fluid lost, eg through NGT; give 2L of dextrose-saline every 24h.
- Consider *furosemide* and central line if output is poor despite adequate hydration.
- Give 20mmol of K^+/L of fluid after 24h post-op if urine output good.

Surgery in those on steroids

Patients on steroid therapy need extra cover to cope with stress of surgery—their endogenous adrenal hormone levels will be suppressed, even for a period after cessation of a course of treatment. The amount of extra cover needed depends on the type of the surgery and the pre-op dose of steroids. For routine surgery, aim to ↓ the dose of steroid as much as possible. Consider steroid cover for anyone who has had high-dose glucocorticoid therapy in the last year. ***Major surgery:*** Typically give **hydrocortisone** 50–100mg IV with the pre-med and then every 6–8h IV/IM for 3d, then wean to previous medication. ***Minor surgery:*** Prepare as for major surgery except that **hydrocortisone** is given for 24h only.

The major risk with adrenal insufficiency is hypotension, so if this is encountered without an obvious cause, it may be worthwhile giving a stat dose of 50mg *hydrocortisone* IV. See *BNF* section 6.3 for steroid dose equivalences.

Surgery in those on anticoagulants

►Contact your lab, and inform the surgeon and anaesthetist. ***Very minor surgery*** has been undertaken without stopping *warfarin* (do INR within 24h: it may be safe to proceed if <3.5).[65] In ***major surgery***, drugs may be stopped for 2–5d pre-op. Risks and benefits are individual to each patient, so exact rules are impossible. Discuss these issues when arranging consent. *Vitamin K* (eg 10mg IV) ± *FFP* may be needed in emergency surgery. ►**Monitor clotting meticulously.**

One elective option is conversion to *heparin* (stop 6h prior to surgery, and monitor APTT perioperatively): unfractionated heparin's short $t_{1/2}$ allows swift reversal with *protamine* (p344).[66] When re-warfarinizing, don't stop heparin cover until the INR is therapeutic, as warfarin is prothrombotic in the early stages.

The bleeding tendency effects of *aspirin* are reversed by 5d after stopping, but check with local policy to see if cessation is required.[67] The alteration of antiplatelet agents (and NSAIDs) is a complex business and is best discussed with an expert.[68]

Thyroid disease and surgery

Thyroid surgery for hyperthyroidism If severe, give *carbimazole* until euthyroid (p210). Arrange operation date and 10–14d before this, start aqueous iodine oral solution (Lugol's solution), 0.1–0.3mL/8h PO well diluted with milk or water. Continue until surgery.

Mild hyperthyroidism Start *propranolol* 80mg/8h PO and Lugol's solution as above at the 1st consultation. Stop Lugol's solution on the day of surgery but continue *propranolol* for 5d post-op.

⏩**Thyrotoxic storm** A rare but potentially fatal consequence of thyroid surgery (mortality 50%). See p845.

Non-thyroid surgery *Thyroxine* has a long $t_{½}$ (~7d) so omitting a dose while nil by mouth will not have any major effects.

Surgery in the obese

(see also p628)

It has long been believed that obesity delays wound healing and increases the risk of post-operative complications.[1] Indeed, 50 years ago obesity was considered a contraindication to elective surgery.

One study has suggested, however, that obesity in itself may not be a risk factor for most complications.[69] Overall incidence of complications after elective general surgery did not differ significantly between obese and non-obese patients, though only 1.7% of the 6336 patients in the trial had a BMI >40kg/m^2. The only post-operative complication found to have an increased incidence in the obese was wound infection after open surgery. Overall it would seem that the practice of forcing patients to lose weight prior to elective general surgery may be inappropriate.

1 Obesity has been shown to increase risks of cardiac and spinal surgery.

The terms 'keyhole surgery' or minimal access surgery may be preferred, because these procedures can be as invasive as any laparotomy, having just the same set of side-effects—plus some new ones. It is the size of the incision and the use of laparoscopes which marks out this branch of surgery. Laparoscopy has been well established in gynaecology for many years where initially a purely optical telescope, held by the surgeon, was used for visualization. The development of miniaturized video cameras was the impetus to the widespread use of laparoscopy, as it allowed an assistant to have the same view as the surgeon. The surgeon could therefore operate with both hands, while his assistant held the laparoscope and retracted the viscera. Laparoscopic cholecystectomy was shown to be possible, and became the method of choice. Laparoscopy is now in widespread use for diagnostic purposes and for other conditions, such as appendicectomy,[70] fundoplication, splenectomy, and adrenalectomy. It is currently under evaluation for hernia repair,[71] colectomy,[72] nephrectomy (in renal transplants), parathyroidectomy, sentinel node biopsy, and perforated peptic ulcer repair.[73]

As a rule of thumb, whatever can be done by laparotomy can also be done with the laparoscope. This does not mean that it **should** be done, but if the patient feels better sooner, has less post-operative pain, and can return to work earlier, and have fewer complications, then these specific techniques will gain ascendency—provided hospitals can afford the equipment. Laparoscopic surgery may also have the benefit of a less suppressive effect on the immune system.[74]

It is worth noting that advantages do not always include time. In upper GI surgery, laparoscopic surgery may take longer than open procedures. Also, the patient needs to spend a night in hospital, usually. This has economic implications when comparing laparoscopic inguinal hernia repair with open surgery done under local anaesthesia (after which the patient can go home the same day). On the other side of the economic equation for hernia repair is that pain >24h post-op is less after laparoscopic procedures, and the patient can return to full employment after a week. In addition, laparoscopic repair allows detection of a previously undiagnosed contralateral hernia. Which method makes economic sense depends on who is doing the calculation; NICE concluded that open hernia repair was cheaper, but their calculations did not include out of hospital costs.[75]

Problems with minimal access surgery: for the surgeon

Inspection: Anatomy looks different due to the different surgical approach.

Palpation is impossible during laparoscopic procedures. This may make it hard to locate colon lesions prior to cutting them out. This means that pre-operative tests may need to be more extensive (eg colonoscopy **and** barium enema).

Skill: Here the problem is not just that a new skill has to be learned and taught. Old skills may become attenuated if operations are done laparoscopically, and new surgeons may not achieve optimal skill in either sphere if they try to do both.

Problems for patients and GPs

- *Post-operative complications:* What may be easily managed on a well-run surgical ward (eg haemorrhage) may be a challenge for a GP and terrify the patient, who may be all alone after early discharge.
- *Loss of tell-tale scars:* Afterwards there may only be a few abdominal wounds, so future carers have to guess at what has been done. The answer here is to communicate carefully with the patient, so that he knows what has been done—see BOX.

Problems for hospitals Just because minimal access surgery is often cost-effective, it does not follow that hospitals can afford the procedures. Instruments are continuously being refined, and quickly become obsolete—so that many are now produced in disposable single-use form. Because of budgeting boundaries, hospitals cannot use the cash saved, by early return to work or by freeing-up bed use, to pay for capital equipment and extra theatre time that may be required.

Who is not suitable for day-case surgery?

Over the years peri-operative care has evolved from the inpatient setting, with better results for the patient.[1] A number of operations are performed as day-cases, including varicose vein surgery, cataracts and inguinal hernia repairs. Even traditionally more demanding surgery is now being performed as day-cases (eg laparoscopic cholecystectomy). Theoretically any procedure is suitable, provided the time under general anaesthetic does not exceed ~1h. The use of regional anaesthesia helps to avoid the SE of nausea and disorientation that may accompany a general anaesthetic, thus facilitating discharge. To avoid putting the patient at unnecessary risk, it is important to identify those who are **not** suitable for day-case surgery:

• Severe dementia. • Severe learning difficulties • Living alone (and no helpers). • Children if supervision difficult—changes in expectation, delays & pain relief can be problematic.[76] • BMI >32 (see p237) • ASA category ≥III (see p569) thus potentially unstable co-morbidities—discuss with the anaesthetist as category III may be suitable with appropriate optimisation. • Infection at the site of the operation.

Exclusions from local regional anaesthesia: Poor communication (if require cooperation during anaesthetic procedure), severe claustrophobia.

Discharge checklist for use after day-case surgery ('Leap-frog')

Lucid, not vomiting, and cough reflex established.
Easy breathing; easy urination.
Ambulant without fainting.
Pain relief + post-op drugs dispensed + given. Does he understand doses?
Follow-up arranged.
Rhythm, pulse & BP checked: is trend satisfactory? Check no postural drop.
Operation site checked and explained to patient.
GP letter sent with patient or carer; he/she *must* know what has happened.

Exposing patients to our learning curves? the jury is still out...

All surgeons get better over time (for a while), as they perform new techniques with increasing ease and confidence. When Wertheim did his first hysterectomies, his first dozen patients died—but then one survived. He assumed it was a good operation, and pressed ahead. He was a brave man, and thousands of women owe their lives to him. But had he tried to do this today, he would have been stopped. The UK's General Medical Council (GMC), and other august bodies tell us that we must protect the public by reporting doctors whose patients have low survival rates. The reason for this is partly ethical, and partly to preserve self-regulation.

We have the toughest codes of practice and disciplinary procedures of any group of workers. It is assumed that doctors are loyal to each other out of self-interest, and that this loyalty is bad. This has never been tested formally, and is not evidence-based. We can imagine two clinical worlds: one of constant 'reportings' and recriminatory audits, and another of trust and team-work. Both are imperfect, but we should not assume that the first world would be better for our patients.

When patients are sick with fear, they do not, perhaps, want to know everything. We may tell to protect ourselves. We may **not** tell to protect ourselves. Perhaps what we should do is, in our hearts, appeal to those 12 dead women-of-Wertheim—a jury as infallible as sacrificial—and try to hear their reply. And to those who complain that in doing so we are playing God, it is possible to reply with some humility that, whatever it is, it does not seem like play.

'It is amazing what little harm doctors do when one considers all the opportunities they have.' M Twain

1 Advantages: shorter waiting lists, fewer infections, fewer days off work, and ↑patient satisfaction.

►Examine the regional lymph nodes as well as the lump. If the lump is a node, examine its area of drainage. Always examine the circulation & nerve supply distal to any lump.

History How long has it been there? Does it hurt? Any other lumps? Is it getting bigger? Ever been abroad? Otherwise well?

Physical exam Remember the '6 S's: site, size, shape, smoothness (consistency), surface (contour/edge/colour), and surroundings. ***Other questions:*** Does it transilluminate (see below)? Is it fixed/tethered to skin or underlying structures (see BOX)? Is it fluctuant/compressible? Temperature? Tender? Pulsatile (US duplex may help)?

Transilluminable lumps After eliminating as much external light as possible, place a bright, thin 'pen' torch on the lump, from behind (or at least to the side), so the light is shining through the lump towards your eye. If the lump glows red it is said to transilluminate—a fluid-filled lump such as a hydrocele is a good example.

Lipomas These benign fatty lumps, occurring wherever fat can expand (ie **not** scalp or palms), have smooth, imprecise margins, a hint of fluctuance, and are not fixed to skin or deeper structures. Only cause symptoms via pressure. Malignant change very rare (suspect if rapid growth/hardening/vascularization). Multiple scattered lipomas, which may be painful, occur in Dercum's disease, typically in postmenopausal women.[77]

Sebaceous cysts These are intradermal, so you cannot draw the skin over them. Look for the characteristic punctum marking blocked sebaceous outflow. Infection is quite common, and foul pus exits through the punctum. They are common on the scalp but may occur anywhere there are sebaceous glands (ie neither soles nor palms). ***Treatment:*** excision of cyst and contents.

Lymph nodes (fig 1) Causes of enlargement: ***Infection:*** Glandular fever; brucellosis; TB; HIV; toxoplasmosis; actinomycosis; syphilis. ***Infiltration:*** Malignancy (carcinoma, lymphoma); sarcoidosis.

Cutaneous abscesses Staphylococci are the most common organisms. Haemolytic streptococci only common in hand infections. *Proteus* is a common cause of non-staphylococcal axillary abscesses. Below the waist faecal organisms are common (aerobes & anaerobes). ***Treatment:*** Incision & drainage usually cures. ***Boils (furuncles)*** are abscesses involving a hair follicle and associated glands. ***A carbuncle*** is an area of subcutaneous necrosis which discharges itself on to the surface through multiple sinuses. Think of ***hidradenitis suppuritiva*** if recurrent inguinal or axillary abscesses.

Rheumatoid nodules are collagenous granulomas which appear in established rheumatoid arthritis on the extensor aspects of joints—especially the elbows.

Ganglia Degenerative cysts from an adjacent joint or synovial sheath commonly seen on the dorsum of the wrist or hand and dorsum of the foot. May transilluminate. 50% disappear spontaneously. Aspiration may be effective, especially when combined with instillation of steroid and **hyaluronidase**.[78] For the rest, treatment of choice is excision rather than the traditional blow from your bible (the *Oxford Textbook of Surgery*!).

Fibromas These may occur anywhere in the body, but most commonly under the skin. These whitish, benign tumours contain collagen, fibroblasts, and fibrocytes.

Dermoid cysts contain dermal structures; found at the junction of embryonic cutaneous boundaries, eg in the midline or lateral to the eye.

Malignant tumours of connective tissue Fibrosarcomas, liposarcomas, leiomyosarcomas (smooth muscle), & rhabdomyosarcomas (striated muscle). Staged using modified TNM system including tumour grade. Needle-core (Trucut®) biopsies of large tumours precede excision. Any lesion suspected of being a sarcoma should not be simply enucleated. ►Refer to a specialist.

Neurofibromas see p518

Keloids Caused by irregular hypertrophy of vascularised collagen forming raised edges at sites of previous scars that extend outside the scar. Treatment is excision ± topical/injected corticosteroids.

In or under the skin?

Intradermal	Subcutaneous
• Sebaceous cyst	• Lipoma
• Abscess	• Ganglion
• Dermoid cyst	• Neuroma
• Granuloma	• Lymph node

If a lump is intradermal, you cannot draw the skin over it, while if the lump is subcutaneous you should be able to manipulate it independently from the skin.

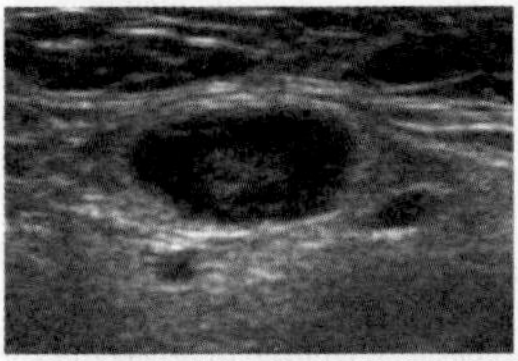

Fig 1. Ultrasound image of a normal lymph node showing a normal echogenic fatty hilum within, which is lost with malignant infiltration. Duplex mode can also be used to check for abnormal vascular patterns found in malignant lymph nodes.

Both images courtesy of Norwich Radiology Dept.

Salivary gland pathology

There are 3 pairs of major salivary glands: parotid, submandibular, and sublingual (there are many minor glands). ***History:*** Lumps; swelling related to food; pain; taste; dry eyes. ***Examination:*** Note external swelling; look for secretions; bimanual palpation for stones. Examine VIIth nerve and regional lymph nodes. ***Cytology:*** This may be ascertained by FNA.

Acute swelling Think of mumps & HIV. ***Recurrent unilateral pain and swelling*** is likely to be from a stone. 80% are submandibular. The classical story is of pain and swelling on eating—with a red, tender, swollen, but uninfected gland. The stone may be seen on plain X-ray or by sialography (**fig 2**). Distal stones are removed via the mouth but deeper stones may require excision of the gland. ***Chronic bilateral symptoms*** may coexist with dry eyes and mouth and autoimmune disease, eg hypothyroidism, Mikulicz's or Sjögren's syndrome (p720 & p724)—also bulimia. ***Fixed swelling*** may be from a tumour/ALL (**fig 4**, p349), sarcoid, amyloid, Wegener's syndrome, or be idiopathic.

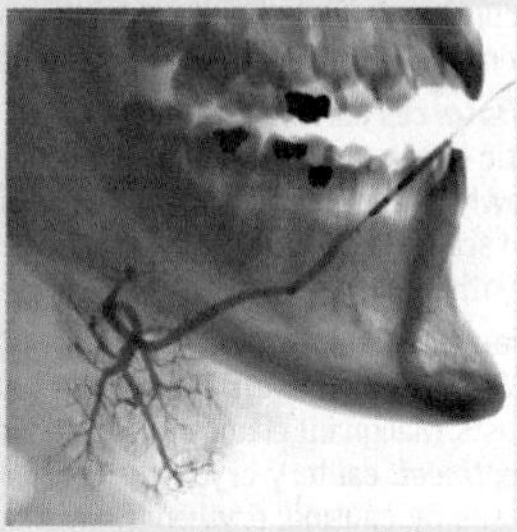

Fig 2. Normal sialogram of the submandibular gland. Wharton's (submandibular) duct opens into the mouth near the frenulum of the tongue. Stensen's (parotid) duct opens into the mouth opposite the 2nd upper molar.

Salivary gland tumours '80% are in the parotid, 80% of these are pleomorphic adenomas, 80% of these are in the superficial lobe.' Deflection of the ear outwards is a classic sign. ►Remove any salivary gland swelling for assessment if present for >1 month. VIIth nerve palsy means malignancy.

Benign or malignant	Malignant	Malignant
Cystadenolymphoma	Mucoepidermoid	Squamous or adeno Ca
Pleomorphic adenoma	Acinic cell	Adenoid cystic Ca

Pleomorphic adenomas often present in middle age and grow slowly. Remove by superficial parotidectomy. Adenolymphomas (Warthin's tumour): usually older men; soft; treat by enucleation. Carcinomas: rapid growth; hard fixed mass; pain; facial palsy. Treatment: surgery + radiotherapy. Surgery complications:

1 Facial palsy. Have a facial nerve stimulator in theatre to aid identification.
2 Salivary fistula (often close spontaneously).
3 Frey's syndrome (gustatory sweating); interposition of a soft-tissue flap at surgery may be preventative.[79] Tympanic neurectomy may also help.

Malignant tumours

1 ***Malignant melanoma*** ♀:♂ ≈ 1.5 : 1. UK incidence: ~10,000/yr, with ~2,000 deaths/yr (up ≥80% in last 20yrs).Metastasise early. Sunlight is a major cause, particularly in the early years and if short periods of intense exposure. May occur in pre-existing moles. If smooth, well-demarcated and regular, it is unlikely to be a melanoma but diagnosis can be tricky so ►if in doubt, refer. Refer if there are ≥3 points on the Glasgow scale (2 for major feature, 1 for minor feature), or with 1 point if suspicious. See **fig 1**.

Major	**Minor**	**Less helpful signs**
• Change in size	• Inflammation, crusting, or bleeding	• Asymmetry
• Change in shape	• Sensory change	• Irregular colour
• Change in colour	• Diameter >7mm (unless growth is in the vertical plane: beware)	• Elevation
		• Irregular border

Superficial spreading melanomas (80%) grow slowly, metastasise later & have better prognosis than **nodular melanomas** which invade deeply & metastasise early. Breslow thickness (depth in mm) is a good indicator of prognosis. Clark's staging stratifies depth by 5 anatomical levels from confinement to epidermis (stage 1) to penetration of the sc fat (stage 5) Neighbouring 'satellite' lesions, amelanosis, ulceration, high mitotic index, & male sex are all poor prognostic indicators. ℞: urgent excision. *OHCS* p592.

2 ***Squamous cell cancer*** Usually presents as an ulcerated lesion, with hard, raised edges, in sun-exposed sites. May begin in solar keratoses (below), or be found on the lips of smokers or in long-standing ulcers (=Marjolin's ulcer). Metastasise to lymph nodes (rare), local destruction may be extensive. ℞: Excision + radiotherapy to treat recurrence/affected nodes. **NB:** the condition may be confused with a keratoacanthoma—a fast-growing, benign, self-limiting papule plugged with keratin. See **fig 2**.

3 ***Basal cell carcinoma*** **(rodent ulcer)** Typically, a pearly nodule with rolled telangiectatic edge, usually on the face on a sun-exposed site. Metastases are very rare. It slowly causes local destruction if left untreated. Lesions on the trunk can appear as red scaly plaques with a raised smooth edge. *Cause*: UV exposure. ℞: Excision is best; cryotherapy/radiotherapy may be used. See **fig 3**.

Pre-malignant tumours

1 ***Solar (actinic) keratoses*** appear on sun-exposed skin as crumbly, yellow-white crusts. Malignant change to squamous cell carcinoma may occur after several years. ***Treatment:*** cautery, cryotherapy or twice-daily 5% 5-fluorouracil (5-FU) cream—this works by causing: erythema → vesiculation → erosion → ulceration → necrosis → healing epithelialization, leaving healthy skin unharmed. Treatment with 5-FU cream is usually for 4wks, but may be prolonged. No significant systemic absorption if the area treated is <500cm^2. Avoid in pregnancy. The hands should be washed after applying the cream. Alternative: diclofenac gel (3%; Solaraze®, use thinly twice-daily for ≤90d).

2 ***Bowen's disease*** Slow-growing red/brown scaly plaque, eg on lower legs. ***Histology:*** Full-thickness dysplasia (carcinoma *in situ*). It infrequently progresses to squamous cell cancer. Penile Bowen's disease is called Queyrat's erythroplasia. ***Treatment:*** Cryotherapy, topical 5-flurouracil (as above) or photodynamic therapy.

Others

Secondary carcinoma Most common metastases to skin are from breast, kidney, or lung. Usually a firm nodule, most often on the scalp. See acanthosis nigricans (p564).
Mycosis fungoides Cutaneous T-cell lymphoma usually confined to skin. Causes itchy, red plaques. (Sézary syndrome-variant also associated with erythroderma).
Leucoplakia This appears as white patches (which may fissure) on oral or genital mucosa (where it may itch). Frank carcinomatous change may occur.
Leprosy Suspect in any anaesthetic hypopigmented lesion (p428).
Syphilis Any genital ulcer is syphilis until proved otherwise. Secondary syphilis: papular rash—including, unusually, on the palms[1] (p431).

3 **Also** Kaposi's sarcoma (p716); Paget's disease of the breast (p722).

1 *Other causes:* Stevens-Johnson syn.; hand, foot & mouth disease; palmar erythema in liver disease.

ABCDE criteria for diagnosis of melanoma
Asymmetry
Border—irregular
Colour—non-uniform
Diameter >7mm
Elevation

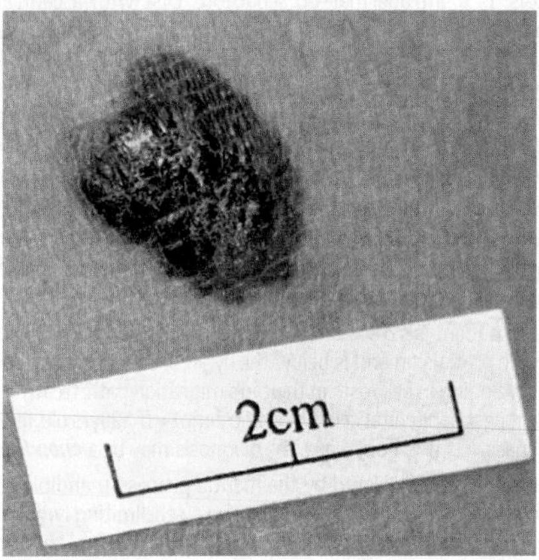

Fig 1. Melanoma

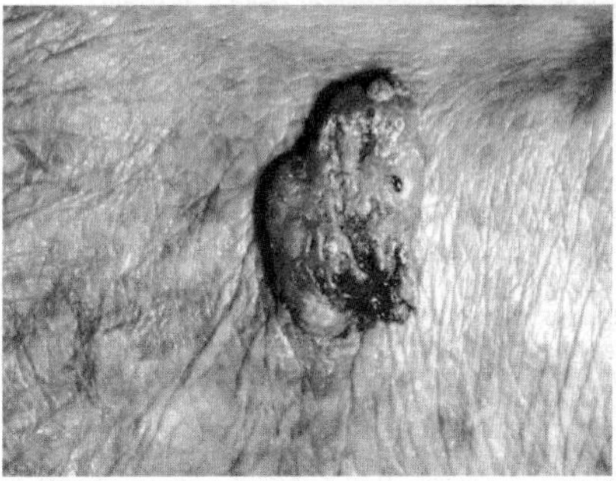

Fig 2. Squamous cell cancer

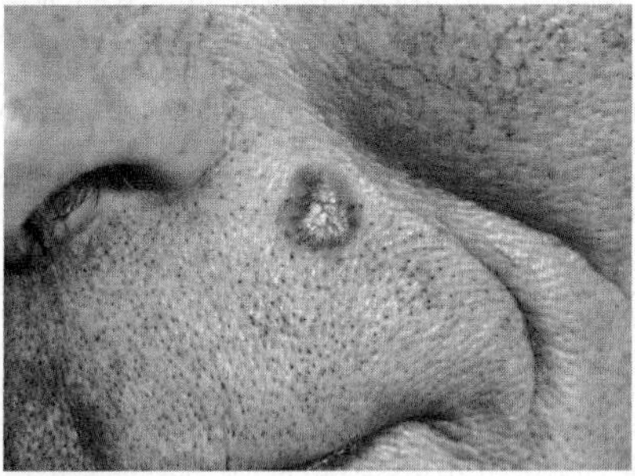

Fig 3. Basal cell carcinoma (BCC)

►Don't biopsy lumps until tumours within the head and neck have been excluded by an ENT surgeon. Culture all biopsied lymph nodes for TB.

Diagnosis First, ask how long the lump has been present. If <3wks, self-limiting infection is the likely cause and extensive investigation is unwise. Next ask yourself where the lump is. Is it intradermal—eg sebaceous cyst with a central punctum (p596)? Is it a lipoma (p596)? If the lump is not intradermal, and is not of recent onset, you are about to start a diagnostic hunt over complicated terrain. **85% of neck swellings are lymph nodes** (examine areas which they serve). Consider TB, viruses such as HIV or EBV (infectious mononucleosis), any chronic infection or, if >20yrs, consider lymphoma (hepatosplenomegaly?) or metastases eg from GI or bronchial or head and neck neoplasia.[1]), 8% are goitres (p602), and other diagnoses account for 7%.

Tests Ultrasound shows lump consistency: cystic, solid, complex, vascular. CT defines masses in relation to their anatomical neighbours. Do virology and Mantoux test. CXR may show malignancy or reveal bilateral hilar lymphadenopathy; here you should consider sarcoid. Consider fine-needle aspiration (FNA)

Midline lumps: • If patient is <20yrs old, likely diagnosis is *dermoid cyst* (p596). • If it moves **up** on tongue protrusion and is below the hyoid, likely to be a *thyroglossal cyst* (fluctuant lump developing in cell rests in thyroid's migration path; treatment: surgery; they are the commonest congenital cervical cystic lump). • If >20yrs old, it is probably a *thyroid isthmus* mass. • If it is bony hard, the diagnosis may be a *chondroma*.

Submandibular triangle: (Bordered by the mental process, mandible, and the line between the two angles of the mandible.) • If <20yrs, self-limiting lymphadenopathy is likely. If >20yrs, exclude *malignant lymphadenopathy* (eg firm and non-tender). ►Is TB likely? • If it is not a node, think of submandibular *salivary stone*, *sialadenitis*, or *tumour* (See BOX on p597 for *Salivary gland pathology*)

Anterior triangle: (Between midline, anterior border of sternocleidomastoid, and the line between the two angles of the mandible). • *Branchial cysts* emerge under the anterior border of sternocleidomastoid where the upper third meets the middle third (age <20yrs). Due to non-disappearance of the cervical sinus (where 2nd branchial arch grows down over 3rd & 4th). Lined by squamous epithelium, their fluid contains cholesterol crystals. Treat by excision. There may be communication with the pharynx in the form of a fistula • If lump in the supero-posterior area of the anterior triangle, is it a *parotid tumour* (more likely if >40yrs)? • *Laryngoceles* are an uncommon cause of anterior triangle lumps. They are painless and may be made worse by blowing. These cysts are classified as external, internal, or mixed, and may be associated with laryngeal cancer. If *pulsatile* may be: • *Carotid artery aneurysm* • *Tortuous carotid artery* or • *Carotid body tumours* (chemodectoma). These are very rare, move from side to side but not up and down, and splay out the carotid bifurcation. They are usually firm and occasionally soft and pulsatile. They do not usually cause bruits. They may be bilateral, familial, and malignant (5%). Suspected in any mass just anterior to the upper third of sternomastoid. Diagnose by duplex USS (splaying at the carotid bifurcation) or digital computer angiography. ℞: extirpation by vascular surgeon.

Posterior triangle: (Behind sternocleidomastoid, in front of trapezius, above clavicle.) • *Cervical ribs* may intrude into this area. These are enlarged costal elements from C7 vertebra. The majority are asymptomatic but can cause Raynaud's syndrome by compressing subclavian artery and neurological symptoms (eg wasting of 1st dorsal interosseous) from pressure on lower trunk of the brachial plexus • *Pharyngeal pouches* can protrude into the posterior triangle on swallowing (usually left-sided)—see **fig 1**. • *Cystic hygromas* (usually infants) arise from jugular lymph sac. These macrocystic lymphatic malformations transilluminate brightly. Treat by surgery/hypertonic saline sclerosant injection. Recurrence can be troublesome. • *Pancoast's tumour* (see p722) • *Subclavian artery aneurysm* will be pulsatile.

1 In young Asian women **Kikuchi's disease** (necrotising lymphadenitis) is a rare and benign cause of cervical lymphadenopathy. Diagnosis is made on excision biopsy.

The distribution of lymph nodes in the head and neck

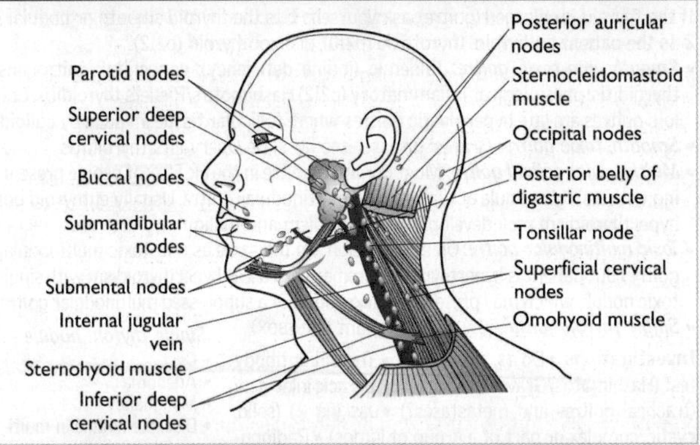

Important relations to the carotid artery and internal jugular vein in the neck

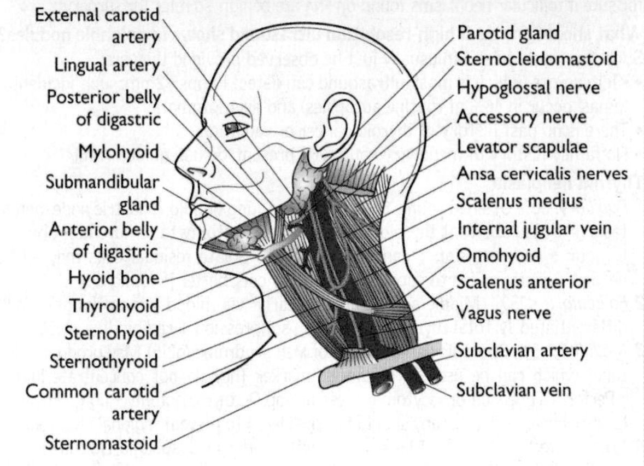

Both line drawings after RCSI website.

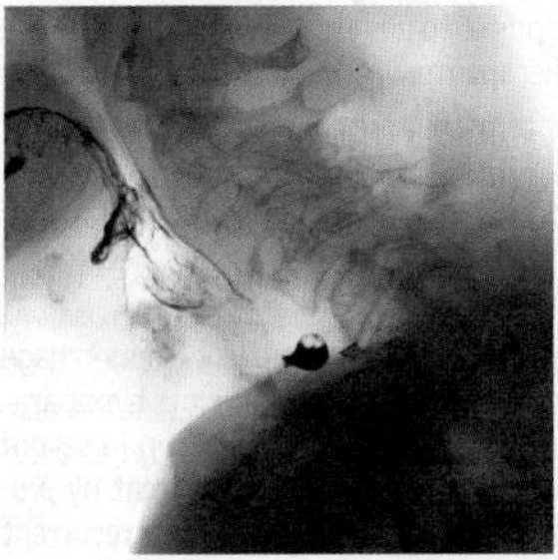

Fig 1. Contrast swallow study showing a pharyngeal pouch (arrow). It is a pulsion diverticulum caused by cricopharyngeus spasm that protrudes between the fibres of the inferior pharyngeal constrictor muscle. The patient may have a history of halitosis, sore throats and regurgitation of undigested food. As the pouch enlarges, there may be dysphagia as it presses against the oesophagus. These symptoms usually precede a palpable swelling in the neck which, if felt, would emanate from behind the trachea and sternocleidomastoid.

Courtesy of Norwich Radiology Department

If the thyroid is enlarged (goitre), ask yourself: **1** Is the thyroid smooth or nodular? **2** Is the patient euthyroid, thyrotoxic (p210), or hypothyroid (p212)?

- *Smooth, non-toxic goitre:* Endemic (iodine deficiency); congenital; goitrogens; thyroiditis; physiological; inflammatory (p212) Hashimoto's/Riedel's thyroiditis. Colloid goitres are late hyperplastic goitres where follicular tissue invaded by colloid.
- *Smooth, toxic goitre:* Graves' disease—see **fig 1**, De Quervain's thyroiditis
- *Multinodular colloid goitre:* Most common goitre in the UK. 50% of people presenting with a single nodule actually have a multinodular goitre. Usually euthyroid but hyperthyroidism may develop. Hypothyroidism and malignancy are rare
- *Toxic multinodular goitre:* On examination are the same as non-toxic multinodular goitres but patient is hyperthyroid. Plummer's disease is hyperthyroidism with single toxic nodule which may present in background of a suppressed multinodular goitre.
- *Single thyroid lump* ~10% are malignant (MINIBOX)

Single thyroid nodule
• Cyst • Adenoma • Malignancy • Discrete nodule in multinodular goitre

Investigations • Do T3, T4 and TSH • Thyroid antibody test (Hashimoto's/Graves?) • CXR with thoracic inlet view (tracheal goitres and metastases?) • USS (**fig 2**) (solid, cystic, complex or part of a group of lumps). • Radionuclide scans may show malignant lesions as hypofunctioning or 'cold', whereas a hyperfunctioning 'hot' lesion suggests adenoma. • FNA (fine-needle aspiration) and cytology on the fluid. ►No clinical/lab test good enough to tell for sure if follicular neoplasms found on FNA are benign, so refer for surgery.[81]

What should you do if high-resolution ultrasound shows impalpable nodules? Such thyroid nodules can usually just be observed provided they are:

- <1cm across (which is most; ultrasound can detect lumps <2mm; such 'incidentalomas' occur in 46% of routine autopsies) and asymptomatic.
- There is no past history of thyroid cancer or radiation.
- No family history of medullary cancer. (If present, do USS-guided FNA.)

Thyroid neoplasia[82]

1 *Papillary:* 60%. Often in young. Spread: nodes & lung (jugulo-digastric node metastasis is 'lateral aberrant thyroid'). ℞: total thyroidectomy to remove non-obvious tumour ± node excision ± radioiodine (^{131}I) to ablate residual cells may all be needed. Give thyroxine to suppress TSH. Prognosis: better if young & ♀.

2 *Follicular:* ≤25%. Middle-aged, spreads early via blood (bone, lungs). Well-differentiated. ℞: total thyroidectomy + T_4 suppression + radioiodine ablation.

3 *Medullary:* 5%. Sporadic (80%) or part of MEN syndrome (p215). May produce calcitonin which can be used as a tumour marker. They do not concentrate iodine. ►Perform a phaeochromocytoma screen pre-op. Do thyroidectomy + node clearance. External beam radiotherapy should be considered to prevent regional recurrence.

4 *Lymphoma:* 5%. ♀:♂ ≈3:1. May present with stridor or dysphagia. Do full staging pre-treatment (chemoradiotherapy). Assess histology for mucosa-associated lymphoid tissue (MALT) origin (associated with a good prognosis).

5 *Anaplastic:* Rare. ♀:♂ ≈3:1. Elderly, poor response to any treatment. In the absence of unresectable disease, excision + radiotherapy may be tried.

Thyroid surgery *Indications:* Pressure symptoms, relapse hyperthyroidism after >1 failed course of drug treatment, carcinoma, cosmetic reasons, symptomatic patients planning pregnancy. Render euthyroid pre-op with antithyroid drugs (but stop 10 days prior to surgery as these increase vascularity) and/or *propranolol*. Check vocal cords by indirect laryngoscopy pre- and post-op.

Complications: Also see p582. *Early:* Recurrent laryngeal nerve palsy, haemorrhage (►►if compresses airway, instantly remove sutures for evacuation of clot); hypoparathyroidism (check plasma Ca^{2+} daily; there is commonly a transient drop in serum concentration); thyroid storm (symptoms of severe hyperthyroidism—treat by *propranolol* PO or IV, antithyroid drugs, and iodine, p844). *Late:* Hypothyroidism; recurrent hyperthyroidism.

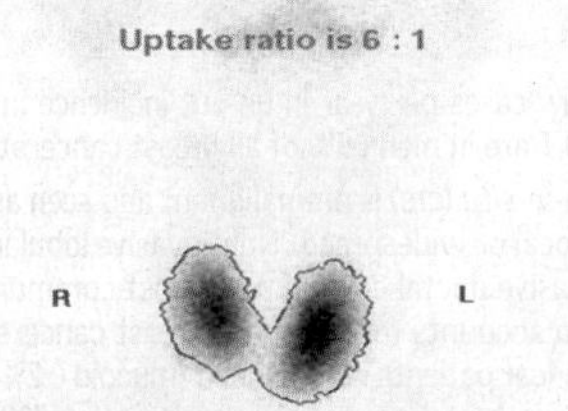

Fig 1. Radionuclide study of the thyroid showing changes consistent with Graves' disease (see also *hot and cold nodules* (p209) and *nuclear medicine*, p752). There is increased uptake of the radionuclide trace diffusely throughout both lobes of the gland (uptake ratio =6:1).

Image courtesy of Norwich Radiology Department

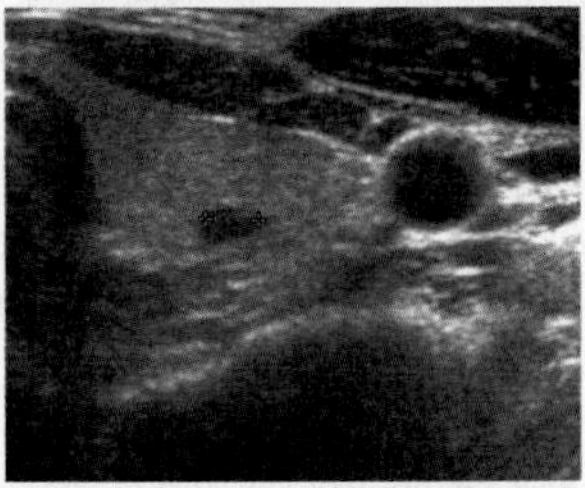

Fig 2. Transverse ultrasound of the left lobe of the thyroid showing a small low-reflectivity cyst within higher-reflectivity thyroid tissue. Note the proximity to the gland of the common carotid artery and internal jugular vein (the latter compressed slightly by pressure from the probe), both seen beneath the body of sternocleidomastoid muscle.

Image courtesy of Norwich Radiology Department

The anatomy of the region of the thyroid gland

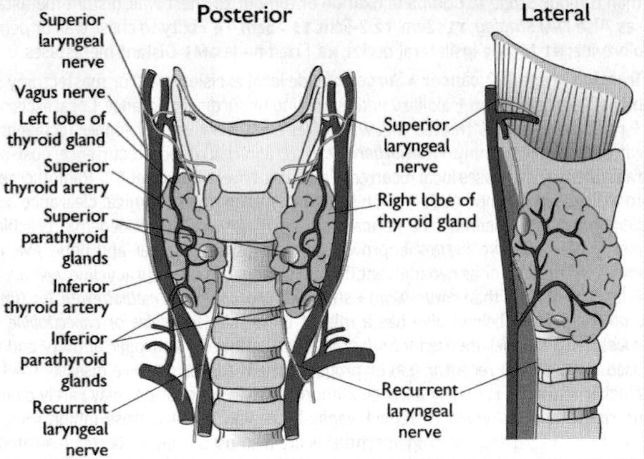

The important structures that must be considered when operating on the thyroid gland include:

- Recurrent laryngeal nerve
- Superior laryngeal nerve
- Parathyroid glands
- Trachea
- Common carotid artery
- Internal jugular vein (not depicted-see **fig 2**).

Epidemiology Affects 1 in 11 ♀, ~20,000 new cases per year in UK but incidence increasing (especially in developed countries). Rare in men (~1% of all breast cancers).

Pathology Non-invasive ductal carcinoma-*in-situ* (CIS) is premalignant and seen as microcalcification on mammography (unifocal or widespread). Non-invasive lobular CIS is rarer and tends to be multifocal. Invasive ductal carcinoma is most common (~70%) whereas invasive lobular carcinoma accounts for 10-15% of breast cancers. Medullary cancers (~5%) tend to affect younger patients while colloid /mucoid (~2%) tend to affect the elderly. Others: papillary, tubular, adenoid-cystic and Paget's (p722)

Risk factors Risk is related to family history, age and uninterrupted oestrogen exposure, hence: nulliparity; 1st pregnancy >30yrs old, early menarche; late menopause; HRT; obesity; BRCA genes (p 524); not breast-feeding; the Pill (possibly); past breast cancer (metachronous rate ≈2%, synchronous rate ≈1%).

The patient (p66) Lump, nipple discharge/inversion, skin change (*peau d'orange*).

Investigations ►All lumps should undergo *'triple' assessment:* Clinical examination + histology/cytology (C1-aspirate inadequate, C2-benign, C3-probably benign, C4-probably carcinoma, C5-carcinoma) + mammography/ultrasound; see FLOWCHART.

Staging: *Stage 1:* Confined to breast, mobile *Stage 2:* Growth confined to breast, mobile, lymph nodes in ipsilateral axilla *Stage 3:* Tumour fixed to muscle (but not chest wall), ipsilateral lymph nodes matted and may be fixed, skin involvement larger than tumour *Stage 4:* Complete fixation of tumour to chest wall, distant metastases. Also *TNM staging*: **T1**<2cm, **T2** 2-5cm, **T3** >5cm, **T4** Fixity to chest wall or *peau d'orange*; **N1** Mobile ipsilateral nodes; **N2** Fixed nodes; **M1** Distant metastases.

Treating stage 1-2 cancer • *Surgery:* Wide local excision (WLE) or mastectomy ± breast reconstruction + axillary node sampling or surgical clearance. Local excision + radiotherapy (80% treated this way) gives equal survival, but higher recurrence rates, than mastectomy. • *Radiotherapy:* If at high risk of local recurrence, post-op radiotherapy decreases local recurrence and may ↑overall survival.[83] [84] Radiotherapy to axilla used if lymph node +ve on sampling and complete surgical clearance not performed. SE: pneumonitis, pericarditis, rib fractures, lymphoedema, brachial plexopathy. • *Chemotherapy* improves survival (esp. if younger and node +ve, in recurrent disease, or as neoadjuvant if large tumour), eg an anthracycline (*epirubicin* is less cardiotoxic than *doxorubicin*) + 5FU + *cyclophosphamide* ± *methotrexate*. *Trastuzumab* (Herceptin®, below) also has a role. If these fail, *vinorelbine* or *capecitabine* + *docetaxel* (a taxane) are used. • *Endocrine agents* aim to ↓oestrogen activity, and is used in oestrogen receptor (ER) or progesterone receptor (PR) +ve disease. The ER blocker *tamoxifen* is widely used, eg 20mg/d PO for 5yrs post-op (may rarely cause uterine cancer so warn to report vaginal bleeding).[85] Aromatase inhibitors (eg *anastrozole*) targeting oestrogen synthesis are also used (may be better tolerated). They are often used if post-menopausal. If pre-menopausal and an ER+ve tumour, ovarian ablation (via surgery or radiotherapy), or GnRH analogues (eg *goserelin*) ↓recurrence and ↑survival. • *Support:* Breastcare nurses • *Reconstruction options:* eg implants, latissimus dorsi flap, TRAM flap. (Transverse rectus abdominis myocutaneous)

Treating distant disease (Stage 3–4) Assess LFT, Ca^{2+}, CXR, skeletal survey, bone scan, CT/MRI or PET-CT (p752), liver US. DXT (p530) to painful bony lesions (*bisphosphonates*, p696, may ↓pain & fracture risk). *Tamoxifen* is often used in ER+ve; if relapse after initial success, consider chemotherapy (1st-line docetaxel, 2nd vinorelbine or capecitabine). Tumours +ve for HER2 protein metastasizing to brain may respond to the monoclonal antibody *trastuzumab* (Herceptin®).[86] CNS surgery for solitary (or easily accessible) metastases may be possible; if not—radiotherapy. Get specialist help for arm lymphoedema (try decongestive methods before compressive methods).[NICE 2009]

Preventing deaths • *Exercise*; good *diet* (p236)[87] • Promote *awareness* • *Screening:* 2-view mammography every 3yrs for women aged 50-70 in UK MRI may be better); ↓ breast cancer deaths by 25%. *Raloxifene* may prevent some ER+ve cancers (*OHCS* p256).

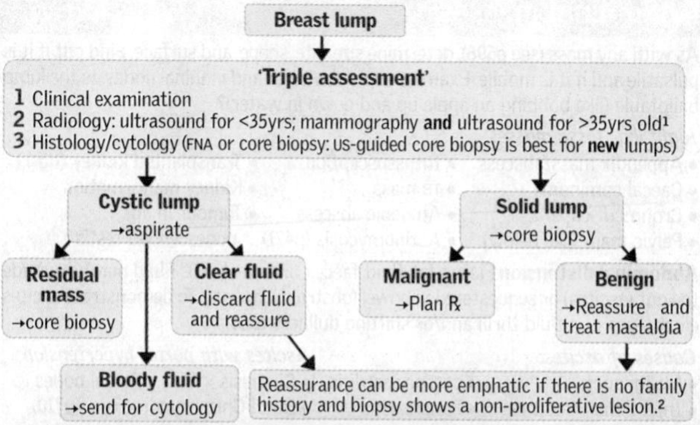

Breast lump
'Triple assessment'
1 Clinical examination
2 Radiology: ultrasound for <35yrs; mammography and ultrasound for >35yrs old[1]
3 Histology/cytology (FNA or core biopsy: US-guided core biopsy is best for new lumps)
Cystic lump →aspirate
Solid lump →core biopsy
Residual mass →core biopsy
Clear fluid →discard fluid and reassure
Malignant →Plan ℞
Benign →Reassure and treat mastalgia
Bloody fluid →send for cytology
Reassurance can be more emphatic if there is no family history and biopsy shows a non-proliferative lesion.[2]

Sentinel node biopsy

Decreases needless axillary clearances in lymph node -ve patients.

- Patent blue dye and/or radiocolloid injected into periareolar area or tumour.
- A gamma probe/visual inspection is used to identify the sentinel node.
- The sentinel node is biopsied and sent for histology ± immunohistochemistry.

Trials suggest sentinel node identified in 90% of patients. False-negative rates are 9-14% (drop to <5% as surgeons become more experienced).

Prognostic factors in breast cancer

Tumour size, grade, lymph node status, ER/PR status, presence of vascular invasion all help assess prognosis. Nottingham Prognostic Index (NPI) is widely used to predict survival & risk of relapse, and to help select appropriate adjuvant systemic therapy:[3] NPI = *0.2 × tumour size (cm) + histological grade + nodal status.*
If treated with surgery alone, 10yr survival rates are: NPI <2.4: 95%; NPI 2.4–3.4: 85%; NPI 3.4–4.4: 70%; NPI 4.4–5.4: 50%; NPI >5.4: 20%.

Benign breast disease

Common benign lumps
• Fibroadenoma & cysts • Fibroadenosis (focal or diffuse nodularity)
Rare lumps
• Periductal mastitis • Galactocoele • Abscess • 'Non-breast' lipoma, fat necrosis, or seb. cyst

Congenital absence of breast: Hypoplasia is more common than amastia (some asymmetry is common).
Accessory nipples: From failure of regression of primitive milk line from axilla (most common) to groin.
Benign mammary dysplasia: Pre-menstrual breast nodularity and pain often in upper outer quadrant. ANDI (Aberration of Normal Development and Involution) includes fibrosis, adenosis, cysts, epitheliosis and papillomatosis. ℞: Reassurance, analgesia, good bra ± evening primrose oil.
Cystic disease: Cysts common peri-menopause. ℞: Aspiration and reassurance.
Fibroadenomas: From overgrowth of collagenous mesenchyme. Firm, smooth, mobile ('the breast mouse'), multiple. ⅓ regress, ⅓ stay same, ⅓ get bigger. ℞: Observation but if in doubt FNA ± excision.
Infective mastitis/breast abscesses: often associated with lactation (usually *Staphylococcus aureus*). ℞: Antibiotics/incision and drainage if abscess.
Duct ectasia: Duct dilatation with age. Nipple discharge (green/brown/bloody).
Fat necrosis: Fibrosis and calcification after trauma forms a mass.

1 US has become more accurate at detecting invasive breast cancer, though mammography remains most accurate at detecting ductal carcinoma *in situ* (DCIS). MRI is used in the assessment of multifocal/bilateral disease and patients with cosmetic implants who are identified as high risk.
2 There is a relatively ↑risk of malignancy if there is atypical hyperplasia or a proliferative lesion.
3 Nodal status is scored **1-3**: **1** = node -ve; **2** = 1-3 nodes +ve; **3** = >3 nodes +ve for breast cancer. Histological grade is also scored 1-3.

As with any mass (see p596), determine size, site, shape, and surface. Find out if it is pulsatile and if it is mobile. Examine supraclavicular and inguinal nodes. Is the lump ballotable (like bobbing an apple up and down in water)?

Right iliac fossa masses:		
• Appendix mass/abscess	• Intussusception	• Transplanted kidney (**fig 1**)
• Caecal carcinoma	• TB mass	• Kidney malformation
• Crohn's disease	• Amoebic abscess	• Tumour in an undescended testis
• Pelvic mass (see below)	• Actinomycosis (p421)	

Abdominal distension Flatus, fat, fluid, faeces, or fetus (p57)? Fluid may be outside the gut (ascites) or sequestered in bowel (obstruction; ileus). To demonstrate ascites elicit signs of a fluid thrill and/or shifting dullness (p60).

Causes of ascites:		*Ascites with portal hypertension:*	
• Malignancy★	• CCF; pericarditis	• Cirrhosis	• Portal nodes
• Infections★—esp TB	• Pancreatitis★	• Budd-Chiari syndrome★ (p710)	
• ↓Albumin (eg nephrosis)	• Myxoedema	• IVC or portal vein thrombosis	

Tests: Aspirate ascitic fluid (paracentesis, p779) for cytology, culture, & protein level (≥30g/L in diseases marked★) with a 21G needle in RIF (p778); ultrasound. Protein level rarely helps diagnostically; it tends to rise with diuretic therapy.

Left upper quadrant mass Is it spleen, stomach, kidney, colon, pancreas, or a rare cause (eg neurofibroma)? Pancreatic cysts may be true (congenital; cystadenomas; retention cysts of chronic pancreatitis; cystic fibrosis) or pseudocysts (fluid in lesser sac from acute pancreatitis).

Splenomegaly Causes are often said to be **infective**, **haematological**, **neoplastic**, etc, but grouping by **associated feature** is more useful clinically:

Splenomegaly with fever	*With lymphadenopathy*	*With purpura*
• Infection^HS (malaria, SBE/IE hepatitis,^HS EBV,^HS TB, CMV, HIV) • Sarcoid; malignancy^HS	• Glandular fever^HS • Leukaemias; lymphoma • Sjögren's syndrome	• Septicaemia; typhus • DIC; amyloid^HS • Meningococcaemia
With arthritis	*With ascites*	*With a murmur*
• Sjögren's syndrome • Rheumatoid arthritis; SLE • Infection, eg Lyme (p430) • Vasculitis/Behçet's (p558)	• Carcinoma • Portal hypertension^HS	• SBE/IE • Rheumatic fever • Hypereosinophilia • Amyloid^HS (p364)
With anaemia	*With weight↓ + CNS signs*	*Massive splenomegaly*
• Sickle-cell;^HS thalassaemia^HS • Leishmaniasis;^HS leukaemia^HS • Pernicious anaemia (p328) • POEM (p212)	• Cancer; lymphoma • TB; arsenic poisoning • Paraproteinaemia^HS	• Malaria; leishmaniasis • Myelofibrosis; CML^HS • Gaucher's syndrome^HS
HS=causes of hepatosplenomegaly.		

Smooth hepatomegaly Hepatitis, CCF, sarcoidosis, early alcoholic cirrhosis (a small liver is typical later); tricuspid incompetence (→ pulsatile liver).

Craggy hepatomegaly Secondaries or 1° hepatoma. (Nodular cirrhosis typically causes a small, shrunken liver, not an enlarged craggy one.)

Pelvic masses
• Fibroids
• Fetus
• Bladder
• Ovarian cysts or malignancies

Pelvic masses *Is it truly pelvic?*—Yes, if by palpation you cannot get 'below it'.

Investigating lumps There is much to be said for performing an early *CT* to save time and money compared with leaving the test to be the last in a long chain. If unavailable, *ultrasound* is the first test (transvaginal approach may be useful—**fig 2**). *Others:* IVU; liver and spleen radioisotope scans; Mantoux test (p398). Routine tests: FBC (with film); ESR; U&E; LFT; proteins; Ca^{2+}; CXR; AXR; biopsy tests—a tissue diagnosis may be made using a fine needle guided by ultrasound or CT control. MRI also has a role.

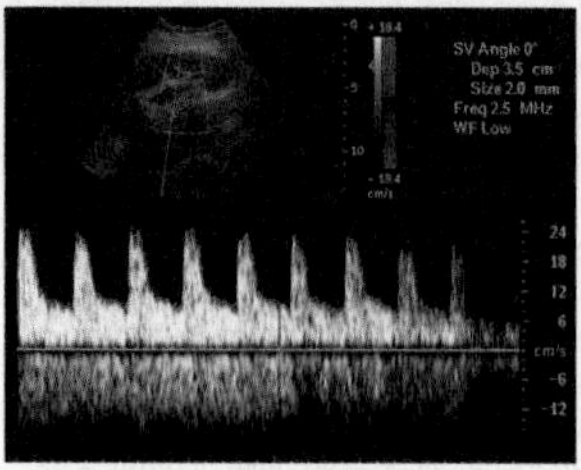

Fig 1. Ultrasound of a transplanted kidney with colour duplex imaging and Doppler mode (below) showing flow in the graft vessels. Venous and arterial thrombosis are serious early post-operative complications in organ transplantation and ultrasound assessment is an invaluable investigative tool.

Image courtesy of Norwich Radiology Department

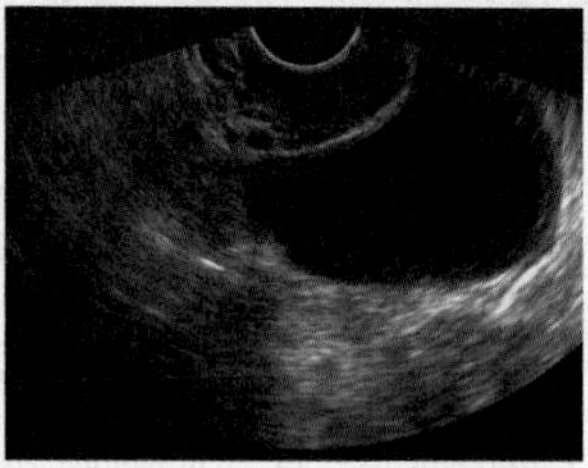

Fig 2. Transvaginal ultrasound showing a cystic lesion in the left ovary. Ovarian masses can grow to fill the abdomen and therefore may be seen in general surgical clinics. The fan-shaped view of this ultrasound image is produced by the curved footplate of the transvaginal probe.

Image courtesy of Norwich Radiology Department

In 1809 an American surgeon by the name of Ephraim McDowell performed an astonishing operation: the first successful elective laparotomy for an abdominal tumour. It was an ovariotomy for an ovarian mass in a 44-year-old who, prior to physical examination by McDowell, was believed to be gravid. Not only was this feat performed in the age before anaesthesia and antisepsis, but it was also performed on a table in the front room of McDowell's Kentucky home, at that time on the frontier of the West in the United States. His account of the operation makes fascinating reading.[1] Whilst the strength of his diagnostic convictions combined with his speed and skill at operating is to be admired (the operation took 25 minutes), there is an even more laudable part played in this story. The patient, Mrs Jane Todd-Crawford, was fully willing to be involved with what can only be described as experimental surgery in the face of uncertainty. She defied pain simply by reciting psalms and hymns, and was back at home within 4 weeks with no complications. We would be well served in remembering the commitment of Mrs Todd-Crawford as most exceptional. In the rush and hurry of our daily tasks perhaps it is all to easy to forget that the undertaking of surgery today may be no less fear-provoking for patients than it was 200 years ago.

1 *A History of Surgery*, H. Ellis, Greenwich Medical Media Limited, 2001, ISBN 1841100234

Someone who becomes acutely ill and in whom symptoms and signs are chiefly related to the abdomen has an acute abdomen. Prompt laparotomy is sometimes essential: **repeated examination is the key to making the decision.**

Clinical syndromes that usually require laparotomy:

1 *Rupture of an organ* (Spleen, aorta, ectopic pregnancy) Shock is a leading sign—see TABLE for assessment of blood loss. Abdominal swelling may be seen. Any history of trauma: blunt trauma → spleen; penetrating trauma → liver. **Delayed** rupture of the spleen may occur weeks after trauma. Peritonism may be mild.

2 *Peritonitis* (Perforation of peptic ulcer/duodenal ulcer – eg diverticulum, appendix, bowel, or gall bladder) Signs: prostration, shock, lying still, +ve cough test (p62), tenderness (± rebound/percussion pain, p62), board-like abdominal rigidity, guarding, and no bowel sounds. Erect CXR may show gas under the diaphragm (**fig 2**). **NB:** acute pancreatitis (p638) causes these signs, but does **not** require a laparotomy so don't be caught out and ►*always check serum amylase.*

Syndromes that may not require a laparotomy:

Local peritonitis: Eg diverticulitis, cholecystitis, salpingitis, and appendicitis (the latter **will** need surgery). If abscess formation is suspected (swelling, swinging fever, and WCC↑) do ultrasound or CT. Drainage can be percutaneous (ultrasound or CT-guided), or by laparotomy. Look for 'a sentinel loop' on plain AXR (p740).

Colic is a regularly waxing and waning pain, caused by muscular spasm in a hollow viscus, eg gut, ureter, salpinx, uterus, bile duct, or gall bladder (in the latter pain is often dull and constant). Colic, unlike peritonitis, causes restlessness and the patient may well be pacing around when you go to see him!

Obstruction of the bowel See p612.

Tests U&E; FBC; amylase; LFT; CRP; ABG (is there mesenteric ischaemia?); urinalysis. Erect CXR (**fig 2**), AXR may show Rigler's sign (p740) Laparoscopy may avert open surgery. CT can be helpful provided it is readily available and causes no delay (**fig 2**, p747); USS is becoming more popular and may identify perforation or free fluid immediately, but appropriate performer training is important.

Pre-op ►Don't rush to theatre. **Anaesthesia compounds shock**, so resuscitate properly first (p805) unless blood being lost faster than can be replaced, eg ruptured ectopic pregnancy, (*OHCS* p262), aneurysm leak (p656), trauma.

Plan: **Put to bed—then:**
- Treat shock (p804)
- Crossmatch, eg 2U or just group and save
- Blood culture; then...
- Antibiotics[1]
- Relieve pain (p576)
- IVI (0.9% saline)
- Plain abdominal film
- CXR if peritonitic or >50yrs
- ECG if >50yrs
- Consent
- NBM for 2h pre-op

The medical acute abdomen Irritable bowel syndrome (p276) is the chief cause, so always ask about episodes of pain associated with loose stools, relieved by defecation, bloating, and urgency (but **not** blood—this may be UC). Other causes:

►►Myocardial infarction	Pneumonia (p160)	Sickle-cell crisis (p334)
Gastroenteritis or UTI	Thyroid storm (p844)	Phaeochromocytoma (p846)
Diabetes mellitus (p198)	Zoster (p400)	Malaria (p394)
Bornholm disease (p66, p376)	Tuberculosis (p398)	Typhoid fever (p426)
Pneumococcal peritonitis	Porphyria (p706)	Cholera (p426)
Henoch-Schönlein (p716)	Narcotic addiction	*Yersinia enterocolitica* (p422)
Tabes dorsalis (p431)	PAN (p558)	Lead colic

Hidden diagnoses ►►Mesenteric ischaemia (p622), ►►acute pancreatitis (p638) and ►►a leaking AAA (p600) are the *Unterseebooten* of the acute abdomen—unsuspected, undetectable unless carefully looked for, and underestimatedly deadly. They may have non-specific symptoms and signs that are surprisingly mild, so always think of them when assessing the acute abdomen and hopefully you will 'spot' them! ►Finally: *always exclude pregnancy (± ectopic?) in females.*

1 Give antibiotics if peritonitic, eg **cefuroxime** 1.5g/8h IV + **metronidazole** 500mg/8h IV/PR.

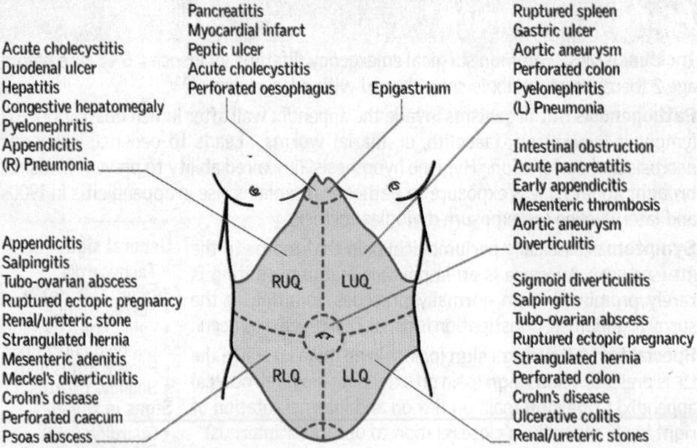

Fig 1. Causes of abdominal pain.

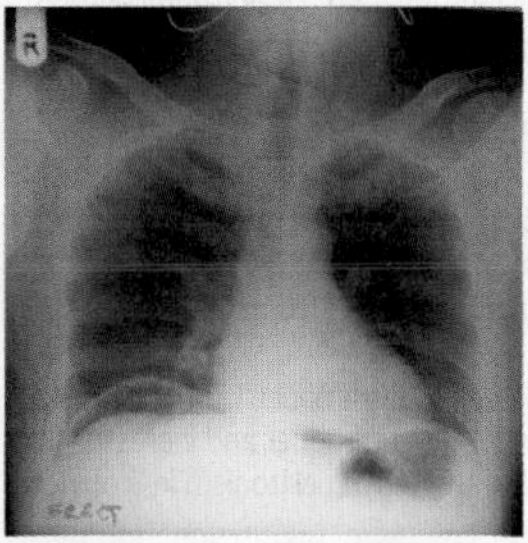

Fig 2. Erect CXR showing a sliver of air beneath the right hemidiaphragm (arrow), indicating presence of a pneumoperitoneum. *Causes:*
- Perforation of the bowel (visible only in 75%)
- Gas-forming infection, eg *C. perfringens*
- Iatrogenic, eg open or laparoscopic surgery (Gas under the diaphragm can be still detected on CXR up to 10 days post-op).
- *Per vaginam* (prolonged intercourse)
- Interposition of bowel between liver & diaphragm

Image courtesy of Mr P. Paraskeva

Assessing hypovolaemia from blood loss

The most likely cause of shock in a surgical patient is hypovolaemia (but don't forget the other causes—p804). The chief physiological parameters for assessing shock assess target organ perfusion rather than the direct measurement of BP and pulse, which may be 'normal' in one individual and yet totally abnormal for another. The most perfused organs in a normal state are the kidney, brain, and skin, so check **urine output**, **GCS** and **capillary refill** (CR). ▶▶*The best quick test is:* "do you feel dizzy if you sit up?"

Of course, BP, pulse, and respirations are still **vital** signs, but the message here is: ▶▶treat suspected shock rather than wait for BP to fall. When there is any blood loss (eg a trauma situation), assess the status of the following:

Parameter	Class I	Class II	Class III	Class IV
Blood loss	<750mL	750-1500mL	1500-2000mL	>2000mL
	<15%	15-30%	30-40%	>40%
Pulse	<100bpm	>100bpm	>120bpm	>140bpm
BP	↔	↔	↓	↓
Pulse pressure	↔ or ↑	↓	↓	↓
Respirations	14-20/min	20-30/min	30-40/min	>35/min
Urine output	>30mL/h	20-30mL/h	5-15mL/h	Negligible
Mental state	Slightly anxious	Mildly anxious	Confused →	→Lethargic
Fluid to give	Crystalloid	Crystalloid	Crystalloid + blood	

Assumes a body mass of 70kg and a circulating blood volume of 5L.

Acute appendicitis

Incidence Most common surgical emergency (lifetime incidence = 6%), rare before age 2 (because appendix is cone shaped with a larger lumen)

Pathogenesis Gut organisms invade the appendix wall after lumen obstruction by lymphoid hyperplasia, faecolith, or filarial worms. Leads to oedema, ischaemic necrosis and perforation. 'Hygiene hypothesis' (impaired ability to prevent invasion, brought about by less exposure to pathogens) explains rise in appendicitis in 1900s and later decline (as exposure dwindles further).

Symptoms Classically periumbilical pain that moves to the RIF (see BOX). Anorexia is an important feature; vomiting is rarely prominent—pain normally precedes vomiting in the surgical abdomen. Constipation is usual. Diarrhoea may occur.

Special tests: Rovsing's sign (pain > in RIF than LIF when the LIF is pressed). **Psoas sign** (pain on extending hip if retrocaecal appendix) **Cope sign** (pain on flexion and internal rotation of right hip if appendix in close relation to obturator internus).

Investigations: Blood tests may reveal neutrophil leucocytosis and elevated CRP. USS may help.[89] In one USS series the location of the appendix tip was abdominal in 9.5%, pelvic in 75%, retrocecal in 6%, and there was midline extension in 9.5%.[90] CT (if diagnosis unclear: reduces -ve appendicectomy rate, but may cause fatal delay).[91]

General signs
- Tachycardia
- Fever 37.5-38.5°C
- Furred tongue
- Lying still
- Coughing hurts, p62
- Foetor ± flushing
- Shallow breaths

Signs in the RIF
- Guarding (p62)
- Rebound + percussion tenderness, p62
- PR painful on right (sign of low-lying pelvic appendix)

Variations in the clinical picture
- Inflammation in a retrocecal/retroperitoneal appendix (2.5%) may cause flank[92] or RUQ pain;[93] its only sign may be ↑tenderness on the right on PR.
- The boy with vague abdominal pain who will not eat his favourite food.
- The shocked, confused octogenarian who is not in pain.
- Appendicitis occurs in ~1/1000 pregnancies. It is not commoner, but mortality is higher, especially from 20wks gestation. Perforation is commoner, and increases fetal mortality from. Pain is often less well localized, and signs of peritonism less obvious.

Hints
- If the child is anxious, use his hand to press his belly—see also p629 for tips.
- Check for recent viral illnesses and lymphadenopathy—mesenteric adenitis?
- Don't **start** palpating in the RIF (makes it difficult to elicit pain elsewhere).
- Expect diagnosis to be wrong half the time. If diagnosis uncertain re-examine often; don't give antibiotics as this can cloud findings.

Treatment Prompt *appendicectomy*. *Antibiotics:* **Metronidazole** 500mg/8h + **cefuroxime** 1.5g/8h, 1 to 3 doses IV starting 1h pre-op, reduces wound infections. Give a longer course if perforated. *Laparoscopy:* Useful because of its diagnostic and therapeutic advantages (when done by an experienced surgeon), especially in women and the obese. It is not recommended in cases suspected of gangrenous perforation as the rate of abscess formation may be higher.[94]

ΔΔ
- Ectopic (➧do a pregnancy test!)
- UTI (test urine!)
- Mesenteric adenitis
- Cystitis
- Cholecystitis
- Diverticulitis
- Salpingitis/PID
- Dysmenorrhoea
- Crohn's disease
- Perforated ulcer
- Food poisoning
- Meckel's diverticulum

Complications
- *Perforation* is commoner if a faecolith is present[95] and in young children, as diagnosis is more often delayed.[96] Doesn't cause infertility in girls.[97]
- *Appendix mass* may result when an inflamed appendix becomes covered with omentum. US/CT may help with diagnosis. Some advocate early surgery. Alternatively, initial conservative management—NBM and antibiotics. If the mass resolves, some perform an **interval** (ie delayed) **appendicectomy**. Exclude a colonic tumour (laparotomy or colonoscopy), which can present as early as the 4th decade.
- *Appendix abscess* May result if an appendix mass fails to resolve but enlarges and the patient gets more unwell. Treatment usually involves drainage, either surgical or percutaneous (under US/CT-guidance). Antibiotics alone may bring resolution.

Explaining the pattern of abdominal pain in appendicitis

A viscus and its visceral peritoneum have no somatic innervation, so the brain attributes the visceral (splanchnic) signals to a physical location whose dermatome corresponds to the same entry level in the spinal cord. Importantly, there is no laterality to the visceral unmyelinated C-fibre pain signals, which enter the cord bilaterally and at multiple levels. Division of the gut according to embryological origin is the important determinant here:

Gut	Division points	Somatic referral	Arterial supply
Fore	Proximal to 2nd part of duodenum	Epigastrium	Coeliac axis
Mid	Above to ⅔ along transverse colon	Periumbilical	Superior mesenteric
Hind	Distal to above	Suprapubic	Inferior mesenteric

Early inflammation irritates the structure and walls of the appendix, so a colicky pain is referred to the mid-abdomen—classically periumbilical. As the inflammation progresses and irritates the parietal peritoneum (especially on examination!) the somatic, lateralized pain settles at McBurney's point, ⅔ of the way along from the umbilicus to the right anterior superior iliac spine.

These principles also help us understand patterns of ***referred pain***. In pneumonia, the T9 dermatome is shared by the lung and the abdomen. Also, irritation of the underside of the diaphragm (sensory innervation is from above through the phrenic nerve, C3–5) by an inflamed gallbladder or a subphrenic abscess refers pain to the right shoulder: dermatomes C3–5!

The open appendicectomy

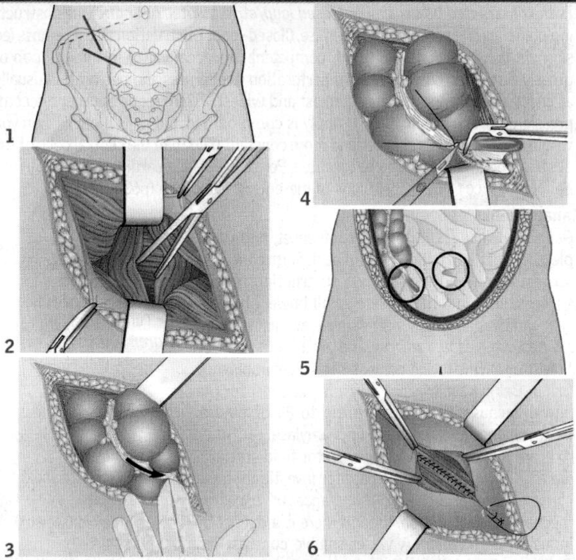

1. Traditional approach is Gridiron incision over McBurney's point, at 90° to line from umbilicus to the anterior superior iliac spine. Lanz incision is more horizontal in Langer's lines (skin creases) & gives a better scar. **2.** Divide subcutaneous fat & superficial/Scarpa's fascia. Fibres of external oblique, internal oblique & transversus abdominus divided with muscle splitting incision. **3.** Incise pre-peritoneal fat & peritoneum to reveal caecum. Deliver caecum through incision. Appendix located at convergence of taenia coli. **4.** Mesoappendix (blood vessels & mesentery) & appendix divided, ligated and excised (stump may be inverted). **5.** In case of a normal-looking appendix, excise (may be histologically if not macroscopically inflamed); look for Meckel's diverticulum. **6.** Wash, close in layers, dress wound.

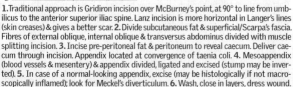

Cardinal features of intestinal obstruction
• Vomiting
• Colic
• Constipation
• Distension

Features of obstruction Vomiting, nausea and anorexia. Fermentation of the intestinal contents in established obstruction causes 'faeculent' vomiting ('faecal' vomiting is found when there is a colonic fistula with the proximal gut). **Colicky** pain is seen in early obstruction and may be absent in long-standing complete obstruction. **Constipation** need not be absolute (ie no faeces or flatus passed) if obstruction is high, though in distal obstruction nothing will be passed. Abdominal **distension** becomes more marked as the obstruction progresses. There are active, 'tinkling' bowel sounds.

The key decisions:

1 *Is the obstruction of the small or large bowel?* In small bowel obstruction, vomiting occurs earlier, distension is less, and pain is higher in the abdomen. **The AXR plays a key role in diagnosis—see** p740. In small bowel obstruction, AXR shows central gas shadows with *valvulae conniventes* that completely cross the lumen and no gas in the large bowel. In large bowel obstruction, pain is more constant; AXR shows peripheral gas shadows proximal to the blockage (eg in caecum) but not in the rectum, unless you have done a PR examination ►which is always essential! Large bowel haustra do **not** cross all the lumen's width. If the ileocaecal valve is competent (ie doesn't allow reflux) pain may be felt over a distended caecum (see below).

2 *Is there an ileus or mechanical obstruction?* In ileus (**fig 3**, p740; ie functional obstruction from reduced bowel motility) there is no pain & bowel sounds are absent.

3 *Is the obstructed bowel simple/closed loop/strangulated?* **Simple:** One obstructing point and no vascular compromise. **Closed-loop:** Obstruction at two points (eg sigmoid volvulus, distension with competent ileocaecal valve) forming a loop of grossly distended bowel at risk of perforation (tenderness and perforation usually at caecum where the bowel is thinnest and widest, >12cm requires urgent decompression). **Strangulated:** Blood supply is compromised and he is more ill than you would expect. There is sharper and more constant pain than the central colic of the obstruction and it tends to be localized. Peritonism is the cardinal sign. There may be fever + WCC↑ with other signs of mesenteric ischaemia (p622).

Management

Typical causes
• Constipation (p248)
• Hernias (p614)
• Adhesions (p567)
• Tumours (p618)
Rarer causes
• Crohn's disease
• Gallstone ileus (p636)
• Intussusception (p628)
• Diverticular stricture
• TB (developing world)
• Volvulus:
• Gastric (see BOX)
• Caecal
• Sigmoid (see BOX)
• Foreign body

- *General principles:* Site, speed of onset, and completeness of obstruction determine definitive therapy: strangulation and large bowel obstruction require surgery; ileus and incomplete small bowel obstruction can be managed conservatively, at least initially.
- *Immediate action:* ►'Drip and suck'—NGT and IV fluids to rehydrate and correct electrolyte imbalance (p680). Being NBM does not give adequate rest for the bowel because it can produce up to 9L of fluid/d. (Also: analgesia, blood tests (inc. amylase, FBC, U&E), AXR, erect CXR, catheterise to monitor fluid status)
- *Further imaging:* There is a case for investigating the cause by colonoscopy in some instances of suspected mechanical obstruction, though there is a danger of inducing perforation. A water-soluble contrast (eg Gastrografin®) follow-through study may be helpful in determining the level of obstruction—it also has some therapeutic action against mild mechanical obstruction. CT may show dilated, fluid-filled bowel and a transition zone at the site of obstruction (**figs 1 & 2**).
- *Surgery:* ►Strangulation needs emergency surgery, as does 'closed loop obstruction'. For less urgent large bowel obstruction, there is time for a water-soluble enema to try to clear the obstruction and to correct fluid imbalance. Small bowel obstruction secondary to adhesions should rarely lead to surgery—see BOX, p583.

Paralytic ileus or pseudo-obstruction?

Paralytic ileus is adynamic bowel due to the absence of normal peristaltic contractions. Contributing factors include abdominal surgery, pancreatitis (or any localized peritonitis), spinal injury, hypokalaemia, hyponatraemia, uraemia, peritoneal sepsis and drugs (eg tricyclic antidepressants).

Pseudo-obstruction is like mechanical GI obstruction but with no cause for obstruction found. **Acute** colonic pseudo-obstruction is called Ogilvie's syndrome (p720), and clinical features are similar to that of mechanical obstruction.[98] Predisposing factors: puerperium; pelvic surgery; trauma; cardiorespiratory disorders. *Treatment: **Neostigmine*** or colonoscopic decompression are sometimes useful. In **chronic** pseudo-obstruction weight loss from malabsorption is a problem.[99]

Sigmoid volvulus

Sigmoid volvulus occurs when the bowel twists on its mesentery, which can produce severe, rapid, strangulated obstruction. There is a characteristic AXR with an 'inverted U' loop of bowel that looks a bit like a coffee bean. It tends to occur in the elderly, constipated and co-morbid patient, and is often managed by sigmoidoscopy and insertion of a flatus tube. Sigmoid colectomy is sometimes required. ►If not treated successfully, it can progress to perforation and fatal peritonitis.

Volvulus of the stomach

The classical triad of gastro-oesophageal obstruction may occur: vomiting (then retching), pain, and failed attempts to pass an NG tube. Regurgitation of saliva also occurs. Dysphagia and noisy gastric peristalsis (relieved by lying down) may occur in chronic volvulus.

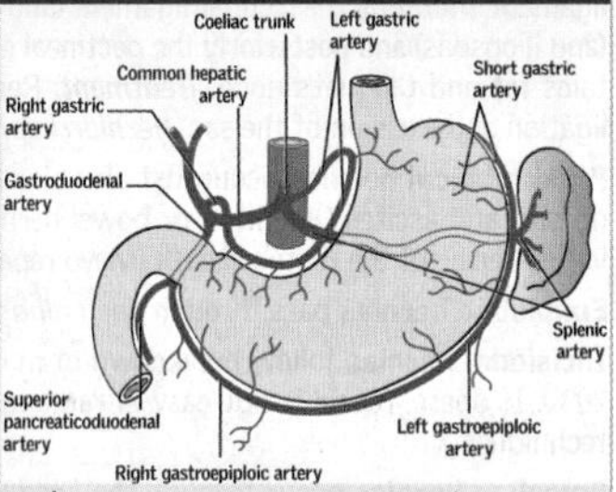

Risk factors ***Congenital:*** Paraoesophageal hernia; congenital bands; bowel malformations; pyloric stenosis. ***Acquired:*** Gastric/oesophageal surgery.

Tests Look for gastric dilatation and a double fluid level on erect films.

Treatment If acutely unwell arrange prompt resuscitation and laparotomy. In organoaxial volvulus, rotation is typically 180° left to right, about a line joining the relatively fixed pylorus and oesophagus. Mesenteroaxial rotation is at 90° to this line (and from right to left). Laparoscopic management may be possible.[100]

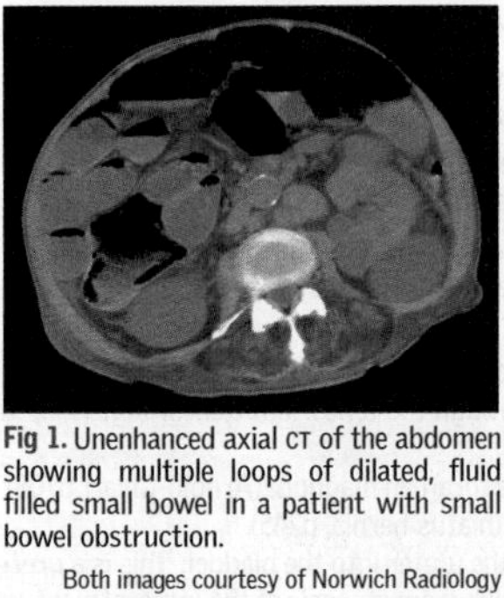

Fig 1. Unenhanced axial CT of the abdomen showing multiple loops of dilated, fluid filled small bowel in a patient with small bowel obstruction.

Both images courtesy of Norwich Radiology Department.

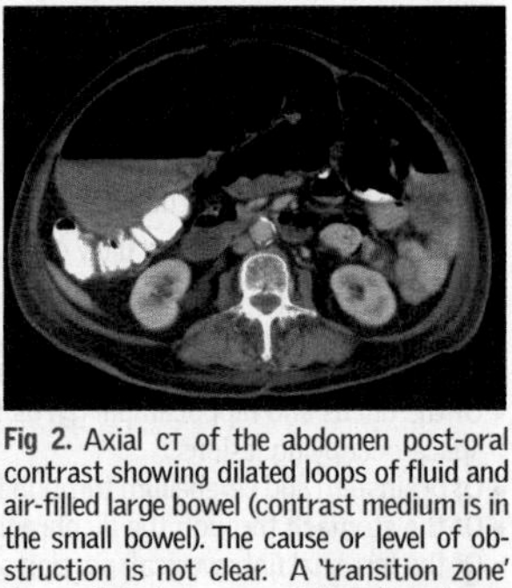

Fig 2. Axial CT of the abdomen post-oral contrast showing dilated loops of fluid and air-filled large bowel (contrast medium is in the small bowel). The cause or level of obstruction is not clear. A 'transition zone' from dilated to non-dilated bowel can sometimes be seen at the obstruction point.

Definition *The protrusion of a viscus or part of a viscus through a defect of the walls of its containing cavity into an abnormal position.* Hernias involving bowel are said to be **irreducible** if they cannot be pushed back into the right place. This does not mean that they are either necessarily obstructed or strangulated. **Incarceration** implies that the contents of the hernial sac are stuck inside by adhesions. Gastrointestinal hernias are **obstructed** if bowel contents cannot pass through them—the classical features of intestinal obstruction soon appear (p612). They are **strangulated** if ischaemia occurs—the patient becomes toxic and requires urgent surgery. Care must be taken when attempting reduction (see p616 for the technique) as it is possible to perform **reduction** *en masse*, pushing the strangulated bowel and hernial sac back into the abdominal cavity, but giving the initial appearance of successful reduction.

Inguinal hernia The commonest kind (far more common in men), described on p616.

Femoral hernia Bowel enters the femoral canal, presenting as a mass in the upper medial thigh or above the inguinal ligament where it points down the leg, unlike an inguinal hernia which points to the groin. They occur more often in women especially in middle age and the elderly. They are likely to be irreducible and to strangulate due to the rigidity of the canal's borders. ***Anatomy:*** The neck of the hernia is felt **inferior and lateral to the pubic tubercle** (inguinal hernias are superior and medial to this point). The boundaries of the femoral canal are **anteriorly** the inguinal ligament; **medially** the lacunar ligament (and pubic bone); **laterally** the femoral vein (and iliopsoas) and **posteriorly** the pectineal ligament and pectineus. The canal contains fat and Cloquet's node. ***Treatment:*** Repair is recommended. (*Herniotomy* is ligation and excision of the sac, *Herniorrhaphy* is repair of the hernial defect).

Paraumbilical hernias occur just above or below the umbilicus. Risk factors are obesity and ascites. Omentum or bowel herniates through the defect. Surgery involves repair of the rectus sheath (Mayo repair). Also see BOX.

Epigastric hernias pass through *linea alba* above the umbilicus.

Incisional hernias follow breakdown of muscle closure after surgery (seen in 11-20%). If obese, repair is not easy. A randomized trial favoured mesh over suture techniques.[101]

Spigelian hernias occur through the *linea semilunaris* at the lateral edge of the rectus sheath, below and lateral to the umbilicus.

Lumbar hernias occur through 1 of the 2 lumbar triangles.

Richter's hernias involve bowel wall only—not the whole lumen.

Maydl's hernias involve a herniating 'double loop' of bowel. The strangulated portion may reside as a single loop **inside** the abdominal cavity.

Littre's hernias are hernial sacs containing strangulated Meckel's diverticulum.

Obturator hernias occur through the obturator canal. Typically there is pain along the medial side of the thigh in a thin woman.

Sciatic hernias pass through the lesser sciatic foramen (a way through various pelvic ligaments). GI obstruction + a gluteal mass suggests this rare possibility.[102]

Sliding hernias contain a partially extraperitoneal structure (eg caecum on the right, sigmoid colon on the left). The sac does not completely surround the contents.

Other examples of hernias:
- Of the nucleus pulposus into the spinal canal (slipped disc).
- Of the uncus and hippocampal gyrus through the tentorium (tentorial hernia) in space-occupying lesions.
- Of brainstem and cerebellum through the foramen magnum (Arnold-Chiari, p708).
- Of the stomach through the diaphragm (hiatus hernia, p245).
- Of the terminal (intravesical) portion of the ureter into the bladder. This is a *ureterocele* (*kēlē* is Greek for hernia), and results from stenosis of the ureteral meatus. *Causes:* congenital, or rarely from schistosomiasis or phaeochromocytoma.

Some examples of hernias

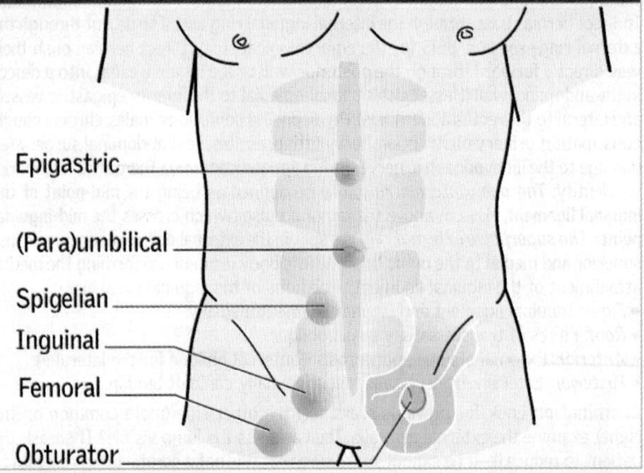

Abdominal wall defects in children

(see *OHCS*, p130)

During embryonic development, the testis is led down from its original position on the posterior abdominal wall into the scrotum by the gubernaculum. If the connection between the peritoneal cavity and the tunica vaginalis fails to close behind the testis, then there is a ***patent processus vaginalis***. It is through this that an indirect inguinal hernia occurs. About 4% of all male infants have an indirect inguinal hernia (prematurity is a risk factor), whereas it is very uncommon in female infants and, if found, should prompt thoughts of testicular feminisation. If the patent *processus vaginalis* contains peritoneal fluid only, then it is a ***communicating hydrocele***. Repair is the same for both, involving high ligation and division of the protruding peritoneal sac. Reinforcement of the posterior wall (eg with a mesh) is not needed as the internal ring has not been chronically dilated.

True umbilical hernias (3% of live births) are a result of a persistent defect in the transversalis fascia—the umbilical ring, through which the umbilical vessels passed to reach the foetus (more common in Afro-Caribbeans, trisomy 21 and congenital hypothyroidism)—whereas ***paraumbilical hernias*** are found in adults in a canal bordered by the umbilical fascia posteriorly, the linea alba anteriorly and the rectus sheath laterally. True umbilical hernias can recur in adulthood, eg in pregnancy (3rd trimester) or gross ascites (**fig 2**, p261). Surgical repair is rarely needed in children (3 in 1000) as most resolve by the age of 3.

Protrusion of the abdominal contents through a defect in the anterior abdominal wall to the right of the umbilicus is seen in ***gastroschisis***, with the protruding bowel covered by a thin 'peel'. Prompt surgical repair is performed after fluid resuscitation.[103] Concomitant congenital abnormalities are rare.

Exomphalos (also called ***omphalocele***),[1] however, is associated with other congenital abnormalities, such as anencephaly, cardiac defects, hydrocephalus and spina bifida. In this condition the abdominal contents are found outside the abdomen, covered in a three-layer membrane consisting of peritoneum, Wharton's jelly and amnion. Surgical repair is less urgent than in gastroschisis because the bowel is protected by these membranes. The challenge of surgery is to fit the contents back into the relatively small abdominal cavity without compromising venous return and lung ventilation. ***Meckel's diverticulum:*** p720.

1 The *omphalos* is the centre-stone at the Temple of Apollo in Delphi, centre of the ancient world—hence its umbilical association. Here Apollo persuaded Pan (the god of wild places, music, and syrinxes, p520) to reveal the art of prophesy, without which we would be without our most mysterious tool: *prognosis*.

Indirect hernias pass through the internal inguinal ring and, if large, out through the external ring—see BOX, p615 for the embryological story. Direct hernias push their way directly forward through the posterior wall of the inguinal canal, into a defect in the abdominal wall (Hesselbach's triangle; medial to the inferior epigastric vessels and lateral to the rectus abdominus). Predisposing conditions: males, chronic cough, constipation, urinary obstruction, heavy lifting, ascites, past abdominal surgery (eg damage to the iliohypogastric nerve during appendicectomy). There are 2 landmarks to identify: ***The deep/internal ring*** may be defined as being the **mid-point of the inguinal ligament**, ~1½ cm above the femoral pulse (which crosses the **mid-inguinal point**). ***The superficial/external ring*** is a split in the external oblique aponeurosis just superior and medial to the pubic tubercle (the bony prominence forming the medial attachment of the inguinal ligament). Relations of the inguinal canal are:

- *Floor:* Inguinal ligament and lacunar ligament medially.
- *Roof:* Fibres of transversalis, internal oblique.
- *Anterior:* External oblique aponeurosis + internal oblique for the lateral ⅓.
- *Posterior:* Laterally, transversalis fascia; medially, conjoint tendon.

Examination Look for previous scars; feel the other side (more common on the right); examine the external genitalia. Then ask: • Is the lump visible? If so, ask the patient to reduce it—if he cannot, make sure that it is not a scrotal lump. Ask him to cough. Appears **above and medial to the pubic tubercle**. • If no lump is visible, feel for a cough impulse. • Repeat the examination with the patient standing. ***Distinguishing direct from indirect hernias:*** This is loved by examiners but is of little clinical use—not least because repair is the same for both (see below). The best way is to reduce the hernia and occlude the deep/internal ring with two fingers. Ask the patient to cough or stand—if the hernia is restrained, it is indirect; if not, it is direct. (The 'gold standard' for determining whether an inguinal hernia is direct or indirect is at surgery with reference to the inferior epigastric vessels.)

Indirect hernias:	*Direct hernias:*	*Femoral hernias:*
• Common (80%) • Can strangulate	• Less common (20%) • Reduce easily • Rarely strangulate	• More frequent in females • Frequently irreducible • Frequently strangulate

Irreducible hernias You may be called because a long-standing hernia is now irreducible and painful. It is always worth trying to reduce these yourself to prevent strangulation and necrosis (demanding prompt laparotomy). Learn how to do this from an expert, ie one of your patients who has been reducing his hernia for years. Then you will know how to act correctly when the incipient emergency presents. Notice that such patients use the flat of the hand, directing the hernia from below, up towards the contralateral shoulder. Sometimes, as the hernia obstructs, reduction requires perseverance, which may be rewarded by a gurgle from the retreating bowel and a kiss from the attending spouse who had thought that surgery was inevitable.

Repairs Advise to diet (if over-weight) and stop smoking pre-op. Warn that hernias may recur. Mesh techniques (eg Lichtenstein repair) have replaced methods such as the 'Shouldice' repair, with its multilayered suture involving both anterior and posterior walls of the inguinal canal. In mesh repairs, a polypropylene mesh reinforces the posterior wall. Recurrence rate is less than with other methods (eg <2% *vs* 10%). (CI: strangulated hernias, contamination with pus/bowel contents). Local anaesthetic techniques and day-case 'ambulatory' surgery may halve the price of surgery. This is important because this is one of the most common operations (>100,000 per year in the UK). ***Laparoscopic repair*** is also possible, and gives similar recurrence rates.[104] Benefits include less post-op. pain, an earlier return to work and identification of undiagnosed contralateral hernias, though the set-up may cost more than conventional surgery (p594).

Return to work: We used to advise 4 weeks' rest and convalescence over 10 weeks, but with new mesh (or laparoscopic) repairs, if comfortable, return to manual work (& driving) after ≤2 weeks is OK; explain this pre-operatively.

The anatomy of the inguinal canal

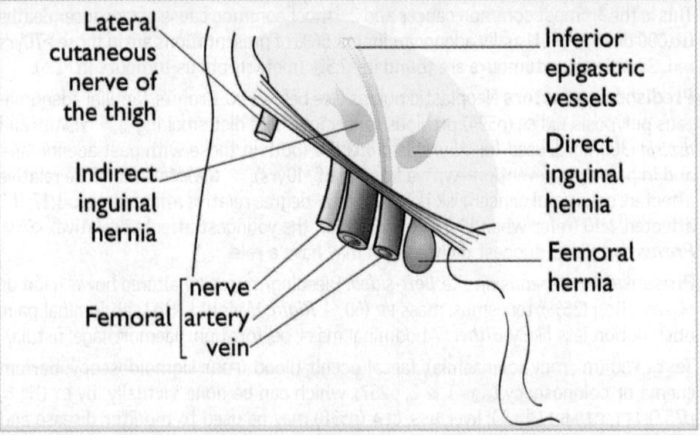

Inguinal hernia mesh repair

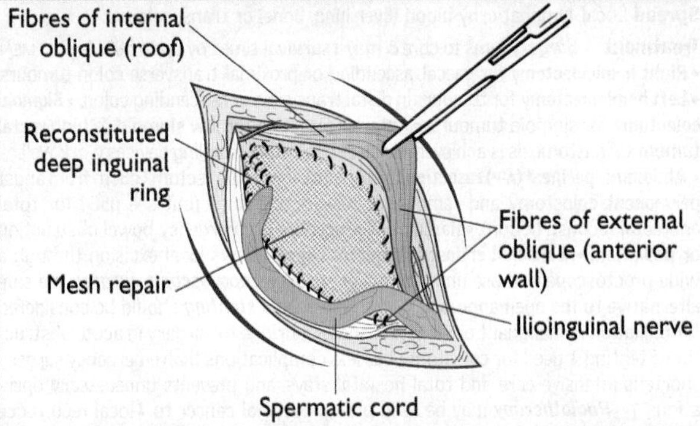

After RCSI website.

The contents of the inguinal canal in the male

- The external spermatic fascia (from external oblique), cremasteric fascia (from internal oblique and transverses abdominus) and internal spermatic fascia (from transversalis fascia) covering the cord
- The spermatic cord:
  - Vas deferens, obliterated processus vaginalis, and lymphatics
  - Arteries to the vas, cremaster, and testis
  - The pampiniform plexus and the venous equivalent of the above
  - The genital branch of the genitofemoral nerve and sympathetic nerves
- The ilioinguinal nerve, which enters the inguinal canal via the anterior wall and runs anteriorly to the cord.

NB: in the female the round ligament of the uterus is in place of the male structures. A hydrocele of the canal of Nuck is the female equivalent of a hydrocele of the cord.

Colorectal carcinoma

This is the 3rd most common cancer and 2nd most common cause of UK cancer deaths (16,000 deaths/yr). Usually adenocarcinoma. 56% of presentations are in those >70yrs old. Synchronous tumours are found in ~2.5% (metachronous tumours in ~1%).

Predisposing factors Neoplastic polyps (see below), UC, Crohn's, familial adenomatous polyposis, HNPCC (p524), previous cancer, low-fibre diet, smoking.[105] NSAIDs and *aspirin* (300mg/d, used for ≥5yrs) is ***protective*** (both in those with past adenomas—and in primary prevention—with a latency of ~10yrs).[106] *Genetics:* No close relative affected: colorectal cancer risk is 1:50. One 1st degree relative affected: risk=1:17; if 2 affected, 1:10 (refer when 10yrs younger than the youngest affected relative). ♂=♀. *Prevention:* Trials suggest daily aspirin may have a role.[107] [108]

Presentation depends on site: ***Left-sided:*** Bleeding/mucus PR; altered bowel habit or obstruction (25%); tenesmus; mass PR (60%). ***Right:*** Weight↓; Hb↓; abdominal pain; obstruction less likely. ***Either:*** Abdominal mass; perforation; haemorrhage; fistula.

Tests FBC (microcytic anaemia); faecal occult blood (FOB); sigmoidoscopy; barium enema or colonoscopy (**figs 1 & 2**, p257), which can be done 'virtually' by CT (**fig 5**, p757); LFT, CT/MRI (**fig 1**); liver USS. CEA (p538) may be used to monitor disease and effectiveness of treatment. If polyposis in family, refer for DNA test once >15yrs old. DNA test may also help determine who will benefit from chemotherapy—see p524.

Spread Local, lymphatic, by blood (liver, lung, bone) or transcoelomic.

Treatment[109] *Surgery* aims to cure & may ↑survival times by up to 50% (eg in TME[1]). • **Right hemicolectomy** for caecal, ascending or proximal transverse colon tumours. • **Left hemicolectomy** for tumours in distal transverse or descending colon. • **Sigmoid colectomy** for sigmoid tumours. • **Anterior resection** for low sigmoid or high rectal tumours. Anastomosis is achieved at the 1st operation—stapling devices work well.[110] • **Abdomino-perineal (A-P) resection** for tumours low in the rectum (≤8cm from anus): permanent colostomy and removal of rectum and anus (but see p584 for total anorectal reconstruction). • **Hartmann's procedure** in emergency bowel obstruction or palliation. • **Transanal endoscopic microsurgery** allows local excision through a wide proctoscope in those unfit for major surgery. ***Laparoscopic surgery*** is a safe alternative to the open approach.[111] [112] ***Endoscopic stenting*** should be considered for palliation in malignant obstruction and as a bridge to surgery in acute obstruction. Stenting ↓ need for colostomy, has less complications than emergency surgery, shortens intensive care and total hospital stays, and prevents unnecessary operations.[113] ***Radiotherapy*** may be used pre-op in rectal cancer to ↓local recurrence and ↑5yr survival.[114] It may be associated with a higher rate of post-operative complication eg DVT, pathological fractures, fistulization.[115] Pre-op radiotherapy ± *5-FU* is also used to downstage initially unresectable rectal tumours. Post-op radiotherapy is only used in patients with rectal tumours at high risk of local recurrence. ***Chemotherapy*** Good evidence adjuvant *5-FU* ±other agents (eg ***folinic acid, levamisole***) reduce Dukes' C mortality ~25%.[116] Role of chemotherapy in Dukes' B under investigation. Chemotherapy also used in palliation of metastatic disease; newer agents (eg ***irinotecan, oxaliplatin***) may give more options. Surgery with liver resection may be curative if single-lobe hepatic metastases and no extrahepatic spread.[117]

Prognosis 60% amenable to radical surgery, 75% of these will be alive at 7yrs (or dead from another cause). Post-op anastomotic leakage shown to ↓survival rates in otherwise potentially curative surgery.[118] Imaging suspected leaks (↑T°, abdominal pain, peritonism) is with water-soluble contrast enema or CT (+ rectal contrast).

Polyps are lumps that appear above the mucosa. **1** ***Inflammatory:*** Ulcerative colitis, Crohn's, lymphoid hyperplasia. **2** ***Hamartomatous:*** Juvenile polyps, Peutz-Jeghers syndrome (p722). **3** ***Neoplastic:*** Tubular or villous adenomas: malignant potential, esp. if >2cm. ***Symptoms:*** Passage of blood/mucus PR. Should be biopsied and removed if show malignant change. Most can be reached by flexible colonoscope and diathermy can avoid morbidity of colectomy. Check resection margins are clear of tumour.

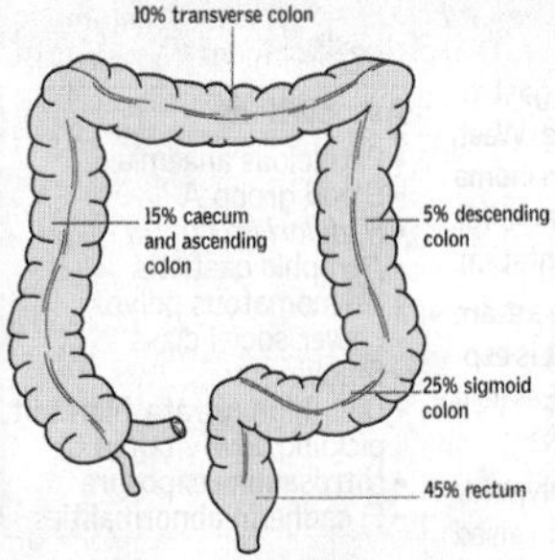

Fig 1. Locations of colorectal carcinomas. These are averages: black females tend to have more proximal neoplasms. White men tend to have more distal neoplasms.

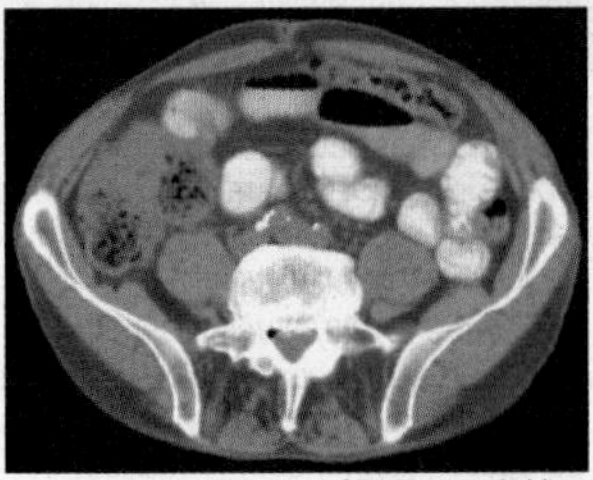

Courtesy of Dr Stephen Golding.

Fig 2. Axial CT of the abdomen with oral contrast medium showing thickening of the wall of the caecum (lying in the right iliac fossa) from adenocarcinoma.

Dukes' classification for the staging of colorectal cancer

(see also TNM staging p621)

Stage	Description	Treated 5yr survival rate (%)
A	Confined to beneath muscularis mucosae	~90
B	Extension through muscularis mucosae	~65
C	Involvement of regional lymph nodes	~30
D	Distant metastases	<10

Examples of scenarios prompting urgent referral for surgeon's assessment within 2 weeks

- Rectal bleeding and a persistent change in bowel habit for >6wks.
- Persistent rectal bleeding without anal symptoms in those over 45yrs, with no obvious external evidence of benign anal disease.
- Iron-deficiency anaemia without an obvious cause and Hb <10g/dL.
- A palpable abdominal or rectal mass.
- Recent onset of looser stools and/or ↑frequency of defecation, persisting for >6wks. See p537 for review of the logic behind '2-week rules'.

Universal adult screening for colorectal cancer

►A number of screening methods have been proposed.[119]

- *FOB* screening every 2yrs with home tests reduces mortality by 15-33%, but false +ve rates are high (up to 10%) and there are problems with acceptability.
- *Sigmoidoscopy* can be used to screen for left-sided lesions with 90% sensitivity and 99% specificity within the region of the scope. One recent RCT reported good tolerability and a pick-up rate of any cancer or adenoma of up to 8% in women and up to 12% in men.[120] Limitations include acceptability, cost, and not picking up right-sided lesions.
- *Colonoscopy* examines the **entire** colon and is the most accurate test. It is already used in those at ↑risk of colorectal cancer due to personal or family history, adenoma, or IBD. Perforation rate is higher than sigmoidoscopy (0.2% *vs* 0.01%) and limitations include cost, need for sedation, acceptability to patients, and the availability of trained endoscopists.

The **NHS Bowel Cancer Screening Programme** introduced in the UK in July 2006 offers screening every 2 years to all men and women aged 60-69 (may be requested by those older) using FOB testing. Those with abnormal results are offered an appointment with a specialist nurse and further investigation (usually a colonoscopy).[121]

1 TME = total mesorectal excision. It entails sharp dissection to yield an intact mesorectal envelope.

Carcinoma of the stomach

Associations
• Pernicious anaemia • Blood group A • *H. pylori* (p242) • Atrophic gastritis • Adenomatous polyps • Lower social class • Smoking • Diet (high nitrate, high salt, pickling, low vitamin C) • Nitrosamine exposure • E. cadherin abnormalities

Incidence of adenocarcinoma at the gastro-oesophageal junction is increasing in the West, though incidence of distal & body gastric carcinoma has fallen sharply. It remains a tumour notable for its gloomy prognosis and non-specific presentation.

Incidence 23/100,000/yr in the UK, but there are unexplained wide geographical variations; it is especially common in Japan, as well as Eastern Europe, China, and South America.. ♂:♀ ≈2:1

Pathology Borrmann classification: i) Polypoid/fungating ii) Excavating iii) Ulcerating and raised iv) Linitis plastica (leather bottle-like uniform thickening of stomach wall). Some are confined to mucosa and submucosa—'early' gastric carcinoma.

Presentation *Symptoms:* Often non-specific. Dyspepsia (p59; for >1 month & age ≥50yrs demands investigation), weight ↓, vomiting, dysphagia, anaemia. *Signs* suggesting incurable disease: epigastric mass, hepatomegaly; jaundice, ascites (p606); large left supraclavicular (Virchow's) node (=Troisier's sign); acanthosis nigricans (p564). *Spread* is local, lymphatic, blood-borne, and transcoelomic eg to ovaries (Krukenberg tumour).

Tests Gastroscopy + multiple ulcer edge biopsies. ►*Aim to biopsy all gastric ulcers as even malignant ulcers may appear to heal on drug treatment.* Endoscopic ultrasound (EUS) and CT/MRI help staging (**fig 1**). Staging laparoscopy is recommended for locally advanced tumours if metastases are not detected on other investigations.[122]

Treatment See p624 for a description of surgical resections. For tumours in the distal ⅔, a partial gastrectomy may suffice, but, if more proximal, total gastrectomy may be needed. Combination chemotherapy (eg **epirubicin**, **cisplatin** & **5-fluorouracil**) appears to increase survival in advanced disease.[123] Endoscopic mucosal resection is used for early tumours confined to the mucosa.[124] Palliation is often needed for obstruction, pain, or haemorrhage. In metastatic disease, chemotherapy increases quality of life and survival. Judicious use of surgery and radiotherapy may also help.

5yr survival <10% overall, but nearly 20% for patients undergoing radical surgery. The prognosis is much better for 'early' gastric carcinoma.

Carcinoma of the oesophagus

Incidence Australia <5/100,000/yr; UK <9; Brittany >50; Iran >100. *Risk factors:* Diet, alcohol excess, smoking, achalasia, Plummer-Vinson syndrome (p240), obesity, diet low in vitamin A & C, nitrosamine exposure, reflux oesophagitis ± Barrett's oesophagus (p708; 44-fold ↑risk of adenocarcinoma if severe reflux for >10 years). ♂:♀ ≈5:1

Site 20% occur in the upper part, 50% in the middle, and 30% in the lower part. They may be squamous cell or adenocarcinomas (incidence rising).

The patient Dysphagia; weight↓; retrosternal chest pain; lymphadenopathy (rare). *Signs from upper from the upper third of the oesophagus:* Hoarseness; cough (may be paroxysmal if aspiration pneumonia). **ΔΔ**: See **Dysphagia**, p240.

Tests Barium swallow, CXR, oesophagoscopy with biopsy/brushings/EUS, CT/MRI. Staging laparoscopy if significant infra-diaphragmatic component. *Staging:* TABLE.

Treatment Survival rates are poor with or without treatment. If localized T1/T2 disease, radical curative oesophagectomy may be tried. Transhiatal oesophagectomy causes less morbidity than extended transthoracic resection, though the latter may be associated with ↑long-term survival. Pre-op chemotherapy (*cisplatin* + *5-FU*) improves survival but causes some morbidity.[125] Surgery alone may be preferable.[126]

If surgery is **not** indicated, then chemo-radiotherapy may be better than radiotherapy alone.[127] Palliation in advanced disease aims to restore swallowing with chemo/radiotherapy, stenting, and laser use.

Multi-disciplinary cancer meetings

These essential meetings aim to improve quality of life for cancer sufferers by standardising and optimising screening, early detection and treatment of cancer.[128] At any meeting you should be able to spot:

- Paired surgeons and physicians (eg upper GI surgeon and gastroenterologist).
- Radiologists
- Pathologists
- Oncologists
- Specialist care nurses
- Meeting administrators

This expert forum aims to provide the most up-to-date and relevant options for treatment individualised for each patient. However, despite everyone's best efforts, there can still remain an inherent uncertainty as to what is *exactly* the best treatment for the patient—something which in the end may only be known to the patient themself when given the options.

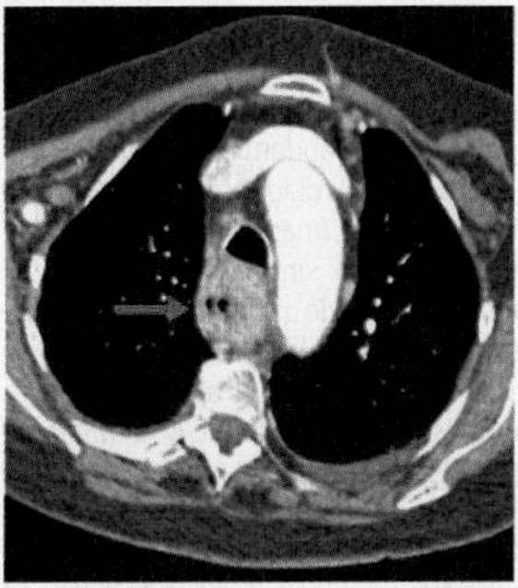

Fig 1. Axial CT of the chest after IV contrast medium showing concentric thickening of the oesophagus (arrow); the diagnosis here is oesophageal carcinoma. Loss of the fatty plane around the oesophagus suggests local invasion. Anterior to the oesophagus is the trachea and next to it is the arch of the aorta.

Image courtesy of Dr. Stephen Golding

TNM staging in oesophageal cancer

Spread of oesophageal cancer is direct, by submucosal infiltration and local spread—or to nodes, or, later, via the blood.

T_{is}	Carcinoma *in situ*	**Nx**	Nodes cannot be assessed
T1	Invading lamina propria/submucosa	**N0**	No node spread
T2	Invading muscularis propria	**N1**	Regional node metastases
T3	Invading adventitia	**M0**	No distant spread
T4	Invasion of adjacent structures	**M1**	Distant metastasis

Oesophageal rupture

Causes: • *Iatrogenic* eg endoscopy/biopsy/dilatation (accounts for 85-90% of perforations) • *Trauma* eg penetrating injury/ingestion of foreign body • *Carcinoma* • *Boerhaave syndrome* is rupture due to violent emesis • *Corrosive ingestion* **Clinical features:** odynophagia, tachypnoea, dyspnoea, fever, shock, surgical emphysema (a crackling sensation felt on palpating the skin over the chest or neck caused by air tracking from the lungs; ΔΔ: pneumothorax.)

℞ Iatrogenic perforations are less prone to mediastinitis and sepsis and may be managed conservatively with NG tube, PPI and antibiotics. Others require resuscitation, PPI, antibiotics, antifungals and surgery (debridement of mediastinum and placement of T-tube for drainage and formation of a controlled oesophago-cutaneous fistula).

►AF with abdominal pain should always prompt thoughts of mesenteric ischaemia.

Acute mesenteric ischaemia[129] almost always involves the small bowel and may follow superior mesenteric artery (SMA) thrombosis or embolism, mesenteric vein thrombosis, or non-occlusive disease (see MINIBOX). Arterial thrombosis is becoming the commonest cause of acute ischaemia as embolism becomes rarer. Venous thrombosis is more common in younger patients with hypercoagulable states and tends to affect smaller lengths of bowel. Non-occlusive ischaemia occurs in low-flow states and usually reflects poor cardiac output, though there may be other factors such as recent cardiac surgery or renal failure.[130] Presentation is **a classical clinical triad:** ►Acute severe abdominal pain; no abdominal signs; rapid hypovolaemia → shock. Pain tends to be constant and central, or around the right iliac fossa. The degree of illness is often far out of proportion with clinical signs.

Acute ischaemia

• Arterial
  • Thrombotic(35%)
  • Embolic(35%)
• Non-occlusive(20%)
• Venous(5%)
• Other
  • Trauma
  • Vasculitis (p558)
  • Radiotherapy
  • Strangulation eg volvulus or hernia

Chronic ischaemia
Usually a combination of a low-flow state with atheroma. Classified as either small or large bowel.

- *Tests:* There may be Hb↑ (due to plasma loss), WCC↑, modestly raised plasma amylase, and a persistent metabolic acidosis. Early on the abdominal x-ray shows a 'gasless' abdomen. Arteriography (**fig 1**) helps but many diagnoses are only made on finding a nasty necrotic bowel at laparotomy. CT/MR (magnetic resonance) angiography may provide a non-invasive alternative to simple arteriography.[131] Measurement of mucosal oxygen tension and MR oximetric measurements of superior mesenteric vein flow are emerging as diagnostic tools.[132]
- *Treatment:* The main life-threatening complications secondary to acute mesenteric ischaemia are **1** septic peritonitis and **2** progression of a systemic inflammatory response syndrome (SIRS) into a multi-organ dysfunction syndrome (MODS), mediated by bacterial translocation across the dying gut wall. Resuscitation with fluid, antibiotics (***gentamicin*** + ***metronidazole***, p381) and, usually, ***heparin*** are required. If arteriography is done, thrombolytics may be infused locally via the catheter. At surgery dead bowel must be removed. Revascularization may be attempted on potentially viable bowel but it is a difficult process and often needs a 2nd laparotomy.
- *Prognosis:* Poor for arterial thrombosis and non-occlusive disease (<40% survive), though not so bad for venous and embolic ischaemia.[133]

Chronic small bowel ischaemia This presents quite a different picture to acute ischaemia, with severe, colicky post-prandial abdominal pain ('gut claudication') with PR bleeding ± ↓weight (food hurts) and malabsorption. It is difficult to diagnose but, following angiography, surgery may be helpful. Angioplasty is an appropriate treatment if the bowel is viable.

Chronic colonic ischaemia This usually follows low flow in the inferior mesenteric artery (IMA) territory. *Presentation:* Lower left-sided abdominal pain and bloody diarrhoea. There may be pyrexia, tachycardia, PR bleeding, and a leucocytosis. Usually this 'ischaemic colitis' resolves, but it may progress to gangrenous ischaemic colitis with the development of peritonitis and hypovolaemic shock. *Tests:* Barium enema may show 'thumb-printing' indentation of the barium due to submucosal swelling. Doppler USS may be useful in detection of coeliac artery and SMA stenoses.[134] MR angiography is being used increasingly.[135] *Treatment:* This is usually conservative with fluid replacement and antibiotics. Most recover but strictures are common. Percutaneous transluminal angioplasty and endovascular stent insertion are alternatives to revascularization surgery that show good results with lower mortality.[136] Gangrenous ischaemic colitis requires prompt resuscitation followed by resection of the affected bowel and stoma formation.

The arterial supply to the colon

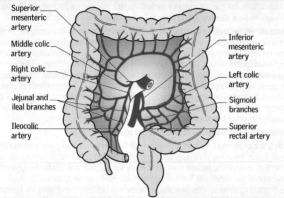

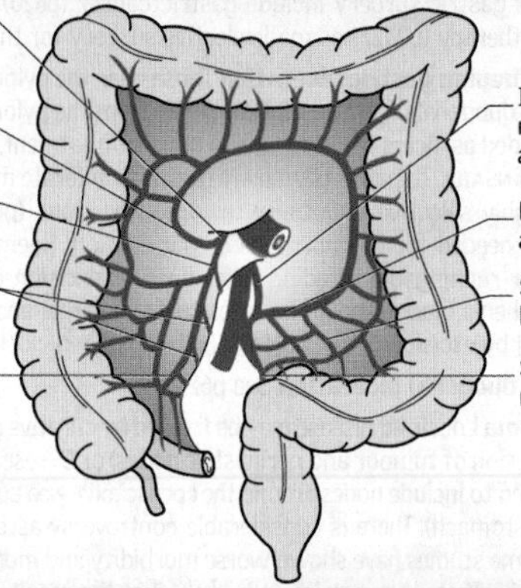

There are two **potential watershed areas** in the arterial supply of the colon. The first is at the splenic flexure where the superior and inferior mesenteric circulations meet as the 'Marginal artery of Drummond'—it has also been called Griffith's point. The significance of good blood flow at this point to ensure adequate colonic supply after surgical ligation of the IMA has long been a point of debate.[137] The 2nd contentious watershed area is at the origin of the superior rectal artery—also known as Sudeck's point (**fig 1**). When ligated, flow to the rectum is maintained by the sigmoidal branches that arise from the left colic artery.[138] Remember that the arterial supply to the gut does have a large number of anatomical variations.

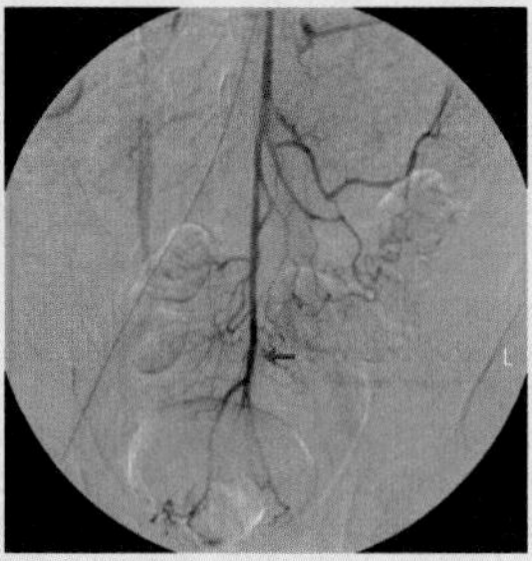

Fig 1. Digital subtraction angiogram (DSA) of the inferior mesenteric artery and the superior rectal artery (arrow).
Image courtesy of Norwich Radiology Department

►Indications for gastric surgery include gastric cancer (p620) and peptic ulcers, though medical therapy (p242) has made elective surgery for the latter rare.

Operations for benign gastric ulceration Those near the pylorus may be considered similarly to duodenal ulceration (p626). Away from the pylorus, elective operation is rarely needed as ulcers respond well to medical treatment, stopping smoking, and avoidance of NSAIDs. In patients who are unable to tolerate medical treatment, a laparoscopic highly selective vagotomy (HSV) can be done (p626). ►►*Emergency surgery* may be needed for haemorrhage or perforation. Haemorrhage is usually treated by under-running the bleeding ulcer base or excision of the ulcer. If the former is done, then a biopsy should be taken to exclude malignancy. Perforation is usually managed by excision of the hole for histology, then closure.

Operations for duodenal ulceration See p626.

Gastric carcinoma Localized disease may be treated by curative gastrectomy, either D_1 resection (excision of tumour and perigastric nodes) or D_2 resection (basically a D_1 resection extended to include nodes around the coeliac axis—see BOX for the lymphatic drainage of the stomach). There is considerable controversy as to which should be performed, as some studies have shown worse morbidity and mortality for D_2 resections performed in Western countries. It is likely that the results reflect the lack of dedicated specialists such as those in Japan, where gastric carcinoma is particularly common. D_2 resections should therefore only be performed in specialist centres.[139]

Surgery *Billroth I:* Partial gastrectomy with simple re-anastomosis (rejoining). *Billroth II (=Polya) gastrectomy* (**fig 1**) Partial gastrectomy. The duodenal stump is oversewn (leaving a blind loop), and anastomosis is achieved by a longitudinal incision further down (into the proximal jejunum). *Roux-en-Y* (**fig 2**) is replacing the Billroth operations. Following total or subtotal gastrectomy, the proximal duodenal stump is oversewn, the proximal jejunum is divided from the distal duodenum and connects with the oesophagus (or proximal stomach after subtotal gastrectomy) whilst the distal duodenum is connected to distal jejunum.

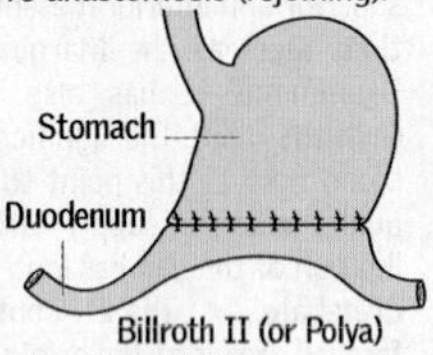

Fig 1 Billroth II.

Physical complications of gastrectomy and peptic ulcer surgery.

- *Recurrent ulceration:* Symptoms are similar to those experienced pre-operatively but complications are more common and response to medical treatment is poor. Further surgery is difficult.
- *Abdominal fullness:* Feeling of early satiety (± discomfort and distension) improving with time. Advise to take small, frequent meals.
- *Bilious vomiting:* This is difficult to treat—but often improves with time.
- *Diarrhoea:* May be disabling after vagotomy. *Codeine phosphate* may help.
- *Gastric tumour:* A rare complication of any surgery which ↓acid production.
- *Amylase↑:* If with abdominal pain, this may indicate afferent loop obstruction after Billroth II surgery and requires emergency surgery.[140]

Metabolic complications

- *Dumping syndrome:*[141] Fainting and sweating after eating due to food of high osmotic potential being dumped in the jejunum, causing oligaemia from rapid fluid shifts. 'Late dumping' is due to rebound hypoglycaemia and occurs 1-3h after meals. Both tend to improve with time but may be helped by eating less sugar, and more guar and pectin (slows glucose absorption). *Acarbose* (p200) may also help to reduce the early hyperglycaemic stimulus to insulin secretion.[142]
- *Weight loss:* Often due to poor calorie intake.
- *Bacterial overgrowth ± malabsorption* (blind loop syndrome) may occur.
- *Anaemia:* Usually from lack of iron, hypochlorhydria and stomach resection. B_{12} levels are frequently low but megaloblastic anaemia is rare.
- *Osteomalacia:* There may be pseudofractures which look like metastases.

Complications of peptic ulcer surgery

	Partial gastrectomy	Vagotomy & pyloroplasty	Highly selective vagotomy
Recurrence	2%	7%	>7%
Dumping	20%	14%	6%
Diarrhoea	1%	4%	<1%
Metabolic	++++	++	0

(These values are approximate and depend on the skill of the surgeon.)

The Roux-en-Y bypass/reconstruction

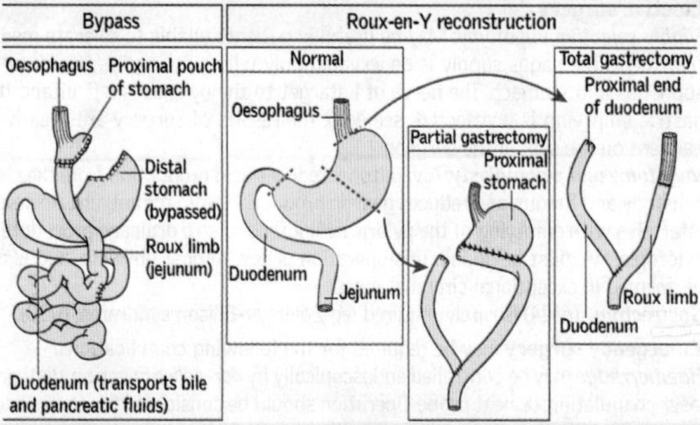

Lymphatic drainage of the stomach

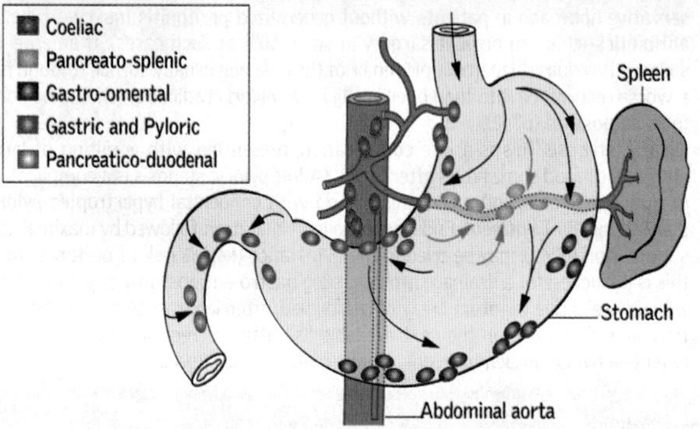

After RCSI website.

Theodor Billroth was a surgeon of German-Austrian origin, whose name lives on as a set of operations on the stomach. He was a pioneer of abdominal surgery and the use of aseptic techniques, performing the first Billroth I procedure in 1881 for the resection of a pyloric gastric carcinoma. Among the many of his remarkable achievements is included the first laryngectomy. He was also a talented musician (a close friend of Brahms) and a dedicated educator with something of a realist's view of the world: *The pleasure of a physician is little, the gratitude of patients is rare, and even rarer is material reward, but these things will never deter the student who feels the call within him.* Theodor Billroth (1829–94)[143] [144]

Operations for peptic ulcers

Peptic ulcers usually present as epigastric pain and dyspepsia (p242). There is no reliable method of distinguishing clinically between gastric and duodenal ulcers. Although management of both is usually medical in the 1st instance (eg with *H. pylori* eradication, p242), surgery still has a role.

Surgery is usually only required for complications such as ***haemorrhage, perforation***, and ***pyloric stenosis***, though may be considered for the few patients who are not responsive to or tolerant of medical therapy.

Several types of operation have been tried but, as whenever considering an operation, one must consider efficacy, side effects, and mortality.

1 Elective surgery (fig 1)

- *Highly selective vagotomy:* May be useful in patients unable to tolerate medical treatment. The vagus supply is denervated only where it supplies the lower oesophagus and stomach. The nerve of Latarget to the pylorus is left intact; thus, gastric emptying is unaffected (see BOX). The results of surgery are greatly dependent on the skill of the surgeon.
- *Vagotomy and pyloroplasty:* A vagotomy reduces acid production from the stomach body and fundus, and reduces gastrin production from the antrum. However, it interferes with emptying of the pyloric sphincter and so a drainage procedure (eg pyloroplasty) must be added. This operation is now almost obsolete, and is only performed in exceptional circumstances.
- *Gastrectomy* (p624) is rarely required (eg Zollinger-Ellison syndrome, p730).

2 Emergency surgery may be required for the following complications:

- *Haemorrhage* may be controlled endoscopically by ***adrenaline*** injection, diathermy, laser coagulation, or heat probe. Operation should be considered for severe haemorrhage or rebleeding, especially in the elderly—see p254 for indications. At surgery, the bleeding ulcer base is underrun or oversewn.
- *Perforation* Most patients undergo surgery, though some advocate an initial conservative approach in patients without generalized peritonitis (NBM, NG tube, IV antibiotics—this can prevent surgery in up to 50% of such cases). If emergency surgery is required, laparoscopic repair of the hole will usually suffice (though has a worse recurrence rate than open repair).[145] *H. pylori* eradication should be commenced post-op (p242).
- *Pyloric stenosis* This is a late complication, presenting with vomiting of large amounts of food some hours after meals. (Adult pyloric stenosis is a complication of duodenal ulcers, and has nothing to do with congenital hypertrophic pyloric stenosis, p628.) *Treatment:* Endoscopic balloon dilatation, followed by maximal acid suppression (p242), may be tried in the 1st instance (**NB:** 5% risk of perforation). If this is unsuccessful, a drainage procedure (eg gastro-enterostomy or pyloroplasty) ± highly selective vagotomy may be performed, often laparoscopically. The operation should be done on the next available list, after correction of the metabolic defect—a hypochloraemic, hypokalaemic metabolic alkalosis.

Fundoplication for gastro-oesophageal reflux

The goal 1 Repair the defect in the diaphragm **2** Prevent reflux.

The procedure Involves wrapping the gastric fundus around the lower oesophagus, closing the hiatus, and securing the wrap in the abdomen—see **fig 2**. There are various types of procedure eg Nissen (360° wrap), Toupet (270° posterior wrap), Watson (anterior hemifundoplication).

Access Usually laparoscopic, which in specialist centres is at least as effective at controlling reflux as open surgery but with a lower mortality. Wound infections and respiratory complications are also more common in open surgery, though the incidence of dysphagia is similar for the two procedures—but see p594.

Complications 'Gas-bloat syndrome' (inability to belch/vomit) or dysphagia if too tight.

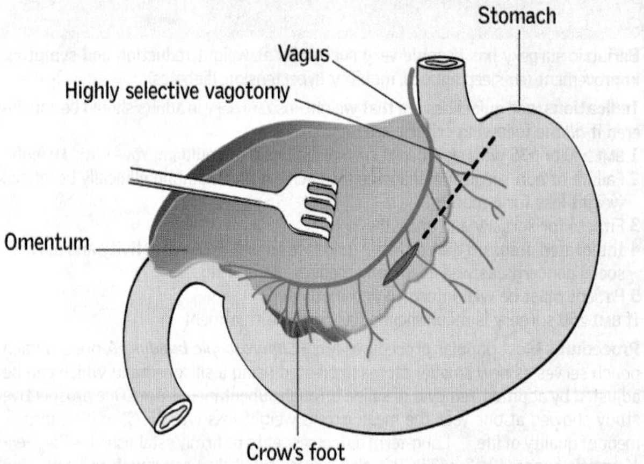

Fig 1. Highly selective vagotomy

After RCSI website.

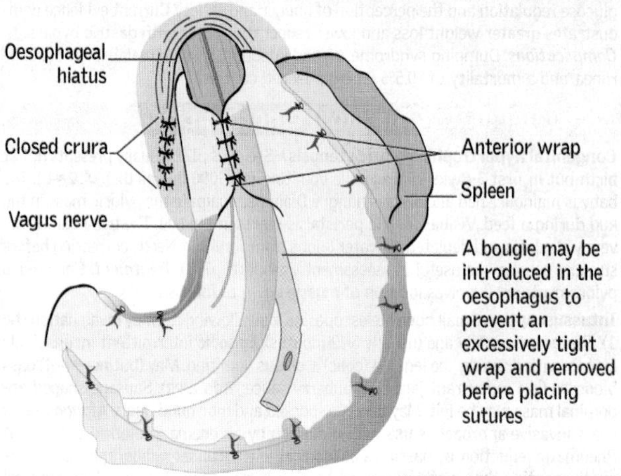

Fig 2. Nissen fundoplication.

After Corine Sandone, MA.

Bariatric surgery

Bariatric surgery has become very successful at weight reduction **and** symptom improvement (eg sleep apnoea, mobility, hypertension, diabetes).[146]

Indications NICE guidelines are that weight-loss surgery in adults should be considered if *all* the following criteria are met:

1 BMI ≥40 or ≥35 with significant co-morbidities that could improve with ↓weight.
2 Failure of non-surgical management to achieve and maintain clinically beneficial weight loss for 6 months.
3 Fitness for surgery and anaesthesia.
4 Integrated program that provides guidance on diet, physical activity, and psychosocial concerns, as well as lifelong medical monitoring.
5 Patient must be well-informed and motivated.

If BMI ≥50 surgery is recommended as first-line treatment.

Procedures Most popular procedures are: • ***Laparoscopic banding:*** A pre-stomach pouch serves as new smaller stomach created using a silicone band which can be adjusted by addition/removal of saline through subcutaneous port. One prospective study showed at one year the mean **excess** weight loss was 45.7%, with improvement of quality of life.[147] Long-term outcomes yet to be firmly established. • ***Roux-en-Y gastric bypass*** (**fig 2**, p625): This also creates small stomach pouch, but a portion of the jejunum is attached to the pouch to allow food to bypass distal stomach, duodenum, and proximal jejunum. May alter secretion of hormones that influence glucose regulation and the perception of hunger and satiety. Current evidence demonstrates greater weight loss and lower reoperation rates with gastric bypass.[148] *Complications:* Dumping syndrome, wound infection, hernias, malabsorption, diarrhoea, and a mortality of ~0.5% (at experienced centres).

Some paediatric surgical emergencies

Congenital hypertrophic pyloric stenosis ►See *OHCS* p172. Usually presents not at birth but in first 3–8wks as projectile vomiting (4 in1000 live births). ♂:♀≈4:1. The baby is malnourished and always hungry. Diagnosis: palpate the pyloric mass in the RUQ during a feed. Visible gastric peristalsis starts in the LUQ. The baby can be severely alkalotic and depleted of water & ions from vomiting. Needs correcting **before** surgery. USS may be useful in assessment. Pass NGT (p773). *Treatment:* Ramstedt's pyloromyotomy (involves incision of muscle down to mucosa).

Intussusception Small bowel telescopes, as if swallowing itself by invagination (**fig 1**). *Presentation:* Any age (usually 5–12 months). **Episodic** intermittent inconsolable crying, with drawing the legs up (colic) ± bilious vomiting. May (but need not) pass blood PR (like redcurrant jam or cranberry sauce:[149] do a PR). Sausage-shaped abdominal mass may be felt. May become shocked and moribund. *Tests/Management:* Least invasive approach is USS with reduction by air enema (preferred to barium). Pneumatic reduction, by passing a balloon catheter PR under radiographic control, is another option that is effective in up to 80%. If reduction by enema fails, surgical reduction is needed. Prompt treatment may avoid necrosis of the intussuscepting bowel, which if present, will need to be excised at surgery. *Pre-op care:* ►►Resuscitate, crossmatch blood, pass NGT. **NB:** children >4yrs present differently: rectal bleeding less common, more likely to have a long history (>3wks) and some sort of contributing pathology, eg Henoch–Schönlein purpura, cystic fibrosis, Peutz–Jeghers' syndrome or tumours, eg lymphomas—in the latter, obstructive symptoms caused by intussusception are the chief mode of presentation. Recurrence rate: ~5%.

Midgut malrotation During embryonic development, the mid-gut undergoes 270° anticlockwise rotation. If malrotated the gut is prone to undergo volvulus upon its abnormally-pedicled mesentery. Usually presents in neonatal period with dark green bilious vomiting, distension, and rectal bleeding. Can be asymptomatic for years before acute presentation. *Treatment:* ►►Resuscitation, then surgery (involves broadening the mesentery and replacing bowel in a non-rotated position).

Tips on examining the abdomen in children

Examining the abdomen of a child or infant can prove extremely difficult and requires patience, practice and opportunism. So:

- An age-directed approach will help develop your relationship with the child.
- Remember that the parents will be closely involved in what you do.
- Play specialists may be able to provide distraction.
- Examining the abdomen may require an unorthodox approach, eg whilst sitting in mum's lap.
- There is no hope of eliciting any signs whilst the child is crying and tensing their tummy—everyone will be better off if you return when the child has settled down!
- Examining for rebound tenderness in young children is probably of little use for us and definitely uncomfortable for them.
- You should always examine the scrotum and inguinal regions in young boys to exclude the possibility of testicular torsion or a strangulated hernia.
- Performing a PR examination, if required, is best left to a specialist.
- Unless you have a magical way with children, don't be surprised to get the cold shoulder once in a while!

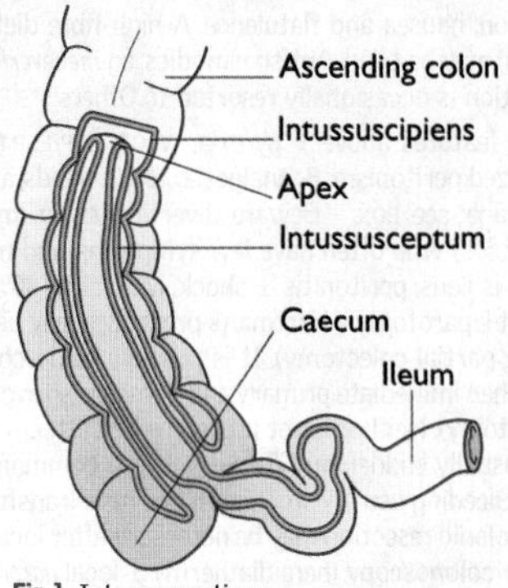

Fig 1. Intussusception.

Adapted with permission from McKee, C. www.yoursurgery.com

Diverticular disease

A GI **diverticulum** is an outpouching of the gut wall, usually at sites of entry of perforating arteries. These are false pulsion diverticula composed of mucosa (true diverticula consist of all layers of parent viscus). **Diverticulosis** means that diverticula are present, and **diverticular disease** implies they are symptomatic. **Diverticulitis** refers to inflammation of a diverticulum. Although diverticula may be congenital or acquired and can occur in any part of the gut, by far the most important type are acquired colonic diverticula, to which this page refers.

Pathology Most occur in the sigmoid colon with 95% of complications at this site, but right-sided and massive single diverticula can occur. Lack of dietary fibre is thought to lead to high intraluminal pressures which force the mucosa to herniate through the muscle layers of the gut at weak points adjacent to penetrating vessels. 30% of Westerners have diverticulosis by 60 years of age.

Diagnosis *PR examination* (may reveal a pelvic abscess, or colorectal cancer, the chief competing diagnosis); ***sigmoidoscopy*, *barium enema*, *colonoscopy*** (**fig 6**, p257); CT may be more useful than ***ultrasound***, and ***plain films*** may only be useful in showing vesical fistulae (air in the bladder).

Complications of diverticulosis There may be altered bowel habit ± left-sided colic relieved by defecation; nausea and flatulence. A high-fibre diet (wholemeal bread, fruit and vegetables) may be tried. Antispasmodics, eg *mebeverine* 135mg/8h PO may help. Surgical resection is occasionally resorted to. Others:

Diverticulitis—with features above + pyrexia, WCC↑, CRP/ESR↑, a tender colon, ± localized or generalized peritonism. ℞: analgesia, NBM, IV fluids, antibiotics, CT-guided percutaneous drainage: see BOX. ►Beware diverticulitis in immunocompromised patients (eg on steroids) who often have few symptoms, and may present late.

- ►►*Perforation* There is ileus, peritonitis ± shock. Mortality: 40%. Manage as for an acute abdomen. At laparotomy a Hartman's procedure may be performed (temporary colostomy + partial colectomy). It is possible to do colonic lavage via the appendix stump, then immediate primary anastomosis (so avoiding repeat surgery to close the colostomy). Neither is yet proven to be better.150
- *Haemorrhage* is usually sudden and painless. It is a common cause of big rectal bleeds. ►See BOX. Bleeding usually stops with bed rest. Transfusion may be needed. Embolization or colonic resection may be necessary after locating bleeding points by angiography or colonoscopy (here diathermy ± local *adrenaline* injections may obviate the need for surgery).
- *Fistulae* Enterocolic, colovaginal, or colovesical (pneumaturia ± intractable UTIs). Treatment is surgical, eg colonic resection.
- *Abscesses* eg with swinging fever, leucocytosis, and localizing signs, eg boggy rectal mass (pelvic abscess—drain rectally). If no localizing signs, remember the aphorism: *pus somewhere, pus nowhere = pus under the diaphragm*. A subphrenic abscess is a horrible way to die, so do an urgent ultrasound. Antibiotics ± ultrasound/CT-guided drainage may be needed.
- *Post-infective strictures* may form in the sigmoid colon.

Angiodysplasia

Angiodysplasia refers to submucosal arteriovenous malformations that typically present as fresh PR bleeding in the elderly. The underlying cause is unknown. *Pathology:* 70-90% of lesions occur in right colon, though angiodysplasia can affect anywhere in the GI tract. *Diagnosis:* PR examination, Ba enema, colonoscopy (**fig 5**, p257) may exclude competing diagnoses; ^{99m}Tc radionuclide-labelled red-cell imaging (p753) is useful in identifying lesions during active bleeding (if >0.1mL/min). Mesenteric angiography is very helpful in diagnosing angiodysplasia (shows early filling at the lesion site, then extravasation), and allows therapeutic embolization during bleeding—it detects bleeding >1mL/min. CT angiography offers a non-invasive alternative. *Treatment options:* Embolization, endoscopic laser electrocoagulation, resection.

Managing diverticulitis [151]

Initial management

- Mild attacks can be treated at home with bowel rest (fluids only) + *co-amoxiclav* (*ciprofloxacin* if allergic) ± *metronidazole* (p378-381).[152]
- If oral fluids cannot be tolerated or pain cannot be controlled, admit to hospital for analgesia, NBM, IV fluids and antibiotics eg *cefuroxime* 1.5g/8h IV with *metronidazole* 500mg/8h IV/PR, until the results of cultures are available. Most settle on this regimen but there may be abscess formation (necessitating drainage—usually CT-guided percutaneous drainage) or perforation—see *complications of diverticulosis*, p630, for management.
- **Imaging** Erect CXR. USS can detect perforation, free fluid, and collections, though CT with contrast is probably more accurate, especially in complicated disease. If a contrast enema is performed, then water-soluble contrast should be used (see p762). ►In an acute attack colonoscopy should not be done.[153]

Surgery The need for surgery is reflected by the degree of infective complications:

Stage 1	Small confined pericolonic abscesses	Surgery rarely needed
Stage 2	Larger abscesses	May resolve without surgery
Stage 3	Generalized suppurative peritonitis	Surgery required
Stage 4	Faecal peritonitis	Surgery required

- For severe or recurrent diverticulitis ~20% will require surgery.
- Elective sigmoid resection after medical management as a 1-stage open procedure has been performed (also laparoscopically);[154] interestingly no evidence exists to support elective surgery after ≥2 acute attacks of diverticulitis.[155]
- For emergency colonic resection see *complications of diverticulosis*, p630.

Rectal bleeding—an acute management plan

The causes of rectal bleeding are covered elsewhere (MINIBOX). Here let's make an **acute management plan** for this common surgical event:

Typical causes
- Diverticulitis, p630
- Colorectal cancer, p618
- Haemorrhoids, p634
- Crohn's, UC, p272-274
- Perianal disease, p632
- Angiodysplasia, p630
- Rarities—trauma, also:
  - ischaemic colitis, p622
  - radiation proctitis
  - aorto-enteric fistula

»**ABC** resuscitation, if necessary.

»**History and examination.**

»**Blood tests:** FBC, U&E, LFT, clotting, amylase (always thinking of pancreatitis), CRP, group & save serum—await Hb result before cross-matching unless unstable and bleeding.

»**Imaging** May only need plain AXR, but if there are signs of perforation (eg sepsis, peritonism) or if there is cardiorespiratory co-morbidity, then request an erect CXR. See *angiodysplasia*, p630, for more imaging options.

»**Fluid management** Insert 2 cannulae (≥18G) into the antecubital fossae. Insert a urinary catheter if there is a suspicion of haemodynamic compromise—there is no absolute indication, but remember that you are weighing up the risks and benefits. Give crystalloid as replacement and maintenance IVI. Blood transfusion is rarely needed in the acute setting.

»**Antibiotics** may occasionally be required if there is evidence of sepsis or perforation, eg *cefuroxime* 1.5g/8h IV + *metronidazole* 500mg/8h IV.

»**PPI** Consider *omeprazole* 40mg/d IV as ~15% are from upper GI causes (p252-4).

»**Keep bedbound** The patient may feel the need to get out of bed to pass stool, but this could be another large bleed, resulting in collapse if they try to walk. ►Don't allow them to mobilise and inform the nursing staff of this.

»**Start a stool chart** to monitor volume and frequency of motions. Send a sample for MC+S (3 if known to have compromising co-morbidity such as IBD).

»**Diet** Keep on clear fluids so that they can have something, yet the colon will be clear for colonoscopy (which is of little value until bleeding has stopped).

»**Surgery** The main indication for this is unremitting, massive bleeding.

Surgery

Pruritus ani Itch occurs if the anus is moist/soiled; fissures, incontinence, poor hygiene, tight pants, threadworm, fistula, dermatoses, lichen sclerosis, anxiety, contact dermatitis (perfumed goods). ℞: Careful hygiene, anaesthetic cream, moist wipe post-defecation, no spicy food, no steroid/antibiotic cream. Capsaicin may help.[156]

Fissure-in-ano Tear in the squamous lining of the lower anal canal—often, if chronic, with a 'sentinel pile' or mucosal tag at the external aspect. 90% are posterior (anterior ones follow parturition). ♂:♀ is >1. *Causes:* Most are due to hard faeces, which makes defecation painful. Spasm may constrict the inferior rectal artery, causing ischaemia, making healing difficult and perpetuating the problem.[157] Rare causes (multiple ± lateral): syphilis; herpes; trauma; Crohn's; anal Ca; psoriasis. Groin nodes suggest a complicating factor (eg immunosuppression/HIV). ℞: 5% ***lidocaine*** ointment, ↑dietary roughage & fluids, hygiene advice. GTN ointment (0.2–0.4%) (SE: headache). Trials suggest ***botulinum toxin*** injection or topical diltiazem (2%) are at least as effective as GTN with fewer side effects.[158] If conservative measures fail, try ***lateral partial internal sphincterotomy***; (manual anal dilatation is no longer used due to ↑ risk of post-op incontinence).[159] [160] Pre-operative assessment with anorectal USS and manometry is recommended, especially for postpartum fissures.

Fistula-in-ano A track communicates between the skin and anal canal or rectum. Blockage of deep intramuscular gland ducts is thought to predispose to the formation of abscesses, which then discharge to form the fistula. ***Goodsall's rule*** determines the path of the fistula track between openings: if anterior, the track is in a straight line (radial); if posterior, the internal opening is **always** at the 6 o'clock position. *Causes:* perianal sepsis, abscesses (see below); Crohn's disease, TB, diverticular disease, rectal carcinoma, immunocompromise *Tests:* MRI;[161] endoanal US scan.[162] ℞: Fistulotomy + excision (fistula laid open to heal by secondary intention). High fistulae (involving continence muscles of anus) require 'seton suture' tightened over time to maintain continence; for low fistulae, division of sphincters poses no risk to continence.

Anorectal abscesses usually caused by gut organisms (rarely staphs or TB). ♂:♀ ≈1.8. Perianal (~45%), ischiorectal (≤30%), intersphincteric (>20%), supralevator (~5%). ℞: incision & drainage under GA. *Associations:* DM, Crohn's, malignancy..

Perianal haematoma (also called thrombosed external pile—see BOX, p635). Strictly, it is actually a clotted venous saccule. It appears as a 2–4mm 'dark blueberry' under the skin. It may be evacuated under LA or left alone to resolve spontaneously.

Pilonidal sinus Obstruction of natal cleft hair follicles ~6cm above the anus, with ingrowing of hair, excites a foreign body reaction, and may cause secondary tracks to open laterally ± abscesses, with foul-smelling discharge. (Barbers get these between fingers.) ♂:♀ ≈10:1. Obese Caucasians and those from Asia, the Middle East, and Mediterranean at ↑risk. ℞: excision of the sinus tract ± primary closure. Consider pre-op antibiotics. Complex tracks can be laid open and packed individually, or skin flaps can be used to cover the defect.[163] Offer hygiene and hair removal advice.

Rectal prolapse The mucosa (type 1), or all layers (type 2—more common), may protrude through the anus. Incontinence in 75%. It is due to a lax sphincter, prolonged straining, and related to chronic neurological and psychological disorders. ℞ *Abdominal approach*: fix rectum to sacrum (rectopexy) ± mesh insertion ± rectosigmoidectomy, or *perineal approach*: Delorme's procedure (resect close to dentate line and suture mucosal boundaries), anal encirclement with a Thiersch wire.[164]

Perianal warts Condylomata acuminata (viral warts) treated with podophyllin paint/cryotherapy/surgical excision. Confluent nodules (giant condylomata acuminata of Bushke & Loewenstein) may evolve into verrucous cancers (low-grade, non-metastasizing). Condylomata lata secondary to syphilis, treated with penicillin.

Proctalgia fugax Idiopathic, intense, brief, stabbing/crampy rectal pain, often worse at night. Treat with reassurance. Inhaled salbutamol may shorten attacks.

Anal ulcers are rare. Consider Crohn's disease, anal cancer, TB, and syphilis.

Skin tags seldom cause trouble but are easily excised.

Examination of the rectum and anus

►It is necessary to have a chaperone present for the examination. Explain what you are about to do. Make sure curtains are pulled and doors are closed. The patient (and passers-by!) will appreciate it. Have the patient on his left side, his knees brought up towards the chest. Use gloves and lubricant. Part the buttocks and **inspect the anus**: • A gaping anus suggests a neuropathy or megarectum. • Symmetry (a tender unilateral bulge suggests an abscess) • Prolapsed piles • A subanodermal clot may peep out. • Prolapsed rectum (descent of >3cm when asked to strain, as if to pass a motion) • Anodermatitis (from frequent soiling). The anocutaneous reflex tests sensory and motor innervation—on lightly stroking the anal skin, does the external sphincter briefly contract?

Press your index finger against the side of the anus. Ask the patient to breathe deeply and insert your finger slowly; press with the pad of the finger first then twist and push in the tip. Feel for masses (haemorrhoids are not palpable) or impacted stool. Twist your arm so that the pad of your finger is feeling anteriorly. Feel for the cervix or prostate. Note consistency, size, and symmetry of the prostate. Obliteration of its midline sulcus is a sign (unreliable) of prostate cancer. If there is faecal incontinence or concern about the spinal cord, ask the patient to squeeze your finger and note the tone. This is best done with your finger pad facing posteriorly, so the upward and anterior action of puborectalis can be appreciated (it attaches to the symphysis pubis and loops around the rectum proximal to the external sphincter).[165] Note stool or blood on the glove and test for occult blood.

Wipe the anus. Consider proctoscopy (for the anus) or sigmoidoscopy (which mainly inspects the rectum). Reassure that all is well (if this is the case).

Anatomy of the anal canal

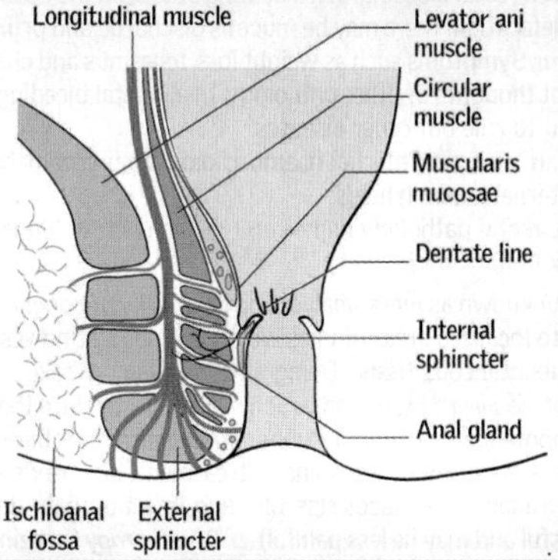

Perianal abscesses present as tender, inflamed, localized swellings at the anal verge. Ischiorectal abscesses are also tender but cause a diffuse, indurated swelling in the ischioanal fossa area.

You will find your patient waiting anxiously for you, pacing about, or on the edge of his chair: avoiding all pressure is his imperative.

Anal cancer

Incidence: 300/yr.[UK] *Risk*↑*:* Syphilis, anal warts (HPV 16, 6, 11, 18, 31 & 33 implicated), anoreceptive homosexuals (often young). *Histology:* Squamous cell (80%); rarely basaloid, melanoma, or adenocarcinoma. Anal margin tumours are usually well-differentiated, keratinising lesions with a good prognosis. Anal canal tumours arise above dentate line, are poorly differentiated and non-keratinising with a poorer prognosis. *Spread:* Tumours above the dentate line spread to pelvic lymph nodes; those below spread to the inguinal nodes. *The patient* may present with bleeding, pain, bowel habit change, pruritus ani, masses, stricture. **ΔΔ***:* Perianal warts; leucoplakia; lichen sclerosis; Bowen's disease; Crohn's disease. *Treatment:* Radiotherapy + *5-fluorouracil* + *mitomycin/cisplatin* is usually preferred to anorectal excision & colostomy; 75% retain normal anal function.[166]

Definition 'Disrupted and dilated anal cushions.' The anus is lined mainly by discontinuous masses of spongy vascular tissue—the anal cushions, which contribute to anal closure. Viewed from the lithotomy position, their positions are at 3, 7, & 11 o'clock (where the 3 major arteries that feed the vascular plexuses enter the anal canal). They are attached by smooth muscle and elastic tissue, but are prone to displacement and disruption, either singly or together. The effects of gravity (our erect posture), increased anal tone (?stress), and the effects of straining at stool may make them become both bulky and loose, and so to protrude to form piles (Latin *pila*, meaning a ball). They are vulnerable to trauma (eg from hard stools) and bleed readily from the capillaries of the underlying lamina propria, hence their other name, haemorrhoids (≈*running blood* in Greek). Because loss is from capillaries, it is bright red. **NB:** piles are **not** varicose veins.

As there are no sensory fibres above the dentate line (squamomucosal junction), piles are not painful unless they thrombose when they protrude and are gripped by the anal sphincter, blocking venous return.

Differential diagnosis: Perianal haematoma; anal fissure; abscess; tumour; proctalgia fugax. ►Never ascribe rectal bleeding to piles without adequate examination or investigation.

Causes Constipation with prolonged straining is a key factor. In many the bowel habit may be normal. Congestion from a pelvic tumour, pregnancy, CCF, or portal hypertension are important in only a minority of cases.

Pathogenesis There is a vicious circle: vascular cushions protrude through a tight anus, become more congested, so hypertrophying to protrude again more readily. These protrusions may then strangulate. See TABLE for classification.

The patient notices bright red rectal bleeding, often coating stools, on the tissue, or dripping into the pan after defecation. There may be mucous discharge and pruritus ani. Severe anaemia may occur. Symptoms such as weight loss, tenesmus and change in bowel habit should prompt thoughts of other pathology. In all rectal bleeding do:

- An abdominal examination to rule out other diseases.
- PR exam: prolapsing piles are obvious. Internal haemorrhoids are not palpable.
- Proctoscopy to see the internal haemorrhoids.
- Sigmoidoscopy to identify rectal pathology higher up (you can get no higher up than the rectosigmoid junction).

Treatment Best treatment unknown as meta-analyses differ. ***Infra-red coagulation*** applied for 1.5–2s, 3–8 times to localized areas of piles works by coagulating vessels, and tethering mucosa to subcutaneous tissue. Doing all the piles may take a few sessions. ***Sclerosants:*** 2mL of 5% ***phenol*** in almond/arachis oil is injected into the pile above the dentate line; SE: impotence; prostatitis). ***Rubber band ligation:*** SE: bleeding; infection. Do <3 band-treatments per session; a cheap treatment, but needs skill. Banding produces an ulcer to anchor the mucosa (SE: bleeding, infection; pain—infra-red coagulation is as successful and may be less painful).[167] ***Cryotherapy*** (freezing) is also used but can produce a lot of watery discharge after the procedure. A high-fibre diet may also help, as well as laxatives, eg lactulose (stool softener), Fybogel® (ease bowel opening), and topical analgesics, anaesthetics &astringents.

In all but 4th degree piles, these measures may obviate need for ***haemorrhoidectomy*** (excision of piles ± ligation of vascular pedicles, as day-case surgery, needing ~2wks off work). SE: haemorrhage or stenosis. Stapled haemorrhoidectomy may result in less pain, a shorter hospital stay and quicker return to normal activity than conventional surgery, provided the surgeon has the technical experience.[168] 1 week's ***lactulose*** + ***metronidazole*** (p381) starting pre-op reduces pain and time off work.[169]

Complications: Constipation; infection; stricture; bleeding.

Prolapsed, thrombosed piles are treated with analgesia, ice packs, stool softeners and bed rest (raise the foot of the bed). Pain usually resolves in 2-3 weeks and surgery is seldom necessary.

Classification of haemorrhoids

1st degree	Remain in the rectum
2nd degree	Prolapse through the anus on defecation but spontaneously reduce
3rd degree	As for second-degree but require digital reduction
4th degree	Remain persistently prolapsed

Internal and external haemorrhoids

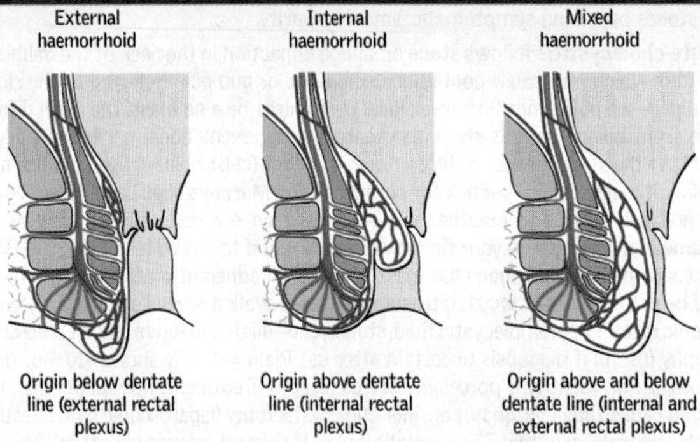

Gallstones

Bile contains cholesterol, bile pigments (from broken down Hb), and phospholipids. If the concentrations vary, different stones may form.[170] ***Pigment stones:*** (<10%) Small, friable, and irregular. Causes: haemolysis. ***Cholesterol stones:*** Large, often solitary. Causes: ♀, age, obesity (Admirand's triangle: ↑risk of stone if ↓lecithin, ↓bile salts, ↑cholesterol). ***Mixed stones:*** Faceted (calcium salts, pigment, and cholesterol). ***Gallstone prevalence:*** 8% of those over 40yrs. 90% remain asymptomatic. Risk factors for stones becoming symptomatic: smoking; parity.

Acute cholecystitis follows stone or sludge impaction in the neck of the gallbladder (GB), which may cause continuous epigastric or RUQ pain (referred to the right shoulder—see p611), vomiting, fever, local peritonism, or a GB mass. The main difference from biliary colic is the inflammatory component (local peritonism, fever, WCC↑). If the stone moves to the common bile duct (CBD), obstructive jaundice and cholangitis may occur—see BOX for complications. **Murphy's sign**: Lay 2 fingers over the RUQ; ask patient to breathe in. This causes pain & arrest of inspiration as an inflamed GB impinges on your fingers. It is only +ve if the same test in the LUQ does not cause pain. A **phlegmon** (RUQ mass of inflamed adherent omentum and bowel) may be palpable. *Tests:* WCC↑, ultrasound—a thick-walled, shrunken GB (also seen in chronic disease), pericholecystic fluid, stones, CBD—dilated if >6mm), HIDA cholescintigraphy (useful if diagnosis uncertain after US). Plain AXR only shows ~10% of gallstones; it may identify a 'porcelain' GB (?cancer).[171] *Treatment:* NBM, pain relief, IVI, and, eg **cefuroxime** 1.5g/8h IV; consider cholecystectomy (laparoscopic if no question of GB perforation) within 72h; mortality: <1%. If delayed, relapse occurs in 18% and may be associated with more complications, so early surgery is often advised.[172] Otherwise, operate after 6-12wks. If elderly or high risk/unsuitable for surgery, consider percutaneous cholecystostomy; cholecystectomy can still be done later. Cholecystostomy is also the preferred treatment for acalculous cholecystitis.[173]

Chronic cholecystitis Chronic inflammation ± colic. 'Flatulent dyspepsia' :vague abdominal discomfort, distension, nausea, flatulence, and fat intolerance (fat stimulates cholecystokinin release and GB contraction). US to image stones and assess CBD diameter. MRCP (p757) is used to find CBD stones. ℞: Cholecystectomy. If US shows a dilated CBD with stones, ERCP (p756) + sphincterotomy before surgery. No comparative trials favour lithotripsy. (If symptoms persist post-cholecystectomy consider hiatus hernia/IBS/peptic ulcer/relapsing pancreatitis/tumour).

Biliary colic Gallstones are symptomatic with cystic duct obstruction or bypassing into the CBD. RUQ pain (radiates → back) ± jaundice. ℞: Analgesia (see p638), rehydrate, NBM. Elective cholecystectomy. **ΔΔ**: The above may overlap as part of a spectrum of gallstone disease. Urinalysis, CXR, and ECG help exclude other diseases.

Other presentations:

- *Obstructive jaundice with CBD stones* (see p250)—if LFT worsening, ERCP with sphincterotomy ± biliary trawl, then cholecystectomy may be needed, or open surgery with CBD exploration. If CBD stones are suspected pre-operatively, intraoperative fluoroscopic cholangiography can be done, though they can now be successfully identified with pre-operative MRCP, p762.[174]
- *Cholangitis* (bile duct infection) causing RUQ pain, jaundice, and rigors (Charcot's triad'). Treat with eg *cefuroxime* 1.5g/8h IV and *metronidazole* 500mg/8h IV/PR.
- *Gallstone ileus:* A stone erodes through the GB into the duodenum; it may then obstruct the terminal ileum. X-ray: air in CBD (=pneumobilia), small bowel fluid levels, and a stone. Duodenal obstruction is rarer (Bouveret's syndrome).[175]
- *Pancreatitis* (p638)
- *Mucocoele/empyema* Obstructed GB fills with mucus (secreted by GB wall)/pus.
- *Silent stones:* Do elective surgery on those with sickle cell, immunosuppression (debatably diabetes) as well as all calcified/porcelain GBs.[176] [177]
- *Mirizzi's syndrome:* A stone in the GB presses on the bile duct causing jaundice.
- *Gallbladder perforation:* Rare because of dual blood supply (hepatic artery via cystic artery, and from small branches of the hepatic artery in the GB fossa).

Complications of gallstones

In the gall bladder:
- Biliary colic
- Acute and chronic cholecystitis
- Empyema
- Mucocoele
- Carcinoma
- Mirizzi's syndrome

In the bile ducts:
- Obstructive jaundice
- Pancreatitis
- Cholangitis

In the gut:
- Gallstone ileus

Diseases having biliary complications

Causes of cholecystitis and biliary symptoms, other than gallstones, are rare, eg:
- Infections: typhoid, cyptosporidiosis, brucellosis, ascariasis, opisthorchiasis
- Complications of parenteral nutrition
- Cystic duct structural abnormality
- Hormonal: release of cholecystokinin
- High-pressure sphincter of Oddi.
- Polyarteritis nodosa (p558)

Is it possible to perform double-blind RCTs in surgery?

In 2005 a double-blinded randomized controlled trial (RCT) looked at the differences between open and laparoscopic cholecystectomy.[178] This raises issues on both the place and validity of double-blinded RCTs in surgery.

Overcoming established treatments always has difficulties. When faced with either surgery or non-operative management, everyone's preference would be to avoid surgery especially if there is ambivalence about which treatment is superior. The negative influence of the learning curve for a new treatment must be considered and this may take time to overcome (p595). Furthermore, controlling the bias introduced by interperformer and patient variance is not least because each patient is different. There are also inherent difficulties in double-blinding surgical treatment:; 'sham' surgery remains a contentious issue.[179]

The laparoscopic cholecystectomy

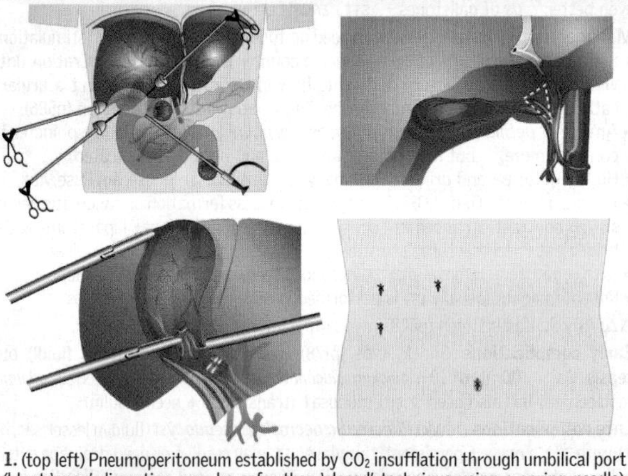

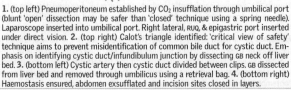

1. (top left) Pneumoperitoneum established by CO_2 insufflation through umbilical port (blunt 'open' dissection may be safer than 'closed' technique using a spring needle). Laparoscope inserted into umbilical port. Right lateral, RUQ, & epigastric port inserted under direct vision. **2.** (top right) Calot's triangle identified: 'critical view of safety' technique aims to prevent misidentification of common bile duct for cystic duct. Emphasis on identifying cystic duct/infundibulum junction by dissecting GB neck off liver bed. **3.** (bottom left) Cystic artery then cystic duct divided between clips. GB dissected from liver bed and removed through umbilicus using a retrieval bag. **4.** (bottom right) Haemostasis ensured, abdomen exsufflated and incision sites closed in layers.

Acute pancreatitis

This unpredictable disease (mortality ~12%) is managed on surgical wards, but because surgery is often not involved, it's easy to think that there's no acute problem. There is: self-perpetuating pancreatic inflammation (and of other retroperitoneal tissues). Oedema and fluid shifts cause hypovolaemia as extracellular fluid is trapped in the gut, peritoneum, and retroperitoneum (worsened by vomiting). Progression may be rapid from mild oedema to necrotizing pancreatitis by enzyme-mediated autodigestion. ~50% of cases that advance to necrosis are further complicated by infection. Contributory factors include protease-induced activation of complement, kinin, and fibrinolytic and coagulation cascades. Oxidant stress may be important.[180] Congenital abnormality (eg pancreas divisum or annular pancreas) can predispose to pancreatitis.[181]

Causes 'GET SMASHED'

Gallstones (38%)
Ethanol (35%)
Trauma (1.5%)
Steroids
Mumps
Autoimmune (PAN)
Scorpion venom
Hyperlipidaemia, hypothermia, hypercalcaemia
ERCP (5%) and emboli
Drugs
Also pregnancy and neoplasia or no cause found (10–30%)

Symptoms Gradual or sudden severe **epigastric** or **central abdominal pain** (radiates to back, sitting forward may relieve); vomiting prominent.
Signs may be mild in serious disease! Tachycardia, fever, jaundice, shock, ileus, rigid abdomen ± local/general tenderness, periumbilical bruising (**Cullen's sign**) or flanks (**Grey Turner's sign**) from blood vessel autodigestion & retroperitoneal haemorrhage
Tests Raised serum *amylase* (>1000U/mL or around 3-fold upper limit of normal range); cholecystitis, mesenteric infarction, and GI perforation can cause lesser rises (usually). It is excreted renally so renal failure will ↑ levels. ►Amylase may be normal even in severe pancreatitis (levels starts to fall within the 1st 24–48h). Serum *lipase* is more sensitive and specific for pancreatitis.[182] *ABG* to monitor oxygenation and acid-base status. *AXR:* No psoas shadow (retroperitoneal fluid↑), 'sentinel loop' of proximal jejunum from ileus (solitary air-filled dilatation). *Erect CXR* helps exclude other causes (eg perforation). *CT* to assess severity (low-density changes) —*MRI* may be even better.[183] *US* (if gallstones + AST↑). *ERCP* if LFT worsen.

Management Nil by mouth, likely to need NG tube (decrease pancreatic stimulation).
- Set up IVI and give lots of 0.9% saline, to counter third-space sequestration, until vital signs are satisfactory and urine flow stays at >30mL/h. Insert a urinary catheter and consider CVP monitoring. Think about nutrition early on (p586).
- Analgesia: ***pethidine*** 75–100mg/4h IM, or ***morphine*** (may cause Oddi's sphincter to contract more,[184] but it is a better analgesic and not contraindicated).[185]
- Hourly pulse, BP, and urine output; daily FBC, U&E, Ca^{2+}, glucose, amylase, ABG.
- If worsening: ITU, O_2 if P_aO_2↓. In suspected abscess formation or pancreatic necrosis (on contrast-enhanced CT), consider parenteral nutrition ± laparotomy & debridement ('necrosectomy'). Antibiotics may help in specific severe disease.[186]
- ERCP + gallstone removal may be needed if there is progressive jaundice.
- Repeat imaging (usually CT) is performed in order to monitor progress.

ΔΔ: Any acute abdomen (p608), myocardial infarct. **Prognosis** See BOX.

Early complications: Shock, ARDS (p178), renal failure (►**give lots of fluid!**), DIC, sepsis, Ca^{2+}↓, (10mL of 10% *calcium gluconate* IV slowly is, rarely, needed; *albumin* replacement has also been tried), glucose↑ (transient; 5% need insulin).

Late complications (>1wk) *Pancreatic necrosis* & *pseudocyst* (fluid in lesser sac, **fig 1**), with T°↑, a mass ± persistent ↑amylase/LFT; may resolve or need drainage externally or into stomach (eg laparoscopically). *Abscesses* need draining. *Bleeding* from elastase eroding a major vessel (eg splenic artery); embolization may be life-saving. *Thrombosis* may occur in the splenic/gastroduodenal arteries, or colic branches of the superior mesenteric artery, causing bowel necrosis. *Fistulae* normally close spontaneously. If purely pancreatic they do not irritate the skin. Some patients suffer ***recurrent oedematous pancreatitis*** so often that near-total pancreatectomy is contemplated. ►It can all be a miserable course.

Modified Glasgow criteria for predicting severity of pancreatitis

►3 or more positive factors detected within 48h of onset suggest severe pancreatitis, and should prompt transfer to ITU/HDU. Mnemonic: **PANCREAS**.187

P$_a$O$_2$	<8kPa
Age	>55yrs
Neutrophilia	WBC >15 x 10^9/L
Calcium	<2mmol/L
Renal function	Urea >16mmol/L
Enzymes	LDH >600iu/L; AST >200iu/L
Albumin	<32g/L (serum)
Sugar	blood glucose >10mmol/L

Courtesy of Mr Etienne Moore FRCS

Moore EM. A useful mnemonic for severity stratification in acute pancreatitis. *Ann R Coll Surg Engl* 2000; **82**: 16-17. © The Royal College of Surgeons of England. Reproduced with permission

These criteria have been validated for pancreatitis caused by gallstones and alcohol; Ranson's criteria are valid for alcohol-induced pancreatitis, and can only be fully applied after 48h, which does have its disadvantages.

Other methods of severity assessment: Severity can be assessed with the help of CT.[1] CRP can also be a helpful marker.188

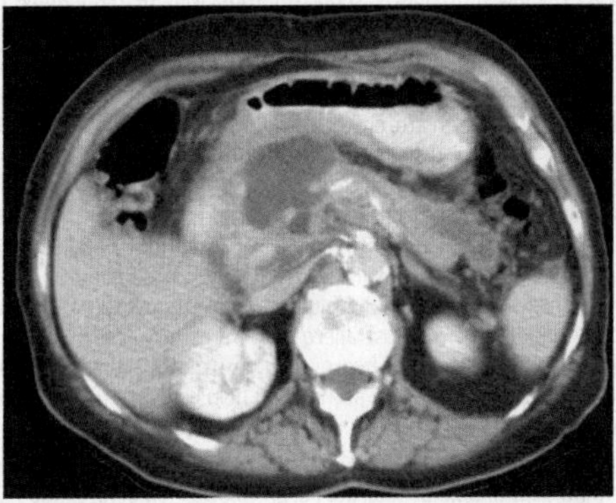

Fig 1. Axial CT of the abdomen (with IV and PO contrast media) showing a pancreatic pseudocyst occupying the lesser sac of the abdomen posterior to the stomach. It is called a 'pseudocyst' because it is not a true cyst, rather a collection of fluid in the lesser sac (ie not lined by epi/endothelium). It develops at ≥6wks. The cyst fluid is of low attenuation compared with the stomach contents because it has not been enhanced by the contrast media.

Image courtesy of Dr Stephen Golding.

1 For a useful exposition on imaging in pancreatitis see www.emedicine.com/radio/topic521.htm

Renal stones (calculi) consist of crystal aggregates. Stones form in collecting ducts and may be deposited anywhere from the renal pelvis to the urethra though classically at **1** Pelviureteric junction **2** Pelvic brim **3** Vesicoureteric junction.

Prevalence Common: lifetime incidence up to 15%. ***Peak age:*** 20–40yr. ♂:♀≈3:1.

Types • Calcium oxalate (75%) • Magnesium ammonium phosphate (struvite; 10–20%) • Also: urate (5%), hydroxyapatite (5%), brushite, cystine (1%), mixed.

The patient Asymptomatic or: **1** ***Renal colic:*** excruciating spasms 'loin to groin' (or genitals/inner thigh), often with nausea/vomiting. Often cannot lie still (differentiates from peritonitis). ***Renal obstruction*** felt in the loin, between rib 12 and lateral edge of lumbar muscles (like intercostal nerve irritation pain; the latter is not colicky, and is worsened by specific movements/pressure on a trigger spot). ***Obstruction of mid-ureter*** may mimic appendicitis/diverticulitis. ***Obstruction of lower ureter*** may lead to symptoms of bladder irritability and pain in scrotum, penile tip, or labia majora.[189] ***Obstruction in bladder or urethra*** causes pelvic pain, dysuria, strangury (desire but inability to void[190]) ± interrupted flow. **2** *UTI* can co-exist (↑risk if voiding impaired); ***pyelonephritis*** (fever, rigors, loin pain, nausea, vomiting), ***pyonephrosis*** (infected hydronephrosis) **3** Haematuria **4** Proteinuria **5** Sterile pyuria **6** Anuria.

Examination: Usually no tenderness on palpation. May be renal angle tenderness especially to percussion if there is retroperitoneal inflammation

Tests: FBC, U&E, Ca^{2+}, PO_4^{3-}, glucose, bicarbonate, urate. ***Urine dipstick:*** Usually +ve for blood (90%). ***MSU:*** MC&S. ***Further tests for cause:*** Urine pH (on dipstick); 24h urine for: calcium, oxalate, urate, citrate, sodium, creatinine; stone biochemistry.
Imaging: **KUB XR** (kidneys+ureters+bladder). Look along ureters for calcification over the transverse processes of the vertebral bodies: 80% of stones are visible (99% on CT). **IVU**: radio-opaque contrast injected & serial films taken until contrast seen down to level of obstruction. Cannot be interpreted without a plain control. *Abnormal findings*: failure of contrast to flow to bladder, dense nephrogram (contrast unable to flow from kidney), clubbed/blunted renal calyces (back pressure), filling defects in the bladder. (CI: contrast allergy, severe asthma, pregnancy, metformin) **USS** to look for hydronephrosis or hydroureter. **Spiral non-contrast CT** is superior to and is replacing IVU for imaging stones, and helps exclude differential causes of an acute abdomen. ►A ruptured abdominal aortic aneurysm may present similarly.

℞: ***Initially:*** Analgesia eg **diclofenac** 75mg IV/IM, or 100mg suppository.[191] (If CI: **opioids**) + IV fluids if unable to tolerate PO; antibiotics (eg **cefuroxime** 1.5g/8h IV) if infection. ***Stones <5mm in lower ureter:*** ~90–95% pass spontaneously. ↑fluid intake. Sieve urine for analysis. ***Stones >5mm/pain not resolving:*** **Medical expulsive therapy: nifedipine** 10mg/8h PO[192] or α-blockers (**tamsulosin** 0.4mg/d[193]) ± **prednisolone** (↓inflammation) promote expulsion: ►start at presentation.[194] Most pass within 48h (>80% after ~30d). If not, try ESWL (if <1cm), or ureteroscopy using 'Dormier basket'.[195] **Shockwave lithotripsy (ESWL):** US waves shatter stone. *SE:* renal injury, may also cause ↑BP and DM.[196] **Percutaneous nephrolithotomy (PCNL)**: keyhole surgery to remove stones, when large, multiple, or complex.[197] Open surgery is rare.

►*Indications for urgent intervention (delay may lead to permanent loss of renal function):* Presence of infection + urinary tract obstruction (percutaneous nephrostomy may be needed to relieve obstruction), urosepsis, intractable pain or vomiting, impending ARF, obstruction in a solitary kidney, bilateral obstructing stones.[198]

Prevention ***General:*** Drink plenty. *Normal* Ca^{2+} intake is now recommended, as low Ca^{2+} diets increase oxalate excretion. ***Specifically:*** • *Calcium stones:* in hypercalciuria, a thiazide diuretic is used to ↓ Ca^{2+} excretion • *Oxalate:* ↓oxalate intake; pyridoxine may be used (p312) • *Struvite:* treat infection promptly • *Urate:* allopurinol (100–300mg/24h PO). Urine alkalinization may also help, as urate is more soluble at pH>6 (eg with potassium citrate or sodium bicarbonate) • *Cystine:* vigorous hydration to keep urine output >3L/day and urinary alkalinization (as above). D-penicillamine is used to chelate cystine, given with pyridoxine to prevent vitamin B_6 deficiency.

Questions to address when confronted by a stone

What is its composition?

Type	Causative factors	Appearance on XR
Calcium oxalate (**fig 1**)	Metabolic or idiopathic	Spiky, radio-opaque
Calcium phosphate	Metabolic or idiopathic	Smooth, may be large, radio-opaque
Magnesium ammonium phosphate	UTI (proteus causes alkaline urine and calcium precipitation and ammonium salt formation)	Large, horny, 'staghorn' radio-opaque
Urate (p694, **fig 2**)	Hyperuricaemia	Smooth, brown, radiolucent
Cystine (**fig 3**)	Renal tubular defect	Yellow, crystalline, semi-opaque

Why has he or she got this stone now?

"What do you eat?" Chocolate, tea, rhubarb, strawberries, nuts and spinach ↑oxalate levels.

Is it summer? Seasonal variations in calcium and oxalate levels are thought to be mediated by vitamin D synthesis via sunlight on skin."

"What's your job?" Can he/she drink freely? Is there dehydration?

Are there any precipitating drugs? These include:

Loop diuretics, antacids, acetazolamide, corticosteroids, theophylline, aspirin, thiazides, allopurinol, vitamin C & D, indinavir.

Are there any predisposing factors? For example:

Recurrent UTIs (in magnesium aluminium phosphate calculi).

Metabolic abnormalities:

- Hypercalciuria/hypercalcaemia (p690): hyperparathyroidism, neoplasia, sarcoidosis, hyperthyroidism, Addison's, Cushing's, lithium, vit D excess.
- Hyperuricosuria/↑plasma urate: on its own, or with gout.
- Hyperoxaluria (p312).
- Cystinuria (p312).
- Renal tubular acidosis (p310).

Urinary tract abnormalities: eg pelviureteric junction obstruction, hydronephrosis (renal pelvis or calyces), calyceal diverticulum, horseshoe kidney, ureterocele, vesicoureteric reflux, ureteral stricture, medullary sponge kidney.[1]

Foreign bodies: eg stents, catheters.

Is there a family history? ↑risk of stones × 3-fold. Specific diseases include X-linked nephrolithiasis and Dent's disease: proteinuria, hypercalciuria and nephrocalcinosis.

►*Is there infection above the stone?* eg fever, loin tender, pyuria? This needs urgent intervention.

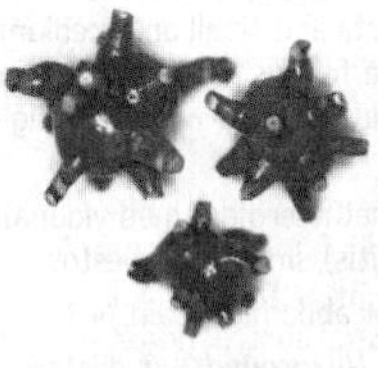

Fig 1. Calcium oxalate monohydrate.

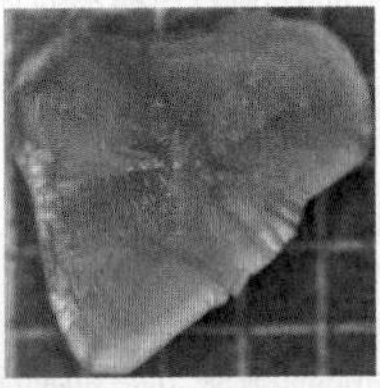

Fig 2. Struvite stone.

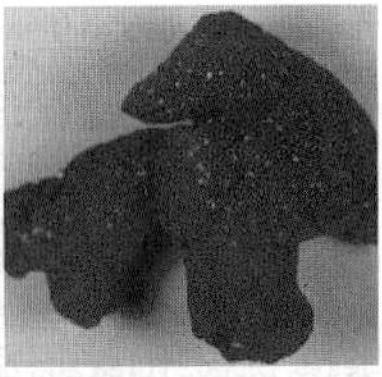

Fig 3. Cystine stone.

Figs 1-3 courtesy Dr Glen Austin

1 Medullary sponge kidney is a typically asymptomatic developmental anomaly of the kidney mostly seen in adult females, where there is dilatation of the collecting ducts, which if severe leads to a sponge-like appearance of the renal medulla. *Complications/associations:* UTIs, nephrolithiasis, haematuria and hypercalciuria, hyperparathyroidism (if present, look for genetic markers of MEN type 2A, see p215).

Urinary tract obstruction

►*Urinary tract obstruction is common and should be considered in any patient with impaired renal function.* Damage can be permanent if the obstruction is not treated promptly. It occurs anywhere from the renal calyces to the urethral meatus, and may be *partial* or *complete, unilateral* or *bilateral.* Obstructing lesions are *luminal* (stones, blood clot, sloughed papilla, tumour: renal, ureteric, or bladder), *mural* (eg congenital or acquired stricture, neuromuscular dysfunction, schistosomiasis), or *extra-mural* (abdominal or pelvic mass/tumour, retroperitoneal fibrosis). Unilateral obstruction may be clinically silent (normal urine output and U&E) if the other kidney is functioning. ►Bilateral obstruction or obstruction with infection requires urgent treatment. See EMERGENCY BOX p645.

Clinical features

- ***Acute upper tract obstruction:*** Loin pain radiating to the groin. There may be superimposed infection ± loin tenderness, or an enlarged kidney.
- ***Chronic upper tract obstruction:*** Flank pain, renal failure, superimposed infection. Polyuria may occur owing to impaired urinary concentration.
- ***Acute lower tract obstruction:*** Acute urinary retention typically presents with severe suprapubic pain, often preceded by symptoms of bladder outflow obstruction (as below). Clinically: distended, palpable bladder, dull to percussion.
- ***Chronic lower tract obstruction:*** *Symptoms:* urinary frequency, hesitancy, poor stream, terminal dribbling, overflow incontinence. *Signs:* distended, palpable bladder ± large prostate on PR. *Complications:* UTI, urinary retention.

Tests *Blood:* U&E, creatinine. *Urine:* MC&S. ***Ultrasound*** (p758) is the imaging modality of choice. If there is hydronephrosis or hydroureter (distension of the renal pelvis and calyces or ureter), the next test is ***antegrade or retrograde ureterograms*** (pyelograms; p759): it offers a therapeutic option of drainage. **NB:** In ~5% of cases of obstruction, no distension is seen on ultrasound. ***Radionuclide imaging*** enables functional assessment of the kidneys. *CT & MRI* also have a role.

Treatment *Upper tract obstruction:* Nephrostomy or ureteric stent. Pyeloplasty, to widen the PUJ, may be performed if obstruction is at this level.

Lower tract obstruction: Urethral or suprapubic catheter (p776). Treat the underlying cause if possible. Beware of a large diuresis after relief of obstruction; a temporary salt-losing nephropathy may occur resulting in the loss of several litres of fluid a day. Monitor weight, fluid balance, and U&E closely.

Peri-aortitis (retroperitoneal fibrosis *et al*)

Causes include idiopathic retroperitoneal fibrosis (RPF), inflammatory aneurysms of the abdominal aorta, and perianeurysmal RPF. Idiopathic RPF is an autoimmune disorder, where there is B-cell and CD4(+) T-cell associated vasculitis. This results in fibrinoid necrosis of the vasa vasorum, affecting the aorta and small and medium retroperitoneal vessels. The ureters get embedded in dense, fibrous tissue resulting in progressive bilateral ureteric obstruction. Secondary causes of RPF include malignancy, typically lymphoma.

Associations: Drugs (eg β-blockers, bromocriptine, methysergide, methyldopa), autoimmune disease (eg thyroiditis, SLE, ANCA+ve vasculitis), smoking, asbestos.

Typical patient: Middle-aged ♂ with vague loin, back or abdominal pain, BP↑.

Tests: *Blood:* ↑urea and creatinine; ↑ESR; ↑CRP; anaemia. *Ultrasound/IVU:* dilated ureters (hydronephrosis) + medial deviation of ureters. *CT/MRI:* peri-aortic mass (this allows biopsy, to rule out malignancy).

Treatment: Retrograde stent placement to relieve obstruction ± ureterolysis (dissection of the ureters from the retroperitoneal tissue). Immunosuppression with steroids or other agents is controversial, but some studies show benefit.[200]

Problems of ureteric stenting (depend on site)	
Common	*Rare*
Trigonal irritation	Obstruction
Haematuria	Kinking
Fever	Ureteric rupture
Infection	Stent misplacement
Tissue inflammation	Stent migration (especially if made of silicone)
Encrustation	Tissue hyperplasia
Biofilm formation	

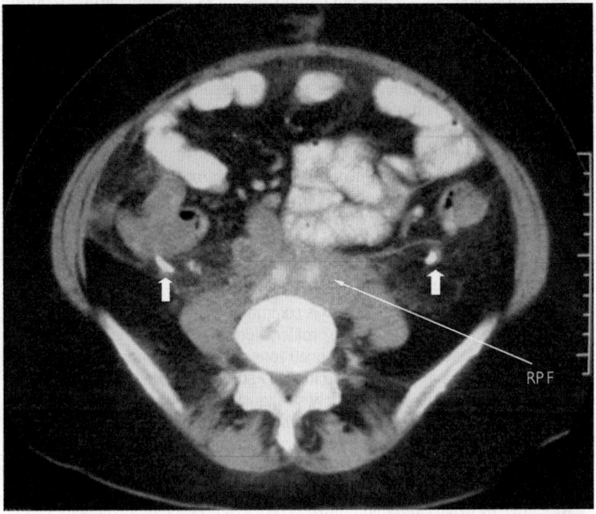

Fig 1. CT scan of retroperitoneal fibrosis (RPF), with subsequent obstruction and dilatation of the ureters (thick arrows). *Oxford Textbook of Nephrology*, 2465,OUP.

Retention means not emptying the bladder (∵ **obstruction** or ↓**detrusor power**).

- **Acute retention** Bladder usually tender, containing ~600mL. *Causes:* prostatic obstruction (usual cause in ♂), urethral strictures, anticholinergics, 'holding', alcohol, constipation, post-op (pain/inflammation/anaesthetics), infection (p292), neurological (cauda equina syndrome), carcinoma. *Examine:* Abdomen, PR, perineal sensation (cauda equina compression). *Tests:* MSU, U&E, FBC, and prostate-specific antigen (PSA, p538).[1] Renal ultrasound if renal impairment. *Tricks to aid voiding:* Analgesia, privacy on hospital wards, ambulation, standing to void, voiding to the sound of running taps—or in a hot bath. *If the tricks fail:* Catheterize (p776) and try a prostate procedure (below). If in clot retention will require 3-way catheter and bladder washout. After eg 7 days, trial without catheter (p777) may work (esp. if <75yrs old and <1L drained or retention was triggered by a passing event, eg GA), p751. *Prevention: Finasteride* reduces prostate size and retention risk. *Tamsulosin* reduces risk of needing recatheterization after acute retention.[201]
- **Chronic retention** More insidious. Bladder capacity may be >1.5L. May be painless. *Presentation:* overflow incontinence, acute on chronic retention, lower abdominal mass, UTI, or renal failure (eg bilateral obstructive uropathy—see EMERGENCY BOX) *Causes:* Prostatic enlargement is common, pelvic malignancy; rectal surgery; DM; CNS disease eg transverse myelitis/MS; zoster (S2–S4). ►Only catheterize patient if there is pain, urinary infection, or renal impairment (urea >12mmol/L). Institute definitive treatment promptly. Intermittent self-catheterization is sometimes required (p776). **Catheters** p776. **Prostate ca** p620.

Benign prostatic hyperplasia (BPH) is common (24% if aged 40–64; 40% if older). *Pathology:* Benign nodular or diffuse proliferation of musculofibrous and glandular layers of the prostate. Inner (transitional) zone enlarges in contrast to peripheral layer expansion seen in prostate carcinoma. *Features:* Nocturia, frequency, post-micturition dribbling, poor stream/flow, strangury, hesitancy, overflow incontinence, haematuria, bladder stones, UTI. *Management:* Assess severity of symptoms and impact on life. PR exam. *Tests:* MSU; U&E; ultrasound (residual volume↑, hydronephrosis—**fig 1**). 'Rule out' cancer: PSA,[1] transrectal USS ± biopsy. Then consider:

- *Self-help:* Avoid caffeine, alcohol (to ↓urgency/nocturia). Relax when voiding. Void twice in a row to aid emptying. Control urgency by practising distraction methods (eg breathing exercises). Train the bladder by 'holding on' to ↑time between voiding.
- *Transurethral resection of prostate* (TURP) ≤14% become impotent—see BOX). Crossmatch 2U. Beware bleeding, clot retention & TUR syndrome: absorption of washout causing hyponatraemia & fits. ~20% need redoing within 10yrs.[202]
- *Transurethral incision of the prostate* (TUIP) involves less destruction than TURP, and less risk to sexual function, but gives similar benefit.[203] It achieves this by relieving pressure on the urethra. It is perhaps the best surgical option for those with small glands <30g—ie ~50% of those operated on in some areas.
- *Retropubic prostatectomy* is an open operation (if prostate very large).
- *Transurethral laser-induced prostatectomy* (TULIP) may be as good as TURP.[204]
- *Drugs* may be useful in mild disease, and while awaiting TURP, eg: **α-blockers**: 1st line eg *tamsulosin* 400μg/d PO; also *alfuzosin, doxazosin, terazosin*. ↓smooth muscle tone (prostate & bladder). SE: drowsiness, depression; dizziness; BP↓; dry mouth; ejaculatory failure; extra-pyramidal signs; nasal congestion; weight↑. **5α-reductase inhibitors**: *finasteride* 5mg/d PO (↓testosterone's conversion to dihydrotestosterone).[2] Excreted in semen, so warn to use condoms; females should avoid handling. SE: impotence; ↓libido. Effects on prostate size are limited and slow.
- *Phytotherapy* (pharmacological use of plants) *Saw palmetto* (*Serenoa repens*) is said to help symptoms of BPH (no more than drugs[205]); trials are disappointing.
- *Wait and see* is an option, but risks incontinence, retention, and renal failure.

1 Do venepuncture for PSA **before** PR, as PR can ↑total PSA by ~1ng/mL (free PSA ↑by 10%). It's difficult to know if acute retention raises PSA, but relieving obstruction does cause it to drop.

2 *Finasteride* can prevent retention but has odd effects on risk of prostate cancer. The PCPT trial showed ↓risk of indolent cancers, but ↑risk of Gleason >7 (p647).

Advice for patients concerning transurethral prostatectomy

Pre-op consent issues may centre on risks of the procedure, eg:

- Haematuria/haemorrhage
- Haematospermia
- Hypothermia
- Urethral trauma/stricture
- Post TURP syndrome (T° ↓; Na^+↓)[206]
- Infection; prostatitis
- Erectile dysfunction ~10%
- Incontinence ≤10%
- Clot retention near strictures
- Retrograde ejaculation (common)

Post-operative advice:

- Avoid driving for 2 weeks after the operation.
- Avoid sex for 2 weeks after surgery. Then get back to normal. The amount ejaculated may be reduced (as it flows backwards into the bladder—harmless, but may cloud the urine). It means you may be infertile. Erections may be a problem after TURP, but do not expect this: in some men, erections improve. Rarely, orgasmic sensations are reduced.
- Expect to pass blood in the urine for the first 2 weeks. A small amount of blood colours the urine bright red. Do not be alarmed.
- At first you may need to urinate **more** frequently than before. Do not be despondent. In 6 weeks things should be much better—but the operation cannot be guaranteed to work (8% fail, and lasting incontinence is a problem in 6%; 12% may need repeat TURPs within 8yrs, compared with 1.8% of men undergoing open prostatectomy).
- If feverish, or if urination hurts, take a sample of urine to your doctor.

Obstructive uropathy

In chronic urinary retention, an episode of **acute** retention may go unnoticed for days and, because of their background symptoms, may only present when overflow incontinence becomes a nuisance—pain is not necessarily a feature. After diagnosing acute on chronic retention and placing a catheter, the bladder residual can be as much as 1.5L of urine. Don't be surprised to be called by the biochemistry lab to be told that the serum creatinine is 1500μmol per L! The good news is that renal function usually returns to baseline after a few days (there may be mild background impairment). Ask for an urgent renal US (**fig 1**) and consider the following in the acute plan to ensure a safe course:

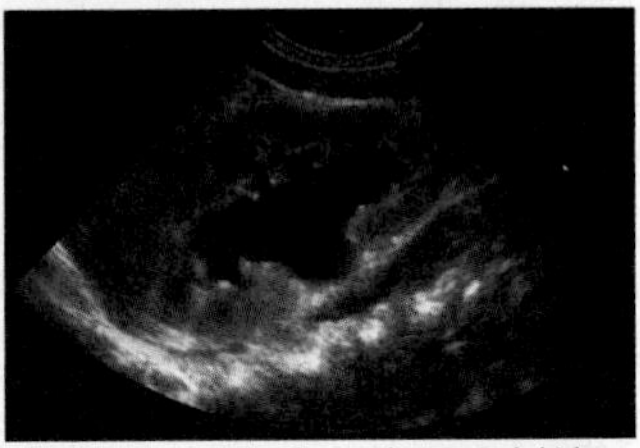

Fig 1. Ultrasound of an obstructed kidney showing hydronephrosis. Note dilatation of renal pelvis and ureter, and clubbed calyces.
Image courtesy of Norwich Radiology Department

- **Hyperkalaemia:** See p849.
- **Metabolic acidosis:** On ABG there is likely to be a respiratory compensated metabolic acidosis. Concerns should prompt discussion with a renal specialist (a good idea anyway), in case haemodialysis is required (p304).
- **Post-obstructive diuresis:** In the acute phase after relief of the obstruction, the kidneys produce **a lot** of urine—as much as a litre in the first hour. It is vital to provide resuscitation fluids and then match input with output.

►Fluid depletion rather than overload is the danger here.

- **Sodium- and bicarbonate-losing nephropathy:** As the kidney undergoes diuresis, Na^+ and bicarbonate are lost in the urine in large quantities. Replace 'in for out' (as above) with isotonic 1.26% sodium bicarbonate solution—this should be available from ITU. Some advocate using 0.9% saline, though the chloride load may exacerbate acidosis. Withhold any nephrotoxic drugs.
- **Infection:** Treat infection, bearing in mind that the WCC↑ and CRP↑ may be part of the stress response. Send a sample of urine for MC+S.

Renal cell carcinoma (RCA, hypernephroma, Grawitz tumour) arises from proximal renal tubular epithelium. *Epidemiology:* 90% of renal cancers; mean age 55yrs. ♂:♀≈2:1. 15% of haemodialysis patients develop RCA. *Features:* 50% incidental findings. Haematuria, loin pain, abdominal mass, anorexia, malaise, weight loss, PUO—often in isolation. Rarely, invasion of left renal vein compresses left testicular vein causing a varicocele. Spread may be direct (renal vein), via lymph, or haematogenous (bone, liver, lung). *Tests:* BP: ↑from renin secretion **Blood:** FBC (polycythaemia from erythropoietin secretion); ESR; U&E, ALP (bony mets?). **Urine:** RBCs; cytology. **Imaging:** US (p758); CT/MRI (including 3D 208) renal angiography (if partial nephrectomy/palliative embolization being considered); IVU (filling defect ± calcification); CXR ('cannon ball' metastases). *℞:* Radical nephrectomy (possible role for nephron-sparing surgery in tumours ≤4cm). 209 In low & intermediate-risk patients with clear cell renal cell carcinoma and prior nephrectomy, progression-free survival is augmented by 3 angiogenesis-targeted agents: sunitinib, bevacizumab and sorafenib. As a 1st-line treatment for patients with multiple poor-risk factors, temsirolimus (inhibits mTOR) improves survival compared with INF. 210 (Interferon-α and interleukin-2 were formerly used on their own.) 211 *Robson staging:* **I** confined to kidney **II** involves perinephric fat but not beyond Garota's fascia **III** spread to renal vein **IV** spread to adjacent/distant organs *Prognosis:* 5yr survival: 45%.

Transitional cell carcinoma (TCC) may arise in the bladder (50%), ureter, or renal pelvis. *Epidemiology:* Age >40yrs; ♂:♀ = 4:1. *Risk factors:* p648. *Presentation:* Painless haematuria; frequency; urgency; dysuria; urinary tract obstruction. *Diagnosis:* Urine cytology; IVU; cystoscopy + biopsy; CT/MRI scan. *℞:* See **Bladder tumours**, p648. *Prognosis:* Varies with clinical stage/histological grade: 10–80% 5yr survival.

Wilms' tumour (nephroblastoma) is a childhood tumour of primitive renal tubules and mesenchymal cells. *Prevalence:* 1:100 000—the chief abdominal malignancy in children. It presents with an abdominal mass and haematuria. *℞:* *OHCS* p133.

Prostate cancer 2nd commonest male malignancy. *Incidence:* ↑with age: 80% in men >80yrs (autopsy studies). *Associations:* ↑testosterone, +ve family history (p524). Most are adenocarcinomas arising in peripheral prostate. Spread may be local (seminal vesicles, bladder, rectum) via lymph, or haematogenously (sclerotic bony lesions). *Symptoms:* Asymptomatic or nocturia, hesitancy, poor stream, terminal dribbling, or obstruction. Weight↓ ± bone pain suggests mets. *PR exam:* May show hard, irregular prostate. *Diagnosis:* ↑PSA (normal in 30% of small cancers); transrectal USS & biopsy; bone x-rays; bone scan; CT/MRI. *Staging:* MRI. If contrast-enhancing magnetic nanoparticles used, sensitivity for detecting affected nodes rises from 35% to 90%. 212 *℞:* **Local disease:** Which is better: radical prostatectomy (+ immediate *goserelin* if node +ve; a widely used regimen), radiotherapy or watchful waiting with serial PSA monitoring? One trial found at 10 yrs, radical prostatectomy only improved disease-specific mortality and local progression compared with watchful waiting in those <75 yrs old. 213 (but radical surgery doubles erectile dysfunction & incontinence rates). Radiotherapy combined with hormone therapy improves survival in advanced local disease. 214 Do transurethral resection for obstruction. Brachytherapy is being assessed for local disease. **Metastatic disease:** Hormonal drugs may give benefit for 1–2yrs. Gonadotrophin-releasing analogues, eg 12-weekly *goserelin* (10.8mg SC as Zoladex LA®) first stimulate, then inhibit pituitary gonadotrophin. Also: *cyproterone acetate*; *flutamide*; *diethylstilboestrol*. *Symptomatic ℞:* Analgesia; treat hypercalcaemia; radiotherapy for bone mets/spinal cord compression. *Prognosis:* 10% die in 6 months, 10% live >10yrs. *Screening:* PR exam; PSA; transrectal USS.

Penile cancer *Epidemiology* rare in UK, more common in Far East & Africa, very rare in circumcised. Related to chronic irritation, viruses, smegma. *Presentation:* chronic fungating ulcer, bloody/purulent discharge, 50% spread to lymph at presentation *℞:* DXT & irridium wires if early; amputation & lymph node dissection.

Advice to asymptomatic men asking for a PSA blood test

- Many men over 50 consider a PSA test to detect prostatic cancer. *Is this wise?*
- The test is not very accurate, and we cannot say that those having the test will live longer—even if they turn out to have prostate cancer. Most men with prostate cancer die from an unrelated cause.
- If the test is falsely positive, you may needlessly have more tests eg prostate sampling via the back passage (causes bleeding and infection in 1-5% of men).
- Only one in three of those with a high PSA level will have cancer.
- You may also be worried needlessly if later tests put you in the clear.
- If a cancer is found, there's no way to tell *for sure* if it will impinge on health. You might end up having a bad effect from treatment which wasn't needed.
- There is much uncertainty on treating those who **do** turn out to have prostate cancer: options are radical surgery to remove the prostate (this treatment may be fatal in 0.2-0.5% of patients), radiotherapy, or hormones.
- There is indirect evidence of benefit of screening from the USA where fewer radical prostatectomies reveal cancer-affected lymph nodes than those done before widespread PSA-based screening. Intensive screening and treatment for prostate cancer does not, however, appear to be associated with lower prostate-specific mortality in retrospective studies.[215]

►Ultimately, you must decide for yourself what you want.

Prognostic factors in prostate cancer

A number of prognostic factors help determine if 'watchful waiting' or aggressive therapy should be advised: •Age •Pre-treatment PSA level •Tumour stage (as measured by the TNM system),[216] and tumour grade—as measured by its Gleason score. Gleason grading is from 1 to 5, with 5 being the highest grade, and carrying the poorest prognosis. A pathologist determines Gleason grades by analysing histology from two separate areas of tumour specimen, and adding them to get the total Gleason score for the tumour, from 2 to 10. Scores 8-10 suggest an aggressive tumour; 5-7: intermediate; 2-4: indolent. In one recent (provisional) study, 15yr prostate cancer mortality for conservative treatment of PSA-detected cancers was 0-2% for Gleason scores <7, 9-31% for score 7, and 28-72% for scores >7.[217]

Patients with high Gleason scores are more likely to be treated aggressively (eg if younger and/or have higher-stage disease). If 55-59yrs old at diagnosis, the predicted absolute 15yr survival benefit from radical (curative) treatment is about 0, 12, and 26% for Gleason scores <7, 7, and >7, respectively.[218]

Benign diseases of the penis

Balanitis Acute inflammation of the foreskin and glans. Associated with strep and staph infections. More common in diabetics. Often seen in young children with tight foreskins *Rx:* Antibiotics, circumcision, hygiene advice

Phimosis The foreskin occludes the meatus. In young boys this causes recurrent balanitis and ballooning but time (+ trials of gentle retraction) may obviate the need for circumcision. In adulthood presents with painful intercourse, infection, ulceration and is associated with balanitis xerotica obliterans.

Paraphimosis Occurs when a tight foreskin is retracted and becomes irreplaceable, preventing venous return leading to oedema and even ischaemia of the glans. Can occur if the foreskin is not replaced after catheterisation. ►► *Rx:* Ask patient to squeeze glans. Try applying a 50% dextrose soaked swab (oedema may follow osmotic gradient). Ice packs and lignocaine jelly may also help. May require aspiration/dorsal slit/circumcision

Prostatitis

May be acute or chronic, usually those >35yrs. Caused mostly by *S. faecalis* & *E. coli*, also chlamydia (previously TB). ***Features:*** UTIs, retention, pain, haematospermia, swollen/boggy prostate on PR. *Rx:* Analgesia, levofloxacin 500mg/24h PO for 28d.

Bladder tumours

What appear as benign papillomata rarely behave in a purely benign way. They are almost certainly indolent transitional cell (urothelial) malignancies. Adenocarcinomas and squamous cell carcinomas are rare in the West (the latter may follow schistosomiasis). UK incidence ≈ 1:5000/yr. ♂:♀ ≈ 4:1. Histology is important for prognosis: **Grade 1**—differentiated; **Grade 2**—intermediate; **Grade 3**—poorly differentiated. 80% are confined to bladder mucosa, and only ~20% penetrate muscle (increasing mortality to 50% at 5yrs).

Presentation Painless haematuria; recurrent UTIs; voiding irritability.

Associations Smoking; aromatic amines (rubber industry); chronic cystitis; schistosomiasis (↑risk of squamous cell carcinoma); pelvic irradiation.

Tests
- Urine: microscopy/cytology (cancers may cause sterile pyuria).
- IVU may show filling defects ± ureteric involvement.
- Cystoscopy with biopsy is diagnostic.
- Bimanual EUA helps assess spread.
- CT/MRI or lymphangiography may show involved pelvic nodes.

Staging: See TABLE.

Treatment of transitional cell carcinoma (TCC) of the bladder
- *Tis/Ta/T1:* (80% of all patients.) Diathermy via transurethral cystoscopy/transurethral resection of bladder tumour (TURBT). Consider intravesical chemotherapeutic agents (eg ***mitomycin C***) for multiple small tumours or high-grade tumours. Immunotherapy with intravesical *BCG* (which stimulates a non-specific immune response) is useful in high-grade tumours and carcinoma *in situ*, and may be better at preventing tumour progression than **mitomycin C** in superficial disease.[219] 5yr survival ≈ 95%.
- *T2–3:* Radical cystectomy is the 'gold standard'. Radiotherapy gives worse 5yr survival rates than surgery, but preserves the bladder. 'Salvage' cystectomy can be performed if radiotherapy fails, but yields worse results than primary surgery. Post-op chemotherapy (eg M-VAC: ***methotrexate***, ***vinblastine***, ***adriamycin***, and ***cisplatin***) is toxic but effective, and there may also be a role for neoadjuvant chemotherapy.[220] Methods to preserve the bladder with transurethral resection/partial cystectomy + systemic chemotherapy have been tried, but long-term results are disappointing. If the bladder neck is not involved, orthotopic reconstruction rather than forming a urostoma is an option (both using ~40cm of the patient's ileum), but adequate tumour clearance must not be compromised. ►The patient should have all these options explained by a urologist and an oncologist.
- *T4:* Usually palliative chemo/radiotherapy. Chronic catheterization and urinary diversions may help to relieve pain.

Follow-up History, examination, and regular cystoscopy: • ***High-risk tumours:*** Every 3 months for 2yrs, then every 6 months; • ***Low-risk tumours:*** First follow-up cystoscopy after 9 months, then yearly.

Tumour spread Local → to pelvic structures; lymphatic → to iliac and para-aortic nodes; haematogenous → to liver and lungs.

Survival This depends on age at surgery. For example, the 3yr survival after cystectomy for T2 and T3 tumours is 60% if 65–75yrs old, falling to 40% if 75–82yrs old (in whom the operative mortality is 4%). With unilateral pelvic node involvement, only 6% of patients survive 5yrs. The 3yr survival with bilateral or para-aortic node involvement is nil.

Complications: Cystectomy can result in sexual and urinary malfunction. Massive bladder haemorrhage may complicate treatment; consider ***alum*** solution bladder irrigation (safer than formalin): it is an in-patient procedure.[221]

TNM staging of bladder cancer

Tis	Carcinoma *in situ*	Not felt at EUA
Ta	Tumour confined to epithelium	Not felt at EUA
T1	Tumour in lamina propria	Not felt at EUA
T2	Superficial muscle involved	Rubbery thickening at EUA
T3	Deep muscle involved	EUA: mobile mass
T4	Invasion beyond bladder	EUA: fixed mass

EUA = examination under anaesthetic

Is asymptomatic microscopic haematuria significant?

Dipstick tests are often done routinely for new admissions. If microscopic haematuria is found, but the patient has no related symptoms, what does this mean? Before rushing into a barrage on investigations, consider:

- One study found incidence of urogenital disease (eg bladder cancer) was no higher in those with asymptomatic microhaematuria than in those without.[222]
- Asymptomatic microscopic haematuria is the sole presenting feature in only 4% of bladder cancers, and there is no evidence that these are less advanced than malignancies presenting with macroscopic haematuria.
- When monitoring those with treated bladder cancer for recurrence, microscopic haematuria tests have a sensitivity of only 31% in those with superficial bladder malignancy, in whom detection would be most useful.
- Although 80% of those with flank pain due to a renal stone have microscopic haematuria, so do 50% of those with flank pain but no stone.[223]

The conclusion is not that urine dipstick testing is useless, but that results should not be interpreted in isolation. Take a holistic view. Smokers and those with +ve family history for urothelial cancer may be investigated differently from those with no risk factors (eg ultrasound, cystoscopy ± referral to a renal physician in some patients), but in a young fit athlete, the diagnosis is more likely to be exercise-induced haematuria.[224] Wise doctors liaise with their patients. "Shall we let sleeping dogs lie?" is a reasonable question for **some** patients. Give the facts and let him decide, reserving to yourself the right to present the facts in certain ways, depending on your instincts, and those of a trusted colleague. Remember that medicine is for gamblers (p672), and wise gamblers assess the odds against a shifting set of circumstances.

►Think twice before inserting a urinary catheter.
►Carry out rectal examination to exclude faecal impaction.
►Is the bladder palpable after voiding (retention with overflow)?
►Is there neurological co-morbidity: eg MS; Parkinson's disease; stroke; spinal trauma?

Anyone might 'wet themselves' on a long coach ride (we all would if it was long enough). Don't think of people as either dry or incontinent but as incontinent in some circumstances. Attending to these is as important as focusing on the physiology. Get good at treating incontinence and you will do wonders for quality of life.

Incontinence in men Enlargement of the prostate is the major cause of incontinence: urge incontinence (see below) or dribbling may result from the partial retention of urine. TURP & other pelvic surgery may weaken the bladder sphincter and cause incontinence. Troublesome incontinence needs specialist assessment.

Incontinence in women (See also **Voiding difficulty**, *OHCS* p307.)

- *Functional incontinence,* ie when physiological factors are relatively unimportant. The patient is 'caught short' and too slow in finding the toilet because of immobility or unfamiliar surroundings, for example.
- *Stress incontinence:* Leakage from an incompetent sphincter, eg when intra-abdominal pressure rises (eg coughing, laughing). There may be slippage of the proximal ⅓ of the urethra and the bladder neck out of the abdominal cavity. Increasing age and obesity are risk factors. The key to diagnosis is the loss of small (but often frequent) amounts of urine when coughing etc. Examine for pelvic floor weakness/prolapse.[225] Look for cough leak on standing and with full bladder. Stress incontinence is common in pregnancy and following birth. It occurs to some degree in ~50% of post-menopausal women. In elderly women, pelvic floor weakness, eg with uterine prolapse or urethrocele (*OHCS* p290) is the chief cause.
- *Urge incontinence/overactive bladder syndrome* is the main type seen in hospital. The urge to urinate is quickly followed by uncontrollable and sometimes complete emptying of the bladder as detrusor contracts. Large amounts of urine flow down the legs. Urgency/leaking is precipitated by: arriving home (latchkey incontinence, a conditioned reflex); cold; the sound of running water; coffee, tea or cola in the diet (may cause leak without urgency); obesity. Δ: urodynamic studies. Cause: detrusor instability, eg from central inhibitory pathway malfunction or sensitisation of peripheral afferent terminals in the bladder or bladder muscle problem. Check for organic brain damage (eg stroke; Parkinson's; dementia). Other causes: urinary infection; diabetes; diuretics; 'senile' vaginitis; urethritis.

In both sexes incontinence may result from diminished awareness due to confusion or sedation. Occasionally incontinence may be purposeful (eg preventing admission to an old people's home) or due to anger.

Management *Check for:* UTI; DM; diuretic use; faecal impaction; palpable bladder; GFR.

Stress incontinence: Pelvic floor exercises may help. Intravaginal electrical stimulation may also be effective, but is not acceptable to many women. A ring pessary may help uterine prolapse, eg while awaiting surgical repair. *Duloxetine* 40mg/12h PO is a new treatment; the main SE is nausea.[226] Surgical options include **Burch colposuspension** and **sling procedures.**[227] A variety of minimal access techniques (eg tension-free vaginal tape) are also available. *Urge incontinence:* The patient (or carer) should complete an 'incontinence' chart for 3 days to define the pattern of incontinence. Examine for spinal cord and CNS signs (including cognitive test, p70 & p85); and for vaginitis—treat with *estriol* 0.1% cream (eg Ovestin®, 1 applicator dose twice-weekly for a few months)—consider cyclical *progesterone* if for prolonged use and no hysterectomy, to avoid risk of uterine cancer. Bladder training[1] (may include pelvic floor exercises) and weight loss are important. Drugs may help reduce night-time incontinence (see BOX) but can be disappointing. Consider aids (absorbent pad; Paul's tubing if ♂).

►Do urodynamic assessment (cystometry & urine flow rate measurement) before any surgical intervention to exclude detrusor instability or sphincter dyssynergia.

Managing detrusor instability

Agents for detrusor instability	Symptoms which are improved
Antimuscarinics: *eg tolterodine* 1-2mg/12h PO; SE: dry mouth, eyes/skin, drowsiness, constipation, tachycardia, abdominal pain, urinary retention, sinusitis, oedema, weight↑, glaucoma precipitation.[228] Up to 4mg/12 may be needed (unlicensed).[229]	Frequency, urgency. Alternatives: *solifenacin* 5mg/24h (max 10mg); *oxybutynin*, but more SE unless transdermal route or modified release used; *trospium* or *fesoterodine* (prefers M3 receptors).[230] Avoid in myasthenia, and if glaucoma or UC are uncontrolled.
Imipramine 50mg PO at night	Nocturia, enuresis, coital incontinence
Oestrogens	Post-menopausal urgency, frequency + nocturia may occasionally be improved by raising the bladder's sensory threshold.
Surgery, eg clam ileocystoplasty	Reserved for troublesome or intractable symptoms. The bladder is bisected, opened like a clam, and 25cm of ileum is sewn in.
Neuromodulation via transcutaneous electrical stimulation[231]	(Stimulates afferent nerve fibres to modulate bladder reflexes, suppressing involuntary detrusor contractions.)
Modulation of afferent input from bladder	Gabapentin (unlicensed).[232]
Hypnosis, psychotherapy, bladder training[1]	(These all require good motivation.)

NB: *desmopressin* nasal spray 20μg as a night-time dose has a role in ↓urine production, but is unsuitable if elderly (SE: fluid retention, heart failure, Na^+↓).

A reminder about urinary symptoms

See also p64

Filling/storage symptoms
- Nocturia
- Urgency
- Urge incontinence
- Frequency

Voiding symptoms
- Poor stream ± terminal dribbling
- Strangury
- Hesitancy
- *Pis en deux*=going twice.

Not all male storage and voiding symptoms are prostate-related!

Detrusor overactivity Men get this as well as women.[233] See above. Pressure-flow studies help diagnose this (as does detrusor thickness ≥2.9mm on US).[234]

Primary bladder neck obstruction[235] is a condition in which the bladder neck does not open properly during voiding. Studies in men and women with voiding dysfunction show that it is common. The cause may be muscular or neurological dysfunction or fibrosis. *Diagnosis:* Video-urodynamics, with simultaneous pressure-flow measurement, and visualization of the bladder neck during voiding. *Treatment:* Watchful waiting; α-blockers (p644); surgery.[236]

Urethral stricture This may follow trauma or infection (eg gonorrhoea)—and frequently leads to voiding symptoms, UTI, or retention. Malignancy is a rare cause. *Imaging:* Retrograde urethrogram or antegrade cystourethrogram if the patient has an existing suprapubic catheter. *Internal urethrotomy* involves incising the stricture transurethrally using endoscopic equipment—to release scar tissue. The expectation is that epithelialization ends before wound contraction still further reduces the urethral diameter.[237] *Stents* incorporate themselves into the wall of the urethra and keep the lumen open. They work best for short strictures in the bulbar urethra (anterior urethral anatomy, from distal to proximal: meatus←fossa navicularis←penile or pendulous urethra←bulbar urethra←posterior urethra (membranous urethra←prostatic urethra).

1 Mind-over-bladder: • Void when you DON'T have urge; DON'T go to the bathroom when you do have urge • Gradually extend the time between voiding • Schedule your trips to toilet • Stretch your bladder to normal capacity • When urge comes, calm down and make it go using *mind over bladder* tricks.

►Scrotal lump = cancer until proved otherwise.
►Acute, tender enlargement of testis = torsion (p654) until proved otherwise

Diagnosing scrotal masses (figs 2, 3):
1 *Can you get above it?* 2 *Is it separate from the testis?* 3 *Cystic/solid (transluminates)?*

- Cannot get above ≈ inguinoscrotal hernia (p616) or hydrocele extending proximally
- Separate and cystic ≈ epididymal cyst.
- Separate and solid ≈ epididymitis/orchitis/ varicocele
- Testicular and cystic ≈ hydrocele

► Testicular and solid—**tumour**, orchitis, haematocele, granuloma (p186), gumma (p431). USS may help (**fig 1**).

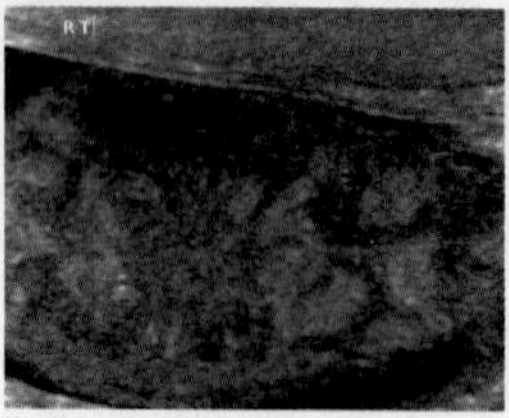

Fig 1. USS testis. Heterogeneity suggests tumour (ΔΔ: chronic inflammation). Courtesy of Norwich Radiology Department

Epididymal cysts usually develop in adulthood and contain clear or milky (spermatocele) fluid. They lie above and behind the testis. Remove if symptomatic.

Hydroceles (fluid within the tunica vaginalis). *Primary* (associated with a patent processus vaginalis, which typically resolves during the 1st year of life) or *secondary* to testis tumour/trauma/infection. Primary hydroceles are more common, larger, and usually in younger men. Can resolve spontaneously. ℞: aspiration (may need repeating) or surgery: plicating the tunica vaginalis (Lord's repair)/ inverting the sac (Jaboulay's repair) ►Is the testis normal after aspiration? If *any* doubt, do USS.

Epididymo-orchitis *Causes*: *Chlamydia* (eg if >35yrs); *E. coli*; mumps; *N. gonorrhoea*; TB. *Features:* Sudden onset tender swelling, dysuria, sweats/fever. Take urine sample; look for urethral discharge. '1st catch' may be more helpful than an MSU. Consider STI screen. Warn of possible infertility[238] & symptoms worsening before improving. ℞: If <35yrs; *doxycycline* 100mg/12h PO for 10d (covers chlamydia; treat sexual partners).[239] If >35yrs old, associated UTI is common so try *ciprofloxacin* 300mg/12h PO for 10d.[240] Also: analgesia, bed rest, scrotal support, drainage of any abscess.

Varicocele Dilated veins of pampiniform plexus. Left side more commonly affected. Often visible as distended scrotal blood vessels that feel like 'a bag of worms'. Patient may complain of dull ache. Associated with subfertility, but repair (via surgery or embolization) seems to have little effect on subsequent pregnancy rates.

Haematocele Blood in tunica vaginalis, follows trauma, may need drainage/ excision

Testis tumours Commonest malignancies in ♂ aged 15–44. *Varieties:* Seminoma (30–65yrs);[241] teratoma (20-30yrs); tumours of Sertoli (→ oestrogens) or Leydig cells (→ androgens); lymphoma. ~10% of malignancies occur in undescended testes, even after orchidopexy. A contralateral tumour is found in 5%. *Presentation:* Typically painless testicular lump, noticed after trauma/infection, may also present with haematospermia, secondary hydrocele, pain, SOB (lung mets), abdominal mass (enlarged lymph nodes), or effects of secreted hormones. *Risk factors:* Undescended testis; infant hernia; infertility. *Staging* **1** No evidence of metastasis. **2** Infradiaphragmatic node involvement (spread via the para-aortic nodes **not** inguinal nodes). **3** Supradiaphragmatic node involvement. **4** Lung involvement (haematogenous). *Tests:* (allow staging) CXR, CT, excision biopsy. α-fetoprotein (eg >3iu/mL)[1] and β-human chorionic gonadotrophin (β-hCG) are useful tumour markers and help monitor treatment; check **before** & **during** treatment. ℞: Orchidectomy (inguinal incision; occlude the spermatic cord before mobilization to ↓risk of intra-operative spread). Options are constantly updated (surgery, radiotherapy, chemotherapy). Seminomas are exquisitely radiosensitive. Stage I seminomas: orchidectomy + radiotherapy cures ~95%. Do close follow-up to detect relapse. Cure of teratomas, even if metastases are present, is achieved by 3-4 cycles of *bleomycin* + *etoposide* + *cisplatin*. Prevention of late presentation: self-examination. 5yr survival >90% in all groups.

1 AFP is **not** ↑ in pure seminoma; may also be ↑ in: hepatitis, cirrhosis, liver cancer, open neural tube defect.

Diagnosing groin lumps: lateral to medial thinking

- Psoas abscess—may present with back pain, limp and swinging pyrexia
- Neuroma of the femoral nerve
- Femoral artery aneurysm
- Saphena varix—like a hernia, it has a cough impulse
- Lymph node
- Femoral hernia
- Inguinal hernia
- Hydrocele or varicocele
- Also consider an undescended testis (cryptorchidism)

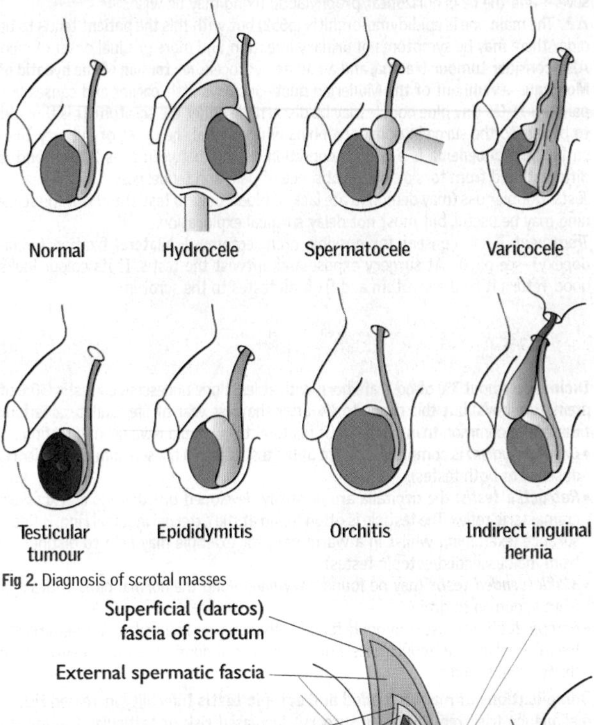

Fig 2. Diagnosis of scrotal masses

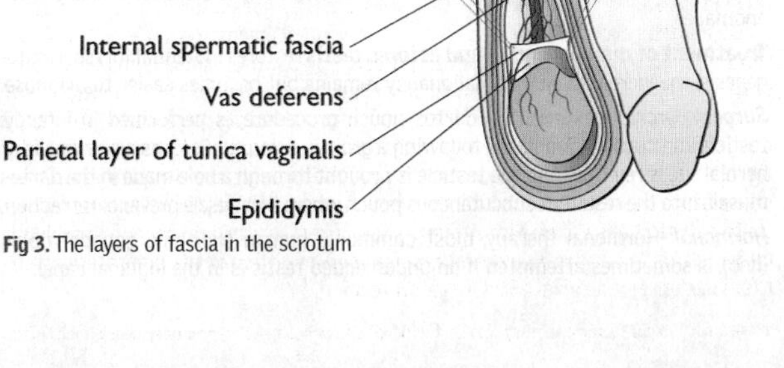

Fig 3. The layers of fascia in the scrotum

The aim is to recognize this condition before the cardinal signs and symptoms are fully manifest, as prompt surgery saves testes.

▸**If in any doubt, surgery is required**.

Symptoms: Sudden onset of pain in one testis, which makes walking uncomfortable. Pain in the abdomen, nausea, and vomiting are common.

Signs: Inflammation of one testis—it is tender, hot, and swollen. The testis may lie high and transversely. Torsion may occur at any age but is most common at 11-30yrs. With **intermittent torsion** the pain may have passed on presentation, but if it was severe, and the lie is horizontal, prophylactic fixing may be wise.[242]

ΔΔ: The main one is epididymo-orchitis (p652) but with this the patient tends to be older, there may be symptoms of urinary infection, and more gradual onset of pain. Also consider tumour, trauma, and an acute hydrocele. **NB: torsion of the hydatid of Morgagni**—a remnant of the Müllerian duct—occurs a little earlier, and causes less pain (**fig 1**). Its tiny blue nodule may be discernible under the scrotum. It is thought to be due to the surge in gonadotrophins which signal the onset of puberty. **Idiopathic scrotal oedema** is a benign condition usually between ages 2-10yrs, and is differentiated from torsion by the absence of pain and tenderness.

Tests: Doppler USS (may demonstrate lack of blood flow to testis) and isotope scanning may be useful, but must not delay surgical exploration.

Treatment: ▸Ask consent for possible orchidectomy + **bilateral** fixation (orchidopexy)—see p570. At surgery expose and untwist the testis. If its colour looks good, return it to the scrotum and fix **both** testes to the scrotum

Undescended testes

Incidence About 3% of boys are born with at least one undescended testis (30% of premature boys) but this drops to 1% after the first year of life. Unilateral is four times more common than bilateral. (If bilateral then should have genetic testing).

- *Cryptorchidism* is complete absence of the testicle from the scrotum (anorchism is absence of both testes).
- *Retractile testis***:** the genitalia are normally developed but there is an excessive cremasteric reflex. The testicle is often found at the external inguinal ring. ℞ Reassurance (examining whilst in a warm bath for example may help to distinguish from maldescended/ectopic testes).
- *Maldescended testis* may be found anywhere along the normal path of descent from abdomen to groin.
- *Ectopic testis* is most commonly found in the superior inguinal pouch (anterior to the external oblique aponeurosis) but may also be abdominal, perineal, penile and in the femoral triangle

Complications of maldescended and ectopic testis Infertility, increased risk of malignancy (risk remains after surgery), increased risk of testicular trauma, increased risk of testicular torsion, associated with hernias (90%) or urinary tract anomalies.

Treatment of maldescended and ectopic testis restores (potential for) spermatogenesis; the increased risk of malignancy remains but becomes easier to diagnose.

Surgery: Orchidopexy, usually dartos pouch procedure, is performed in infancy: testicle and cord are mobilised following a groin incision, any processus vaginalis or hernial sac is removed and the testicle is brought through a hole made in the dartos muscle into the resultant subcutaneous pouch where the muscle prevents retraction.

Hormonal: Hormonal therapy, most commonly human chorionic gonadotrophin (HCG), is sometimes attempted if an undescended testis is in the inguinal canal.

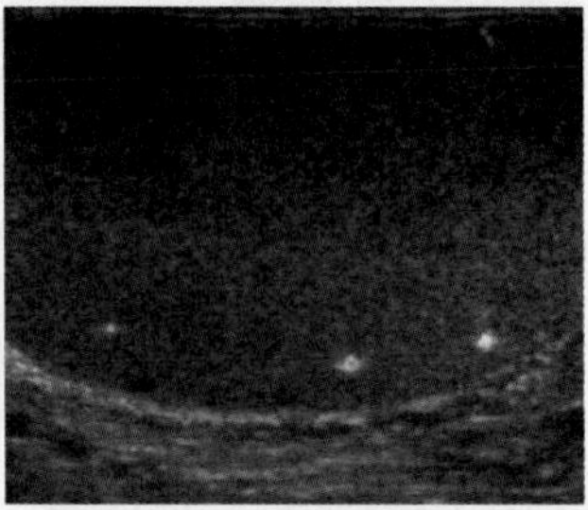

Fig 1. Ultrasound of the testis showing microlithiasis—the focal areas of reflectivity within the parenchyma of the testis. It is unknown (and difficult to prove) whether this condition is linked to an increased risk of malignancy.

Torsion of a hydatid of Morgagni would appear as a focal area of low reflectivity at the superior pole separate from the normal head of the epididymis.

Image courtesy of Norwich Radiology Dept.

Testicular self-examination: advice for patients (& male readers)

Why? Cancers which are detected early are the most easily treated so it makes sense to check yourself regularly. It will help you know what is normal for you and enable you to detect changes.

When? Regularly; at least once a month. Ideally in the shower/bath when the muscle in the scrotum is relaxed.

How?

- Gently feel each testicle individually. You should feel a soft tube at the top and back of the testicle. This is the epididymis which carries and stores sperm. It may feel slightly tender. Don't confuse it with an abnormal lump. You should be able to feel the firm, smooth tube of the spermatic cord which runs up from the epididymis.
- Feel the testicle itself. It should be smooth with no lumps or swellings. It is unusual to develop cancer in both testicles at the same time, so if you are wondering whether a testicle is feeling normal or not you can compare it with the other.
- Remember—if you do notice a change in size/weight or find any abnormal lumps or swellings in your testicle, make an appointment and have it checked by your doctor as soon as possible
- Note—most abnormalities are not cancer but collections of fluid, infection, or cysts. Cancer usually starts as a small hard painless lump. Even if it is cancer, treatment is often effective. In more than 9 in 10 cases, treatment can result in a complete cure. However, the earlier it is detected the easier it is to treat. More than a third of people with this cancer consult their doctor after the cancer has spread, which makes treatment more difficult. Often this is because of unfounded fears, or just hoping it will go away

Adapted from www.cancerhelp.org.uk
Also see "Don't just scratch 'em" leaflet from www.actioncancer.org

▸▸ Aneurysms of arteries

Typical causes
• Atheroma • Trauma • Infection eg mycotic aneurysm in endocarditis, tertiary syphilis (esp. thoracic aneurysms) • Connective tissue disorders (eg Marfan's, Ehlers-Danlos) • Inflammatory eg Takayasu's aortitis

An aneurysm is a >150% dilatation of its original diameter; remember this is an ongoing process. *True* aneurysms are abnormal dilatations of arteries that involve all layers of the wall. *False* aneurysms (pseudo-aneurysms) are collections of blood around a vessel wall (eg after trauma) communicating with the lumen. Aneurysms may be fusiform (eg AAA or sac-like (eg Berry aneurysms; p483, **fig 2**)).

Common sites Aorta (infrarenal most common), iliac, femoral & popliteal arteries.

Complications Rupture; thrombosis; embolism; fistulae; pressure on other structures.

Ruptured abdominal aortic aneurysm (AAA) Death rates/year from ruptured AAAs rise with age: 125/million in those aged 55–59; 2728/million if over 85yrs. *Symptoms & signs:* Intermittent or continuous abdominal pain (radiates to back, iliac fossae, or groins—▸don't dismiss this as renal colic), collapse, an **expansile** abdominal mass (it expands and contracts: swellings that are pulsatile just transmit the pulse, eg nodes overlying arteries), and shock. If in doubt, assume a ruptured aneurysm. *Prevention:* Treat BP. ***Regular universal ultrasound*** for men ≥65yrs. See BOX.

Unruptured AAA *Definition:* >3cm across. ***Prevalence:*** 3% of those >50yrs. ♂:♀ >3:1. *Less* common in diabetics. ***Cause:*** Degeneration of elastic lamellae and smooth muscle loss.[243] There is a genetic component. ***Symptoms:*** Often none, they **may** cause abdominal/back pain, often discovered incidentally on abdominal examination (see BOX). ***Monitoring:*** The UK Small Aneurysm Trial suggested aneurysms <5.5cm might safely be monitored by regular examination and ultrasound/CT,[244] though endovascular repair for these may be better than surveillance.[245] Risk of rupture below this size is <1%/yr, compared to ~25%/yr for aneurysms >6cm across. ~75% of aneurysms so monitored eventually need repair. Rupture is more likely if: • BP↑ • Smoker • Female • Strong family history. Modify risk factors if possible at diagnosis. ***Elective surgery:*** Reserve for aneurysms ≥5cm[246] or expanding at >1cm/yr, or symptomatic aneurysms. Operative mortality: ~5%; complications include spinal or mesenteric ischaemia and distal trash from dislodged thrombus debris.[247] Studies show that age >80yrs is **not** a reason to decline surgery. ***Stenting (EVAR):*** Big operations can be avoided by inserting an endovascular stent via the femoral artery. Failure of the stent-graft to totally exclude blood flow to the aneurysm sac may occur—'endoleak'. When successfully positioned, such stents can lead to a shorter hospital stay and fewer transfusions than with conventional surgery, but see **fig 1** & footnote.

▸▸ Thoracic aortic dissection

Blood splits the aortic media with sudden tearing chest pain (± radiation to back). As the dissection unfolds, branches of the aorta occlude sequentially leading to hemiplegia (carotid artery), unequal arm pulses and BP or acute limb ischaemia, paraplegia (anterior spinal artery), and anuria (renal arteries). Aortic incompetence and inferior MI may develop if dissection moves proximally. *Type A* (70%) dissections involve the ascending aorta, irrespective of site of the tear, whilst if the ascending aorta is not involved it is called *type B* (30%) **▸▸All patients with type A thoracic dissection should be considered for surgery: get urgent cardiothoracic advice.** Definitive treatment for type B is less clear, may be managed medically, surgery reserved for distal dissections that are leaking, ruptured, or compromising vital organs ***Management:*** • Crossmatch 10U blood; ECG & CXR (expanded mediastinum is rare). • CT/MRI or transoesophageal echocardiography (TOE).[248] Take to ITU; hypotensives: keep systolic at ~100–110mmHg: **labetalol** (p134) or **esmolol** (p120; $t_{1/2}$ is ultra-short) by IVI is helpful here (calcium channel blockers may be used if β-blockers contraindicated). Acute operative mortality: <25%.

Emergency management of a ruptured abdominal aneurysm

Mortality—treated: 41% and improving; untreated: ~100%.[249]
- ⏩Summon a vascular surgeon and an experienced anaesthetist; warn theatre.
- ⏩Do an ECG, and take blood for amylase, Hb, crossmatch (10-40U may eventually be needed). Catheterize the bladder.
- ⏩Put up 2 large IVIs. Treat shock with ORh−ve blood (if desperate), but keep systolic BP ≤100mmHg (NB: **raised** BP is common early on).
- ⏩Take the patient straight to theatre. Don't waste time on X-rays: fatal delay may result, though CT can help in a stable patient with an uncertain diagnosis.
- ⏩Give prophylactic antibiotics eg *cefuroxime* 1.5g + *metronidazole* 500mg IV.
- ⏩Surgery involves clamping the aorta above the leak, and inserting a Dacron® graft (eg 'tube graft' or, if significant iliac aneurysm also, a 'trouser graft' with each 'leg' attached to an iliac artery).

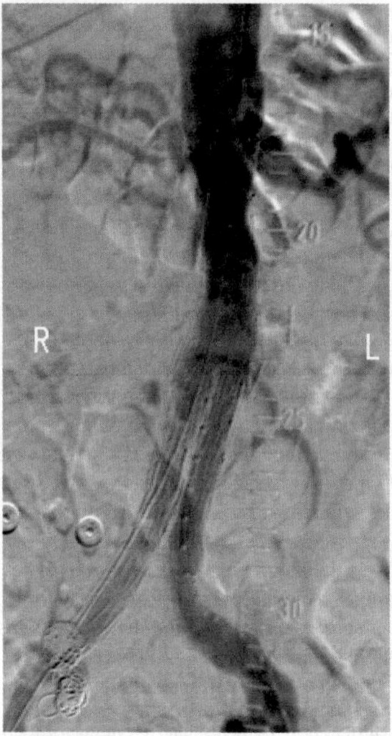

Fig 1. Stenting: not an open or closed case...this is a digital subtraction angiogram showing correct positioning of an endovascular stent at the end of the procedure. Although less invasive than open repair, many are unsuited to this method, owing to the anatomy of their aneurysm. Lifelong monitoring is needed: stents may leak and the aneurysm progress (the risk can be reduced by coiling the internal iliac arteries, as shown).[250]

Figure courtesy of Norwich Radiology Dept.

The bomb inside you?!

A wise doctor might reframe a patient's fear of unexploded bomb inside them to deepen their view of his or her own health: health is not simply a question of being of sound body and mind, but entails a process of adaptation to changing environments, to growing up, to ageing, and to healing when damaged (*OHCS*, p470).

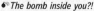

▸▸ Limb ischaemia

Acute ischaemia—See EMERGENCY BOX

Chronic ischaemia This is 'always' due to atherosclerosis (fibromuscular dysplasia and vasculitis are very rare). Its chief feature is intermittent claudication.

Symptoms Cramping pain is felt in the calf, thigh, or buttock after walking for a fairly fixed distance (the **claudication distance**) and relieved by rest (calf claudication suggests femoral disease while buttock claudication suggests iliac disease). Ulceration, gangrene (p662), and foot pain **at rest**—eg burning pain at night relieved by hanging legs over side of bed—are the cardinal features of *critical ischaemia*. Buttock claudication ± impotence imply Leriche's syndrome (p718). Young, heavy smokers are at risk from Buerger's disease (thromboangiitis obliterans, p710).[251]

Fontaine classification: **1** Asymptomatic **2** Intermittent claudication **3** Ischaemic rest pain **4** Ulceration/gangrene (critical ischaemia).

Signs*:* Absent pulses; cold, white leg(s); atrophic skin; punched out ulcers (often painful); postural/dependent colour change; a vascular (Buerger's) angle[1] of <20° and capillary filling time >15s are found in severe ischaemia.

Tests*:* Exclude DM, arteritis (ESR/CRP). FBC (anaemia, infection); U&E (renal disease); lipids (dyslipidaemia); syphilis serology; ECG (cardiac ischaemia). Check platelets, clotting, do group & save if planning arteriography. *Ankle–brachial Pressure Index (ABPI):* Normal ≥ 1. Claudication ≈ 0.9–0.6. Rest pain ≈ 0.3–0.6. Impending gangrene ≤0.3 or ankle systolic pressure <50mmHg. Beware falsely high results from incompressible vessels in severe atherosclerosis, DM, CRF. Do *contrast arteriography, digital subtraction arteriography (DSA,* **fig 2***)* or *colour duplex imaging* to assess extent and location of stenoses and quality of distal vessels (*'run-off'*). Stop *metformin* before angiography to avoid metabolic acidosis. *MR angiography* has a developing role (p749).[252] If only distal obliterative disease seen, and little proximal atheroma, suspect arteritis, previous embolus, or DM.

℞ *Conservative measures*—ie exercise, quit smoking, ↓weight.[253] ~⅓ of claudicants improve with exercise, ⅓ remain the same, and ⅓ deteriorate. Results may be better with a supervised exercise programme.[254] Mainstay of treatment is energetic risk factor reduction: encourage cessation of smoking, and treat diabetes, hypertension (avoid β-blockers) and dyslipidaemia. Antiplatelet agents have a role (usually *aspirin*).

Percutaneous transluminal angioplasty (PTA) is good for short stenoses in big arteries (a balloon is inflated in the narrowed segment). Stents maintain artery patency after angioplasty, and are beneficial for iliac artery disease.

Surgical reconstruction If atheromatous disease is extensive but distal run-off is good (ie distal arteries filled by collateral vessels), he may be a candidate for arterial reconstruction by a bypass graft. Procedures include above knee femoral-popliteal bypass, femoral-femoral crossover and aorto-bifemoral bypass grafts. Vein grafts are often used but prosthetic grafts (eg polytetrafluoroethylene, PTFE) are an option.[255] *Aspirin* helps prosthetic grafts to remain patent; *warfarin* may be better after vein grafts and in high-risk patients.[256]

Sympathectomy (chemical or surgical) may help relieve rest pain if revascularization is impossible. It may not be wise in diabetic patients with neuropathy.

Amputation may relieve intractable pain and death from sepsis and gangrene. A decision to amputate must be made by the patient, usually against a background of failed alternative strategies. The level of amputation must be high enough to ensure healing of the stump. Above knee amputation (AKA) tends to heal better, but has worse rehabilitation potential, whereas the reverse is true of below knee amputation (BKA). Having to perform the above knee procedure can also be the herald of a much poorer overall prognosis—the 5-yr survival for AKA in one retrospective study was 22.5% compared to 37.8% for BKA.[257] Rehabilitation should be started early with a view to limb fitting. *Gabapentin* (regimen on p508) can be used to treat the gruelling post-operative complication of phantom limb pain.[258] It may be more effective if started prior to surgery. *Diabetes & amputations*: see p204.

1 Leg goes pale when raised eg by 20° off the couch; compare sides

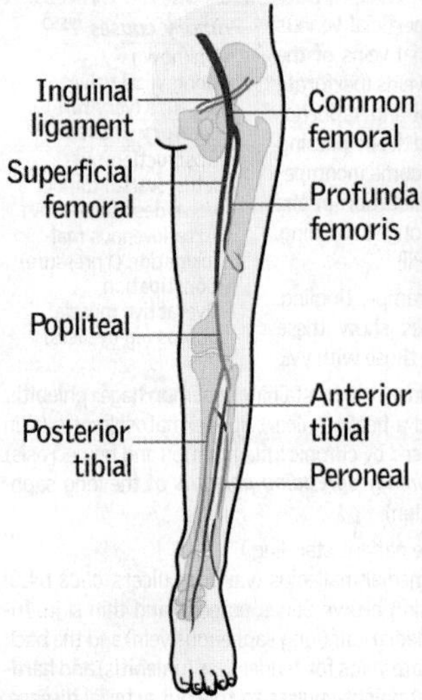

Fig 1.
Leg arteries

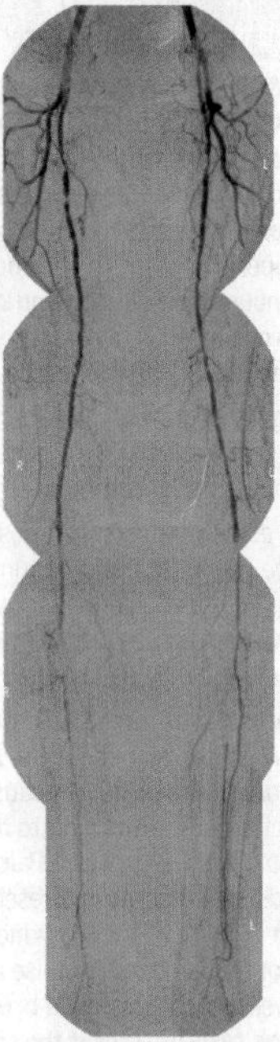

Fig 2. Digital subtraction angiogram (DSA): diffuse bilateral superficial femoral artery disease and an occlusion in the popliteal artery with one vessel run-off on the right. Also only one vessel run-off in the left calf (on right of this image).

Courtesy of Norwich Radiology Department

Acute limb ischaemia

▸▸Surgical emergency requiring revascularisation within 4-6h to save the limb. May be due to thrombosis *in situ* (~40%), emboli (38%), graft/angioplasty occlusion (15%), or trauma. Thrombosis more likely in known 'vasculopaths'; emboli are sudden, eg in those without previous vessel disease; they can effect multiple sites, and there may be a bruit. Mortality: 22%. Amputation rate: 16%.

- *Symptoms & signs:* The part is **p**ale, **p**ulseless, **p**ainful, **p**aralysed, **p**araesthetic, and '**p**erishingly cold'. Onset of fixed mottling implies irreversibility. Emboli commonly arise from the heart (infarcts, AF) or aneurysms. ►Limb may be red, but only when dependent, leading to disastrous misdiagnosis of gout/ cellulitis.
- *Management:* ►This is an emergency and may require urgent open surgery or angioplasty. If diagnosis is in doubt, do urgent arteriography. If the occlusion is embolic, the options are surgical embolectomy (Fogarty catheter) or local thrombolysis, eg *tissue plasminogen activator* (t-PA, p339), balancing the risks of surgery with the haemorrhagic complications of thrombolysis.[259]
- Anticoagulate with *heparin* after either procedure. Later, look for emboli's source: echo; USS of aorta, popliteal and femoral arteries. Ischaemia after trauma and acute thrombosis may needs urgent reconstruction. ►Be aware of possible post-op **reperfusion injury** & subsequent **compartment syndrome**.

Carotid artery disease

Carotid artery disease accounts for 20% of strokes and TIAs. Symptomatic patients with ipsilateral stenosis ≥70% should have ***carotid endarterectomy***.[NASCET trial] (see also p480). ***Complications:*** 7.5% risk of stroke and death within 30 days of endarterectomy.

NB: there is no benefit to treating completely occluded vessels.

Primary causes (95%)
• Unknown • Congenital valve absence (very rare)
Secondary causes (5%)
• Obstruction: DVT, fetus, ovarian tumour • Valve destruction: DVT • Arteriovenous malformation (↑pressure) • Constipation • Overactive muscle pumps (eg cyclists)

Long tortuous & dilated veins of the superficial venous system. **Pathology** Blood from superficial veins of the leg passes into deep veins via perforator veins (perforate deep fascia) and at the sapheno-femoral and sapheno-popliteal junctions. Valves prevent blood from passing from deep to superficial veins. If they become incompetent there is venous hypertension and dilatation of the superficial veins occurs. Risk factors: prolonged standing, obesity, pregnancy, family history, & the Pill. 260

Symptoms "My legs are ugly". Pain, cramps, tingling, heaviness, and restless legs. But studies show these symptoms are only slightly commoner in those with VVs.

Signs Oedema; eczema; ulcers; haemosiderin skin staining; haemorrhage; phlebitis; *atrophie blanche* (white scarring around a healing ulcer); lipodermatosclerosis (skin hardness from subcutaneous fibrosis caused by chronic inflammation and fat necrosis). On their own VVs don't cause DVTs (***proximally spreading phlebitis*** of the long saphenous vein in the thigh may be an exception).

Method of examination (Start with the patient standing.)

1 Inspect for: ulcers usually above the medial malleolus (varicose ulcers, *OHCS* p410) with deposition of haemosiderin causing brown edges, eczema, and thin skin. Inspect the legs from anterior thigh to medial calf (long saphenous vein) and the back of the calf (short saphenous vein). Palpate veins for tenderness (phlebitis) and hardness (thrombosis). If ulceration present palpate pulses to rule out arterial disease.

2 Feel for ***cough impulse*** at the SFJ (≈incompetence). ***Percussion test:*** Tap VVs distally and palpate for transmitted impulse at the SFJ (interrupted by competent valves).

3 Auscultate over varicosities for a bruit, indicating arteriovenous malformation.

4 ***Trendelenburg's test*** assesses if the saphenofemoral junction (SFJ) valve is competent: lie the patient down and raise the leg to empty the vein. Place 2 fingers on the SFJ (5cm below and medial to femoral pulse). Ask him to stand keeping the fingers in place. If the varicosities are controlled, they will not rapidly fill. Release the fingers to confirm that they then fill. This shows that there is SF incompetence and the operation of SF disconnection (Trendelenburg's operation) should help. If the varicosities are not controlled, then there must be incompetence at a lower level.

5 ***Tourniquet test*** is similar to Trendelenburg's test, but instead of controlling varicosities with fingers, use a tourniquet tied around the thigh at the level of the SFJ. If the varicosities are not controlled, repeat test with the tourniquet just above, then just below, the knee until the level at which there is incompetence is identified.

6 ***Perthes' test*** determines if the deep femoral veins are competent. With the patient standing and veins filled, a tourniquet is placed around the mid-thigh and the patient walks for 5min. If the saphenous veins collapse below the tourniquet, the deep veins are patent and the communicating veins are competent; if unchanged, both saphenous and communicating veins are incompetent; if the veins increase in prominence and pain occurs, the deep veins are occluded.

7 ***Doppler ultrasound probes*** have overtaken the above tests. They listen for flow in incompetent valves, eg the SFJ, or the short saphenous vein behind the knee (the calf is squeezed: flow on release lasting over ½–1 seconds indicates significant reflux). If incompetence is not identified and treated, varicosities will return.

For completion, examine the abdomen, the pelvis in females and external genitalia in males (for masses).

►Before surgery and after venous mapping, ensure that all varicosities are indelibly marked **to either side** (to avoid tattooing if the incision is made through inked skin).

Saphena varix Dilatation in the saphenous vein at its confluence with the femoral vein (the SFJ). It transmits a cough impulse and may be mistaken for an inguinal or femoral hernia, but on closer inspection it may have a bluish tinge.

The superficial veins of the leg

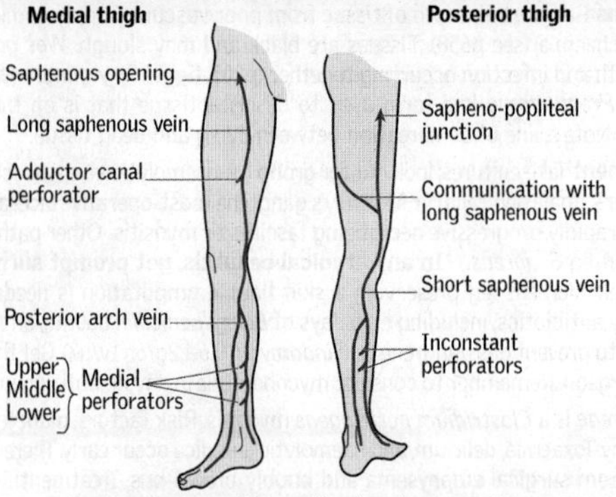

Treating varicose veins

►NICE guidelines suggest that the criteria for specialist referral of patients with VVs should be bleeding, pain, ulceration, superficial thrombophlebitis, or 'a severe impact on quality of life'.

- Treat any underlying cause.
- *Education:* Avoid prolonged standing; support stockings (compliance is a problem); lose weight; regular walks (calf muscle action aids venous return).
- *Injection sclerotherapy:* Especially for varicosities below the knee if there is no gross saphenofemoral incompetence. Sclerosant (eg *ethanolamine*) is injected at multiple sites and the vein compressed for a few weeks to avoid thrombosis (intravascular granulation tissue obliterates the lumen). It is unsuitable for perforation sites. A novel development of this technique involves mixing the sclerosant with air to form a foam that is injected at a single site, and spreads rapidly throughout the veins. Ultrasound monitoring prevents inadvertent spread of foam into the femoral vein.[261]
- *Laser coagulation:* Especially for small varicosities and thread veins.
- *Surgery:* There are several choices, depending on vein anatomy and surgical preference, eg saphenofemoral ligation (Trendelenburg procedure); multiple avulsions; stripping from groin to upper calf (stripping to the ankle is not needed, and may damage the saphenous nerve). ***Post-op:*** Bandage legs tightly, and elevate for 24h. Then encourage regular walking eg 3miles/d, taken as many short walks. Surgery is more effective than sclerotherapy in the long term.[262]

When do varicose veins become an illness?

The obvious answer is that they do so when they hurt, but for some patients, this is too simple. Thanks to Albert Camus, we know that 'certain illnesses are desirable: they provide a compensation for a functional disorder which, in their absence, would express itself in a more serious disturbance'; *this is known to be common with VVs.*[263] Perhaps many opt for surgery as a displacement activity to confronting deeper problems. ►We adopt the sickness role when we want sympathy. Somatization is hard to manage: here is one general approach to consider: Give time; don't dismiss these patients as 'just the "worried well"'.

- Explore the factors perpetuating illness behaviour (disordered physiology, misinformation, unhelpful 'coping' behaviour, social stressors).
- Agree a plan that makes sense to the patient's holistic view of himself.

Treat any underlying depression (drugs & cognitive therapy, *OHCS* p374).

Gangrene and necrotizing fasciitis

Definitions Gangrene is death of tissue from poor vascular supply and is a sign of critical ischaemia (see p658). Tissues are black and may slough. ***Wet gangrene*** is tissue death and infection occurring together (p205, **fig 1**). ***Dry gangrene*** means no infection. ***Pregangrene*** is a term used to describe tissue that is on the brink of gangrene. Note a line of demarcation between living and dead tissue.[1]

Management Take cultures; look out for group A β-haemolytic streptococci—a cause of Fournier's (male genitalia) or Meleney's gangrene (post-operative ulceration), both a form of rapidly progressive necrotizing fasciitis or myositis. Other pathogens can be involved, eg *S. aureus*. ►**In any atypical cellulitis, get prompt surgical help.** Radical debridement (eg preserving a skin flap) ± amputation is needed, always covered by antibiotics, including eg 5 days of ***benzylpenicillin*** 600mg/6h IV starting 1h pre-op, to prevent gas gangrene (± ***clindamycin*** 0.6-1.2g/6h IV/IM). Get the help of a plastic surgeon. Remember to consider mycobacteria in any necrotizing infection.[264]

Gas gangrene is a *Clostridium perfringens* myositis. Risk factors: diabetes; trauma; malignancy. Toxaemia, delirium, and haemolytic jaundice occur early. There is oedema, crepitus from surgical emphysema and bubbly brown pus. Treatment: Remove all dead tissue (eg amputation); ***benzylpenicillin***; ***hyperbaric*** O_2, ***clindamycin*** & ***metronidazole*** have a role.[265]

Skin ulcers

see also *OHCS*, p604

Ulcers are abnormal breaks in an epithelial surface. Leg ulcers affect ~2% in developed countries.

Causes: see MINIBOX– there may be multiple causes. For leg ulcers, venous disease accounts for 70%, mixed arterial and venous disease for 15% and arterial disease alone for 2%. Pressure sores: see **fig 1**, p477.

Causes
• Venous disease
• Arterial disease Large vessel Small vessel
• Neuropathy Diabetes Neuropathic, arterial or both
• Lymphoedema
• Vasculitis
• Malignancy (p598)
• Infection TB, syphilis
• Trauma (pressure)
• Pyoderma gangrenosum
• Drugs

History Ask about number, pain, trauma. Go over co-morbidities—eg varicose veins, peripheral arterial disease, diabetes, vasculitis etc. Is the history long or short? Is the patient taking steroids? Is the patient a bit odd? (remember self-induced ulcers: *dermatitis artefacta*). Has a biopsy been taken?

Examination Note features such as site, number, surface area, depth, edge, base, discharge, lymphadenopathy, sensation, and healing. See BOX. If in the legs, note features of venous insufficiency or arterial disease and if possible, apply a BP cuff to perform ankle–brachial pressure index (ABPI).

Tests Skin and ulcer biopsy may be necessary—eg to assess for vasculitis (will need immunohistopathology) or malignant change in an established ulcer (Marjolin's ulcer). If ulceration is the first presentation of a suspected systemic disorder then further screening tests will be required accordingly.

Management Managing ulcers is often difficult and expensive. Treat the cause(s) and focus on prevention. Optimize nutrition. Are there adverse risk factors (drug addiction, or risk factors for arteriopathy, eg smoking etc)? Get expert nursing care. Consider referral to community nurse, varicose leg ulcer clinic: 'Charing-cross' 4-layer compression bandaging may help (only if arterial pulses OK: ABPI (p658) should be >0.8) and is better than standard bandages. Treating ulcers with systemic antibiotics rarely helps, though topical agents such as ***silver sulfadiazine*** and ***gentamicin*** may be effective.[266]

1 'The first sign of his approaching end was when one of my old aunts, while undressing him, removed a toe with one of his old socks'. Graham Greene, *A Sort of Life*, 1971, Simon & Schuster.

Features of skin ulceration to note on examination

Site Above the medial malleolus is the favourite place for *gravitational ulcers* (mostly related to superficial venous disease, but may reflect venous hypertension via damage to the valves of the deep venous system, eg 2° to DVT). Venous hypertension leads to the development of superficial varicosities and skin changes (*lipodermatosclerosis* = induration, pigmentation, and inflammation of the skin). Minimal trauma to the leg leads to ulceration which often takes many months to heal. Ulcers on the sacrum or greater trochanter, or heel suggest *pressure sores* (*OHCS* p605), particularly if the patient is bed-bound with suboptimal nutrition.

Temperature The ulcer and surrounding tissues are cold in an ischaemic ulcer. If the skin is warm and well perfused then local factors are more likely.

Surface area Draw a map of the area to quantify and time any healing (a wound >4weeks old is a chronic ulcer as distinguished from an acute wound).

Shape Oval, circular (cigarette burns), serpiginous (*granuloma inguinale*, p416); unusual morphology can be secondary to mycobacterial infection, eg cutaneous tuberculosis or scrofuloderma (*tuberculosis colliquativa cutis*, where an infected lymph node ulcerates through to the skin).[267]

Edge Eroded ≈ active and spreading; shelved/sloping ≈ healing; punched-out ≈ syphilis or ischaemic; rolled/everted ≈ malignant; undermined ≈ TB.

Base Any muscle, bone, or tendon destruction (malignancy; pressure sores; ischaemia)? There may be a grey-yellow slough, beneath which is a pale pink base. **Slough** is a mixture of fibrin, cell breakdown products, serous exudate, leucocytes and bacteria—it need not imply infection, and can be part of the normal wound healing process. **Granulation tissue** is a deep pink gel-like matrix contained within a fibrous collagen network and is evidence of a healing wound.

Depth If not uncomfortable for the patient (eg in neuropathic ulceration) a probe can be used gauge how deep the ulceration extends.

Discharge Culture before starting any antibiotics (which usually don't work). A watery discharge is said to favour TB; bleeding can ≈ malignancy.

Associated lymphadenopathy suggests infection or malignancy.

Sensation Decreased sensation around the ulcer implies neuropathy.

Position in phases of extension/healing Healing is heralded by granulation, scar formation, and epithelialization. Inflamed margins ≈ extension.

Contents

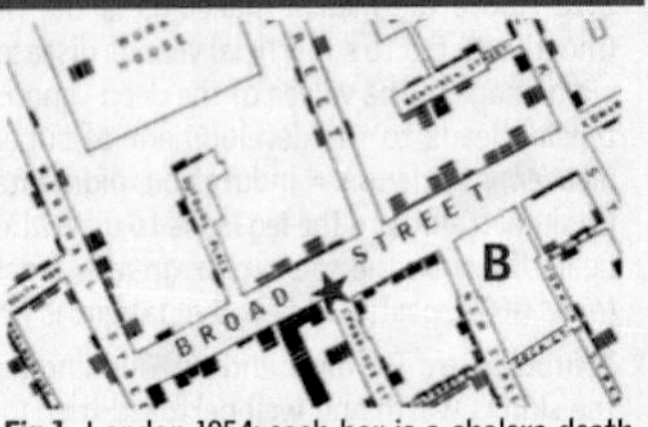

Fig 1. London 1854; each bar is a cholera death. Is the Broad Street pump (★) spreading cholera? But why no deaths at the brewery (B)? John Snow's spine must have tingled (p427) when he found it had its own separate water supply.[1]

Adapted from Snow's map of cholera deaths, 1854.

An example of epidemiology at work

Some decades ago, epidemiologists tested the hypothesis that smoking and hypertension were associated with vascular disease. Painstaking cohort studies confirmed that these were indeed ***risk markers*** (a term that does *not* imply causality). Over the years, as evidence accumulates, the term 'risk marker' may upgrade to ***risk factor***, which *does* imply causation, and the separate idea that risk-factor modification will cause a reduction in disease. Demonstrating a dose-response relationship (with the correct time sequence) is good evidence of a causal relationship, eg showing that the greater the number of cigarettes smoked, or the higher the blood pressure, the greater the cardiovascular mortality. It is still possible that BP is a risk marker of some other phenomenon, but this is less likely if the relationship between BP and cardiovascular mortality is found to correlate *while keeping other known risk factors constant*. The work of the epidemiologist does not stop here. He or she can use actuarial statistics to weigh the relative merits and interactions of a number of risk factors, to give an overall estimate of risk for an individual. It is then possible to say things like: "If the 5yr risk of a serious cardiac event in people with no overt cardiac disease is >15%, then drug treatment of hyperlipidaemia may begin to be cost-effective—and a 10% 5yr risk may be a sufficient point to trigger antihypertensive treatment in someone with, say, a BP of 150/90". These figures are a guide only: only ~60% of those in the top 10% of the risk distribution will have an adverse coronary event in the 5yr period. Nevertheless, this is more accurate than taking into account risk factors singly—and so we are led to our first important conclusion: ***epidemiology improves and informs our dialogue with our patients***. We can give patients good evidence on which to base their choices.

Risk equations: Computerized records allow algorithms derived from millions of UK patients to stratify individual risk of vascular events (QRISK2 qrisk.org/index.php) using age, sex, BMI, cholesterol/HDL, family history (1° relative<60yrs), BP, smoking & medical history (IHD, rheumatoid arthritis, AF, hypertension, renal disease), and social deprivation (via postcode).[2][3][4] In the UK, QRISK2 is more reliable than Framingham data even when refined for UK populations. *Accuracy:* QRISK2 classifies one in 10 UK men as high risk (10yr vascular risk ≥20% if ~30-74yrs old—the threshold recommended by NICE for statin ℞).[6] ►Only 30% of subsequent vascular events occur in this high risk group![7] NB: ~80% of participants in QRISK had some missing data, eg cholesterol:HDL.

The essence of epidemiology

(see Dr John Snow, fig 1 & p427)

Epidemiology is the study of the distribution of clinical phenomena in populations. It is essential to public health research and preventive medicine (p666). For example, it analyses disease outbreaks in terms of **host**, **agent**, and **environment** (the 'epidemiologist's triad')—eg starting by measuring **prevalence** and **incidence.**

Definitions The *period prevalence* is the number of cases, at any time during the study period, divided by the population at risk. If the population at risk is unclear, then the population must be specified, eg the prevalence of uterine cancer varies widely, depending on whether you specify the general population (men, women, boys, girls) or only women, or women who have not already had a hysterectomy. *Incidence* is the number of new cases within the pre-specified study period, eg annual incidence. *Point prevalence* is the prevalence at a point in time. The *lifetime prevalence* of hiccups is ~100%; the (UK) incidence is millions/year—but the point prevalence may be 0 at 3AM today if no one is actually having hiccups.

Association Epidemiology is concerned with comparing rates of disease in different populations, eg rates of lung cancer in a population of men who smoke compared with men who don't. A difference in rates points to an association (or dissociation) between the disease and factors distinguishing the populations (in this case, smoking or not). If the rates are equal, association is still possible, with a confounding variable (eg both groups share the same smoky environment).

Ways of accounting for associations: *A* may cause *B*; *B* cause *A*; a 3rd unknown agent, *P*, causes *A* and *B*; or it may be a chance finding. If it looks as if *A* might cause *B*, bear in mind the **Bradford Hill 'criteria'** (he did not claim any were essential):

1 Consistent findings: the same results are got by different people and studies.
2 Temporality: the effect must occur after the cause.
3 Biological gradient: greater exposure leading to greater incidence of the effect.
4 A plausible mechanism linking cause to effect is reassuring, but not essential.[1]
5 Coherence between epidemiological and lab findings ↑ likelihood of an effect.
6 Analogy: The effect of similar factors may be considered.
7 Use of *direct experiment*. Other criteria relate to *specificity* and *strength of association*. Global scores of causation-likelihood can be calculated.[6]

There are 2 types of studies which explore causal connections

Case–control (retrospective) studies: The study group consists of those with the disease (eg lung cancer); the control group consists of those without the disease. The previous occurrence of the putative cause (eg smoking) is compared between each group. Case–control studies are retrospective in that they start after the onset of the disease (although cases may be collected prospectively).

Cohort (prospective) studies: The study group consists of subjects exposed to the putative cause (eg smoking); the control group comprises unexposed subjects. The incidence of the disease is compared between the groups over time.

►A cohort study generates incidence data, whereas a case–control study does not.

Matching An association between *A* and *B* may be due to another factor *P*. To eliminate this possibility, matching for *P* is often used in case–control studies. One powerful (but unreliable, if numbers are small) way to do this in clinical trials is for the subjects to be allocated to groups randomly; check important *P*s have been distributed evenly between groups.

Overmatching If unemployment causes low income, and low income causes depression, then matching study and control groups for income would mask the genuine causal link between unemployment and depression. ►Avoid matching factors that may intervene in the causal chain linking *A* and *B*.

Blinding If the subject does not know which of two trial treatments she is having, the trial is single blind. To further reduce risk of bias, the experimenter should also not know (double blind). ►In a good trial, the blind lead the blind.

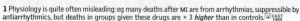

1 Physiology is quite often misleading: eg many deaths after MI are from arrhythmias, suppressible by antiarrhythmics, but deaths in groups given these drugs are × 3 *higher* than in controls. CAST 1989

Epidemiology

Examples of prevention
Primary prevention: (preventing occurrence) • Vaccination • Advice on smoking, alcohol or healthy eating • Safe(r) sex advice (HIV) • Screening for hypertension • Preconception folic acid to prevent spina bifida • Fluoride in water (caries)
Secondary prevention: (screening for 1st stages) • Cervical cytology • Mammography • Proteinuria in pre-eclampsia • Microalbuminuria in DM • Colonoscopy for polyps • Densitometry (osteoporosis) • Diet advice in impaired fasting glycaemia
Tertiary prevention: (preventing complications) • Aspirin after a stroke • Retinal photography in DM • 'Don't go barefoot' in those with diabetic neuropathy • Vitamin D in osteoporosis
Quaternary prevention: (preventing medicalization) • Prioritizing preventive actions • Shielding from ruthless targets (eg easing a diabetic's BP target so he feels better or is less prone to falls).

Two questions: *Is the only good medicine preventive medicine?* and *If preventable... why not prevented?* Prevention is one of the core aims of epidemiology, and during life on the wards you will have many opportunities for preventive medicine. You will pass most of them over, unconsciously, in favour of more glamorous or urgent (but less important) tasks, such as diagnosis, and clever interventions, involving probes, scalpels, and imaging. But if we imagine a ward where scalpels remain sheathed and the only thing being probed is our commitment to health, then preventive medicine comes to the fore, and it is our contention that such a ward might produce more health than some entire hospitals. The first step is to motivate your patient to take steps to benefit their own health by asking Socratic questions. "Do you want to smoke?" "What does your family think about smoking?" "Do you want your children to smoke?" "Would there be any advantages in giving up?" "Why is your health important to you?" "Is there anything more important we can help with?" These motivational questions with specific strategies in prevention (p87, plus when and where to turn up to get help) produce more change than withering looks and lectures on lung cancer or legs dropping off.

The law of unintended consequences (Sod's law, p359) decrees that those whom you have to persuade the hardest to accept prevention will be those to whom a complication befalls, eg colon perforation during colonoscopy to prevent cancers in those with UC or polyps. With this in mind, concentrate on those preventive activities which are simple, cheap, have a complication rate of about zero, and which do not interfere (much) with how the patient runs his life.

When drugs aren't the answer: the laws of quaternary prevention

1 Prevention is better than cure. (Not all prevention is good, though: see above.)
2 Don't treat symptoms without working out underlying pathologies.[7]
3 Don't treat just pathology, and go beyond the biopsychosocial straitjacket (p9).
4 Don't feel you must treat all diseases: agree with patients about what's important.
5 When you can, work *with* Nature: don't try to pull cures like rabbits out of hats.
6 Think graded *exercise* (or *bed rest*), *diet* and *hygiene* before *drugs, drugs, drugs*.
7 All interventions have unintended consequences. Don't delude yourself about this.
8 Find something to measure to monitor disease progression and your treatment.
9 All laws have exceptions (if he's doing well on the wrong drug, it's the right drug).

Individualized risk communication Risk communication done thoughtlessly and only dwelling on positive aspects can lead to bitterness, anger, and litigation.[8] If communication is based on a person's individual risk factors for a condition (eg age, family history, smoking status, cholesterol level, eg using formulae such as that on p664), is risk communicated in ways that change behaviour? A 2003 Cochrane meta-analysis[9] suggests 'not necessarily' (although uptake of screening tests *is* improved). At least this technique promotes dialogue, and dialogue opens doors, minds, and possibilities for choice. *Informed participation* is the aim, not passive acceptance of advice. It does not make much difference whether information is given as an absolute risk, or as a risk score, or categorized as high, medium, or low risk. See also 'Consent' on p570.

Screening (secondary prevention)

Modified Wilson criteria for screening (1-10 spells IATROGENIC[1]—to remind us that in treating healthy populations we have an especial duty to do no harm.)

1 The condition screened for should be an important one.
2 There should be an acceptable treatment for the disease.
3 Diagnostic and treatment facilities should be available.
4 A recognizable latent or early symptomatic stage is required.
5 Opinions on who to treat as patients must be agreed.
6 The test must be of *high discriminatory power* (see below), *valid* (measuring what it purports to measure, not surrogate markers which might not correlate with reality), and be *reproducible*—with safety guaranteed.
7 The examination must be acceptable to the patient.
8 The untreated natural history of the disease must be known.
9 A simple inexpensive test should be all that is required.
10 Screening must be continuous (ie not a 'one-off' affair).

Conclusion: screening tests must be cost-effective.

Problems *All screening programs do harm; some do good as well.* J Muir Gray 2004 Brit J Gen Pr 54 292

1 Those most at risk do not present for screening, thus increasing the gap between the healthy and the unhealthy—the *inverse care law* (p10).
2 The 'worried well' overload services by seeking repeat screening.
3 Services for investigating those testing positive are inadequate.
4 Those who are false positives suffer stress while awaiting investigation, and remain anxious about their health despite reassurance.

►Before screening, the chances of harming a patient (by anxiety or subsequent invasive tests), as well as any benefits must be quantified: this is *Rees' rule* 10

Examples of effective screening	Unproven/ineffective screening
Cervical smears (cervical cancer)	Mental test score (dementia)
Mammography (breast cancer)	Urine tests (diabetes; kidney disease)
Finding smokers (+quitting advice)	Antenatal procedures (*OHCS* p8)
Looking for malignant hypertension	PSA screening (prostate cancer, p647)

NB: screening for cervical cancer and mammography are far from perfect: both are liable to false negatives (p674), and a negative result is interpreted as "I'm fine" (and may be seen as a licence to take risks). So signs of interval cancers (arising between screenings) may be ignored by patients who assume they are in the clear.

Public health advice and other useful contacts

Central Public Health Lab: 020 8200 4400. www.hpa.org.uk
Committee on Safety of Medicines: (part of the MHRA) www.mhra.gov.uk/committees/...
.../MedicinesAdvisoryBodies/CommitteeonSafetyofMedicines/index.htm
Communicable Disease Surveillance Centre: 020 8200 6868. www.hpa.org.uk
Disabled Living Foundation: (advice on aids etc for the disabled) 020 7289 6111. www.dlf.org.uk
Health Information Line: (incl addresses of disease-specific organizations) 0800 665544
Liverpool School of Tropical Medicine: 0151 705 3100. www.liv.ac.uk/lstm
London School of Hygiene and Tropical Medicine: 020 7636 8636. www.lshtm.ac.uk
Medical Foundation for the Care of Victims of Torture: 020 7813 7777. www.torturecare.org.uk
National Counselling Service for Sick Doctors: 0870 241 0535.
National Travel Health Network and Centre: (travel advice) 0845 602 6712. www.nathnac.org
Medic-Alert Foundation: 0800 581 420. www.medicalert.org.uk
Poisons information services: see p850.
Patients' Association: (patient advisory line) 0845 608 4455. www.patients-association.org.uk
Transplant Service (UK) (can these organs be used?) 0845 60 60 400.

1 From Greek: *iatros* (physician) + genic, denoting illness caused by us doctors. You will find this word etched on all our soles, producing a malign imprint however lightly we try to tread. *Ways to reduce iatrogenic illness:* • Use EBM if possible. • Involve patients in all decisions. • Check drug labels/dosages by reading them aloud. • Be aware of drug interactions: look it up—don't assume you know. • Explain to patients how to tell if things are going wrong, and what action to take ("if ... tell me...").

This is the conscientious and judicious use of current best evidence from research to optimize management plans and integrate them with patients' values.[12] EBM includes 6 steps: **1** Asking answerable questions. **2** Finding the best information. **3** Information appraisal for validity and relevance. **4** Dialogue to find out what the patient wants. **5** Data application to patient care. **6** Evaluation of the performance.

The problem More than 2,000,000 papers are published each year. Patients benefit directly from a tiny fraction of these papers. How do we find them?

A partial solution Journals are scanned not by experts in a specialized field, but by searchers trained to identify papers which have a direct message for clinical practice and meet predefined criteria of rigour (below). Summaries are then published, eg in *Evidence-based Medicine*.[13] ***Questions used to evaluate papers:***

- Are the results valid? Randomized? Blinded? Were all patients accounted for who entered the trial? Was follow-up complete? Were the groups similar at the start? Was everyone treated equally, apart from the experimental intervention? NB: randomized trials are now recognised as blunt instruments: adaptive (Bayesian) designs may sometimes be a more efficient way to get to the truth (p674).[14]
- What are the results? How large (and precise) was the treatment effect?
- Will the results help my patients (cost/benefit sum)?[15]

Problems with the solution ▶ *The concept of scientific rigour is opaque*. What do we want? The science, the rigour, the truth, or what will be most useful to patients? These may overlap, but they are not the same.

- Will the best be the enemy of the good? Are useful papers rejected due to some blemish? Answer: appraise *all* evidence (often impossible).
- By insisting on *answerable* questions, EBM may subvert a patient's aims. He may only want to share his fears, not be used as a substrate for an intellectual exercise.
- Is the standard the same for the evidence for *all* changes to our practice? We might avoid prescribing drug X for constipation if there is any chance that it might cause colon cancer, as the choice of drugs is wide. More robust evidence is needed to persuade us to do something rather counterintuitive, eg giving heparin in DIC (p346). There is no science to tell us how robust the data need to be: we decide off the top of our head (albeit a wise head, we hope).
- What about the correspondence columns of the journals from which the winning papers are extracted? It takes years for unforeseen but fatal flaws to surface here.
- There is a danger that by always asking "What is the evidence…" we will divert resources from hard-to-prove areas (eg physiotherapy, which may be very valuable) to easy-to-prove services. The unique personal attributes of the therapist may be as important as the objective regimen.
- EBM is never 100% up-to-date, and reworking meta-analyses takes time and money, so specialists may ostensibly reject a new trial due to a tiny flaw, when the real reason is that they dread it might flip their once-perfect formulation.
- 'My increased knowledge gradually permeated or repressed the world of intuitive premonitions…' Carl Jung These premonitions may be vital!
- If EBM is prescriptive, patient choice declines: not all patients are amenable to rational dialogue. Does our zeal for EBM make us arrogant and inflexible?
- The patient before us may not quite fit the type of patient who provided the research basis—and we may be tempted to ignore these small differences, which may then have major unforeseen adverse effects.

Advantages of EBM This is mainly that patients get better faster—also:

- Our reading habits improve, and we can offer more rational choices to patients.
- EBM leads us to ask questions, and then to be sceptical of the answers.
- As taxpayers, we should like it (wasteful practices can be abandoned).

EBM may not have as much impact as we hope, as gaining evidence is time-consuming and expensive, and sometimes impossible. Despite these caveats, EBM is here to stay, so we may as well subscribe to its ideals—and to its journals.

Medicine and the internet

During the time it takes you to read this page, your better-connected patients may have checked out your latest prescription and be wondering why it does not tally with the recommendations of Guatemalan Guidelines on Gynaecomastia, or the National Institute for Health and Clinical Excellence's Treatise on Toxoplasmosis. Our patients have time and motivation, whereas we have little time and our motivation may be flickering. This can seem threatening to the doctor who sees himself/herself as a dispenser of wisdom and precious remedies. It is less threatening if we consider ourselves to be in partnership with our patients. The evidence is that those who use the internet to question their therapy receive a better service.

For the doctor, the role of the internet is to answer your clinical questions. Can tetanus toxoid cause purpura? Is there a connection between knee pain and constipation? Frame your questions as simply as possible. You are not asking if it is likely that this patient's purpura is due to last week's tetanus vaccine, just if it is a reported happening. You maintain clinical responsibility and use the knowledge you are given to frame appropriate management.

Some useful online resources:

- ***Drugs:*** eMIMS (more up to date than *eBNF*, but see the *What's new* section at www.bnf.org); *eMIMS* contains many data-sheets—free and updated monthly.
- ***Differential diagnoses,*** eg 'what causes chest pain, knee pain, and ↑urea?', and *rare diseases*—try Mentor (www.webmentorlibrary.com)
- ***Research:*** PubMed (MedLine) is free at www.ncbi.nlm.nih.gov/pubmed. The *Advanced Search* function can be used to refine searches to reduce the number of hits produced. Be sure to check your spelling carefully.
- ***Meta-analyses:*** (p670) eg the Cochrane Library at www.cochrane.org. Other similar resources are available through Update Software (www.update-software.com).

When a randomized controlled trial might not be the best method

- Generating new ideas beyond current paradigms (case reports may be better).
- Researching causes of illnesses and prognoses (cohort studies may be better).
- Evaluating diagnostic tests is best done with a cohort study and decision model.
- Where the researcher has no idea of the effective dose of a drug. An dose-ranging adaptive design where the next dose given depends on the effects of previous doses is a more efficient methodology,[16] as there can be a dynamic termination rule allowing for early discontinuation either for efficacy or futility.
- When recruiting of patients would be impossible or unethical.[17]
- If the unique gifts of the therapist might have a bigger effect than the drug used.
- When personalized medicine is the aim. For example, new cancer drugs seek to match effective treatments with patients' biomarker profiles. This may be better accomplished by adaptive designs.[18]

►In the end all randomized trials have to submit to the ultimate test when the statistical collides with the personal *"Will this treatment help me?" "Will this procedure help you?"* No randomized trial is complete until real-life decisions taken in the light of its findings are scrutinized and a narrative is compiled to suggest when results should be applied and when they should be ignored.[19] So do not ask for definitive trials: everything is provisional.

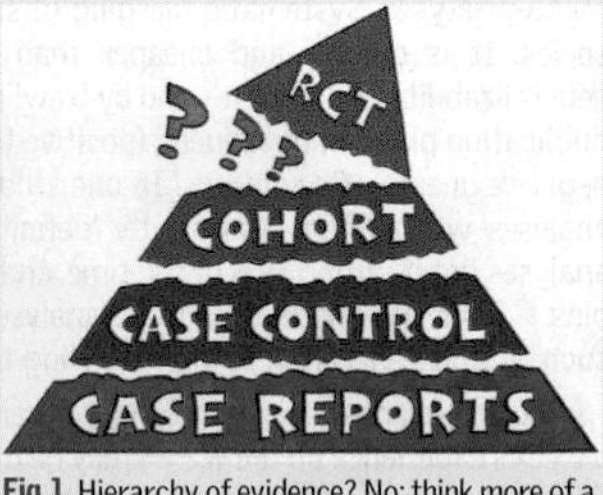

Fig 1. Hierarchy of evidence? No: think more of a network of evidence that takes into account epidemiology, lab work and experiential data. RCT=randomized controlled trial.

Anyone who has conducted a simple randomized trial will know how seductive they are: to eliminate bias and get at the truth as to whether this drug is any good or not is brilliant. But remember that Sod's law (p359) never sleeps, and if something can go wrong with a trial, it will—in at least 8 realms.

Types of study
- Simple randomized trial
- Randomized adaptive design (see below)
- Historical (retrospective) trial
- Non-randomized contemporaneous trial
- Case-control study
- Before and after designs
- N=1 trial (the patient acts as his own control)
- Case series
- Case reports
- Narrative: "What did it feel like when you took digoxin?"

1 There may be no true or false answer to the question.
2 The question being asked may be the wrong one.
3 The patients invited into the trial may be the wrong ones, eg all from a country where a gene conferring resistance to a treatment is prevalent. Or there may be under-representation of elderly people or those with other illnesses.
4 Randomization may give 2 groups that are quite dissimilar (the play of chance)—eg the group having the new antihypertensive may have lower cholesterol levels.
5 Blinding may be subverted if the patients can guess whether they are having the active or placebo treatment—for example by the side effects.
6 The design may allow for rejection of the null hypothesis (that there is no difference between the two treatments)—but the null hypothesis may be irrelevant if previous studies show that the new treatment has some benefits. 73% of randomized trials made this mistake in one analysis.[20]
7 Not enough patients may have been recruited to show a small but valuable effect. Also, if a small trial that lacks power (the ability to detect true differences) *does* give 'positive' results, the size of the difference between the groups is likely to be exaggerated. (This is type I error; a type II error applies to results which indicate that there is no effect, when in fact there is.) ►So beware even quite big trials that purport to show that a new drug is as effective as an established agent.
8 Subgroup analysis may seem to show that a drug works in a subset of patients. But trawling of data will often produce these 'effects' if repeated often enough.

What to do about these shortcomings? Sometimes Bayesian probabilistic approaches will help. These ask about the probability of a range of hypotheses conditional on the data. The best dose, for example, may be found during an experiment as a Bayesian protocol (an *adaptive design*) allows for learning during the experiment. This makes asking the wrong question less of a problem, and allows conclusions using far fewer patients (eg 50% less).[21]

In summary, no single methodology is uniquely valid and there is no coherent hierarchy of evidence. Just making do with what is available, and applying it sensibly.

Meta-analyses Systematic merging of similar trials *may* explain data inconsistencies. It is quicker and cheaper than doing new studies, and can establish generalizability of research[22] and by trawling for unpublished trials ('grey literature') publication bias can be reduced (positive trials are more likely to be published than negative ones).[23] *Be cautious!* In one study looking at recommendations of meta-analyses where there was a later 'definitive' big trial, it turned out that meta-analyses got it wrong 30% of the time, and 20% of good meta-analyses fail to avoid bias.[24] Don't assume that all meta-analyses, even those from the cleanest stables, such as Cochrane, are free of bias owing to pharmaceutical funding.[25]

►A big well-planned trial may be worth centuries of uncritical medical practice; but a week's experience on the wards may be more valuable than years reading journals. This is the paradox in medical education: How can we trust our own experiences knowing they are all anecdotal? How can we be open to novel ideas but avoid being merely fashionable? A stance of wary open-mindedness may serve us best.

Number needed to treat (NNT)

Statistical analysis is the glue that holds together the conclusions of a study. It is also the mask behind which the shortcomings of a study may hide. Having an understanding of what the statistical terms mean, and what they can be used for, will help you to decide for yourself whether a study's conclusions are valid. Some other important statistical definitions are given on p765.

If the risk of dying from an MI after 'standard treatment' is 10%, and a new treatment reduces this to 8%, the new drug can be made to look very effective by quoting the ***relative risk reduction***, which is 20% ([10–8]/10 × 100%; ie the new drug is 20% more effective). However, the ***absolute risk reduction*** is 2% (10–8%; ie only an extra 2% of patients would derive benefit from the new treatment). In terms of the ***number needed to treat***, we might say therefore that 50 patients would need treating to save one additional life ([1/absolute risk reduction] × 100). NNTs provide a useful way of quantifying benefit. In some preventive studies of mild hypertension in the young, ~800 people may need treating according to a certain regimen to prevent one stroke—when expressed like this, the treatment seems less wonderful. However, they do not take into account treatment *costs* or the *degree* of potential benefit.

The converse of NNT is ***number needed to harm***. This is the number of people who must receive a treatment in order to produce one adverse event.

Strengths: NNTs are context-dependent. Thus if a new antihypertensive regimen is being compared with an old regimen where the NNT was 800 and the new regimen is only marginally better, the NNT to prevent one death or stroke *by adopting the new regimen in place of the old* may run into many thousands, as will your drugs bill if the new drug is more expensive.

Weaknesses: • NNTs are difficult to interpret if there is a large *placebo effect*, eg in pain relief. Say the placebo response rate is 40% and that of a new analgesic is 60%, then the NNT is 5. Perhaps it is better to say to patients starting the new drug that 60% respond. • *Keep your eye on the question:* NNTs can vary markedly if the question is slightly rephrased—eg from being about primary prevention to being about secondary prevention (as in the statin example above).[26] • Also, one needs to be clear whether the mean or median is given as the length of follow-up. For further examples, see www.nntonline.net.

NNT confidence intervals Get these by taking reciprocals of the values defining the confidence interval for the absolute risk reduction (ARR). If ARR ≈ 10% with a 95% confidence interval of 5-15%, NNT ≈ 10 (ie 100/10) and the 95% NNT-confidence interval ≈ 6.7-20 (ie 100/15 to 100/5). Non-significant treatment effects are problematic as NNTs can only be positive; here, give NNT *without* confidence intervals (Altman's rule).[27]

Examples of NNTs

Study	*Outcome*	*NNT*
Statins (p109) for primary prevention[1]	Death (MI)	931 (78) for 5yrs
Statins for secondary prevention (4S)	Death (MI)	30 (15) for 5.4yrs
Mild hypertension (MRC trial)	Stroke	850 for 1yr
Systolic hypertension in elderly (SHEP)	Stroke	43 for 4.5yrs
Aspirin in acute MI (ISIS-1)	Death	40
Streptokinase in acute MI (ISIS-2)	Death	40
ACE-i for CCF (NYHA class IV, p131)	Death	6 for 1yr

1 Meta-analysis *Bandolier* 17(7), 41(3), 50(8)

Six to five against (*Odds ratios*)

Your surgical tutor asks whether Gobble's disease is commoner in women or men. You have no idea, and make a guess. What is the chance of getting it right? Common sense decrees that it is even chances; 'Sod's law' (p359) predicts that whatever you guess, you will always be wrong. A less pessimistic view is that the balance is slightly tipped against you: according to Damon Runyon, 'all life is 6 to 5 against'.[28]

Do new symptoms suggest a new disease or are they from an existing disease? The answer is often counter-intuitive. Suppose **s** is quite a rare symptom of Gobble's disease (seen in 5% of patients), but that it is a very common symptom of disease **A** (seen in 90%). If we have a man whom we already know has Gobble's disease and who goes on to develop symptom **s**, is not **s** more likely to be due to disease **A**, rather than Gobble's disease? The answer is usually no: *it is generally the case that* **s** *is due to a disease that is already known, and does not imply a new disease.*

The 'odds ratio' makes this clearer, ie the ratio of [***the probability of the symptom, given the known disease***] to [***the probability of the symptom given the new disease*** × ***the probability of developing the new disease***]. Usually this is vastly in favour of the symptom being due to the old disease, because of the prior odds of the two diseases.

Doctors as gamblers (**fig 1**). To the average mind it is distasteful to learn that doctors gamble with patients' lives. One of us (JML) has just finished consulting with 23 patients. Not too many, perhaps: it might be argued that each symptom, especially if *serious*, should be investigated until the cause is found.

Let us look at this critically. What counts as a serious symptom? One that might mean death, disfigurement, or disability. Some of these patients offered 5 symptom groups before being gently dissuaded from going on. During elucidation of these symptoms others emerged, yielding a potentially endless cycle of investigation. Certainly some of their symptoms might not seem serious ("this pain in my toe..."). But toe pain might be mortal if caused by emboli or osteomyelitis. Fingernail problems with a slight rash might mean arsenic poisoning, lethargy may mean cancer, and so on. So medicine is not for pessimists—almost anything can be made to seem fatal, so that a pessimistic doctor would never get any sleep at night for worrying about the meanings of his patients' symptoms.

Medicine is not for blind optimists either, who too easily embrace a fool's paradise of false reassurance. Rather, ***medicine is for gamblers***: gamblers who are happy to use subtle clues to change their outlook from pessimism to optimism and *vice versa*. Sometimes the gambling is scientific, rational, and methodical (odds-ratio analysis): sometimes it is not, as when the gambling is based on prior knowledge (vital but ill-defined) of one's patient, or the faint apprehension of terror in this new patient's eyes that shows you that there is something wrong, and that you don't yet know what it is.

Being lucky in both types of gambling is a requisite for being a successful doctor: after all we would all rather have a lucky doctor than a wise one. In this game, especially when it gets deadly serious, the chips are not just financial (the most cost-effective next step). They betoken time (for you are spending yourself as surely as you are spending money, as you walk the wards), your reputation, and the health or otherwise of your patient. So do not worry about the fact of gambling: ***gambling is your job***. If you cannot gamble you cannot cure. But try hard to assemble sufficient evidence to maximize the chances of being lucky. Professions allied to medicine often seem similar to medicine, but typically without this central role of risk-taking (midwifery is among the notable exceptions).

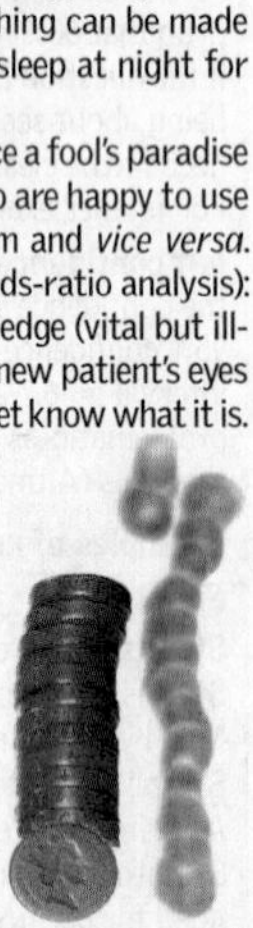

Fig 1. Her ESR is 21. Is it normal? Heads or tails? Play rouleaux-roulette to find out (p322).

The foregoing explains why courage is the cardinal clinical virtue: without it we would not follow our hunches and take justified risks—and all our other clinical virtues and skills (holistic care, diagnostic acumen, and operative dexterity) would not be deployed to their full advantage, while we pass the buck.

An example of the odds ratio at work

A 50-yr-old man with known carcinoma of the lung has some transient neurological symptoms and a normal CT scan. Are these symptoms due to secondaries in the brain or to transient ischaemic attacks (TIAs)?

- The chance of secondaries in the brain which cause transient neurological symptoms is 0.045 given carcinoma of the lung.
- The chance of such secondaries not showing up on a CT scan is 0.1. Therefore the chance of this cluster of symptoms is 0.0045 (ie 0.045 × 0.1).
- The chance of a normal CT + transient CNS symptoms given a TIA is 0.9.
- The chance of a 50-yr-old man developing TIA is 0.0001.
- Therefore the odds ratio is 0.0045/(0.9 × 0.0001). This equals 50.

That is, the odds ratio is ~50 to 1 in favour of secondaries in the brain.

NB: It is only very rarely that the prior odds of a new disease are so high that the new disease is more likely, eg someone presenting with anaemia already known to have breast cancer, who lives in an African community where 50% of people have hookworm-induced anaemia, is likely to have anaemia due to hookworm *as well as* breast carcinoma.

Odds ratio and relative risk compare the relative likelihood of an event occurring in two distinct groups. Relative risk (p671) is easier to interpret and often consistent with our intuitions. Some study designs, however, such as case-control studies, prevent the calculation of the relative risk (due to a pre-selected population). Which to use when? See childrensmercy.org/stats/journal/oddsratio.asp.

Investigations change the odds

Only rarely does a single test provide a definitive diagnosis. More often tests alter the odds of a diagnosis. When taking a history and examining patients, we make various wagers with ourselves (often barely consciously) as to how likely various diagnoses are. Further test results simply affect these odds. A test is worthwhile if it alters diagnostic odds in a clinically useful way.

The effect of an investigation on the diagnostic odds To work this out you need to know the *sensitivity* and *specificity* of the test. All tests have false-positive and false-negative rates, as summarized below:

Test result	Patients with the condition	Patients without the condition
Result +ve for the condition	True +ve (*a*)	*False* +ve (*b*)
Result -ve for the condition	*False* -ve (*c*)	True -ve (*d*)

Specificity: How often is the test -ve in health? *d/d+b*. ***Sensitivity:*** How often is the test +ve in the disease? *a/a+c*. ***Positive predictive value:*** How often will someone with a +ve result have the disease? *a/a+b*. ***Negative predictive value:*** How often will someone with a -ve result really not have the disease? *d/d+c*. Screening tests need to have a high sensitivity, to include everyone with the disease (at a cost of including some without), while diagnostic tests need a high specificity, to be certain the disease is present. For example, we know that 3–6% of chest pain patients sent home from casualty departments on the basis of a single ECG actually have myocardial infarction (MI). A single ECG is *specific* (77–100%), but not very sensitive for MI (56%). Troponin tests (p112) are very *sensitive*. So if history and ECG suggest MI, admit (thrombolysis, p782). If story and ECG are not typical of MI, do a troponin test ≥6h after onset of chest pain—only send home if 'normal'.[1] This strategy reduces inappropriate discharge to 0.3%.[2] Note that studies showing these effects are *very* dependent on the local prevalence of MI. A few more MIs in the 'troponin normal' group would radically alter these results.

The ***likelihood ratio*** of the disease given a +ve result (LR+) is the ratio of the chance of having a +ve test if the disease is present to the chance of having a +ve test if the disease is absent: LR+=sensitivity/(1–specificity). Conversely the likelihood ratio given a -ve result, LR-, is (1–sensitivity)/specificity. Suppose we have a test of sensitivity 0.8 and specificity 0.9. LR+ will be 8:1 [ie 0.8/(1–0.9)], and LR- will be 2:9 [(1–0.8)/0.9].

Is there any point to this test? Work out the **posterior odds** assuming first a +ve and then a -ve test result—via the equation: *posterior odds* = (*prior odds*) × (*likelihood ratio*). If your clinical assessment of a man with exercise-induced chest pain is that the odds of this being due to coronary artery disease (CAD) are 4:1 (80%), is it worth his doing an exercise tolerance test (sensitivity 0.72; specificity 0.8)?[30] If the test were +ve, the odds in favour of CAD would be 4 × (0.72)/(1–0.8) = 14:1 (93%). If -ve, they would be 4 × (1 - 0.72)/0.8 = 1.4:1 (58%), so the test has not in any way 'ruled out' CAD.

Experienced doctors are likely to have higher prior odds for the most likely diagnosis. The above shows that with high prior odds, a test must have high sensitivity and specificity for a negative result to bring the odds below 50%.

Another example is John, who is a 40-yr-old (not on NSAIDs, with no prior peptic ulcer) referred for '?endoscopy' because of dyspepsia. Before the result of a bedside test for *Helicobacter pylori* is known, he has a 50% chance of harbouring this organism, which, if present, is the probable cause of an ulcer.[31] The likelihood ratio for a -ve test result is 0.13[32] (sensitivity 0.88, specificity 0.91). *If the test is -ve*, the chance of John having *H. pylori* is <11%—and it may be OK to send him home with symptomatic treatment (eg ranitidine) without endoscopy—if there are no 'cancer (alarm) symptoms' (weight loss, dysphagia, etc, p242).[33] *If the test is +ve*, the probability of *H. pylori* is >90%, strongly suggesting the need for specific anti-ulcer (anti-*Helicobacter*) therapy (p242), and endoscopy if this does not cure his symptoms.

1 Troponin T ≤0.1μg/L (or troponin I ≤0.2μg/L; labs vary); what is normal is itself a statistical issue, p652—as is what counts as an MI.

2 Sensitivity: 97%; specificity: 93%; -ve predictive value: 99.6%; +ve predictive value: 66%; LR+: 13.9; LR-: 0.03.

"I did an ESR to exclude giant cell arteritis..."

William Osler wrote that 'Variability is the law of life, and as no two faces are the same, so no two bodies are alike, and no two individuals react alike and behave alike under the abnormal conditions which we know as disease. This is the fundamental difficulty of the physician, and one which he may never grasp.'[34] So whenever you hear the word 'exclude' on ward-rounds or in consulting rooms, wink at Osler—for you have discovered another one of his cases of a doctor who does not understand variability and probability. ►***Nothing is ever excluded and everything is always provisional***—even death, for a while. (We have all been caught out by the last gasp not being the last.)

So isn't all this morass of nebulous uncertainty (**fig 1**) depressing? No. It's beautiful, for luckily the human brain is brilliantly constructed to solve these very problems, because life itself (off the wards, and since the beginning of time) is full of them. Medical education gets itself into a pickle when it tries to teach us too much—as if a mother would try to teach her daughter what to do on day 38 of marriage (yet this is exactly what we do with trypanosomiasis—see past editions). So, as Osler pointed out, if we give ourselves 'good methods and a proper point of view, all other things will be added as [our] experience grows.'[35] Then, if on day 38, we find our patient is in labour, for example, we may recognise that other priorities may apply.

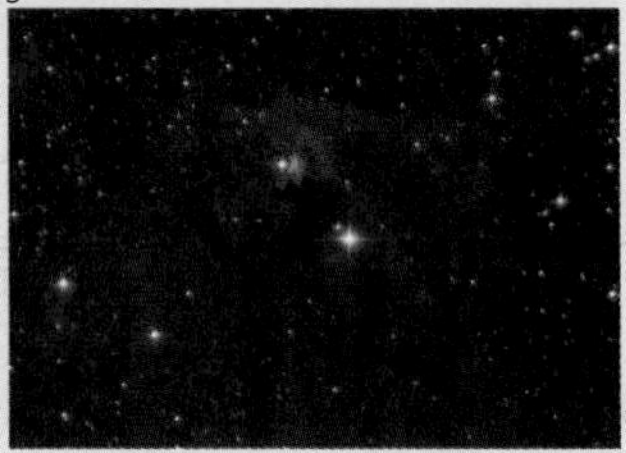

Fig 1. Like the chair you are sitting in, and your last ward round, Hind's Variable Nebula probably contains what we call a 'very young stellar object.' Learning to shine is only a matter of time.

Contents

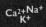

Relevant pages elsewhere: Reference intervals (p770); acute renal failure (p298).

On being normal in the society of numbers

Laboratory medicine reduces our patients to a few easy-to-handle numbers: this is the discipline's great attraction—and its greatest danger. The normal range (reference interval) is usually that which includes 95% of a given population (given a Normal distribution, see p765). If variation is randomly distributed, 2.5% of our results will be 'too high', and 2.5% 'too low' on an average day, when dealing with apparently normal people. This statistical definition of normality is the simplest. Other definitions may be *normative*—ie stating what an upper or lower limit *should* be. The upper end of the reference interval for plasma cholesterol may be given as 6mmol/L because this is what biochemists state to be the *desired* maximum. 40% of people in some populations will have a plasma cholesterol greater than 6mmol/L and thus may be at increased risk. The WHO definition of anaemia in pregnancy is an Hb of <11g/dL, which makes 20% of mothers anaemic. This 'lax' criterion has the presumed benefit of triggering actions which result in fewer deaths from haemorrhage. So do not just ask "What is the normal range?"—also enquire about who set the range, for what population, and for what reason.

►Normal values can have hidden historical, social, and political desiderata—just like the normal values novelists ascribe to their characters: '*Conventions and traditions, I suppose, work blindly but surely for the preservation of the normal type; for the extinction of proud, resolute and unusual individuals... Society must go on, I suppose, and society can only exist if the normal, if the virtuous, and the slightly deceitful flourish, and if the passionate, the headstrong, and the too-truthful are condemned to suicide and to madness. Yes, society must go on; it must breed, like rabbits. That is what we are here for ... But, at any rate, there is always Leonora to cheer you up; I don't want to sadden you. Her husband is quite an economical person of so normal a figure that he can get quite a large proportion of his clothes ready-made. That is the great desideratum of life.*' Ford Maddox Ford 1915 *The Good Soldier*. Penguin. 214,228

We thank Dr Johann Graggaber who is our Specialist Reader for this chapter.

The essence of laboratory medicine

General principles

- Laboratory testing may contribute to four aspects of medicine:
  - diagnosis;
  - prognosis (eg clotting in liver failure);
  - monitoring disease activity or progression (eg creatinine in chronic kidney disease);
  - screening (eg phenylketonuria in newborn babies).
- Only do a test if the result will influence management. Make sure you look at the result.

►Laboratory staff like to have contact with you. They are an excellent source of help and information for both requests and results.

- Do not interpret laboratory results except in the light of clinical assessment (unless forced to by examiners!).
- If a result does not fit with the clinical picture, trust clinical judgment and repeat the test. Could it be an artefact? The 'normal' range for a test (reference interval) is usually defined as the interval, symmetrical about the mean, containing 95% of results in a given population (p765). The more tests you run, the greater the probability of an 'abnormal' result of no significance.

►Involve the patient. Don't forget to explain to them where the test fits into their overall management plan.

Getting the best out of the lab—a laboratory decalogue

1. Interest someone from the laboratory in your patient's problem.
2. Fill in the request form fully.
3. Give clinical details, not your preferred diagnosis.
4. Ensure that the lab knows who to contact.
5. Label specimens as well as the request form.
6. Follow the hospital labelling routine for cross-matching.
7. Find out when analysers run, especially batched assays.
8. Talk with the lab before requesting an unusual test.
9. Be thoughtful: at 1630h the routine results are being sorted.
10. Plot results graphically: abnormalities show sooner.

Artefacts and pitfalls in laboratory tests

- Do not take blood sample from an arm which has IV fluid running into it.
- Repeat any unexpected and inconsistent result before acting on it.
- For clotting time do not sample from a heparinized IV catheter.
- Serum K^+ is overestimated if sample is old or haemolysed (this occurs if venepuncture is difficult).
- If using Vacutainers, fill *plain* tubes first—otherwise, anticoagulant contamination from previous tubes can cause errors.
- Total calcium results are affected by albumin concentration (p690).
- INR may be overestimated if citrate bottles are under-filled.
- Drugs may cause *analytic* errors (eg prednisolone cross-reacts with cortisol). Be suspicious if results are unexpected.
- Food may affect result, eg bananas raise urinary HIAA (p278).

Dehydration: ↑urea (disproportionate relative to smaller ↑ in creatinine),[1] ↑albumin (also useful to plot change in a patient's condition), ↑haematocrit (PCV); also ↓urine volume and ↓skin turgor.

Abnormal kidney function: There are two major biochemical pictures:

- ***Low GFR:*** ↑urea, ↑creatinine, ↑K^+, ↑H^+, ↑urate, ↑PO_4^{3-}, ↑anion gap, ↓Ca^{2+}, ↓HCO_3^- oliguria. *Causes:* early acute oliguric renal failure (p298), chronic kidney disease (p300). In chronic kidney disease also ↓Hb, ↑PTH and renal bone disease.
- ***Tubular dysfunction*** (damage to tubules): ↓K^+, ↓urate, ↓PO_4^{3-}, ↓HCO_3^-, ↑H^+, normal urea and creatinine. Other possible findings include polyuria with urinary glucose, amino acids, proteins (lysozyme, β_2-microglobulin), or phosphate. Diagnosis is made by testing renal concentrating ability (p233). *Causes:* recovery from acute renal failure, hypercalcaemia, hyperuricaemia, myeloma, pyelonephritis, hypokalaemia, Wilson's disease, galactosaemia, and heavy metal poisoning.

Thiazide and loop diuretics: ↓Na^+, ↓K^+, ↑ HCO_3^-, ↑urea.

Bone disease:

	Ca^{2+}	*PO_4^{3-}*	*Alk phos*
Osteoporosis (p696)	Normal	Normal	Normal
Osteomalacia (p698)	↓	↓	↑
Paget's	Normal	Normal	↑↑
Myeloma	↑	↑, normal	Normal
Bone metastases	↑	↑, normal	↑
1° Hyperparathyroidism	↑	↓, normal	Normal, ↑
Hypoparathyroidism	↓	↑	Normal
Renal failure (low GFR)	↓	↑	Normal, ↑

Hepatocellular disease: ↑bilirubin, ↑AST, alk phos ↑ slightly, ↓albumin. Also ↑clotting times. For details of the differences between AST and ALT, see p283.

Cholestasis: ↑bilirubin, ↑↑γGT, ↑↑alk phos, ↑AST.

Excess alcohol intake: Evidence of hepatocellular disease. Early evidence in ↑γGT, ↑MCV, and ethanol in blood before lunch.

Myocardial infarction: ↑troponin T/I, ↑CK, ↑AST, ↑LDH (p112).

Addison's disease: ↑K^+, ↓Na^+.

Cushing's syndrome: May show ↓K^+, ↑HCO_3^-, ↑Na^+.

Conn's syndrome: May show ↓K^+, ↑HCO_3^-. Na^+ normal or ↑. (Also hypertension.)

Diabetes mellitus: ↑glucose, (↓HCO_3^- if acidotic).

Diabetes insipidus: ↑Na^+, ↑plasma osmolality, ↓urine osmolality. (Both hypercalcaemia and hypokalaemia may cause nephrogenic diabetes insipidus.)

Inappropriate ADH secretion (SIADH): (see p687) ↓Na^+ with normal or low urea and creatinine, ↓plasma osmolality. ↑urine osmolality (and > than plasma osmolality), ↑urine Na^+ (>20mmol/L).

Some immunodeficiency states: Normal serum albumin but *low* total protein (because immunoglobulins are missing. Also makes cross-matching difficult because expected haemagglutinins are absent; *OHCS* p198).

1 Dehydration affects urea more than creatinine because in dehydration a greater proportion of filtered urea is reabsorbed by the kidney. Creatinine is hardly absorbed at all.

Laboratory results: ▸▸when to take action NOW

- On receiving a dangerous result, first check the name and date.
- Go to the bedside. If the patient is conscious, turn off any IVI (until fluid is checked: a mistake may have been made) and ask the patient how he or she is. *Any fits, faints, collapses, or unexpected symptoms?*
- Be sceptical of an unexpectedly wildly abnormal result with a well patient. Compare with previous values. Could the specimens have got muddled up? Is there an artefact? Was the sample taken from the 'drip' arm? Is a low calcium due to a low albumin (p690)? Perhaps the lab is using a new analyser with a faulty wash cycle? ►*When in doubt, seek help and repeat the test.*

The values chosen below are somewhat arbitrary and must be taken as a guide only. Many results less extreme than those below will be just as dangerous if the patient is old, immunosuppressed, or has some other pathology such as pneumonia.

Plasma biochemistry

▸▸The main risks when plasma electrolytes are dangerously abnormal are of cardiac arrhythmias and CNS events such as seizures.

Electrolyte	Lower limit	Upper limit	Relevant pages
Na^+	< 120 mmol/L	> 155 mmol/L	p686
K^+	< 2.5 mmol/L	> 6.5 mmol/L	p688 p849
Corrected Ca^{2+}	< 2.0 mmol/L	> 3.5 mmol/L	p690, p692
Glucose	< 2 mmol/L	> 20 mmol/L	p842, p844

Blood gases

- **P_aO_2 <8.0kPa** = *Severe hypoxia. Give O_2.* See p180.
- **pH <7.1** = *Dangerous acidosis. See* p684 *to determine the cause.*

Haematology results

- **Hb <7g/dL** with low mean cell volume (<75fL) or history of bleeding. This patient may need urgent transfusion (no spare capacity). See p318ohcm chapter08FINAL.doc - p358.
- **Platelets <40×10⁹/L** May need a platelet transfusion; call a haematologist.
- ***Plasmodium falciparum* seen on blood film** *Start antimalarials now.* See p396.
- **ESR >30mm/h + headache** *Could there be giant cell arteritis?* See p558.

CSF results

▸▸Never delay treatment when bacterial meningitis is suspected.

- **>1 neutrophil/mm³** *Is there meningitis: usually >1000 neutrophils?* See p832.
- **Positive Gram stain** *Talk to a microbiologist; urgent blind therapy.* See p832.

Conflicting, equivocal, or inexplicable results ►Get prompt help.

Fluid requirement in a normal person over 24h is roughly 2500mL. Normal daily losses are through urine (1500mL), stool (200mL), and insensible losses (800mL). This requirement is normally met through food (1000mL) and drink (1500mL).

Intravenous fluids are given if sufficient fluids cannot be given orally. About 2500mL fluid containing roughly 100mmol Na^+ and 70mmol K^+ per 24h are required. Thus, a good regimen is 2L of 5% dextrose and 1L of 0.9% saline every 30h with 20mmol of K^+ per litre of fluid. Alternative routes are via a central venous line or subcutaneously. However, remember that all cannulae carry a risk of MRSA infection: femoral > jugular > subclavian > peripheral, so always resume oral fluid intake as soon as possible.

►In a sick patient, don't forget to include additional sources of fluid loss when calculating daily fluid requirements, such as drains, fevers, or diarrhoea (see BOX 2). Daily weighing helps to monitor overall fluid balance, as will fluid balance charts.

►Examine patients regularly to assess fluid balance (see BOX 1).

Fluid compartments & types of IV fluid

For a 70kg man *total bodily fluid* is approximately 42L (60% body weight). Of this ⅔ is intracellular (28L), and ⅓ is extracellular (14L). Of the extracellular compartment, ⅓ is intravascular (5L blood). Different types of IV fluid will equilibrate with the different fluid compartments depending on the osmotic content of the given fluid.

5% dextrose (=glucose) is isotonic, but contains only a small amount of glucose (50g/L) and so provides little energy (~10% daily energy per litre). The liver rapidly metabolizes all the glucose leaving only water, which rapidly equilibrates throughout all fluid compartments. It is therefore useless for fluid resuscitation (only 1/9 will remain in the intravascular space), but suitable for maintaining hydration. Excess 5% dextrose IV may lead to water overload and hyponatraemia (p686).

0.9% saline ('normal saline') has about the same Na^+ content as plasma (150mmol/L) and is isotonic with plasma. 0.9% saline will equilibrate rapidly throughout the extracellular compartment only, and takes longer to reach the intracellular compartment than 5% dextrose. It is therefore appropriate for fluid resuscitation, as it will remain predominantly in the extracellular space (and thus ⅓ of the given volume in the intravascular space), as well as for maintaining hydration. Hypertonic and hypotonic saline solutions are also available, but are for specialist use only.

Colloids (eg Gelofusine® or Haemaccel®) have a high osmotic content similar to that of plasma and therefore remain in the intravascular space for longer than other fluids, making them appropriate for fluid resuscitation, but not for general hydration. Colloids are expensive, and may cause anaphylactic reactions. In reality, effective fluid resuscitation will use a combination of colloid and 0.9% saline.

Hypertonic dextrose (10% or 50%) may be used in the treatment of hypoglycaemia. It is irritant to veins, so care in its use is needed. Infusion sites should be inspected regularly, and flushed with 0.9% saline after use.

Dextrose-saline (one-fifth 'normal saline') is isotonic, containing 0.18% saline (30mmol/L of Na^+) and 4% glucose (222mmol/L). It has roughly the quantity of Na^+ required for normal fluid maintenance, when given 10 hourly in adults, but is now most commonly used in a paediatric setting.

Hartmann's solution contains Na^+ 131mmol, Cl^- 111mmol, lactate 29mmol, K^+ 5mmol, HCO_3^- 29mmol, and Ca^{2+} 2mmol per litre of fluid. It is an alternative to 0.9% saline, and some consider it more physiological. [1]

Assessing fluid balance

Underfilled	Overfilled
• Tachycardia	• ↑JVP (p40)
• Postural drop in BP (low BP is a late sign of hypovolaemia)	• Pitting oedema of the sacrum, ankles, or even legs and abdomen
• ↓capillary refill time	• Tachypnoea
• ↓urine output	• Bibasal crepitations
• Cool peripheries	• Pulmonary oedema on CXR
• Dry mucous membranes	See also p128 for signs of heart failure
• ↓skin turgor	
• Sunken eyes	

The JVP is a substitute marker of central venous pressure, and in cases where assessing fluid balance is difficult a CVP line may be necessary to guide fluid management.

Special cases

Acute blood loss Resuscitate with colloid or 0.9% saline via large bore cannulae until blood is available.

Children Use dextrose-saline for fluid maintenance: 100mL/kg for the first 10kg, 50mL/kg for the next 10kg, and 20mL/kg thereafter—all per 24h.

Elderly These patients are more prone to fluid overload, so use IV fluids with care.

GI losses (diarrhoea, vomiting, NG tubes, etc) Replace lost K^+ as well as lost fluid volume.

Heart failure Use IV fluids with care to avoid fluid overload (p128).

Liver failure These patients often have a raised total body sodium, so use salt-poor albumin or blood for resuscitation, and avoid 0.9% saline for maintenance.

Pancreatitis Aggressive fluid resuscitation is required in acute pancreatitis due to large amounts of sequestered 'third space' fluid (p638).

Poor urine output Aim for > 1 mL/kg/h; the minimum is > ½ mL/kg/h. Give a fluid challenge, eg 500ml 0.9% saline over 1h (or half this volume in heart failure or the elderly), and recheck the urine output. If not catheterized exclude retention; if catheterized, ensure the catheter is not blocked!

Post-operative Check the operation notes for intraoperative losses, and ensure you chart and replace added losses from drains, etc.

Shock Resuscitate with colloid or 0.9% saline via large bore cannulae. Identify the type of shock (p804).

Transpiration losses (fever, burns) Beware the large amounts of fluid that can be lost unseen through transpiration. Severe burns in particular may require aggressive fluid resuscitation (p858).

Potassium in IV fluids

- Potassium ions can be given with 5% dextrose or 0.9% saline, usually 20mmol/L or 40mmol/L.
- K^+ may be retained in renal failure, so beware giving too much IV.
- Gastrointestinal fluids are rich in K^+, so increased fluid loss from the gut (eg diarrhoea, vomiting, high-output stoma, intestinal fistula) will need increased K^+ replacement.

►The maximum concentration of K^+ that is safe to infuse via a peripheral line is 40mmol/L, at a maximum rate of 20mmol/h. Fluid-restricted patients may require higher concentrations or rates in life-threatening hypokalaemia. Faster rates risk cardiac dysrhythmias and asystole, and higher concentrations thrombophlebitis, depending on the size of the vein, so give concentrated solutions >40mmol/L via a central venous catheter, and use ECG monitoring for rates over >10mmol/h. For symptoms and signs of hyper- and hypokalaemia see p688.

Electrolyte physiology and the kidney

The kidney controls the homeostasis of a number of serum electrolytes (including Na^+, K^+, Ca^{2+} and PO_4^{3-}), helps to maintain acid-base balance, and is responsible for the excretion of many substances. It also makes erythropoietin and renin, and hydroxylates 25-hydroxyvitamin D to 1,25-dihydroxyvitamin D (see p690 for Ca^{2+} and PO_4^{3-} physiology). All of these functions can be affected in chronic kidney disease (p300) but it is the biochemical effects of kidney failure that are used to monitor disease progression.

The Renin-Angiotensin-Aldosterone system Plasma is filtered by the glomeruli, and Na^+, K^+, H^+ and water are reabsorbed from this filtrate under the control of the renin-angiotensin-aldosterone system. *Renin* is released from the juxtaglomerular apparatus (**fig 3**, p295) in response to low renal blood flow and raised sympathetic tone, and catalyses the conversion of *angiotensinogen* (a peptide made by the liver) to *angiotensin I*. This is then converted by angiotensin-converting enzyme (ACE), which is located in the lung (mainly) and blood vessels to *angiotensin II*. The latter has several important actions including efferent renal arteriolar constriction (thus ↑ perfusion pressure), peripheral vasoconstriction, and stimulation of the adrenal cortex to produce *aldosterone*, which activates the Na^+/K^+ pump in the distal renal tubule leading to reabsorption of Na^+ and water from the urine, in exchange for K^+ and H^+. Glucose spills over into the urine when the plasma concentration > renal threshold for reabsorption (≈10mmol/L, but varies between people, & is ↓ in pregnancy).

Control of sodium is through the action of aldosterone on the distal convoluted tubule (DCT) and collecting duct to increase Na^+ reabsorption from the urine. The natriuretic peptides ANP, BNP and CNP (p131) contribute to Na^+ homeostasis by reducing Na^+ reabsorption from the DCT and inhibiting renin. A *high GFR* (below) results in increased Na^+ loss, and *high renal tubular blood flow* and haemodilution decrease Na^+ reabsorption in the proximal tubule.

Control of potassium Most K^+ is intracellular, and thus serum K^+ levels are a poor reflection of total body potassium. The concentrations of K^+ and H^+ in extracellular fluid tend to vary together. This is because these ions compete with each other in the exchange with Na^+ that occurs across most cell membranes and in the distal convoluted tubule of the kidney, where Na^+ is reabsorbed from the urine. Thus, if the H^+ concentration is high, fewer K^+ will be excreted into the urine. Similarly K^+ will compete with H^+ for exchange across cell membranes and extracellular K^+ will accumulate. Insulin and catecholamines both stimulate K^+ uptake into cells by stimulating the Na^+/K^+ pump.

Serum osmolality is a laboratory measurement of the number of osmoles per *kilogram* of solvent. It is approximated by ***serum osmolarity*** (the number of osmoles per *litre* of solution) using the equation *2(Na⁺ + K⁺) + Urea + Glucose*, since these are the predominant serum electrolytes. Normal serum osmolarity is 280–300mmol/L, which will always be a little less than the laboratory-measured osmolality—the ***osmolar gap***. However, if the osmolar gap is greater than 10mmol/L, this indicates the presence of additional solutes: consider diabetes mellitus or high blood ethanol, methanol, mannitol, or ethylene glycol.

Control of water is mainly via serum Na^+ concentration, since water intake and loss are regulated to hold the extracellular concentration of Na^+ constant. Raised plasma osmolality (eg dehydration or ↑glucose in diabetes mellitus) causes thirst through the hypothalamic thirst centre and the release of antidiuretic hormone (ADH) from the posterior pituitary. ADH increases the passive water reabsorption from the renal collecting duct by opening water channels to allow water to flow from the hypotonic luminal fluid into the hypertonic renal interstitium. Low plasma osmolality inhibits ADH secretion, thus reducing renal water reabsorption.

Glomerular filtration rate (GFR) is the volume of fluid filtered by the glomeruli per minute (units mL/min), and is one of the primary measures of disease progression in chronic kidney disease. It can be estimated in a number of different ways (see BOX).

Estimating GFR

Calculating GFR is useful because it is a more sensitive indication of the degree of renal impairment than serum creatinine. Subjects with low muscle mass (eg the elderly, women) can have a 'normal' serum creatinine, despite a significant reduction in GFR. This can be important when prescribing nephrotoxic drugs, or drugs that are renally excreted, which may therefore accumulate to toxic levels in the serum.

A number of methods for estimating GFR exist, all relying on a calculation of the clearance of a substance that is renally filtered and then not reabsorbed in the renal tubule. For example, the rate of clearance of creatinine can be used as a marker for the rate of filtration of fluid and solutes in the glomerulus because it is only slightly reabsorbed from the renal tubule. The more of the filtered substance that is reabsorbed, however, the less accurate the estimate of GFR.

The **MDRD** (*Modification of Diet in Renal Disease Study Group*) equation provides an estimate of GFR from 4 simple parameters: *serum creatinine, age, gender* and *race (black/non-black).* It is one of the best validated for monitoring patients with established moderately severe renal impairment,[2] and most labs now routinely report estimated GFR (eGFR) using the MDRD equation on all U&E reports.

$$\text{eGFR} = 32788 \times \text{serum creatinine}^{-1.154} \times \text{age}^{-0.203} \times [1.212 \textit{ if black}] \times [0.742 \textit{ if female}]$$

However, a number of caveats exist, so that it is best used in monitoring declining renal function rather than labelling elderly patients with mild renal impairment:

- it is not validated for mild renal impairment, and therefore it's use for screening *general* populations is questionable;
- inter-individual variations (and thus confidence intervals) are wide, although for each individual variations are small so that a decline in eGFR over a number of serum samples is always significant;
- single results may be affected by variations in serum creatinine, such as after a protein-rich meal.

The **Cockcroft-Gault equation** provides an estimate of creatinine clearance. It is an improvement on the MDRD equation because it also takes into account the patient's weight. However, small amounts of creatinine are reabsorbed in the distal renal tubule, and therefore creatinine clearance underestimates the GFR (and overestimates renal impairment). Moreover, the equation assumes ideal body weight and is thus unreliable in the obese or oedematous. For an example of adjusting for ideal body weight, see p446. Also unreliable in unstable renal function.

$$\text{Creat clearance} = \frac{(140 - \text{age}) \times \text{weight (kg)} \times [0.85 \textit{ if female}] \times [1.212 \textit{ if black}]}{0.813 \times \text{serum creatinine } (\mu\text{mol/L})}$$

Creatinine clearance can also be calculated by measuring the excreted creatinine in a **24h urine collection** and comparing it with the serum creatinine concentration. However, the accuracy of collection is vital but often poor, making this an unreliable and inconvenient method.

GFR can also be measured by injection of a radioisotope followed by sequential blood sampling (**^{51}Cr-EDTA**) or by an isotope scan (eg DTPA ^{99}Tc, p190). These methods allow a more accurate estimate of GFR than creatinine clearance, since smaller proportions of these substances are reabsorbed in the tubules. They also have the advantage of being able to provide split renal function.

Inulin clearance (not insulin) is the gold standard for calculating GFR, because 100% of filtered inulin is retained in the luminal fluid and therefore reflects exactly the rate of filtration of water and solutes in the glomerulus. However, measuring inulin clearance again requires urine collection over several hours, and also a constant IV infusion of inulin, and is therefore inconvenient to perform.

Arterial blood pH is closely regulated in health to 7.40 ± 0.05 by various mechanisms including bicarbonate, other plasma buffers such as deoxygenated haemoglobin, and the kidney. Acid-base disorders needlessly confuse many people, but if a few simple rules are applied, then interpretation and diagnosis are easy. The key principle is that primary changes in HCO_3^- are ***metabolic***, and in CO_2 ***respiratory***. See **fig 1**.

A simple method

1 ***Look at the pH:*** is there an acidosis or alkalosis?
- pH < 7.35 is an acidosis; pH > 7.45 is an alkalosis.

2 ***Is the CO_2 abnormal?*** (Normal concentration 4.7–6.0kPa)
If so, is the change in keeping with the pH?
- CO_2 is an acidic gas—is CO_2 raised with an acidosis, lowered with an alkalosis? If so, it is in keeping with the pH and thus caused by a ***respiratory*** problem. If there is no change, or an opposite one, then the change is compensatory.

3 ***Is the HCO_3^- abnormal?*** (Normal concentration 22–28mmol/L)
If so, is the change in keeping with the pH?
- HCO_3^- is alkaline—is HCO_3^- raised with an alkalosis, lowered with an acidosis? If so, the problem is a ***metabolic*** one.

An example

Your patient's blood gas shows: pH 7.05, CO_2 2.0kPa, HCO_3^- 8.0mmol/L.
There is an *acidosis*. The CO_2 is low, and thus it is a compensatory change. The HCO_3^- is low and is thus the primary change, ie a *metabolic* acidosis.

The anion gap estimates unmeasured plasma anions ('fixed' or organic acids such as phosphate, ketones, and lactate, which are hard to measure directly). It is calculated as the difference between plasma cations (Na^+ & K^+) and anions (Cl^- & HCO_3^-). Normal range: 10–18mmol/L. It is helpful in determining the cause of a metabolic acidosis.

Metabolic acidosis pH↓, HCO_3^-↓

Causes of metabolic acidosis and an increased anion gap:
Due to increased production, or reduced excretion, of fixed/organic acids. HCO_3^- falls and unmeasured anions associated with the acids accumulate.
- Lactic acid (shock, infection, tissue ischaemia)
- Urate (renal failure)
- Ketones (diabetes mellitus, alcohol)
- Drugs/toxins (salicylates, biguanides, ethylene glycol, methanol)

Causes of metabolic acidosis and a normal anion gap:
Due to loss of bicarbonate or ingestion of H^+ ions (Cl^- is retained).
- Renal tubular acidosis
- Diarrhoea
- Drugs (acetazolamide)
- Addison's disease
- Pancreatic fistula
- Ammonium chloride ingestion

Metabolic alkalosis pH↑, HCO_3^-↑
- Vomiting
- K^+ depletion (diuretics)
- Burns
- Ingestion of base

Respiratory acidosis pH↓, CO_2↑

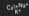

Ca^{2+} Na^+ K^+

- Type 2 respiratory failure due to any lung, neuromuscular, or physical cause (p180).
- Most commonly chronic obstructive pulmonary disease (COPD). Look at the P_aO_2. It will probably be low. Is oxygen therapy required? Use controlled O_2 (Venturi connector) if COPD is the underlying cause, as too much oxygen may make matters worse (p181).

▸▸Beware exhaustion in asthma, pneumonia and pulmonary oedema, which can present with this picture when close to respiratory arrest. These patients require urgent ITU review for ventilatory support.

Respiratory alkalosis pH↑, CO_2↓

A result of hyperventilation of any cause.
CNS causes: Stroke; subarachnoid bleed; meningitis. ***Others:*** Anxiety; altitude; T°↑; pregnancy; pulmonary emboli (reflex hyperventilation); drugs, eg salicylates.

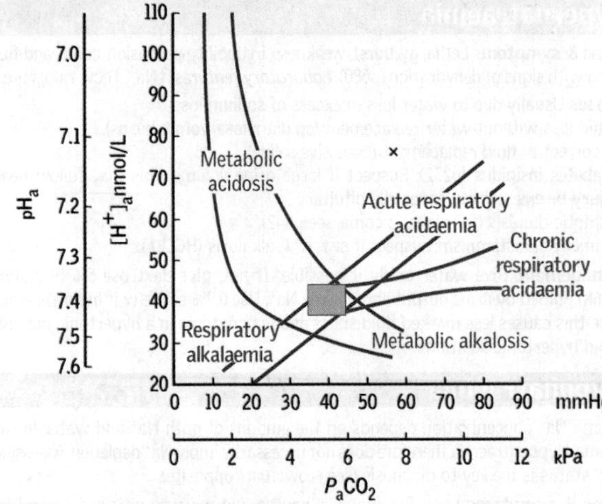

Fig 1. The shaded area represents normality. This method is very powerful. The result represented by point ×, for example, indicates that the acidosis is in part respiratory and in part metabolic. Seek a cause for each.

Terminology To aid understanding, we have used the terms acidosis and alkalosis, where a purist would sometimes have used acidaemia and alkalaemia.

Hypernatraemia

Signs & symptoms Lethargy, thirst, weakness, irritability, confusion, coma, and fits, along with signs of dehydration (p680). ***Laboratory features:*** ↑Na^+, ↑PCV, ↑alb, ↑urea.

Causes Usually due to water loss in excess of sodium loss:

- Fluid loss without water replacement (eg diarrhoea, vomit, burns).
- Incorrect IV fluid replacement (excessive saline).
- Diabetes insipidus (p232). Suspect if large urine volume. This may follow head injury, or CNS surgery, especially pituitary.
- Osmotic diuresis (for diabetic coma, see p842).
- Primary aldosteronism: suspect if BP↑, K^+↓, alkalosis (HCO_3^-↑).

Management Give water orally if possible. If not, give dextrose 5% IV slowly (1L/6h) guided by urine output and plasma Na^+. Use 0.9% saline IV if hypovolaemic, since this causes less marked fluid shifts and is hypotonic in a hypertonic patient. Avoid hypertonic solutions.

Hyponatraemia

Plasma Na^+ concentration depends on the amount of both Na^+ and water in the plasma. Hyponatraemia therefore does not necessarily imply Na^+ depletion. Assessing fluid status is the key to diagnosis (see FLOWCHART opposite).

Signs & symptoms Look for anorexia, nausea and malaise initially, followed by headache, irritability, confusion, weakness, ↓GCS and seizures, depending on the severity and rate of change in serum Na^+. Cardiac failure or oedema may help to indicate the cause. Hyponatraemia also increases the risk of falls in the elderly.[3]

Causes See the FLOWCHART opposite. Artefactual causes include: • Blood sample was from a drip arm; • High serum lipid/protein content causing ↑ serum volume, with ↓Na^+ concentration but normal plasma osmolality; • If hyperglycaemic (≥20mmol/L) add ~4.3mmol/L to plasma Na^+ for every 10mmol/L rise in glucose above normal.

Iatrogenic hyponatraemia If 5% dextrose is infused continuously without adding 0.9% saline, the dextrose is quickly used, rendering the fluid hypotonic and causing hyponatraemia. Those especially at risk include those on thiazide diuretics, women (especially pre-menopausal) and those undergoing physiological stress (eg post-operative, septic). In some patients, only marginally low plasma Na^+ levels cause serious effects (eg ~128mmol/L)—don't attribute odd CNS signs to non-existent strokes/TIAs if Na^+↓.

Management

- Correct the underlying cause; never base treatment on Na^+ concentration alone.
- The presence of symptoms, the chronicity of the hyponatraemia, and state of hydration are all important. Replace Na^+ and water at the same rate they were lost: • In ***asymptomatic chronic hyponatraemia*** **fluid restriction** is often sufficient if asymptomatic, although **demeclocycline** (ADH antagonist) may be required. If hypervolaemic (cirrhosis, CCF) treat the underlying disorder first. • In ***acute*** or ***symptomatic hyponatraemia***, or if ***dehydrated***, cautious rehydration with 0.9% saline may be given, but do not correct changes rapidly as *central pontine myelinolysis*[1] may result. Maximum rise in serum Na^+ 15mmol/L per day if chronic, or 1mmol/L per hour if acute. Consider using furosemide when not hypovolaemic to avoid fluid overload.
- **Vasopressor receptor antagonists** ('vaptans', eg conivaptan, tolvaptan, lixivaptan and satavaptan) promote water excretion without loss of electrolytes, and appear to be effective in treating hypervolaemic and euvolaemic hyponatraemia.[4]

▸▸***In emergency*** (seizures, coma) seek expert help. Consider hypertonic saline (eg 1.8% saline) at 70mmol Na^+/h ± furosemide. Aim for a gradual increase in plasma Na^+ to ≈125mmol/L. Beware heart failure and central pontine myelinolysis.[1]

1 **Central pontine myelinolysis:** irreversible and often fatal pontine demyelination seen in malnourished alcoholics or rapid correction of ↓Na^+. There is subacute onset of lethargy, confusion, pseudobulbar palsy, para- or quadriparesis, 'locked-in' syndrome or coma.

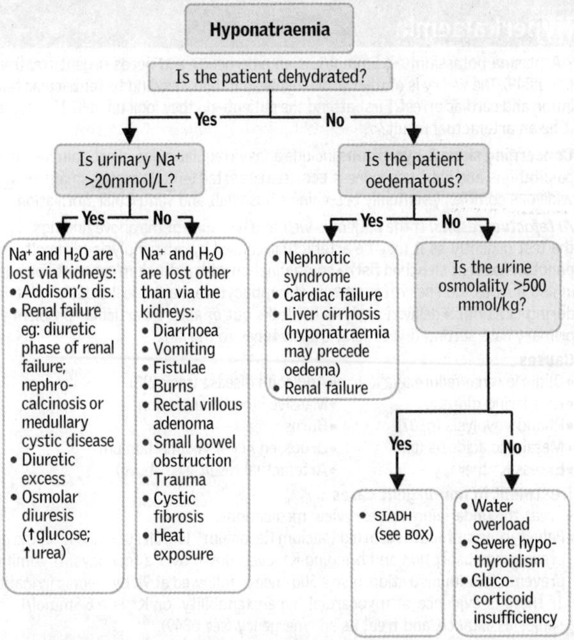

Syndrome of inappropriate ADH secretion (SIADH)

An important, but over-diagnosed, cause of hyponatraemia. The diagnosis requires concentrated urine (Na^+ >20mmol/L and osmolality >500mosmol/kg) in the presence of hyponatraemia (plasma Na^+ <125mmol/L) or low plasma osmolality (< 260mosmol/kg), and the absence of hypovolaemia, oedema, or diuretics.

Causes • *Malignancy:* lung small-cell, pancreas, prostate, thymus, or lymphoma.
• *CNS disorders:* meningoencephalitis, abscess, stroke, subarachnoid or subdural haemorrhage, head injury, neurosurgery, Guillain-Barré, vasculitis or SLE.
• *Chest disease:* TB, pneumonia, abscess, aspergillosis, small-cell lung cancer.
• *Endocrine disease:* hypothyroidism (not true SIADH, but perhaps due to excess ADH release from carotid sinus baroreceptors triggered by ↓ cardiac output).[5]
• *Drugs:* opiates, psychotropics, SSRIs, cytotoxics.
• *Other:* acute intermittent porphyria, trauma, major abdominal or thoracic surgery, symptomatic HIV.

Treatment Treat the cause and restrict fluid. Consider salt ± loop diuretic if severe. Demeclocycline is used rarely. Vasopressin receptor antagonists ('vaptans', p686) are an emerging class of drug used in SIADH and other types of hyponatraemia.

Hyperkalaemia

▸▸A plasma potassium >6.5mmol/L is an emergency and needs urgent treatment (see p849). The worry is of myocardial hyperexcitability leading to ventricular fibrillation and cardiac arrest. First attend the patient—do they look unwell? If not, could it be an artefactual result?

Concerning signs & symptoms include a fast irregular pulse, chest pain, weakness, palpitations, and light-headedness. **ECG:** (see ECG 9) tall tented T waves, small P waves, a wide QRS complex (eventually becoming sinusoidal), and ventricular fibrillation.

Artefactual results: If the patient is well, and has none of the above findings, repeat the test urgently as it may be artefactual, caused by: • haemolysis (difficult venepuncture; patient clenched fist); • contamination with potassium EDTA anticoagulant in FBC bottles (do FBCs *after* U&Es); • thrombocythaemia (K^+ leaks out of platelets during clotting); • delayed analysis (K^+ leaks out of RBCs; a particular problem in a primary care setting due to long transit times to the lab).

Causes

- Oliguric renal failure
- K^+-sparing diuretics
- Rhabdomyolysis (p307)
- Metabolic acidosis (DM)
- Excess K^+ therapy
- Addison's disease (see p218)
- Massive blood transfusion
- Burns
- Drugs, eg ACE-i, suxamethonium
- Artefactual result (see above)

Treatment in non-urgent cases

- Treat the underlying cause; review medications.
- **Polystyrene sulfonate resin** (eg Calcium Resonium® 15g/8h PO) binds K^+ in the gut, preventing absorption and bringing K^+ levels down over a few days. If vomiting prevents PO administration, give a 30g enema, followed at 9h by colonic irrigation.
- ▸▸If there is evidence of myocardial hyperexcitability, or K^+ is >6.5mmol/L, get senior assistance, and treat as an emergency (see p849).

Hypokalaemia

If K^+ <2.5mmol/L, urgent treatment is required. Note that hypokalaemia exacerbates digoxin toxicity.

Signs & symptoms Muscle weakness, hypotonia, hyporeflexia, cramps, tetany, palpitations, light-headedness (arrhythmias).

ECG Small or inverted T waves, prominent U waves (after T wave), a long PR interval, and depressed ST segments.

Causes

- Diuretics
- Vomiting and diarrhoea
- Pyloric stenosis
- Rectal villous adenoma
- Intestinal fistula
- Cushing's syndrome/steroids/ACTH
- Conn's syndrome
- Alkalosis
- Purgative and liquorice abuse
- Renal tubular failure (p310 & p678)
- If on diuretics, ↑HCO_3^- is the best indication that hypokalaemia is likely to have been long-standing. Mg^{2+} may be low, and hypokalaemia is often difficult to correct until Mg^{2+} levels are normalized.
- Suspect Conn's syndrome if hypertensive, hypokalaemic alkalosis in someone not taking diuretics (p220).
- In ***hypokalaemic periodic paralysis***, intermittent weakness lasting up to 72h appears to be caused by K^+ shifting from extra- to intracellular fluid. See *OHCS* p652.

Treatment *If mild:* (>2.5mmol/L, no symptoms) give oral K^+ supplement (≥80mmol/24h, eg Sando-K® 2 tabs/8h). Review K^+ after 3 days. If taking a thiazide diuretic, hypokalaemia >3.0mmol/L rarely needs treating. ***If severe:*** (<2.5mmol/L, and/or dangerous symptoms) give IV potassium cautiously, not more than 20mmol/h, and not more concentrated than 40mmol/L. Do not give K^+ if oliguric. ▸▸**Never** give K^+ as a fast stat bolus dose.

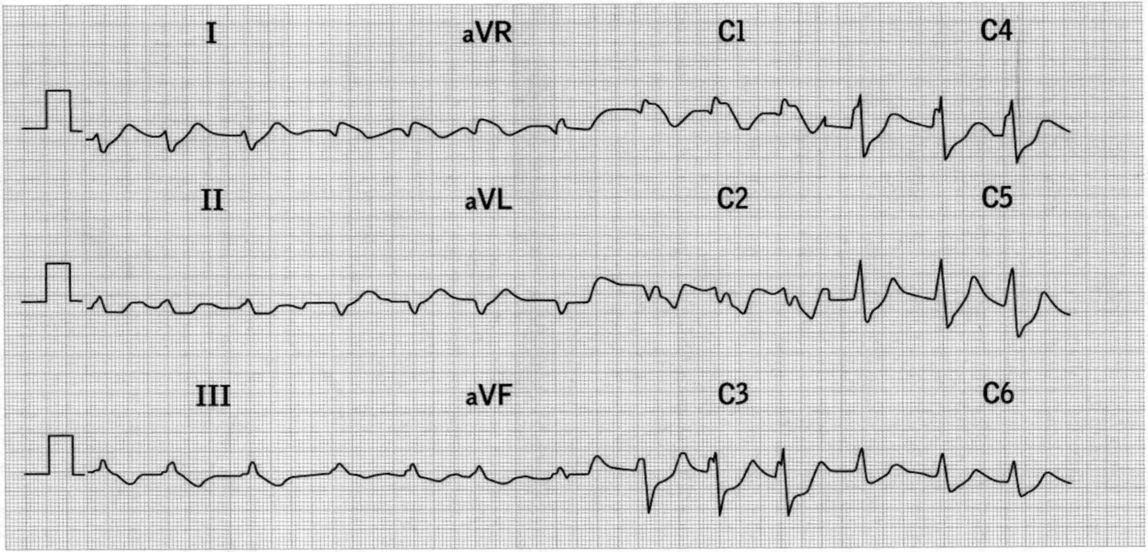

ECG 9. Hyperkalaemia—note the flattening of the P waves, prominent T waves, and widening of the QRS complex.

Calcium and phosphate physiology

Calcium and phosphate homeostasis is maintained through:

Parathyroid hormone (PTH): Overall effect is ↑Ca^{2+} & ↓PO_4^{3-}. Secretion by 4 parathyroid glands is triggered by ↓serum ionized Ca^{2+}; controlled by -ve feedback loop. *Actions* are: • ↑osteoclast activity releasing Ca^{2+} & PO_4^{3-} from bones; • ↑Ca^{2+} & ↓PO_4^{3-} reabsorption in the kidney; • ↑renal production of 1,25dihydroxy-vitamin D_3.

Vitamin D and calcitriol: Vit D is hydroxylated first in the liver to 25hydroxy-vit D, and again in the kidney to 1,25dihydroxy-vit D (**calcitriol**) the biologically active form, and 24,25hydroxy-vit D (inactive). Calcitriol production is stimulated by ↓Ca^{2+}, ↓PO_4^{3-}, and PTH. *Actions* are: • ↑Ca^{2+} and ↑PO_4^{3-} absorption from the gut; • inhibition of PTH release; • Enhanced bone turnover; • ↑Ca^{2+} and ↑PO_4^{3-} reabsorption in the kidney. **Cholecalciferol** (vit D_3—from animal sources) and **ergocalciferol** (vit D_2—from vegetables) are biologically identical in their activity. Disordered regulation of calcitriol underlies familial normocalcaemic hypercalciuria, which is a major cause of calcium oxalate renal stone formation (p640).

Calcitonin: Made in C-cells of the thyroid, this causes ↓Ca^{2+} and PO_4^{3-}, but its physiological role is unclear. It can be used as a marker of recurrence or metastasis in medullary carcinoma of the thyroid.

Magnesium: ↓Mg^{2+} prevents PTH release, and may cause hypocalcaemia.

Plasma binding: ~40% of plasma Ca^{2+} is bound to albumin. Labs usually measure total plasma Ca^{2+}, although it is unbound, ionized Ca^{2+} that is important. Therefore, **correct total Ca^{2+} for albumin as follows:** Add 0.1mmol/L to Ca^{2+} level for every 4g/L that albumin is below 40g/L, and a similar subtraction for raised albumin. However, many other factors affect binding (eg other proteins in myeloma, cirrhosis, individual variation) so be cautious in your interpretation. If in doubt over a high Ca^{2+}, take blood specimens uncuffed (remove tourniquet after needle in vein, but before taking blood sample), and with the patient fasted.

Hypercalcaemia

Signs & symptoms 'Bones, stones, groans, and psychic moans'. Abdominal pain; vomiting; constipation; polyuria; polydipsia; depression; anorexia; weight loss; tiredness; weakness; hypertension, confusion; pyrexia; renal stones; renal failure; ectopic calcification (eg cornea—see MINIBOX); cardiac arrest. *ECG:* QT interval↓.

Causes (See FLOWCHART) Most commonly malignancy (eg from bone metastases, myeloma, PTHrP) or primary hyperparathyroidism. Others include sarcoidosis, vit D intoxication, thyrotoxicosis, lithium, tertiary hyperparathyroidism, milk-alkali syndrome, and familial benign hypocalciuric hypercalcaemia (rare; defect in calcium-sensing receptor). HIV can cause both ↑ & ↓ Ca^{2+} (perhaps from PTH-related bone remodelling).[17]

Investigations The main distinction is malignancy vs 1° hyperparathyroidism. Pointers to malignancy are ↓albumin, ↓Cl^-, alkalosis, ↓K^+, ↑PO_4^{3-}, ↑alk phos. ↑PTH indicates hyperparathyroidism. Also FBC, protein electrophoresis, CXR, isotope bone scan, 24h urinary Ca^{2+} excretion (for familial hypocalciuric hypercalcaemia).

Causes of metastatic (ectopic) calcification 'PARATHORMONE'
Parathormone (PTH)↑ (p214) & other causes of Ca^{2+}↑, eg sarcoidosis[7]
Amyloidosis
Renal failure (relates to ↑PO_4^{3-})
Addison's disease (adrenal calcification)[8]
TB nodes; **T**oxoplasmosis (CNS)
Histoplasmosis (eg in lung)[9]
Overdose of vitamin D[10]
Raynaud's-associated diseases, eg SLE; CREST[11] (p554; calcification in skin or CNS vessels); dermatomyositis[12] [13]
Muscle primaries/leiomyosarcomas)[14]
Ossifying metastases (**o**steosarcoma) or **o**varian mets (to peritoneum)[15]
Nephrocalcinosis
Endocrine tumours (eg gastrinoma)[16]

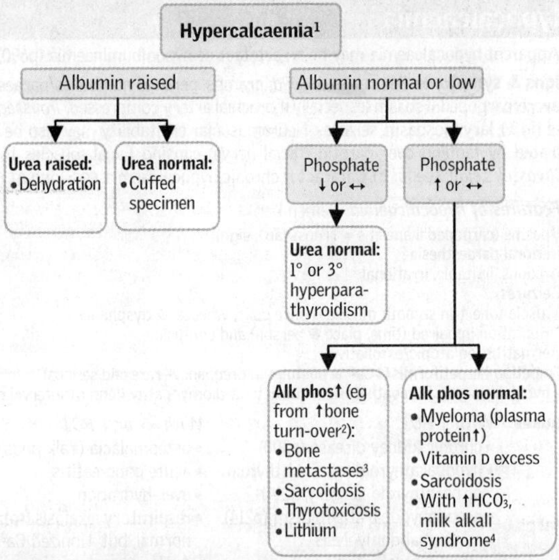

Treating acute hypercalcaemia

Diagnose and treat the underlying cause. If Ca^{2+} >3.5mmol/L and symptomatic:

1 *Correct dehydration* if present with IV 0.9% saline.

2 *Bisphosphonates* prevent bone resorption by inhibiting osteoclast activity. A single dose of **pamidronate** lowers Ca^{2+} over 2-3d; maximum effect is at 1wk. *Infuse slowly*, eg 30mg in 300mL 0.9% saline over 3h via a largish vein. Max dose 90mg (see TABLE below). *SE:* 'Flu symptoms, ↓PO_4^{3-}, bone pain, myalgia, nausea, vomiting, headache, lymphocytopenia, ↓Mg^{2+}, ↓Ca^{2+}, seizures.

3 *Further management* **Chemotherapy** may help in malignancy. **Steroids** are used in sarcoidosis, eg prednisolone 40-60mg/d. **Salmon calcitonin** acts similarly to bisphosphonates, and has a quicker onset of action, but is now rarely used. NB: The use of **furosemide** is contentious, as supporting RCT evidence is scant.[18 19] It helps to promote renal excretion of Ca^{2+}, but can exacerbate hypercalcaemia by worsening dehydration. Thus it should only be used once fully rehydrated, and with concomitant IV fluids (eg 0.9% saline 1L/4-6h). Avoid thiazides.

Disodium pamidronate doses

Calcium (mmol/L; corrected)[20]	Single-dose pamidronate (mg)
<3	15-30
3-3.5	30-60
3.5-4	60-90
>4	90

Other bisphosphonates include zoledronic acid, sodium clodronate and ibandronic acid. **Zoledronic acid** is significantly more effective in reducing serum Ca^{2+} than previously used bisphosphonates.[21] Usually, a single dose of 4mg IVI over 2h will normalize plasma Ca^{2+} within a week. A higher dose should be used if corrected Ca^{2+} is >3mmol/L. *SE:* Flu symptoms, bone pain, PO_4^{3-}↓, confusion, thirst, taste disturbance, nausea, pulse↓, WCC↓, creatinine↑.

1 This diagram is only a guide: take in conjunction with the clinical picture.
2 Increased alkaline phosphatase from increased bone turnover.
3 Most common primary: breast, kidney, lung, thyroid, prostate, ovary, colon.
4 Ingesting too much calcium and alkali (eg in milk) can cause hypercalcaemia with metastatic calcification and renal failure. Thyrotoxicosis causes alkalaemia because of hyperventilation.

Hypocalcaemia

►Apparent hypocalcaemia may be an artefact of hypoalbuminaemia (p690).

Signs & symptoms See MINIBOX. *Mild:* cramps, perioral numbness/paraesthesiae. *Severe:* carpopedal spasm (especially if brachial artery compressed, *Trousseau's sign;* see **fig 1**), laryngospasm, seizures. Neuromuscular excitability may also be demonstrated by tapping over parotid (facial nerve) causing facial muscles to twitch (*Chvostek's sign;* see **fig 2**). Cataract if chronic hypocalcaemia. *ECG:* long QT interval.

Features of hypocalcaemia: Remember '**SPASMODIC**'[22]
Spasms (carpopedal spasms = Trousseau's sign)
Perioral paraesthesiae
Anxious, irritable, irrational
Seizures
Muscle tone ↑ in smooth muscle—hence colic, wheeze, & dysphagia[23]
Orientation impaired (time, place & person) and confusion
Dermatitis (eg atopic/exfoliative)[24]
Impetigo herpetiformis (↓Ca^{2+} & pustules in pregnancy—rare and serious)
Chvostek's sign; **c**horeoathetosis; **c**ataract; **c**ardiomyopathy (long QT interval on ECG)

Causes *With ↑ PO_4^{3-}*
- chronic kidney disease (p300)
- hypoparathyroidism (incl thyroid or parathyroid surgery, p214)
- pseudohypoparathyroidism (p214)
- acute rhabdomyolysis
- vitamin D deficiency
- hypomagnesaemia

With ↔ or ↓ PO_4^{3-}
- osteomalacia (↑alk phos)
- acute pancreatitis
- over-hydration
- respiratory alkalosis (total Ca^{2+} is normal, but ↓ionized Ca^{2+} due to ↑pH ∴ symptomatic)

Treatment
- *Mild symptoms:* give calcium 5mmol/6h PO, with daily plasma Ca^{2+} levels.
- *In chronic kidney disease*: see p300. May require **alfacalcidol**, eg 0.5-1μg/24h PO.
- *Severe symptoms:* give 10mL of **10% calcium gluconate** (2.25mmol) IV over 30min, and repeat as necessary. If due to respiratory alkalosis, correct the alkalosis.

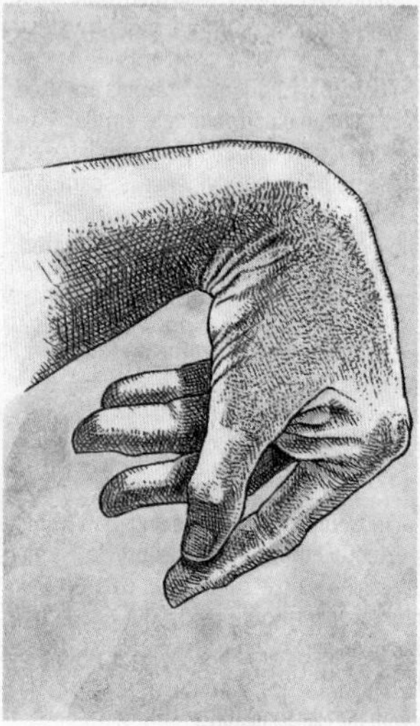

Fig 1. Trousseau's sign: on inflating the cuff, the wrist and fingers flex and draw together (carpopedal spasm).

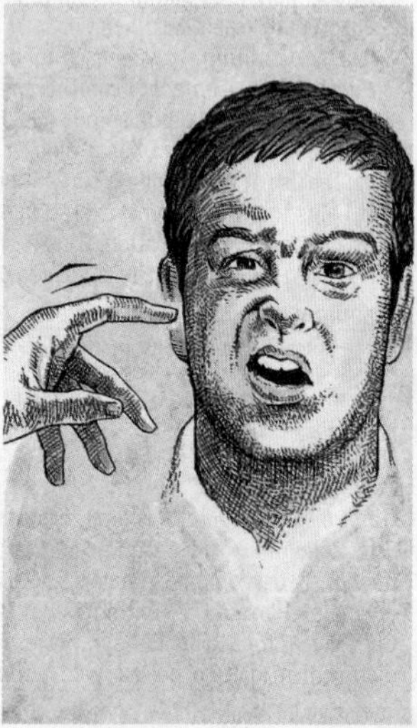

Fig 2. Chvostek's sign: the corner of mouth twitches when the facial nerve is tapped over the parotid.

Phosphate

Hypophosphataemia is common and of little significance unless severe (< 0.4mmol/L). *Causes* include vitamin D deficiency, alcohol withdrawal, refeeding syndrome (p5789, inadequate oral intake, severe diabetic ketoacidosis, renal tubular dysfunction and 1° hyperparathyroidism. *Signs & symptoms* include muscle weakness or rhabdomyolysis, red cell, white cell and platelet dysfunction, and cardiac arrest or arrhythmias. *Treatment* is by oral or parenteral phosphate supplementation, eg Phosphate Polyfusor® IVI (100mmol PO_4^{3-} in 500mL). Never give IV phosphate to a patient who is hypercalcaemic or oliguric.

Hyperphosphataemia is most commonly due to chronic kidney disease, when it is treated with phosphate binders, eg sevelamer 800mg/8h PO during meals. Also catabolic states such as tumour lysis syndrome (p526).

Magnesium

Magnesium is distributed 65% in bone and 35% in cells; plasma concentration tends to follow that of Ca^{2+} and K^+.

Hypomagnesaemia causes paraesthesiae, ataxia, seizures, tetany, arrhythmias. Digitalis toxicity may be exacerbated. *Causes* include diuretics, severe diarrhoea, ketoacidosis, alcohol abuse, total parenteral nutrition (monitor weekly), ↓Ca^{2+} and ↓K^+ and ↓PO_4^{3-}. *Treatment:* If needed, give magnesium salts, PO or IV (eg 8mmol $MgSO_4$ IV over 3min to 2h, depending on severity, with frequent Mg^{2+} levels).

Hypermagnesaemia rarely requires treatment unless severe (>7.5mmol/L). *Causes* are renal failure or iatrogenic (eg excessive antacids). *Signs* if severe include neuromuscular depression, ↓BP, ↓pulse, hyporeflexia, CNS & respiratory depression, coma.

Zinc

Zinc deficiency This may occur in parenteral nutrition or, rarely, from a poor diet (too few cereals and dairy products; anorexia nervosa; alcoholism). Rarely it is due to a genetic defect. *Symptoms:* Alopecia, dermatitis (look for red, crusted skin lesions especially around nostrils and corners of mouth), night blindness, diarrhoea. *Diagnosis:* Therapeutic trial of zinc (plasma levels are unreliable as they may be low, eg in infection or trauma, without deficiency).

Selenium

An essential element present in cereals, nuts, and meat. Low soil levels in some parts of Europe and China cause deficiency states. Required for the antioxidant glutathione peroxidase, which ↓ harmful free radicals. This is said to explain why selenium (200mg/d) helps in HIV (CD4↑; viral load↓).[25] Selenium is also antithrombogenic, and is required for sperm motility proteins. Deficiency may increase risk of neoplasia and atheroma, and may lead to a cardiomyopathy or arthritis. Serum levels are a poor guide. Toxic symptoms may also be found with over-energetic replacement.

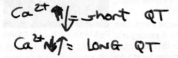

Ca^{2+} ↑ = short QT
Ca^{2+} ↓ = LONG QT

Ca^{2+} Na^+ K^+

Causes of hyperuricaemia High levels of urate in the blood (hyperuricaemia) may result from increased turnover (15%) or reduced excretion of urate (85%). Either may be drug induced.

- *Drugs:* Cytotoxics, thiazides, loop diuretics, pyrazinamide.
- *Increased cell turnover:* Lymphoma, leukaemia, psoriasis, haemolysis, muscle death (rhabdomyolysis, p307; tumour lysis syndrome, p526).
- *Reduced excretion:* Primary gout (p550), chronic kidney disease, lead nephropathy, hyperparathyroidism, pre-eclampsia (*OHCS* p48).
- *Other:* Hyperuricaemia may be associated with hypertension and hyperlipidaemia. Urate may be raised in disorders of purine synthesis such as the *Lesch–Nyhan syndrome* (*OHCS* p648).

Hyperuricaemia and renal failure Severe renal failure from any cause may be associated with hyperuricaemia, and rarely this may give rise to gout. Sometimes the relationship of cause and effect is reversed so that it is the hyperuricaemia that causes the renal failure. This can occur following cytotoxic treatment (tumour lysis syndrome, p526), and in muscle necrosis.

How urate causes renal failure: Urate is poorly soluble in water, so overexcretion can lead to crystal precipitation. Renal failure occurs most commonly because urate precipitates in the renal tubules. This may occur at plasma levels ≥1.19mmol/L. In some instances ureteric obstruction from urate crystals may occur. This responds to retrograde ureteric catheterization and lavage.

Prevention of renal failure: Before starting chemotherapy, ensure good hydration and initiate **allopurinol** (xanthine oxidase inhibitor) or **rasburicase** (recombinant urate oxidase), which prevent a sharp rise in urate following chemotherapy (see p526). There is a remote risk of inducing xanthine nephropathy.

Treatment of hyperuricaemic acute renal failure: Exclude bilateral ureteric obstruction, then give prompt **rehydration ± loop diuretic** to wash uric acid crystals out of the renal tubules, and correct electrolyte abnormalities. Once oliguria is established, **haemodialysis** is required (in preference to peritoneal dialysis). There is no evidence for either preventing (above) or treating hyperuricaemic renal failure.

Gout See p550.

Urate renal stones Urate stones (**fig 1**) comprise 5–10% of all renal stones and are radiolucent.

Incidence: ~5–10% in temperate climates (double if confirmed gout),[27] but up to 40% in hot, arid climates. ♂:♀ ≈4:1. But most urate stone formers have no detectable abnormalities in urate metabolism.

Risk factors: Acidic or strongly concentrated urine; ↑urinary excretion of urate; chronic diarrhoea; distal small bowel disease or resection (regional enteritis); ileostomy; obesity; diabetes mellitus; chemotherapy for myeloproliferative disorders; inadequate caloric or fluid intake.

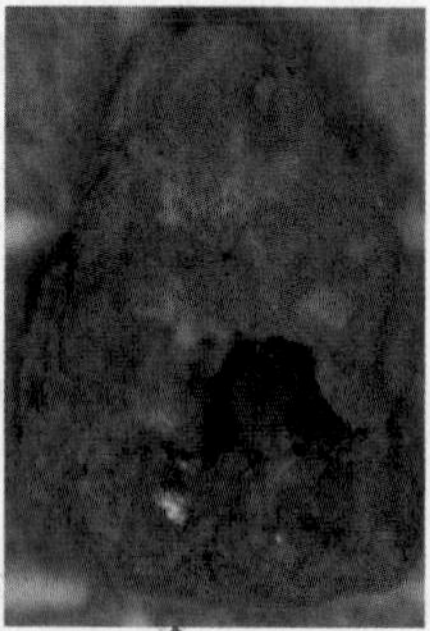

Fig 1. Urate stone.[26] ©Dr G Austin

Treatment: **Hydration** to increase urine volume (aim >2L/d). Unlike most other renal calculi, existing uric acid stones can often be dissolved with either systemic or topical alkalinizing agents. **Potassium citrate** or **potassium bicarbonate** at a dose titrated to alkalinize the urine to a pH of 6–7 dissolves some urate stones. If hyperuricosuria, consider dietary management ± allopurinol (xanthine oxidase inhibitor).

Metabolic bone diseases: osteoporosis

Osteoporosis implies reduced bone mass. It may be 1° (age-related) or 2° to another condition or drugs. If trabecular bone is affected, crush fractures of vertebrae are common (hence the 'littleness' of little old ladies and their dowager's hump); if cortical bone is affected, long bone fractures are more likely, eg femoral neck: the big cause of death and [illegible] (orthopaedic [illegible]) in the elderly [illegible].

Prevalence (in those >50yrs): ♂ 6%; ♀ 18%. Women [illegible] bone with age [illegible] constant [illegible] [illegible] bone formation [illegible] [illegible] and their lifetime risk of fracture is [illegible].

Risk factors: Age-independent risk factors for osteoporosis: parental history, alcohol >4 units daily, rheumatoid arthritis, BMI <22, prolonged immobility and untreated menopause. See MINIBOX for other risk factors (including for 2° osteoporosis).

Investigations: X-ray (low sensitivity, specificity, often with fractures after a fracture). Bone densitometry (DEXA—see BOX). Bloods: Ca²⁺, PO₄, alk phos normal. Consider specific investigation for 2° causes if suggestive history. Biopsy is unsuitable and unnecessary with non-invasive techniques available.

Management: Lower bone mineral density may not be [illegible] reversible. Age, number of risk factors and bone mineral density (DEXA scan, see BOX) guide the clinical approach (eg FRAX, which is a WHO assessment tool for estimating the 10yr risk of osteoporotic fractures in untreated patients; see www.shef.ac.uk/FRAX, although DEXA is not necessary [illegible]). Lifestyle measures should apply to all (including those at risk but not yet osteoporotic):

Lifestyle measures:
- Quit smoking and reduce alcohol consumption.
- Weight-bearing exercise may increase bone mineral density.
- Balance exercises [illegible] tai chi [illegible] risk of falls.
- [illegible]
- Home-based [illegible] intervention [illegible] with [illegible] assessment and [illegible] visit [illegible] for preventing fractures.

Pharmacological measures:
- Bisphosphonates: alendronate [illegible] if eGFR >35. [illegible]
- Calcium and vitamin D: Calcium 1.2–1.5g/day and vitamin D 800–2000U/day. Calcium [illegible] Target serum 25-hydroxy-vitamin D level >75nmol/L. Exposure to sunlight is usually more good than harm.
- Strontium ranelate: ↓ fracture rate [illegible] as effective as bisphosphonates. Strontium [illegible] calcium and reduces reabsorption and may [illegible] bone formation.
- Hormone replacement therapy (HRT) can prevent [illegible] postmenopausal women [illegible] breast cancer [illegible]
- Raloxifene is a selective oestrogen receptor modulator (SERM) that acts similarly to HRT, but with ↓ breast cancer risk.
- Teriparatide (recombinant PTH) is used in those who suffer further fractures despite treatment with other agents. There is a potential risk of [illegible] malignancy.
- Calcitonin may reduce pain after vertebral fracture.
- Testosterone may help in hypogonadal men by promoting trabecular connectivity.

Osteoporosis risk factors

Family history
[illegible]
7.5mg/day of prednisolone
Hyperthyroidism
[illegible]
Hypogonadism
Alcohol and tobacco use
BMI <22
[illegible]
[illegible]
Chronic liver failure
[illegible]
[illegible]
[illegible]
Diabetes mellitus (type 1)

Osteoporosis implies reduced bone mass. It may be 1° (age-related) or 2° to another condition or drugs. If trabecular bone is affected, crush fractures of vertebrae are common (hence the 'littleness' of little old ladies and their dowager's hump); if cortical bone is affected, long bone fractures are more likely, eg femoral neck: *the* big cause of death and orthopaedic expense (80% hip fractures in the UK occur in women >50yrs).

Prevalence (in those >50yrs): ♂ 6%, ♀ 18%. Women lose trabeculae with age, but in men, although there is reduced bone formation, numbers of trabeculae are stable and their lifetime risk of fracture is less.[28]

Osteoporosis risk factors
Family history +ve, or old and **SHATTERED**...
Steroid use of >5mg/day of prednisolone
Hyperthyroidism; **h**yperparathyroidism; **h**ypercalciuria
Alcohol and tobacco use↑
Thin (BMI <22)
Testosterone↓ (eg anti-androgen ca prostate ℞)
Early menopause
Renal or liver failure
Erosive/inflammatory bone disease (eg myeloma or rheumatoid arthritis)
Dietary Ca^{2+}↓/malabsorption; **d**iabetes mellitus type 1

Risk factors Age-independent risk factors for 1° osteoporosis: parental history, alcohol >4 units daily, rheumatoid arthritis, BMI <22, prolonged immobility, and untreated menopause. See MINIBOX for other risk factors, including for 2° osteoporosis.

Investigations X-ray (low sensitivity/specificity, often with hindsight after a fracture). Bone densitometry (**DEXA**—see BOX). **Bloods:** Ca^{2+}, PO_4^{3-} & alk phos normal. Consider specific investigations for 2° causes if suggestive history. **Biopsy** is unreliable and unnecessary with non-invasive techniques available.

Management Loss of bone mineral density may not be entirely irreversible. Age, number of risk factors and bone mineral density (DEXA scan; see BOX) guide the pharmacological approach (eg FRAX, which is a WHO risk assessment tool for estimating 10-yr risk of osteoporotic fracture in untreated patients; see www.shef.ac.uk/frax),[29] [30] although DEXA is not necessary if age >75yrs. Lifestyle measures should apply to all (including those at risk but not yet osteoporotic).

Lifestyle measures:

- Quit smoking and reduce alcohol consumption.
- Weight-bearing exercise may increase bone mineral density.[31]
- Balance exercises such as tai chi reduce risk of falls.
- Calcium and vitamin D-rich diet (use supplements if diet is insufficient—see below).
- Home-based fall-prevention program, with visual assessment and a home visit. NB: hip-protectors are unreliable for preventing fractures.[32]

Pharmacological measures:

- **Bisphosphonates:** alendronate is 1st line (10mg/d or 70mg/wk; not if eGFR <35). Use also for prevention in long-term steroid use. If intolerant, try etidronate or risedronate. Say to swallow pills with *plenty* of water while remaining upright for >30min and wait 30min before eating or other drugs. (SE: photosensitivity; GI upset; oesophageal ulcers—stop if dysphagia or abdo pain; rarely, jaw osteonecrosis).
- **Calcium** and **vitamin D**: Calcium 1.2–1.5g/d + vit D 800–2000U/d, eg Calcium D3 Forte 1 tab/12h. Target serum 25-hydroxy-vitamin D level ≥75nmol/L. Exposure to sunlight may do more good than harm.[33]
- **Strontium ranelate** helps ↓ fracture rates, and is an alternative in those intolerant of bisphosphonates. Strontium is in the same periodic group as calcium and reduces reabsorption, and may promote new bone formation.
- **Hormone replacement therapy** (HRT) can prevent (not treat) osteoporosis in postmenopausal women. Relative risk of breast cancer is 1.4 if used >10yrs.
- **Raloxifene** is a selective oestrogen receptor modulator (SERM) that acts similarly to HRT, but with ↓ breast cancer risk.
- **Teriparatide** (recombinant PTH) is useful in those who suffer further fractures despite treatment with other agents. There is a potential ↑ risk of renal malignancy.
- **Calcitonin** may reduce pain after a vertebral fracture.
- **Testosterone** may help in hypogonadal men by promoting trabecular connectivity.[34]

DEXA bone densitometry: WHO osteoporosis criteria

DUAL ENERGY X-RAY ABSORPTIOMETRY

It is better to scan the hip than the lumbar spine. Bone mineral density (g/cm^2) is compared with that of a young healthy adult. The 'T-score' is the number of standard deviations (SD, p765) the bone mineral density (BMD) is from the youthful average. Each decrease of 1 SD in bone mineral density ≈ 2.6-fold ↑ in risk of hip fracture.

T-score > 0	BMD is better than the reference.
0 to -1	BMD is in the top 84%: no evidence of osteoporosis.
-1 to -2.5	Osteopenia. Risk of later osteoporotic fracture. Offer lifestyle advice.
-2.5 or worse	Osteoporosis. Offer lifestyle advice and treatment (p696). Repeat DEXA in 2yrs.

Some indications for DEXA:

- NICE suggest DEXA if previous low-trauma fracture, or for women ≥65yrs with one or more risk factors for osteoporosis, or younger if two or more. The benefits of universal screening for osteoporosis remain unproven, but some authorities recommend this for men and women over 70—and earlier if risk factors are present.[35]
- DEXA is not needed pre-treatment for women over 75yrs if previous low-trauma fracture, or ≥2 present of rheumatoid arthritis, alcohol excess, or positive family history.
- Prior to giving long-term prednisolone (eg ≥3 months at >5mg/d). Steroids cause osteoporosis by promoting osteoclast bone resorption, ↓muscle mass, and ↓Ca^{2+} absorption from the gut.
- Men or women with osteopenia if low-trauma non-vertebral fracture.[36]
- Bone and bone-remodelling disorders (eg parathyroid disorders, myeloma, HIV, esp if on protease inhibitors).[37]

In osteomalacia there is a normal amount of bone but its mineral content is low (there is excess uncalcified osteoid and cartilage). This the reverse of osteoporosis in which mineralization is unchanged, but there is overall bone loss. Rickets is the result if this process occurs during the period of bone growth; osteomalacia is the result if it occurs after fusion of the epiphyses.

Signs & symptoms

Rickets: Growth retardation, hypotonia, apathy in infants. Once walking: knock-kneed, bow-legged and deformities of the metaphyseal-epiphyseal junction (eg the rachitic rosary). Features of ↓Ca^{2+}—often mild (p692). Children with rickets are ill.

Osteomalacia: Bone pain and tenderness; fractures (esp femoral neck); proximal myopathy (waddling gait), due to ↓PO_4^{3-} and vitamin D deficiency *per se*.

Causes

- ***Vitamin D deficiency:*** Due to malabsorption (p280), poor diet, or lack of sunlight.
- ***Renal osteodystrophy:*** Renal failure leads to 1,25-dihydroxy-cholecalciferol deficiency [1,25$(OH)_2$-vitamin D deficiency]. See also renal bone disease (p302).
- ***Drug-induced:*** Anticonvulsants may induce liver enzymes, leading to an increased breakdown of 25-hydroxy-vitamin D.
- ***Vitamin D resistance:*** A number of mainly inherited conditions in which the osteomalacia responds to high doses of vitamin D (see below).
- ***Liver disease:*** Due to reduced hydroxylation of vitamin D to 25-hydroxy-cholecalciferol and malabsorption of vitamin D, eg in cirrhosis (p260).
- ***Tumour-induced osteomalacia*** (oncogenic hypophosphataemia): mediated by raised tumour production of phosphatonin fibroblast growth factor 23 (FGF-23) which causes hyperphosphaturia. ↓ serum PO_4^{3-} often causes myalgia and weakness.[38]

Investigations

Plasma: Mildly ↓Ca^{2+} (but may be severe); ↓PO_4^{3-}; alk phos↑; PTH high; 25(OH)-vitamin D↓, except in vitamin D resistance. In renal failure 1,25$(OH)_2$-vitamin D↓ (p302).

Biopsy: Bone biopsy shows incomplete mineralization. Muscle biopsy (if proximal myopathy) is normal.

X-ray: In osteomalacia there is a loss of cortical bone; also, apparent partial fractures without displacement may be seen especially on the lateral border of the scapula, inferior femoral neck and medial femoral shaft (Looser's zones; see **fig 1**). Cupped, ragged metaphyseal surfaces are seen in rickets (**fig 2**).

Treatment

- In dietary insufficiency, give vitamin D, eg as one **Calcium D_3 Forte** tablet/12h PO.
- In malabsorption or hepatic disease, give vitamin D_2 (ergocalciferol), up to 40,000U (=1mg) daily, or **parenteral calcitriol**, eg 7.5mg monthly.
- If due to renal disease or vitamin D resistance, give **alfacalcidol** (1α-hydroxy-vitamin D_3) 250ng–1μg daily, or **calcitriol** (1,25-dihydroxy-vitamin D_3) 250ng–1μg daily, and adjust dose according to plasma Ca^{2+}. ►►Alfacalcidol and calcitriol can cause dangerous hypercalcaemia.
- Monitor plasma Ca^{2+}, initially weekly, and if nausea/vomiting.

Vitamin D-resistant rickets exists in 2 forms. Type I has low renal 1α-hydroxylase activity, and type II has end-organ resistance to 1,25-dihydroxy-vitamin D_3, due to a point mutation in the receptor. Both are treated with large doses of calcitriol.

X-linked hypophosphataemic rickets Dominantly inherited—due to a defect in renal phosphate handling (due to mutations in the PEX or PHEX genes which encode an endopeptidase). Rickets develops in early childhood and is associated with poor growth. Plasma PO_4^{3-} is low, alk phos is high, and there is phosphaturia. Treatment is with high doses of oral phosphate, and calcitriol.

Metabolic bone diseases: Paget's disease of bone

Also called *osteitis deformans*, there is increased bone turnover associated with increased numbers of osteoblasts and osteoclasts with resultant remodelling, bone enlargement, deformity, and weakness. Rare in the under-40s. Incidence rises with age (3% over 55yrs old). Commoner in temperate climates, and in Anglo-Saxons.

Clinical features Asymptomatic in ~70%. Deep, boring pain, and bony deformity and enlargement—typically of the pelvis, lumbar spine, skull, femur, and tibia (classically a bowed *sabre* tibia; **fig 3**). *Complications* include pathological fractures, osteoarthritis, ↑Ca^{2+}, nerve compression due to bone overgrowth (eg deafness, root compression), high-output CCF (if >40% of skeleton involved) and osteosarcoma (<1% of those affected for >10yrs—suspect if sudden onset or worsening of bone pain).[39]

Radiology X-ray: localized enlargement of bone. Patchy cortical thickening with sclerosis, osteolysis, and deformity (eg *osteoporosis circumscripta* of the skull). Affinity for axial skeleton, long bones, and skull. **Bone scan** may reveal 'hot spots'.

Blood chemistry: Ca^{2+} and PO_4^{3-} normal; alk phos markedly raised.

Treatment If analgesia fails, **alendronate** may be tried to reduce pain and/or deformity. It is more effective than etidronate or calcitonin, and as effective as IV pamidronate. Follow expert advice.

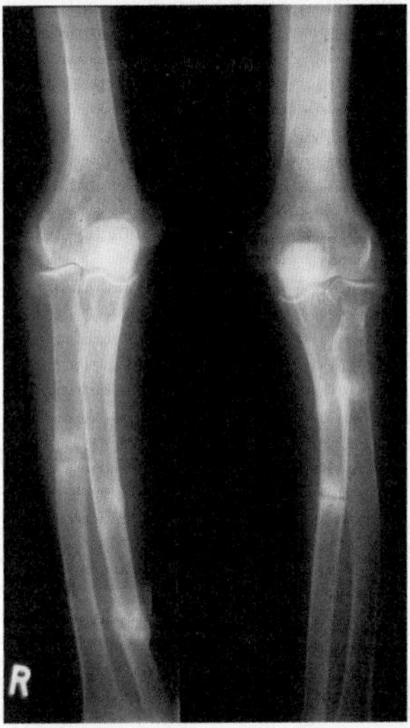

Fig 1. Osteomalacia.

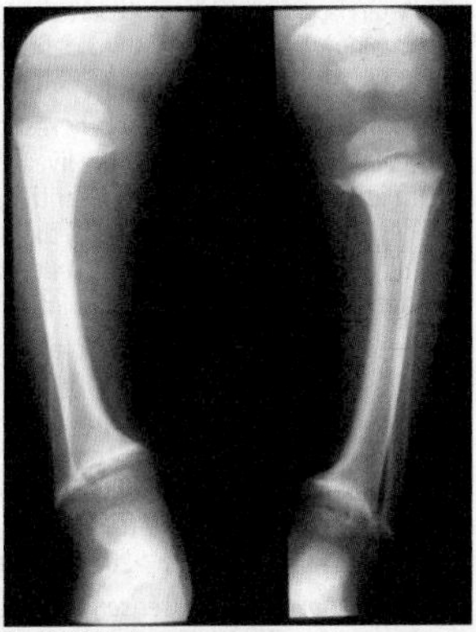

Fig 2. Rickets.

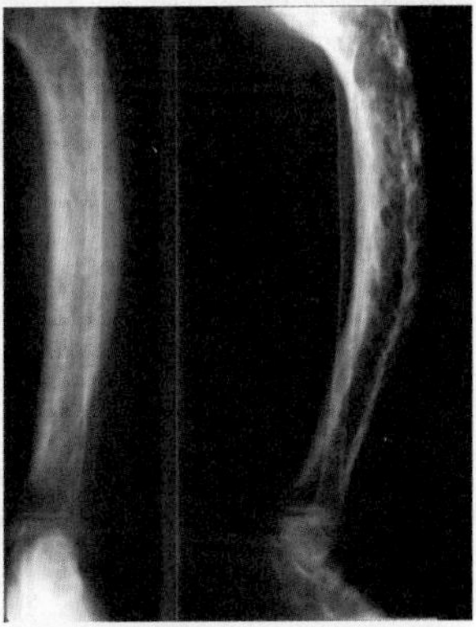

Fig 3. Paget's disease.

Cortical bone lucency and Looser's zones are seen in both forearms of a patient with osteomalacia (**fig 1**). Typical ragged metaphyseal surfaces are seen in the knee and ankle joints of a child with rickets, with bowing of the long bones (**fig 2**). The 'sabre tibia' seen in Paget's disease, with multiple sclerotic lesions (**fig 3**).

Images courtesy of Dr Ian Maddison.

Plasma proteins

Electrophoresis distinguishes a number of bands (**fig 1**).

Albumin is synthesized in the liver; $t_{½}$≈20d. It binds bilirubin, free fatty acids, Ca^{2+}, and some drugs. *Low albumin* results in oedema, and is caused by: • ↓*synthesis:* liver disease, acute phase response (due to ↑vascular permeability—eg sepsis, trauma, surgery), malabsorption, malnutrition, malignancy; • ↑*loss:* nephrotic syndrome, protein-losing enteropathy, burns; • *haemodilution:* late pregnancy, artefact (eg from 'drip' arm). Also posture (↑5g/L if upright) and genetic variations. *High albumin:* Dehydration; artefact (eg stasis).

α1 zone: α_1-antitrypsin, thyroxine-binding globulin, and high-density lipoprotein (HDL). α_1-antitrypsin deficiency leads to cirrhosis and emphysema (see p264).

α2 zone: α_2-macroglobulin, caeruloplasmin, very low density lipoprotein (VLDL, p704), and haptoglobin (p330).

β zone: Transferrin, low-density lipoprotein (LDL), fibrinogen, C3 and C4 complement. Reduced in active nephritis, glomerulonephritis, and SLE.

γ zone: Immunoglobulins, factor VIII, C-reactive protein (CRP), and α-fetoprotein. *Specific monoclonal band* in paraproteinaemia (see p364). *Diffusely raised* in chronic infections, TB, bronchiectasis, liver cirrhosis, sarcoidosis, SLE, RA, Crohn's disease, 1° biliary cirrhosis, hepatitis, and parasitaemia. *Low* in nephrotic syndrome, malabsorption, malnutrition, and immune deficiency states (eg severe illness, renal failure, diabetes mellitus, malignancy, or congenital).

Acute phase response The body responds to a variety of insults with, amongst other things, the synthesis, by the liver, of a number of proteins (normally present in serum in small quantities)—eg α_1-antitrypsin, fibrinogen, complement, haptoglobin, and CRP. An increased density of the α_1- and α_2-fractions, often with a reduced albumin level, is characteristic of conditions such as infection, malignancy (especially α_2-fraction), trauma, surgery, and inflammatory disease.

CRP So-called because it binds to a polysaccharide (fraction C) in the cell wall of pneumococci. Levels help monitor inflammation/infection (normal <8mg/L). Like the ESR, it is raised in many inflammatory conditions, but changes more rapidly. It increases in hours and begins to fall within 2-3d of recovery; thus it can be used to follow disease activity (eg Crohn's disease) or the response to therapy (eg antibiotics). CRP values in mild inflammation 10-50mg/L; active bacterial infection 50-200mg/L; severe infection or trauma >200mg/L; see BOX.

CRP in cardiovascular disease: CRP levels also predict outcome in patients with cardiovascular disease if measured using a highly sensitive assay. Low risk <1mg/L; moderate risk 1-3; and high risk >3mg/L. Furthermore, the JUPITER trial suggests that treating these patients with a statin reduces cardiovascular risk, even in the absence of hypercholesterolaemia.[40]

Urinary proteins

Urinary protein loss >150mg/d is pathological (p286).

Albuminuria is usually caused by renal disease (p286). *Microalbuminuria* is urinary protein loss between 3 and 300mg/d (so not visible on dipstick) and may be seen with diabetes mellitus, ↑BP, SLE and glomerulonephritis (see p309 for role in DM).

Bence Jones protein consists of light chains excreted in excess by some patients with myeloma (p362). They are not detected by dipsticks and may occur with normal serum electrophoresis.

Haemoglobinuria is caused by intravascular haemolysis (p330).

Myoglobinuria is caused by rhabdomyolysis (p307).

C-reactive protein (CRP)

Marked elevation	*Normal-to-slight elevation*
Bacterial infection	Viral infection
Abscess	Steroids/oestrogens
Crohn's disease	Ulcerative colitis
Connective tissue diseases (except SLE)	SLE
	Atherosclerosis
Neoplasia	Morbid obesity
Trauma	
Necrosis (eg MI)	

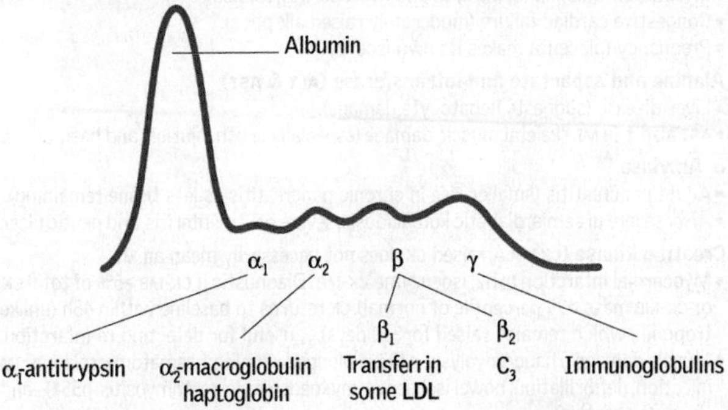

Fig 1. A normal electrophoretic scan.

►Reference intervals vary between laboratories. See p770 for guide normal values.

Raised levels of specific enzymes can be a useful indicator of a disease. However, remember that most can be raised for other reasons too. Levels may be raised due to cellular damage, ↑cell turnover, cellular proliferation (malignancy), enzyme induction, and ↓clearance. The major causes of *raised enzymes* are given below.

Alkaline phosphatase

- Liver disease (suggests cholestasis; also cirrhosis, abscess, hepatitis or malignancy).
- Bone disease (isoenzyme distinguishable, reflects osteoblast activity) especially Paget's, growing children, healing fractures, bone metastases, osteomalacia, osteomyelitis, chronic kidney disease and hyperparathyroidism.
- Congestive cardiac failure (moderately raised alk phos).
- Pregnancy (placenta makes its own isoenzyme).

Alanine and aspartate aminotransferase (ALT & AST)

- Liver disease (suggests hepatocyte damage).
- AST also ↑ in MI, skeletal muscle damage (especially crush injuries) and haemolysis.

α-Amylase

- Acute pancreatitis (smaller rise in chronic pancreatitis as less tissue remaining).
- *Also:* severe uraemia, diabetic ketoacidosis, severe gastroenteritis, and peptic ulcer.

Creatine kinase (CK) ►A raised CK does not necessarily mean an MI.

- Myocardial infarction (p112; isoenzyme 'CK-MB'. Diagnostic if CK-MB >6% of total CK, or CK-MB mass >99 percentile of normal). CK returns to baseline within 48h (unlike troponin, which remains raised for ~10 days), ∴ useful for detecting re-infarction.
- Muscle damage (rhabdomyolysis, p307; prolonged running; haematoma; seizures; IM injection; defibrillation; bowel ischaemia; myxoedema; dermatomyositis, p554)—and *drugs* (eg statins).

Gamma-glutamyl transferase (GGT, γGT)

- Liver disease (particularly alcohol-induced damage, cholestasis, drugs).

Lactate dehydrogenase (LDH)

- Myocardial infarction (p112).
- Liver disease (suggests hepatocyte damage).
- Haemolysis (esp sickle cell crisis), pulmonary embolism, and tumour necrosis.

Troponin

- Subtypes troponin T and troponin I are used clinically.
- Cardiac damage or strain (MI—p112, pericarditis, myocarditis, PE, sepsis, CPR).
- Chronic kidney disease (troponin T only; elevation less marked; aetiology unknown).

Enzyme inducers and inhibitors

Hepatic drug metabolism is either by conjugation or oxidation. The oxidative pathways are catalysed by the family of cytochrome P450 isoenzymes, the most important of which is the CYP 3A4 isoenzyme. The cytochrome P450 pathway may be either induced or inhibited by a range of commonly used drugs and foods:

Enzyme inducers	Enzyme inhibitors	
Phenytoin	SSRIs	Amiodarone
Rifampicin	Ciprofloxacin	Diltiazem
Carbamazepine	Isoniazid	Verapamil
Alcohol	Macrolides	Omeprazole
St John's wort	HIV protease inhibitors	Grapefruit juice
Barbiturates	Imidazole & triazole antifungal agents	

This can lead to important interactions or side-effects. For example phenytoin reduces the effectiveness of the Pill due to more rapid oestrogen metabolism, and ciprofloxacin retards the metabolism of methylxanthines (aminophylline) which leads to higher plasma levels and potentially more side-effects. The *BNF* contains a list of the major interactions between drugs.

Ca^{2+} Na^{+} K^{+}

Hyperlipidaemia

Lipids travel in blood packaged with proteins as lipoproteins. There are 4 classes: chylomicrons and VLDL (mainly triglyceride), LDL (mainly cholesterol) and HDL (mainly phospholipid). The evidence that cholesterol is a major risk factor for cardiovascular disease (CVD) is now incontrovertible (table 14.[illegible]). Studies [illegible] HEART PROTECTION STUDY [illegible] and it may even be [illegible] alone [illegible] other risk factors. Half the UK population have a serum cholesterol putting them at significant risk of CVD [illegible] appears to correlate inversely with CVD.

Who to screen for hyperlipidaemia

Note: full screening requires a fasting lipid profile.

Those at risk of hyperlipidaemia: • Family history of hyperlipidaemia • Corneal arcus <50yrs old • Xanthomata or xanthelasmata (fig [illegible])

Those at risk of CVD: see CVD risk equation (p[illegible]) • Known CVD • Family history of CVD <55yrs old • DM or impaired glucose tolerance • Hypertension • Smoker • ↑BMI • Low socioeconomic or Indian Asian background

Types of hyperlipidaemia

Common primary hypercholesterolaemia accounts for 70% of hypercholesterolaemia. *Familial primary hypercholesterolaemias* comprise multiple phenotypes [illegible]. Risk of CVD↑↑, although evidence suggests protection from CVD achieved with lower doses of statin than for common primary hypercholesterolaemia.

Secondary hyperlipidaemia may be caused by Cushing's syndrome, thiazide diuretics, hypothyroidism, nephrotic syndrome, or cholestasis. Treat the cause first.

Mixed hyperlipidaemia results in ↑ both LDL and triglycerides. Caused by type 2 diabetes mellitus, metabolic syndrome, alcohol abuse, and chronic renal failure.

Management

• *Lifestyle advice:* Aim for BMI of 20–25. Diet with <10% of calories from saturated fat. [illegible] fresh fruit & vegetables, omega-3 fatty acids. ↑Exercise.

• Identify familial or 2° hyperlipidaemias. Treat any other set [illegible].

• *Who to treat?* [illegible] statins for primary prevention causes side-effects and is expensive [illegible]. Treat those with known CVD (there is no need to calculate their risk—they already have high risk) =2° prevention. Treat all those with DM (especially if [illegible], even [illegible]). Treat those with a 10-yr risk of CVD >20% [illegible]. Current guidelines suggest a target [illegible] cholesterol of [illegible]. There is not yet enough data to support [illegible] statins to women over 70 and women under 65.

• [illegible] therapeutic (eg simvastatin 40mg at night) [illegible] synthesis. [illegible]

[illegible]

• *Other therapy:* [illegible] ezetimibe [illegible] or mixed hyperlipidaemias [illegible] cholesterol absorption inhibitors, eg ezetimibe 10mg/d can combine with a statin to enhance the reduction (it is not known if the additional [illegible]). [illegible] nicotinic acid [illegible]

• Hypertriglyceridaemia responds best to fibrates, nicotinic acid, or fish oil.

Xanthomata These yellow lipid deposits may be eruptive (itchy nodules in crops in hypertriglyceridaemia), tuberous [illegible] or palmar [illegible], diagnostic of remnant hyperlipidaemia [illegible] corneal arcus [illegible].

Abbreviations: VLDL = very low density lipoprotein; IDL = intermediate density lipoprotein; LDL = low density lipoprotein; chylo = chylomicrons; TG = triglycerides.

Lipids travel in blood packaged with proteins as lipoproteins. There are 4 classes: chylomicrons and VLDL (mainly triglyceride), LDL (mainly cholesterol), and HDL (mainly phospholipid). The evidence that cholesterol is a major risk factor for cardiovascular disease (CVD) is now incontrovertible ('4S' STUDY,[41] WOSCOPS,[42] CARE STUDY,[43] HEART PROTECTION STUDY[44]) and indeed it may even be the 'green light' that allows other risk factors to act.[45] Half the UK population have a serum cholesterol putting them at significant risk of CVD. HDL appears to correlate *inversely* with CVD.

Who to screen for hyperlipidaemia

►NB: full screening requires a fasting lipid profile.

Those at risk of hyperlipidaemia: • Family history of hyperlipidaemia; • Corneal arcus < 50yrs old; • Xanthomata or xanthelasmata (**fig 1**).

Those at risk of CVD: (see *risk equation*, p642) • Known CVD; • Family history of CVD < 65yrs old; • DM or impaired glucose tolerance; • Hypertension; • Smoker; • ↑BMI; • Low socioeconomic or Indian Asian background.

Types of hyperlipidaemia

Common primary hyperlipidaemia accounts for 70% of hyperlipidaemia. ↑LDL only.

Familial primary hyperlipidaemias comprise multiple phenotypes (see TABLE). *Risk of CVD*↑↑, although evidence suggests protection from CVD achieved with lower doses of statin than for common primary hyperlipidaemia.[46]

Secondary hyperlipidaemia may be caused by Cushing's syndrome, thiazide diuretics, hypothyroidism, nephrotic syndrome, or cholestasis. ↑LDL. Treat the cause first.

Mixed hyperlipidaemia results in ↑ both LDL and triglycerides. Caused by type 2 diabetes mellitus, metabolic syndrome, alcohol abuse, and chronic renal failure.

Management[47] ★[48]

- *Lifestyle advice.* Aim for BMI of 20-25. Diet with <10% of calories from saturated fats; ↑fibre, fresh fruit & vegetables, omega-3 fatty acids. ↑Exercise.
- Identify familial or 2° hyperlipidaemias. Treat may differ—see above.
- *Treatment priorities:* Using statins in primary prevention causes side-effects and is expensive. • *Top priority:* Treat those with known CVD (there is no need to calculate their risk: *ipso facto* they already have high risk). • *2nd priority:* Treat all those with DM (especially if risk of cardiac event >2%/yr). • *3rd priority:* Those with a 10-year risk of CVD >20%, *irrespective of baseline lipid levels.*[49] Current guidelines suggest a target plasma cholesterol of ≤4mmol/L.[50] There is not yet enough data to support a 4th priority of giving statins to all men over 50 and women over 65.
- *1st-line therapy:* **statins**, eg **simvastatin** (40mg PO at night), ↓cholesterol synthesis in the liver. CI: porphyria, cholestasis, pregnancy. SE: myalgia ± myositis (stop if ↑CK ≥10-fold; if any myalgia, check CK; risk is 1 per 100,000 treatment-years),[51] abdominal pain, and ↑LFTs (stop if AST ≥100U/L). Cytochrome P450 inhibitors (p702) ↑ serum concentrations (eg 200mL of grapefruit juice may ↑ simvastatin concentration by 300%, and atorvastatin ↑80%, but pravastatin is almost unchanged).[52] [53] [54]
- *2nd-line therapy:* **fibrates**, eg **bezafibrate** (useful in mixed hyperlipidaemias), or cholesterol absorption inhibitors, eg **ezetimibe** (useful combined with a statin to enhance LDL reduction (it is not known if the additional 12-19% drop in LDL translates into lives saved);[55] anion exchange resins, eg cholestyramine; also consider nicotinic acid (HDL↑; LDL↓; SE: severe flushes; aspirin 300mg ½h pre-dose helps this).
- Hypertriglyceridaemia responds best to fibrates, nicotinic acid, or fish oil.

Xanthomata These yellow lipid deposits may be: **eruptive** (itchy nodules in crops in hypertriglyceridaemia); **tuberous** (plaques on elbows & knees); or **planar**—also called palmar (orange streaks in palmar creases), 'diagnostic' of remnant hyperlipidaemia; or in tendons p36, eyelids (**xanthelasma**, see **fig 1**), or cornea (**arcus**, p36).

Abbreviations (V)LDL = (very) low-density lipoprotein; IDL = intermediate density lipoprotein; HDL = high density lipoprotein; chol = cholesterol; trig = trigylcerides.

Primary hyperlipidaemias

Blue numbers = WHO phenotype; chol/trig levels given in mmol/L.

Familial hyperchylomicronaemia (lipoprotein lipase deficiency or apoCII deficiency)[I]	Chol <6.5 Trig 10–30 Chylomicrons ↑		Eruptive xanthomata; lipaemia retinalis; hepatosplenomegaly
Familial hypercholesterolaemia[II] (LDL receptor defects)	Chol 7.5–16 Trig <2.3	LDL↑	Tendon xanthoma; corneal arcus; xanthelasma
Familial defective apolipoprotein B-100[IIa]	Chol 7.5–16 Trig <2.3	LDL↑	Tendon xanthoma; arcus; xanthelasma
Common hypercholesterolaemia[IIa]	Chol 6.5–9 Trig <2.3	LDL↑	*The commonest 1° lipidaemia*; may have xanthelasma or arcus
Familial combined hyperlipidaemia[IIb, IV or V]	Chol 6.5–10 Trig 2.3–12	LDL↑ VLDL↑ HDL↓	*Next commonest 1° lipidaemia*; xanthelasma; arcus
Dysbetalipoproteinaemia (remnant particle disease)[III]	Chol 9–14 Trig 9–14	IDL↑ HDL↓ LDL↓	Palmar striae; tubero-eruptive xanthoma
Familial hypertriglyceridaemia[IV]	Chol 6.5–12 Trig 3.0–6.0	VLDL↑	
Type V hyperlipoproteinaemia	Trig 10–30; chylomicrons		Eruptive xanthomata; lipaemia retinalis; hepatosplenomegaly

Primary HDL abnormalities

- Hyperalphalipoproteinaemia: ↑HDL, chol >2.
- Hypoalphalipoproteinaemia (Tangier disease): ↓HDL, chol <0.92.

Primary LDL abnormalities

- Abetalipoproteinaemia (ABL): trig <0.3, chol <1.3, missing LDL, VLDL and chylomicrons. Autosomal recessive disorder of fat malabsorption causing vitamin A & E deficiency, with retinitis pigmentosa, sensory neuropathy, ataxia, pes cavus and acanthocytosis.
- Hypobetalipoproteinaemia: chol <1.5, LDL↓, HDL↓. Autosomal codominant disorder of apolipoprotein B metabolism. ↑ longevity in heterozygotes. Homozygotes present with a similar clinical picture to ABL.

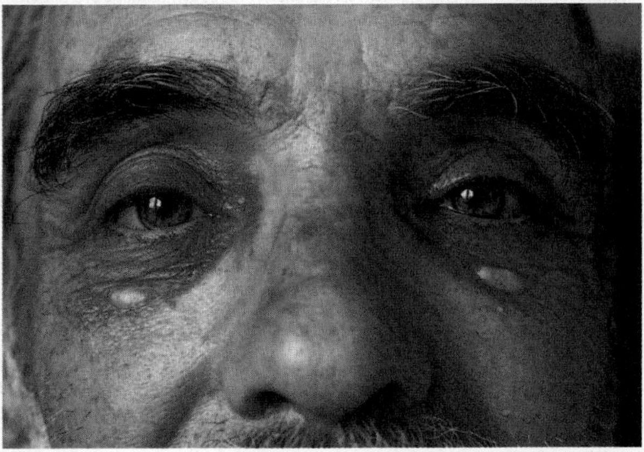

Fig 1. Xanthelasma. *Xanthos* is Greek for yellow, and *elasma* means plate. Xanthelasmata are lipid-laden yellow plaques, typically a few mm wide. They congregate around the lids, or just below the eyes, and signify hyperlipidaemia.

The porphyrias are a heterogenous group of rare diseases caused by various errors of haem biosynthesis (produced when iron is chelated into protoporphyrin IXα), which may be genetic or acquired. Depending on the stage in haem biosynthesis that is faulty, there is accumulation of either porphyrinogens, which are unstable and oxidize to porphyrins, or their precursors, porphobilinogen and δ-aminolaevulinic acid. Porphyrin precursors are neurotoxic, while porphyrins themselves induce photosensitivity and the formation of toxic free radicals.

- Alcohol, lead, and iron deficiency cause abnormal porphyrin metabolism.
- Genetic counselling (*OHCS* p154) should be offered to all patients and their families.

Acute porphyrias occur when the accumulation of porphyrinogen precursors predominates, and are characterized by acute neurovisceral crises, though some forms have additional photosensitive cutaneous manifestations.

Acute intermittent porphyria *('the Madness of King George')* A low-penetrant autosomal dominant condition (porphobilinogen deaminase gene); 28% have no family history (*de novo mutations*). ~10% of those with the defective gene have neurovisceral symptoms. Attacks are intermittent, more common in women and those aged 18–40, and may be precipitated by drugs. Urine porphobilinogens are raised during attacks (the urine may go deep red on standing) and also, in ~50%, between attacks. Faecal porphyrin levels are normal. There is never cutaneous photosensitivity. It is the commonest form of porphyria—prevalence in UK: 1-2/100,000.

Variegate porphyria and hereditary coproporphyria Autosomal dominant, characterized by photosensitive blistering skin lesions and/or acute attacks. The former is prevalent in Afrikaners in South Africa. Porphobilinogen is high only during an attack, and other metabolites may be detected in faeces.

Triggers of an acute attack include infection, starvation (including pre-operative 'nil-by-mouth'), reproductive hormones (pregnancy, premenstrual), smoking, anaesthesia, and cytochrome P450 enzyme inducers (alcohol, and other drugs—see BOX).

Features of an acute attack:

- *Gastrointestinal:* abdominal pain, vomiting, constipation.
- *Neuropsychiatric:* peripheral neuropathy (weakness, hypotonia, pain, numbness), seizures (often associated with severe ↓Na^+), psychosis (or other odd behaviour).[1]
- *Cardiovascular:* hypertension, tachycardia, shock (due to sympathetic overactivity).
- *Other:* fever, ↓Na^+, ↓K^+, proteinuria, urinary porphobilinogens, discoloured urine. Rare but serious complications include bulbar and respiratory paralysis.

►► Beware the 'acute abdomen' in acute intermittent porphyria: colic, vomiting, fever and ↑WCC—so mimicking an acute surgical abdomen. Anaesthesia could be disastrous.

Treatment of an acute attack

- Remove precipitants (review medications; treat intercurrent illness/infection).
- IV **fluids** to correct electrolyte imbalance.
- High **carbohydrate** intake (eg Hycal®) by NG tube, or IV if necessary.
- IV **haematin** is 1st-line (inhibits production of porphyrinogen precursors).
- Nausea controlled with **prochlorperazine** 12.5mg IM.
- Sedate if necessary with **chlorpromazine** 50–100mg PO/IM.
- Pain control with opiate or opioid **analgesia** (avoid oxycodone).
- Seizures can be controlled with **diazepam** (although this will prolong the attack).
- Treat tachycardia and hypertension with a **β-blocker**.

Non-acute porphyrias

Porphyria cutanea tarda **(PCT)**, ***erythropoietic protoporphyria***, and ***congenital erythropoietic porphyria*** are characterized by cutaneous photosensitivity alone, as there is no overproduction of porphyrinogen precursors, only porphyrins. PCT presents in adults with blistering skin lesions ± facial hypertrichosis and hyperpigmentation. Total plasma porphyrins and LFTs are ↑. Screen for associated disorders: hep C, HIV, iron overload, hepatocellular ca. ℞: phlebotomy, iron chelators, chloroquine, sunscreens.

Drugs to avoid in acute intermittent porphyria

There are many, many drugs that may precipitate an acute attack ± quadriplegia, and this is by no means an exhaustive list (see *BNF/OTM*).

- For an up-to-date list of drugs considered *safe* in acute porphyria see **www.wmic.wales.nhs.uk/porphyria_info.php**

• Diclofenac	• Metoclopramide	• Furosemide
• Alcohol	• ACE-inhibitors	• Sulphonylureas
• Oral contraceptive pill[56] & HRT	• Ca^{2+}-channel blockers	• Lidocaine
• Tricyclic antidepressants	• Statins	• Gold salts
• Benzodiazepines	• Anticonvulsants	• Antihistamines
• Anaesthetic agents (barbiturates, halothane)		• Amphetamines
• Antibiotics (cephalosporins, sulphonamides, macrolides, tetracyclines, rifampicin, trimethoprim, chloramphenicol, metronidazole)		

1 Be sure I looked at her eyes
Happy and proud; at last I knew
Porphyria worshipped me; surprise
Made my heart swell, and still it grew
While I debated what to do.
That moment she was mine, mine, fair,
Perfectly pure and good: I found
A thing to do, and all her hair
In one long yellow string I wound
Three times her little throat around,
And strangled her ...

From *Porphyria's Lover* by Robert Browning

Alice in Wonderland syndrome (Todd's syndrome) Disturbance of one's view of oneself ± fast-forwarding of intrapsychic time, seen in epilepsy, migraine & encephalitis.

Arnold-Chiari malformation The cerebellar tonsils and medulla are malformed and herniate through the foramen magnum. This may cause infantile hydrocephalus with mental retardation, optic atrophy, ocular palsies and spastic paresis of the limbs. Spina bifida, syringomyelia (p520), or focal cerebellar and brainstem signs may occur eg ataxia, dysphagia, oscillopsia, nystagmus (p503). There may be bony abnormalities of the base of the skull (basilar impression). MRI is better than CT in aiding diagnosis.

Baker's cyst Fluid from a knee effusion escapes to form a popliteal cyst (often swollen/painful) in a sub-gastrocnemius bursa.[1] It may rupture (→compartment syndrome). **ΔΔ**: DVT; sarcoma. ***Imaging:*** Ultrasound; MRI. **℞**: If painful or from knee derangement, consider arthroscopic correction of any derangement + cystectomy or a non-absorbable purse-string to close the orifice of the posterior joint capsule.[2]

Barrett's oesophagus In chronic reflux oesophagitis (p244), columnar gastric epithelium extends upwards replacing normal oesophageal squamous epithelium (the squamocolumnar junction migrates upwards). Metaplasia occurs in these cells. The length affected may be a few cm or all the oesophagus, and can be continuous or patchy (on endoscopy). ►There is a 40-fold ↑risk of oesophageal adenocarcinoma. In fact, most distal oesophageal adenocarcinomas are believed to be Barrett's-associated.[3] There is no clear association with *H. pylori*. ***Management*** depends on biopsy. If pre-malignant/high-grade dysplasia, ***oesophageal resection*** or ***eradicative mucosectomy,***[4][5] eg if young & fit. Endoscopic ***targeted mucosectomy,***[6] or mucosal ablation by ***epithelial laser, radiofrequency*** (HALO),[7] or ***photodynamic ablation*** (PD) is used in others. PD involves light-induced activation of an oral photosensitizer, eg 5-aminolaevulinic acid, which ↑protoporphyrin IX in GI mucosa. Local laser light then causes necrosis (confirm by finding squamous re-epithelialization). PD is limited by side effects: strictures, cutaneous photosensitivity, chest pain, vomiting.[8] If no pre-malignant changes are found, regular endoscopy + biopsy, and intensive antireflux measures (high-dose long-term proton pump inhibitors) are used. Who to screen and how often is unclear. Shorter endoscopic intervals for surveillance of low-grade dysplasia associate with ↑detection of high-grade dysplasia & adenocarcinoma.[9]

Bazin's disease Localized areas of fat necrosis with ulceration and an indurated rash, characteristically on adolescent girls' calves. Originally thought to be a form of skin TB, but cases unrelated to tuberculosis have been seen.

Behçet's disease A systemic vasculitis of unknown cause, associated with HLA-B51. It is most commonly found in Turkey, the Mediterranean and Japan. ***Features:*** recurrent oral and genital ulceration, ocular inflammation (eg anterior or posterior uveitis), skin lesions (eg erythema nodosum, papulopustular lesions), neurological (eg aseptic meningitis, encephalitis, CN palsies, confusion), vasculitis, joints (non-erosive large joint oligoarthropathy), GI: diarrhoea, colitis. ***Diagnosis*** is mainly clinical. Pathergy test: needle prick leads to papule formation within 48 hours. **℞**: Steroids, ciclosporin, azathioprine or cyclophosphamide are used in severe disease, eg with ocular involvement.[10] Colchicine may be effective in treating ulceration.

Berger's disease (IgA nephropathy, p294) is the commonest glomerulonephritis causing renal failure. Episodic haematuria is triggered by viral infections (risk factors: alcoholic liver disease, ankylosing spondylitis, coeliac disease, HIV). Genetic abnormalities in glycosylation of IgA are important.[11] Renal survival rate: 61% after 20yrs. Proteinuria, hypoalbuminaemia & haematuria predict deterioration. Tonsillectomy can improve proteinuria and stabilize renal function.[12]

Bickerstaff's brainstem encephalitis (related to Miller-Fisher syndrome, p717): as well as ophthalmoplegia, ataxia, and areflexia, there are extensor plantars ± tetraplegia ± coma, and a reversible brain death picture (but there is *no* structural damage). MRI: hyperintense brainstem signals. GQ1b antibodies +ve.[13] Plasmapheresis may help.

Eponyms are so-called because they take their names from their chief protagonists (either doctors or patients). They are our sole route to an exotic variety of obscure fame: 'if one was a drunkard and one's name was Johnny Walker one could form a society called *Alcoholics Eponymous*'. Alan Bennett

Monochromatic doctors may try to abolish eponyms seeking to replace them with histologically driven disease titles. But classifications vary as more becomes known, so renaming of non-eponyms becomes essential. Eponyms carry on for ever, because they imply nothing about causes. We like eponyms—and, where possible, the use of the term ***syndrome*** rather than ***disease***. A syndrome is a collection of phenomena and is neutral on whether the collection is a disease. To tell someone with Gilles de La Tourette's syndrome that they have a disease is a slap in the face—when the condition is bound up with who they are ("I tic therefore I am", p714). Syndromes can sound dire to patients, or falsely glamorous. When, for an earlier edition, we requested from interlibrary loan *The Carcinoid Syndrome* (by D Graham-Smith) we were delighted when it arrived from 'The Wigan Pleasure Library' where presumably it had been filed next to *The Thanatos Syndrome* and other exotic-sounding novels.

Brugada syndrome

Note right bundle branch block and the unusual morphology of the raised ST segments in V1-3. This genetic condition causing faulty sodium channels predisposes to fatal arrhythmias, eg ventricular fibrillation, typically in young males (eg triggered by a fever).[14] It is preventable by implanting a defibrillator. ►*Consider primary electrical cardiac disease in all with unexplained syncope.* Programmed electrical stimulation may be needed.[15] Relatives of those with sudden unexplained death may undergo unmasking of arrhythmias by IV ajmaline tests—but some results are false +ve.[16] Use judgment in subjecting those with ST abnormalities but no symptoms to electrophysiological tests, right ventricular myocardial biopsy, and MRI. Sequencing SCN5A loci may identify R367H missense mutations in affected families.

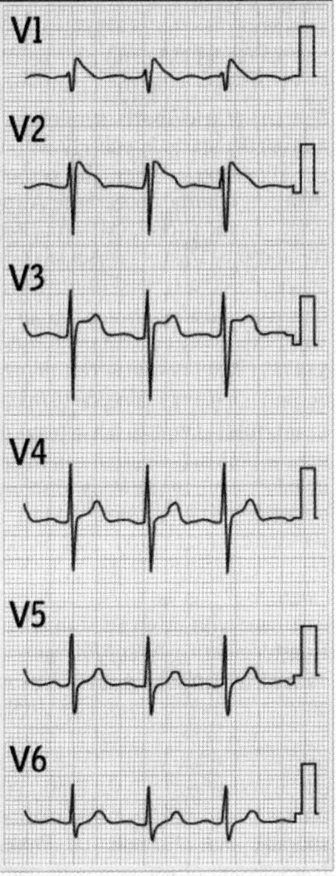

ECG 10. Note right bundle branch block and ST morphology in leads V1-3. According to some authorities, these ST-segment elevations should not be seen as a marker of a specific syndrome, but as an electrical expression of structural abnormalities in the right ventricle that have genetic, infective, or inflammatory origins.

Courtesy of Dr Shayashi.[17]

See also *OHCS* p638-p655 concerning further unusual eponymous syndromes.
Consult the index for eponyms covered in other chapters. Biographical details: www.whonamedit.com

Brown-Séquard syndrome A lesion in one half of the cord (due to hemisection or unilateral cord lesion) causes • Ipsilateral UMN weakness below the lesion (severed corticospinal tract, causing spastic paraparesis, brisk reflexes, extensor plantars) • Ipsilateral loss of proprioception and vibration (l dorsal column severed) • Contralateral loss of pain and T° sensation (severed spinothalamic tract which has crossed over; **fig 1** p520). *Causes:* Bullet, stab, dart, kick, tumour, disc hernia, cervical spondylosis, MS, neuroschistosomiasis, myelitis,[18] septic emboli (eg meningococcal).[19] Do MRI.

Budd-Chiari syndrome Hepatic vein obstruction by thrombosis or tumour causes ischaemia and hepatocyte damage, presenting with liver failure or insidious cirrhosis. Abdominal pain, hepatomegaly, ascites and ↑ALT occur. Portal hypertension occurs in chronic forms. *Causes:* include hypercoagulable states (the Pill, pregnancy, malignancy, paroxysmal nocturnal haemoglobinuria, polycythaemia rubra vera, thrombophilia) or liver, renal or adrenal tumour. *Tests:* Ultrasound + hepatic vein Dopplers, CT or MRI. Angioplasty, transjugular intrahepatic portosystemic shunt (TIPS) or a surgical shunt may be needed. Anticoagulate (lifelong) unless there are varices. Consider liver transplant in fulminant hepatic necrosis or cirrhosis.[20]

Buerger's disease (thromboangiitis obliterans) Smoking-related inflammation of veins, nerves, and middle-sized arteries (which thrombose, causing gangrene). Cause: unknown. Stopping smoking is vital. Most patients are men (or giants, see BOX 2).

Caplan's syndrome This is multiple lung nodules in coal workers with rheumatoid arthritis, caused by an inflammatory reaction to external allergen. CXR: bilateral peripheral nodules (0.5-5cm). CT ± needle biopsy may be needed for diagnosis. **ΔΔ:** TB. *Risk↑ if:* Silica, asbestos, or anthracite exposure. **℞:** Symptomatic, only (p192).

Charcot-Marie-Tooth syndrome (peroneal muscular atrophy) This inherited neuropathy starts in puberty with weak legs and foot drop, with variable loss of sensation and reflexes. The peroneal muscles atrophy, leading to an inverted champagne bottle appearance. Atrophy of hand and arm muscles also occurs. The most common form, CMT1A (caused by mutations in the PMP22 myelin gene on chromosome 17), has autosomal dominant inheritance. Quality of life is good;[21] *total* incapacity is rare. Hand pain/paraesthesiae may respond to nerve release.

Churg-Strauss syndrome A triad of late-onset asthma, eosinophilia, and granulomatous small vessel vasculitis (±vasospasm ± MI ± DVT), affecting lungs, nerves, heart, and skin. A septic-shock picture/systemic inflammatory response syndrome may occur (with glomerulonephritis/renal failure, esp. if ANCA+ve). **℞:** Steroids; INFα.[22] [23]

Creutzfeldt-Jakob disease (CJD) The cause is a prion (PrPSc), a misfolded form of a normal protein (PrPc), that can transform other proteins into prion proteins (hence its infectivity). ↑PrPSc leads to spongiform changes (tiny cavities ± tubulovesicular structures) in the brain.[24] Most cases are *sporadic* (incidence: 1-3/million/yr). *Variant CJD* (vCJD; ≤200 cases worldwide)[25] 2009 DATA is transmitted via meat contaminated by CNS tissue affected by bovine spongiform encephalopathy BSE; see BOX 3). In *inherited* forms (eg Gerstmann-Sträussler-Scheinker syndrome, P102L mutation in PRNP gene with ataxia ± self-mutilation), the 'normal' protein is too unstable, readily transforming to PrPSc. *Iatrogenic* causes: contaminated surgical instruments, corneal transplants, growth hormone from human pituitaries, and blood (vCJD only).[26] Prion protein resists sterilisation. *Signs:* Progressive dementia, focal CNS signs, myoclonus (present in 95%),[27] depression, eye signs (diplopia, supranuclear palsies, complex visual disturbances, homonymous field defects, hallucinations, cortical blindness).[28] *Tests:* Tonsil/olfactory mucosa biopsy;[29] CSF gel electrophoresis; MRI (esp. caudate/putamen). *Treatment*: None proven. Death occurs in ~6 months in sporadic and iatrogenic CJD. *Prevention:* Regulations aimed at ↓spread of BSE, transmission of BSE prions to humans, and iatrogenic transmission are limiting spread of this disease.[30]

ABC

Crigler-Najjar syndrome An inherited cause of unconjugated hyperbilirubinaemia presenting in the 1st days of life with jaundice ± CNS signs. Cause: mutation leading to abolition of bilirubin UDP-glucuronosyltransferase (UGT) activity. **℞:** Liver transplant before irreversible kernicterus (*OHCS* p115) develops.[31]

Fame and infamy in the search for lost youth

After his neurological experiments, Charles-Edouard Brown-Séquard (1817-94), the most visionary of all neuroanatomists and the grandfather of HRT, proclaimed he had found the secret of perpetual youth after injecting himself with a concoction of testicular blood, semen, and testicular extracts from dogs and guinea pigs. In the 1880s over 12,000 doctors were queuing up for his special extracts, which they used on their patients in various ways. He gave the extracts away free, provided results were reported back to him. 314 out of 405 cases of spinal syphilis improved, and his own urinary flow rate rose by 25%. Endocrinologists never forgave him for bringing their science into disrepute. To this day, no one really knows if his (literally) seminal work has given us anything of any practical value.[32] But he might be pleased to know that testosterone is now known to have the urodynamic benefits he anticipated, at least in men with hypogonadism.[33]

Like many brilliant men, he had a cruel streak, backing clitoridectomy for preventing blindness and other imaginary complications of 'masturbatory melancholia.' Had he not been blinded by 19th-century ideas about female sexuality, could he have found a marvellous use for his concoctions, for 21st century 'hypoactive sexual desire disorder'? Possibly, but only if he relied on placebo responses.[34] [35]

Poisoning your boss

In 1931, Buerger's disease caused gangrene in the toes of Harvey Cushing (p216)—the most cantankerous (and greatest) neurosurgeon ever. He had to be wheeled to the operating theatre to carry on his brilliant art (and to continue terrifying his assistants).[36] He had to retire partially, whereupon his colleagues presented him with a magnificent silver cigarette box, containing 2000 cigarettes (to which he was addicted)—one for each brain tumour he had removed during his long career, so verifying the truth that although we owe everything to our teachers, we must eventually kill them to move out from under their shadow.[1]

Hermann Hesse *Demian*; 1917

Signs which may distinguish variant CJD from sporadic CJD (sCJD)

- An earlier age at presentation (median 29yrs vs 60yrs in sporadic CJD).
- Longer survival and later dementia (median 14 months *vs* 4 for sporadic CJD).
- Psychiatric features are an early sign (anxiety, withdrawal, apathy, agitation, a permanent look of fear in the eyes, depression, personality change, insomnia). Hallucinations and delusions may occur—before akinetic mutism.
- Painful sensory symptoms are commoner (eg foot pain hyperaesthesia).
- More normal EEG (sporadic CJD has a characteristic spike and wave pattern).
- Mean CSF tau-pT181/tau protein ratio is 10-fold higher in vCJD than in sCJD.[37]
- Homozygosity for methionine at codon 129 of the PRP gene is typical.

Why bother studying rare diseases? The Liberski imperative...

For centuries, kuru was no bigger than a man's hand: a cloud barely visible on our horizon: a rare disease in cannibals beyond the Pacific. But meticulous work on kuru led to knowledge of prion diseases *before* the 1990s epidemic of vCJD. If in 1950s, Gajdusek and Zigas had not been intrigued as to why kuru affected women and children more than men (their strange neural diet was the culprit), the discovery of vCJD would have been delayed, as no surveillance would have been in place. Neural tissue might still be in our food chain, with dreadful consequences. But further than this, the notion of 'protein-misfolding diseases'[2] would have been delayed by decades. So this is the lesson: ►*let curiosity flourish*. This is Liberski's imperative.[38] So now let's scan our horizon for other intriguing clouds.

1 Der Vogel kämpft sich aus dem Ei. Das Ei ist die Welt. Wer geboren werden will, muss eine Welt zerstören. The bird struggles out of the egg. The egg is the world. Whoever will be born, must first destroy a world.
2 Cystic fibrosis (misfolded CFTR protein), Marfan's (misfolded fibrillin), Fabry's (misfolded α-galactosidase), Gaucher's (misfolded β-glucocerebrosidase), retinitis pigmentosa 3 (misfolded rhodopsin); some cancers may be caused by misfolding of tumour suppressor proteins (von Hippel-Lindau protein).

Curtis–Fitz-Hugh syndrome is inflammation of the liver capsule (perihepatitis) due to chlamydial or gonococcal infection, often with pelvic inflammatory disease (in women). Right upper quadrant pain occurs.

Devic's syndrome (neuromyelitis optica; NMO) Inflammatory demyelination causes attacks of optic neuritis ± myelitis. ΔΔ: MS (BOX); SLE. Abnormal CSF (may mimic bacterial meningitis) & serum NMO-IgG antibody (in 65%) help distinguish it from classical MS.[39] ℞: IV steroids, plasma exchange and azathioprine aim to suppress attacks. *Prognosis:* Variable; complete remission may occur.

Dressler's syndrome This develops 2–10wks after an MI, heart surgery (or even pacemaker insertion). It is thought that myocardial injury stimulates formation of autoantibodies against heart muscle. *The Patient:* He or she may suffer recurrent fever and chest pain ± pleural or pericardial rub (from serositis). Cardiac tamponade may occur, so avoid anticoagulants. ℞: Aspirin, NSAIDs or steroids.

Dubin–Johnson syndrome An autosomal recessive disorder, causing defective hepatocyte excretion of conjugated bilirubin. It is caused by a point mutation in a gene coding for a canalicular transport protein. There is intermittent jaundice with pain in the right hypochondrium. There is no hepatomegaly. *Tests:* Alk phos ↔; bilirubinuria on dipstick. Liver biopsy: diagnostic pigment granules.[40]

Dupuytren's contracture (fig 1). Palmar fascia contracts disabling finger (often 5th finger) extension. There is nodular thickening of the connective tissue over the 4th & 5th fingers. *Prevalence:* ~10% of ♂ >65yrs (↑ if +ve family history). *Associations:* Smoking, alcohol use, heavy manual labour, trauma, DM, phenytoin, HIV. Peyronie's may coexist (p722). It is thought to be caused by local hypoxia: ischaemia (the primary event)→ ↑xanthine oxidase activity→reduced oxygen→superoxide free radicals→fibroblast proliferation→type III collagen→palmar fibrosis. Surgery may be needed.

Ekbom's syndrome (Restless legs) Criteria: **1** Compelling desire to move legs **2** Worse at night **3** Relieved by movement **3** Unpleasant leg sensations (eg shootings or tinglings) worse at rest. *Mechanism:* Endogenous opioid system fault causes altered central processing of pain. *Prevalence:* 1–3%. ♀:♂ ≈2:1. *Associations:* Iron deficiency, uraemia, pregnancy, DM, polyneuropathy, rheumatoid arthritis, COPD, persistent genital arousal disorder.[41] *Exclude:* Cramps, positional discomfort, and local leg pathology. ℞: Tramadol, dopamine agonists, clonazepam (1–4mg PO nocte) have been tried. Ekbom also described delusional parasitosis: "I am invaded by parasites".[42]

Fabry disease X-linked lysosomal storage disorder caused by abnormalities in the GLA gene, which leads to a deficiency in α-galactosidase A. There is accumulation of glycosphingolipids in skin (angiokeratoma corporis diffusum ± hypohidrosis), eyes (lens opacities), heart (angina/MI, syncope, dyspnoea, LVH, conduction defects, eg VT), kidneys (renal failure), CNS (stroke) and nerves (neuropathy/acroparaesthesia) ± corneal verticillata (whorls). Most die in the 5th decade due to renal failure, stroke or MI. ℞: 2-weekly infusions of recombinant human agalsidase α and β are available.

Fanconi anaemia Autosomal recessive; HLA-DRB1*04 Defective stem cell repair and chromosomal fragility leads to aplastic anaemia, ↑risk of AML & breast ca (BRCA2 defects), skin pigmentation, absent radii, short stature, microcephaly, syndactyly), deafness, IQ↓, hypopituitarism, and cryptorchidism. ℞: Stem-cell transplant. *[Guido Fanconi, 1927]*

Felty's syndrome Rheumatoid arthritis + WCC↓ + splenomegaly (±hypersplenism, eg anaemia & platelets↓), recurrent infections, skin ulcers and lymphadenopathy. Rh factor ↑↑. Splenectomy may raise the WCC. ℞: DMRDs (p549) including rituximab.[43]

Foster Kennedy syndrome Optic atrophy of one eye with papilloedema of the other, due respectively to optic nerve compression and ↑ICP from a mass (eg meningioma, hydatid, plasmacytoma) on the side of the optic atrophy. *[Foster Kennedy 1911]*

Friedreich's ataxia This is an autosomal recessive disorder, with expansions of the trinucleotide repeat GAA in the X25 (frataxin) gene. There is degeneration of many nerve tracts: spinocerebellar tracts degenerate causing cerebellar ataxia, dysarthria, nystagmus, and dysdiadochokinesis. Loss of corticospinal tracts occurs (weakness and plantars ↑↑) with peripheral nerve damage, so tendon reflexes are paradoxically

Signs distinguishing Devic's syndrome from multiple sclerosis[44]

	Devic's syndrome	Multiple sclerosis
Course	Monophasic or relapsing	Relapsing usually; see p500
Attack severity	Usually severe	Often mild
Respiratory failure	~30%, from cervical myelitis	Rare
MRI head	Usually normal	Many periventricular white-matter lesions
MRI cord lesions	Multiple, small, peripheral	Extensive central lesions
CSF oligoclonal bands	Absent	Present
Permanent disability	Unusual, and attack-related	In late progressive disease
Other autoimmunities	In ≤50% (eg Sjögren's)	Uncommon

Diagnostic criteria for Devic's Optic neuritis, myelitis, and ≥2 out of 3 of:
• MRI evidence of a continuous cord lesion for ≥3 segments • Onset brain MRI changes non-diagnostic for MS • NMO-IgG seropositivity.
NB: CNS involvement beyond the optic nerves and cord is compatible with NMO.

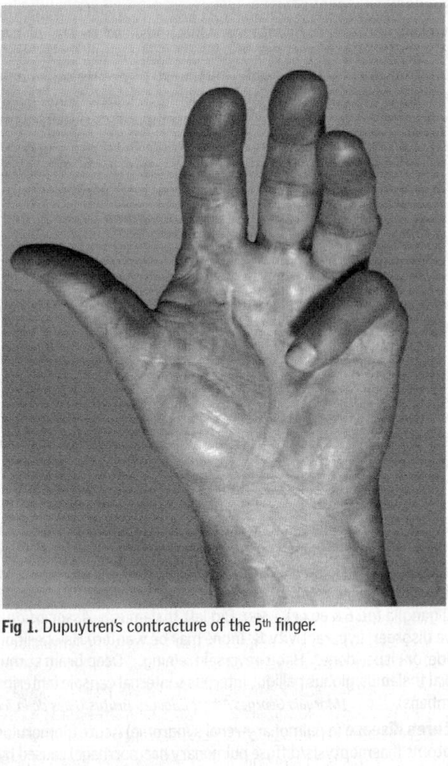

Fig 1. Dupuytren's contracture of the 5th finger.

depressed (differential diagnosis p351). There is also dorsal column degeneration, hence loss of positional and vibration sense. Pes cavus and scoliosis occur. Cardiomyopathy may cause CCF. Typical age at death: ~50yrs. ℞: There is no cure; surgery may provide symptomatic relief for musculoskeletal problems.

Froin's syndrome CSF protein↑ and xanthochromia with normal cell count, a sign of blockage in CSF flow in the spine, eg from a spinal tumour. *[Georges Froin, 1874]*

Gardner's syndrome Autosomal dominant Variant of familial adenomatous polyposis, caused by mutations in the APC gene (5q21). *Signs:* 100s of colon polyps (which 'inevitably', given time, become malignant, eg before 40yrs old),[45] benign bone osteomas, epidermal cysts, dermoid tumours, fibromas, and neurofibromas. *Fundoscopy:* Black spots (congenital hypertrophy of retinal pigment epithelium); this helps pre-symptomatic detection. *Onset:* 2–70yrs, eg mass effect (eg obstructed ureters) or bloody diarrhoea. Careful follow-up is needed. Subtotal colectomy + removal of polyps may prevent malignancy. Endoscopic polypectomy with long-term sulindac therapy has been tried to postpone prophylactic colectomy.[46] *[EJ Gardner 1950]*

Gélineau's syndrome (narcolepsy) The patient, usually a young man, succumbs to irresistible attacks of inappropriate sleep ± vivid hallucinations, cataplexy (sudden hypotonia), and sleep paralysis (paralysis of speech + willed movement on waking, while fully alert, *OHCS* p392). *Hypothesis:* Mutations lead to loss of hypothalamic hypocretin-containing neurons, via autoimmune destruction.[47] 95% are +ve for HLA DR2. ℞: Stimulants (eg methylphenidate, 10–15mg PO after breakfast and lunch) may cause dependence ± psychosis. Modafinil (~200mg/d PO, before noon) may be better. SE: anxiety, aggression, dry mouth, euphoria, insomnia, BP↑, dyskinesia, alk phos↑.

Gerstmann's syndrome Finger agnosia (inability to identify fingers by name), left/right disorientation, agraphia (inability to write), acalculia (to calculate) & alexia (to read). These symptoms together suggest a dominant parietal lesion.

Gilbert's syndrome is a common cause of *unconjugated* hyperbilirubinaemia ∵ ↓ bilirubin UDP-glucuronosyl-transferase activity. Prevalence is estimated at 1–2%. The onset is shortly after birth, but it may be unnoticed for many years. Jaundice occurs during intercurrent illness, and bilirubin rises on fasting. Liver biopsy is normal, but should rarely be required clinically. It is a benign condition. *[Nicolas Gilbert 1901]*

Gilles de la Tourette syndrome Tonic, clonic, dystonic, or phonic tics: jerks, blinks, sniffs, nods, spitting, stuttering, irrepressible explosive obscene verbal ejaculations (coprolalia, in 20%) or gestures (coprophilia, 6%),[48] grunts, squeaks, burps, twirlings, and nipping others ± tantrums. There may be a witty, innovatory, phantasmagoric picture, with mimicry (echopraxia), antics, impishness, extravagance, "audacity, dramatizations, surreal associations, uninhibited affect, speed, 'go', vivid imagery and memory, and hunger for stimuli." *The tic paradox:* Tics are *voluntary*, but often *unwanted*: the desire to tic stems from the relief of the odd sensation that builds up prior to the tic and is relieved by it, "like scratching a mosquito bite, tics lead to more tics."[49] Tics may be controlled though the medium of dance, or when concentrating, or having sex,[50] but note: ►"tics aren't just little annoyances now and then, they form an integral part of my existence. I tic therefore I am."[51] *Mean age of onset:* 6yrs. ♂:♀ ≈4:1 *Molecular mimicry hypothesis:* Anti-streptococcal antibodies cross-react with basal ganglia (p136 & BOX 2).[52] *MRI:* Big left thalamus.[53] *Association:* Obsessive-compulsive disorder; hyperactivity. ℞: (none may be wanted) Haloperidol ~1.5mg/8h PO, pimozide, or risperidone. Habit-reversal training.[54] Deep brain stimulation may help—medial thalamus, globus pallidus internus & internal capsule (anterior limb/nucleus accumbens).[55] [56] *[Marquis Georges Albert Edouard Brutus Gilles de la Tourette, 1885]*

Goodpasture's disease (a pulmonary-renal syndrome) Acute glomerulonephritis + lung symptoms (haemoptysis/diffuse pulmonary haemorrhage) caused by antiglomerular basement membrane antibodies (binding kidney's basement membrane and alveolar membrane). *Tests:* CXR: infiltrates due to pulmonary haemorrhage, often in lower zones. Kidney biopsy: crescentic glomerulonephritis. ℞: ►►Treat shock. Vigorous immunosuppressive treatment & plasmapheresis. *[Ernest Goodpasture, 1919]*

ABC

Cataplexy is highly specific for narcolepsy/Gélineau's syndrome

Daytime sleepiness has many causes, but if it occurs with cataplexy the diagnosis 'must' be narcolepsy. Cataplexy is bilateral loss of tone in antigravity muscles provoked by emotions such as laughter, startle, excitement, or anger. Associated phenomena include: falls, mouth opening, dysarthria, mutism, and phasic muscle jerking around the mouth. Most attacks are brief, but injury can occur (eg if several attacks per day). It is comparable to the atonia of rapid eye movement sleep *but without loss of awareness.* **ΔΔ:** bradycardia, migraine, atonic/akinetic epilepsy,[57 58] delayed sleep phase syndrome, conversion disorder, malingering, and psychosis.[59]

Don't confuse cata**plex**y with cata**leps**y—a waxy flexibility where involuntary statue-like postures are effortlessly maintained (frozen) despite looking most uncomfortable (this motor-perceptual dissociative phenomenon may be induced by hypnosis, psychosis, antipsychotics, or a thalamic lesion).[60] **Catalepsy** is one of the signs of **catatonia**[61]—a neuropsychiatric syndrome of catalepsy, negativism, mutism, muscular rigidity, mannerisms, autonomic instability, and fever.[62]

Post-streptococcal autoimmune CNS disorders (eg Tourettism)

Group A streptococci can (rarely) induce autoimmune diseases of the heart, joints, and brain, eg movement disorders (chorea, tics/Tourettism, dystonia, and Parkinsonism), emotional disorders, and sleep disorders. MRI and pathological studies suggest that the most vulnerable CNS region is the basal ganglia. Immunopathogenesis is poorly understood: there is some support for autoantibody-mediated disease, but studies are conflicting.[63]

The lung and its various vasculitides (eg Goodpasture's)[1]

Lung vasculitis is most commonly seen with the primary idiopathic, small-vessel or ANCA (p555) associated vasculitides (Wegener's granulomatosis, microscopic polyangiitis, and Churg-Strauss syndrome).[64] Medium-vessel vasculitis (classic polyarteritis nodosa), large-vessel vasculitis (Takayasu arteritis), primary immune complex-mediated vasculitis (Goodpasture's disease), and secondary vasculitis (SLE) can all affect the lung. Hepatitis C is a rare cause of lung vasculitis—usually associated with glomerulonephritis and cryoglobulinaemia.[65]

1 Should it be Goodpasture's **disease** or **syndrome**? The latter might refer to any pulmonary-renal vasculitis (eg caused by cryoglobulinaemia or SLE). Goodpasture's **disease** is reserved for the clinical condition characterised by lung haemorrhage, and crescentic glomerulonephritis associated with linear deposition of antibodies along the glomerular basement membrane.

Guillain–Barré syndrome (Acute autoimmune inflammatory demyelinating polyneuropathy)[66] ***Incidence:*** 1-2/100,000/yr. ***Signs:*** A few weeks after an infection a symmetrical ascending muscle weakness starts. ***Triggers:*** *Campylobacter jejuni*, CMV, mycoplasma, zoster, HIV, EBV, vaccinations. The trigger causes antibodies which attack nerves. In 40%, no cause is found. It may advance quickly, affecting all limbs at once, and can lead to paralysis. There is a progressive phase of up to 4 weeks, followed by recovery. Unlike other neuropathies, *proximal* muscles are more affected, eg trunk, respiratory, and cranial nerves (esp. VII). Pain is common (eg back, limb) but sensory signs may be absent. Autonomic dysfunction: sweating, ↑pulse, BP changes, arrhythmias. ***Nerve conduction studies:*** Slow conduction. ***CSF:*** protein↑ (eg >5.5g/L), normal CSF white cell count. Respiratory involvement (the big danger) requires transfer to ITU. Do forced vital capacity (FVC) 4 hourly. ►*Ventilate sooner rather than later*, eg if FVC <1.5L, P_aO_2 <10kPa, P_aCO_2 >6kPa. **℞:** IV immunoglobulin 0.4g/kg/24h for 5d. Plasma exchange is good too (?more SE).[67] Steroids have no role. ***Prognosis:*** Good; ~85% make a complete or near-complete recovery. 10% are unable to walk alone at 1yr. *Complete paralysis is compatible with complete recovery.* ***Mortality:*** 10%.

Henoch–Schönlein purpura (HSP) (**fig 2**) is a small vessel vasculitis, which presents with purpura (purple nodules which do not disappear on pressure—signifying intradermal bleeding) often over buttocks and extensor surfaces, typically affecting young ♂. There may be glomerulonephritis (p294), joint involvement, and abdominal pain (±intussusception), which may mimic an 'acute abdomen'.

Horner's syndrome Pupil constriction (*miosis*, **fig 1**), sunken eye (*enophthalmos*), *ptosis* + ipsilateral loss of sweating (*anhidrosis*) due to interruption of the face's sympathetic supply, eg at the brainstem (demyelination, vascular disease), cord (syringomyelia), thoracic outlet (Pancoast's tumour, p722), or on the sympathetic's trip on the internal carotid artery into the skull (**fig 3**, carotid aneurysm), and thence to the orbit. *[Johann Horner, 1869]*

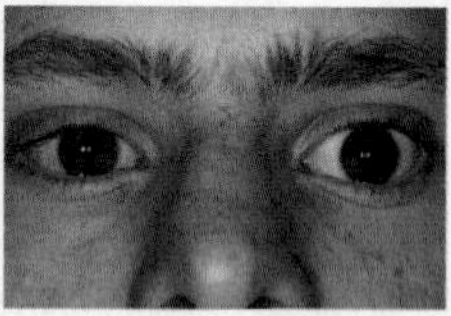

Fig 1. Right Horner's: everything reduces: pupil, eye, sweating etc.[68]

Huntington's chorea Autosomal dominant gene on chromsome 4 Onset is usually in middle age, so the child of an affected parent lives under a Damocles' sword, with a 50% chance of being affected. Genetic tests are available. Signs are insidious, then progressive: chorea → irritability→dementia ± fits→death (within ~15yrs of diagnosis). ***Pathology:*** Cerebral atrophy with loss of corpus striatum GABA-nergic & cholinergic neurons. **℞:** (p81) None prevents progression. Offer counselling to patient & family.[69] *[George Huntington, 1872]*

Jervell-Lange-Nielsen syndrome Autosomal recessive Aberrant ventricular repolarization with a long QTc interval (p90, hence syncope, seizures, torsade de pointes ± sudden death) and bilateral deafness. Mutations in a K^+ channel subunit may be responsible.[70]

Kaposi's sarcoma (KS) is a multicentric neoplasm derived from capillary endothelial cells or from fibrous tissue, caused by human herpes virus (KSHV = HHV-8; also causes other malignancies: primary effusion lymphoma and multicentric Castleman disease). It presents as purple papules (½-1cm) or plaques on skin (**figs 4, 5**) & mucosa (any organ). It metastasizes to nodes. 3 types: **1** Classic, especially elderly Jewish or Mediterranean ♂ (esp. in Po Valley and Sardinia, ?related to blood-sucking insects). **2** Endemic (Central Africa). In forms 1 & 2, peripheral, slow-growing skin lesions are found, visceral involvement is rare, but node involvement may cause oedema. **3** KS in immunosuppression, eg organ transplant recipients. Taper immunosuppressives to the lowest level that keeps the graft functional.[71] Sirolimus has a role.[72] In HIV, KS is diagnostic of AIDS (p408; and may be life-threatening with many skin, gut and lung lesions), affecting mostly homo- or bi-sexual men (but ♂:♀ ≈1 in HIV-KS in S. Africa).[73] Prevalence is less with HHART (p414).[74] Lung KS may present in HIV+ve men and women as dyspnoea and haemoptysis.[75] Bowel KS may cause nausea, abdominal pain. ***Rare sites:*** CNS, larynx, eye, glands, heart, breast, wounds or biopsy sites. **Δ:** Biopsy. **℞:** Optimize HHART;[76] consider radiotherapy for skin lesions. Chemotherapy example: pegylated liposomal doxorubicin ± interleukin-12.[77] *[Moricz Kaposi, 1887]*

ABC

Diagnostic criteria in typical Guillain-Barré polyneuritis[78]

Features required for diagnosis:
Progressive weakness of all 4 limbs
Areflexia

Features excluding diagnosis:
Purely sensory symptoms
Diagnosis of:
- Myasthenia
- Botulism
- Poliomyelitis
- Diphtheria
- Porphyria
- Toxic neuropathy

Features supporting diagnosis:
Progression over days, up to 4wks
Near symmetry of symptoms
Sensory symptoms/signs only mild
CN involvement (eg bilateral facial weakness)
Recovery starts ~2wks after the period of progression has finished
Autonomic dysfunction
Absence of fever at onset
CSF protein ↑ with CSF WCC $<10\times10^6$/L
Typical electrophysiological tests

Variants of Guillain-Barré syndrome include:
Chronic inflammatory demyelinating polyradiculopathy: (CIDP) characterized by a slower onset and recovery.
Miller-Fisher syndrome which comprises of ophthalmoplegia, ataxia and areflexia. Associated with anti-GQ1b antibodies in the serum.

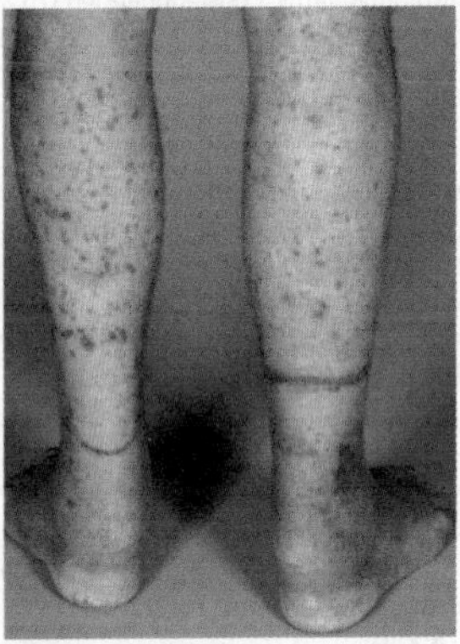

Fig 2. Henoch-Schönlein vasculitis.

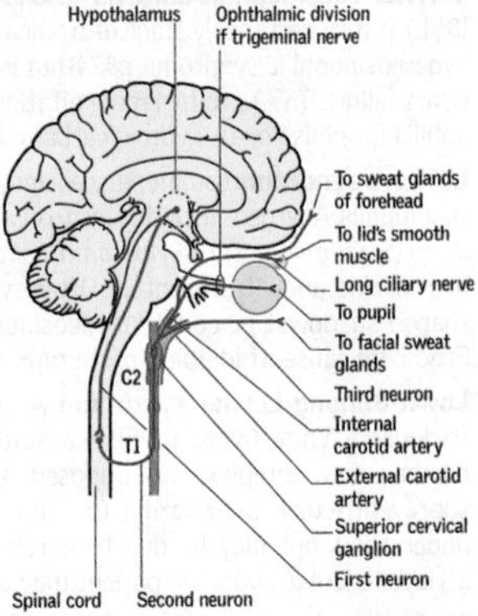

Fig 3. Pathways in Horner's syndrome.

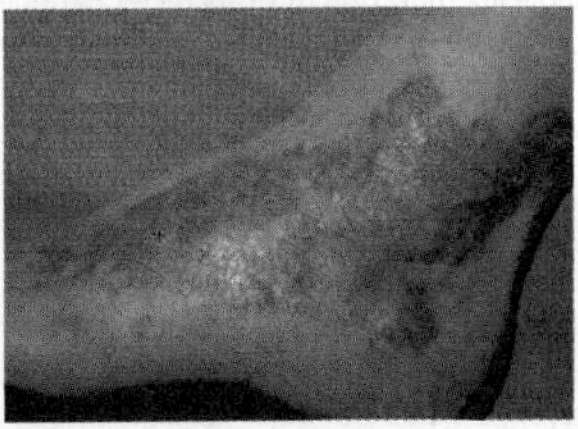

Fig 4. Kaposi's sarcoma.[79]

Courtesy of Prof. Thomas Habif

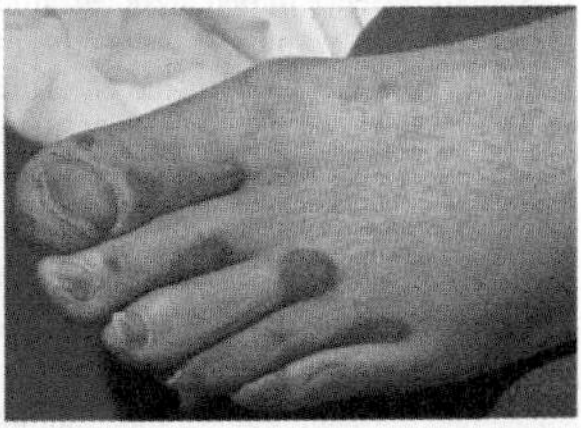

Fig 5. Another image of Kaposi's sarcoma.[80]

Courtesy of The Crookston collection

Klippel-Trénaunay syndrome A triad of port wine stain, varicose veins, and limb hypertrophy, due to vascular malformation. Usually sporadic, though a few families exhibiting autosomal dominant inheritance have been reported.[81]

Korsakoff's syndrome ↓Ability to acquire new memories, eg after Wernicke's encephalopathy, due to thiamine deficiency (eg in alcoholics). The patient may have to relive his grief each time he hears of the death of a friend. He confabulates to fill in gaps in his memory owing to retrograde amnesia. ℞: See *Wernicke's*, p728. Donepezil may have a role.[82] *[Sergei Korsakoff, 1887, better transliterated as 'Korsakov']*

Langerhans cell histiocytosis (histiocytosis X**)** A group of disorders, either single- (in 73%, eg bone) or multi-system (in 27%; at risk organs are liver, lung, spleen, marrow) with infiltrating granulomas containing dendritic (Langerhans) cells. ♂:♀≈1.5:1. Pulmonary Langerhans cell histiocytosis presents with pneumothorax or pulmonary hypertension. CXR/CT: nodules and cysts and honeycombing in upper and middle zones. **Δ**: Biopsy (skin, lung): characteristic Birbeck granules on electron microscopy. ℞: Local excision, steroids, vinblastine ± etoposide if severe. *OHCS* p644.[83]

Leriche's syndrome Absent femoral pulse, claudication/wasting[84] of the buttock, a pale cold leg, and erectile dysfunction from aorto-iliac occlusive disease, eg a saddle embolus at the aortic bifurcation. Surgery may help.[85] *[René Leriche, 1940]*

Löfffler's eosinophilic carditis Restrictive cardiomyopathy + eosinophilia (eg 120 × 10^9/L). It may be an early stage of tropical endomyocardial fibrosis (and overlaps with hypereosinophilic syndrome, p324) but is distinct from eosinophilic leukaemia. ***Signs:*** Heart failure (75%) ± mitral regurgitation (49%) ± heart block. ℞: Suppress the eosinophilia (prednisolone ± hydroxycarbamide), and then anti-heart failure ℞ may work.

Löffler's syndrome (pulmonary eosinophilia**)** An allergic infiltration of the lungs by eosinophils. Allergens include: *Ascaris lumbricoides, Trichinella spiralis, Fasciola hepatica, Strongyloides, Ankylostoma, Toxocara, Clonorchis sinensis,*[86] sulfonamides, hydralazine, and nitrofurantoin. Often symptomless with incidental CXR (diffuse fan-shaped shadows), or cough, T°↑, eosinophilia (in ~20%) & larval migrans (p442). ℞: Eradicate cause. If idiopathic, steroids are effective. *[Wilhelm Löffler, 1887-1972]*

Lown-Ganong-Levine syndrome A pre-excitation syndrome, similar to Wolf-Parkinson-White (WPW, p120), characterized by a short PR interval (<0.12sec), a normal QRS complex (as opposed to the δ-waves of WPW), and risk of supraventricular tachycardia (but not AF/flutter). The cause is not completely understood, but may be due to paranodal fibres that bypass all or part of the atrioventricular node. The patient may complain of intermittent palpitations.[87]

McArdle's glycogen storage disease (type V) Autosomal recessive pure myopathy caused by absence of glycolytic enzymes (eg R50X mutation of PYGM gene). Fatigue and crises of cramps ± hyperthermia, rhabdomyolysis/myoglobinuria follow exercise. *Tests:* CK↑↑. Muscle biopsy is diagnostic (necrosis & atrophy). *In vitro* lack of lactate in the presence of glycogen (as muscle phosphorylase↓). ℞: Moderate aerobic exercise helps. Avoid heavy exertion and statins. Sucrose ~37g 5min pre-exercise make life better.[88] [89] Creatine (~60mg/kg/d) may have a role.[90] *[Brian McArdle, 1951]*

Mallory-Weiss tear Vomiting *causes* haematemesis via an oesophageal tear.

Marchiafava-Bignami syndrome Alcohol-induced corpus callosum necrosis (±extrapontine myelinolysis) causing left-handed deficit of constructional ability, agraphia, mutism, ataxia, poor bimanual coordination, gaze apraxia/pseudo-hallucinated look, dysarthria, epilepsy, paucity of vocal and facial expression modulation,[91] ↓consciousness, coma. **Δ:** MRI.[92] ℞: As for Wernicke's, p728.

Marchiafava-Micheli syndrome (paroxysmal nocturnal haemoglobinuria, PNH**)** an acquired clonal expansion of a multipotent stem cell carrying a somatic mutation in the X-linked PIG-A gene. Glycosylphosphatidylinositol (GPI)-anchored proteins are lacking on blood cells derived from these mutated stem cells, predisposing to haemolysis, thrombosis, sepsis, and marrow failure.[93] See p332; see **fig 1**.

ABC

Fatal effects of alcohol on the CNS
• Inhibitions↓ (unsafe sex↑ etc etc)[1]
• Wernicke's encephalopathy
• Hepatic encephalopathy
• Cerebral atrophy (dementia)
• Central pontine myelinolysis
• Cerebellar atrophy (falls etc)
• Stroke (all varieties)
• Seizures
• Marchiafava–Bignami syndrome

Fig 1. PNH. As always, the darkest hour is before dawn (in this 24h urine sample). NB: this phenomenon is not all that reliable. A much better test even than a marrow biopsy (right-hand panel, showing a clone of PNH cells) is flow cytometric analysis of GPI-anchored proteins on peripheral blood cells. This can determine the size of the PNH clone and type of GPI deficiency (complete or partial). ℞: Most benefit from supportive measures—but allogeneic stem cell transplantation is the only cure. Courtesy of Crookston Collection

1 Alcohol is frequently fatal to fetuses—in the UK *thousands* of terminations are carried out *every month* out from conceptions related to binge drinking. Also, fewer inhibitions lead to more sex, and hence more deaths from cervical cancer (human papilloma virus-associated, HIV etc).

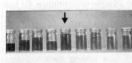

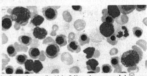

Marfan's syndrome Autosomal dominant fibrillin gene, FBN1 There is ↓extracellular microfibril formation, with poor elastic fibres.[96] ~25% occur with no family history. *Major criteria* (diagnostic if >2): Lens dislocation (*ectopia lentis*; **fig 1**); aortic dissection or dilatation; dural ectasia; skeletal features: arachnodactyly (long spidery fingers), armspan > height, pectus deformity, scoliosis, pes planus. *Minor signs:* Mitral valve prolapse, high-arched palate, joint hypermobility. Diagnosis is clinical; MRI for dural ectasia (enlargement of the neural canal) may be helpful. ℞: The danger is aortic dissection: beta-blockers are used to slow dilatation of the aortic root. Do annual echos, with elective surgical repair when maximal aortic diameter is >5cm. In pregnancy, the risk of dissection rises. Homocystinuria has similar skeletal deformities:

Marfan's autosomal dominant vs	*Homocystinuria* cystathione β-synthetase deficiency; autosomal recessive with early vasculopathy
• Upwards lens dislocation	• Downwards lens dislocation
• Aortic valve incompetence	• Heart rarely affected
• *Normal* intelligence	• Mental retardation
• Scoliosis, flat feet, herniae	• Recurrent thromboses, osteoporosis
• Life expectancy is lower from cardiovascular risks	• Positive urine cyanide-nitroprusside test
	• Response to pyridoxine

[Antoine Marfan, 1896]

Meckel's diverticulum *Prevalence:* ≤2%. ≤2 inches long, and >2 feet from the ileocaecal valve, it contains gastric and pancreatic tissue. There may be gastric acid secretion, causing occult GI pain and bleeding. *Diagnosis:* Radionucleotide scan; laparotomy. Acute inflammation may present like appendicitis.

Meigs' syndrome Ovarian fibroma or thecoma + ascites + pleural transudate (usually right side; rarely bloody[97]). Despite appearances, it's benign.[98] *[Joseph Meigs, 1937]*

Ménétrier's disease Giant gastric mucosal folds up to 4cm high, in the fundus, with atrophy of the glands + ↑mucosal thickness + hypochlorhydria + protein-losing gastropathy (hence hypoalbuminaemia ± oedema). Causes: CMV, streps,[99] *H. pylori*. There may be epigastric pain, vomiting ± ↓weight. It is premalignant. ℞: Try *H. pylori* eradication; surgery if intractable symptoms or malignant change. Drugs targeting ↑epidermal growth factor receptor signalling show promise.[100] *[Pierre Ménétrier, 1859]*

Meyer-Betz syndrome (paroxysmal myoglobinuria) This idiopathic condition causes necrosis of exercising muscles. There is muscle pain, weakness, and discoloured urine: pink→brown (as ↑myoglobin is excreted). Acute renal failure can result from myoglobinuria (p307). DIC is associated. *Tests:* WCC↑, LFT↑, LDH↑, CPK↑, urine myoglobin↑. *Diagnosis:* Muscle biopsy. Exertion should be avoided.

Mikulicz's syndrome Diagnostic criteria: symmetric, persistent swelling of lacrimal and parotid (or submandibular) glands with exclusion of diseases mimicking these signs: (sarcoidosis, TB, viral infection, lymphoproliferative disorders). It is a variant of Sjögren's syndrome and is usually self-limiting.[101] *[Johann von Mikulicz-Radecki, 1892]*

Milroy's syndrome Autosomal dominant Mutations in the gene vascular endothelial growth factor receptor 3, VEGFR3 (FLT4), cause lymphatic malfunction with asymmetric leg swelling (usually in young girls). **Δ**: Isotopic lymphoscintigraphy ℞ (**fig 2**) • Good foot hygiene • Surgery (rarely needed). • Treat comorbid cellulitis actively.[102]

Münchausen's syndrome Vivid liars, who are addicted to institutions, flit from hospital to hospital, feigning illness, eg hoping for a laparotomy (*laparotimophilia migrans*) or mastectomy (*mammomania non-neoplastica*), or they complain of awful bleeding (*haemorrhagica histrionica*), odd eye movements (*nystagmus confabulus*), curious fits (*neurologica diabolica*), sexual assaults (*phantasmorotica penetrans*), throat closings (*otolaryngologica prevarica*), false asthma (*bronchospasmus absurdum*) or heart attacks (*cardiopathia fantastica*). Münchausen-by-proxy entails injury to a dependent person by a carer (eg mother) to gain medical attention. Covert video surveillance is an ethically problematic tool which may aid diagnosis.

Ogilvie's syndrome Acute functional ('pseudo') colonic obstruction caused by: malignant retroperitoneal infiltration, spine fracture, or electrolyte imbalance. ℞: Correct U&E, conservative measures. Contrast enema or colonoscopy allows decompression, and excludes mechanical causes. Neostigmine is also effective, suggesting parasympathetic suppression is to blame.[103] Surgery is rarely needed.

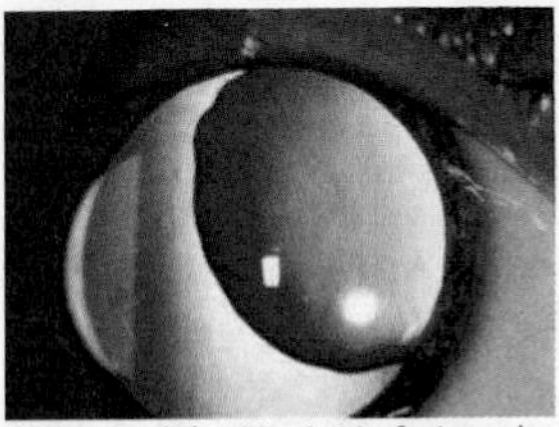

Fig 1. Lens dislocation in Marfan's syndrome: here the lens is dislocated superiorly and medially. 104
Courtesy of Prof Jonathan Trobe

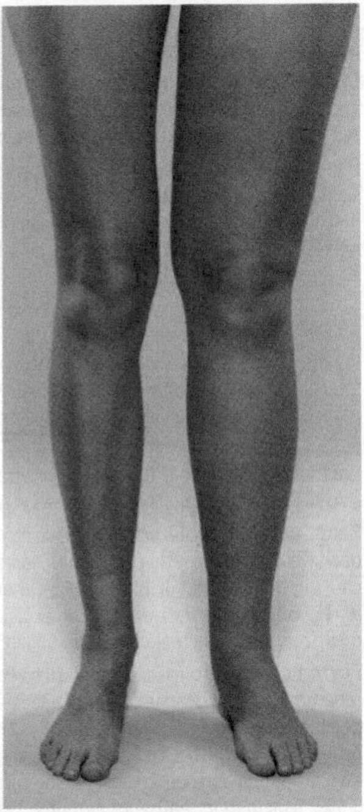

Fig 2. Milroy's syndrome is benign (but ≤10% cross to the other leg). It is possible to reroute lymph via remaining functional lymphatics by elevation, exercises, compression garments, various devices, and manual lymph drainage.

Who was Baron Münchausen?

Baron Karl Münchausen was an 18th-century German aristocrat and fabulist, whose tall tales became first a popular book, then a byword for circular logic, and finally a medical syndrome of self-delusion. He is famous for pulling himself out of a swamp by his own hair. ►►In emergencies (we've all had that sinking feeling....) this method may save your life, for example in your final exams (**fig 3**). *Examiner:* "What is ITP?"

You: "ITP is idiopathic thrombocytopenic purpura." (you have scored 50% already).

Examiner: "And what is idiopathic thrombocytopenic purpura?"

You: "It's when a cryptogenic cause of a low platelet count leads to purpura."

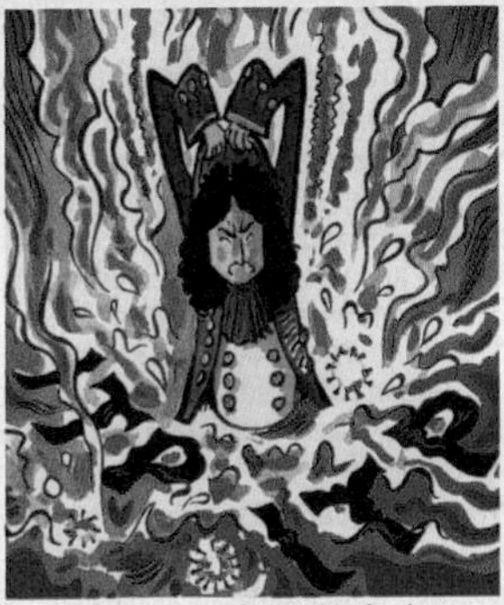

Fig 3. Münchausen during his finals.

You have deployed your skills with logical brilliance, without adding a single insight. For this Münchausen circularity you may be awarded 100%—unless your examiner is a philosopher, when the right answer would be "What is ITP? I don't know—and nor do you"—but don't try this too often. You see, you must *never* forget that medicine is marvellously scientific, and no-one is popular who dares cast doubt on this article of faith.

Ortner's cardiovocal syndrome Recurrent laryngeal nerve palsy from a large left atrium (eg from mitral stenosis) or aortic dissection.

Osler-Weber-Rendu syndrome (hereditary telangiectasia) Telangiectasia on the skin and mucous membranes (causing epistaxis and GI bleeds), see **fig 2**. It is associated with pulmonary, hepatic and cerebral AVMs. Inheritance: autosomal dominant.[105]

Paget's disease of breast is intra-epidermal spread of an intraductal cancer, which can look just like eczema. ►Any red, scaly lesion at the nipple (see **fig 1**) *must* suggest PDB: do a biopsy. ℞: Mastectomy + node clearance. *[Sir James Paget, 1874]*

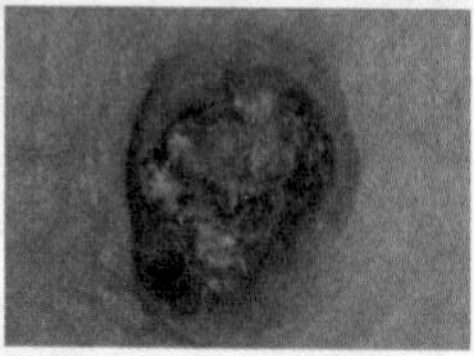

Fig 1 Paget's disease of breast.

Pancoast's syndrome Apical lung cancer invades sympathetic plexus in the neck (→ipsilateral Horner's, p716) ± brachial plexus (→arm pain) ± recurrent laryngeal nerve (→hoarse voice/bovine cough from vocal cord palsy). *[Henry Pancoast, 1932]*

Parinaud's syndrome (dorsal midbrain syndrome) Upward gaze palsy + pseudo-Argyll Robertson pupils (p79). Causes: hydrocephalus, pineal tumours, stroke.

Peutz-Jeghers' syndrome Germline mutations of gene LKB1 cause mucocutaneous dark freckles on lips (**fig 4**), oral mucosa, palm and soles ± GI polyps (hamartomas), causing obstruction or bleeds. *Malignant change:* ≤3%, typically duodenal polyps. ℞: Usually conservative or local excision. **NB:** hamartomas are excessive focal overgrowths of normal cells in an organ composed of the same cell type.

Peyronie's disease (penile angulation) *Pathogenesis:* Microtrauma during coitus→inflammation (under tunica albuginea)→fibroblast proliferation/immortalization→penile plaque→faulty compression of cavernosal venules[106] between engorging corporal tissue and the tunica albuginea→painful erectile dysfunction (in 50%) + angulation, making coitus most inconvenient (esp. if ossification occurs).[107] *Prevalence:* 3-9%. *Typical age:* >40. *Associations:* Dupuytren's (p712); endothelial dysfunction; atheroma; radical prostatectomy. **ΔΔ**: Haemangioma. *Tests:* Ultrasound.[108] ℞: Find out exactly what he wants: "How straight do you want to be?"[109] See p222. Manage associated depression (seen in 48%). Topical verapamil 15% gel,[110] N=57 intralesional interferon α2B, vitamin E, tamoxifen, and colchicine have variable success, even in early disease.[111] radiotherapy, lasers, surgery (eg tunica plication ± prostheses aid may help penetration). Penile rehabilitation can help (p222).[112] *[Francois de la Peyronie, 1687]*

Pott's syndrome (spinal TB). Rare in the West, this is usually spread from an extra-spinal source, eg lungs. *Features:* Backache, and stiffness of *all* back movements. T°↑, night sweats and weight loss occur. Progressive bone destruction leads to vertebral collapse and gibbus (sharply angled spinal curvature). Abscess formation may lead to cord compression, causing paraplegia, and bowel and bladder dysfunction (p470). *X-rays:* (**fig 3**) Narrow disc spaces and vertebral osteoporosis early, leading to destruction with wedging of vertebrae. Lesions in the thoracic spine often lead to kyphosis. Abscess formation in the lumbar spine may track down to the psoas muscle, and erode through the skin. ℞: Anti-TB drugs (p398). *[Sir Percival Pott, 1779]*

Prinzmetal (variant) angina Angina from coronary artery spasm: ECG: ST *elevation*. ℞: Use Ca^{2+}-channel blockers (p110), not β-blockers.[113] Association: Circle of Willis occlusion from intimal thickening (moyamoya disease). *[Myron Prinzmetal, 1908]*

ABC

Raynaud's syndrome This is peripheral digital ischaemia due to vasospasm, precipitated by cold or emotion. Fingers or toes ache and change colour: pale→blue→red. It may be idiopathic (Raynaud's *disease*—prevalence: 3-20%; ♀:♂ >1:1) or have an underlying cause (Raynaud's *phenomenon*; **fig 5**). *Tests:* Exclude an underlying cause (see BOX). ℞: Keep warm (eg electrically heated mittens); stop smoking. Nifedipine 5-20mg/8h PO helps, as may losartan, prazosin, or fluoxetine. Sympathectomy may help in those with severe disease. Iloprost, as a nebulized solution, may salvage digits with ulcers ± near-gangrene; effects last up to 16 weeks. Relapse is common.

Prinzmetal angina and vascular hyperreactivity

Coronary spasm causes Prinzmetal angina and also contributes to coronary heart disease in general, eg acute coronary syndrome (esp. in Japan).[114] Coronary spasm can be induced by ergonovine, acetylcholine, and methacholine (the former is used diagnostically).[1] These cause vasodilatation by endothelium-derived relaxing factor when vascular endothelium is functioning normally, whereas they cause vasoconstriction if the endothelium is damaged. In the light of these facts, patients with coronary spasm are thought to have a disturbance in endothelial function as well as local hyperreactivity of the coronary arteries.

If full anti-anginal therapy does not reduce symptoms, stenting[115] or intra-coronary radiation (20Gy brachytherapy) to vasospastic segments may be tried.[116]

Prognosis is good (especially if non-smoker, no past MI, and no diabetes; progress to infarction is quite rare);[117] there is some evidence that prognosis may be better with the new calcium channel blockers such as benidipine.[118]

Prinzmetal angina is associated with vascular hyperreactivity/vasospastic disorders such as Raynaud's phenomenon and migraine.

β-blockers and large doses of aspirin are contraindicated.

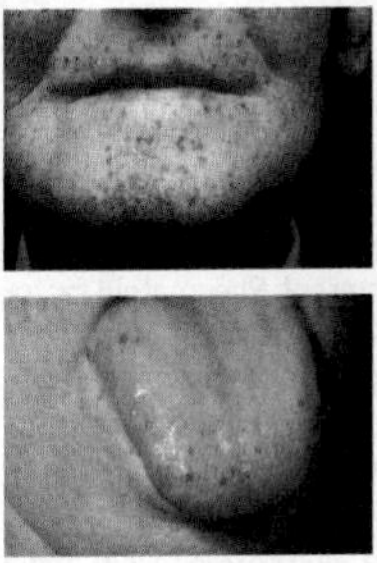

Fig 2. Telangiectasia in Osler-Weber-Rendu syndrome

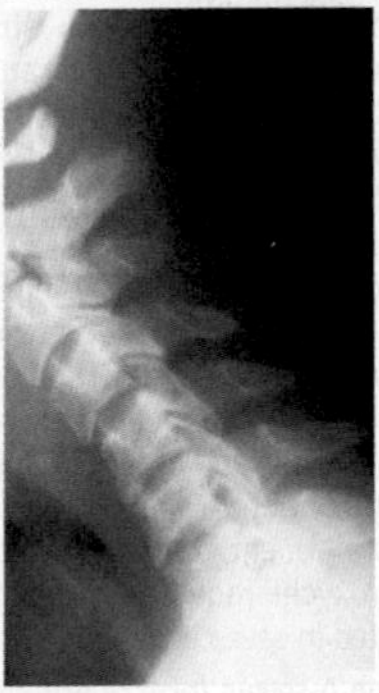

Fig 3. TB of axis: soft tissue swelling displaces the retro-pharyngeal air-tissue boundary forwards. There is an anterior defect in the vertebra, below the axis peg.

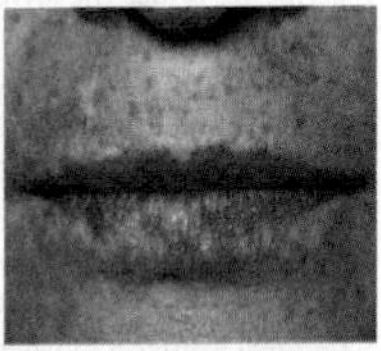

Fig 4. Perioral pigmentation, seen in Peutz-Jegher's syn.

Figures courtesy of: Figs 2 &4: Clinical Skills, Oxford Core Text, p411; Fig 3: Dr Ian Maddison myweb.lsbu.ac.uk; Fig 5 the Crookston Collection

Conditions in which Raynaud's phenomenon may be exhibited[2]

Connective tissue disorders: Systemic sclerosis, SLE, rheumatoid arthritis, dermatomyositis/polymyositis.
Occupational: Using vibrating tools.
Obstructive: Thoracic outlet obstruction, Buerger's disease, atheroma.
Blood: Thrombocytosis, cold agglutinin disease, polycythaemia rubra vera (p360), monoclonal gammopathies.
Drugs: β-blockers.
Others: Hypothyroidism.

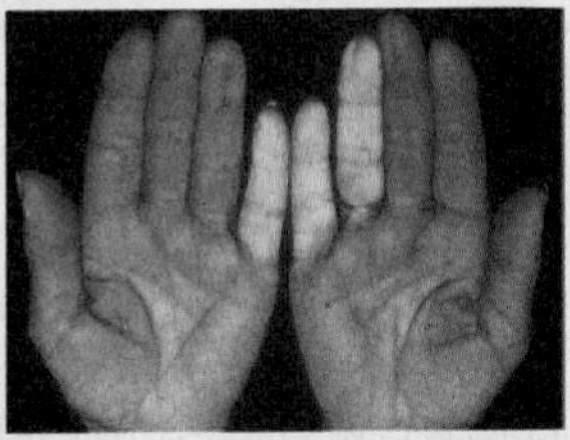

Fig 5. Raynaud's phenomenon in SLE.[119]

1 Since Prinzmetal angina is not a 'demand-induced' symptom, but a supply (vasospastic) abnormality, treadmill tests don't help. The most sensitive and specific test is IV ergonovine; 50μg at 5min intervals in a specialist lab until a +ve result or 400μg is given. When positive, the symptoms and ↑ST should be present. Nitroglycerin rapidly reverses the effects of ergonovine if refractory spasm occurs.

2 Patient information on Raynaud's is available from **www.raynauds.org.uk**.

Refsum's syndrome Autosomal recessive Phytanic acid accumulates in tissues, due to a mutation of the gene coding for the peroxisomal enzyme phytanoyl-CoA hydroxylase. This leads to a polyneuropathy, nerve deafness, night blindness (retinitis pigmentosa), cerebellar ataxia, ichthyosis, anosmia, and cardiomyopathy. *Tests:* Plasma phytanic acid↑. ↑CSF protein. ℞: Restrict foods containing phytanic acid (animal fats, dairy products, green leafy vegetables); plasmapheresis is used for severe symptoms.[120]

Romano–Ward syndrome Autosomal dominant A mutation in a K^+ channel subunit causes long QT syndrome ± episodic ventricular tachycardia, VF, *torsades de pointes* ± sudden death. (Jervell & Lange-Nielsen syndromes (JLNS) are similar, but cause deafness too. Autosomal recessive)

Rotor syndrome Autosomal recessive ↓Excretion of bilirubin with fluctuating conjugated hyperbilirubinaemia with almost normal liver histology.[121] Cholescintigraphy: 'absent' liver.

Sister Mary Joseph nodule An umbilical metastatic nodule from intra-abdominal malignancy. Sister Mary (1856–1939) was Dr William Mayo's (sharp-eyed) scrub nurse.

Sjögren's syndrome is a chronic inflammatory autoimmune disorder. It may be primary (♀:♂≈9:1, onset 4th–5th decade) or secondary, associated with connective tissue disease (eg RA, SLE, systemic sclerosis). There is lymphocytic infiltration and fibrosis of exocrine glands, especially lacrimal and salivary glands. *Features:* ↓tear production (dry eyes, keratoconjunctivitis sicca), xerostomia (↓salivation—dry mouth, caries), parotid swelling. Other glands are affected causing vaginal dryness, dyspareunia, dry cough and dysphagia. Systemic signs include polyarthritis/arthralgia, Raynaud's, lymphadenopathy, vasculitis, lung, liver and kidney involvement, peripheral neuropathy, myositis and fatigue. It is associated with other autoimmune diseases (eg thyroid disease, autoimmune hepatitis, PBC) and an ↑risk of non-Hodgkin's B-cell lymphoma. *Tests:* Measure conjunctival dryness using Schirmer's test: put a strip of filter paper under the lower lid and measure the distance along the paper that tears are absorbed; <5mm in 5min is +ve. Rose Bengal staining may show keratitis (use a slit-lamp). Anti-Ro (SSA) & anti-La (SSB) antibodies may be present. Rheumatoid factor is usually +ve; there may be +ve ANA and hypergammaglobulinaemia. Gland biopsy shows focal lymphocytic aggregation. ℞: Treat sicca symptoms: eye drops eg hypromellose (artificial tears), gels, ointment, frequent drinks, sugar-free pastilles/gum or pilocarpine. NSAIDs and hydroxychloroquine are used for arthralgia, and immunosuppressants may be indicated in severe systemic disease.[122] *[Henrik Sjögren, 1933]*

Stevens–Johnson syndrome A severe form of erythema multiforme (p564), and a variant of toxic epidermal necrolysis. It is caused by a hypersensitivity reaction, usually to drugs (eg salicylates, sulfonamides, penicillin, barbiturates, carbamazepine, phenytoin), but is also seen with infections or cancer. There is ulceration of the skin and mucosal surfaces (eg mouth, urethra, lungs, conjunctivae); **fig 1**. Typical target lesions develop, often on the palms or soles with blistering in the centre. There may be a prodromal phase with fever, malaise, arthralgia, myalgia ± vomiting and diarrhoea. ℞: The disease is usually self-limiting, so removing any precipitant and supportive care (eg calamine lotion for the skin) may suffice. Steroids (systemic and eye-drops) were used, but trials have been variable, so ask a dermatologist and ophthalmologist. Ciclosporin and thalidomide have been used, but IV immunoglobulin is not helpful.[123] *Prognosis:* Mortality ~5%. The illness may be severe for the first 10d before resolving over 30d. Damage to the eyes may persist and at worst blindness may result.[124]

ABC

Sturge–Weber syndrome (encephalotrigeminal angiomatosis) The association of a port wine stain on the face (often in trigeminal distribution) with contralateral focal seizures, due to a corresponding haemangioma in the brain. There may be glaucoma, hemiplegia and IQ↓. *Tests:* Skull X-ray: cortical calcification, angiography: usually normal; MRI: may show the angioma. ℞: Laser therapy can remove facial stains. Anticonvulsants are for seizures; hemispherectomy may be needed to control seizures.

Causes of a long QT interval (eg Romano-Ward)

Many conditions and drugs (check *BNF*) cause a long QT interval—and Brugada syndrome (p709) is a similar syndrome predisposing to sudden cardiac death.

Congenital: Jervell-Lange-Nielsen syndrome: autosomal recessive with associated deafness.[125] (Romano-Ward syndrome is autosomal dominant).

Cardiac: Myocardial infarction or ischaemia; mitral valve prolapse.

HIV: May be a direct effect of the virus or from protease inhibitors.

Metabolic: $K^+\downarrow$; $Mg^{2+}\downarrow$; $Ca^{2+}\downarrow$; starvation; hypothyroidism; hypothermia.

Toxic: Organophosphates.

Anti-arrhythmic drugs: Quinidine; amiodarone; procainamide; sotalol.

***Antibiotics** et al*: Erythromycin; levofloxacin; pentamidine; halofantrine.

Antihistamines: Terfenadine; astemizole.

Motility drugs: Domperidone.

Psychoactive drugs: Haloperidol; risperidone; tricyclics; SSRIs.

Connective tissue diseases: anti-Ro/SSA antibodies (p554).

Herbalism: Ask about Chinese folk remedies (may contain unknown amounts of arsenic).[126] [127] Cocaine, quinine and artemisinins (and other antimalarials) are examples of herbalism-derived products which can prolong the QT interval.

Herbalism is not a bed of roses...

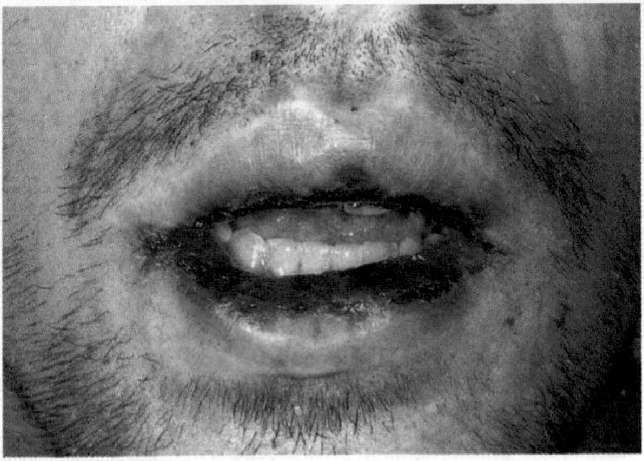

Fig 1. Stevens-Johnson syndrome.[128]

Courtesy of Prof. Thomas Habif

Takayasu's arteritis (aortic arch syndrome, pulseless disease) Rare outside of Japan, this systemic vasculitis affects the aorta and its major branches, causing stenosis and thrombosis. Acute inflammation causes dilatation and aneurysms. It often affects ♀, 20–40yrs old. Symptoms depend on the arteries involved. The aortic arch is often affected, with cerebral, ophthalmological and upper limb symptoms eg dizziness, visual changes, weak arm pulses. Systemic features are common—eg fever, weight loss and malaise. ↑BP is often a feature, due to renovascular involvement. Complications include aortic valve regurgitation, aortic aneurysm and dissection; ischaemic stroke (↑BP and thrombus); and ischaemic heart disease. *Diagnosis:* ↑ESR & CRP; angiography of the aorta (invasive or CT/MRI). ℞: Prednisolone (1mg/kg/day PO). Methotrexate or cyclophosphamide have been used in resistant cases. BP control is essential to ↓risk of stroke. Angioplasty ± stenting, or bypass surgery are done for vascular complications. *Prognosis:* ~95% survival at 15 years. *[Mikito Takayasu, 1908]*

Tietze's syndrome (idiopathic costochondritis) Localized pain/tenderness at the costosternal junction, enhanced by motion, coughing, or sneezing. The 2nd rib is most often affected. The diagnostic key is *localized* tenderness which is marked (flinches on prodding). *Treatment:* Simple analgesia, eg aspirin, NSAIDs. Its importance is that it is a benign cause of what at first seems to be alarming, eg cardiac pain. In lengthy illness, local steroid injections may be used.

Todd's palsy Limb weakness (eg hemiplegia) following a seizure. The patient seems to have had a stroke, but recovers in <24h. *[Robert Todd, 1856]*

Vincent's angina Mouth infection with ulcerative gingivitis from *Borrelia vincentii* (a spirochete) + fusiform bacilli, often affecting young male smokers with poor oral hygiene. Try penicillin V 250mg/6h and metronidazole 400mg/8h PO, with chlorhexidine mouthwashes.

Von Hippel–Lindau syndrome Autosomal dominant A germ-line mutation of a tumour suppressor gene on chromosome 3p (also implicated in sporadic renal cell cancer). It predisposes to bilateral renal cell cancer, retinal and cerebellar haemangioblastoma, and phaeochromocytoma. See **figs 1 & 2.** It may present with visual impairment or cerebellar signs (eg ataxia).

Von Willebrand's disease (VWD) Von Willebrand's factor (VWF) has 3 roles in clotting: to bring platelets into contact with exposed subendothelium, to make platelets bind to each other, and to bind to factor VIII protecting it from destruction in the circulation. There are >22 types of VWD; the commonest are:
Type I: (commonest) Autosomal dominant deficiency (↓levels) of VWF.
Type II: Abnormal VWF, with lack of high molecular weight multimers.
Type III: Undetectable VWF levels (autosomal recessive with gene deletions).
Type Normandy: Impaired VWF-factor VIII binding (mutations in VIII-binding domains of VWF; causes an *autosomal recessive* mimic of haemophilia A).
Signs are of a platelet type disorder (p338): bruising, epistaxis, menorrhagia, ↑bleeding post-tooth extraction. Symptoms are mild in type I and II disease. *Tests:* APTT↑, bleeding time↑, factor VIIIC↓ (clotting activity), VWF Ag↓; INR & platelets ↔. ℞: Get expert help. Vasopressin is used in mild bleeding, VWF rich factor VIII concentrate for surgery or major bleed. Avoid NSAIDs.

Wallenberg's lateral medullary syndrome This relatively common syndrome comprises lesions to multiple CNS nuclei, caused by posterior or inferior cerebellar artery occlusion leading to brainstem infarction (**fig 3**). *Features:* •dysphagia, dysarthria (IX and X nuclei) •vertigo, nausea, vomiting, nystagmus (vestibular nucleus) •ipsilateral ataxia (inferior cerebellar peduncle) •ipsilateral Horner's syndrome (descending sympathetic fibres) •loss of pain and temperature sensation on the ipsilateral face (V nucleus) and contralateral limbs (spinothalamic tract). There is no limb weakness as the pyramidal tracts are unaffected.

In the rarer *medial medullary syndrome*, vertebral or anterior spinal artery occlusion causes ipsilateral tongue paralysis (XII nucleus) with contralateral limb weakness (pyramidal tract, sparing the face) and loss of position sense.

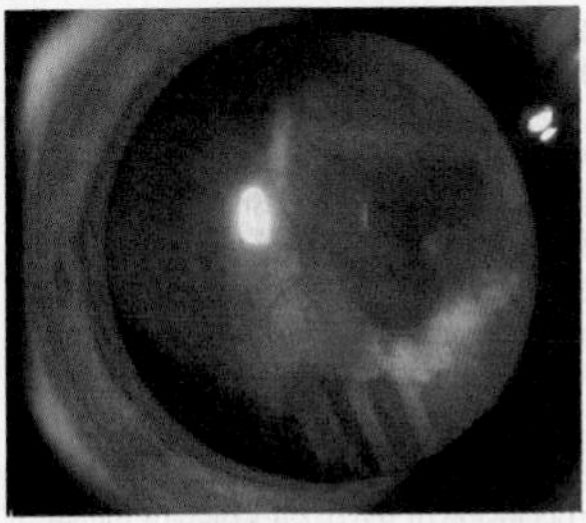

Fig 1. Von Hippel–Lindau syndrome showing retinal detachment.

Reproduced with permission from the National Eye Institute, National Institutes of Health)

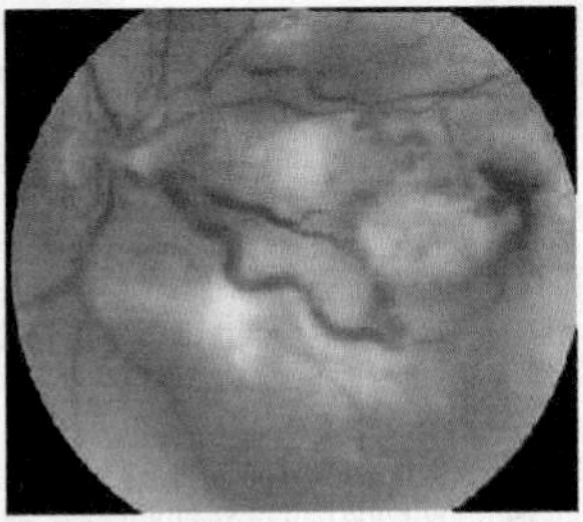

Fig 2. Von Hippel–Lindau syndrome showing a retinal tumour.

Reproduced with permission from the National Eye Institute, National Institutes of Health)

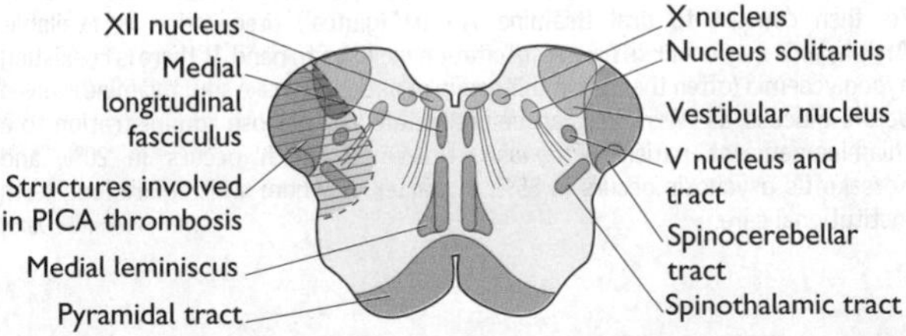

Fig 3. Cross section of the medulla showing structures involved in Wallenberg's lateral medullary syndrome (posterior inferior cerebellar artery thrombosis).

Waterhouse-Friderichsen's (WhF) syndrome Bilateral adrenal cortex haemorrhage, often occurring in rapidly deteriorating meningococcal sepsis, alongside widespread purpura, meningitis, coma, and DIC (**fig 1**). The meningococcal endotoxin acts as a potent initiator of inflammatory and coagulation cascades. Other causes include *H. influenzae*, pneumococcal, streptococcal, and staphylococcal sepsis. Adrenal failure causes shock, as normal vascular tone requires cortisol to set activity of alpha and beta adrenergic receptors, and aldosterone is needed to maintain extracellular fluid volume. ***Treatment:*** ►►Antibiotics eg ceftriaxone 2-4g/24h by IVI over 30min (p832) and hydrocortisone 200mg/4h IV for adrenal support. ICU admission is usually indicated.

Weber's syndrome Ipsilateral 3rd-nerve palsy with contralateral hemiplegia, due to infarction of one half of the midbrain, after occlusion of the paramedian branches of the basilar artery (which supply the cerebral peduncles).

Wegener's granulomatosis is a multisystem disorder of unknown cause characterised by necrotizing granulomatous inflammation and vasculitis of small and medium vessels. It has a predilection for the upper respiratory tract, lungs and kidneys. ***Features:*** Upper airways disease is common, with nasal obstruction, ulcers, epistaxis, or destruction of the nasal septum causing a characteristic 'saddle-nose' deformity[1]. Sinusitis is often a feature. Renal disease causes rapidly progressive glomerulonephritis with crescent formation, proteinuria or haematuria. Pulmonary involvement may cause cough, haemoptysis (severe if pulmonary haemorrhage) or pleuritis. There may also be skin purpura or nodules, peripheral neuropathy, mononeuritis multiplex, arthritis/arthralgia or ocular involvement eg keratitis, conjunctivitis, scleritis, episcleritis, uveitis, proptosis. ***Tests:*** cANCA, confirmed with a raised PR3 in the majority (p555). Urinalysis should be performed to look for proteinuria or haematuria. If these are present, consider a renal biopsy. Do a CXR to look for evidence of pulmonary haemorrhage. Cytology from sputum/BAL may show atypical cells that can be confused with bronchial carcinoma.[129] ***Treatment:*** Depends on the extent of disease. Severe disease (eg biopsy-proven renal disease) should be treated with corticosteroids and cyclophosphamide. Continuous oral cyclophosphamide may be more effective than pulsed IV regimens at inducing sustained remission, but may have more side effects. Co-trimoxazole may be given as prophylaxis against *Pneumocystis jiroveci* and *Staphylococcal* colonisation. Patients with severe renal disease (eg creatinine >500μmol/L) may benefit from plasma exchange in addition. Azathioprine and methotrexate are used as maintenance therapies.

Wernicke's encephalopathy Thiamine (vitamin B_1) deficiency with a classical triad of ophthalmoplegia (nystagmus, lateral rectus or conjugate gaze palsies), ataxia (wide-based gait; **fig 2**) and confusion. Always consider this diagnosis in alcoholics: it may also present with memory disturbance, hypotension, hypothermia, or reduced consciousness. Focal areas of brain damage occur, including periaqueductal punctate haemorrhages. ***Recognised causes:*** Alcoholism, eating disorders, malnutrition, prolonged vomiting eg with chemotherapy, GI malignancy, hyperemesis gravidarum. ***Tests:*** Red cell transketolase↓ (rarely done). ***Treatment:*** Urgent thiamine to prevent irreversible Korsakoff's syndrome (p718). Give IV thiamine (Pabrinex®) if there are any of the above features, 2-3 pairs of high-potency ampoules/8h IV over 30min for up to 7d, then convert to oral thiamine. An IM (gluteal) preparation is available. Anaphylaxis may occur so have resuscitation facilities to hand. If there is coexisting hypoglycaemia (often the case in this group of patients), make sure thiamine is given *before* glucose, as Wernicke's can be precipitated by glucose administration to a thiamine-deficient patient. ***Prognosis:*** Untreated, death occurs in 20%, and Korsakoff's psychosis occurs in 85%, a quarter of whom will require long-term institutional care. *[Karl Wernicke, 1875]*

ABC

1 Common causes of a 'saddle-nose' deformity are trauma and iatrogenic (eg post-rhinoplasty). Rarer causes (popular with some finals examiners): Wegener's, relapsing polychondritis, syphilis, and leprosy.

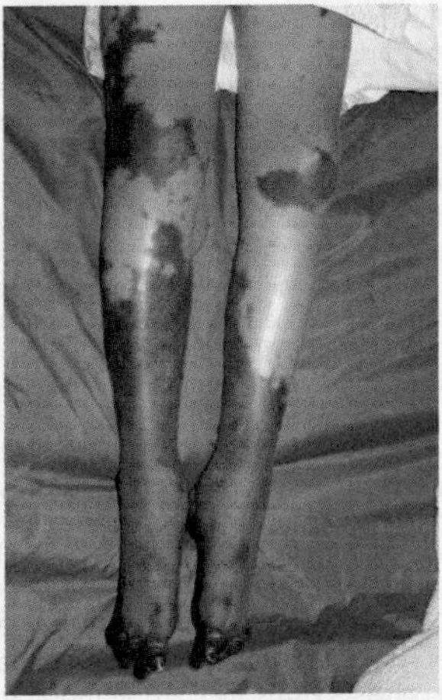

Fig 1. Meningococcal sepsis with purpura.

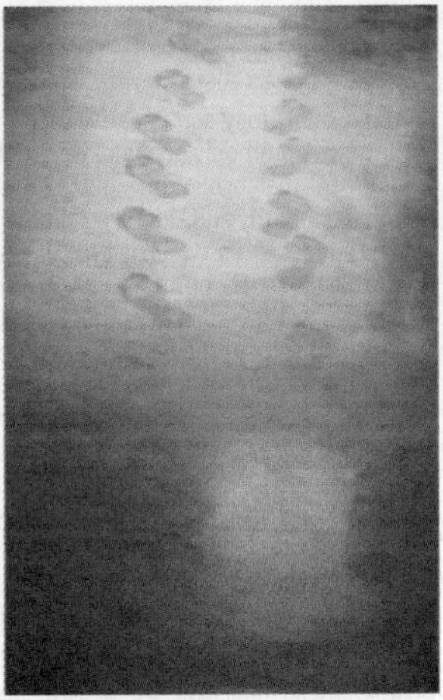

Fig 2. Wide-based gait (footprints), seen in Wernicke's encephalopathy. Before jumping to the conclusion that these footprints are those of an *OHCM* author on the way back from the pub, bear in mind that alcohol is not the only cause of Wernicke's: think of rapidly growing tumours, malabsorption, hyperemesis gravidarum, hyperthyroidism, and prolonged vomiting of any cause.[130]

Whipple's disease[1] A rare cause of GI malabsorption which usually occurs in middle-aged white males, most commonly in Europe. It is caused by *Tropheryma whippelii*, which produces a systemic disease. ***Features:*** often starts insidiously with arthralgia (chronic, migratory, seronegative arthropathy affecting mainly peripheral joints). GI symptoms commonly include weight loss, diarrhoea or colicky abdominal pain, leading to malabsorption (p280). Systemic symptoms such as fever, sweats, lymphadenopathy and skin hyperpigmentation also occur. Cardiac involvement may lead to endocarditis, which is typically blood culture negative. CNS features include a reversible dementia, ophthalmoplegia, and facial myoclonus (if all together, they are highly suggestive)—also hypothalamic syndrome (hyperphagia, polydipsia, insomnia). **NB:** CNS involvement may occur without GI involvement. *Tests:* Jejunal biopsy shows stunted villi. There is deposition of macrophages in the lamina propria containing granules which stain positive for periodic acid-Schiff (PAS). Similar cells may be found in affected samples eg CSF, cardiac valve tissue, lymph nodes, synovial fluid. The bacteria may be seen within macrophages on electron microscopy. MRI may demonstrate CNS involvement. ℞: should include antibiotics which cross the blood-brain barrier. Current recommendations: IV ceftriaxone (or penicillin+streptomycin) for 2wks then oral co-trimoxazole for 1yr. Shorter courses risk relapse with CNS features. A rapid improvement in symptoms usually occurs. *[George Whipple, 1907]*

Zellweger syndrome (cerebrohepatorenal syndrome) A rare autosomal recessive disorder characterized by absent peroxisomes. Peroxisomes are intracellular organelles, required for many cellular activities, including lipid metabolism. The syndrome is a severe form of infantile Refsum's syndrome, and exhibits similar biochemical abnormalities (p724). Clinical features include craniofacial abnormalities, severe hypotonia and mental retardation, glaucoma, cataracts, hepatomegaly and renal cysts. A number of causative genes (eg PEX1) have been identified. Life expectancy is usually a few months only.

Zollinger-Ellison syndrome This is the association of peptic ulcers with a gastrin-secreting adenoma (gastrinoma). Gastrin excites excessive gastric acid production, which may produce multiple ulcers in the duodenum and stomach. The adenoma is usually found in the pancreas, although it may arise in the stomach or duodenum. Most cases are sporadic; 20% are associated with multiple endocrine neoplasia, type 1 (MEN1, p215). 60% are malignant, metastases are found in local lymph nodes and the liver. ***Symptoms:*** Include abdominal pain and dyspepsia, from the ulcer(s), and chronic diarrhoea due to inactivation of pancreatic enzymes (also causes steatorrhoea) and damage to intestinal mucosa. ***Incidence:*** ~0.1% of patients with peptic ulcer disease. Suspect in those with multiple peptic ulcers, ulcers distal to the duodenum, or a family history of peptic ulcers (or of islet cell, pituitary, or parathyroid adenomas). *Tests:* (**fig 1**) ↑Fasting serum gastrin level (>1000pg/mL). Hypochlorhydria (reduced acid production eg in chronic atrophic gastritis) should be excluded as this also causes a raised gastrin level: gastric pH should be <2. The secretin stimulation test is useful in suspected cases with only mildly raised gastrin levels (100-1000pg/mL). The adenoma is often small and difficult to image; a combination of somatostatin receptor scintigraphy, endoscopic ultrasound and CT is used to localise and stage the adenoma. ℞: High-dose proton pump inhibitors (PPIs), eg omeprazole: start with 60mg/d and adjust according to response. Measuring intragastric pH helps determine the best dose (aim to keep pH at 2-7). All gastrinomas have malignant potential—and surgery is better sooner than later (with lymph node clearance is generally recommended if >2cm in size). Surgery may be avoided in MEN1, as adenomas are often multiple, and metastatic disease is rare. If well-differentiated (G1 & G2) somatostatin analogues may be 1st-line and chemotherapy with streptocotozin (if available) + doxorubicine/5-FU is 2nd-line. In G3, etoposide + cisplatin is possible.[31] Selective embolization may be done for hepatic metastases. ***Prognosis:*** 5yr survival: 80% if single resectable lesion, ~20% with hepatic metastases. Screen all patients for MEN1.

ABC

1 For a review of Whipple's disease, see T Marth 2003 *Lancet* **361** 239

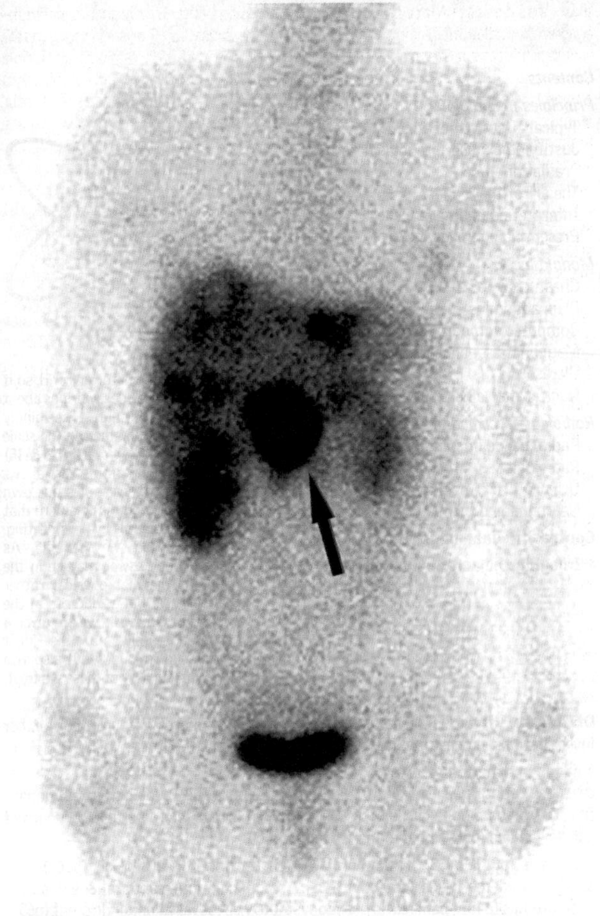

Fig 1. Gastrinoma in a 68-yr-old with Zollinger-Ellison syndrome. Serum gastrin was 158pg/mL (normal, 8-47pg/mL). This rather ghostly anterior ^{111}indium pentetreotide image shows focal radiotracer uptake in the pancreatic head (arrow), the primary tumour. Note multiple liver metastases.[132]

Courtesy of Charles Intenzo. *Scintigraphic Imaging of Body Neuroendocrine tumors.* C Intenzo, S Jabbour, H Lin, J Miller, S Kim, D Capuzzi E Mitchell. RadioGraphics 2007 27 1355-136. RSNA[133]

Epilogue

25% of patients with rare diseases have to wait from 5 to 30 years for a diagnosis. 40% are misdiagnosed resulting in inappropriate drugs or psychological treatments—eg 20% of people with Ehlers-Danlos syndrome had to consult over 20 doctors before the diagnosis was made,[134] causing understandable loss of confidence in our profession. Lack of appropriate referral and rejection because of disease complexity are common problems. Let us cultivate our networks with each other and approach 'unexplained symptoms' with an open mind.

Contents

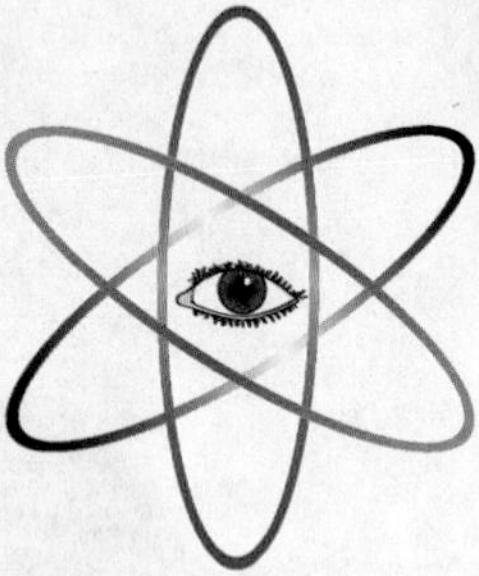

Fig 1. As in the natural world, so it is in the physical: decay brings about new matter through a seemingly endless cycle—whether on the scale of galaxies (p229), stars (p2 & 18), cells (p359) or atoms, as above. Between these scales lies our own orbit—fragile and dimly aware that its own part in this cycle is fleeting.

So how do we benefit? As humans, the answer may lie in the realm of the metaphysical rather than physical, but as doctors, at the nucleus of our work, we are given a vision not only into the inner workings of the body, but also into the colourful lives of those we treat.

Other relevant pages Chest medicine (Chapter 4); echocardiography (p106); further investigations in chest medicine (p158); cerebral artery territories (p452)

Images in other chapters

CXR: Cavitating lung cancer (p154); lung metastasis (p171); idiopathic pulmonary fibrosis (p190); industrial dust diseases (p193); correct PICC line (p589); incorrect subclavian line (p589); pneumoperitoneum (p609).

CT: Stroke (p81 & p453); hiatus hernia (p245); retroperitoneal fibrosis (p643); subarachnoid haemorrhage (p483, with 3DCT reconstruction); subdural & extradural haematomas (p487); pancreatic pseudocyst (p639); endovascular aortic stent (p657); SBO (p613); large bowel obstruction (p613); caecal cancer (p619); oesophageal cancer (p620).

MRI: Pituitary adenoma (p227); stroke (p475); superior sagittal sinus thrombosis (MR venogram, p485); cervical spondylosis (p512); the cauda equina (p783).

US: Liver metastases (p271); compression US/US imaging of DVT (p563); torsion of the hydatid of Morgagni and testis cancer (p655 & p652); hydronephrosis (p645); malignant lymph node (p597); thyroid lesion (p603); renal transplant duplex (p607).

Nuclear medicine: Graves' disease (p603).

ERCP/MRCP: Primary sclerosing cholangitis (p267).

Contrast studies: Oesophageal cancer (p241); parotid sialogram (p597); pharynx (p601).

DSA: Inferior mesenteric artery (p623); lower limb (p659).

We thank Dr Jennie Roberts and Professor Peter Scally, our Specialist Readers for this chapter, and Dr Tom Turmezei, who originated it, and many other facets of OHCM.

Typical effective doses

The effective dose of an examination is calculated as the weighted sum of the doses to different body tissues. The weighting factor for each tissue depends on its sensitivity. The effective dose thus provides a single dose estimate related to the total radiation risk, no matter how the radiation dose is distributed around the body. This table is certainly not to be learnt; rather it serves as a reminder of the relative exposures to radiation that we prescribe in practice.

Procedure	Typical effective dose (mSv)	CXR equivalents	Approx. equivalent period of background radiation[1]
X-ray examinations			
Limbs and joints	<0.01	<0.5	<1.5 days
Chest (PA)	0.02	1	3 days
Abdomen	1	50	6 months
Lumbar spine	1.3	65	7 months
CT head	2.3	115	1 year
IVU	2.5	125	14 months
Barium meal	3	150	16 months
Barium enema	7	350	3.2 years
CT chest	8	400	3.6 years
CT abdo/pelvis	10	500	4.5 years
Radionuclide studies			
Lung ventilation	0.3	15	7 weeks
Lung perfusion	1	50	6 months
Thyroid	1	50	6 months
Bone	4	200	1.8 years
PET head	5	250	2.3 years
Dynamic cardiac	6	300	2.7 years

After *Making the Best Use of Department of Clinical Radiology*, 5e RCOR; with permission.

Justifying exposure to ionising radiation

The very nature of ionising radiation that gives us vision into the human body also gives it lethal properties. The decision to expose patients to radiation must be made with the risks in mind, and even with strict guidelines we still have a tendency to over-exposure in medical practice. So when requesting an examination, the clinical benefits should far outweigh the risks of cancer induction and genetic mutation.

The responsibility lies with us not to rely too heavily on radiology. ►Don't request examinations to comfort patients, or to replace lost images, or when the result will not affect management. ~20% of images do not contribute to decisions.[2] To give an idea of relative doses, a CT of the abdomen and pelvis gives a typical effective dose of 500 times as much radiation as a CXR (see TABLE). This important factor also tells us about the preference of ultrasound over CT when investigating abdominal and pelvic complaints such as acute appendicitis, especially given its youthful demographics. Avoid radiation simply for medico-legal reasons. In the US each year, >600,000 CTs are done on children less than 15. 500 will ultimately die from a cancer attributable to CT radiation.[3]

►Unwitting exposure of the unborn fetus to radiation is inexcusable at any stage of gestation—unless the mother's life is in immediate danger—and it is the responsibility of the referring clinician to ensure that this is avoided. Discuss beforehand with the patient that you would like to do a pregnancy test, explaining why, being broad in your suppositions and tactful in your inquisitions.

One of the most nerve-wracking moments that you can encounter as a recently qualified doctor might be having to request a radiology investigation face-to-face with a seasoned consultant radiologist. Imagine that you have been asked by your team to request an ultrasound examination of the renal tract for one of your patients who has a newly raised creatinine of 300μmol/L. You explain that you aren't quite sure what to write on the request form; however, they have already moved on to the next patient on the busy post-take ward-round. What do you write? How much do you write? Who do you ask? Below are some pointers that will aid you in making a successful request for a radiological investigation.

Before you start...

- Ensure that the investigation has not been done already or recently.
- *Is the patient fit to have the investigation?* An agitated or confused individual is unlikely to stay still for a claustrophobic CT head examination!

The request form ►Get the patient's name right!

- Include all relevant clinical information, blood tests and recent radiology findings on the request form. This is especially important given that there has been an increase in e-based request systems combined with a decrease in direct communication between the radiologist and the requesting clinician. Remember that the aim of radiology is to provide information in order to alter management and the outcome of the disease. Think: "What do I need to know?" (see MINIBOX), *Can radiology help?*
- Include how the investigation will help resolve the clinical problem facing you.
- Include '± intervention' on the request form if you think it may take place (eg CT abdomen ± drainage, for an abdominal collection).

Radiology can help:

- **Confirm** a suspected diagnosis
- **'Exclude'** something important: remember that exclusion is 'never' 100%.
- **Define** the extent of a disease
- **Monitor** the progress of a disease

The verbal request ►Always **request** and never order an investigation.

- Know the patient as fully as possible, but keep your request brief and accurate.
- Know what you need to confirm, exclude, monitor, or define.
- "I was hoping to get your opinion about this interesting patient..." may work.
- Pre-empt by saying how the image will change management (you will be asked!).
- Have past relevant images with you as you make the request, eg a CXR if requesting a CT pulmonary angiogram (CTPA) or ventilation/perfusion (V/Q) scintigram.
- Enquire of the radiologist what he thinks is the correct investigation for the case.
- You may have an easier time requesting an investigation from a radiologist who specialises in that particular technique (eg CT) or who is linked to your clinical team (eg he may lead your clinical radiology meeting).

Stuck in the middle? You may find yourself a go-between, with your team on one side eagerly awaiting the image before the next move and the radiology department on the other side trying to prioritise and fit the image into their overscheduled diary. Here, it is wise to remember that the patient is also caught in the middle, completely unaware of the goings-on around him. Take a few moments to outline your plan to your patient and to air expectations—this will make the experience of being swept away to the radiology department without warning a far less scary experience!

Interpreting an image

You won't always be able to get a radiologist's interpretation (especially at night). ►Make sure the image you are looking at is of your patient. Check its date. Remembering the following points may help hone your own interpreting skills:

- Take every opportunity to look at images so that spotting normal and abnormal variations gets easier: the old adage *practice makes perfect* is very apt here.
- Getting to grips with the science behind radiology makes interpretation easier and will explain the suitability of modalities to different clinical scenarios. Knowing how an investigation is done will also give practical clues to the result produced—eg a routine CXR is performed in the posteroanterior (PA) direction (the source posterior, the cassette anterior) so that the cardiac shadow is minimised.
- Use a systematic approach so that you don't pass anything unnoticed. Don't worry, though—some things can be notoriously difficult to spot.
- Virtually all investigations yield a 2D image from a 3D structure, though there have been recent developments in 3D imaging (fig 3, p745). A basic understanding of anatomical relationships of the area in question will help reconstruct the images in your mind into a clear representation of the reality before you.
- The standard orientation of all axial cross-sectional imaging is as if you are looking up at the supine patient ►*from his feet*. For images with non-conventional orientations (eg MRCP) look on the image for clue markings, or rely on your knowledge of anatomy—it can be tricky to visualise oblique sections!
- Don't rely solely on the investigation, but use it as part of the clinical work-up to help make an informed management decision.
- Go back to see the patient after looking at the investigation and reading the radiologist's report: you might picture them in a different light and notice something that you didn't before.

Presenting an image

Everyone has their own method for presenting, and the right way is **your own way**. As long as you cover everything systematically—because we all get 'hot-seat amnesia' at some point—the particulars will take care of themselves. Continue to polish your own method and remember a few extra tips for when an image is presented expectantly by your consultant/examiner and the floor is yours. A brief silence with a thoughtful expression as you analyse the image is fine, then...

- State the written details: name, date of birth, where and how the imaging was taken. Look for clues: weighting of an MRI, a '**+ c**' indicating that contrast medium has been used, the phase of the investigation (arterial/venous/portal), or even the name of the organ printed on an ultrasound.
- State the type, mode and technical quality of investigation—not always easy!

Going through the above also gives you a bit of thinking time. Then:

- Start with life-threatening or very obvious abnormalities. *Then be systematic:*
- Is the patient's position adequate? Any lines, leads or tubes? Note their position.
- Just like the bedside clues in a physical examination, there are clues in radiology examinations. Note oxygen masks, ECG leads, venous access, infusion apparatus, and invasive devices. Identifying what they are also helps you to look through what may otherwise appear to be a cluttered mess.
- Not everything on the image is inside the subject—some things may be on the surface/outside or not there at all, eg ring artefacts or 'stair-stepping'[1] on CT.
- Giving a differential diagnosis is good practice, as not all findings are diagnostic.
- If there is additional clinical information that would help you to make a diagnosis, don't be afraid to ask. After all, we treat patients and not images!

Remember: • X-ray=*radiodensity* (lucency/opacity) • CT=*attenuation* • US=*echogenicity/reflectivity* • MRI=*signal intensity*

1 Geometry of helical CT causes periodic asymmetries and variable noise distribution, appearing as stripes (**zebra artefact**) or steps (**stair-stepping**) when surfaces are inclined relative to the table translation direction. These distort volume and diameter measurements (taking thinner slices helps).

Images are usually taken on inspiration with the patient standing in front of the cassette and the X-ray source behind (postero-anterior, PA). Emergency mobile images may antero-posterior (AP), so magnifying heart size and elevating the diaphragm. If supine, distribution of air and fluid in lungs and pleural cavities is altered.

Acclimatize yourself to the 4 cardinal elements of the chest radiograph's world, memorably (albeit slightly inaccurately) termed **bone, air, fat,** and **'water'/soft tissue.** Each has its own radiographic density. ►*A border is only seen at an interface of 2 densities,* eg heart (soft tissue) and lung (air); this 'silhouette' is lost if air in the lung is replaced by consolidation ('water'). The silhouette sign localizes pathology (eg middle lobe pneumonia or collapse causing loss of clarity of the right heart border, **fig 1**). When interpreting a CXR use a systematic approach that works for you, eg from outside to inside, or inside-out. Start by assessing technical quality:

- *Rotation:* The sternal ends of the clavicles should symmetrically overlie the transverse processes of the 4th or 5th thoracic vertebrae.
- *Inspiration:* There should be 5 to 7 ribs visible anteriorly (or 10 posteriorly). Hyperinflation can be abnormal, eg COPD.
- *Exposure:* An under-exposed image will be too white and an over-exposed image will be too black. Both cause a loss of definition and quality.
- *Position:* The entire lung margins must be visible, especially costophrenic angles.

Trachea Normally central or just to the right. Deviated by collapse (towards the lesion), tension (away from the lesion), or patient rotation. Check heart position (below).

Mediastinum Widened by mediastinal fat; retrosternal thyroid; unfolded aorta, or aneurysm; lymph node enlargement (sarcoidosis, lymphoma, metastases, TB); tumour (thymoma, teratoma); aortic aneurysm; cysts (bronchogenic cyst, pericardial cyst); paravertebral mass (TB). There are 3 moguls[1] normally visible on the left border of the mediastinum that help identify pathology if abnormal. From superior to inferior they are: **1** Aortic knuckle **2** Pulmonary outflow tract **3** Left ventricle.

The mediastinum may be shifted towards a collapsed lung or way from processes which increase lung volume (eg an effusion).

Hila The left hilum is higher than the right or at the same level (not lower); they should be the same size and density. May be pulled up or down by fibrosis or collapse. **1** *Enlarged hila:* Nodes; pulmonary arterial hypertension (± an enlarged 2nd mogul); bronchogenic ca. **2** *Calcification:* Past TB; silicosis; histoplasmosis (p440). Sarcoidosis, TB & lymphoma can give bilateral hilar + paratracheal lymphadenopathy.

Heart Normally <15cm across—approximately 50% of the width of the thorax. ⅓ should lie to the right of the vertebral column, ⅔ to the left. It may appear elongated if the chest is hyperinflated (COPD) or enlarged if the image is AP, there is failure (**fig 2**), or a pericardial effusion. Are there calcified valves?

Diaphragm The right side is often higher (due to the liver) *Causes of raised hemi-diaphragm:* Trouble above the diaphragm—lung volume loss; stroke; phrenic nerve palsy (causes, p506; any mediastinal mass?). Below the diaphragm—hepatomegaly; subphrenic abscess. NB: subpulmonic effusion (effusions having a similar contour to the diaphragm without a characteristic meniscus) and diaphragm rupture give apparent elevation. **NB:** bilateral palsies (polio, muscular dystrophy) cause hypoxia.

1 It's as if skiing down the left heart border creates these moguls or bumps of radio-opaque 'snow'.

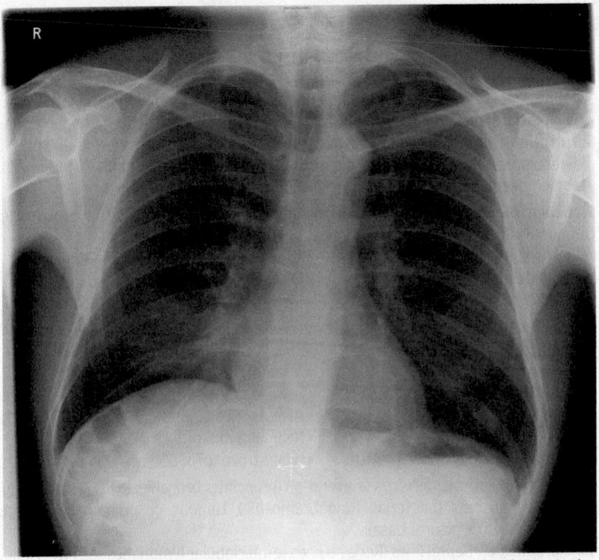

Fig 1. Middle lobe collapse (right lung). The right heart border is obscured and there is also volume loss in the right lower zone.

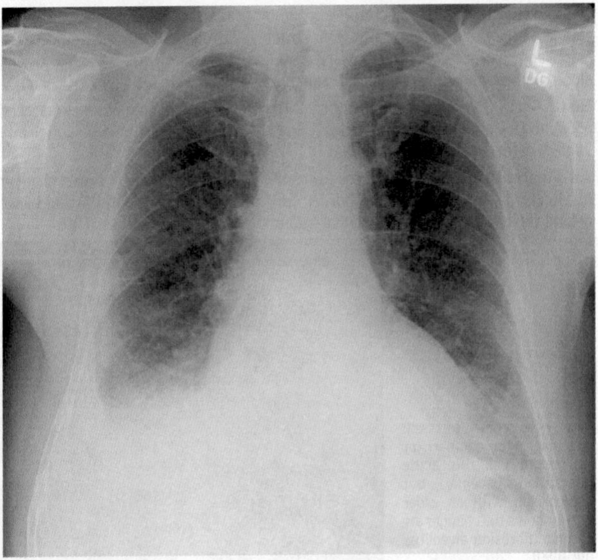

Fig 2. Cardiomegaly and loss of the right costophrenic angle from a pleural effusion: consistent with heart failure.

Lung shadowing is described as nodular, reticular (network of fine lines, interstitial), or alveolar (fluffy). A single nodule may be called a SOL (space-occupying lesion).

Nodules:[1] (if >3cm across, the term pulmonary mass is used instead)

1 Neoplasia: metastases (often missed if small), lung cancer, adenoma, hamartoma.
2 Infections: varicella pneumonia, hydatid, septic emboli, abscess (eg as an SOL).
3 Granulomas: miliary TB, sarcoidosis, histoplasmosis, Wegener's granulomatosis, p728.
4 Pneumoconioses (except asbestosis), Caplan's syndrome (p710).

Reticular shadows: (**fig 1**) Usually acute interstitial changes (cardiac or noncardiac pulmonary interstitial oedema; atypical pneumonia (eg, viral); or:

- Fibrosis; TB; histoplasmosis
- Sarcoidosis; silicosis; asbestosis
- Usual interstitial pneumonitis (UIP)
- Neoplasia (lymphangitis carcinomatosa)
- Fibrosing alveolitis; rheumatoid (p548)
- Wegener's (p728); SLE; PAN; CREST (p554)

Alveolar shadows: Usually pulmonary oedema from LVF (p812). Also:

- Pneumonia
- Haemorrhage
- Drugs (heroin, cytotoxics, p528)
- Smoke inhalation (p859)
- O_2 toxicity
- Fat emboli, ~7 days post-fracture
- Renal or liver failure (p300 & p258)
- ARDS (p178); DIC (p346)
- Head injury, or after neurosurgery
- Alveolar proteinosis
- Near-drowning (*OHCS* p786)
- Heat stroke (p788).

'Ring' shadows: Either airways seen end-on (bronchitis; bronchiectasis) or cavitating lesions, eg abscess (bacterial, fungal, amoebic), tumour, or pulmonary infarct (triangular with a pleural base).

Linear opacities: Septal lines (Kerley B lines, ie interlobular lymphatics seen with fluid, tumour, or dusts); atelectasis; pleural plaques (asbestos exposure). *White-out* of whole hemithorax (**fig 2**): pneumonia, large pleural effusion, ARDS, post-pneumonectomy.

Gas outside the lungs Check for a pneumothorax (hard to spot if apical or in a supine image), surgical emphysema (trauma, iatrogenic) and gas under the diaphragm (surgery, perforated viscus, trauma). Pneumomediastinum: air tracks along mediastinum, into the neck. Pneumopericardium: rare (usually iatrogenic)

Bones Check the *clavicles* for fracture, *ribs* for fractures, notching, absence (surgery, p566), and lesions (eg metastases), *vertebral column* for collapse or destruction and *shoulders* for fracture and arthritis.

An apparently normal CXR? Check for tracheal compression, absent breast shadow (mastectomy), double left heart border (left lower lobe collapse, **fig 3**), fluid level behind the heart (hiatus hernia, achalasia), and paravertebral abscess (TB).

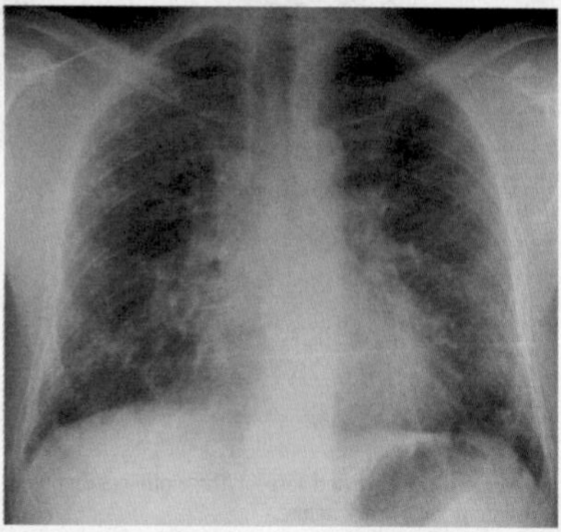

Fig 1. ►Remember to check old images for comparison. You might call this acute interstitial oedema, but comparison with an older image shows the changes are chronic (fibrosing alveolitis/UIP, p190).

Courtesy of Prof Peter Scally.

1 Remember that the apex of the lower lobe rises up to the 4th rib posteriorly, so it is difficult to ascribe the true location of a lesion on a PA image without additional information from a lateral view. It may be better to use the term 'zone' rather than lobe when localising a lesion.

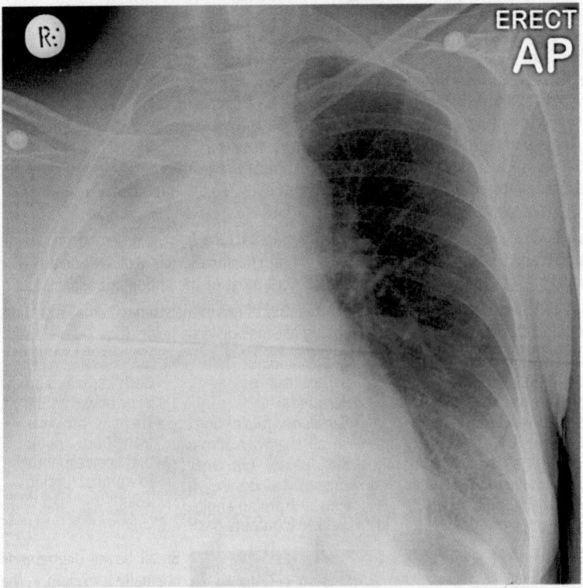

Fig 2. Opacification of the right hemi-thorax from pneumonia; note right-shifted trachea. Complete white-out with no tracheal shift implies increased volume, eg from an effusion.

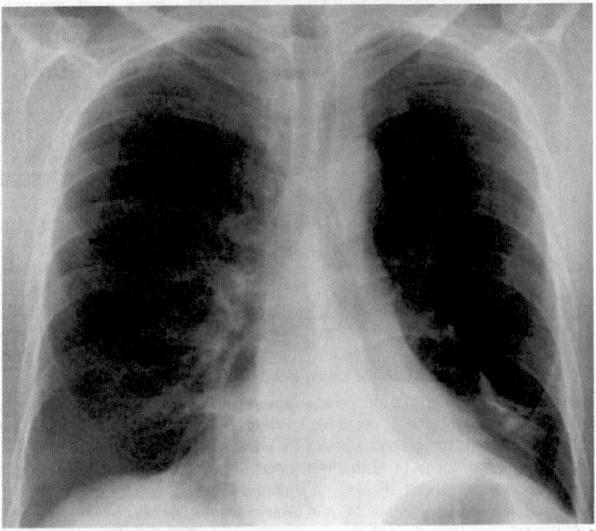

Fig 3. Collapse of the left lower lobe—the triangular opacity behind the heart. Also, the left main bronchus has been pulled down.

Figs 2 & 3 courtesy of Norwich Radiology Department.

Plain abdominal X-ray (AXR)

These are rarely diagnostic, and are non-contributory in most mild or moderate instances of abdominal pain. Indications for AXR with acute abdominal symptoms are:
- Acute abdominal pain warranting admission or surgery.
- Suspicion of perforation, or obstruction (or intussusception, eg in paediatrics).
- Acute exacerbation of inflammatory bowel disease.
- Haematuria, renal failure, or renal colic (but CT urogram is better, if available).
- Ingestion of a sharp or poisonous foreign body (eg lithium battery).
- Blunt or penetrating injury to the abdomen.

Erect AXRs are rarely done, since bowel gas pattern is best assessed on supine images and free intraperitoneal gas (signifying perforation) is best seen on an erect CXR (**fig 1**, p609). The following routine covers most of the important aspects:

Gas patterns: Look for: an abnormal quantity of gas in the stomach, small intestine, or colon. Decide whether you are looking at small or large bowel (**figs 1-3**).

Small bowel:	*Large bowel:*	*Ileus:*
• Smaller calibre • Central; multiple loops • *Valvuli conniventes:* folds that go from wall to wall, all the way across the lumen; more regular and finer than haustra • Grey (contains air & fluid)	• Larger calibre • Peripheral • *Semilunar folds:*[1] don't go all the way across the lumen, but may appear to do so if viewed from an angle • Blacker (contains gas)[2]	• Both small and large bowel visible • There is no clear transition point that corresponds to an obstructing lesion

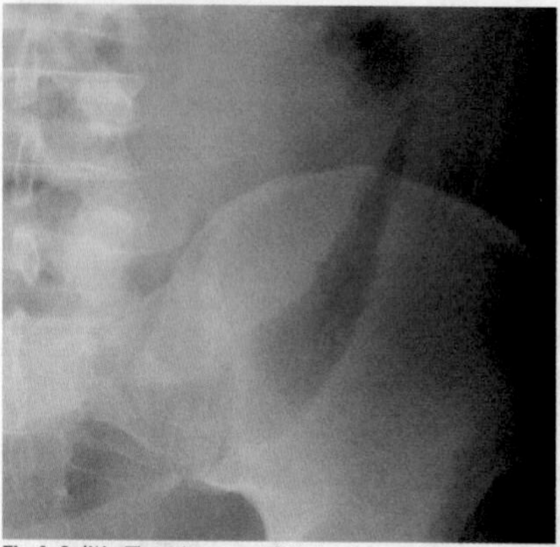

Fig 4. Colitis. There is mucosal thickening and loss of normal haustral pattern in the descending colon. Courtesy P. Scally.

Small bowel diameter is normally ~2.5cm, the colon ~5cm, and the caecum up to 10cm. Dilated small bowel is seen in obstruction and paralytic ileus. Dilated large bowel (≥6cm) is seen in both these, and also in 'toxic dilatation' (ie very sick), and, in the elderly, in benign hypotonicity. Grossly dilated segments of bowel are seen in sigmoid and caecal volvulus. Loss of normal mucosal folds, irregular mucosal islands, and bowel wall thickening are seen in inflammatory colitis (eg IBD)—**fig 4**. 'Thumb-printing' is protrusion of rounded indentations of thickened mural folds into the lumen and is seen in large bowel ischaemia.

Gas outside the lumen You must explain any gas outside the lumen of the stomach, small intestine, and colon. It could be: 1 Pneumoperitoneum; signs visible on the supine AXR include: gas on both sides of the bowel wall (Rigler's sign), a triangle of gas in the RUQ trapped beneath the falciform ligament, and a football-shaped distribution of gas beneath the anterior abdominal wall. 2 Gas in the urinary tract—eg in the bladder from a fistula. 3 Gas in biliary tree (pneumobilia, p742), or rarely 4 Intramural gas, found in bowel necrosis, clostridial infection, necrotizing enterocolitis (neonates) and pneumatosis cystoides intestinalis (rare and benign).

1 Semi-lunar folds (plicae semilunares) lie in between adjacent haustra
2 Also, the ascending colon contains liquid faeces, but the descending colon contains faecal pellets (*scyballa*).

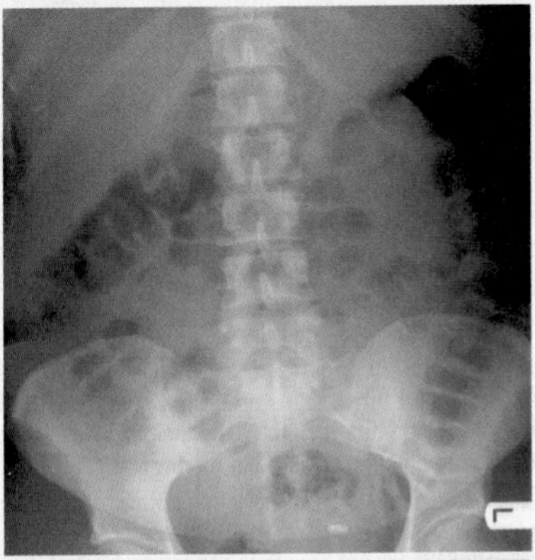

Fig 1. Normal large bowel gas pattern

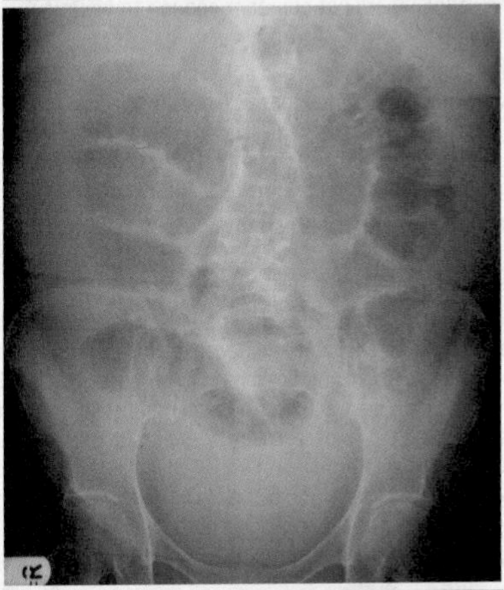

Fig 2. The pattern seen in small bowel obstruction.

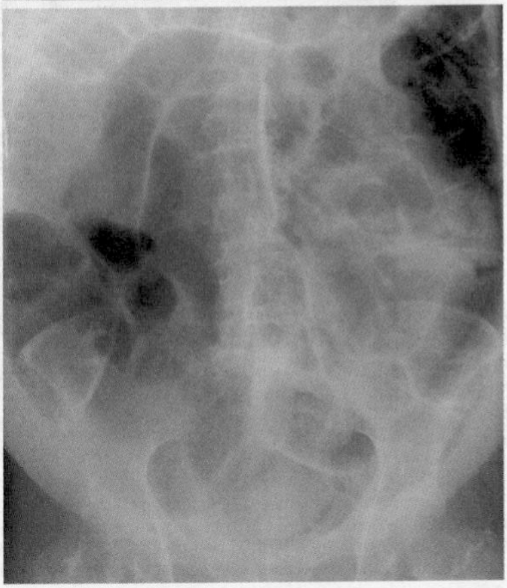

Fig 3. Multiple dilated air filled loops of large and small bowel. This pattern is seen in ileus.

Figures 1-3 courtesy of Norwich Radiology Department.

Pneumobilia:
• Post-ERCP/sphincterotomy
• Post-surgery (eg Whipple's)
• Anaerobic cholangitis (rare)
• Recent stone passage 5
• Gallbladder-bowel fistula[1]

Biliary tree Any stones? ~10% visible on plain AXR. Pneumobilia (air in the biliary system: see MINIBOX).

Urinary tract The kidneys normally have an equivalent length of 2½-3½ vertebral bodies and slope inferolateraly. The right is lower than the left ('pushed down' by the liver). Their outline can usually be seen as they have a surrounding layer of perinephric fat—if this is or has been inflamed (eg perinephric abscess) then the outline is obliterated. The ureters pass near the tips of the lumbar transverse processes, cross the sacroiliac joints, down to the ischial spines, and turn medially to join the bladder. Check the kidneys and ureteric courses for calculi (visible in 90% of cases)—this requires practice! See p758 for intravenous urography (IVU). Don't get confused by other calcifications[2]—eg phleboliths, recognised by their rounded shape and radiolucent centre, are harmless calcifications found in the perivesical veins.

Local peritonitis is said to cause localized ileus (a sentinel loop of intraluminal gas), giving a clue to pathology. *RUQ* ≈ cholecystitis, *LUQ* ≈ pancreatitis, *RLQ* ≈ appendicitis, *LLQ* ≈ diverticulitis. These locations (p567) are not constant enough to be useful.

Other soft tissues Look for size/position of: liver, spleen and bladder. A big liver will push bowel to the left side of the abdomen. An enlarged spleen displaces bowel and stomach bubble to the right. A big bladder elevates these. Liver and spleen shouldn't extend below the level of the 12th rib on a correctly aligned image. A *Riedel's lobe* can arise from the liver's right lobe, and projects like an ominous fin towards the RIF (**fig 2**, p747), simulating a pathological mass (don't worry: it's a normal variant).

Medical devices: Double-J and biliary stents, nephrostomy and gastrostomy tubes, intrauterine devices (eg coil, **fig 3**), laparoscopic sterilisation clips, and chronic ambulatory peritoneal dialysis (CAPD) catheters can all be seen on AXR.

Bones and joints Plain AXR is not the best image, but there may be important abnormalities, In the lumbar spine, look for scoliosis and degeneration (osteophytes, joint space narrowing). Compare the vertebral bodies, spinous processes (lack of arch closure in spina bifida), pedicles (can be destroyed in cancer), facet joints, and transverse processes (**fig 2**). Any osteolytic or osteosclerotic metastases? Paget's disease (unusual bone expansion, sclerosis and/or lysis). Sacroiliac joints pathology? (sclerotic in ankylosing spondylitis). In renal osteodystrophy (p300) there is a 'rugger jersey' spine of alternating bands of sclerosis (opaque) and osteopenia (lucent).

Bringing it all together See **fig 1** for a systematic approach.

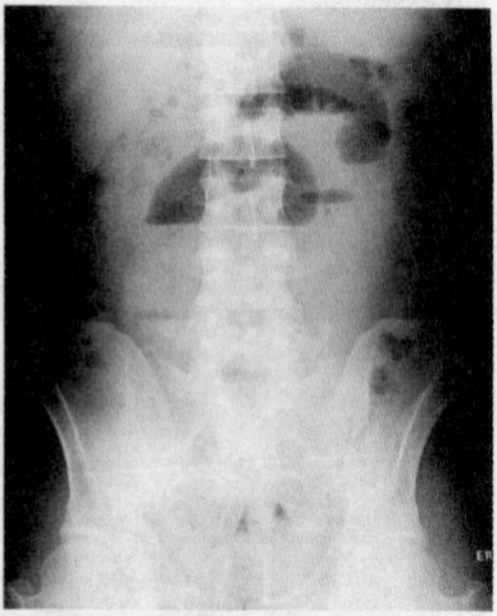

Fig 1. Erect. Gas can be seen from the rectum back to the caecum. The stomach bubble is barely visible. That leaves the obvious fluid levels to explain—note that they are central with few valvulae conniventes—so they are probably in the small intestine. If the large bowel were obstructed, a few peripheral loops often over 5cm would be seen. No sign of calcification in the biliary or urinary tract. The bones and soft tissues appear normal. Note that there are no clues as to the cause of the GI obstruction, ie no hernia, and no surgical clips or signs of past surgery which might now be causing adhesions.

Courtesy of Prof Peter Scally.

1 Gallstone ileus: a big stone migrates directly from an inflamed gallbladder eg to the transverse colon. Rigler's triad (seen in 25%): **1** pneum(at)obilia **2** small bowel obstruction **3** an ectopic gallstone.
2 The aorta may calcify, as may the pancreas (chronic pancreatitis) and gallbladder. (='porcelain gallbladder'), from chronic inflammation from gallstones (associates with gallbladder cancer in 22%).

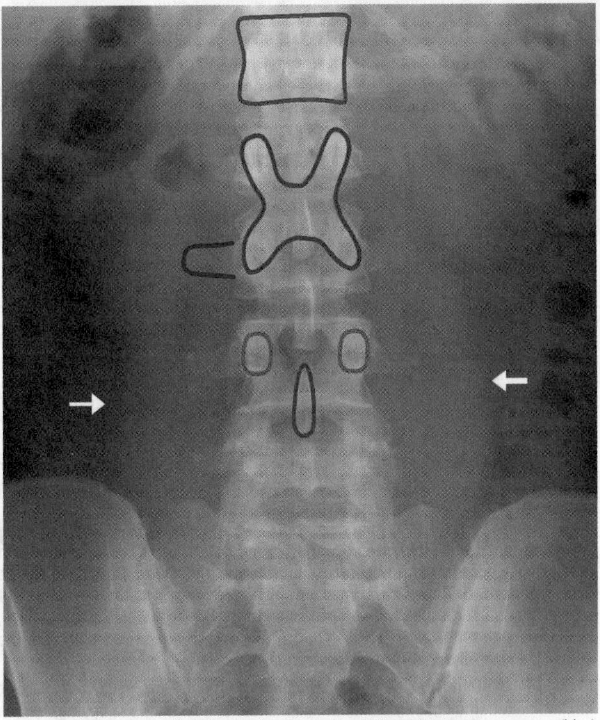

Fig 2. AXR showing: psoas lines (arrows); spinous process (green); transverse process (blue); pedicles (yellow): facet joint processes (outline in red); vertebral body (cyan). ►NB: don't expect too many answers from plain images! Develop and rely on your clinical skills. The most common diagnosis is abdominal pain of unknown origin: think of major pathologies.

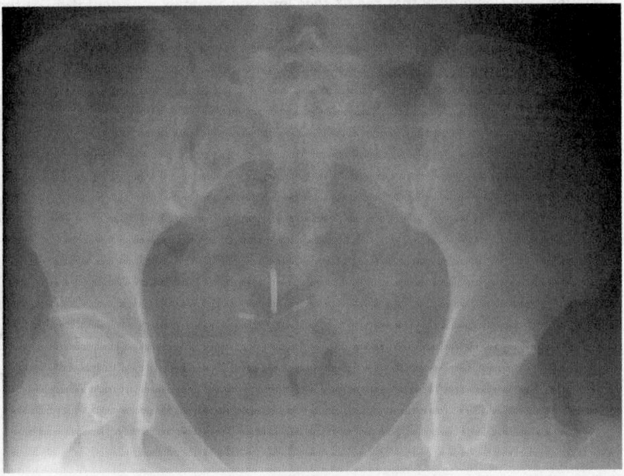

Fig 3. An intrauterine contraceptive device. Figs 2&3 courtesy of Norwich Radiology Department.

Computed tomography (CT)

Since its first use in Atkinson Morley Hospital in 1972, CT has become a speedy and accurate aid to the clinician. Modern systems give whole-body images in under one breath (thanks to continuous, helical rather than sequential, axial data acquisition). Within a single slice (eg 2-5mm thick) CT records the **attenuation**[1] of different tissues to ionising radiation and calculates a mean value for a given volume of tissue, called a **voxel**, in a process called **volume averaging**. This value is represented in greyscale as a single point, called a **pixel**, in the final 2D image, usually 512 by 512 pixels. The greyscale of the image is measured on the Hounsfield scale relative to the attenuation of water, which has a value of 0 Hounsfield units (HU) and ranges from less than -1000 HU (low attenuation) to more than +1000 HU (high attenuation).

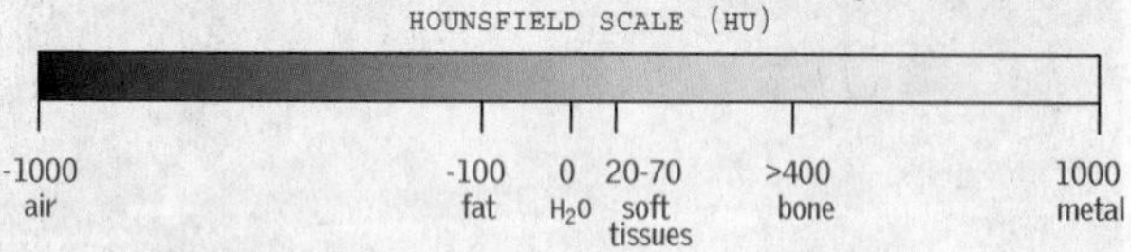

CT is better than humans in picking up subtle variation in attenuation of the tissues so different windows are used to look at tissues of different density, eg bone or lung (**fig 1**).

CT with intravenous iodinated contrast medium gives the ability to image vascular anatomy and vascular structures (ie most organs) in arterial, venous and delayed phases after the injection of contrast (**fig 2**). Contrast is usually given IV for examinations of the chest, abdomen and pelvis. If infection or neoplasia need excluding contrast is often given. CTs of the brain, spine, and musculoskeletal system are normally done without IV contrast. Enhancement of the colonic lumen can be achieved with oral contrast medium given 24h beforehand, or by rectal administration. Air is insufflated for CT colonography or 'virtual colonoscopy'—**fig 5**, p757. Oral contrast or water is given 1h before an examination for definition of the stomach and small bowel. Also see *Contrast in imaging*, p762.

CT as the examination of choice Staging and monitoring malignant disease; intracranial pathology, eg stroke, trauma, ↑ICP, and space-occupying lesions (especially when calcified, eg oligodendroglioma); trauma; pre-operative assessment of complex masses; obese patients (US in thinner individuals); most post-operative complications; visualisation of anatomy for drainage, biopsy, and nerve blocks.

Interference Remember that the CT slice image is a matrix representation of the attenuation produced by rotating the system around the patient—this explains some of the artefacts that can be produced. High-attenuation items such as metal fillings, clips and prostheses (and even bone) can cause interference. Other CT artefacts: p735.

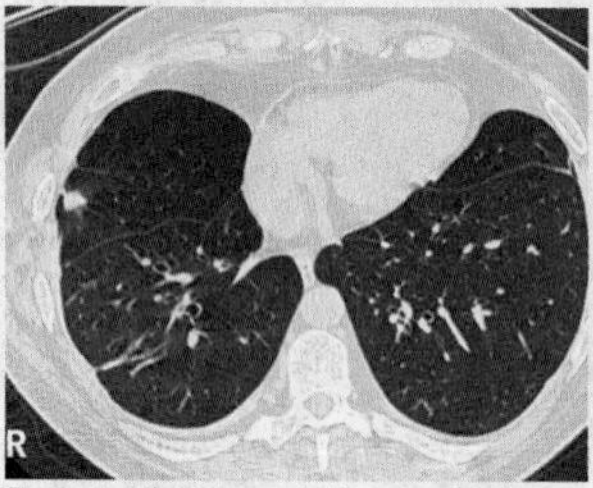

Fig 1. Axial high-resolution CT chest on a lung window algorithm; note solitary lesion in the right lung (Wegener's granulomatosis).

Figs 1-4 courtesy of Norwich Radiology Dept

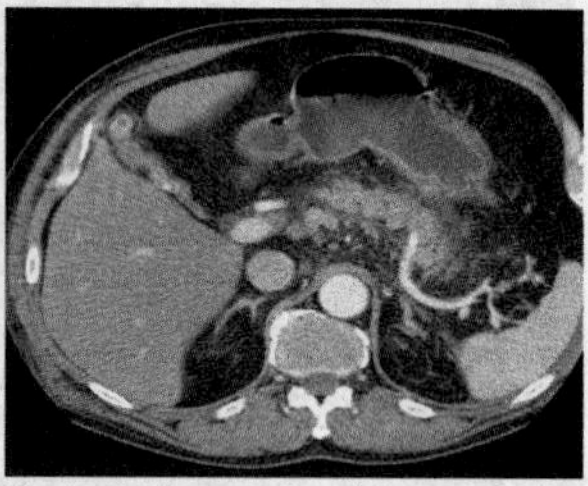

Fig 2. Axial CT of the abdomen after IV contrast (arterial phase). The tortuous splenic artery is enhanced (arrow)—so is the aorta, but not the inferior vena cava.

1 Attenuation is loss of energy of a wave from absorption, refraction, reflection and/or divergence.

The future of CT Multi-detector CT (MDCT) systems (see BOX V/Q *vs* CTPA, p725) are good because they image a volume of tissue, rather than individual slices. Also by decreasing slice thickness, they increase resolution and reduce artefact. Multiplanar (not just axial) slices can be retrieved from one 'sweep', giving thousands of images that are stored digitally and reconstructed, eg into a 3D image (**fig 3**). CT angiography uses MDCT and digital modulation to make 3D colour images. CT urography is becoming the image of choice for the urinary tract. Perfusion CT scanning is a developing technique that maps cerebral blood flow by acquiring images after an IV bolus of contrast. Its role is yet to be established in stroke, but it does have advantages of being less invasive than angiography and more available than MRI.[7] CT combined with PET (see p752) has an increased sensitivity and specificity over each alone.

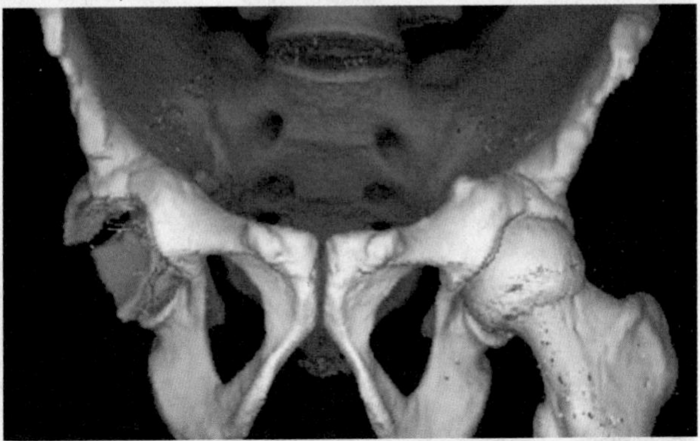

Fig 3. Surface rendered 3D CT reconstruction of the pelvis. The posterior aspect of the right acetabulum is fractured. The right femur has been removed digitally.

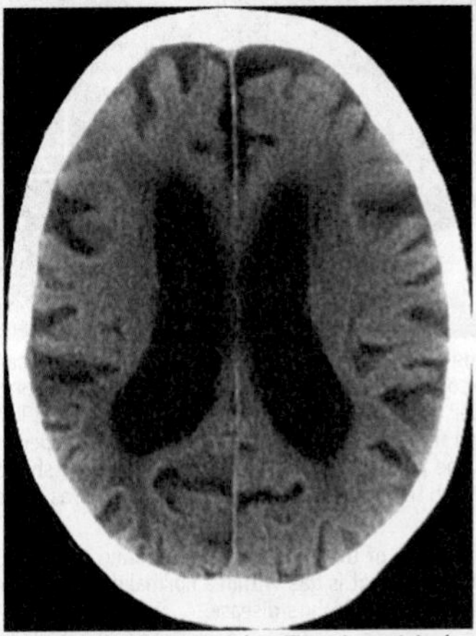

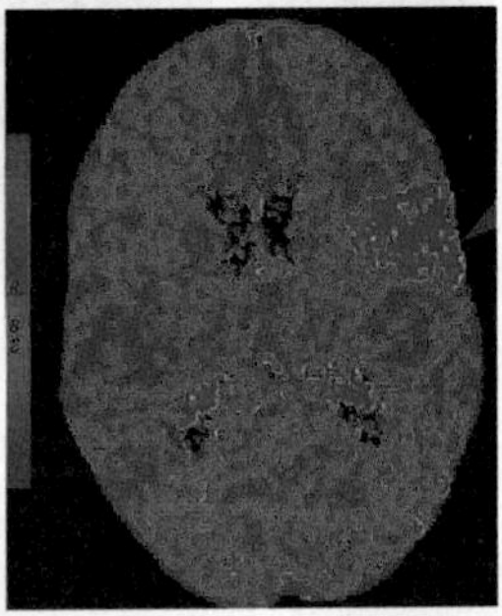

Fig 5. Head perfusion CT showing ischaemia around the Sylvian fissure (arrow). Courtesy of Dr C Cousens.

Fig 4. Axial non-enhanced CT. There is ventricular dilatation with prominent cerebral sulci indicating cerebral atrophy. But remember that morphology does not reflect function.

Too many CTs? (CT≈40% of iatrogenic radiation; ≈1.5% of all cancers)

In one review, no substantial group of patients who were undergoing unnecessary CT could be found.[8] When contemplating CT, balance benefits of CT vs other images with less or no radiation (ultrasound; MRI).[9] To get the best balance, talk to a radiologist. Risk is worst when screening healthy populations, and in children.

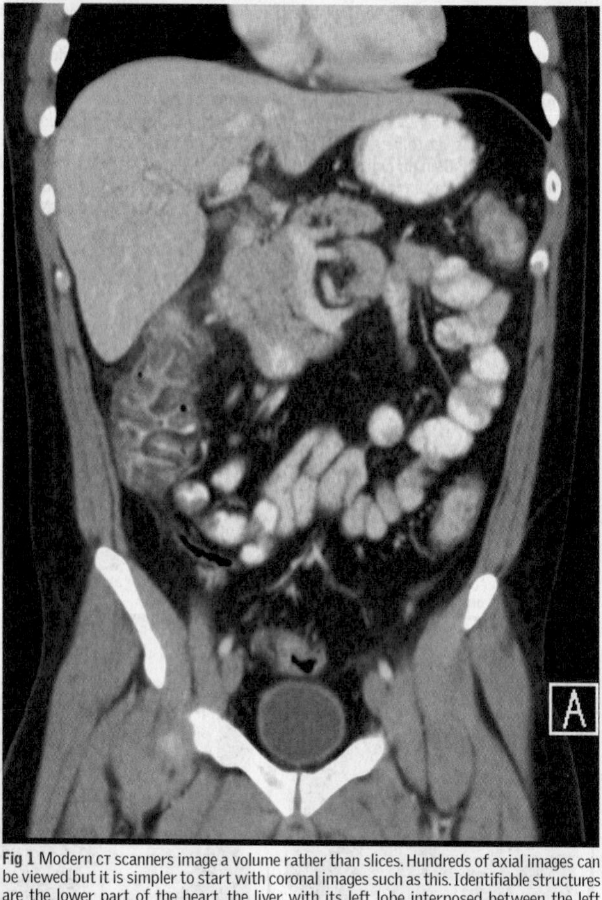

Fig 1 Modern CT scanners image a volume rather than slices. Hundreds of axial images can be viewed but it is simpler to start with coronal images such as this. Identifiable structures are the lower part of the heart, the liver with its left lobe interposed between the left ventricle and the contrast-filled stomach fundus. Between the stomach and the superior mesenteric vein is part of the body of the pancreas—recognized by its lobulated shape. Loops of contrast-filled small intestine with thin (normal) bowel walls are visible, as is the bladder.

The history was 'RIF pain'. Below the right lobe of the liver is the caecum and ascending colon with markedly thickened wall. Inferior to that is gas within a normal appendix. The diagnosis is inflammatory bowel disease, probably Crohn's disease.

Courtesy of Professor Peter Scally and Dr Jennie Roberts.

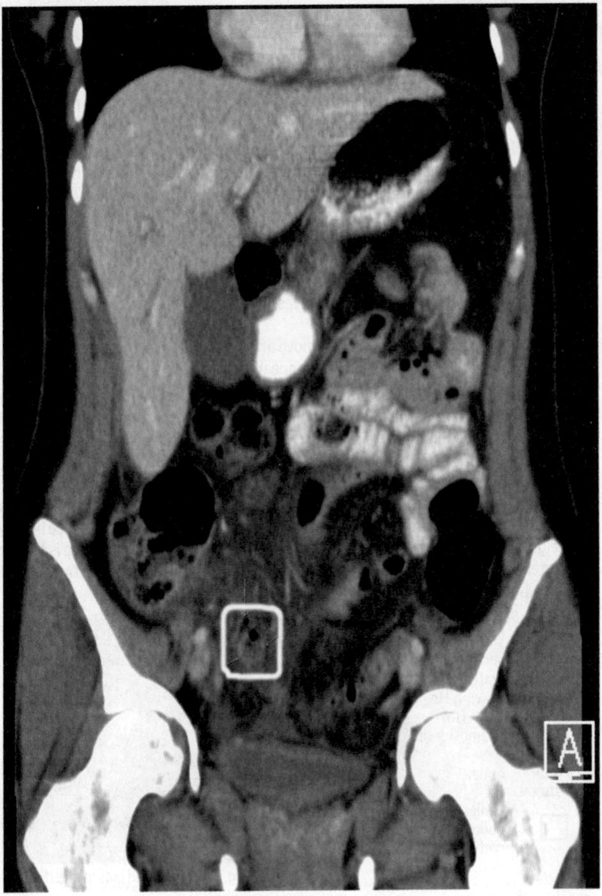

Fig 2. In this coronal CT we can see a long Riedel's lobe of the liver (right) extending past the somewhat darker gallbladder almost into the right iliac fossa. The portal veins are opacified. In this patient, who presented with RIF pain, the caecum is normal. But is the appendix normal? It is usually a gas-filled structure, but here its wall is thickened, a small amount of gas (black) lies outside it, and the surrounding fat is inflamed (whiter than normal). Diagnosis: perforated appendix. Courtesy of Prof P Scally & Dr J Roberts.

The changing role of CT in acute abdominal pain In the days when general surgeons did their rounds towards the end of an on-call day, there would be wards of patients with undiagnosed abdominal pain having 'drip-and-suck' regimens (IVI & NGT) while awaiting improvement or the unequivocal need for surgery. On opening up, the surgeon would be confident that whatever he found he could deal with. But with the waning of the general surgeon, and the waxing of minimally invasive procedures, specialist surgical teams and highly accurate imaging, it is now best (unless immediate surgery is essential) to match the team to the condition diagnosed by imaging. CT is the single best image in adults, unless a gifted ultrasonographer is to hand. So, in this context, drip-and-suck is on the ebb, giving way to imaging, accurate diagnosis, and rapid discharge or referral to the appropriate team.

1 A large proportion of the human body is fat or water (~80%).
2 Fat and water contain a large number of hydrogen nuclei (unpaired protons).
3 The spin of a positively charged hydrogen nucleus gives it magnetic polarity.

Thus...

- Placing the human body in a magnetic field (clinically from 0.2-3 Tesla) aligns its hydrogen nuclei either with (parallel) or against (anti-parallel) the field.
- A radiofrequency (RF) pulse at the resonant frequency flips nuclei away from their original alignment by an angle depending on the amount of energy they absorb.
- When the RF pulse stops, the nuclei flip back (or **relax**) into their original alignment, emitting the energy (called an **echo**) that was absorbed from the RF field.
- Measuring and plotting the energy of the returning signal according to location (provided the nuclei haven't moved) gives a picture of fat, tissue, and water as distributed throughout the body.
- The hydrogen nuclei in flowing blood move after receiving the RF pulses. The echo is not detected, and so the vessel lumen appears black.

Rather than radiodensity or attenuation, the correct descriptive terminology for the greyscale seen in MRI is **signal intensity**: high signal appears white and low signal black (see below). **Weighting** is a quality of MRI that is dependent on the length of the period between the RF pulses (**repetition time**, **TR**) and the time between an RF pulse and the echo (**echo time**, **TE**). MR images are most commonly T1-weighted (good for visualising anatomy) or T2-weighted (good for visualising disease) but can also be a mixture of both, called **proton density** (PD) weighting. **FLAIR** sequences produce heavily T2-weighted images. A good way to determine the weighting of an MR image is to look for water—eg in the aqueous humour of the eye, CSF, or synovial fluid (see TABLE, **fig 1**). See also **figures 1-5**.

	T1-WEIGHTED	T2-WEIGHTED
TR	short (<1000ms)	long (>2000ms)
TE	short (<30ms)	long (>80ms)
LOW SIGNAL ■	**water** flowing Hb fresh Hb haemosiderin	bone flowing Hb deoxyHb haemosiderin melanin
HIGH SIGNAL □	bone fat cholesterol gadolinium (p762) metHb	**water** cholesterol fresh Hb metHb

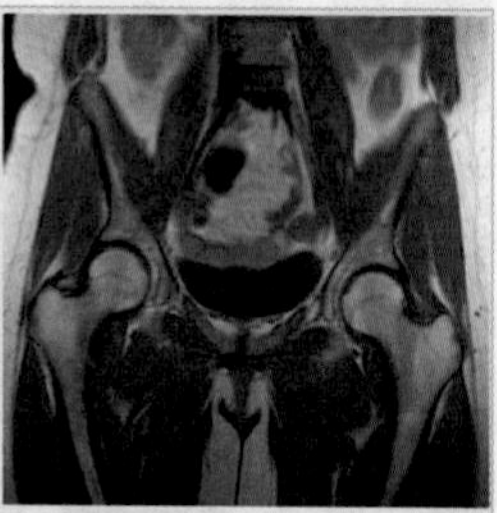

Fig 1. T1 weighted MRI of the hips.[1]

Advantages MRI's great bonus is that it does not involve ionising radiation. It has no known long-term adverse effects, though power is limited by controls on energy deposition into tissue. It is excellent for imaging soft tissues (water- and hence proton-dense). It is preferred over CT for many intracranial, head and neck, spinal, and musculoskeletal disorders. Multiplanar acquisition of images can provide multiple views and 3D reconstruction from one examination.

Disadvantages Poor imaging of lung parenchyma and GI mucosa. More claustrophobic and noisy than CT. High cost combined with limited availability.

Contraindications *Absolute:* • Cardiac pacemakers; other electrical devices. • Intra-ocular metallic foreign bodies. (You may need an X-ray of the orbits to exclude a foreign body) *Relative:* • Intracranial aneurysm clips. • Certain types of artificial heart valves. • If unable to complete the pre-scan questionnaire. • 1st trimester of pregnancy (not currently approved.) • Cochlear implants. **NB:** orthopaedic prostheses and extracranial metallic clips are generally safe. ►If uncertain, ask a radiologist.

1 Coronal T1 weighted MRI of the hips—so normal adult bone marrow is high signal due to fatty yellow marrow, while red marrow gives a lower signal. There is also low signal from urine in the bladder. MRI gives great soft tissue definition.

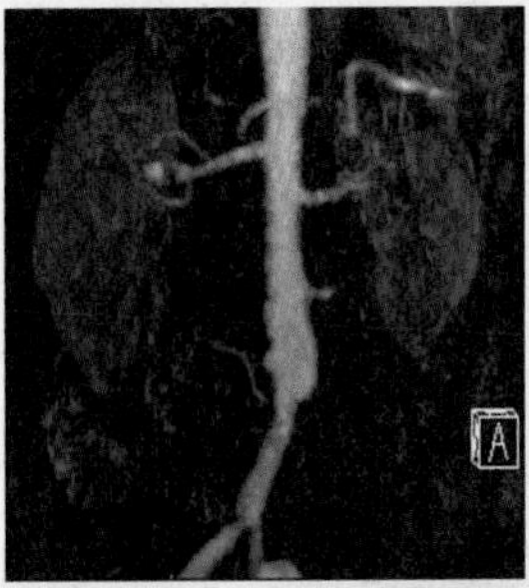

Fig 2. One of the many successful developments in MRI has been magnetic resonance angiography (MRA). It can accurately reconstruct vascular anatomy with or without IV gadolinium. This makes it valuable in the assessment of vascular disease in patients with nephropathy. This also precludes the need for femoral puncture (the usual point of entry for conventional contrast angiography), which can have complications of haemorrhage, pseudoaneurysm formation and arterial thrombosis. This MRA shows complete occlusion of the left common iliac artery.

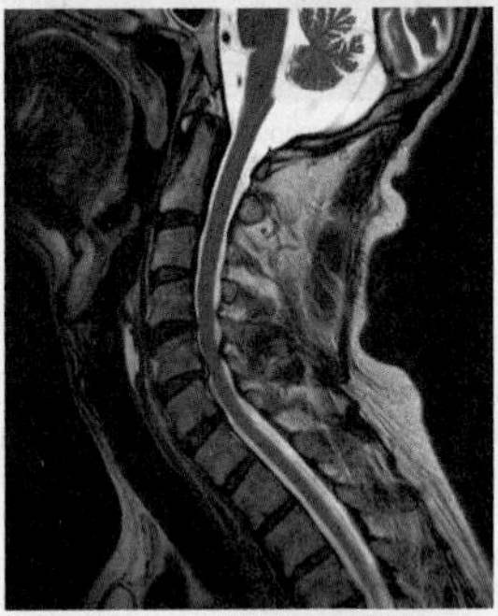

Fig 3. T2-weighted sagittal MRI of the cervical spine. There is impingement of the spinal cord at the C4/5 and C5/6 levels caused by degenerative disease. C2 (axis) is identifiable from the odontoid peg, which is embryologically derived from the body of C1 (atlas).

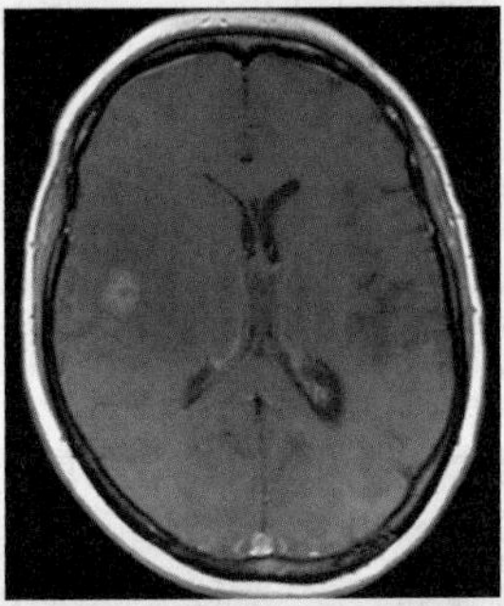

Fig 4. Axial T1 weighted MRI of the brain post-IV gadolinium. In the right temporo-parietal region there is a small area of high signal enhancement with a more central area of low signal, surrounded by a region of low signal (presumably vasogenic cerebral oedema) in comparison to the normal brain tissue. This is all causing mass effect with effacement of the sulci and adjacent right frontal horn of the lateral ventricle. There is very subtle midline shift.

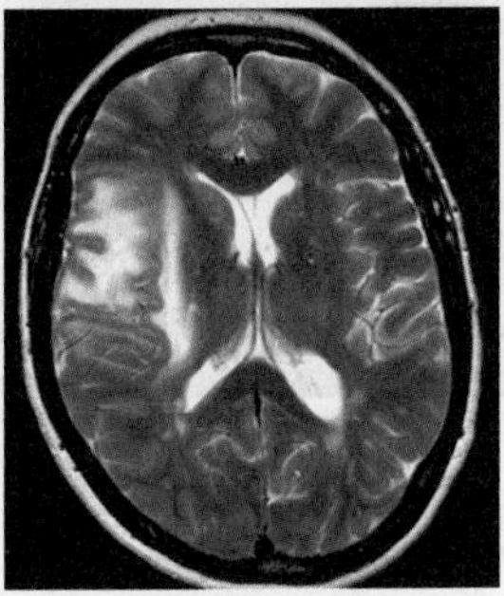

Fig 5. Axial T2-weighted MRI of the same patient at the same level as **fig 4**. The high signal in the temporo-parietal region shows a mass effect. The diagnosis was of a solitary metastasis. Note on this T2-weighted image the cerebrospinal fluid within the ventricles and cortical sulci are of high signal due to their water content.

All figures courtesy of Norwich Radiology Department.

Unlike the other methods of imaging, US doesn't use electromagnetic radiation. Instead, it relies on properties of longitudinal sound waves. This has made it a popular and safe form of imaging (eg in obs & gynae, testes, gallbladders, vessels, fistulae, thyroid, etc). High-frequency sound waves (3-15MHz) are made from a piezo-electric quartz crystal; its size, shape, and resonant frequency determine tissue penetration and image quality. NB: transducers act as transmitter and receiver due to the piezo-electric properties of quartz crystal.[1]

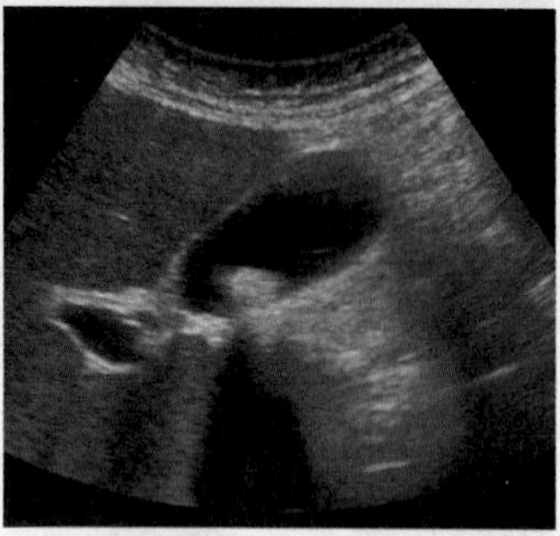

Fig 1. Abdominal US showing a hyperechoic calcified gallstone causing a dense acoustic shadow (**black**) posteriorly. A hypoechoic gallbladder (bile) attenuates few sound waves so that more reach the deep tissues which therefore give more echoes (acoustic enhancement, **white**, within the drawn yellow horseshoe).

Passage of sound waves through tissue is affected by **attenuation** and **reflection**. Attenuation disperses waves out of the receiver's range, but it is the waves reflected to the receiver that determine the image. Its quality depends on the difference in **acoustic impedance** between adjacent soft tissues.

With the help of software a real-time 2D image is made (**fig 1**). During processing an average attenuation value is assumed throughout the tissue examined, so if a higher-than-average attenuation structure is in the superficial tissues, then everything deep to it will be in a low intensity (black) **acoustic shadow**. If a lower-than-average attenuation object is in the superficial tissues then everything deep to it will be high intensity (white) or **enhanced.** If a tissue interface is strongly disparate, then all the waves are reflected back, making it impossible to image beyond it. See also **figures 1-6**.

Modes *B* (brightness) is the most common, giving 2D slices that map the different magnitudes of echo in greyscale. ***M*** (movement) traces the movement of structures within the line of the sound beam. It is used in imaging eg heart valves (p106).

Duplex ultrasonography (flow and morphology) By combining Doppler effects (shifts in wavelength caused by movement of a source or reflecting surface) with B-mode ultrasound technology, flow characteristics of blood can be infered (**fig 2**). This is extremely useful in arterial and venous studies, and echocardiography.

Advantages Portable; fast; non-ionising; cheap; real-time; can be used with intervention; can enter organs, eg rectum, vagina, gut (eg *endoscopic US* to image the heart=transoesophageal echocardiogram, TOE, p106—also used to assess depth of invasion of cancers, eg pancreas, stomach).

Disadvantages of US Inter-performer variance; poor quality if fat; interference from bone, bowel gas, calculi, or superimposed organs.

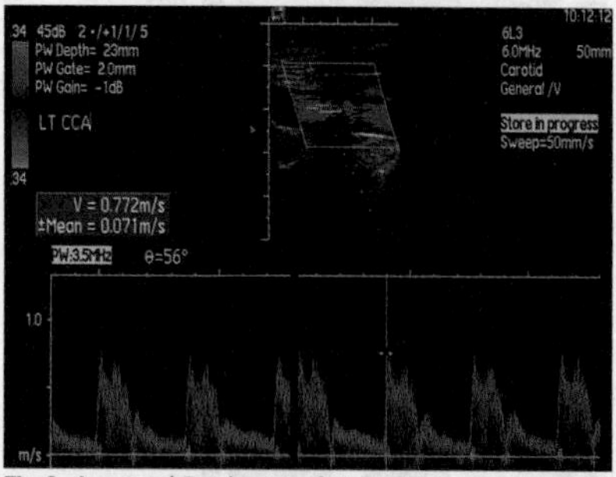

Fig 2. A normal Duplex US of the right common carotid artery with a flow rate=77cm/s. The Doppler trace (orange) is displayed below the main image.

1 When a voltage is applied to a piezo-electric crystal it changes shape, emitting a sound wave when it vibrates. In reverse, when a sound wave physically alters its shape an electrical current is induced.

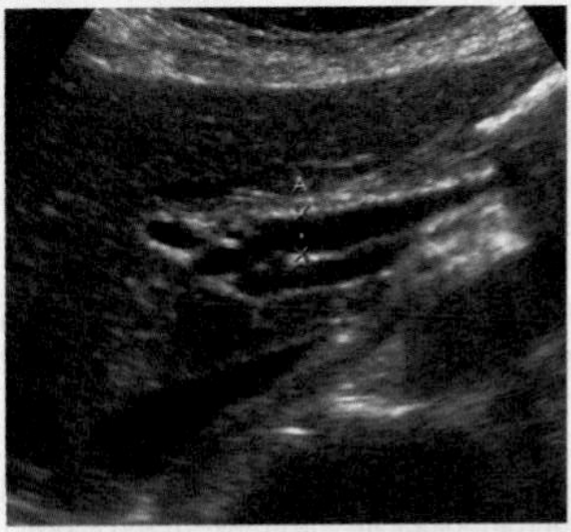

Fig 3. Ultrasound of the liver shows the CBD to be dilated. Distal obstruction of the CBD gives proximal dilatation of the duct. A CBD width >6mm if ≤60yrs is abnormal; after cholecystectomy ~8mm may be OK (up to 14mm in the elderly). It is important to check that the distal CBD tapers as it enters the duodenum. NB: the portal vein lies posterior to the duct (along with the hepatic artery) in the free edge of the lesser omentum. The next questions are "What is causing the obstruction?" and "Where can I get that information?"

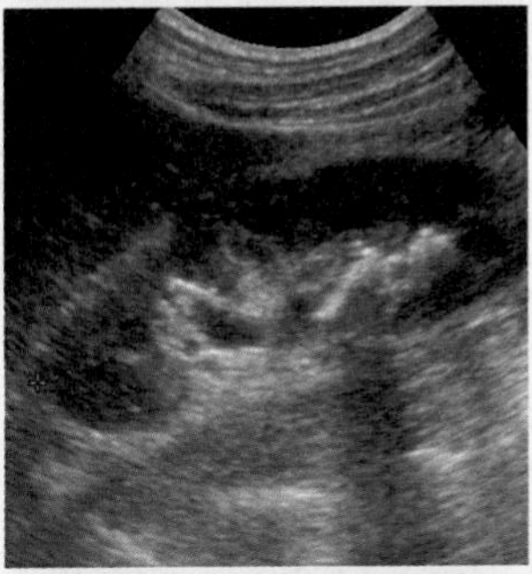

Fig 4. Ultrasound of the kidney. At first the image may seem normal but there is a wedge of posterior acoustic shadow cast by the object which is causing increased echogenicity in the lower pole calyces. Acoustic shadows in the kidney suggest stones—as here—or nephrocalcinosis.

Acoustic shadow
• Fibrous tissue • Calcification • Gas
Acoustic enhancement
• Fluid-filled and cystic structures

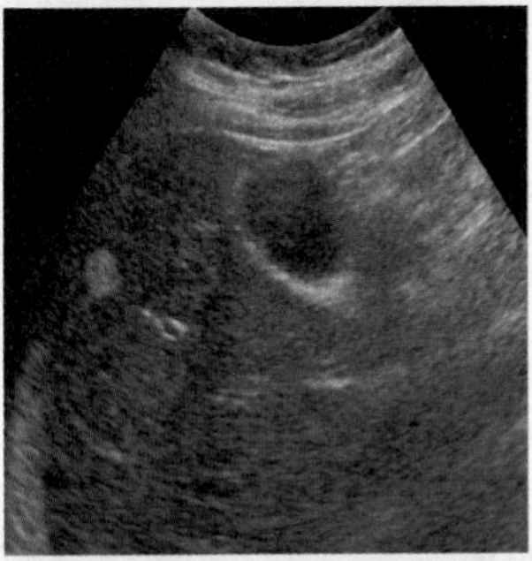

Fig 5. Longitudinal ultrasound of the right lobe of the liver showing a well-defined small area of echogenicity. This is the typical appearance of a liver haemangioma, a very common benign liver lesion.

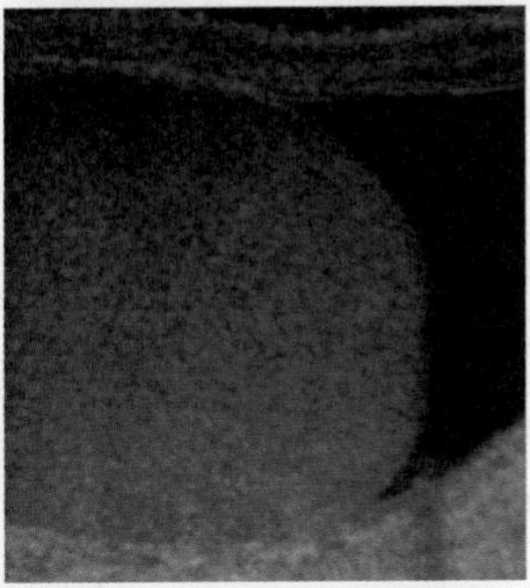

Fig 6. Ultrasound of the testis showing a hydrocele. One of the great advan-tages of ultrasound is that it does not use radiation, and so is ideal for imaging radiosensitive tissues such as the testis, thyroid, and fetus.

Figures 1-6 courtesy of Norwich Radiology Dept.

Nuclear medicine is both diagnostic and therapeutic. The latter is developing rapidly, but here we are mostly concerned with its diagnostic capabilities. Use of molecules labelled with a radioisotope means that there is exposure to ionising radiation, though doses are usually less than those from a CT abdomen (see TABLE, p733).

Positron emission tomography (PET) maps glucose metabolism in the body. ^{18}F fluorodeoxyglucose (FDG), a short half-life glucose analogue (λ=110min), is taken up by metabolically active tissues. It decays rapidly to produce a positron that, after travelling a few mm through tissue, annihilates with an electron to produce a pair of high-energy photons (γ rays), which PET detects. Neoplasms have high uptake of FDG, but so do benign inflammatory and granulomatous lesions—if one is considering false +ves, consider sarcoidosis and TB. Non-pathological high uptake of FDG in brain, liver, kidney, bladder, larynx and lymphoid tissue of pharynx can be confusing. Resolution of lesions can be down to 4mm. 3D analysis increases sensitivity compared with 2D. *Cancer:* PET has a role eg if combined with MRI/CT. It is used in colorectal cancer to see local recurrence ± extrahepatic metastases when considering hepatic resection. Also indicated for staging of: non-small cell lung cancer; lymphoma; melanoma; oesophageal cancer. *Dementia:* PET of no proven value, but is used in research. *Radionuclide imaging in cardiology:* p754.

Ventilation (V) scintigraphy (fig 1) uses technetium (Tc) or xenon-133 (^{133}Xe). Requires a CXR within last 24h for comparison. You can sometimes discern it from a perfusion image by the presence of radioisotope in the upper airway.

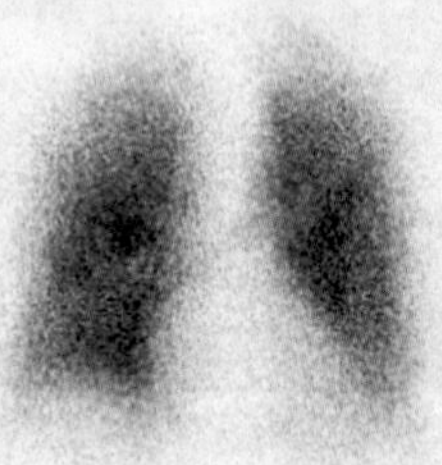

Fig 1. Ventilation scintigram.

Perfusion (Q) scintigraphy (fig 2) uses 99m-technetium(^{99m}Tc)-labelled macroaggregates that block a small proportion of lung capillaries and thus lodge in the pulmonary circulation. Reported as high, intermediate, low probability, or normal according to findings. A normal perfusion scintigram excludes PE, hence its high sensitivity.

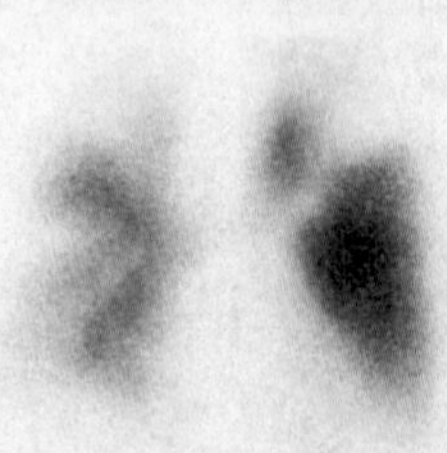

Fig 2. Perfusion scintigram showing mismatches with fig 1.

Bone scintigraphy Important for primary and secondary bone tumours (often -ve in myeloma) and bone disorders such as osteomalacia, stress fractures, avascular necrosis, and the arthropathies. Uses bisphosphonates labelled with ^{99m}Tc. It is more sensitive than X-ray for finding metastases (some lesions may not appear on X-ray if <50% of the bone matrix has been destroyed).

Thyroid disease TcO_4 is commonly used and can differentiate between Graves', toxic multinodular goitre, and subacute thyroiditis (**fig 3** & **fig 1**, p603). Good for identifying ectopic tissue and functioning nodules, and also indicated for detecting residual or recurrent thyroid tissue after surgery. ~15% of cold (non-functioning) nodules are malignant.

Hot nodules are often toxic adenomas. Iodine-131 (^{131}I) is used for therapeutic intervention in thyrotoxicosis.

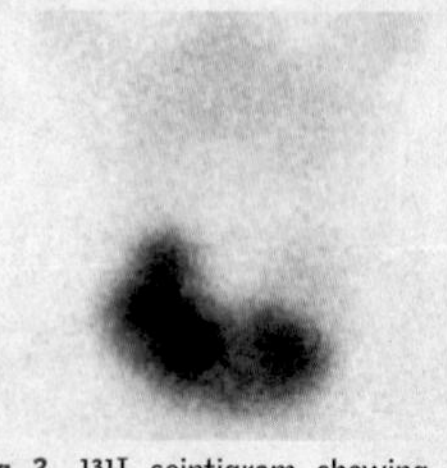

Fig 3. ^{131}I scintigram showing a multinodular goitre.

Phaeochromocytoma Iodine-123 (^{123}I) meta-iodobenzylguanide (MIBG) is taken-up by sympathetic tissues, and indicates functioning, ectopic, and metastatic adrenal medullary (+other neural crest) tumours. ^{131}I-MIBG is also used for treatment.

Hyperparathyroidism ^{99m}Tc-methoxyisobutyl isonitrile (MIBI) scans can detect parathyroid adenomas (**fig 4**).

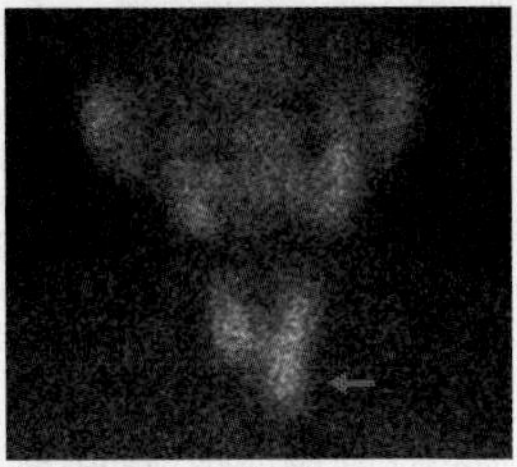

Fig 4. MIBI study showing a parathyroid adenoma.

Adrenal cortical disease Radionuclide imaging is used to differentiate adenoma from diffuse hyperplasia.

GI haemorrhage Scans performed after endoscopy and CT for *acute bleeding*. Uses a red-cell-labelled technique. More sensitive than angiography and useful in cases of intermittent GI bleeding. In *chronic bleeding*, done when all other investigations are negative, using red cell (^{99m}Tc-pertechnetate) techniques if ectopic gastric mucosa or Meckel's diverticulum is suspected.

Crohn's disease White-cell-labelled techniques (indium-111) can pinpoint areas of small bowel activity and extent of disease in conjunction with barium studies and MRI. Also indicated to assess acute flare-up of colonic disease for Crohn's and UC.

Renal studies Chromium-51 (^{51}Cr) EDTA or DTPA (^{99m}Tc, p683) is used to assess GFR. ^{99m}Tc-mercapto-acetyltriglycine (MAG3) technique assesses relative renal function and renal transit time (eg in obstructive nephropathy or renovascular disease). Dynamic renal mapping gives quantifiable information about renal function and the degree of obstruction which is not available from other modalities. ^{99m}Tc-dimercaptosuccinic acid (DMSA) scanning (**fig 5**) is the gold standard for evaluation of renal scarring that occurs eg in reflux nephropathy.

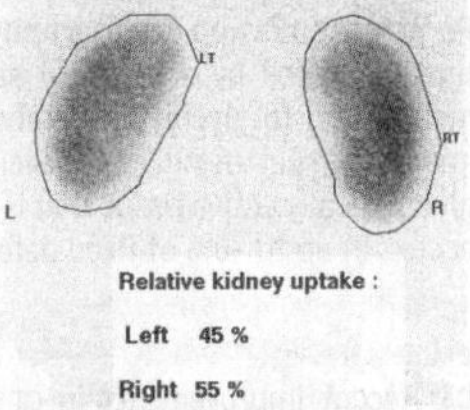

Fig 5. DMS showing relative renal function of each kidney.

V/Q scintigram or CTPA?[1]

This question has no clear answer (so far). Standard procedure has been CXR then V/Q scintigraphy: positive predictive value≈96% if high probability, and reliably excludes PE if 'normal'. CTPA (**fig 6**) is sensitive and specific (≥90%) if the embolus is in a pulmonary artery, but its bane has been the subsegmental PE (making CTPA only 60% sensitive and 70% specific if included in total lung analysis). New multidetector CT (MDCT) systems have up to 64 detectors, giving thinner slices (0.6–1.25mm) and a faster scanning time that reduces respiratory motion artefacts and gives good subsegmental imaging. Faster data acquisition also requires less IV contrast, beneficial for patients with renal and cardiac impairment. Results from the PIOPED II trial (a prospective study) gave CTPA alone a sensitivity & specificity of 83% and 96% respectively.[12] Complete data are awaited, but so far we recommend as 1st-line CTPA and venous phase CT of the leg veins and pelvis.[13] CTPA's advantages are that it is more readily available and that it can show other lesions.

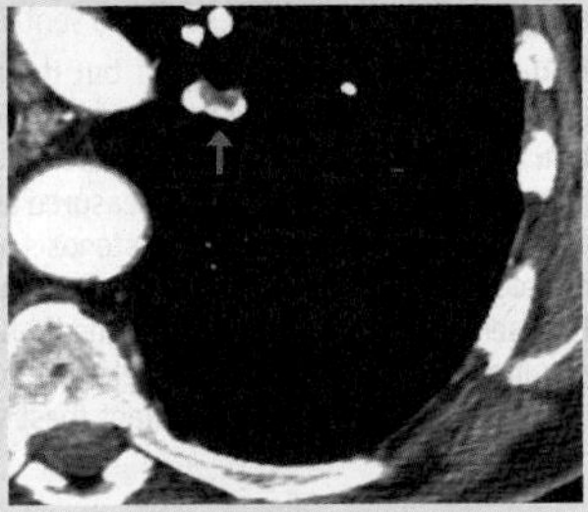

Fig 6. CT pulmonary angiogram (CTPA) with a grey filling defect (presumed embolus in a branch of a left pulmonary artery).

1 V/Q = ventilation/perfusion; CTPA=CT pulmonary angiography. All images ©Norwich Radiology Dept.

Radionuclide imaging in cardiology

Myocardial perfusion imaging A non-invasive method of assessing regional myocardial blood flow and the cellular integrity of myocytes. The technique uses radionuclide tracers which cross the myocyte membrane and are trapped intracellularly. **Thallium-201** (^{201}Tl), a K^+ analogue, is distributed via regional myocardial blood flow and requires cellular integrity for uptake. Newer **technetium-99** (^{99}Tc) based agents are similar to ^{201}Tl but have improved imaging characteristics, and can be used to assess myocardial perfusion and LV performance in the same study. Myocardial territories supplied by unobstructed coronary vessels have normal perfusion whereas regions supplied by stenosed coronary vessels have poorer relative perfusion, a difference that is accentuated by exercise. For this reason, exercise tests are used in conjunction with radionuclide imaging to identify areas at risk of ischaemia/infarction. Exercise scans are compared with resting views: ***reperfusion*** (ischaemia, see BOX, 'Cardiac perfusion scintigraphy') or ***fixed defects*** (infarct) can be seen and the coronary artery involved reliably predicted. Drugs (eg ***adenosine***, ***dobutamine*** and ***dipyridamole***) can also be used to induce perfusion differences between normal and underperfused tissues.

Myocardial perfusion imaging adds information in patients presenting with acute MI (to determine the amount of myocardium salvaged by thrombolysis) and in diagnosing acute chest pain in those without classical ECG changes (to define the presence of significant perfusion defects).

Positron emission tomography (PET) Severely underperfused tissues, such as those supplied by a critically stenotic coronary artery, switch from fatty acid metabolism to glycolytic metabolism. Such altered cellular biochemistry may be imaged by pet using ^{18}F-labelled fluorodeoxyglucose (FDG), which identifies the glycolytically active tissue that is viable. This phenomenon, severe resting ischaemia, occurs in up to 40% of fixed defects seen on ^{201}Th scans.

Cardiac CT and MRI

CT Recent improvements in CT technology have made routine cardiac imaging possible. 16 or 64 slice CT, because of its speed and resolution, can image coronary arteries and exclude significant disease with a negative predictive value (NPV) of 97-99%. It can also visualise CABG patency, provide coronary artery Ca^{2+} scoring (a risk factor for coronary artery disease, p103), demonstrate cardiac anatomy including congenital anomalies, and estimate ventricular function.

MRI has less resolution than CT but its lack of ionising radiation make it a good choice for congenital heart disease in children and adults. MRI is superior to CT for functional assessment although resolution limits its imaging of coronary artery disease. Flow velocities can be measured and, because the flow is proportional to the pressure differences, degrees of stenosis and regurgitation across heart valves can be calculated. Myocardial infarction, perfusion and viability can also be imaged with the use of IV gadolinium contrast medium (p762). Both CT and MR use ECG-gating to acquire the imaging data and relate it to the position in the cardiac cycle, thus minimising the movement artefact (best when the patient is in sinus rhythm).

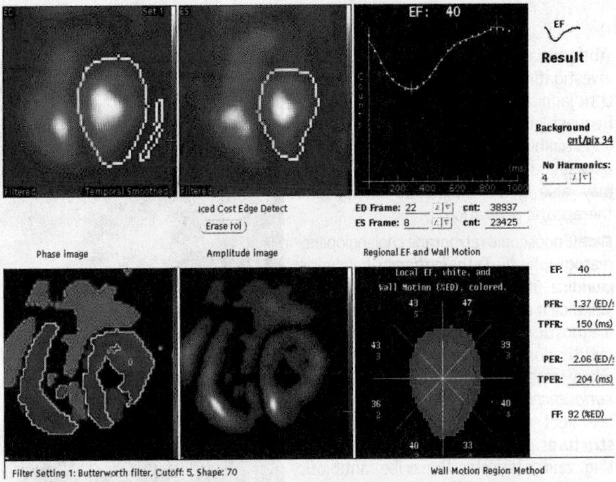

Multiple gated acquisition (MUGA) scanning is a non-invasive way to measure left ventricle ejection fraction (EF, 40% in the study above). After injection of ^{99m}Tc, a dynamic image of the left ventricle is obtained a few hundred heartbeats by gamma camera. A widespread use for MUGA scanning has been in the pre-op assessment of patients for vascular surgery. However, one review suggested that it was an accurate predictor of long-term prognosis but not of operative risk. Stress echocardiography and perfusion scintigraphy may have more clinical relevance in this role. Image courtesy of Dr Chris Cousens. This image was prepared using the HERMES FUGA preprocessing application. HERMES Medical Solutions. www.hermesmedical.com

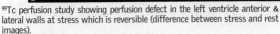

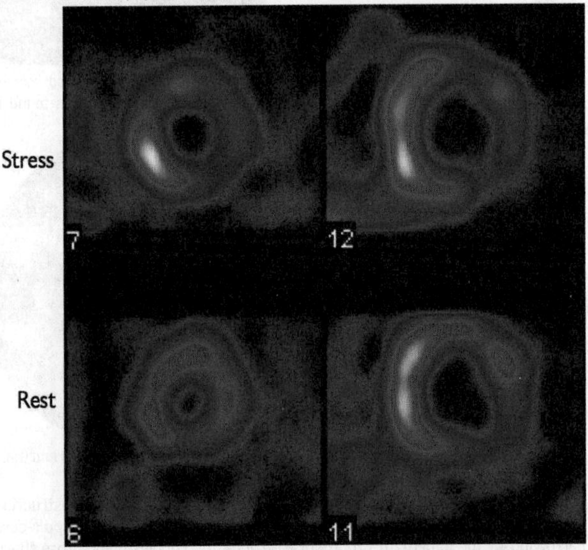

^{99}Tc perfusion study showing perfusion defect in the left ventricle anterior & lateral walls at stress which is reversible (difference between stress and rest images).

Abdominal ultrasound (US) is used for investigating abdominal pain, abnormal LFTs, jaundice, hepatomegaly, and masses. Request 'nil by mouth' for 4h beforehand (aids gallbladder filling, **fig 1**, p750). Pelvic ultrasound needs a full bladder. Ultrasound may also guide diagnostic biopsy and therapeutic aspiration.

ERCP (Endoscopic retrograde cholangiopancreatography, **fig 1**) *Indications:* Cholangitis; jaundice if dilated intrahepatic ducts; jaundice if normal calibre ducts and a non-diagnostic liver biopsy; recurrent pancreatitis; post-cholecystectomy pain. Useful when MRCP (p757) is unavailable. *Therapeutic ERCP:* Sphincterotomy for common bile duct stones; stenting of malignant strictures. *Pre-procedure:* Check LFTs clotting and platelets. Prescribe antibiotic prophylaxis (eg *ciprofloxacin* 750mg PO 2h before), analgesia (eg *morphine* 5mg and *metoclopramide* 10mg IV 1h before) and sedation (eg *midazolam* 2.5–10mg IV). *Method:* A catheter is advanced from a side-viewing duodenoscope via the ampulla into the common bile duct. Contrast medium is injected and X-rays taken to show lesions in the biliary tree and pancreatic ducts. *Complications:* Pancreatitis; bleeding; cholangitis; perforation. Mortality <0.2% overall; 0.4% if performing stone removal.

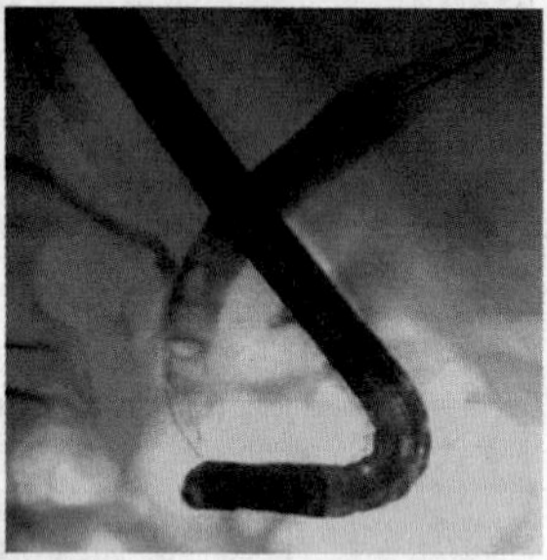

Fig 1. The ERCP shows a dilated common bile duct. The multiple filling defects are calculi within and obstructing the duct.

Contrast swallows (fig 2) can help in dysphagia (p240). Realtime fluoroscopic imaging studies assess swallowing function.

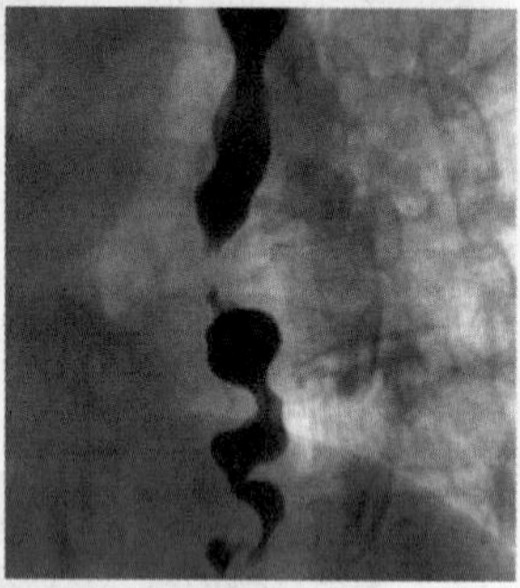

Fig 2. Barium swallow: note 'corkscrew' appearance of the oesophagus found in some motility disorders.

Small bowel follow-through (fig 3) After bowel prep, barium is drunk and images taken every ~½h until it fills the caecum. Spot images are taken of areas of interest, eg terminal ileum.

Small bowel enema After bowel prep, the duodenum is intubated and barium is introduced. It is harder to do than Ba follow-through, but gives better mucosal definition.

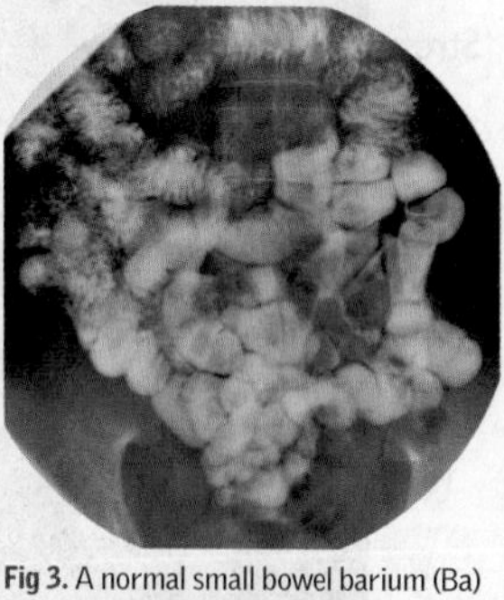

Fig 3. A normal small bowel barium (Ba) follow-through study.

Barium enema Done less commonly, as CT colonography is better. Always do a PR first ± rigid sigmoidoscopy & biopsy. Preparation is as for colonoscopy (p256). For a double-contrast barium enema (**fig 4**), barium and air or CO_2 are introduced rectally. Iodinated contrast medium may be used instead of barium in suspected colonic obstruction. The enema may show diverticular disease or cancers (eg an irregular 'apple-core' narrowing of the lumen). In Crohn's disease, look for 'cobblestoning', 'rose thorn' ulcers, and colonic strictures with rectal sparing. *Disadvantages:* Big radiation dose; no biopsy possible.

CT (figs 5 & 6) is indicated if barium enema is difficult or non-diagnostic. It allows better visualization of the gut and retroperitoneal areas. Oral or IV contrast medium enhances definition (p744). The big disadvantage is the radiation dose. CT colonography ('virtual colonoscopy') is popular, giving good mucosal definition but interpretation takes time and has inter-observer variability.[14] For polyps >9mm specificity is 97% but sensitivity is 85% and drops to 48% if <6mm.[15]

Magnetic resonance imaging (MRI) gives good soft tissue imaging, helping diagnose many benign and malignant lesions. Often used to image the liver. **MRCP** (magnetic resonance cholangiopancreatography) gives detail of the biliary system and the pancreatic duct (**fig 7**). The technique is limited by poor spatial resolution.[16] MRCP has a sensitivity of 83% (specificity 99%) for diagnosing common bile duct stones (p636), and, according to some, is the image of choice (esp. as few SEs).[17]

Wireless capsule endoscopy p256.

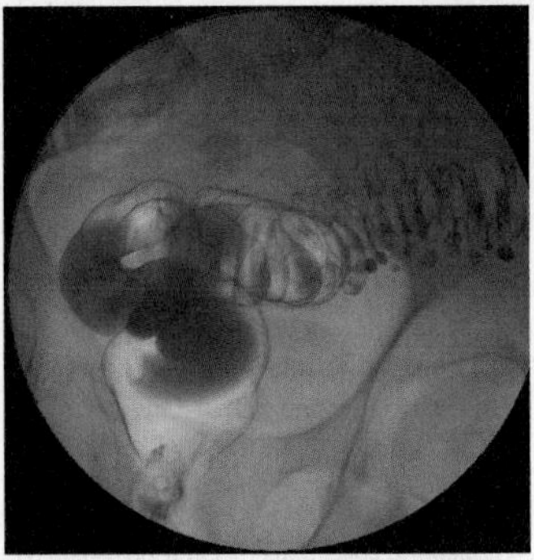

Fig 4. Double-contrast enema improves definition of this sigmoid diverticulum.

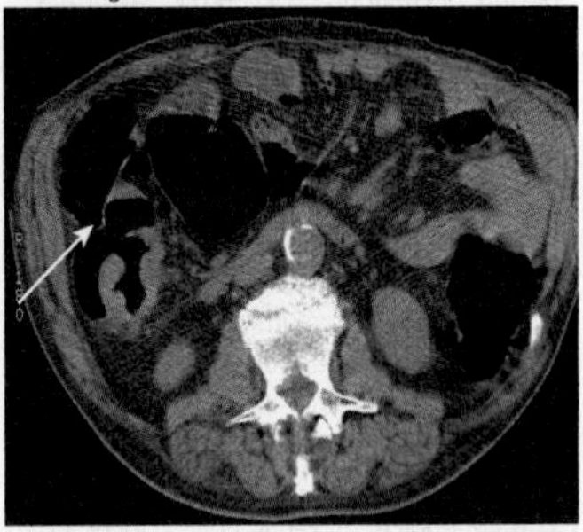

Fig 5. Axial CT colonogram: mural thickening (?ascending colon tumour).

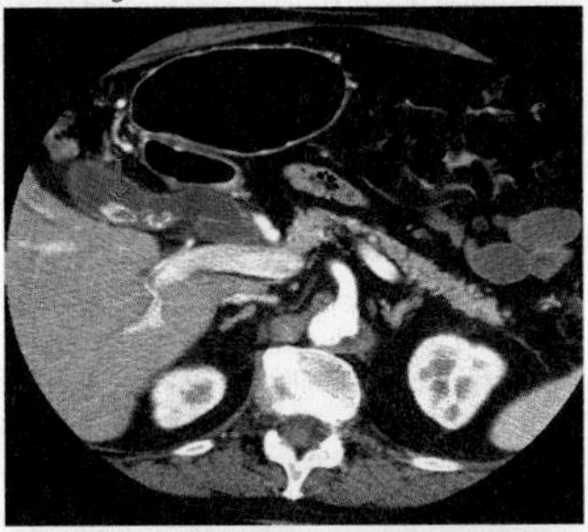

Fig 6. Axial CT of the abdomen post IV and oral contrast medium. The gallbladder contains gallstones (arrow). Lateral to the vertebral column are the kidneys. Anterior to the vertebrae are the IVC and the aorta.

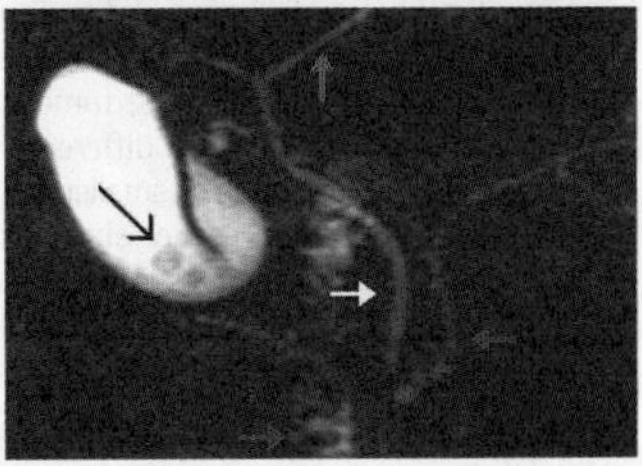

Fig 7. MRCP of the biliary system showing: left hepatic duct (yellow arrow); multiple gallstones in the gallbladder (black arrow); common bile duct (white arrow); pancreatic duct (red arrow); duodenum (green arrow).

Fig 6 courtesy of Dr S Golding; figs 1-5 & 7 courtesy of Norwich Radiology Department.

AXR Look at kidneys, paths of the ureters, and bladder. Note any abnormal calcification—related to which of these 3 processes?

1 Calculi (10–50% are missed on plain films).
2 Dystrophic calcification, eg cancers or TB.
3 Nephrocalcinosis (parenchymal).

Ultrasound is best initial image, showing:

- *Renal size—small* in chronic renal failure, *large* in renal masses, cysts,[1] hypertrophy if other kidney missing, polycystic kidney disease (**fig 1**), and rarities (eg amyloidosis, p364).
- *Hydronephrosis*, which may indicate ureteric obstruction or reflux (**fig 1**, p645).
- *Perinephric collections* (trauma, post-biopsy).
- *Transplanted kidneys* (collections, obstruction, perfusion—**fig 1**, p607).
- *Bladder residual volume:* useful in assessment of the need to catheterise.
- *Prostate*: transrectal ultrasound enables US-guided biopsy of focal lesions. **NB:** prostate size does not correlate with symptoms.

Advantages: Fast; cheap; independent of renal function; no IV contrast or radiation risk. *Disadvantages:* Intraluminal masses (transitional cell ca) in the upper tracts may not be seen; not a functional study; only suggests obstruction if there is dilatation of the collecting system (95% of obstructed kidneys).

CT is 1st-choice in renal colic. Unenhanced images miss only 3% of stones, and show other pathologies (**fig 2**). It delineates masses (cystic or solid, contrast enhancement, calcification, local/distant extension, renal vein involvement); renal trauma (presence of 2 kidneys; haemorrhage; devascularization; laceration; urine leak); retroperitoneal lesions. CT has all but replaced IVU. Radiation dose is similar.

IVU; IVP (intravenous urogram) defines anatomy (esp. pelvicalyceal) and detects pathology distorting collecting systems. It is giving way to CT. It gives some functional data. Images are taken before and after IV contrast. This is filtered by the kidney, reaching the tubules at ~1min (***nephrogram phase***). At this stage look for indentations (scarring) and protrusions (cysts, tumour). Decide which kidney is normal if different in size or nephrogram delayed. The smaller may be normal (other side enlarged) or abnormal (chronic disease). The larger may be normal (compensatory) or abnormal (eg tumour, cysts, obstruction). Later images show contrast in the renal pelvis (***pyelogram***), ureters, and bladder ± filling defects (**fig 7**) and obstruction (**fig 3**)?

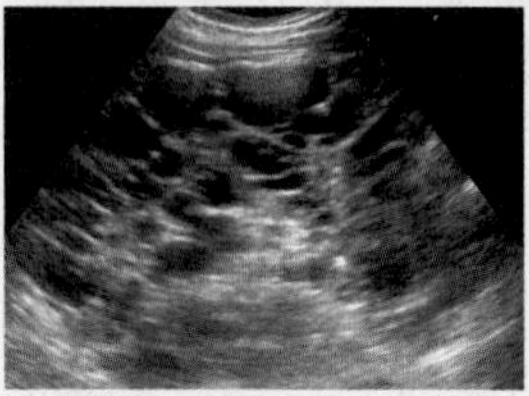

Fig 1. Ultrasound of the kidney showing multiple simple cysts.

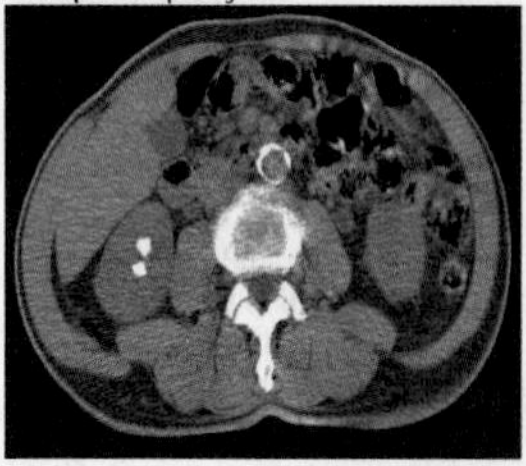

Fig 2. Axial unenhanced abdominal CT: note right calyceal calculus occupying calyces, suggesting it may develop into a staghorn calculus. Most calculi <7mm across pass spontaneously. A bone window algorithm highlights calcium-dense objects within the abdomen.

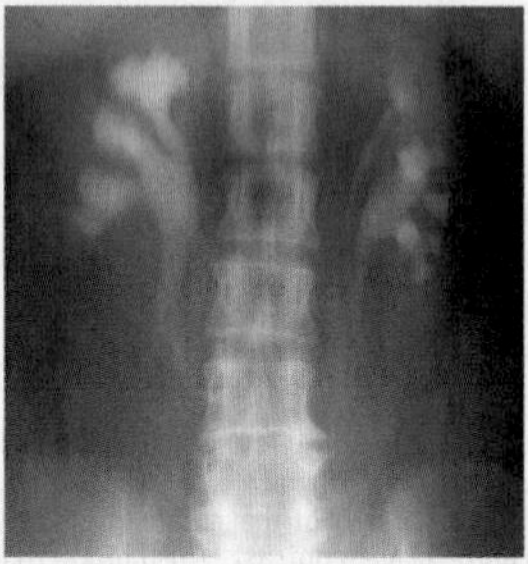

Fig 3. Tomographic IVU: note left duplex system. The superior ureter moiety is usually ectopic and enters the bladder, urethra or vagina more inferiorly than the normally placed inferior moiety. The superior ureter may be associated with a ureterocele and is more likely to obstruct; reflux nephropathy/scarring is more common in the inferior moiety. There appears to be uretero-calyceal system obstruction on the right.

1 Examples of cysts: polycystic kidney disease, medullary sponge kidney, multicystic dysplastic kidney, medullary cystic disease, tuberous sclerosis, renal sinus cysts, von Hippel-Lindau syndrome.

Retrograde pyelography/ureterograms are good at showing pelvicalyceal, ureteric anatomy, and transitional cell carcinomas (TCC). Contrast is injected via a ureteric catheter.

Percutaneous nephrostomy The renal pelvis is punctured (with imaging guidance). Images are got following contrast injection (antegrade pyelogram, **fig 4**). A nephrostomy tube may then be placed to allow drainage.

Renal arteriography (**fig 5**). Therapeutic indications: angioplasty; stenting; selective embolization (bleeding tumour, trauma, or AV malformation).

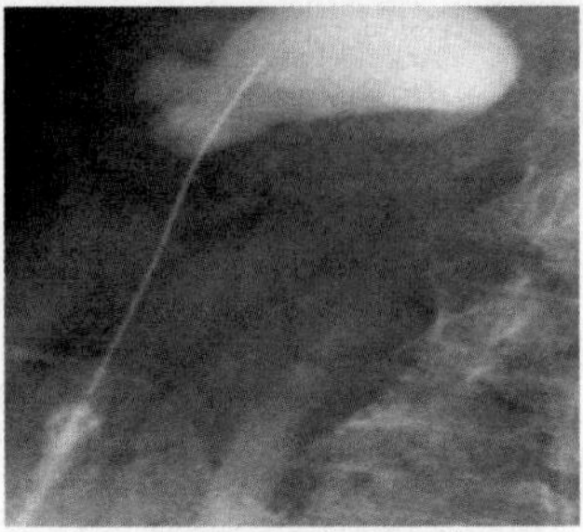

Fig 4. Antegrade pyelogram (fine-needle percutaneous puncture of a dilated renal pelvis; contrast is injected to outline the calyces).

Magnetic resonance imaging (MRI), with its good soft tissue resolution, may be used to clarify equivocal CT findings. Magnetic resonance angiography (MRA) helps image renal artery anatomy/stenosis (**fig 6**).

Radionuclide imaging See p753.

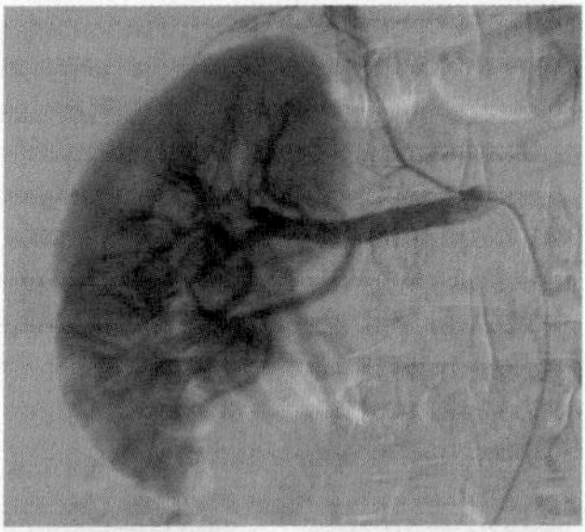

Fig 5. Renal artery digital subtraction angiogram (DSA; DSA is the final arbiter of renal artery stenosis). It is possible to tell that this is a DSA as no other structure has any definition or contrast in the image. There is, however, some interference from overlying bowel gas, which is not an uncommon problem. GI tract peristalsis can be diminished during the examination by using IV *buscopan* or *glucagon*.

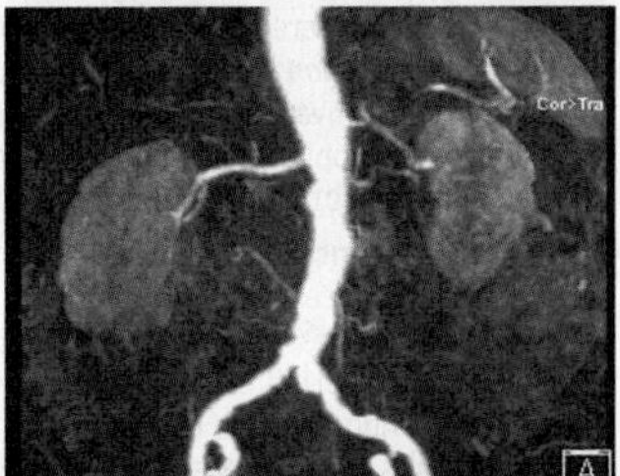

Fig 6. Coronal 3D MRA of the kidneys showing two renal arteries supplying the left kidney. This is important information pre-transplant. Anomalous renal arteries are common and, like the normal renal arteries, are end arteries, hence the consequence of infarction if tied at surgery.

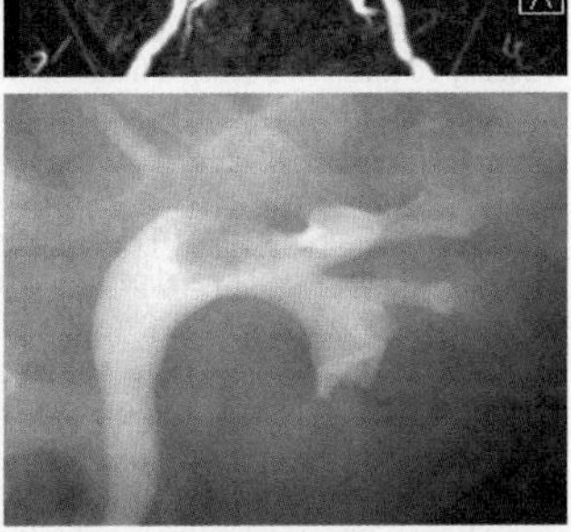

Fig 7. IVU: filling defect in the renal pelvis—eg urothelial tumour (as here), or from stones, haematomas, fungal balls or sloughed papillae (from renal papillary necrosis). The filling defect can sometimes have the impressive multi-faceted appearance of a staghorn calculus that can occupy the entire pelvi-calyceal system.

Figs 1-7 courtesy of Norwich Radiology Dept.

Computed tomography (CT) The attenuation of biological soft tissues is in a narrow range from about +80 for blood and muscle, to 0 for CSF, and down to -100 for fat (Hounsfield units, p744). IV contrast medium may be given, initially giving an angiographic effect as high-attenuation contrast in the vessels whitens them. Later, if there is a defect in the blood-brain barrier, as with tumours or infection, contrast will opacify a lesion's margins, giving enhancing white areas. Some CNS areas have no blood-brain barrier and enhance normally, eg pituitary gland and choroid plexus. Compared with MRI, CT is good at showing acute haemorrhage and fractures, and is much easier to do in ill or anaesthetized patients, and so is good in emergencies. Fresh blood is of higher attenuation (∴ whiter) than brain tissue. Attenuation of haematomas declines as Hb breaks down so that a subacute subdural haematoma at 2wks may have an attenuation the same as adjacent brain, making it difficult to detect. A chronic subdural haematoma will be of relatively low attenuation.

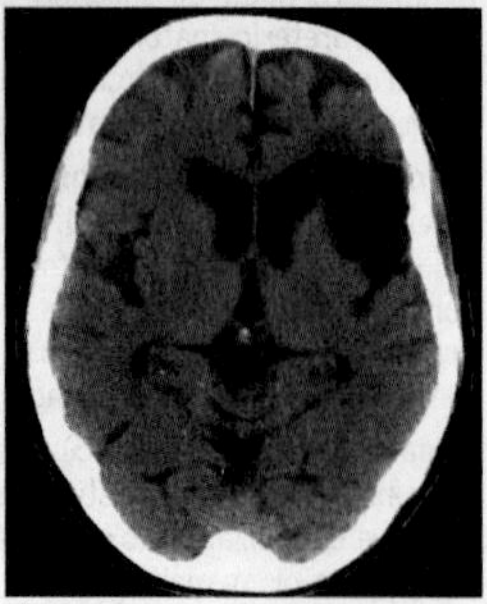

Fig 1. Unenhanced axial CT head: note the old stroke in the left middle cerebral artery territory.

CT is often used in acute stroke to exclude haemorrhage (eg pre-thrombolysis/anticoagulation). The actual area of infarction/ischaemia will not show up for a day or so, and will be low-attenuation **cytotoxic oedema** (intracellular oedema including both white and grey matter—look for loss of grey matter definition).

Tumours and abscesses appear similar, eg a ring enhancing mass, surrounding vasogenic oedema, and mass effect. **Vasogenic oedema** (from leaky capillaries) is extracellular and spreads through the white matter. Mass effect causes compression of the sulci and ipsilateral ventricle, and may also cause herniation (subfalcine, transtentorial, or tonsillar). ►On p487 (& see also **fig 2**) there are images of this.

One indication for CT is acute, severe headache. If concern is about subarachnoid haemorrhage, a non-contrast CT may show acute blood. Even if it does not, it will show if the basal cisterns are normal and therefore lumbar puncture is (probably!) safe.

Cranial CT perfusion is a developing technique that assesses cerebral blood flow without need for invasive angiographic techniques (**fig 5**, p745). *3D CT angiography* gives excellent mapping of the cerebral circulation (**fig 4**), and can be done directly after non-contrast CT if there is subarachnoid haemorrhage, looking for an aneurysm.

Magnetic resonance imaging (MRI) See p748. Example of MRI in stroke: p475. The chief image sequences are:

- *T1-weighted images:* Give good anatomical detail to which the T2 image can be compared. Fat is brightest (signal intensity↑); other tissues are darker to varying degrees. Flowing blood is low signal. Gadolinium-DTPA contrast medium (p762) usually results in an increase in signal intensity.
- *T2-weighted images:* These provide the best detection of most lesions as they usually contain some oedema fluid and therefore appear white (eg **fig 4**, p749). Fat and fluid appear brightest. Flowing blood is again low signal.

Magnetic resonance angiography (MRA) maps carotid, vertebrobasilar and cerebral arterial circulations (+sinuses and veins). *Functional MRI* can image local blood flow.

Contrast angiography (**fig 4**) is less common as a diagnostic tool since the advent of MRA and CT angiography and perfusion techniques, though it has the advantage of being therapeutic—eg coil embolization of saccular aneurysms.

Radionuclide imaging See p752. PET is mostly used as a research tool in dementia, but perfusion scintigraphy can be used in the assessment of Alzheimer's disease, other dementias (**fig 5**), and localising epileptogenic foci. Dopamine scintigraphy can be used to assess local cerebral uptake in Parkinson's disease.

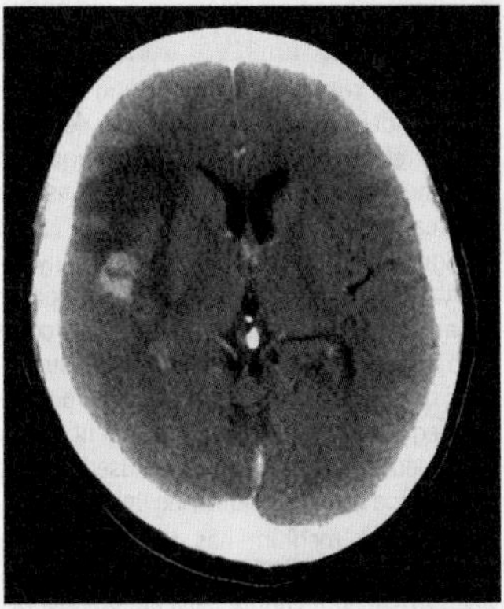

Fig 2. Axial CT of the brain with intravenous contrast. There is a homogenously enhancing well-defined, small mass in the right cerebral hemisphere, that has a central area of non-enhancement. There is a mild mass effect (the corpus callosum is displaced to the left and the right frontal ventricular horn is slightly effaced). Low attenuation (vasogenic oedema) surrounds the mass. Vasogenic oedema respects the grey-white matter junction, whereas cytotoxic oedema (eg from acute infarction) does not. Compare this image with **figs 3 & 4**, p 749...is it the same patient?

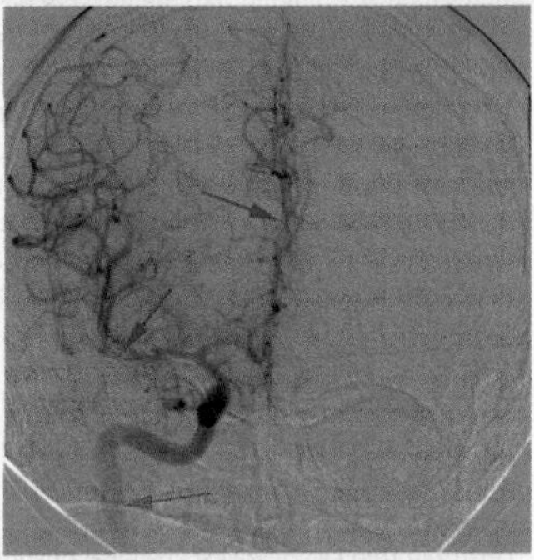

Fig 3. Digital subtraction angiogram (DSA). The right internal carotid artery (yellow arrow), anterior cerebral artery (green arrow) and middle cerebral artery (red arrow) are shown.

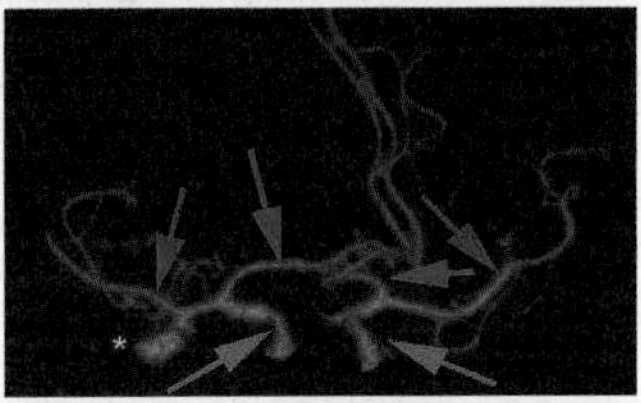

Fig 4. A 3D reconstruction of a CT angiogram of the paired internal carotid arteries (yellow arrows) and their branches (anterior cerebral arteries—green arrows, middle cerebral arteries—red arrows), seen from the front and slightly to the right. There is an aneurysm of the right middle cerebral artery (*).

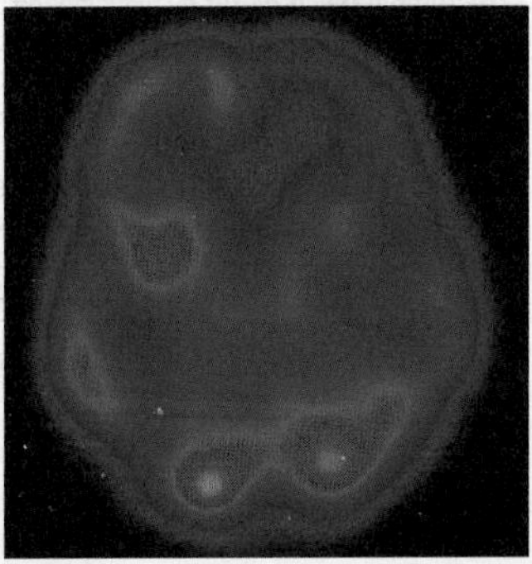

Fig 5. Selected axial image from a cerebral perfusion SPECT study showing hypoperfusion in the left parietal & frontal lobes.

Fig 1 & 2 courtesy of Norwich Radiology Department; figs 3 & 4 courtesy of Dr Chris Cousens; fig 5 courtesy of Dr John Andersen, Princess Alexandra Hospital.

Contrast in imaging

The use of X-irradiation in imaging relies on the principle that tissues of different electron densities produce different degrees of attenuation. Two adjacent tissues of a similar electron density are indistinguishable on plain X-ray. Increasing electron density increases attenuation and makes tissues appear more radio-opaque. Although this can occur pathophysiologically (eg calcification in chronic pancreatitis or malignancy) it can be induced artificially by the use of a contrast medium and thus create a visible interface. Most of the body consists of hydrogen (1 electron), oxygen (8), and carbon (6) atoms. Conventional contrast agents contain iodine (53 electrons) or barium (56). Contrast medium is usually administered by the following routes:

- PO: barium or iodine based agents for swallow, meal, or follow-through.
- PR: eg barium or iodine based agent enema.
- Inhaled: technetium or xenon used in ventilation scintigraphy.
- IV: iodine or gadolinium (see below) based contrast agents (p762).

IV contrast medium has the most widespread clinical application. The ideal intravenous contrast medium should be non-ionic, hydrophilic, iso-osmolar and non-chemotoxic and should have no adverse reactions.

Iodine-based contrast agents Iodine is used because of its relatively high electron density and good physiological tolerance. When used with CT, the examination is said to be **contrast enhanced**—look for '**+ c**' amongst the scan details. Caution should be exercised in patients with the following because of the increased risk of adverse reactions (have latest renal function to hand): renal or cardiac impairment; atopy; myeloma; diabetes; sickle cell disease; the elderly and infants; a history of allergy. Minor reactions include nausea, vomiting and a sensation of warmth. Moderate reactions include urticaria, bronchospasm, angioedema and ↓BP (1:250); theoretical risk of death for 1:150 000 ►*Metformin* must be withheld before and for 48h after IV contrast administration because of risk of lactic acidosis. ►Avoid iodine-based agents in patients with active hyperthyroidism.

Barium sulfate is the most common contrast medium used in examination of the GI tract. Water-insoluble particles of 0.6-1.4μm diameter are mixed with large organic molecules such as pectin and gum to promote good flow, mucosal adherence and high density in thin layers. Risks: chemical pneumonitis or peritonitis.

Water-soluble **iodine based** contrast agents are used instead of barium where there is a risk of peritoneal contamination (eg fistula, megacolon, ulceration, diverticulitis, bowel anastomosis, acute intestinal haemorrhage). ►Contains iodine so establish allergy history and thyroid status.

Air In a double-contrast enema, air (or CO_2) is insufflated as a **negative contrast medium** after barium administration to enhance mucosal definition (**fig 4**, p757).

Gadolinium is a lanthanide series element with paramagnetic qualities that is administered intravenously (as gadolinium-DTPA) to enhance the contrast of certain structures in MRI. It works by reducing the time to relaxation (TR) of hydrogen nuclei in its proximity and appears as high signal on T1 weighted scans. It does not cross the blood-brain barrier so is useful in enhancing isointense extra-axial tumours such as meningiomas. It can also highlight areas where the blood-brain barrier has broken down secondary to inflammatory or neoplastic processes. It is renally excreted: ►check eGFR: if ↓, up to 30% may develop ***progressive nephrogenic systemic fibrosis/nephrogenic fibrosing dermopathy*** which causes generalized fibrosis which impairs movement and breathing—and which may be fatal. Aberrations in calcium-phosphate metabolism and erythropoietin treatment seem to ↑risk.[19]

Other adverse reactions include headache, nausea and local irritation at the site of injection, with idiosyncratic reaction reported in less than 1%.

Imaging the acutely unwell patient

Asking yourself *"Does this investigation need to be done right now?"* will often yield the answer *"No!"*, yet there are a few occasions when early imaging can provide vital diagnostic information and influence the prognosis for a patient:

- Acute cauda equina syndrome (p470): ►►MRI lumbar spine.
- Suspected thoracic aorta dissection (p656): ►►CT thorax + IV contrast, MRI or transoesophageal echo (TOE). The mediastinum is rarely widened on CXR.
- Acute renal failure (p298 & p848): ►►US of renal tract to exclude obstruction.
- Acute pulmonary oedema: ►►Portable CXR: don't delay to get an ideal film.
- Acute abdomen with signs of peritonism: ►►Erect CXR to find intraperitoneal free gas (**fig 1**, p609; ≈GI perforation). Remember: post-op there will be detectable gas (air/CO_2) in the abdomen for ~10 days.[20] Early CT (<6h after onset of symptoms) in addition to plain films appears not to give added diagnostic information in peptic perforation.[21] In one study, performing a US technique (the scissors manoeuvre) to look for sub-diaphragmatic free air had 94% sensitivity and 100% specificity.[22]
- Any patient with post-traumatic midline cervical spine tenderness—not just for the emergency department! ►►Hard collar and backboard immobilisation followed by a lateral C-spine X-ray, then full C-spine series. All the vertebrae down to the top of T1 must be visualised and cleared before it is safe to take the collar off. CT may be required if the plain radiographs are inadequate or inconclusive.
- Sudden onset focal neurology, worst-ever headache, deteriorating GCS: ►►CT head, then LP if no evidence of ↑ICP. Once an examination has been reported as normal, the nursing team can take a rest from work-intensive 'neuro' observations.

Remember that imaging—or re-imaging for a poor quality film—should never delay the definitive treatment of an emergency condition, eg:

- Tension pneumothorax (p824 and **fig 1**): ►►decompression **not** CXR.
- Intra-abdominal haemorrhage or viscus rupture (p608): ►►laparotomy.
- High clinical suspicion of torsion of testis (p654): ►►surgery **not** Doppler US. Collapse, acute abdomen, shock, moribund: ►►laparotomy. A ruptured aneurysm has an extremely poor prognosis that tails off by the minute (p656).

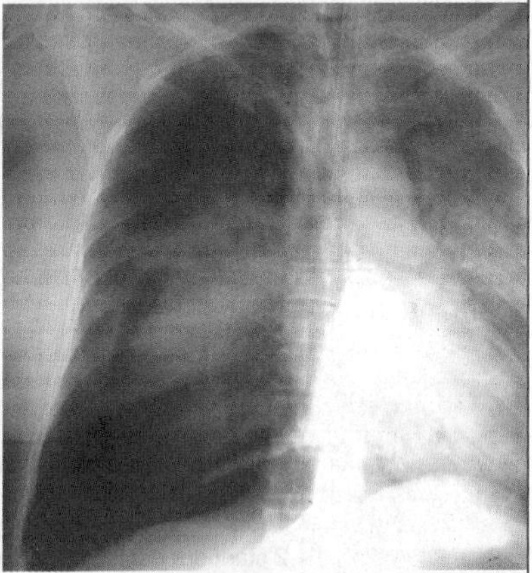

Fig 1. This is a great educational image from ITU. The inexperienced doctor could be distracted by the poor quality, badly centred image: technicians do their best under difficult conditions. To ask for a new CXR here would be a mistake. There is adequate information for a life-saving decision. After checking the name, see that the tubes and lines are well-positioned—the endotracheal & NG tubes and the right subclavian line. **Lungs:** The left lung shows consolidation. The right is too black and the right hemidiaphragm is depressed. **Pleura:** The pleural recess is seen at the right base. **Mediastinum:** Left-shifted, obstructing venous return—so cardiac output↓, and a threat to life. Is it being pushed or pulled? Check hila, bones and soft tissues. Is the ET tube down the right main bronchus, inflating the right lung and collapsing the left? No. Is the right lung collapsed? Yes. ►►Right tension pneumothorax. Needle thoracocentesis decompression and a chest tube are needed now. The left lung consolidation could be a result of any of the causes of ARDS (p178). If intubated, consolidation/collapse often occurs at the left base: suction catheters pass down the ET tube and preferentially into the right main bronchus.

Contents

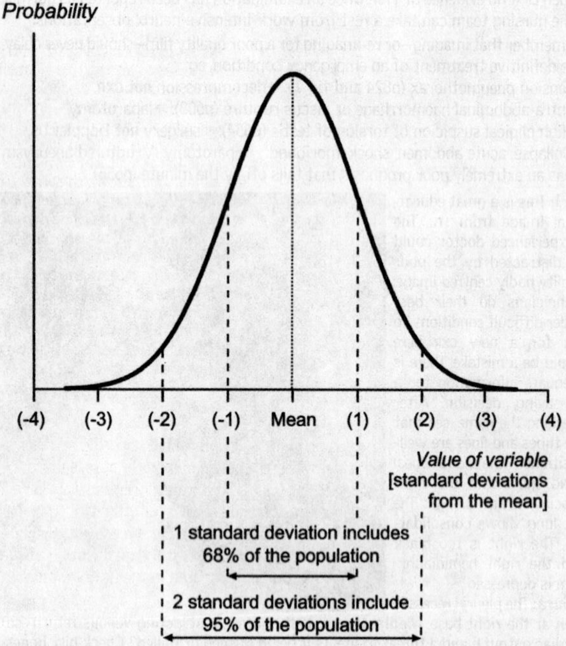

Reproduced with permission from *Concepts of Epidemiology*; Bhopal R, Oxford University Press 2008.

The Gaussian ('Normal') distribution

Once upon a time, in a famous hospital named R– in the middle of England, there lived a crusty old surgeon and a brilliant young house officer. The surgeon issued infallible and peremptory edicts such as "All my patients with a haemoglobin less than 10 must be transfused." Everyone did as the surgeon said (this was a long time ago) except for the wily house officer who understood statistics, sampling error, and the play of chance. One day she was rung up by the haematologist who asked her "Why have you requested 3 blood counts on Mrs Wells today? One is enough. You are wasting our resources!" "Not so," said the house officer. "The first Hb was 9.8, the second was 9.7 and the third was 10.1g/dL. I knew if I was persistent, I stood a good chance of preventing an unnecessary transfusion. She is a patient of Mr X." The two conspirators smiled at each other down the telephone, and no more was said. Of course the right way of dealing with this problem is through clinical governance and dialogue with the surgeon. But the point remains: numbers are elastic, despite, on occasion, being given to 3 decimal places. Don't believe in them as absolute entities, and don't believe that the normal range is anything other than arbitrary; think before you act: think statistically. *Think like Gauss.*

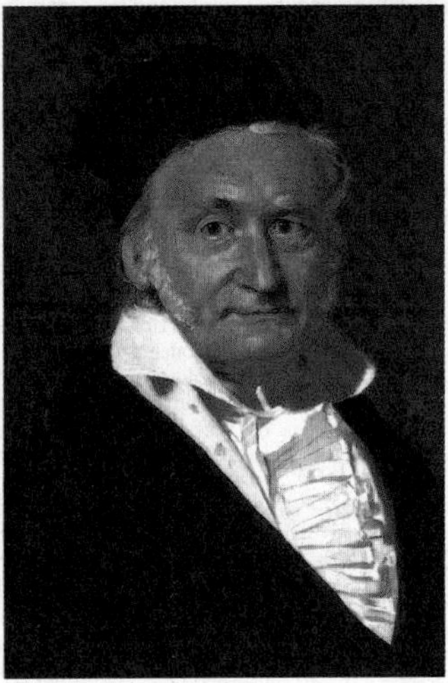

Fig 1. Carl Friedrich Gauss (1777-1855) and his Gaussian ('Normal') distribution. This bell-shaped graph is the theoretical basis of reference intervals (normal values—see below). In some ways Gauss would have made an ideal handbook author: he left behind him a tiny notebook of just 19 pages which solved 146 problems in mathematics including non-Euclidean geometry—his motto being *pauca sed matura* (few but ripe). His messages were brief and perhaps *too* much to the point (not surprisingly, since he invented the first telegraph in 1833)—on being disturbed during deep thought to be told that his wife was dying it is reported that he replied "Tell her to wait a moment until I'm through..." [1]

Image courtesy of Axel Wittman

Some definitions

- ***Range:*** The lowest and highest value of all observations in the set being studied.
- ***Arithmetic mean:*** The sum of all observations ÷ by the number of observations.
- ***Median:*** The median is the middle value (eg 9 data points are higher and 9 are lower). If their distribution is Normal, then the median coincides with the mean.
- ***Standard deviation (SD):*** The square root of the variance (the average of the square of the distance of each data point from the mean). When the distribution of the observations is Normal, 95% of observations are located in the interval 'mean ± 1.96 SD.' This is the basis of the reference interval.
- ***Standard error of the mean:*** This gives an estimate of the reliability of the mean of a sample representing the mean of the population from which the sample was taken, and is the SD of the sample ÷ by the square root of the number of observations in the sample. Thus the larger the sample size, the smaller the standard error of the mean. Sample means are always Normally distributed, even if the underlying population they are taken from is not, thus you would expect 95% of those sample means to fall within the range '*population* mean ± 1.96 × *population* SD.'

►Ranges should only be used as a guide to treatment. A drug in an apparently too low concentration may still be clinically useful.[2] Some patients require (and tolerate) levels in the 'toxic' range.

►The time since the last dose should be specified on the request form.

Amikacin Peak (1h post IV dose): 20–30mg/L. Trough: <10mg/L.

Carbamazepine Optimal concentration: 20–50μmol/L (4–12mg/L).

*† **Digoxin** (6–12h post dose) 1–2.6nmol/L (0.8–2μg/L). <1.3nmol/L may be toxic if there is hypokalaemia. *Signs of toxicity*—CVS: arrhythmias, heart block. CNS: confusion, insomnia, agitation, seeing too much yellow (xanthopsia), delirium. GI: nausea. *NB:* in those over 65yrs, 0.5–0.9ng/mL may be sufficient and if the indication is CCF.[3]

*† ***Gentamicin*** (p381) and ***tobramycin*** The potential for oto- and nephrotoxicity is high if aminoglycosides are used inappropriately, so use local expert advice/guidelines. *Signs of toxicity:* tinnitus, deafness, nystagmus, vertigo, renal failure. Although historically given two or three times daily, many now favour **once-daily dosing**, such as the Hartford protocol (**fig 1**),[4] with fewer SEs, and better bactericidal activity. They are suitable only for short therapeutic courses, and are contraindicated in severe renal or liver failure, ascites, burns, high cardiac output states (eg anaemia, Paget's disease), children, and pregnancy. In endocarditis, dosing 8-hourly increases the synergistic bactericidal effect of prescribing gentamicin with other agents (see p145). **Divided daily dosing** in such cases may be calculated as 1mg/kg/8h (or 12-hourly in renal failure), or more accurately using a nomogram such as that shown in **fig 2**. Peak (1h post-dose) and trough (just before dose) levels should be monitored daily—*peak:* 5–10mg/L (3–5mg/L in IE); *trough:* <2mg/L (<1mg/L in IE). Adjust the **dose** if peak level is out of range, and dose **interval** if trough level is out of range.

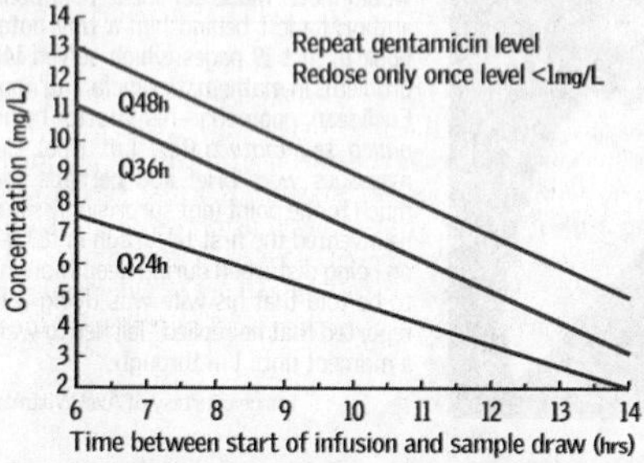

Fig 1. Hartford protocol for 7mg/kg once-daily gentamicin dosing IVI over 15min. Adjust the dosing interval depending on the zone into which the level falls. Q48h means give every 48h; Q24h means give once daily. Above the blue line repeat the gentamicin level and redose only once level <1mg/L. Use lean body weight (p446).

Antimicrobial Agents and Chemotherapy, 1995, Vol 39, pages 650–655, with permission from American Society for Microbiology.

† ***Lithium*** (12h post dose). Guidelines vary: 0.4–0.8mmol/L is reasonable. *Early* signs of toxicity (Li^+ >1.5mmol/L): tremor. *Intermediate:* lethargy. *Late:* (Li^+ >2mmol/L) spasms, coma, fits, arrhythmias, renal failure (haemodialysis may be needed). See *OHCS* p354.

Phenobarbital Trough: 60–180μmol/L (15–40mg/L).

*† ***Phenytoin*** Trough: 40–80μmol/L (10–20mg/L). Beware if ↑↓ albumin, as the assay is for bound phenytoin, while it is free phenytoin that is pharmacologically important. *Signs of toxicity:* ataxia, diplopia, nystagmus, sedation, dysarthria.

Theophylline 10–20mg/mL (55–110μmol/L). (►see p821) Take sample 4–6h after starting an infusion (which should be stopped for ~15min just before the specimen is taken). *Signs of toxicity:* arrhythmias, anxiety, tremor, convulsions.

Vancomycin Trough: 5–10 mg/L (10–15mg/L in SBE/IE and less-sensitive MRSA infections). Start monitoring 48h after 1st dose.

* Trough levels should be taken just before the next dose.

† Drugs for which *routine* monitoring is indicated.

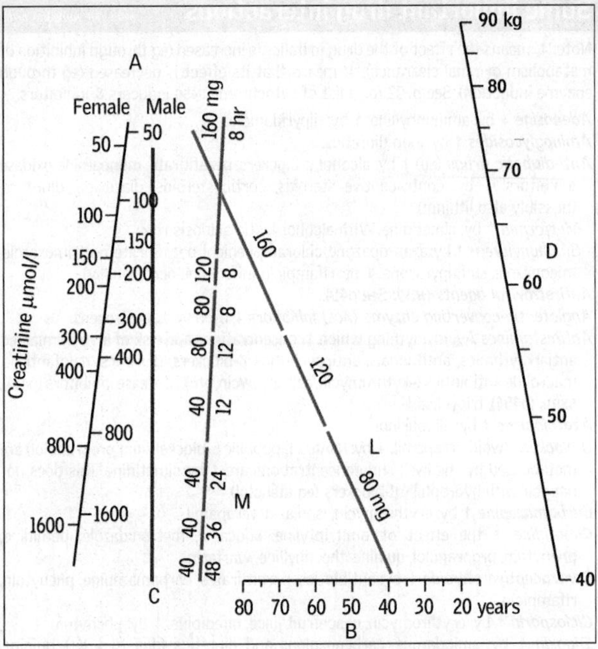

Fig 2. Nomogram for divided daily dosing of gentamicin.

1 Join with a straight line the serum creatinine concentration appropriate to the sex on scale A and the age on scale B. Mark the point at which this line cuts line C.

2 Join with a line the mark on line C and the body weight on line D. Mark the points at which this line cuts lines L and M, to get loading & maintenance doses, respectively.

3 Confirm the appropriateness of this regimen at an early stage by measuring serum levels, especially in severe illness and renal impairment.

4 Adjust dose if peak concentration (1h after IM dose; ½h after IV dose) outside the range 5-10mg/L. A trough concentration (just before dose) above 2mg/L indicates the need for a longer dosage interval.

Note: '↑' means the effect of the drug in italics is increased (eg through inhibition of metabolism or renal clearance). '↓' means that its effect is decreased (eg through enzyme induction). See p702 for a list of cytochrome P450 inducers & inhibitors.

Adenosine ↓ by: aminophylline. ↑ by: dipyridamole.

Aminoglycosides ↑ by: loop diuretics.

Anti-diabetic drugs (all) ↑ by: alcohol, β-blockers, bezafibrate, monoamine oxidase inhibitors. ↓ by: contraceptive steroids, corticosteroids, diazoxide, diuretics, (possibly also lithium).

Metformin ↑ by: cimetidine. With alcohol: lactic acidosis risk.

Sulphonylureas ↑ by: azapropazone, chloramphenicol, bezafibrate, co-trimoxazole, miconazole, sulfinpyrazone. ↓ by: rifampicin (nifedipine occasionally).

Antiretroviral agents (HIV): See p414.

Angiotensin-converting enzyme (ACE) inhibitors ↓ by: NSAIDs, oestrogens.

Antihistamines Avoid anything which ↑ concentrations and risk of arrhythmias, eg antiarrhythmics, antifungals, antipsychotics, β-blockers, diuretics, halofantrine, macrolide antibiotics (erythromycin, azithromycin, etc), protease inhibitors (p414), SSRIs (p454), tricyclics.

Azathioprine ↑ by: allopurinol.

β-blockers Avoid verapamil. ↓ by: NSAIDs. Lipophilic β-blockers (eg propranolol) are metabolized by the liver, and concentrations are ↑ by cimetidine. This does not happen with hydrophilic β-blockers (eg atenolol).

Carbamazepine ↑ by: erythromycin, isoniazid, verapamil.

Cimetidine ↑ the effect of: amitriptyline, lidocaine, metronidazole, pethidine, phenytoin, propranolol, quinine, theophylline, warfarin.

Contraceptive steroids ↓ by: antibiotics, barbiturates, carbamazepine, phenytoin, rifampicin.

Ciclosporin ↑ by: erythromycin, grapefruit juice, nifedipine. ↓ by: phenytoin.

Digoxin ↑ by: amiodarone, carbenoxolone and diuretics (due to ↓ K^+), quinine, verapamil.

Diuretics ↓ by: NSAIDs—particularly indometacin.

Ergotamine ↑ by: erythromycin (ergotism may occur).

Fluconazole: Avoid concurrent astemizole.

Lithium ↑ by: thiazide diuretics.

Methotrexate ↑ by: aspirin, NSAIDs. Many antibiotics (check *BNF*).

Phenytoin ↑ by: chloramphenicol, cimetidine, disulfiram, isoniazid, sulfonamides. ↓ by: carbamazepine.

Potassium-sparing diuretics with ACE-inhibitors: Hyperkalaemia.

Theophyllines ↑ by: cimetidine, ciprofloxacin, erythromycin, contraceptive steroids, propranolol. ↓ by: barbiturates, carbamazepine, phenytoin, rifampicin. See p821.

Valproate ↓ by: carbamazepine, phenobarbital, phenytoin.

Warfarin and ***nicoumalone*** (=acenocoumarol) ↑ by: alcohol, allopurinol, amiodarone, aspirin, chloramphenicol, cimetidine, ciprofloxacin, co-trimoxazole, danazol, dipyridamole, disulfiram, erythromycin (and broad-spectrum antibiotics), gemfibrozil, glucagon, ketoconazole, metronidazole, miconazole, nalidixic acid, neomycin, NSAIDs, phenytoin, quinidine, simvastatin (but not pravastatin), sulfinpyrazone, sulfonamides, tetracyclines, thyroxine.

Warfarin and ***nicoumalone*** ↓ by: aminoglutethimide, barbiturates, carbamazepine, contraceptive steroids, dichloralphenazone, griseofulvin, rifampicin, phenytoin, vitamin K.

Zidovudine (AZT) ↑ by: paracetamol (increased marrow toxicity).

IVI solutions to avoid

Dextrose: Avoid furosemide, ampicillin, hydralazine, insulin, melphalan, phenytoin, and quinine.

0.9% saline: Avoid amphotericin, lidocaine, nitroprusside.

Haematology reference intervals

(For B_{12}, folate, Fe, and TIBC, see p770–1)

Measurement	**Reference interval**	**Your hospital**
White cell count (WCC)	$4.0\text{–}11.0 \times 10^9$/L	
Red cell count	♂ $4.5\text{–}6.5 \times 10^{12}$/L	
	♀ $3.9\text{–}5.6 \times 10^{12}$/L	
Haemoglobin	♂ 13.0–18.0g/dL	
	♀ 11.5–16.0g/dL	
Packed red cell volume (PCV) or haematocrit	♂ 0.4–0.54L/L	
	♀ 0.37–0.47L/L	
Mean cell volume (MCV)	76–96fL	
Mean cell haemoglobin (MCH)	27–32pg	
Mean cell haemoglobin concentration (MCHC)	30–36g/dL	
Neutrophils	$2.0\text{–}7.5 \times 10^9$/L; 40–75% WCC	
Lymphocytes	$1.3\text{–}3.5 \times 10^9$/L; 20–45% WCC	
Eosinophils	$0.04\text{–}0.44 \times 10^9$/L; 1–6% WCC	
Basophils	$0.0\text{–}0.10 \times 10^9$/L; 0–1% WCC	
Monocytes	$0.2\text{–}0.8 \times 10^9$/L; 2–10% WCC	
Platelet count	$150\text{–}400 \times 10^9$/L	
Reticulocyte count	0.8–2.0%[1] $25\text{–}100 \times 10^9$/L	
Erythrocyte sedimentation rate	Depends on age (p366)	
Prothrombin time (citrated bottle) (factors I, II, VII, X)	10–14s	
Activated partial thromboplastin time (VIII, IX, XI, XII)	35–45s	
D-dimer (citrated bottle, as for INR)[2]	<0.5mg/L	

Proposed therapeutic ranges for prothrombin time: See p345

1 Only use percentages as reference interval if red cell count is normal; otherwise, use the absolute value. Express as a ratio *vs* control.

2 D-dimer assay is useful for *excluding* thromboembolic disease if the assay is normal. The D-dimer is so non-specific, however, that a raised level is unhelpful, thus the assay should only be requested if the probability of thromboembolic disease is low (eg Wells score; see p581).

See p676 *for the philosophy of the normal range*; see OHCS p222 *for children.* Drugs (and other substances) may interfere with any chemical method; as these effects may be method dependent, it is difficult for the clinician to be aware of all the possibilities. If in doubt, discuss with the lab.

Substance	**Specimen**	**Reference interval** *(labs vary, so a guide only)*	**Your hospital**
Adrenocorticotrophic hormone	P	<80ng/L	
Alanine aminotransferase (ALT)	P	5–35U/L	
Albumin[1]	P	35–50g/L	
Aldosterone[2]	P	100–500pmol/L	
Alkaline phosphatase	P	30–150U/L (adults)	
α-amylase	P	0–180 Somogyi U/dL	
α-fetoprotein	S	<10kU/L	
Angiotensin II[2]	P	5–35pmol/L	
Antidiuretic hormone (ADH)	P	0.9–4.6pmol/L	
Aspartate transaminase	P	5–35U/L	
Bicarbonate[1]	P	24–30mmol/L	
Bilirubin	P	3–17µmol/L	
BNP (see p689)	P	<50ng/L	
Calcitonin	P	<0.1µg/L	
Calcium (ionized)	P	1.0–1.25mmol/L	
Calcium[1] (total) See p690 to correct for albumin	P	2.12–2.65mmol/L	
Chloride	P	95–105mmol/L	
Cholesterol[3] (see p704)	P	<5.0mmol/L	
VLDL (see p704)	P	0.128–0.645mmol/L	
LDL	P	<2.0mmol/L	
HDL	P	0.9–1.93mmol/L	
Cortisol	P	AM 450–700nmol/L midnight 80–280nmol/L	
Creatine kinase (CK)	P	♂ 25–195U/L ♀ 25–170U/L	
Creatinine[1] (∝ to lean body mass)	P	70–150µmol/L	
Ferritin	P	12–200µg/L	
Folate	S	2.1µg/L	
Follicle-stimulating hormone (FSH)	P/S	2–8U/L in ♀ (luteal); >25U/L in menopause	
Gamma-glutamyl transpeptidase	P	♂ 11–51U/L ♀ 7–33U/L	
Glucose (fasting)	P	3.5–5.5mmol/L	
Growth hormone	P	<20mU/L	
HbA_{1c} = glycosylated Hb (DCCT)	B	4–6%. 7% ≈ good DM control	
HbA_{1c} IFCC (more specific than DCCT)	B	20–42mmol/mol; 53 ≈ good DM control	
Iron	S	♂ 14–31µmol/L ♀ 11–30µmol/L	
Lactate	P ABG	Venous 0.6–2.4mmol/L Arterial 0.6–1.8mmol/L	
Lactate dehydrogenase (LDH)	P	70–250U/L	
Lead	B	<1.8mmol/L	
Luteinizing hormone (LH) (premenopausal)	P	3–16U/L (luteal)	

1 See *OHCS* p15 for reference intervals in pregnancy.
2 The sample requires special handling: contact the laboratory.
3 Desired upper limit of cholesterol would be <6mmol/L. In some populations, 7.8mmol/L is the top end of the distribution.

Magnesium	P	0.75–1.05mmol/L
Osmolality	P	278–305mosmol/kg
Parathyroid hormone (PTH)	P	<0.8–8.5pmol/L
Potassium	P	3.5–5.0mmol/L
Prolactin	P	♂ <450u/L ♀ <600u/L
Prostate specific antigen (PSA)	P	0–4µg/ml, age specific, see p538
Protein (total)	P	60–80g/L
Red cell folate	B	0.36–1.44µmol/L (160–640µg/L)
Renin[2] (erect/recumbent)	P	2.8–4.5/ 1.1–2.7pmol/mL/h
Sodium[1]	P	135–145mmol/L
Thyroid-binding globulin (TBG)	P	7–17mg/L
Thyroid-stimulating hormone (TSH)	P	0.5–5.7mU/L widens with age, p208
Thyroxine (T4)	P	70–140nmol/L
Thyroxine (free)	P	9–22pmol/L
Total iron-binding capacity	S	54–75µmol/L
Triglyceride	P	0.55–1.90mmol/L
Triiodothyronine (T3)	P	1.2–3.0nmol/L
Troponin T (see p112)	P	<0.1µg/L
Urate[1]	P	♂ 210–480µmol/L ♀ 150–390µmol/L
Urea[1]	P	2.5–6.7mmol/L
Vitamin B_{12}	S	0.13–0.68nmol/L (>150ng/L)
Vitamin D	S	60–105nmol/L

Arterial blood gases reference intervals

pH: 7.35–7.45 P_aCO_2: 4.7–6.0kPa

P_aO_2: >10.6kPa   Base excess: ±2mmol/L

Note: 7.6mmHg = 1kPa (atmospheric pressure ≈ 100kPa)

Urine reference intervals	Reference interval	Your hospital
Cortisol (free)	<280nmol/24h	
Hydroxyindole acetic acid	16–73µmol/24h	
Hydroxymethylmandelic acid (HMMA, VMA)	16–48µmol/24h	
Metanephrines	0.03–0.69µmol/mmol creatinine (or <5.5µmol/day)	
Osmolality	350–1000mosmol/kg	
17-oxogenic steroids	♂ 28–30µmol/24h ♀ 21–66µmol/24h	
17-oxosteroids (neutral)	♂ 17–76µmol/24h ♀ 14–59µmol/24h	
Phosphate (inorganic)	15–50mmol/24h	
Potassium	14–120mmol/24h	
Protein	<150mg/24h	
Sodium	100–250mmol/24h	

P=plasma (eg citrate bottle); **S**=serum (clotted; no anticoagulant); **B**=whole blood (edetic acid EDTA bottle)

Contents

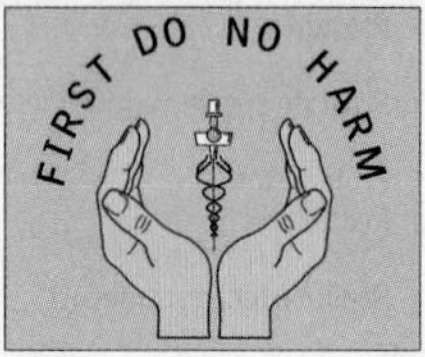

Fig 1. Hands-on experience is a vital part of the learning process in medicine—without it we could never hope to improve our skills, and they would gently drift away from us on a current of inadequacy. But a golden rule to remember is: ▶*first do no harm.* We must know when we are out of our depth. A call for senior help may be one of the most important that you ever make.

▶Always keep your skills in emergency procedures well-honed by going on courses etc. It is often wiser to wait for someone else to come and carry out an urgent procedure than to try for the first time by oneself (**fig 1**)—but some procedures must occasionally be performed at once—see EMERGENCY BOX, p775.

Relevant pages in other chapters: Arrhythmias (p118); bone marrow biopsy (p358); cardiogenic shock (p814); consent, (p570); intravenous fluid therapy (p680); liver failure (p258); local anaesthetics (TABLE, p575); meningitis (p832); pleural effusion (p184); pneumothorax (p182, p824); renal biopsy (p303); subarachnoid haemorrhage (p482); tension pneumothorax (p824); the venous system of the thoracic inlet (BOX, p589).

Nasogastric tubes

These tubes are passed into the stomach via the nose—orogastric if via the mouth—and drain externally. Sizes: 16 = large, 12 = medium, 10 = small. **Uses**:

- To empty the stomach: eg pre-op, acute pancreatitis, intestinal obstruction, paralytic ileus, gastric outflow obstruction, risk of aspiration.
- For gastric lavage following overdose.
- Intra-operatively: eg to inflate/deflate the stomach to give easier access to the upper abdomen, to decompress the bowel or to test an anastomosis.
- For irreversible dysphagia: eg motor neuron disease.
- For feeding ill patients: use a special fine-bore tube.

Passing the tube Nurses are experts and will ask you (who may never have passed one) to do so only when they fail—so the first question to ask is: "Have you asked the charge-nurse from the ward next door?"

- Wear non-sterile gloves and an apron to protect from those 'rich encrustations' so often found on our clothes after a few days on the wards.[1]
- Explain the procedure. Take a new, cool (hence less flexible) tube. Have a cup of water to hand. Lubricate well with aqueous gel.
- Use the tube, by holding it against the patient's head, to estimate the length required to get from the nostril to the back of the throat.
- Place lubricated tube in nostril with its natural curve promoting passage down, rather than up. The right nostril is often easier than the left. Advance directly backwards (not upwards).
- When the tip is estimated to be entering the throat, rotate the tube by ~180° to discourage passage into the mouth.
- Advance the tube into the oesophagus during a swallow and thence to the stomach. It may be easier to swallow with a sip of water and easier to advance if rotating rather than pushing. **If this fails:** Try the other nostril, then oral insertion.
- The tube has distance markings along it: the stomach is at ~35–40cm in adults, so advance > this distance, preferably 10–20cm beyond. Tape securely to the nose.
- Check placement: use pH paper (pH gradations of 0.5 and a pH range of 0–6 or 1–11) to test that you are in the stomach: aspirated gastric contents are acid (pH ≤5.5). Turning the patient on the left side helps dip the tube in gastric contents. Aspirates should be >0.5mL and tested directly on unhandled pH paper. Allow 10s for the colour change to occur. Litmus paper is less reliable, as is the 'woosh test'—listening over the stomach for bubbling (=*borborygmi*) with a stethoscope whilst pushing 5–10mL of air down the tube.[2] If a CXR is to be used to check positioning (not always needed)—the whoosh test may be a useful screening test in some hands: if negative, a disruptive CXR may be avoided, as the tube is most unlikely to be in the stomach.[3] (It is more likely to be in lung, oesophagus, or coiled in the pharynx.) Aspirates are harder to get from fine-bore tubes, and a CXR is more likely to be needed. *Additional tip:* If the patient is alert with intact swallowing, ask him to sip a coloured drink, and aspirate the tube; if you get the coloured fluid back, the tube must be in the stomach.[4]
- Either spigot the tube, or allow to drain into a dependent catheter bag secured to clothing (zinc oxide tape around tube to form a flap, safety pin through flap).

►Do not pass a tube nasally if there is any suspicion of a facial fracture.

►Get senior help if the patient has recently had upper GI surgery—it is not good news to have pushed the tube through a fresh anastomosis!

Complications: • Pain, or, rarely: • Loss of electrolytes • Oesophagitis • Tracheal or duodenal intubation • Necrosis: retro- or nasopharyngeal • Stomach perforation.

Weaning When planning removal of an NGT *in situ* for decompression or relief of obstruction, it is wise to wean it so that the patient manages well without it:

- First it should be on free drainage with eg 4hrly aspirations;
- Then spigot with 4hrly aspirations;
- Then spigot only. If this is tolerated along with oral intake then it is probably safe to remove the tube; if not, then take a step backwards.

►Although siting a cannula has almost become *de rigueur* for hospital admissions, try to avoid IVIs, as infections/MRSA at the IVI site can cause real problems, especially in the elderly. Insertion skill is best shown at the bedside by an expert:

1 **Set up a tray** Swab to clean skin; cannula(e); syringe + 1mL 1% *lidocaine*; cotton-wool/gauze swab to stop bleeding from unsuccessful attempts; tape/ Tegaderm® to fix cannula; Elastoplast; saline flush; portable sharps bin: ►**needlestick injuries do happen**. Take multiple items for brave but failed attempts.
2 **Set up a drip-stand** with first bag of fluid (carefully checked with a nurse); 'run through' a giving set (a nurse will show you how).
3 **Wash hands and ask a nurse to help** until you are experienced. Nurses prefer helping rather than changing the bed clothes because of spilt blood.
4 **Explain** the procedure to the patient, including that only the tube and **not** the needle remains in the arm. Place the tourniquet around the arm.
5 **Have the patient lying down** This prevents most faints.
6 **Search hard for the best vein** (palpable, not merely visible). Don't be too hasty. Rest the arm below the level of the heart to aid filling. Ask them to clench and unclench their fist. Feel with your most sensitive finger—a golden touch will come with practice.
7 ►**Stay away from** arms with AV dialysis fistulae and the ipsilateral side to axillary surgery. Also avoid sites crossing a joint, if possible.
8 **Get comfortable** It makes all the difference when learning.
9 **Place a paper towel** under arm to soak up any blood.
10 **Tap the vein** to make it prominent.
11 **Clean the skin** Use local anaesthetic (or *Emla*® cream or **tetracaine** 4% gel[5]): it is kinder, it **does** work, but takes ~¾h to work. Consider using a fine needle to raise a bleb of *lidocaine*, like a nettle sting, just to the vein's side. Wait 15s.

After it is in: 1 Take blood with a syringe or adapter, if you are going to. 2 Remove the tourniquet. 3 Flush the cannula checking flow. 4 Fix cannula firmly with tape. 5 Connect fluid tube. 6 Bandage a loop of the tube to the arm. If the drip is across a joint, use a splint. 7 Check the flow speed. Write a fluid chart (p680). 8 When the drip comes down, remove the cannula. (A patient once asked at follow-up if he still needed 'this green plastic thing in my hand'.) NB: Adding heparin to the IVI has not been shown to maintain patency (unlike arterial lines).[6]

If you fail after 3 attempts ►Shocked patients need fluid quickly: if you are having trouble putting in a drip, call your senior. The advice below assumes that the drip is not immediately life-saving. ►►If it is, see EMERGENCY BOX.

Experienced doctors can forget they had to learn. Ask to be taught and for help when you need it. Is this the right needle for the right job? What is the drip for? If the patient may need blood quickly, use a large size (eg grey; green is suitable for slow IVIs—or even pink if the veins are fragile (see TABLE). Other measures:

- Try submerging the arm in a bowl of warm water for 2min.
- Use a blood pressure cuff at 80mmHg as a tourniquet.
- Try putting a small amount of GTN paste over the vein.
- Ultrasound may be used to identify a suitable vein and to guide insertion.

If you still cannot get the drip in You are now downcast, so call your senior—it may hurt your pride but perhaps this was not your time. Calling him could make him, you and your patient happy and not many things do that! If you are afraid to ask your senior, ask another colleague—they are much more likely to succeed than you at this juncture. If you cannot find anyone to help, have a coffee and return an hour later. Veins are capricious: they come and go.

Re-siting Inflamed drip sites need prompt re-siting of the drip. If site is healthy, gently infuse a 5mL syringe of 0.9% saline through the cannula. If resistance and/or pain prevents this, the drip needs re-siting. If the drip has 'tissued' (subcutaneous leakage), re-siting is also required (see BOX).

'The drip has tissued'

If you are called about this, ask yourself:

• Is there fluid in bag and giving set? • Inspect the cannula: take bandage off. • Is the drip still needed? • Are the control taps open? • Are there kinks in the tube? • Is a venous valve blocking the cannula end?

Intravenous cannulae sizes and UK colour conventions

Gauge	Colour	Diameter (mm)	Length (mm)	Flow rate (mL/min[V])
14G		2.0	45	250
16G		1.7	42	170
18G		1.2	40	90
20G		1.0	32	55
22G		0.28	25	25
24G		0.7	19	24

V=Maximum flow rate under gravity.

According to Poiseuille's law[1] the flow rate (Q) of a fluid through a tubular structure is inversely proportional to viscosity (η) and length (l) and proportional to the pressure difference across it ($P_i - P_o$) and the radius to the power of 4. Hence:

$$Q \propto \frac{(P_i - P_o)\, r^4}{\eta\, l}$$

A last throw of the dice

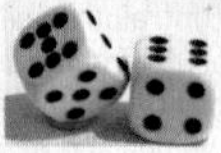

Just once it may come down to you. For some, this is one of the challenges and thrills in medicine. There may be no one else available to help when there is an absolute and urgent indication for IV drugs/fluids/blood—and all of the above measures have been tried, and have failed. Think of lonesome night shifts, overrun emergency departments, a disaster scene, war, or medicine in the field. The following measures are not recommended for non-life-threatening scenarios.

⏩ Don't worry. Have a good look again. Feet? Inside of the forearm? Upper arm?

⏩ Have you really exhausted all of your options for help from a colleague? Maybe the ITU registrar is approachable—they do have remarkable skills.

⏩ Is the patient familiar with his/her own veins (eg previous IV drug abuser)?

⏩ If there is only a small amount IV medication required and a small, short vein, you may be able to gain access with a carefully placed butterfly needle that is taped down. Some drugs cannot be passed this way (eg **amiodarone**, K^+).

⏩ The external jugular vein may become prominent when the patient is head down (Trendelenberg) by 5-10° (▶not in situations of fluid overload, LVF, ↑ICP) Only attempt cannulation of this vein if you are not going to jeopardise future central line insertion, and if you can clearly determine the surrounding anatomy.

Only do the following if you have had the appropriate training/experience:

⏩ Options in children: **1** Inserting an intraosseous needle 2-3cm inferior and just medial to the tibial tuberosity (indicated after 2 failed peripheral cannulations in an emergency). This is not generally done in adults (off the battlefield)[7] as the bone is far less forgiving and far more painful. **2** Cannulating a scalp vein.

⏩ Central venous catheterisation (p789). This may be just as hard in a profoundly hypovolaemic arrest patient, and a good knowledge of local anatomy and of the procedure (± ultrasound guidance) will be invaluable.

NB: **A cut down to the long saphenous** vein may (must!) be attempted, *in extremis*,[8] *even if you have no prior experience* (at this site you won't kill by being ham-fisted). ⏩Make a transverse incision 1-2cm anterior and superior to the medial malleolus ⏩Free the vein with forceps ⏩Cannulate it under direct vision. **▶Here, 'first do no harm' is trumped by 'nothing ventured, nothing gained'.**

Hopefully, it shouldn't ever have to come to these measures, but one day...

1 Poiseuille's law is a neat piece of physiology and worth remembering—it is applicable in some form to almost every system in the body.

Catheters *Size:* (in French gauge): 12=small; 16=large; 20=very large (eg 3-way). Use the smallest you can. ***Material:*** Latex is soft (►ask about allergy); Simplastic firmer. A silastic (silicone) catheter may be used long term, but costs more. Silver alloy coating reduces infections[9]. ***Shape:*** **Foley** is typical (**fig 1**); *coudé* **(elbow)** catheters have an angled tip to ease around prostates but are more risky; **Teeman** catheters have tapered ends for a similar reason; **3-way** catheters are used in clot or debris retention and have an extra, separate lumen for irrigation fluid that is attached to the irrigation set via an extra port on the distal end (**fig 2**)—call the urology ward for advice on how to set this up. **Condom** (Conveen®) catheters♂ (Paul's tubing) have no indwelling parts, and are preferred by nurses and patients (less pain) even though they may leak and fall off.[10]

Catheter problems: •*Infection* ~5% develop bacteraemia (don't use antibiotics unless systemically unwell—discuss with microbiology). Consider bladder irrigation, eg 0.9% saline or chlorhexidine 0.02% (may irritate). •***Bladder spasm*** may be painful —try reducing the water in the balloon or an anticholinergic drug, eg *oxybutinin*.

Methods of catheterizing bladders

Checklist:
•Gloves
•Catheter
•*Lidocaine* jelly
•10mL 0.9% saline
•Prep, eg Savlon®
•Drape
•Kidney dish
•Gauze swabs
•Forceps
•Drainage bag
•Specimen container

1 ***Per urethram:*** This route is used to relieve urinary retention, to monitor urine output in critically ill patients, or to collect urine for diagnosis uncontaminated by urethral flora. ►It is contraindicated in urethral injury (eg pelvic fracture) and acute prostatitis. Catheterization introduces bacteria into the bladder, so **aseptic technique is vital**.[1] Nurses can catheterize women and men; you too should be able to catheterize both.

- Explain the procedure, and consider analgesia. If you don't have a catheterisation pack, make up your own (see BOX).
- Lie the patient supine in a well-lit area: women with knees flexed and hips abducted with heels together. Use a gloved hand to prep urethral meatus in a pubis-to-anus direction, holding the labia apart with the other hand. With uncircumcised men (ask the patient beforehand if they have been circumcised to make sure), retract the foreskin to 'prep' the glans; use a gloved hand to hold the penis still and off the scrotum. The hand used to hold the penis or labia should not touch the catheter (use forceps if needed). A sterile drape with a hole in the middle may help asepsis. **Remember:** left hand dirty, right hand sterile.
- Put sterile *lidocaine* 1-2% gel on the catheter tip and ≤10mL into the urethra (≤5mL if ♀). In men, stretch the penis perpendicular to the body to eliminate any urethral folds that may lead to false passage.
- Use steady **gentle** pressure to advance the catheter. ►**Never force the catheter**. In men, mild resistance in the first ~10cm may be from a urethral stricture from previous catheterisation. Insert to the hilt; wait until urine emerges before inflating the balloon. Remember to check the balloon's capacity before inflation (written on the outer end). Collect a sterile specimen and attach a drainage bag. Pull the catheter back so that the balloon comes to rest at the bladder neck.
- If you are having trouble getting past the prostate try: more lubrication; a larger catheter; a *coudé* catheter—or call the urologists, who may use a guide-wire.

► Remember to reposition the foreskin in uncircumcised men after the catheter is inserted to prevent massive oedema of the glans and paraphimos.

2 ***Suprapubic catheterization*** Ensure the bladder is distended so that there is no risk of peritoneal penetration; you may have to wait for it to fill up. Clean the skin, infiltrate with local anaesthetic down to the bladder, nick the skin, and then insert trocar down vertically above the symphysis pubis. When urine is draining, advance the catheter over the trocar and tape it down securely.

►Have all the kit ready beforehand and a helping hand as it can get messy!

1 Routine antibiotic prophylaxis can be used at the time of insertion/removal of a urinary catheter to prevent transient bacteraemia—eg *gentamicin* 2.5mg/kg IV stat. Evidence is scarce, so check local policy.

Self-catheterisation

This is a good, safe way of managing chronic retention from a neuropathic bladder (eg in multiple sclerosis, diabetic neuropathy, spinal tumour or trauma). Never consider a patient in difficulties from a big residual volume to be too old, young, or disabled to learn. 5-yr-old children can learn the technique, and can have their lives transformed—so motivation may be excellent. There may be fewer UTIs as there is no residual urine—and less reflux obstructive uropathy. Assessing suitability entails testing sacral dermatomes: a 'numb bum' implies ↓ sensation of a full bladder; higher sensory loss may mean catheterization will be painless. Get help from your continence adviser who will be in a position to teach the patient or carer that catheterizations must be gentle (the catheter is of a much smaller calibre), particularly if sensation is lacking, and must number >4/d ('always keep your catheter with you; don't wait for an urge before catheterizing'). See **fig 3**.

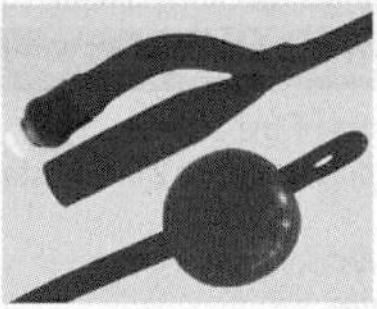

Fig 1. A size 14F latex Foley catheter with the balloon inflated via the topmost port of the outer end (green).[1]

Images © Dr Tom Turmezei (they are not to scale).

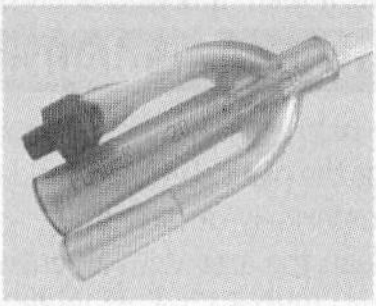

Fig 2. The external end of a size 20F 3-way catheter. The lowest port is for the bladder irrigation fluid and the uppermost port (yellow) is for balloon inflation.

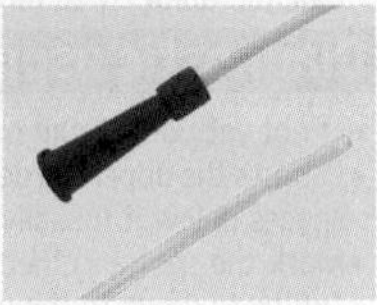

Fig 3. A size 10F catheter for self-catheterisation. They are usually smaller than indwelling catheters eg 10F compared to 14F. Note that this catheter also has no balloon.

"The catheter is not draining..."

You will be asked to check catheters that are not draining. Possibilities are:

- The catheter is bypassing: a condom catheter may be more appropriate.
- The catheter is blocked: with aseptic technique flush and withdraw 20mL of sterile 0.9% saline with a bladder syringe. This may get the flow going again. A 3-way catheter may be needed if there is clot or debris retention.
- The catheter has slipped into the proximal (prostatic♂) urethra, possible even if the balloon is fully inflated. This is may be the case if a flush enters but cannot be withdrawn: with aseptic technique deflate the balloon, advance and reinflate, then flush and withdraw again.
- Renal hypoperfusion: in a dehydrated/post-op patient a fluid challenge of 250mL Gelofusine® STAT (slowly if renal/cardiac comorbidity) may help. Check all other parameters (eg pulse, BP, CVP) and increase rate of IV fluids if appropriate.

►► Acute renal failure (p848): this is unlikely, though most probably from renal hypoperfusion (ie pre-renal failure), but there may be other factors involved causing acute tubular necrosis, eg nephrotoxic drugs.

►► The catheter has perforated the lower urinary tract on insertion and is not lying in the bladder or urethra. If suspected, call the urologists immediately.

Remember: urine output should be >400mL in 24h or >0.5mL/kg/h (see p578).

Trial without catheter (TWOC)

When it is time to remove a catheter, the possibility of urinary retention must be considered. If very likely, arrange for a urology outpatient TWOC in 2 weeks, or start an α-blocker first; otherwise remove the catheter first thing one morning. If retention does occur, insert a long-term catheter (eg silicone) and arrange urology clinic follow-up.

1 We would like to thank Addenbrooke's Hospital Urology Department for supplying the catheters.

Tapping ascites

Ascites may be sampled to give a cytological or bacterial diagnosis, eg to exclude spontaneous bacterial peritonitis (SBP; p260). Before starting, know the patient's platelets + clotting times. If they are abnormal, seek help before proceeding.

- Place the patient flat and tap out the ascites, marking a point where fluid has been identified, avoiding vessels, stomas and scars (adhesions to the anterior abdominal wall). Usually around the level of the umbilicus and the anterior superior iliac spine (the left side may be safer—less chance of nicking liver).
- Clean the skin. Infiltrate some local anaesthetic, eg 1% *lidocaine* (see p575).
- Insert a 21G needle on a 20mL syringe into the skin and advance while aspirating until fluid is withdrawn.
- Remove the needle and apply a sterile dressing.
- Send fluid for ***microscopy***, ***culture***, ***chemistry*** (protein, see p359, p184), and ***cytology***. Call microbiology to forewarn them if urgent analysis of the specimen is required.

Diagnostic aspiration of a pleural effusion

- If not yet done, a CXR may help evaluate the side and size of the effusion.
- Percuss the upper border of the pleural effusion and choose a site 1 or 2 intercostal spaces below it (usually posteriorly or laterally).
- Mark the spot and then clean the area with an antiseptic solution.
- Infiltrate down to the pleura with 5-10mL of 1% **lidocaine**.
- Attach a 21G needle to a syringe and insert it just above the upper border of the rib below the mark to avoid the neurovascular bundle (see BOX). Aspirate whilst advancing the needle. Draw off 10-30mL of pleural fluid. Send fluid to the lab for ***chemistry*** (protein, glucose, pH, LDH, amylase); ***bacteriology*** (microscopy and culture, auramine stain, TB culture); ***cytology*** and, if indicated, ***immunology*** (rheumatoid factor, antinuclear antibodies, complement).
- If any cause for concern, arrange a repeat CXR.

Pleural biopsy

This is usually performed in patients with a pleural effusion when analysis of pleural fluid has not provided an underlying diagnosis. It should not be performed on the ward in patients without an effusion as this requires a different approach. This procedure requires some practice, so if you are inexperienced, ask a senior doctor to assist you.

- Place the patient in an upright position on the edge of the bed, arms resting on a pillow on a bed-table to provide support.
- Identify the upper border of the pleural effusion posteriorly or laterally and mark an intercostal space 1-2 ribs below this.
- Clean the skin with an antiseptic solution and apply sterile drapes.
- Infiltrate down to the pleura with 5-10mL of 1% **lidocaine**.
- Check that you are in the correct space by aspirating pleural fluid.
- Make a deep skin incision 0.5cm wide immediately above the upper border of the rib below the chosen intercostal space (avoids neurovascular bundle).
- Carefully advance the Abrams' needle through the incision until a 'give' is felt as you enter the pleural space.
- Open the needle by twisting the trocar. Check that fluid can be aspirated.
- Manoeuvre the open needle so that the cutting notch is pointing inferiorly (to avoid the neurovascular bundle) and caught on the pleura—pull the needle back slightly at an angle to the chest wall—then close the needle and withdraw. A slight tug may be required at this stage.
- Withdraw the needle in expiration and repeat.
- Place the tissue samples in the appropriate media for histological and microbiological examination. Send to the lab for ***microscopy***, ***culture***, and ***histology***.
- Withdraw the needle, and apply a sterile dressing; occasionally a single suture may be required. Perform a post-procedure CXR.

Abdominal paracentesis (draining ascites)

For patients with refractory or recurrent ascites that is symptomatic, it is possible to drain the ascites using a Bonnano® catheter (initially designed for suprapubic catheterisation), or a long pig-tail catheter. Paracentesis in such patients even in the presence spontaneous bacterial peritonitis may be safe.[11] The procedure is best done supervised before attempting it alone. ***Contraindications:*** End-stage cirrhosis; coagulopathy; hyponatraemia (≤126mmol/L); sepsis. The main complication of the procedure is severe hypovolaemia secondary to reaccumulation of the ascites, so intravascular replenishment with a plasma expander is required—eg 100mL 20% *human albumin* IV for each litre of ascites drained.[12] You may need to call the haematology lab to request this in advance.

- Ensure you have good IV access—eg 18G cannula in the antecubital fossa.
- Examine the abdomen carefully, evaluating the ascites and checking for organomegaly. Mark where you are going to enter. Approach from the left side unless previous local surgery/stoma prevents this—call a senior for support and advice if this is the case.
- Prepare the patient as if for an ascitic tap (see p778), taking extra care to keep the procedure aseptic (use a sterile drape). Infiltrate the local anaesthetic.
- Perform an ascitic tap first so that you know you are in the correct place.
- Carefully thread the catheter over the (large and long) needle using the guide so that the pig-tail has been straightened out. Remove the guide.
- With the left hand hold the needle ~1 inch from the tip—this will stop it from advancing too far (and from performing an aortic biopsy!). With the right hand, hold the other end.
- Gently insert the needle perpendicular to the skin at the site of the ascitic tap up to your hold with your left hand—ascites should now drain easily. If necessary advance the needle and catheter a short distance until good flow is achieved.
- Advance the catheter over the needle with your left hand, keeping the needle in exactly the same place with your right hand. ►Do not re-advance the needle because it will go through the curled pig-tail and do not withdraw it because you won't be able to thread in the catheter.
- When fully inserted, remove the needle, connect the catheter to a drainage bag (keep it below the level of the abdomen) and tape it down securely to the skin.
- The patient should stay in bed as the ascites drains.
- Replenish intravascular volume with human albumin (see above).
- Ask the nursing staff to remove the catheter after 6h or after a pre-determined volume has been drained. (Up to 20L can come off in 6 hours!)
- Send a sample of ascitic fluid to the lab for MC+S.
- Check U&E after the procedure and re-examine the patient.

Safe approach to entering the pleura by the intercostal route

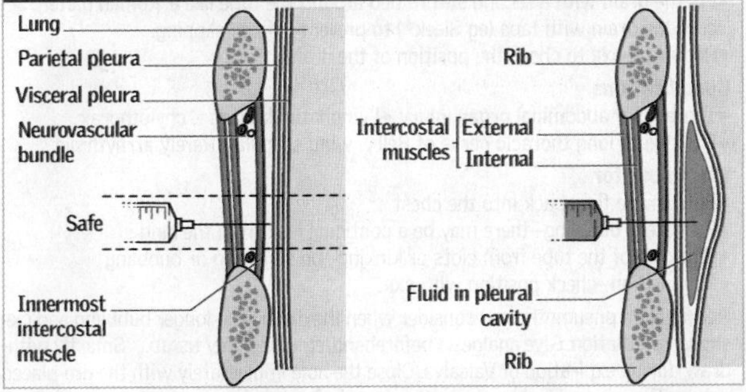

 ►see p824

Indications:

- Pneumothorax: ventilated; tension; persistent/recurrent (eg <24h after 1st aspiration); large 2nd spontaneous pneumothorax if >50yrs old)
- Malignant pleural effusion
- Empyema or complicated parapneumonic effusion
- Traumatic haemopneumothorax; • Air transfer
- Post-operatively: eg thoracotomy; oesophagectomy; cardiothoracic surgery.

►Many effusions are now drained using ultrasound guidance and a Seldinger technique to insert a small pig-tailed drain.

Sterile procedure[13]

- Identify the point for drainage from CXR/CT, or ask ultrasound to 'mark the spot'.
- Preparation: Trolley with dressing pack; iodine; needles; 10mL syringe; 20mL 1% **lidocaine**; scalpel (*N*°15); suture; chest drain (eg 10-14F, if trauma or haemothorax larger gauge eg 28-30F); underwater drainage bottle; connection tubes; sterile H_2O; tape. Incontinence pad under patient. Swab extensively.
- Choose insertion site:[14] 4th-6th intercostal space, anterior- to mid-axillary line—the 'safe triangle' (see BOX). A more posterior approach, eg the 7th space posteriorly, may be required to drain a loculated effusion, and occasionally the 2nd intercostal space in the mid-clavicular line may be used for apical pneumothoraces—however, both approaches tend to be less comfortable.
- Infiltrate down to pleura with 10-20mL of 1% *lidocaine*. Check that either air or fluid can be aspirated from the proposed insertion site—if not **do not** proceed. Wait 3min.
- Make a 2cm incision above 6th rib, to avoid neurovascular bundle under rib 5. **Bluntly** dissect down to the pleura. Puncture pleura with scissors or forceps. If large bore tube (>24F), then sweep a finger inside chest to clear adherent lung and exclude (eg in blunt abdominal trauma) stomach in the chest! **NB:** some new kits use a Seldinger technique for insertion. ►Before inserting the drain, remove the metal trochar; introduce the drain **atraumatically** using forceps to advance it.
- Advance the tip upwards to the apex (or base if draining an effusion). Stop on meeting resistance. Then attach the drain via the tubing to the underwater seal. Ensure that the longer tube within the bottle is underwater and bubbling with respiration. If the patient is to be moved to another hospital, substitute Heimlich flutter valve or drainage bag with flap valve for underwater drain. ►You should never clamp chest drains inserted for pneumothoraces. Clamping is occasionally used when pleural effusions are being drained to control the rate of drainage and prevent expansion pulmonary oedema.[15]
- With large/medium bore tubes, the incision should be closed with a mattress suture or suture across the incision. Purse string sutures are no longer recommended as they may lead to increased scarring and wound pain.
- Fix the drain with a second suture tied around the tube like a 'Roman gaiter'. Secure the drain with tape (eg Sleek®) to prevent it from slipping.
- Request a CXR to check the position of the drain.

Complications

- Thoracic or abdominal organ injury • Lymphatic damage ∴ chylothorax
- Damage to long thoracic nerve of Bell ∴ wing scapula • Rarely, arrhythmia.[16]

Watch out for

- Retrograde flow back into the chest
- Persistent bubbling—there may be a continual leak from the lung
- Blockage of the tube from clots or kinking—no swinging or bubbling
- Malposition—check position with CXR.

Removal (in pneumothorax) consider when the drain is no longer bubbling and CXR shows re-inflation. Give analgesia beforehand, eg morphine/ NSAID.[17] Smartly withdraw during expiration or Valsalva. Close the hole immediately with the pre-placed suture. There is no need to clamp the drain beforehand as reinsertion is unlikely.[18]

The 'safe triangle' for insertion of a chest drain

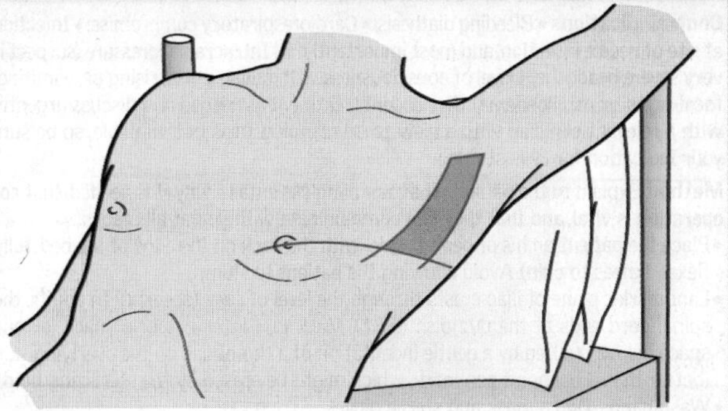

Adapted with permission from Thorax 2003 58 suppl II; ii55.

Relieving a tension pneumothorax

Symptoms Acute respiratory distress, chest pain, ⏩respiratory arrest.

Signs Hypotension; distended neck veins; asymmetrical lung expansion; trachea and apex deviated away from side of reduced air entry and hyperresonance to percussion. ⏩There is no time for a CXR (but see **fig 1**, p763).

Aim To release air from the pleural space. In a tension pneumothorax air is drawn into the intra-pleural space with each breath, but cannot escape due to a valve-like effect of the tiny flap in the parietal pleura. The increasing pressure progressively embarrasses the heart and the other lung.

⏩**100% oxygen.**

⏩**Insert a large bore IV cannula** (eg Venflon®) usually through the 2nd intercostal space in the mid-clavicular line or the 'safe triangle' for chest drain insertion (see BOX). Remove the stylet, which will allow the trapped air to escape, usually with an audible hiss. The tension pneumothorax has now been converted to an open pneumothorax. Tape securely. ►Don't re-cover the cannula as tensioning will recur.

⏩Proceed to formal chest drain insertion (see p780).

Aspiration of a pneumothorax ►p825

Identify the 2nd intercostal space in the midclavicular line (or 4–6th intercostal space in the midaxillary line) and infiltrate with 1% *lidocaine* down to the pleura overlying the pneumothorax.

- Insert a 16G cannula into the pleural space. Remove the needle and connect the cannula to a 3-way tap and a 50mL syringe. Aspirate up to 2.5L of air (50mL×50). Stop if resistance is felt, or if the patient coughs excessively.
- Request a CXR to confirm resolution of the pneumothorax. If successful, consider discharging the patient and repeating the CXR after 24h to exclude recurrence, and again after 7–10d. Advise to avoid air travel for 6 weeks after a normal CXR. Diving should be permanently avoided.
- If aspiration is unsuccessful (in a significant, symptomatic pneumothorax), insert an intercostal drain (see p780).

Contraindications • Bleeding diathesis; • Cardiorespiratory compromise; • Infection at site of needle insertion, and most importantly: • ↑Intracranial pressure (suspect if very severe headache, ↓level of consciousness with falling pulse, rising BP, vomiting, focal signs, or papilloedema). Give urgent treatment as needed and discuss urgently with a relevant clinician with a view to CT scanning. CT is not infallible, so be sure your indication for LP is strong.

Method Explain to the patient **what** sampling CSF entails, **why** it is needed, that **co-operation** is vital, and that they can communicate with you at all stages.

- Place the patient on his or her left side, with the back on the edge of the bed, fully flexed (knees to chin). Avoid allowing the patient to slump.
- Landmarks: plane of iliac crests through the level of L3/4 (see BOX). In adults, the spinal cord ends at the L1/2 disc (**fig 1**). Mark L3/4 intervertebral space (or one space below, L4/5), eg by a gentle indentation of a thumbnail on the overlying skin (better than a ballpoint pen mark, which might be erased by the sterilizing fluid).
- Wash hands. Don a mask and sterile gloves.
- Sterilize the back with tincture of iodine (unless allergic).
- Open the spinal pack. Check manometer fittings. Have 3 plain sterile tubes and 1 fluoride tube (for glucose) ready.
- Inject 0.25–0.5mL 1% **lidocaine** under skin at marked site.
- Wait 1min, then insert spinal needle (22G, stilette in place) through the mark aiming towards umbilicus. Feel resistance of spinal ligaments, and then the dura, then a 'give' as the needle enters the subarachnoid space. **NB:** keep the needle's bevel facing **up**, parallel with dural fibres.
- Withdraw stilette. Wait for CSF.
- Measure CSF 'opening' pressure with a manometer.
- Catch fluid in three sequentially numbered bottles (<5–10mL total). Consider taking and privately reserving a labelled sample in case of an accident!
- Re-insert stilette,[19] and remove needle and apply dressing. Send CSF promptly for ***microscopy, culture, protein, lactate & glucose*** (do plasma glucose too)—call the lab to let them know. If applicable, also send for: cytology, fungal studies, TB culture, virology (± herpes and other PCR), syphilis serology, oligoclonal bands (+serum sample for comparison) if multiple sclerosis suspected. Is there xanthochromia (p482)?
- Lying flat for >1h is traditionally advised (probably unnecessary),[20] checking CNS observations and BP regularly. Post-LP headache is partly preventable by reinserting the stilet before needle withdrawal,[21] and reducing CSF leakage by using finer needles shaped to part the dura rather than cut it: see BOX.
- If you fail; ask for help—try with the patient sitting or with radiology guidance.

CSF composition *Normal values:* Lymphocytes <5/mm^3; no polymorphs; protein <0.4g/L; glucose >2.2mmol/L (or ≥50% plasma level); pressure <200mmCSF. ***In meningitis:*** See p833. ***In multiple sclerosis:*** See p500.

Bloody tap: This is an artefact due to piercing a blood vessel, which is indicated (unreliably) by fewer red cells in successive bottles, and no yellowing of CSF (xanthochromia). To estimate how many white cells (*W*) were in the CSF before the blood was added, use the following:

$$W = \text{CSF WCC} - [(\text{blood WCC} \times \text{CSF RBC}) \div \text{blood RBC}].$$

If the blood count is normal, the rule of thumb is to subtract from the total CSF WCC (per μL) one white cell for every 1000 RBCs. To estimate the true protein level, subtract 10mg/L for every 1000 RBCs/mm^3 (be sure to do the count and protein estimation on the same bottle). **NB:** high protein levels in CSF make it appear yellow.

Subarachnoid haemorrhage: Xanthochromia (yellow supernatant on spun CSF). Red cells in equal numbers in all bottles (unreliable). RBCs will excite an inflammatory response (eg CSF WCC raised), most marked after 48h.

Raised protein: Meningitis; MS; Guillain-Barré syndrome. ***Very raised CSF protein:*** Spinal block; TB; or severe bacterial meningitis.

Post-LP headache

Risk ~30%, typically occurring within 24h of LP, with resolution over hours to 2wks (mean: 3–4d). Patients describe a constant, dull, ache bilaterally which is more frontal than occipital. The most characteristic symptom is of **positional (orthostatic) exacerbation**—worse when upright and usually pain-free when recumbent. There may be mild meningism or nausea. The pathology is thought to be continued leakage of CSF from the puncture site and intracranial **hypo**tension, though there may be other mechanisms involved.[22]

Prevention Use the smallest spinal needle that is practical (22G) and keep the bevel aligned as described on p782. **Blunt** needles (more expensive!) can reduce risk, perhaps from 30% to 5%—and are recommended (ask an anaesthetist about supply).[23] Collection of CSF takes too long (>6min) if needles smaller than 22G are used.[24] Before withdrawing the needle, re-insert the stilette.[25]

Treatment Despite years of anecdotal advice to the contrary, none of the following have ever been shown to be a risk factor: position during or after the procedure; hydration status before, during, or after; amount of CSF removed; immediate activity or rest post-LP.[26] Time is a consistent healer. For severe or prolonged headaches, ask an anaesthetist about a **blood patch**.[27] This is a careful injection of 20mL of autologous venous blood into the adjacent epidural space (said to 'clog up the hole'). Immediate relief occurs in 95%.

NB: post-LP brain MRI scans often show diffuse meningeal enhancement with gadolinium. This is thought to be a reflection of increased blood flow secondary to intracranial hypotension. Interpret these scans with caution and in the context of the patient's clinical situation.

Defining the 3rd - 4th lumbar vertebral interspace

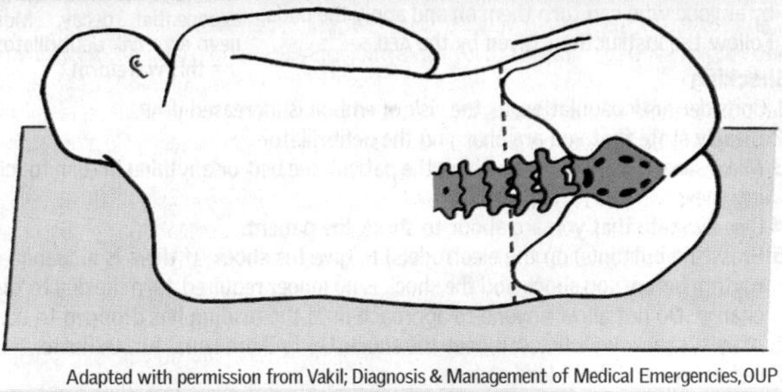

Adapted with permission from Vakil; Diagnosis & Management of Medical Emergencies, OUP

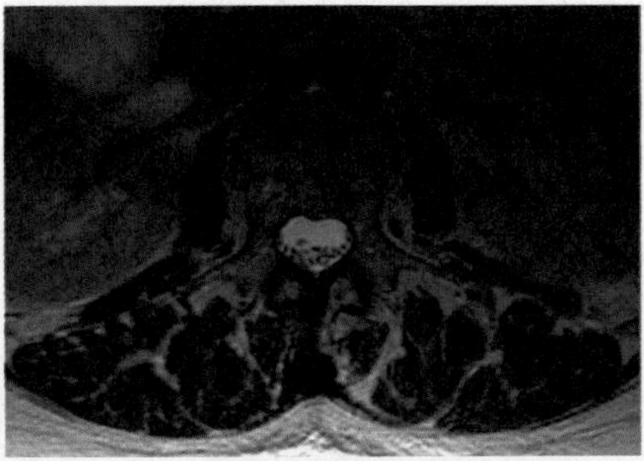

Fig 1. Axial T2-weighted MRI of the lumbar spine. The conus ends at the L1/L2 level with continuation of the cauda equina. Lumbar puncture below the L2 level will not damage the cauda equina as the nerve roots will part around an LP needle.

Image courtesy of Norwich Radiology Dept.

►Do not wait for a crisis before familiarizing yourself with the defibrillator, as there several types. Day 1 on a new ward should include a visit to the 'defib trolley'.

Indications To restore sinus rhythm if VF/VT; AF, flutter, or supraventricular tachycardias if other treatments (p120) have failed, or there is haemodynamic compromise (p124). This may been undertaken as an emergency eg VF/VT or electively eg AF.

Aim To completely depolarize the heart using a direct current.

Procedure

- Unless critically unwell, conscious patients require a general anaesthetic or monitored heavy sedation.
- If elective cardioversion of AF ensure adequate anticoagulation beforehand.
- Almost all defibrillators are now paddle-free and use 'hands-free' pads instead (less chance of skin arc than jelly). Place the pads (eg Littmann™ Defib Pads) on chest, 1 over apex (p39) and 1 below right clavicle. The positions are often given by a diagram on the reverse of the pad.
- ***Monophasic defibrillators*** **(fig 1)**: Set the energy level at 360J for VF/VT; 100J for AF; 50J for atrial flutter.
- ***Biphasic defibrillators*** **(fig 2)**: Impedance is less with a biphasic shock and 150J is used for shocks for VF/VT. They use less energy and are just as effective as monophasic defibrillators in cardioversion of AF, if not better.[28,29,30]
- ***Automatic external defibrillators*** **(AED)**: Can be used by anyone who can turn them on and apply the pads. Follow the instructions given by the AED.

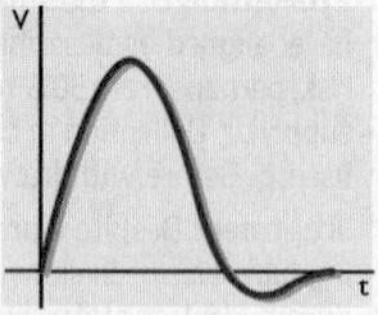

Fig 1. The dampened sine monophasic waveform.

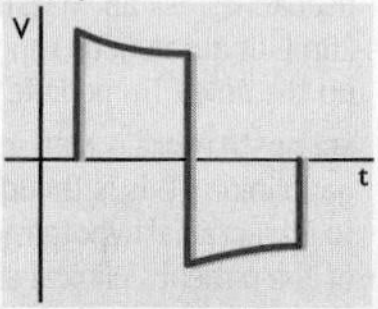

Fig 2. Rectilinear biphasic waveform with truncated exponential decay. Most new external defibrillators use this waveform.

Shocking

1. Consider anticoagulation, as the risk of emboli is increased if AF.
2. Clearly state that you are charging the defibrillator.
3. Make sure no one else is touching the patient, the bed, or anything in turn touching these.
4. Clearly state that you are about to shock the patient.
5. Press the button(s) on the electrode(s) to give the shock. If there is a change in rhythm before you shock and the shock is no longer required, turn the dial to 'discharge'. Do not allow anyone to approach until the reading has dropped to 0J.
6. After a shock: watch ECG; repeat the shock. Up to 3 are usual for AF/flutter.
7. Get an up-to-date 12-lead ECG.

NB: for AF and SVT, it is necessary to synchronize the shock on the R-wave of the ECG (by pressing the 'SYNC' button on the machine; it may be necessary to do this before each shock). This ensures that the shock does not initiate a ventricular arrhythmia. **If the sync mode is engaged in VF, the defibrillator will not discharge!**

►In children, use 2J/kg, then 4J/kg in VF/VT; if monophasic, and if >10kg, use **adult** paddles; *OHCS* p239.

Taking arterial blood gas (ABG) samples

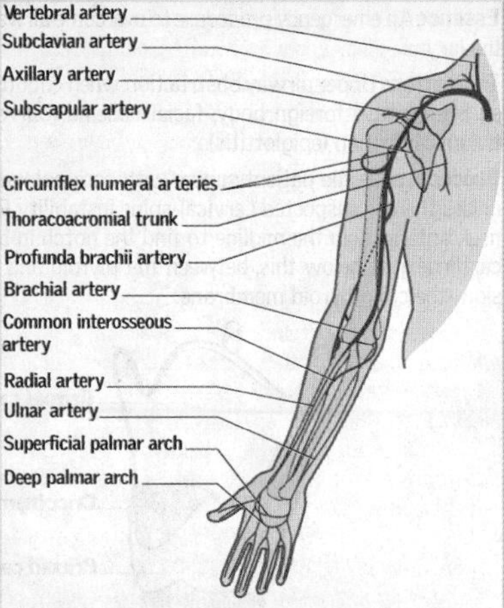

The reaction of a patient to ABG sampling is often very different to when they are subjected to venepuncture, so try to explain that the blood sample you are about to take is going to feel different and is for a different purpose (p156 for indications & analysis). The usual site is the radial artery at the wrist. ►Don't use this site if there is an arteriovenous fistula for haemodialysis.

Procedure:

- Get kit ready; include: portable sharps bin; pre-heparinized syringe; needle—blue size (23G) is good; gloves; alcohol swab; gauze swab; tape.
- Feel thoroughly for the best site. Look at both sides.
- Wipe with an alcohol swab. Let the area dry. Get yourself comfortable.
- Ask an assistant to hold the hand and arm with the wrist slightly extended.
- Before sampling, expel any excess heparin in the syringe. Infiltration over the artery with a small amount of 1% *lidocaine* (p575) through a 25G (orange) needle makes the procedure painless.
- Hold the syringe like a pen, with the needle bevel up. Let the patient know you are about to take the sample. Feel for the pulse with your other hand and enter at 45°, aiming beneath the finger you are feeling with.
- The plunger will move up on its own in a pulsatile manner if you are in the artery; rarely, entry into a vein next to the artery will give a similar result. Colour of the blood is little guide to its source!

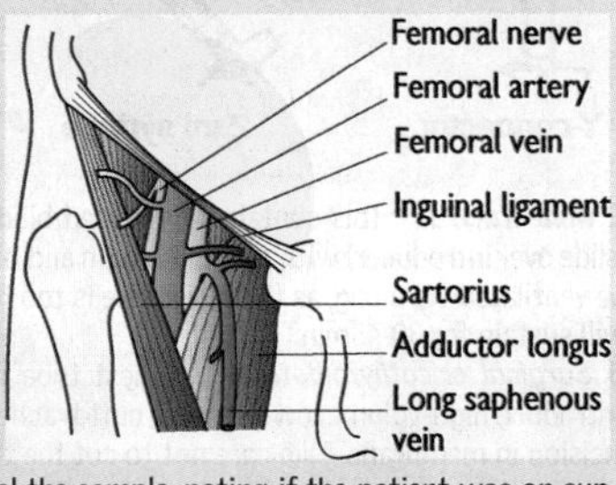

- Remove the needle when enough blood has been taken (1–2mL to allow for spillage or a dud reading from the machine) and apply firm pressure until any leakage is stemmed to avoid a large lump followed by a massive bruise!
- Expel any air from the syringe as this will alter the oxygenation of the blood. Cap and label the sample, noting if the patient was on supplementary oxygen. Take the sample to the nearest analysis machine or send it by express delivery to the lab (which may be by your own feet). If it is going to stand for any foreseeable length of time then put the sample in a bag of ice.
- Syringes and analysis machines differ, so get familiar with the local nuances.

The other site that is amenable to ABG sampling is the femoral artery. Surprisingly this may be less uncomfortable as it is a relatively less sensitive area and because when supine, the patient cannot see the needle and thus may feel less apprehensive. The brachial artery can also be used, but be aware that median nerve sits closely on its medial side and it is an end-artery. Normal values: p771.

Images in this box after RSCI

Essence An emergency procedure to overcome airway obstruction above the level of the larynx.

Indications Upper airway obstruction when endotracheal intubation not possible, eg irretrievable foreign body; facial oedema (burns, angio-oedema); maxillofacial trauma; infection (epiglottitis).

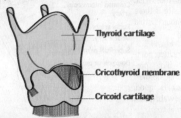

Procedure Lie the patient supine with neck extended (eg pillow under shoulders) unless there is suspected cervical-spine instability. Run your index finger down the neck anteriorly in the midline to find the notch in the upper border of the thyroid cartilage: just below this, between the thyroid and cricoid cartilages, is a depression—the cricothyroid membrane.

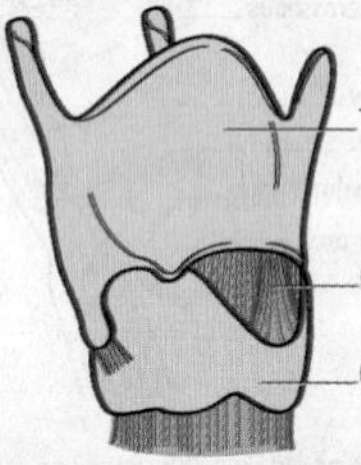

1 *Needle cricothyroidotomy:* Pierce the membrane with large-bore cannula (14G) attached to syringe: withdrawal of air confirms position; *lidocaine* may or may not be required). Slide cannula over needle at 45° to the skin superiorly in the sagittal plane. Use a Y-connector or improvise connection to O_2 supply at 15L/min: use thumb on Y-connector to allow O_2 in over 1s and CO_2 out over 4s ('transtracheal jet insufflation'). This is the preferred method in children <12yrs. This will only sustain life for 30–45min before CO_2 builds up.

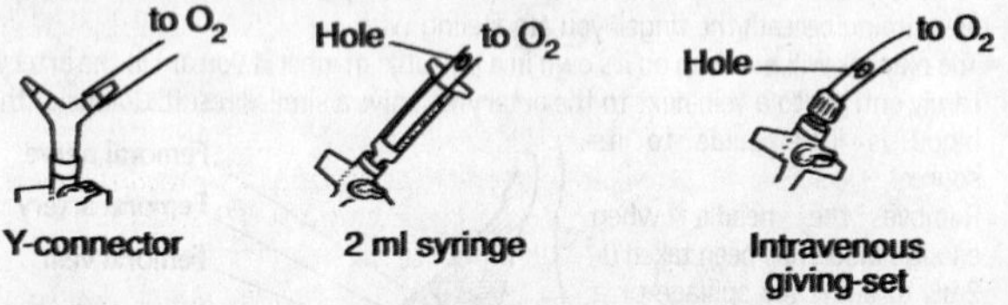

2 *Mini-Trach II®:* This contains a guarded blade, introducer, 4mm uncuffed tube (slide over introducer) with ISO connection and binding tape. The patient will have to be ventilated via a bag, as the resistance is too high to breathe spontaneously. This will sustain for 30–45min.

3 *Surgical cricothyroidotomy:* Smallest tube for prolonged ventilation is 6mm. Introduce high-volume low-pressure cuff tracheostomy tube through a horizontal incision in membrane. Take care not to cut the thyroid or cricoid cartilages.

Complications Local haemorrhage ± aspiration; posterior perforation of trachea ± oesophagus; subglottic stenosis; laryngeal stenosis if membrane over-incised in childhood; tube blockage; subcutaneous tunnelling; vocal cord paralysis or hoarseness (the recurrent laryngeal nerve runs superiorly in the tracheo-oesophageal groove).

►**NB:** needle and Mini-Trach® are temporary measures pending formal tracheostomy.

Emergency needle pericardiocentesis[1]

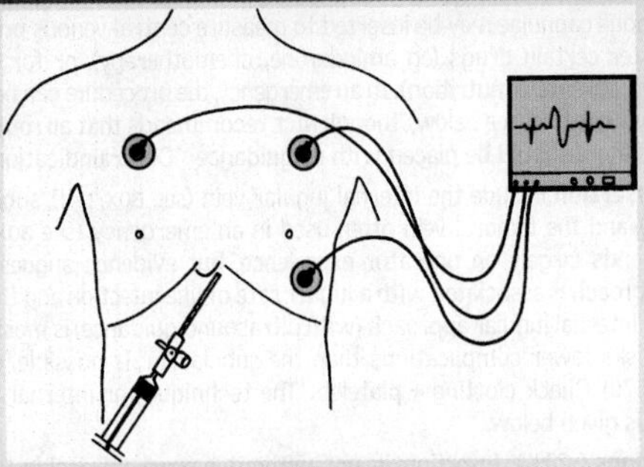

- Get your senior's help (for whom this may serve as an *aide-mémoire*).
- Equipment: 20mL syringe, long 18G cannula, 3-way tap, ECG monitor, skin cleanser. Use echo guidance if time allows.
- If time allows, use aseptic technique, and, if conscious, local anaesthesia and sedation, eg with *midazolam*: titrate up to 0.1mg/kg IV—start with 2mg over 1min, 1mg in elderly—antidote: *flumazenil* 0.2mg IV over 15s, then 0.1mg every 60s, up to 1mg in total.
- Ensure you have IV access and full resuscitation equipment to hand.
- Introduce needle at 45° to skin just below and to left of xiphisternum, aiming for tip of left scapula. Aspirate continuously and watch ECG. Frequent ventricular ectopics or an injury pattern (ST segment↓) on ECG imply that the myocardium has been breached—withdraw slightly. As soon as blood is obtained through the needle, slide the cannula into place.
- Evacuate pericardial contents through the syringe and 3-way tap. Removal of only a small amount of fluid (eg 20mL) can produce marked clinical improvement. If you are not sure whether the fluid you are aspirating is pure blood (eg on entering a ventricle), see if it clots (heavily bloodstained pericardial fluid does not clot), or measure its PCV (though this may be difficult in the acute setting but some blood gas analysers may give this).
- You can leave the cannula *in situ* temporarily, for repeated aspiration. If there is reaccumulation, insert a drain but pericardiectomy may be needed.
- Send fluid for microscopy and culture, as needed, including tests for TB.

Complications: Laceration of ventricle or coronary artery (± subsequent haemopericardium); aspiration of ventricular blood; arrhythmias (ventricular fibrillation); pneumothorax; puncture of aorta, oesophagus (± mediastinitis), or peritoneum (± peritonitis).

1 Procedures used by cardiologists for elective pericardiocentesis may differ, involving the use of guide-wires, screening, and catheters.

Central venous cannulation

Central venous cannulae may be inserted to measure central venous pressure (CVP), to administer certain drugs (eg amiodarone, chemotherapy), or for intravenous access (fluid, parenteral nutrition). In an emergency, the procedure can be done using the landmark method (see below), though NICE recommends that all routine internal jugular catheters should be placed with US guidance[31] Contraindications: TABLE.

Sites of insertion include the internal jugular vein (see BOX, p41), subclavian vein (see below), and the femoral vein often used in an emergency (see BOX, p785). The choice depends largely on operator experience, but evidence suggests that the femoral approach is associated with a higher rate of line infection and thrombosis.[32] Overall, the internal jugular approach (with ultrasound guidance) is most commonly used and risks fewer complications than the subclavian. If possible, get written consent (p570). Check clotting + platelets. The technique for internal jugular and subclavian is given below.

Complications (~20%). Insertion in not without hazard, so decide whether the patient requires one first, and then ask for help if you are inexperienced.

►Bleeding; artery puncture/cannulation; AV fistula formation.
- Air embolism.
- Pneumothorax; haemothorax; chylothorax (lymph).
- Phrenic nerve palsy.[1] The right phrenic nerve passes over the brachiocephalic artery, posterior to the subclavian vein. Hiccups may be a sign of injury.[33]
- Phlebitis; thrombus formation on tip or in vein. If high risk of venous thromboembolism (eg malignancy), a continuous IVI of unfractionated heparin may reduce risk of thrombosis.[34]
- Bacterial colonisation; cellulitis; sepsis. This can be reduced by adherence to a strict aseptic technique, and use of antibiotic- or heparin-coated catheters[35].

►If taking blood cultures in a febrile patient with a central venous line, remember to take samples from the central line and from a new peripheral site (ie not a pre-existing cannula).

Contraindications to central venous cannulation

Absolute	Relative
Infection at insertion site	Coagulopathy
	Ipsilateral carotid endarterectomy
	Newly inserted cardiac pacemaker leads
	Significant tricuspid regurgitation
	Renal cell cancer involving the right atrium

1 Think of phrenic nerve palsy whenever there is orthopnoea (CXR: raised hemidiaphragm). *Other causes:* lung ca; myeloma; thymoma; neck trauma; cervical spondylosis; thoracic surgery; C3-5 zoster; HIV; Lyme dis.; TB; paraneoplastic syndrome.; muscular dystrophy; big left atrium; phrenic nucleus lesion (eg MS).

Subclavian and internal jugular catheterization

- Position the patient flat, with 1 pillow. Head-down tilt may help if volume depleted. NB: ►this can compromise cardiac function and precipitate catastrophic acute LVF.
- Wash hands, don a gown and sterile gloves. This is an aseptic procedure.
- Clean area with chlorhexidine or iodine solution (unless allergic); apply sterile drapes.
- Assemble the catheter, and flush all the lumina with saline.

Subclavian

- Identify the insertion point: 1cm below the junction of the medial third and lateral ⅔ of the clavicle. Nick the skin with a scalpel.
- Using a green needle inject 5–10mL of 1–2% **lidocaine** under the skin and into the subcutaneous tissues, down to the clavicle.
- Using the introducer needle, and an appropriate syringe partly filled with saline, puncture the skin and advance the needle to the clavicle. Once you hit the clavicle, move the needle under the clavicle and aim for the opposite sternoclavicular joint. This method reduces the risk of puncturing the pleura. Aspirate as you advance the needle and you should be able to cannulate the subclavian vein. When in the vein you should be able to easily aspirate blood.
- Order a CXR to check catheter position and exclude a pneumothorax. If a cannula is in the internal jugular vein (**fig 2**, p588), it must be withdrawn and replaced.

Right subclavian vein puncture—infraclavicular approach

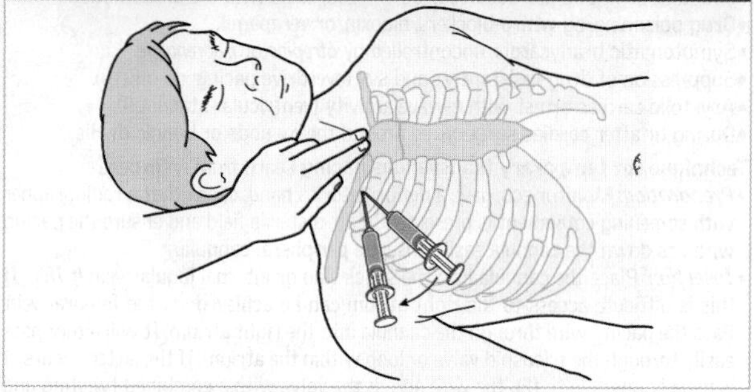

Internal jugular (use ultrasound guidance if possible)

- The technique is very similar to the subclavian approach
- Identify the insertion point - lateral and parallel to the carotid artery at the level of the thyroid cartilage. Ask the subject to turn their head slightly away from you and place the fingers of one hand along the carotid artery and infiltrate the skin and subcutaneous tissues with *lidocaine*, and nick the skin.
- Insert the needle just lateral to the artery at 45° aiming for the ipsilateral nipple or ant. sup. iliac spine. Advance slowly whilst aspirating. The vein is superficial so don't advance too far. Ultrasound will greatly assist if available.
- Then proceed as per subclavian approach.

- Remove the syringe, keeping the needle still and insert the guide-wire. Remove the needle over the wire but **never** let go of the wire or it may all enter the vein, making removal very hard. The wire should advance with ease; if it does not, restart the procedure, as you should not remove the wire through the needle.
- Next, feed the dilator over the wire. Often twisting it slightly will facilitate its insertion. NB: always have one hand on the wire.
- Remove the dilator and feed the catheter over the wire, remembering to have the end of the wire in your hand before the tip of the catheter enters the skin.
- Feed the catheter into the vein, remove the wire, and check that blood can be aspirated through each lumen.
- Flush each lumen, and then stitch the catheter in place.

Often it is wiser to liaise with a specialist pacing centre to arrange prompt, definitive pacing than to try temporary transvenous pacing, which often has complications (see below) which may delay a definitive procedure.

Possible indications in the acute phase of myocardial infarction:

- *Complete AV block:*
  - With inferior MI (right coronary artery occlusion) pacing may only be needed if symptomatic; spontaneous recovery may occur.
  - With anterior MI (representing massive septal infarction).
- *Second-degree block:*
  - Wenckebach (p119 implies decremental AV node conduction; may respond to ***atropine*** in an inferior MI; pace if anterior MI.
  - Mobitz type 2 block is usually associated with distal fascicular disease and carries high risk of complete heart block, so pace in both types of MI.
- *First-degree block:* Observe carefully: 40% develop higher degrees of block.
- *Bundle branch block:* Pace prophylactically if evidence of trifascicular disease (p94) or non-adjacent bifascicular disease.
- *Sino-atrial disease + serious symptoms:* Pace unless responds to ***atropine***.

Other indications where temporary pacing may be needed

- Pre-op: if surgery is required in patients with type 2 or complete heart block (whether or not MI has occurred); do 24h ECG; liaise with the anaesthetist.
- Drug poisoning, eg with β-blockers, digoxin, or verapamil.
- Symptomatic bradycardia, uncontrolled by ***atropine*** or ***isoprenaline***.
- Suppression of drug-resistant VT and SVT (overdrive pacing; do on ITU).
- Asystolic cardiac arrest with P-wave activity (ventricular standstill).
- During or after cardiac surgery—eg around the AV node or bundle of His.

Technique for temporary transvenous pacing Learn from an expert.

- *Preparation:* Monitor ECG; have a defibrillator to hand; check that a radiographer with screening equipment is present.[1] Create a sterile field and ensure the pacing wire fits down the cannula easily. Insert a peripheral cannula.
- *Insertion:* Place the cannula into the subclavian or internal jugular vein (p789). If this is difficult, access to the right atrium can be achieved via the femoral vein. Pass the pacing wire through the cannula into the right atrium. It will either pass easily through the tricuspid valve or loop within the atrium. If the latter occurs, it is usually possible to flip the wire across the valve with a combined twisting and withdrawing movement (**fig 1**). Advance the wire slightly. At this stage the wire may try to exit the ventricle through the pulmonary outflow tract. A further withdrawing and rotation of the wire will aim the tip at the apex of the right ventricle. Advance slightly again to place the wire in contact with the endocardium. Remove any slack to ↓risk of subsequent displacement.
- *Checking the threshold:* Connect the wire to the pacing box and set the 'demand' rate slightly higher than the patient's own heart rate and the output to 3V. A paced rhythm should be seen. Find the pacing threshold by slowly reducing the voltage until the pacemaker fails to stimulate the tissue (pacing spikes are no longer followed by paced beats). The threshold should be less than 1V, but a slightly higher value may be acceptable if it is stable—eg after a large infarction.
- *Setting the pacemaker:* Set the output to 3V or over 3 times the threshold value (whichever is higher) in 'demand' mode. Set the rate as required. Suture the wire to the skin, and fix with a sterile dressing.
- Check the position of the wire (and exclude pneumothorax) with a CXR.
- Recurrent checks of the pacing threshold are required over the next few days. The formation of endocardial oedema can raise the threshold by a factor of 2-3.

Complications Pneumothorax; sepsis; cardiac perforation; pacing failure: from loss of capture, loss of electrical continuity in pacing circuit, or electrode displacement.

1 Balloon-flotation techniques do not need radiographic guidance, have been shown to be quicker and easier to insert, with fewer complications compared to placement of semi-rigid electrode wires.

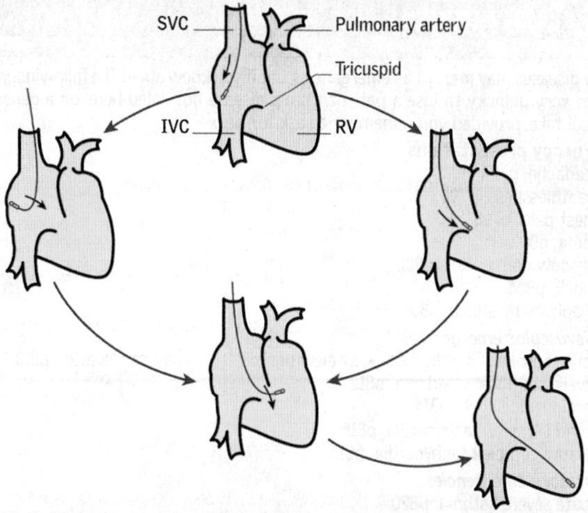

Fig 1. Siting a temporary cardiac pacemaker.

Non-invasive transcutaneous cardiac pacing

This method (performed through a defibrillator with external pacing facility) has the advantages of being quicker, less risky than the transvenous route, and easier to perform. Its main disadvantage is the pain caused by skeletal muscle contraction in the non-sedated patient. Indications for pacing via the transcutaneous route are as OPPOSITE, **plus** if transvenous pacing (or someone able to perform it) is unavailable or non-imminent in an emergency situation.

- ⏩Give sedation and analgesia, eg *midazolam* + *morphine* IV titrated to effect.
- ⏩Clipping chest hair may help improve electrical contact; ►don't shave the skin, as nicks can predispose to electrical burns. Ensure the skin is dry.
- ⏩Almost all modern transcutaneous devices can function through defibrillation 'hands free' pads, and so these can be applied as for defibrillation (see p784). If necessary, the pads can be placed in an AP position: anteriorly over the V_2–V_3 electrode position and posteriorly at the same level, just below the scapula.
- ⏩Select 'demand' mode, (which synchronises the stimulus with the R wave, so avoiding pacing on the T wave—which can provoke VF or VT) and adjust the ECG gain so that QRS complexes can be seen.
- ⏩Select an appropriate pacing rate: eg 60–90bpm in an adult.
- ⏩Set the pacing current at the lowest setting and turn on the pacemaker.
- ⏩Increase the pacing current until electrical capture occurs (normally from 50–100mA), which can be confirmed by seeing a wide QRS complex **and** a T wave on the trace (ventricular electrical capture). This does not necessarily mean that there has been mechanical capture—one clinical trial has described using emergency cardiac ultrasound to assess for this.[36]
- ⏩There will be some interference from skeletal muscle contraction on the ECG trace, as well as possible artefact, which could be mistaken for a QRS complex. The absence of a T wave is an important discriminator between the two.
- ⏩CPR can continue with the pads in place, though only when the pacing unit is **off**.
- ⏩Once adequate cardiac output has been maintained, seek expert help and arrange transvenous pacing.

20 Emergencies[1]

Many diseases may present as emergencies, but if you know about the following, you will be very unlucky to lose a patient from a disease not listed here, on a general medical take, provided you remember to ask for help.

Emergencies covered in other chapters *See inside front cover.*

In OHCS—Paediatrics: Life support and cardiac arrest (*OHCS* p238–p239); is he seriously ill? (*OHCS* p 103); epiglottitis (*OHCS* p158). *Adults:* The major disaster (*OHCS* p806); trauma (*OHCS* chapter 11); drowning (*OHCS* p724); ectopic pregnancy (*OHCS* p262); eclampsia (*OHCS* p48); amniotic fluid embolus (*OHCS* p89); obstetric shock (*OHCS* p55); glaucoma (*OHCS* p430); pre-hospital care/first aid (*OHCS* p790–p814).

Sources include: *BMJ*; *NEJM*; *Oxford Handbook of Acute Medicine*, OUP.

1 "Don't go so fast: we're in a hurry!" Talleyrand to his coachman

We thank Dr S Haydock (Specialist Reader) & Specialist Readers from other chapters.

Introduction to emergencies

There is nothing more intoxicating than spending a day saving lives, but as night creeps on, and you start losing more patients than you should, despair can hit with the force of ice. It is no comfort to know that you are now wiser and older (by 100yrs). So when you find yourself washing your hands between one death and the next, for one second be honest with yourself, and write of your errors and sorrows on the surface of the water—a few temporary ambiguous squiggles framing your thoughts and the life that is lost. This is not about audit and accountability (this comes later: now you need to fortify yourself to survive this onslaught)—so, in case a manager is looking over your shoulder, pull the plug, and as the water flows away, know that it mingles with the rising tide of our own failings at the bedside, through which we have surfaced—no doubt a little faster than we should. At your next bedside you may do better if you can buy time: time to take a history, time to think, and time to ask. How to buy this precious time is described in BOX 2.

The importance of communication between all concerned—colleagues, the relatives, and so on, goes without saying. However, what needs bringing to the fore are those times when communication itself is the emergency. Suppose your patient has end-stage COPD or any of a host of pre-terminal conditions. He may be expecting resuscitation—or dreading it. The family may say "It's kinder not to tell him he's dying...he could not cope with that"—and you may be inclined to agree. If you go along with this collusion you are breaking Pickering's Law which states that whenever relatives offer you an easy way out, you are probably wrong to take it.[1] Don't be tempted! Instead, show leadership. Find out what the patient wants, and then do it, enlarging the vision of sometimes myopic relatives, so they too are reasonably happy. Otherwise you condemn the man to a bad death, and the relatives to a long bereavement, complicated by not saying their good-byes or exchanging messages of love. If the patient is going to die in the next hour, this really is an emergency, and dealing with it is your job, just as much as ordering blood and putting up IVIs.

ABCDE preliminary assessment (primary survey)[2]

Airway	Protect cervical spine, if injury possible. *Assessment:* any signs of obstruction? Ascertain patency. *Management:* establish a patent airway.
Breathing	*Assessment:* determine respiratory rate, check bilateral chest movement, percuss and auscultate. *Management:* if no respiratory effort, treat as arrest[3] (see inside back cover), intubate and ventilate. If breathing compromised, give high-concentration O_2, manage according to findings, eg relieve tension pneumothorax.
Circulation	*Assessment:* check pulse and BP; check if peripherally shut down; check capillary refill; look for evidence of haemorrhage. *Management:* if shocked, treat as on p804 If no cardiac output, treat as arrest (*see* inside back cover).
Disability	Assess 'level of consciousness' with AVPU score (alert? responds to voice? to pain? unresponsive?); check pupils: size, equality, reactions. *Glasgow coma scale*, if time allows.
Exposure	Undress patient, but cover to avoid hypothermia.

Quick history from relatives assists diagnosis: ***Events*** surrounding onset of illness, evidence of overdose/suicide attempt, any suggestion of trauma? ***Past medical history:*** Especially diabetes, asthma, COPD, alcohol, opiate or street drug abuse, epilepsy or recent head injury; recent travel. ***Medication:*** Current drugs. ***Allergies***. Once ventilation and circulation are adequate, proceed to carry out history, examination, investigations, and management in the usual way.

No signs on examination
- Tension headache
- Migraine
- Cluster headache
- Post-traumatic
- Drugs (nitrates, calcium channel antagonists)
- Carbon monoxide poisoning or anoxia
- Subarachnoid haemorrhage

Signs of meningism?
- Meningitis (may not have fever or rash)
- Subarachnoid haemorrhage (examination may be normal)

Decreased conscious level or localizing signs?
- Stroke
- Encephalitis/meningitis
- Cerebral abscess
- Subarachnoid haemorrhage (see p485, **figs 1 & 2**)
- Venous sinus occlusion (focal neurological deficits)
- Tumour
- Subdural haematoma
- TB meningitis

Papilloedema?
- Tumour
- Venous sinus occlusion (focal neurological deficits)
- Malignant (accelerated phase) hypertension
- Idiopathic intracranial hypertension
- Any CNS infection, if prolonged (eg >2wks)—eg TB meningitis

Others
- Giant cell arteritis (ESR↑)
- Acute glaucoma
- Vertebral artery dissection (neck pain and cerebellar/medullary signs)
- Cervical spondylosis
- Sinusitis
- Paget's disease (alk phos ↑↑)
- Altitude sickness

Worrying features or 'red flags'[1]
- First and worst headache—*subarachnoid haemorrhage*
- Thunderclap headache—*subarachnoid haemorrhage;* (p484 for other causes).
- Unilateral headache and eye pain—*cluster headache, acute glaucoma*
- Unilateral headache and ipsilateral symptoms—*migraine, tumour, vascular*
- Cough-initiated headache—*raised ICP/venous thrombosis*
- Worse in the morning or bending forward—*raised ICP/venous thrombosis*
- Persisting headache ± scalp tenderness in over-50s—*giant cell arteritis*
- Headache with fever or neck stiffness—*meningitis*
- Change in the pattern of 'usual headaches'
- Decreased level of consciousness

Two other vital questions:
- Where have you been? (malaria)
- Might you be pregnant? (pre-eclampsia; especially if proteinuria and BP↑)

1 Adapted from C Hawkes 2002 *Hosp Med* **63** 732-42.

Breathlessness: emergency presentations

Wheezing?
- Asthma
- COPD
- Heart failure
- Anaphylaxis

Stridor? (Upper airway obstruction)
- Foreign body or tumour
- Acute epiglottitis
- Anaphylaxis
- Trauma, eg laryngeal fracture

Crepitations?
- Heart failure
- Pneumonia
- Bronchiectasis
- Fibrosis

Chest clear?
- Pulmonary embolism
- Hyperventilation
- Metabolic acidosis, eg diabetic ketoacidosis (DKA)
- Anaemia
- Drugs, eg salicylates
- Shock (may cause 'air hunger', p804)
- Pneumocystis pneumonia
- CNS causes

Others
- Pneumothorax—pain, increased resonance, tracheal deviation (if tension pneumothorax)
- Pleural effusion—'stony dullness'

First exclude any potentially life-threatening causes, by way of history, brief examination, and limited investigation. Then consider other potential causes. For the full assessment of cardiac pain, see p112.

Life-threatening
- Acute myocardial infarction
- Angina/acute coronary syndrome
- Aortic dissection
- Tension pneumothorax
- Pulmonary embolism
- Oesophageal rupture

Others
- Pneumonia
- Chest wall pain:
  - Muscular
  - Rib fractures
  - Bony metastases
  - Costochondritis
- Gastro-oesophageal reflux
- Pleurisy
- Empyema
- Pericarditis
- Oesophageal spasm
- Herpes zoster
- Cervical spondylosis
- Intra-abdominal:
  - Cholecystitis
  - Peptic ulceration
  - Pancreatitis
- Sickle-cell crisis

Before discharging patients with undiagnosed chest pain, be sure in your own mind that the pain is not cardiac (this pain is classically dull, may radiate to the jaw, arm, or epigastrium, and is usually associated with exertion, dyspnoea, sweating, nausea, and lessened by GTN). Discuss options with a [illegible], and if in doubt, do not simply send patients home to the street.

Just because the patient's chest wall is tender to palpation this does not mean the cause of the chest pain is musculoskeletal. Even if palpation reproduces the same [illegible]

Chest pain: differential diagnosis

First exclude any potentially life-threatening causes, by virtue of history, brief examination, and limited investigations. Then consider other potential causes. For the full assessment of cardiac pain, see p88 & p112.

Life-threatening

- Acute myocardial infarction
- Angina/acute coronary syndrome
- Aortic dissection
- Tension pneumothorax
- Pulmonary embolism
- Oesophageal rupture

Others

- Pneumonia
- Chest wall pain:
  - Muscular
  - Rib fractures
  - Bony metastases
  - Costochondritis
- Gastro-oesophageal reflux
- Pleurisy
- Empyema
- Pericarditis
- Oesophageal spasm
- Herpes zoster
- Cervical spondylosis
- Intra-abdominal:
  - Cholecystitis
  - Peptic ulceration
  - Pancreatitis
- Sickle-cell crisis

Before discharging patients with undiagnosed chest pain, be sure in your own mind that the pain is not cardiac (this pain is usually dull, may radiate to jaw, arm, or epigastrium, and is usually associated with exertion). Do CXR, ECG, FBC, U&E, and troponin (p112). Discuss options with a colleague, and the patient. Don't simply turn people out on to the street.

►Just because the patient's chest wall is tender to palpation, this doesn't mean the cause of the chest pain is musculoskeletal. Even if palpation reproduces the same type of pain, ensure that you exclude all potential life-threatening causes. Although chest wall tenderness has discriminatory value against cardiac pain, it may be a feature of a pulmonary embolism.

Definition Unrousable unresponsiveness. Quantify using the Glasgow coma scale.

Causes of coma

Metabolic: Drugs, poisoning, eg carbon monoxide, alcohol, tricyclics
Hypoglycaemia, hyperglycaemia (ketoacidotic or HONK)
Hypoxia, CO_2 narcosis (COPD)
Septicaemia
Hypothermia
Myxoedema, Addisonian crisis
Hepatic/uraemic encephalopathy

Neurological: Trauma
Infection: meningitis (p[illegible]); encephalitis, eg herpes simplex—give IV aciclovir if the slightest suspicion (p[illegible]); tropical: malaria (be quick! do thick films; typhoid, typhus, rabies, trypanosomiasis
Tumour: 1° or 2°

Vascular: stroke, subdural, subarachnoid, hypertensive encephalopathy
Epilepsy: non-convulsive status (p[illegible]) or post-ictal states

Immediate management see FLOWCHART (for GCS see p[illegible])
• Assess airway, breathing, and circulation. Consider intubation if GCS ≤8 (p[illegible]). Support the circulation if required (ie IV fluids). Give O_2 and treat any seizures. Protect the cervical spine unless trauma is known not to be the cause.
• Check blood glucose: give 50mL 50% dextrose IV stat if hypoglycaemia possible. Give thiamine if any suggestion of Wernicke's encephalopathy, see below.
• Naloxone (0.4–2mg IV) for opiate intoxication (may also be given IM or via ET tube); IV flumazenil (p[illegible]) for benzodiazepine intoxication only if airway compromised as risk of seizures especially if concomitant tricyclic intoxication.

Examination • *Vital signs are vital*—obtain full set, including temperature.
• Signs of trauma—haematoma, laceration, bruising, CSF/blood in nose or ears, fracture 'step' deformity of skull, subcutaneous emphysema, 'panda eyes'.
• Stigmata of other illnesses: liver disease, alcoholism, diabetes, myxoedema.
• Skin for needle marks, cyanosis, pallor, rashes (meningitis; typhus), poor turgor.
• Smell the breath (alcohol, hepatic fetor, ketosis, uraemia).
• Opisthotonus (p[illegible])? Meningism (p[illegible])—but do not examine neck unless cervical spine is cleared.
• Pupils (p[illegible]): size, reactivity, gaze.
• [illegible]
• [illegible]
• Is there any focal [illegible]?
• Any features of [illegible]?
• [illegible]

Quick history from family, ambulance staff, bystanders: Abrupt or gradual onset? How found—suicide note, seizure? If injured, suspect cervical spine injury and do not move spine (OHCS p[illegible]). Recent complaints—headache, fever, vertigo, depression? Recent medical history—sinusitis, otitis, neurosurgery, ENT procedure? Past medical history—diabetes, asthma, hypertension, cancer, epilepsy, psychiatric illness? Drug or toxin exposure (especially alcohol or other recreational drugs)? Any travel?

If the diagnosis is unclear:
• Treat the treatable: Consider IV thiamine for Wernicke's encephalopathy (p[illegible]), O_2, naloxone as above, glucose (50mL of 50%), antimicrobials (eg ceftriaxone 2g/12h IV meningitis, p[illegible]), artesunate/quinine (malaria p[illegible]), aciclovir (herpes simplex p[illegible]).
• Do routine biochemistry, haematology, thick films, blood cultures, blood ethanol, drug screen etc.
• Arrange urgent CT head, if normal, and no CI, proceed to LP.

The diagnosis should now be clear, eg hypoglycaemia, alcohol excess, poisoning, malaria, meningitis, subarachnoid, tumour, hypertensive/hepatic encephalopathy.

Coma

Definition *Unrousable unresponsiveness*. Quantify using the *Glasgow coma scale*.

Causes of coma

Metabolic: Drugs, poisoning, eg carbon monoxide, alcohol, tricyclics
Hypoglycaemia, hyperglycaemia (ketoacidotic, or HONK, p844)
Hypoxia, CO_2 narcosis (COPD)
Septicaemia
Hypothermia
Myxoedema, Addisonian crisis
Hepatic/uraemic encephalopathy

Neurological: Trauma
Infection: meningitis (p832); encephalitis, eg herpes simplex—give IV aciclovir if the slightest suspicion (p400), *tropical:* malaria (▸▸p394; do thick films), typhoid, typhus, rabies, trypanosomiasis
Tumour: 1° or 2°
Vascular: stroke, subdural/subarachnoid hypertensive encephalopathy
Epilepsy: non-convulsive status (p489) or post-ictal state

Immediate management see FLOWCHART (and coma CNS exam, p802)

- Assess airway, breathing, and circulation. Consider intubation if GCS <8 (p802). Support the circulation if required (ie IV fluids). Give O_2 and treat any seizures. Protect the cervical spine unless trauma is known not to be the cause.
- Check blood glucose; give 50mL 50% dextrose IV stat if hypoglycaemia possible.
- IV thiamine if any suggestion of Wernicke's encephalopathy; see below.
- IV naloxone (0.4-2mg IV) for opiate intoxication (may also be given IM or via ET tube); IV flumazenil (p854) for benzodiazepine intoxication only if airway compromised as risk of seizures especially if concomitant tricyclic intoxication.

Examination ►*Vital signs are vital—obtain full set, including temperature.*

- Signs of trauma—haematoma, laceration, bruising, CSF/blood in nose or ears, fracture 'step' deformity of skull, subcutaneous emphysema, 'panda eyes'.
- Stigmata of other illnesses: liver disease, alcoholism, diabetes, myxoedema.
- Skin for needle marks, cyanosis, pallor, rash (meningitis; typhus), poor turgor.
- Smell the breath (alcohol, hepatic fetor, ketosis, uraemia).
- Opisthotonus (**fig 1**, p425)≈meningitis or tetanus. Decerebrate/decorticate? p802.
- Meningism (p460) ►but do *not* move neck unless cervical spine is cleared.
- Pupils (p803) size, reactivity, gaze.
- Heart/lung exam for BP, murmurs, rubs, wheeze, consolidation, collapse.
- Abdomen/rectal for organomegaly, ascites, bruising, peritonism, melaena.
- Are there any foci of infection (abscesses, bites, middle ear infection)?
- Any features of meningitis: neck stiffness, rash, focal neurology?
- Note the *absence* of signs, eg *no* pin-point pupils in a known heroin addict.

Quick history from family, ambulance staff, bystanders: Abrupt or gradual onset? How found—suicide note, seizure? If injured, suspect cervical spinal injury and do not move spine (*OHCSP766*). Recent complaints—headache, fever, vertigo, depression? Recent medical history—sinusitis, otitis, neurosurgery, ENT procedure? Past medical history—diabetes, asthma, ↑BP, cancer, epilepsy, psychiatric illness? Drug or toxin exposure (especially alcohol or other recreational drugs)? Any travel?

If the diagnosis is unclear

- Treat the treatable: Pabrinex® IV for Wernicke's encephalopathy, p728; O_2; naloxone as above; glucose (50mL of 50% IV); septic specifics: cefotaxime 2g/12h IV (meningitis, p832), artemether/quinine (malaria, p397), aciclovir (herpes simplex, p834).
- Do routine biochemistry, haematology, thick films, blood cultures, blood ethanol, drug screen etc.
- Arrange urgent CT head, if normal, and no CI, proceed to LP.

The diagnosis should now be clear, eg hyperglycaemia; alcohol excess; poisoning; uraemia; pneumonia; subarachnoid (p482); hypertensive/hepatic encephalopathy.

Managing coma

ABC of life support

↓

IV access

↓

Stabilize the cervical spine (vital if trauma is a possibility)

↓

Blood glucose (ward test & lab)

↓

Control seizures

↓

Treat potential causes, eg IV glucose, thiamine, naloxone (if pupils small or if possible narcotic use). Other antidotes: see p854.

↓

Brief history and examination. Come back to this in detail, later.

↓

Investigations

- ABG, FBC, U&E, LFT, ESR, CRP, ethanol, toxic screen, drug levels
- Blood cultures, urine culture, consider malaria
- CXR, CT head

↓

Reassess the situation and plan further investigations

NB: check pupils every few minutes during the early stages, particularly if trauma is the likely cause. Doing so is the quickest way to find a localizing sign (so helpful in diagnosis, but remember that false localizing signs do occur)—and observing changes in pupil behaviour (eg becoming fixed and dilated) is the quickest way of finding out just how bad things are.

The Glasgow coma scale (GCS)

This gives a reliable, objective way of recording the conscious state of a person. It can be used by medical and nursing staff for initial and continuing assessment. It has value in predicting ultimate outcome. 3 types of response are assessed:

Best motor response. This has 6 grades:

6 *Obeying commands:* The patient does simple things you ask (beware of accepting a grasp reflex in this category).

5 *Localizing response to pain:* Put pressure on the patient's fingernail bed with a pencil, then try supraorbital and sternal pressure: purposeful movements towards changing painful stimuli is a 'localizing' response.

4 *Withdraws to pain:* Pulls limb away from painful stimulus.

3 *Flexor response to pain:* Nailbed pressure causes abnormal flexion of limbs—**decorticate posture** (other signs: arm bent inward on chest, thumb tucked in a clenched fist, legs extended). It means damage above the level of the red nucleus in the midbrain (which mediates antigravity muscles in the upper limb).[1]

2 *Extensor posturing to pain:* The stimulus causes limb extension (adduction, internal rotation of shoulder, pronation of forearm)—**decerebrate posture**. It indicates midbrain damage below the level of the red nucleus.

1 *No response to pain.*

Note that it is the best response of any limb which should be recorded.

Best verbal response. This has 5 grades:

5 *Oriented:* The patient knows who he is, where he is and why, the year, season, and month.

4 *Confused conversation:* The patient responds to questions in a conversational manner but there is some disorientation and confusion.

3 *Inappropriate speech:* Random or exclamatory articulated speech, but no conversational exchange.

2 *Incomprehensible speech:* Moaning but no words.

1 *None.*

Record level of best speech.

Eye opening This has 4 grades:

4 *Spontaneous eye opening.*

3 *Eye opening in response to speech:* Any speech, or shout, not necessarily request to open eyes.

2 *Eye opening in response to pain:* Pain to limbs as above.

1 *No eye opening.*

An overall score is made by summing the score in the 3 areas assessed. Eg: no response to pain + no verbalization + no eye opening = 3. Severe injury, GCS ≤8; moderate injury, GCS 9-12; minor injury, GCS 13-15.

NB: an abbreviated coma scale, AVPU, is sometimes used in the initial assessment ('primary survey') of the critically ill:

- A = alert
- V = responds to vocal stimuli
- P = responds to pain
- U = unresponsive

Some centres score GCS out of 14, not 15, omitting 'withdrawal to pain'. NB: the GCS scoring is different in young children; see *OHCS* p201.

1 Red nucleus output reinforces upper limb antigravity flexion. When its output is damaged, the unregulated reticulospinal and vestibulospinal tracts reinforce extension tone of upper **and** lower limbs.

The neurological examination in coma

This is aimed at locating the pathology in 1 of 2 places. Altered level of consciousness implies either: **1** a diffuse, bilateral, cortical dysfunction (usually producing loss of awareness with normal arousal), or **2** damage to the ascending reticular activating system (ARAS) located throughout the brainstem from the medulla to the thalami (usually producing loss of arousal with unassessable awareness). The brainstem can be affected directly (eg pontine haemorrhage) or indirectly (eg compression from trans-tentorial or cerebellar herniation secondary to a mass or oedema).

- Level of consciousness; describe using *objective* words.
- Respiratory pattern—Cheyne-Stokes (p53), hyperventilation (acidosis, hypoxia, or rarely, neurogenic), ataxic or apneustic (breath-holding) breathing (brainstem damage with grave prognosis).
- Eyes—almost all patients with ARAS pathology will have eye findings.
  1. *Visual fields* In light coma, test fields with visual threat. No blink in 1 field suggests hemianopia and contralateral hemisphere lesion.
  2. *Pupils Normal direct & consensual reflexes present* = intact midbrain. *Midposition (3–5mm) non-reactive ± irregular* = midbrain lesion. *Unilateral dilated & unreactive* ('fixed') = 3rd nerve compression. *Small, reactive* = pontine lesion ('pin-point pontine pupils') or drugs. *Horner's syndrome* (p716) = ipsilateral lateral medulla or hypothalamus lesion, may precede uncal herniation. Beware patients with false eyes or who use eye drops for glaucoma.
  3. *Extraocular movements (EOMS)*—observe resting position and spontaneous movement; then test the vestibulo-ocular reflex (VOR) with either the *doll's-head manoeuvre* (normal if the eyes keep looking at the same point in space when the head is quickly moved laterally or vertically) or *ice water calorics* (normal if eyes deviate towards the cold ear with nystagmus to the other side). If present, the VOR exonerates *most* of the brainstem from the VIIth nerve nucleus (medulla) to the IIIrd (midbrain). *Don't move the head unless the cervical spine is cleared.*
  4. *Fundi*—papilloedema, subhyaloid haemorrhage, hypertensive retinopathy, signs of other disease (eg diabetic retinopathy).
- Examine for CNS asymmetry (tone, spontaneous movements, reflexes). One way to test for hemiplegia in coma is to raise both arms together and compare how they fall under gravity. If one descends fast, like a lead weight, but the other descends more gracefully, you have found a valuable focal sign. The same applies to the legs.

Essence Circulatory failure resulting in inadequate organ perfusion. *Generally* systolic BP is <90mmHg. Signs: pallor, pulse↑, capillary return↓ (press a nailbed), air hunger, oliguria. Causes are either *pump failure* or *peripheral circulation failure*.

Pump failure

- *Cardiogenic shock*
- *Secondary:* pulmonary embolism, tension pneumothorax, cardiac tamponade.

Peripheral circulation failure

- *Hypovolaemia:*
  Bleeding: trauma, ruptured aortic aneurysm, ruptured ectopic pregnancy. *Fluid loss:* vomiting (eg GI obstruction), diarrhoea (eg cholera), burns, pools of sequestered (unavailable) fluids ('third spacing', eg in pancreatitis). ***Heat exhaustion*** may cause hypovolaemic shock (also hyperpyrexia, oliguria, rhabdomyolysis, consciousness↓, hyperventilation, hallucination, incontinence, collapse, coma, pin-point pupils, LFT↑, and DIC, p346).
- *Anaphylaxis*
- *Sepsis:* septic shock from endotoxin-induced vasodilatation may be sudden and severe, with shock and coma but no signs of infection (fever, WCC↑).
- *Neurogenic:* eg post-spinal surgery.
- *Endocrine failure:* Addison's disease or hypothyroidism; see p846.
- *Iatrogenic:* drugs, eg anaesthetics, antihypertensives.

Assessment ►ABC.

- *ECG:* rate, rhythm, ischaemia?
- *General:* cold and clammy suggests cardiogenic shock or fluid loss. Look for signs of anaemia or dehydration, eg skin turgor, postural hypotension? Warm and well perfused, with bounding pulse points to septic shock. Any features suggestive of anaphylaxis—history, urticaria, angio-oedema, wheeze?
- *CVS:* usually tachycardic (unless on β-blocker, or in spinal shock—*OHCS* p772) and hypotensive. But in the young and fit, or pregnant women, the systolic BP may remain normal, although the *pulse pressure* will narrow, with up to 30% blood volume depletion. Difference between arms (>20mmHg)—aortic dissection?
- *JVP or central venous pressure:* If raised, cardiogenic shock likely.
- *Check abdomen:* any signs of trauma, or aneurysm? Any evidence of GI bleed?—check for melaena.

Management[5] ►If BP unrecordable, call the cardiac arrest team.
See FLOWCHART for general management. Specific measures:

- *Anaphylaxis:* p806.
- *Cardiogenic shock:* p814.
- *Septic shock:* Give antibiotics within 1hr (preferably after blood culture). If no clue to source (p382): IV co-amoxiclav 1.2g/8h, or meropenem 1g/8h or gentamicin (p767; do levels; reduce in renal failure) + antipseudomonal penicillin, eg ticarcillin (as Timentin®, p378, max dose 3.2g/4h IVI). Give colloid, or crystalloid, by IVI. Refer to ITU if possible for monitoring ± inotropes; aim for CVP 8-12mmHg, mean arterial pressure >65mmHg. Urine >35ml/h. Low-dose steroids may help if hypotensive despite fluids and vasopressors as may recombinant human-activated protein C.[6]
- *Hypovolaemic shock:* Fluid replacement: saline or colloid initially; if bleeding use blood; risks and benefits: see p358. Titrate against BP, CVP, urine output. Treat the underlying cause. If severe haemorrhage, exsanguinating, or >1L of fluid required to maintain BP, consider using group-specific blood, or O Rh-ve blood (p358). Correct electrolyte abnormalities. Acidosis often responds to fluid replacement.
- *Heat exposure (heat exhaustion):* Tepid sponging + fanning; avoid ice and immersion. Resuscitate with high-sodium IVI, such as 0.9% saline ± hydrocortisone 100mg IV. Dantrolene seems ineffective. Chlorpromazine 25mg IM may be used to stop shivering. Stop cooling when core temperature <39°C.

Management of shock

If BP unrecordable, call the cardiac arrest team

↓

ABC (including high-flow O_2)

↓

Raise foot of the bed Unless cardiogenic)

↓

IV access × 2 (wide bore; get help if this takes >2min)

↓

Identify and treat underlying cause

↓

Infuse crystalloid *fast* to raise BP (unless cardiogenic shock)

↓

Seek expert help early

↓

Investigations
- FBC, U&E, ABG, glucose, CRP
- Cross-match and check clotting
- Blood cultures, urine culture, ECG, CXR
- *Others:* lactate, echo, abdominal CT, USS

↓

Consider arterial line, central venous line, and bladder catheter (aim for a urine flow >30mL/h)

↓

Further management
- Treat underlying cause if possible
- Fluid replacement as dictated by BP, CVP, urine output
- Don't overload with fluids if cardiogenic shock (exclude PE & RV infarct 1st)
- If persistently hypotensive, consider inotropes

NB: remember that higher flow rates can be achieved through peripheral lines than through 'standard' gauge central lines. If cause unclear: ℞ as hypovolaemia—the most common cause, and reversible. Ruptured abdominal aortic aneurysm: aim for a systolic BP of ~90mmHg.

SIRS, sepsis, and related syndromes

The pathogenesis of sepsis and septic shock is becoming increasingly understood. The 'systemic inflammatory response syndrome' (SIRS) is thought to be a central component, involving cytokine cascades, free-radical production, and the release of vasoactive mediators. SIRS is defined as the presence of 2 or more of the following features:[7]
- Temperature >38°C or <36°C
- Tachycardia >90 bpm
- Respiratory rate >20 breaths/min or P_aCO_2 <4.3 kPa
- WBC $>12\times10^9$/L or $<4\times10^9$/L, or >10% immature (band) forms

Related syndromes include:

Sepsis: SIRS occurring in the presence of infection.

Severe sepsis: Sepsis with evidence of organ hypoperfusion, eg hypoxaemia, oliguria, lactic acidosis, or altered cerebral function.

Septic shock: Severe sepsis with hypotension (systolic BP <90mmHg) despite adequate fluid resuscitation, or the requirement for vasopressors/inotropes to maintain blood pressure.

Septicaemia was used to denote the presence of multiplying bacteria in the circulation, but has been replaced with the definitions above.[8]

Type-I IgE-mediated hypersensitivity reaction. Release of histamine and other agents causes: capillary leak; wheeze; cyanosis; oedema (larynx, lids, tongue, lips); urticaria. More common in atopic individuals. An *anaphylactoid reaction* results from direct release of mediators from inflammatory cells, without involving antibodies, usually in response to a drug, eg acetylcysteine.

Examples of precipitants

- Drugs, eg penicillin, and contrast media in radiology
- Latex
- Stings, eggs, fish, peanuts, strawberries, semen (rare)

Signs and symptoms

- Itching, sweating, diarrhoea and vomiting, erythema, urticaria, oedema
- Wheeze, laryngeal obstruction, cyanosis
- Tachycardia, hypotension

Management of anaphylaxis

Secure the airway—give 100% O_2
Intubate if respiratory obstruction

↓

Remove the cause; raising the feet may help restore the circulation

↓

Give adrenaline IM *0.5mg (ie 0.5mL of 1:1000)*
Repeat every 5min, if needed as guided by BP, pulse, and respiratory function, until better

↓

Secure IV access

↓

Chlorphenamine 10mg IV and hydrocortisone 200mg IV

↓

IVI (0.9% saline, eg 500mL over ¼h; up to 2L may be needed)
Titrate against blood pressure

↓

If wheeze, treat for asthma (p820)
May require ventilatory support

↓

If still hypotensive, admission to ITU and an IVI of adrenaline may be needed ± aminophylline (p821) and nebulized salbutamol (p821): get expert help.

↓

Further management:
- Admit to ward. Monitor ECG.
- Continue chlorphenamine 4mg/6h PO if itching.
- Suggest a 'MedicAlert' bracelet naming the culprit allergen (p667).
- Teach about self-injected adrenaline (eg 0.3mg, Epipen®) to prevent a fatal attack.
- Skin-prick tests showing specific IgE help identify allergens to avoid.

▸▸Adrenaline (=epinephrine) is given IM and NOT IV unless the patient is severely ill, or has no pulse. The IV dose is **different:** 100μg/min—titrating with the response. This is 1mL of **1:10,000 solution** per minute. Stop as soon as a response has been obtained.

If on a β-blocker, consider salbutamol IV in place of adrenaline.

Acute coronary syndrome—with ST-elevation

Acute coronary syndrome (ACS) includes unstable angina, STEMI[1] (what most of us mean by acute MI), and NSTEMI (see p112). STEMI is a common medical emergency, and prompt appropriate treatment saves lives. If in doubt, seek immediate help.

Initial treatment Take brief history, do a quick physical exam and take a 12 lead ECG. Blood tests on admission: U&E, troponin, glucose, cholesterol, FBC, CXR. (later on CCU).

- *Aspirin* 300mg PO (if not already given); consider clopidogrel 300mg too. [13]
- *Morphine* 5-10mg IV (repeat after 5min if necessary). Give antiemetic with the 1st dose of morphine: metoclopramide 10mg IV (1st line), cyclizine 50mg IV (2nd line).
- *GTN* 1-2 tablets SL, or spray.
- *Oxygen* must be given for the 1st few hours after acute MI by mask or nasal prongs.
- *Restore coronary perfusion* Either primary PCI (if available) or thrombolysis.
  - *Primary PCI* Now the treatment of choice if ongoing ischaemia and presentation is within 12h. However, not available in all locations.
  - *Thrombolysis* ▸▸The benefit of thrombolysis reduces steadily from the onset of chest pain so start as quickly as possible (target time <30min from admission). Thrombolysis is contraindicated beyond 24h from the time of onset of symptoms. ►Do not thrombolyse ST depression alone, T-wave inversion alone or normal ECG.

Complications

- Recurrent ischaemia or failure to reperfuse (usually detected as persisting pain and ST-segment elevation in the immediate aftermath of thrombolysis): analgesia, GTN, β-blocker, consider re-thrombolysis or PCI.
- Stroke.
- Pericarditis: analgesics, try to avoid NSAIDs.
- Cardiogenic shock: see p814 and heart failure: see p812.

Right ventricular infarction: Confirm by demonstrating ST elevation in rV3/4, and/or echo. NB: rV4 means that V4 is placed in the right 5th intercostal space in the midclavicular line. Treat hypotension and oliguria with fluids (avoid nitrates and diuretics). Monitor BP carefully, and assess early signs of pulmonary oedema. Intensive monitoring and inotropes may be useful in some patients.

Thrombolysis

ECG criteria for thrombolysis

- ST elevation >1mm in 2 or more limb leads or >2mm in 2 or more chest leads.
- LBBB (unless known to have LBBB previously).
- Posterior changes: Deep ST depression and tall R waves in leads V1 to V3.

Contraindications

- Internal (or heavy vaginal) bleeding
- Acute pancreatitis or severe liver disease
- Active lung disease with cavitation
- Recent trauma or surgery (<2wks)
- Severe hypertension (>200/120mmHg)
- Suspected aortic dissection
- Previous allergic reaction
- Recent haemorrhagic stroke
- Oesophageal varices
- Cerebral neoplasm

Relative CI: Severe hypertension; peptic ulcer; history of CVA; bleeding diathesis; pregnancy/recent delivery; anticoagulants SBE; prolonged CPR.

Choice of agent: *Streptokinase* (SK) 1st line for non-anterior MI. Dose: 1.5 million units in 100mL 0.9% saline IVI over 1h. SE: nausea; vomiting; haemorrhage; stroke (1%); dysrhythmias. ↓BP usually responds to slowing down or stopping the infusion. Allergic reactions and anaphylaxis rare. Do not repeat unless within 4d of the 1st dose. *Tenecteplase* is given by bolus injection (useful for paramedics). Indications: • Anterior MI • previous use of SK (ever) • Systolic BP <100mmHg, • New LBBB. *Alteplase* (rt-PA), followed by heparin, may be indicated if the patient has previously received SK (>4d ago) or reacted to SK. Accelerated rt-PA has benefit if given within 6h, especially in younger patients with anterior MI. *Reteplase* is given as 2 IV boluses 2h apart. ►Patients with STEMI who do not receive reperfusion therapy, should be treated immediately with *fondaparinux*. [14]

Management of an acute MI

Attach ECG monitor and record a 12-lead ECG

↓

O_2 2-4L aim for S_aO_2>95% (caution, if COPD)

↓

IV access

Bloods for FBC, U&E, glucose, lipids, cardiac enzymes (p113)

↓

Brief assessment

- History of cardiovascular disease; risk factors for IHD
- Contraindications to thrombolysis?
- Examination: pulse, BP (both arms), JVP, cardiac murmurs, signs of heart failure, upper limb pulses, scars from previous cardiac surgery

↓

Aspirin 300mg (unless already given by GP/paramedics)

↓

Morphine 5-10mg IV + antiemetic, eg metoclopramide 10mg IV

↓

GTN sublingually 2 puffs or 1 tablet as required

↓

Primary PCI or thrombolysis, see p808

↓

β-blocker, eg atenolol 5mg IV (unless asthma or left ventricular failure)

↓

CXR. Do not delay thrombolysis while waiting unless suspected aneurysm (eg interscapular pain; BP different in each arm, p656).

↓

Consider DVT prophylaxis (p580)

↓

Continue medication except calcium channel antagonists (unless specific indication)

↓

For further management: see p114

1 Abbreviations:
STEMI: ST elevation myocardial infarction
NSTEMI: non-ST elevation myocardial infarction
PCI: Percutaneous coronary intervention (eg angioplasty)

NB: ►If pain is uncontrolled, especially if continuing ST elevation, consider re-thrombolysis with rt-PA (no bolus), tenecteplase, or rescue PCI.

Patients should be managed medically until symptoms settle, unless high risk. They are then investigated by angiography with a view to possible percutaneous coronary intervention or surgery (CABG).

Assessment

Brief history: previous angina, relief with rest/nitrates, history of cardiovascular disease, risk factors for IHD.

Examination: pulse, BP, JVP, cardiac murmurs, signs of heart failure, peripheral pulses, scars from previous cardiac surgery.

Investigations ECG: ST depression; flat or inverted T waves; or normal. U&E, CK, glucose, random cholesterol, FBC, CXR (later on CCU, not in A&E, and only if no recent CXR), cardiac troponin. Measurement of cardiac troponins helps to predict which patients are at risk of a cardiac event, and who can be safely discharged early.[16] Note that 2 different forms of troponin are measured: troponin T and troponin I: they have different reference intervals (consult your lab).

Management ►See FLOWCHART for acute management, but p808 if ST elevation. The aim of therapy is to optimize anti-ischaemic and anti-platelet therapy.

Oral antiplatelet therapy: Aspirin 300mg initially followed by 75mg/d **and** *clopidogrel* (300mg initially then 75mg/d PO) should be given to the following groups of patients and continued for 12 months: • ↑troponin • ACS already on aspirin • ↓ST on resting ECG • ACS after recent MI • Patients being transferred for angioplasty • Aspirin intolerant. Clopidogrel should be not be used routinely for patients with suspected cardiac pain in the absence of ECG changes or raised troponin.

Heparin: Usually low molecular weight (LMW), eg enoxaparin 1mg/kg/12h). If unavailable, unfractionated heparin 5000U IV bolus then IVI. Check APTT 6-hourly. Alter IVI rate to maintain APTT at 1.5–2.5 times control.

Glycoprotein IIb/IIIa inhibitors: (see FLOWCHART). Consider in patients with recurrent or persistent chest pain and ECG changes despite standard treatment.[17]

Nitrates (PO or IV) for recurrent chest pain.

Beta-blockers: unless contraindicated in which case diltiazem should be considered.

ACE-i should be given to all patients unless there are CI (monitor renal function).

Lipid management: As for STEMI (p114, p808).

Prognosis Overall risk of death ~1–2%, but ~15% for refractory angina despite medical therapy. Risk stratification can help predict those most at risk and allow intervention to be targeted at those individuals. The following are associated with an increased risk:

- History of unstable angina
- ST depression or widespread T-wave inversion
- Raised troponin (except patients with ST elevation MI)
- Age >70 years
- General comorbidity, previous MI, poor LV function or DM.

►High-risk patients should be considered for inpatient coronary angiography.

Further measures:

- Wean off *glyceryl trinitrate* (GTN) infusion when stabilized on oral drugs.
- Stop heparin when pain-free for 24h, but give at least 3–5 days of therapy.
- Check serial ECGs, and troponin >12h after pain.
- Address modifiable risk factors: smoking, hypertension, hyperlipidaemia, diabetes.
- Gentle mobilization.

►*If symptoms recur; refer to a cardiologist for urgent angiography and PCI or CABG.*

Acute management of ACS without ST-segment elevation

Admit to CCU and monitor closely

↓

O_2 2-4L; aim for S_aO_2>95% (caution in COPD)

↓

Analgesia: eg morphine 5-10mg IV + metoclopramide 10mg IV

↓

Nitrates: GTN spray or sublingual tablets as required

↓

Aspirin: 300mg PO and/or *clopidogrel* 300mg po (unless contraindicated)
Reduces risk of MI and death

↓

Oral β-blocker: eg metoprolol 50-100mg/8h or atenolol 50-100mg/24h
If β-blocker contraindicated (asthma, COPD, LVF, bradycardia, coronary artery spasm), give rate-limiting calcium antagonist (eg verapamil[1] 80-120mg/8h PO, or diltiazem 60-120mg/8h PO)

↓

Heparin: eg enoxaparin 1mg/kg/12h or dalteparin 120U/kg/12h SC

↓

IV nitrate if pain continues
(eg GTN 50mg in 50mL 0.9% saline at 2-10mL/h)
titrate to pain, and maintain systolic BP >100mmHg

↓

Record ECG while in pain

High-risk patients
(persistent or recurrent ischaemia, ST-depression, diabetes, ↑troponin)
- Infusion of a GPIIb/IIIa antagonist (eg tirofiban) and, ideally, urgent angiography.
- Add clopidogrel

↓

Optimize drugs:
- β-blocker; Ca^{2+} channel antagonist; ACE-i; nitrate.
- Intensive statin regimens, *starting at top dosages*, may decrease long- *and* short-term mortality/adverse events, by stabilizing plaques eg atorvastatin 80mg.[2,3]

→ *►If symptoms fail to improve, refer to a cardiologist for urgent angiography ± percutaneous coronary intervention or CABG.*

Low-risk patients
(no further pain, flat or inverted T waves, or normal ECG, and negative troponin)
- May be discharged if a repeat troponin (>12h) is negative.
- Treat medically and arrange further investigation eg stress test, angiogram.

1 Do not use verapamil and a β-blocker together (can cause asystole).
2 Comparing intensive & moderate lipid lowering with statins after ACS. N=4162. Cannon C *NEJM* 2004
3 Intensive statin therapy—a sea change in cardiovascular prevention. Topol E *NEJM* 2004.

Causes

- Cardiovascular, usually left ventricular failure (post-MI or ischaemic heart disease). Also valvular heart disease, arrhythmias, and malignant hypertension.
- ARDS (p178) from any cause, eg trauma, malaria, drugs. Then look for predisposing factors, eg trauma, post-op, sepsis. *Is aspirin overdose or glue-sniffing/drug abuse likely*? Ask friends/relatives.
- Fluid overload.
- Neurogenic, eg head injury.

Differential diagnosis Asthma/COPD, pneumonia, and pulmonary oedema are often hard to distinguish, especially in the elderly, where they may co-exist. Do not hesitate to treat all 3 simultaneously (eg with salbutamol nebulizer, furosemide IV, diamorphine, amoxicillin—p378).

Symptoms Dyspnoea, orthopnoea (eg paroxysmal), pink frothy sputum. NB: note drugs recently given and other illnesses (recent MI/COPD or pneumonia).

Signs Distressed, pale, sweaty, pulse↑, tachypnoea, pink frothy sputum, pulsus alternans, JVP↑, fine lung crackles, triple/gallop rhythm (p42), wheeze (cardiac asthma). Usually sitting up and leaning forward. Quickly examine for possible causes.

Investigations

- CXR (p129, p736): cardiomegaly, signs of pulmonary oedema: look for shadowing (usually bilateral), small effusions at costophrenic angles, fluid in the lung fissures, and Kerley B lines (linear opacities).
- ECG: signs of MI, dysrhythmias.
- U&E, 'cardiac' enzymes, ABG.
- Consider echo.
- Plasma BNP (p131) may be helpful if diagnosis in question (high negative predictive value).

Management

▸▸Begin treatment before investigations. See FLOWCHART.

Monitoring progress: BP; pulse; cyanosis; respiratory rate; JVP; urine output; ABG.

Once stable and improving:

- Daily weights; BP and pulse/6h. Repeat CXR.
- Change to oral furosemide or bumetanide.
- If on large doses of loop diuretic, consider the addition of a thiazide (eg bendroflumethiazide or metolazone 2.5-5mg daily PO).
- ACE-i if left ventricular failure. If ACE-i contraindicated, consider hydralazine and nitrate (may also be more effective in AfroCaribbeans).[18]
- Also consider β-blocker and spironolactone.
- Is the patient suitable for biventricular pacing or cardiac transplantation?
- Consider digoxin ± warfarin, especially if AF.

Nesiritide, recombinant human brain natriuretic peptide, may have a role in the short-term management of decompensated cardiac failure as it improves haemodynamics in such patients.[19] However, it is expensive and further data on safety and outcome are required before it is more widely adopted.

Management of heart failure

Sit the patient upright

↓

Oxygen
100% if no pre-existing lung disease

↓

IV access and monitor ECG
Treat any arrhythmias, eg AF (p116–p124)

↓

Investigations whilst continuing treatment
See p812

↓

Diamorphine 2.5–5mg IV slowly
Caution in liver failure and *COPD*

↓

Furosemide 40–80mg IV slowly
Larger doses required in renal failure

↓

GTN spray 2 puffs SL or 2 × 0.3mg tablets SL
Don't give if systolic BP *<90mmHg*

↓

Necessary investigations, examination, and history

↓

If systolic BP ≥100mmHg, start a nitrate infusion
eg isosorbide dinitrate 2–10mg/h IVI; *keep systolic* BP *≥90mmHg*

↓

If the patient is worsening: further dose of furosemide 40–80mg.
Consider ventilation (invasive or non-invasive eg CPAP; get help)
or increasing nitrate infusion.
Alternatively venesect 500mL blood (rarely done)

↓

If systolic BP <100mmHg, treat as cardiogenic shock (p814),
ie consider a Swan-Ganz catheter and inotropic support

Notes:[20,21]

- If failure to improve, reassess and consider alternative diagnoses, eg hypertensive heart failure, aortic dissection, pulmonary embolism, pneumonia.
- CPAP (5–10 mmHg) in dyspnoeic patients (if no ↓BP or emergent need for intubation) can reduce the need for intubation, and possibly in-hospital mortality.
- Consider IV nitrate therapy for patients with dyspnoea.

▸▸Cardiogenic shock

This has a high mortality. ►Ask a senior physician's help both in formulating an *exact* diagnosis and in guiding treatment.

Cardiogenic shock is a state of inadequate tissue perfusion primarily due to cardiac dysfunction. It may occur suddenly, or after progressively worsening heart failure.

Causes

- Myocardial infarction
- Arrhythmias
- Pulmonary embolus
- Tension pneumothorax
- Cardiac tamponade
- Myocarditis; myocardial depression (drugs, hypoxia, acidosis, sepsis)
- Valve destruction (endocarditis)
- Aortic dissection

Management

If the cause is myocardial infarction prompt revascularization (thrombolysis or acute angioplasty) is vital[1]; ▸▸see p808 for indications and contraindications.

- Manage in Coronary Care Unit, or ITU.
- Investigation and treatment may need to be done concurrently.
- See OPPOSITE for details of management.
- ***Investigations:*** ECG, U&E, cardiac enzymes/troponins, ABG, CXR, echocardiogram. If indicated, CT thorax (aortic dissection/PE) or V/Q scan.
- ***Monitor*** CVP, BP, ABG, ECG, urine output. Do a 12-lead ECG every hour until the diagnosis is made. Consider a Swan-Ganz catheter to assess pulmonary wedge pressure and cardiac output, and an arterial line to monitor pressure. Catheterize for accurate urine output.

Cardiac tamponade

Essence: Pericardial fluid collects → intra-pericardial pressure rises → heart cannot fill → pumping stops.

Causes: Trauma, lung/breast cancer, pericarditis, myocardial infarct, bacteria, eg TB. *Rarely:* Urea↑, radiation, myxoedema, dissecting aorta, SLE. Also coronary artery dissection (secondary to PCI) and/or ruptured ventricle.

Signs: Falling BP, a rising JVP, and muffled heart sounds (Beck's triad); JVP↑ on inspiration (Kussmaul's sign); pulsus paradoxus (pulse fades on inspiration). Echocardiography may be diagnostic. CXR: globular heart; left heart border convex or straight; right cardiophrenic angle <90°. ECG: electrical alternans (p148).

Management: This can be very difficult. Everything is against you: time, physiology, and your own confidence, as the patient may be too ill to give a history, and signs may be equivocal—but bitter experience has taught us not to equivocate for long.

▸▸Request the presence of your senior at the bedside (do not make do with telephone advice). With luck, prompt pericardiocentesis (p787) brings swift relief. While awaiting this, give O_2, monitor ECG, and set up IVI. Take blood for group and save. NB: there may be a role for cardiothoracic surgery (eg CABG, ventricular repair, or pericardial window) as a definitive solution to some causes.

1 SHOCK trial 2003 V Menon *Congest Heart Fail* **9** 35. NNT for acute angioplasty = 5.

Management of cardiogenic shock

Oxygen
Titrate to maintain adequate arterial saturations

↓

Diamorphine 2.5–5mg IV for pain and anxiety

↓

Investigations and *close monitoring*
(see p814)

↓

Correct arrhythmias (p116–p124), U&E abnormalities or acid-base disturbance

↓

Optimize filling pressure
if available measure pulmonary capillary wedge pressure (PCWP)

↓

If PCWP <15mmHg fluid load
↓
Give a plasma expander
100mL every 15min IV
Aim for PCWP of 15–20mmHg

If PCWP >15mmHg
↓
Inotropic support
eg dobutamine
2.5–10µg/kg/min IVI. Aim for a systolic BP >80mmHg

↓

Consider 'renal dose' dopamine
2–5µg/kg/min IV initially *(via central line only)*

↓

Consider intra-aortic balloon pump if you expect the underlying condition to improve, or you need time awaiting surgery

↓

Look for and treat any reversible cause
MI or PE—consider thrombolysis;
surgery for: acute VSD, mitral, or aortic incompetence

ECG shows rate of >100bpm and QRS complexes >120ms (>3 small squares on ECGs done at the standard UK rate of 25mm/s).

Principles of management
If in doubt, treat as ventricular tachycardia (the commonest cause).
Identify the underlying rhythm and treat accordingly.

Differential diagnosis
- *Ventricular tachycardia (VT) including torsade de pointes.* Single ventricular ectopics should not cause confusion; if >3 together at a rate >100, this is VT.
- SVT with aberrant conduction, eg AF, atrial flutter
- Pre-excited tachycardias, eg AF, atrial flutter, or AV re-entry tachycardia with underlying WPW (p120).

Identifying the underlying rhythm may be hard; get help. Diagnosis is based on the history (if IHD/MI likelihood of a ventricular arrhythmia is >95%), 12-lead ECG, and lack of response to IV adenosine (p120). ***ECG findings in favour of VT:***
- Positive QRS concordance in chest leads
- Marked left axis deviation
- AV dissociation (occurs in 25%) or 2:1 or 3:1 AV block
- Fusion beats or capture beats (ECG p123)
- Also bear in mind Brugada's criteria, eg RSR complex in V1 (and +ve QRS in V1): p123.

Management Give high-flow O_2 by mask and monitor O_2 saturations.
- Connect patient to a cardiac monitor and have a defibrillator to hand.
- Correct electrolyte abnormalities.
- Check for adverse signs. Low cardiac output (clammy, consciousness↓, BP <90); oliguria; angina; pulmonary oedema.
- Obtain 12-lead ECG (request CXR) and obtain IV access.

If haemodynamically unstable: ⏩Synchronized DC shock (see inside back cover).
- Correct any hypokalaemia and hypomagnesaemia: up to 60mmol KCl at 30mmol/h, and 4mL 50% **magnesium sulphate** over 30min.
- Follow with **amiodarone** 300mg IV over 20-60min.
- For refractory cases **procainamide** or **sotalol** may be considered.

If haemodynamically stable: Correct hypokalaemia and hypomagnesaemia: as above.
- **Amiodarone** 300mg IV over 20-60 min (avoid if long QT). Alternatively **lidocaine** 50mg (2.5mL of 2% solution) IV over 2min, repeated every 5min up to 200mg.
- If this fails, use synchronized DC shock.

After correction of VT: Establish the cause (via the history and tests above).
- Maintenance anti-arrhythmic therapy may be required. If VT occurs after MI, give IV **amiodarone** or **lidocaine** infusion for 12-24h; if 24h after MI, also start oral anti-arrhythmic: **sotalol** (if good LV function) or **amiodarone** (if poor LV function).
- Prevention of recurrent VT: surgical isolation of the arrhythmogenic area or an implantable cardioverter defibrillator (ICD) may help.

Ventricular fibrillation: (ECG p123) Use non-synchronized DC shock (there is no R wave to trigger defibrillation, p784): see inside back cover.

Ventricular extrasystoles (ectopics): are the commonest post-MI arrhythmia but they are also seen in healthy people (often >10/h). Patients with frequent ectopics post-MI have a worse prognosis, but there is no evidence that antidysrhythmic drugs improve outcome, indeed they may increase mortality.

Torsade de pointes: A form of VT, with a constantly varying axis, often in the setting of long-QT syndromes (ECG p123). Causes (p725): congenital or from drugs (eg some anti-dysrhythmics, tricyclics, antimalarials, antipsychotics). Torsade in the setting of congenital long-QT syndromes can be treated with high doses of β-blockers.

In acquired long-QT syndromes (p725), stop all predisposing drugs, correct hypokalaemia, and give **$MgSO_4$** (2g IV over 10 min). Alternatives include: **overdrive pacing** (pace at a faster rate, then slow reduce) or **isoprenaline** IVI to increase heart rate.

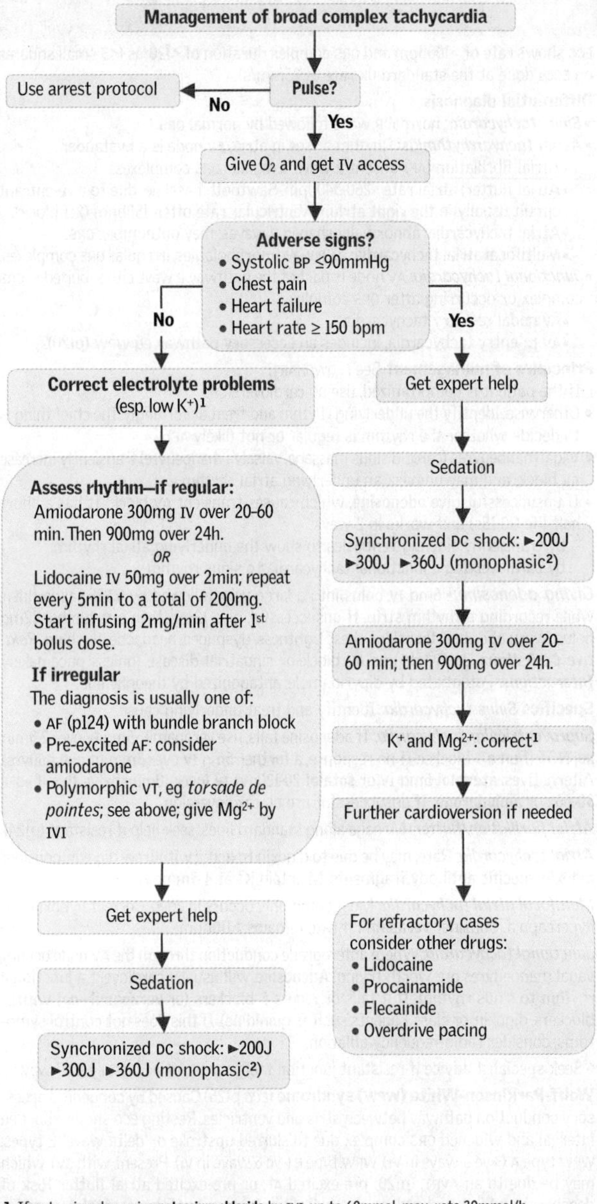
Management of broad complex tachycardia
Use arrest protocol
Pulse?
No
Yes
Give O_2 and get IV access
Adverse signs?
• Systolic BP ≤90mmHg
• Chest pain
• Heart failure
• Heart rate ≥ 150 bpm
No
Yes
Correct electrolyte problems
(esp. low K^+)1
Get expert help
Sedation
Assess rhythm—if regular:
Amiodarone 300mg IV over 20-60 min. Then 900mg over 24h.
OR
Lidocaine IV 50mg over 2min; repeat every 5min to a total of 200mg. Start infusing 2mg/min after 1st bolus dose.
If irregular
The diagnosis is usually one of:
• AF (p124) with bundle branch block
• Pre-excited AF: consider amiodarone
• Polymorphic VT, eg torsade de pointes; see above; give Mg^{2+} by IVI
Synchronized DC shock: ►200J ►300J ►360J (monophasic2)
Amiodarone 300mg IV over 20–60 min; then 900mg over 24h.
K^+ and Mg^{2+}: correct1
Further cardioversion if needed
Get expert help
Sedation
Synchronized DC shock: ►200J ►300J ►360J (monophasic2)
For refractory cases consider other drugs:
• Lidocaine
• Procainamide
• Flecainide
• Overdrive pacing

1 If potassium low: give **potassium chloride** by IVI, up to 60mmol, max. rate 30mmol/h. Give **magnesium sulphate** IVI 5mL 50% in 30min.
2 If biphasic shock used, start at 120-150J.

ECG shows rate of >100bpm and QRS complex duration of <120ms (<3 small squares on ECGs done at the standard UK rate of 25mm/s).

Differential diagnosis

- *Sinus tachycardia:* normal P wave followed by normal QRS.
- *Atrial tachyarrhythmias:* Rhythm arises in atria, AV node is a bystander.
  - Atrial fibrillation (AF): absent P wave, irregular QRS complexes.
  - Atrial flutter: atrial rate ~260-340bpm. Sawtooth baseline, due to a re-entrant circuit usually in the right atrium. Ventricular rate often 150bpm (2:1 block).
  - Atrial tachycardia: abnormally shaped P waves, may outnumber QRS.
  - Multifocal atrial tachycardia: ≥3 P wave morphologies, irregular QRS complexes.
- *Junctional tachycardia:* AV node is part of the pathway. P wave either buried in QRS complex or occurring after QRS complex.
  - AV nodal re-entry tachycardia.
  - AV re-entry tachycardia, includes an accessory pathway, eg WPW (p120).

Principles of management See FLOWCHART.

▸▸If the patient is compromized, use DC cardioversion.

- Otherwise, identify the underlying rhythm and treat accordingly. The chief thing is to decide whether the rhythm is regular or not (likely AF).
- Vagal manoeuvres (carotid sinus massage, Valsalva manoeuvre) transiently increase AV block, and may unmask an underlying atrial rhythm.
- If unsuccessful, give **adenosine**, which causes transient AV block. It has a short half-life (10-15s) and works in 2 ways:
  by transiently slowing ventricles to show the underlying atrial rhythm;
  by cardioverting a junctional tachycardia to sinus rhythm.

Giving adenosine:[1] 6mg IV bolus into a large vein, followed by 0.9% saline flush, while recording a rhythm strip. If unsuccessful, give 12mg, then one further 12mg bolus. Warn about SE: transient chest tightness, dyspnoea, headache, flushing. *Relative CI:* Asthma, 2nd/3rd-degree AV block or sinoatrial disease (unless pacemaker). *Interactions:* Potentiated by dipyridamole; antagonized by theophylline.

Specifics *Sinus tachycardia:* Identify and treat underlying cause.

Supraventricular tachycardia: If adenosine fails, use verapamil ~5mg IV over 2-3min. NB: NOT if on a β-blocker. If no response, a further 5mg IV over 3min (if age <60yrs). Alternatives: **atenolol** 5mg IV or **sotalol** 20-120mg IV (over 10min; halve this if eGFR 30-60); or **amiodarone**. If unsuccessful, use DC cardioversion.

Atrial fibrillation/flutter: Manage along standard lines; seek help if resistant (p124).

Atrial tachycardia: Rare; may be due to digoxin toxicity: withdraw digoxin, consider digoxin-specific antibody fragments. Maintain K^+ at 4-5mmol/L.

Multifocal atrial tachycardia: Most commonly occurs in COPD. Correct hypoxia and hypercapnia. Consider **verapamil** if rate remains >110bpm.

Junctional tachycardia: Where anterograde conduction through the AV node occurs, vagal manoeuvres are worth trying. **Adenosine** will usually cardiovert a junctional rhythm to sinus rhythm. If it fails or recurs, β-blockers (or **verapamil**—*not* with β-blockers, digoxin, or class I agents such as quinidine). If this does not control symptoms, consider radiofrequency ablation.

►Seek specialist advice if resistant junction tachycardia, or accessory pathway.

Wolff-Parkinson-White (WPW) syndrome (*ECG* p125) Caused by congenital accessory conduction pathway between atria and ventricles. Resting ECG shows short PR interval and widened QRS complex due to slurred upstroke or 'delta wave'. 2 types: WPW type A (+ve δ wave in V_1), WPW type B (-ve δ wave in V_1). Present with SVT which may be due to an AVRT, (p120) pre-excited AF, or pre-excited atrial flutter. Risk of degeneration to VF and sudden death. **℞: Flecainide**, **propafenone**, **sotalol**, or **amiodarone**. Refer to cardiologist for electrophysiology and ablation of the accessory pathway.

Emergencies

Management of narrow complex tachycardia (supraventricular tachycardia)

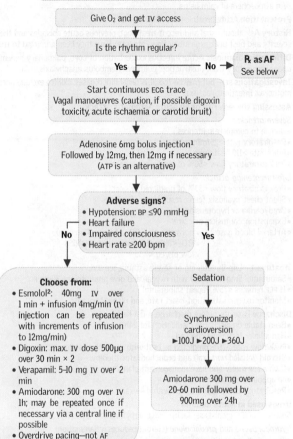

Give O_2 and get IV access

↓

Is the rhythm regular?

- **No** → ℞ as AF. See below
- **Yes** ↓

Start continuous ECG trace
Vagal manoeuvres (caution, if possible digoxin toxicity, acute ischaemia or carotid bruit)

↓

Adenosine 6mg bolus injection[1]
Followed by 12mg, then 12mg if necessary
(ATP is an alternative)

↓

Adverse signs?

- Hypotension: BP ≤90 mmHg
- Heart failure
- Impaired consciousness
- Heart rate ≥200 bpm

No ↓

Choose from:

- Esmolol[2]: 40mg IV over 1 min + infusion 4mg/min (IV injection can be repeated with increments of infusion to 12mg/min)
- Digoxin: max. IV dose 500μg over 30 min × 2
- Verapamil: 5–10 mg IV over 2 min
- Amiodarone: 300 mg over IV 1h; may be repeated once if necessary via a central line if possible
- Overdrive pacing—not AF

Yes ↓

Sedation

↓

Synchronized cardioversion
►100J ►200J ►360J

↓

Amiodarone 300 mg over 20–60 min followed by 900mg over 24h

Irregular narrow complex tachycardia

- Treat as AF—by far the most likely diagnosis.
- Control rate with either β blocker or digoxin.
- If onset <48h consider cardioversion with either amiodarone, 300mg IVI over 20–60 min, then 900mg over 24h; or DC shock, see p784.
- Consider anticoagulation with heparin and/or warfarin to reduce the risk of stroke.

1 Consult *BNF* if on dipyridamole or has had a heart transplant
See Resuscitation Council (UK) guidance for more details (www.resus.org.uk)
2 This dose of esmolol assumes a body weight of 80kg—loading 0.5mg/kg, followed by 0.05mg/kg/min maintenance (max 0.2mg/kg/min). Dilute in 5% dextrose.

►The severity of an attack is easily underestimated.

►An atmosphere of calm helps.

Presentation Acute breathlessness and wheeze.

History Ask about usual and recent treatment; previous acute episodes and their severity and best peak expiratory flow rate (PEF). Have they been admitted to ITU?

Differential diagnosis Acute infective exacerbation of COPD, pulmonary oedema, upper respiratory tract obstruction, pulmonary embolus, anaphylaxis.

Investigations PEF—but may be too ill; arterial blood gases; CXR (to exclude pneumothorax, infection); FBC; U&E.

Assessing the severity of an acute asthmatic attack

Severe attack:

- Unable to complete sentences
- Respiratory rate >25/min
- Pulse rate >110 beats/min
- Peak expiratory flow <50% of predicted or best

Life-threatening attack:

- Peak expiratory flow <33% of predicted or best
- Silent chest, cyanosis, feeble respiratory effort
- Bradycardia or hypotension
- Exhaustion, confusion, or coma
- Arterial blood gases:
  - normal/high P_aCO_2 >4.6kPa (32mmHg)
  - P_aO_2 <8kPa (60mmHg), or S_aO_2<92%
  - low pH, eg <7.35

Treatment ►Life-threatening or severe asthma, see BOX.

- Salbutamol 5mg nebulized with oxygen and give prednisolone 30mg PO.
- If PEF remains <75%, repeat salbutamol.
- Monitor oxygen saturation, heart rate, and respiratory rate.

Discharge Patients, before discharge, must have:

- Been stable on discharge medication for 24h.
- Had inhaler technique checked.
- Peak flow rate >75% predicted or best with diurnal variability <25%.
- Steroid (inhaled *and* oral) and bronchodilator therapy.
- Own a PEF meter and have management plan.
- GP appointment within 1wk.
- Respiratory clinic appointment within 4wks.

Drugs used in acute asthma

Salbutamol (β_2-agonist) *SE:* Tachycardia, arrhythmias, tremor, K^+↓.

Hydrocortisone and ***prednisolone*** (steroid; reduces inflammation)

Aminophylline (Inhibits phosphodiesterase; ↑[cAMP]). *SE:* pulse↑, arrhythmias, nausea, seizures. The amount of IVI aminophylline may need altering according to the individual patient: always check the *BNF*. Monitor ECG.

- ***Factors which may necessitate reduction of dose:*** Cardiac or liver failure, drugs that increase the half-life of aminophylline, eg cimetidine, ciprofloxacin, erythromycin, contraceptive steroids.
- ***Factors which may require↑dose:*** Smoking, drugs which shorten the half-life, eg phenytoin, carbamazepine, barbiturates, rifampicin.

►Aim for plasma concentration of 10–20µg/mL (55–110µmol/L). Serious toxicity (BP↓ arrhythmias, cardiac arrest) can occur at concentrations ≥25µg/mL. Measure plasma K^+: theophyllines may cause K^+↓. Don't load patients already on oral preparations. Stick with one brand (bioavailability varies).

Immediate management of acute severe asthma

Assess severity of attack (see above). Warn ITU if severe attack.

Start treatment immediately (prior to investigations).

- Sit patient up and give high-dose O_2 in 100%, via non-rebreathing bag.
- Salbutamol 5mg (or terbutaline 10mg) plus ipratropium bromide 0.5mg nebulized with O_2.
- Hydrocortisone 100mg IV or prednisolone 40-50mg PO or both if very ill.
- CXR to exclude pneumothorax.

If life-threatening features (above) present:

- Inform ITU and seniors.
- Add magnesium sulphate ($MgSO_4$) 1.2-2g IV over 20min.
- Give salbutamol nebulizers every 15min, or 10mg continuously per hour. Monitor ECG; watch for arrhythmias.

Further management

If improving

- 40-60% O_2.
- Prednisolone 40-50mg/24h PO Continue for at least 5 days.
- Nebulized salbutamol every 4h.
- Monitor peak flow and oxygen saturations.

▸▸If patient not improving after 15-30min

- Continue 100% O_2 and steroids.
- Hydrocortisone 100mg IV or prednisolone 30mg PO if not already given.
- Give salbutamol nebulizers every 15min, or 10mg continuously per hour.
- Continue ipratropium 0.5mg every 4-6h.

▸▸If patient still not improving

- Discuss with seniors and ITU.
- Repeat salbutamol nebulizer every 15min.
- $MgSO_4$ 1.2-2g IV over 20min, unless already given.
- Consider aminophylline; if not already on a theophylline, load with eg 5mg/kg IVI over 20min,[1] then 500μg/kg/h where kg is ideal body weight, p446—eg in a smallish adult: 750mg/24h; large adult 1200mg/24h. Adjust dose according to plasma theophylline, if available. Do levels if infusion lasts >24h. Alternatively, give salbutamol IVI, eg 3-20μg/min. IPPV may be required.
- If no improvement, or life-threatening features are present, consider transfer to ITU, accompanied by a doctor prepared to intubate.

Monitoring the effects of treatment

- Repeat PEF 15-30min after initiating treatment.
- Pulse oximeter monitoring: maintain S_aO_2 >92%.
- Check blood gases within 2h if: initial P_aCO_2 was normal/raised or initial P_aO_2 <8kPa (60mmHg) or patient deteriorating.
- Record PEF pre- and post-β-agonist in hospital at least 4 times.

Once patient is improving

- Wean down and stop aminophylline over 12-24h.
- Reduce nebulized salbutamol and switch to inhaled β-agonist.
- Initiate inhaled steroids and stop oral steroids if possible.
- Continue to monitor PEF. Look for deterioration on reduced treatment and beware early morning dips in PEF.
- Look for the cause of the acute exacerbation and admission.

Emergencies

1 British Thoracic Society advice 2003 *Thorax* 58 sup 1 page 1.

A common medical emergency especially in winter. May be triggered by viral or bacterial infections.

Presentation Increasing cough, breathlessness, or wheeze. Decreased exercise capacity.

History Ask about usual/recent treatments (especially home oxygen), smoking status, and exercise capacity (may influence a decision to ventilate the patient).

Differential diagnosis Asthma, pulmonary oedema, upper respiratory tract obstruction, pulmonary embolus, anaphylaxis.

Investigations
- Peak expiratory flow (PEF)—but may be too ill.
- Arterial blood gases (p785).
- CXR to exclude pneumothorax and infection.
- FBC; U&E; CRP.
- ECG.
- Blood cultures (if pyrexial).
- Send sputum for culture.

Management
- Look for a cause, eg infection, pneumothorax.
- See FLOWCHART for acute management.
- Prior to discharge, liaise with GP regarding steroid reduction, domiciliary oxygen (p176), smoking, and pneumococcal & flu vaccinations (p160).

Treatment of stable COPD: See p176 for further information.

Non-pharmacological:	Stop smoking, encourage exercise, treat poor nutrition or obesity, influenza, vaccination.
Pharmacological:	
• Mild	Short-acting β_2-agonist or ipratropium PRN.
• Moderate	Regular short-acting β_2-agonist and/or ipratropium. Consider corticosteroid trial.
• Severe	Combination therapy with regular short-acting β_2-agonist and ipratropium. Consider corticosteroid trial (p177). Assess for home nebulizers.

More advanced disease:
- Consider pulmonary rehabilitation in moderate/severe disease.
- Consider long-term oxygen therapy if P_aO_2 <7.3kPa (p176).
- Indications for surgery: recurrent pneumothoraces; isolated bullous disease; lung volume reduction surgery (selected patients).
- Assess social circumstances and support required. Identify and treat depression.
- Air travel may be hazardous if P_aO_2 <6.7kPa; check availability of O_2.

Oxygen therapy

- The greatest danger is hypoxia, which probably accounts for more deaths than hypercapnia. *Don't leave patients severely hypoxic.*
- However, in some patients, who rely on their hypoxic drive to breathe, too much oxygen may lead to a reduced respiratory rate and hypercapnia, with a consequent fall in conscious level. Always prescribe O_2 as though it were a drug.
- Therefore care is required with O_2, especially if there is evidence of CO_2 retention. Start with 24–28% O_2 in such patients. Reassess after 30min.
- Monitor the patient carefully. Aim to raise the P_aO_2 above 8.0kPa with a rise in P_aCO_2 <1.5kPa.
- In patients without evidence of retention at baseline use 28–40% O_2, but still monitor and repeat ABG.

Management of acute COPD

↓

Controlled oxygen therapy
Start at 24–28%; vary according to ABG.
Aim for a P_aO_2 >8.0kPa with a rise in P_aCO_2 <1.5kPa

↓

Nebulized bronchodilators
Salbutamol 5mg/4h and ipratropium 500µg/6h

↓

Steroids
IV hydrocortisone 200mg and oral prednisolone 30–40mg (continue for 7–14d)

↓

Antibiotics
Use if evidence of infection, eg amoxicillin 500mg/8h PO, alternatively clarithromycin or doxycycline p381

↓

Physiotherapy to aid sputum expectoration

↓

If no response
Repeat nebulizers and consider IV aminophylline[1]

↓

If no response
1) Consider nasal intermittent positive pressure ventilation[2] (NIPPV) if respiratory rate >30 or pH <7.35. It is delivered by nasal mask and a flow generator

↓

2) Consider intubation[3] & ventilation if pH <7.26 and P_aCO_2 is rising

↓

3) Consider a respiratory stimulant drug, eg doxapram 1.5–4mg/min IV *SE: agitation, confusion, tachycardia, nausea.* In patients who are not suitable for mechanical ventilation. It is a short-term measure, and rarely used now NIPPV available

1 Aminophylline: Do not give a loading dose to patients on maintenance methylxanthines (theophyllines/aminophylline). Load with 250mg over 20min, then infuse at a rate of ~500µg/kg/h, where kg is ideal body weight, p446. Check plasma levels if given for >24h. ECG monitoring is required.
2 This may alone serve as a rescue therapy, be an intermittent step before ventilation, or considered as a 'ceiling of therapy for those deemed not suitable for mechanical ventilation
3 A decision to ventilate will depend on the patient's premorbid state—exercise capacity, home oxygen, and comorbidity. Ask about this information before you need to make this decision.

▸▸Pneumothorax

(see image p763)

▸▸**Tension pneumothorax** requires immediate relief (see below). Do *not* delay management by obtaining a CXR.

Causes Often spontaneous (especially in young thin men) due to rupture of a subpleural bulla. Other causes: asthma; COPD; TB; pneumonia; lung abscess; carcinoma; cystic fibrosis; lung fibrosis; sarcoidosis; connective tissue disorders (Marfan's syndrome, Ehlers-Danlos syndrome); trauma; iatrogenic (subclavian CVP line insertion, pleural aspiration or biopsy, percutaneous liver biopsy, positive pressure ventilation).

Clinical features *Symptoms:* There may be no symptoms (especially in fit young people with small pneumothoraces) or there may be sudden onset of dyspnoea and/or pleuritic chest pain. Patients with asthma or COPD may present with a sudden deterioration. Mechanically ventilated patients may present with hypoxia or an increase in ventilation pressures. *Signs:* Reduced expansion, hyper-resonance to percussion and diminished breath sounds on the affected side. *With a tension pneumothorax, the trachea will be deviated away from the affected side and the patient will be very unwell.*

Tests ►*A CXR should not be performed if a tension pneumothorax is suspected, as it will delay immediate necessary treatment.* Otherwise, request an expiratory film, and look for an area devoid of lung markings, peripheral to the edge of the collapsed lung (see p763). *Ensure the suspected pneumothorax is not a large emphysematous bulla.* Check *ABG* in dyspnoeic patients and those with chronic lung disease.

Management Depends on whether it is a primary or secondary (underlying lung disease) pneumothorax, size and symptoms—see FLOWCHART.

- Pneumothorax due to trauma or mechanical ventilation requires a chest drain.
- Aspiration of a pneumothorax, see p781.
- Insertion and management of a chest drain, see p780.

Surgical advice: Arrange if: bilateral pneumothoraces; lung fails to expand after intercostal drain insertion; 2 or more previous pneumothoraces on the same side; or history of pneumothorax on the opposite side.

▸▸Tension pneumothorax

(see p763)

▸▸This is a medical emergency.

Essence Air drawn into the pleural space with each inspiration has no route of escape during expiration. The mediastinum is pushed over into the contralateral hemithorax, kinking and compressing the great veins. Unless the air is rapidly removed, cardiorespiratory arrest will occur.

Signs Respiratory distress, tachycardia, hypotension, distended neck veins, trachea deviated away from side of pneumothorax. Increased percussion note, reduced air entry/breath sounds on the affected side.

Treatment

▸▸To remove the air, insert a large-bore (14-16G) needle with a syringe, partially filled with 0.9% saline, into the 2nd intercostal interspace in the midclavicular line on the side of the suspected pneumothorax. Remove plunger to allow the trapped air to bubble through the syringe (with saline as a water seal) until a chest tube can be placed. Alternatively, insert a large-bore Venflon in the same location.

▸▸Do this *before* requesting a CXR.

▸▸Then insert a chest drain. See p780.

Acute management of pneumothorax

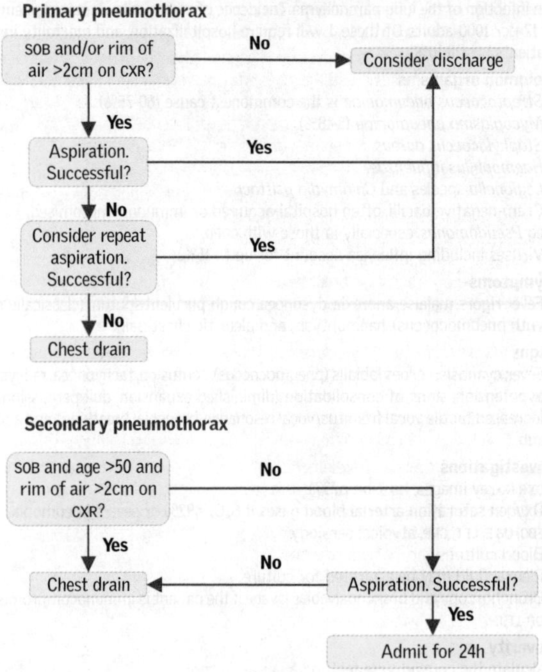

Aspiration of a pneumothorax: ▸▸see p781.

Intercostal tube drainage: For insertion, see p780.

- Use a small tube (10–14F) unless blood/pus is also present.
- Never clamp a bubbling tube.
- Tubes may be removed 24h after the lung has re-expanded and air leak has stopped (ie the tube stops bubbling). This is done during expiration or a Valsalva manoeuvre.
- If the lung fails to re-expand within 48h, or if there is a persistent air leak, specialist advice should be obtained, as suction or surgical intervention may be required.
- If suction is required, high-volume, low-pressure (–10 to –20cm H_2O) systems are required.

An infection of the lung parenchyma. Incidence of community-acquired pneumonia is 12 per 1000 adults. Of these, 1 will require hospitalization, and mortality in these patients is still 10%.

Common organisms

- *Streptococcus pneumoniae* is the commonest cause (60–75%).
- *Mycoplasma pneumoniae* (5–18%).
- *Staphylococcus aureus.*
- *Haemophilus influenzae.*
- *Legionella* species and *Chlamydia psittaci.*
- Gram-negative bacilli, often hospital-acquired or immunocompromised, eg *Pseudomonas*, especially in those with COPD.
- Viruses including influenza account for up to 15%.

Symptoms

- Fever, rigors, malaise, anorexia, dyspnoea, cough, purulent sputum (classically 'rusty' with pneumococcus), haemoptysis, and pleuritic chest pain.

Signs

- Fever, cyanosis, herpes labialis (pneumococcus), confusion, tachypnoea, tachycardia, hypotension, signs of consolidation (diminished expansion, dull percussion note, increased tactile vocal fremitus/vocal resonance, bronchial breathing), and a pleural rub.

Investigations

- CXR (X-ray images, **fig 1** on p737).
- Oxygen saturation arterial blood gases if S_aO_2 <92% or severe pneumonia.
- FBC, U&E, LFT, CRP, atypical serology.
- Blood cultures.
- Pleural fluid may be aspirated for culture.
- Bronchoscopy and bronchoalveolar lavage if the patient is immunocompromised or on ITU.

Severity

Calculate the core adverse features '**CURB-65**' score

- **C**onfusion (abbreviated mental test ≤8)
- **U**rea >7mmol/L
- **R**espiratory rate ≥30/min
- **BP** <90/60mmHg)
- Age≥**65**

Score: 0–1 home treatment if possible; 2 hospital therapy; ≥3 indicates severe pneumonia. Other features increasing the risk of death are: co-existing disease; bilateral/multilobar involvement; P_aO_2 <8kPa or S_aO_2 <92%.

Management See FLOWCHART.

Complications

Pleural effusion, empyema, lung abscess, respiratory failure, septicaemia, pericarditis, myocarditis, cholestatic jaundice, renal failure.

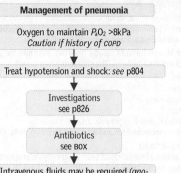

Management of pneumonia

Oxygen to maintain P_aO_2 >8kPa
Caution if history of COPD

↓

Treat hypotension and shock: *see* p804

↓

Investigations
see p826

↓

Antibiotics
see BOX

↓

Intravenous fluids may be required *(anorexia, dehydration, shock)* pneumonia

↓

Analgesia for pleuritic chest pain, eg paracetamol 1g/6h or NSAID

↓

Some patients may need intubation
and a period of ventilatory support

Empirical treatment of severe pneumonia

►Regimens vary, so consult local guidelines—the following are suggestions. For fuller advice see p161.
Co-amoxiclav 1.2g/8h IV or cephalosporin IV (eg cefuroxime 1.5g/8h IV) AND clarithromycin 500mg/12h IVI.

If atypical suspected Legionella pneumophilia add levofloxacin + rifampicin, *Chlamydophila* species (p162) add tetracycline, *Pneumocystis jiroveci* add high-dose co-trimoxazole (p411).

If hospital acquired or neutropenic consider aminoglycoside IV (eg gentamicin, p766) + antipseudomonal penicillin (eg ticarcillin, p378).

►Always suspect pulmonary embolism (PE) in sudden collapse 1-2wks after surgery. Mortality rate in England and Wales: 30,000–40,000/yr.

Mechanism Venous thrombi, usually from DVT, pass into the pulmonary circulation and block blood flow to lungs. The source is often occult.

Risk factors
- Malignancy.
- Surgery—especially pelvic.
- Immobility.
- The Pill (there is also a slight risk attached to HRT).
- Previous thromboembolism and inherited thrombophilia, see p368.

Signs and symptoms
- Acute dyspnoea, pleuritic chest pain, haemoptysis, and syncope.
- Hypotension, tachycardia, gallop rhythm, JVP↑, loud P_2, right ventricular heave, pleural rub, tachypnoea, and cyanosis, AF.

Classically, PE presents 10d post-op, with collapse and sudden breathlessness while straining at stool—but PE may occur after any period of immobility, or with no predisposing factors. Breathlessness may be the only sign. Multiple small emboli may present less dramatically with pleuritic pain, haemoptysis, and gradually increasing breathlessness. ►Look for a source of emboli—especially DVT (is a leg swollen?).

Investigations ►p182
- U&E, FBC, baseline clotting.
- *ECG:* commonly normal or sinus tachycardia; right ventricular strain pattern V1-3 (p94), right axis deviation, RBBB, AF, may be deep S waves in I, Q waves in III, inverted T waves in III ('S_I Q_{III} T_{III}').
- *CXR:* often normal; decreased vascular markings, small pleural effusion. Wedge-shaped area of infarction. Atelectasis.
- *ABG:* hyperventilation + gas exchange↓: P_aO_2↓, P_aCO_2↓, pH often↑, p156.
- *Serum D-dimer:* high sensitivity but low specificity (↑ if thrombosis, inflammation, post-op, infection, malignancy) ∴ excludes PE if normal D-dimer.
- *CT pulmonary angiography* (CTPA) is sensitive and specific in determining if emboli are in pulmonary arteries. If unavailable, a *ventilation-perfusion (V/Q) scan* can aid diagnosis. If V/Q scan is equivocal, pulmonary angiography or bilateral venograms may help (MRI venography or plethysmography are alternatives).

Management See FLOWCHART for immediate management.
- Try to prevent further thrombosis with compression stockings.
- Heparin concurrently with warfarin for ≥5d. Then stop heparin once INR >2.
- If obvious remedial cause, 6 weeks of warfarin may be enough; otherwise, continue for at least 3–6 months (long-term if recurrent emboli, or underlying malignancy).
- Is there an underlying cause, eg thrombophilic tendency (p368), malignancy (especially prostate, breast, or pelvic cancer), SLE, or polycythaemia?

►If good story and signs, make the diagnosis. Start treatment (FLOWCHART) before definitive investigations: most PE deaths occur within 1h.

Prevention Early post-op mobilization is the simplest method; also consider:
- Antithromboembolic (TED) stockings.
- Low molecular weight heparin prophylaxis SC.
- Avoid contraceptive pill if at risk, eg major or orthopaedic surgery.
- Recurrent PEs may be prevented by anticoagulation. Vena caval filters are of limited use, and should be combined with anticoagulation.

⚠ Don't just think of prophylactic low molecular weight heparin (LMWH, p580) for post-op patients. Many acutely ill medical patients are equally at risk (5–15% have DVTs, and >50% of all thromboembolic events are in these patients; prevalence of PE: 0.3–1.5%).[31] Do proper risk analysis—especially in those with MI, pneumonia, malignancy, inflammatory bowel disease, prolonged immobility/on ITU, and stroke (there is no ↑ risk of CNS bleeds if LMWH is used).[32]

Management of large pulmonary embolism

Oxygen, 100%

↓

Morphine 10mg IV with antiemetic
if the patient is in pain or very distressed

↓

►If critically ill with massive PE consider immediate thrombolysis (a 50mg bolus of alteplase) or surgery

↓

IV access and start heparin[1]
either low molecular weight heparin, eg tinzaparin 175U/kg/24h SC
or unfractionated heparin ~10,000U IV bolus
then ~18U/kg/h IVI as guided by APTT (p344)

↓

What is the systolic BP?

<90mmHg
Start rapid colloid infusion[2]

↓

If BP still↓ after 500mL colloid, dobutamine 2.5–10μg/kg/min IV; aim for systolic BP >90mmHg

↓

If BP still low, consider noradrenaline

↓

If the systolic BP <90mmHg after 30-60min of standard treatment, clinically definite PE and no CI (p808), consider thrombolysis (unless already given in step 3).[3]

>90mmHg
Start warfarin
10mg/24h PO (p344)

↓

Confirm diagnosis

1 A bolus of unfractionated heparin may be preferred in massive PE for its faster onset, and unfractionated heparin may also be useful where there may be a need for rapid reversal of anticoagulation.
2 Controversial, but some authorities say it is best to infuse plasma-expanding fluids even if CVP↑, to maintain BP & organ perfusion, see *Concise OTM* (OUP, 2000) p151—but see Task Force on PE, European Society Cardiology *Eur Heart J* 2000 **21** 1301.
3 A standard regimen is: alteplase 50mg bolus IV over 1-2min. See also formulary.

Causes

- Peptic ulcer ~40%.
- Mallory-Weiss tear 15%.
- Gastroduodenal erosions ~10%.
- Oesophagitis ~10%.
- Varices ~7%.
- Other: malignancy, vascular malformations. Consider also facial trauma, nose bleed, or haemoptysis as causes of *swallowed* blood.

Signs & symptoms Haematemesis, or melaena, dizziness (especially postural), fainting, abdominal pain, dysphagia? Postural hypotension, hypotension, tachycardia (not if on β-blocker), ↓JVP, ↓urine output, cool and clammy, signs of chronic liver disease (p260); telangiectasia or purpura; jaundice (biliary colic + jaundice + melaena suggests haemobilia). **NB:** ask about previous GI problems, drug use, and alcohol.

Management:[35]

Is the patient shocked?

- Cool & clammy to touch (especially nose, toes, fingers) ↓capillary refill.
- Pulse >100bpm.
- JVP <1cm H_2O.
- Systolic BP <100mmHg.
- Postural drop (>20mmHg on standing).
- Urine output <30mL/h.

If not shocked: Insert 2 big cannulae; start slow saline IVI to keep lines patent; check bloods and monitor vital signs + urine output. Aim to keep Hb >8g/dL. **NB:** Hb may not fall until circulating volume is restored.

If shocked: See FLOWCHART for management.

CVP line: Consider for high-risk patients, eg ↑age, CV disease, on β-blockers.

Acute drug therapy: Following successful endoscopic therapy in patients with **major** ulcer bleeding, omeprazole (80mg stat IV over 5min followed by 8mg/h for 72h) is recommended. There is no firm evidence to support the use of somatostatin or antifibrinolytic therapy in the majority of patients.

Variceal bleeding: Resuscitate then proceed to urgent endoscopy for banding or sclerotherapy. Give terlipressin 2mg SC qds (caution in PUD). If massive bleed or bleeding continues, pass a Sengstaken-Blakemore tube p255. A bleed is the equivalent of a large protein meal so start treatment to avoid hepatic encephalopathy (p259). Omeprazole 40mg PO may also be helpful in preventing stress ulceration.

Endoscopy: Within 4h if you suspect variceal bleeding; within 12-24h if shocked on admission or significant comorbidity. Endoscopy can identify the site of bleeding, estimate the risk of rebleeding (see FLOWCHART) and be used to administer treatment. ***No site of bleeding identified:*** Bleeding site missed on endoscopy; bleeding site has healed (Mallory-Weiss tear or Dieulafoy's lesion); nose bleed (swallowed blood); site distal to 3rd part of the duodenum (Meckel's diverticulum, colonic site).

Helicobacter pylori: Check status in all patients; eradicate if positive.

Rebleeds Serious event: 40% of patients who rebleed will die. If 'at risk' maintain a high index of suspicion. If a rebleed occurs, check vital signs every 15min and call senior cover. To prevent rebleeding in endoscopically proven high-risk cases, IVI omeprazole has been tried, eg 80mg over 5min followed by an infusion of 8mg/h for 72h, then 20mg/24h PO for 8wks.[36]

Signs of a rebleed:

- Rising pulse rate.
- Falling JVP ± decreasing hourly urine output.
- Haematemesis or melaena.
- Fall in BP (a late and sinister finding) and decreased conscious level.

Immediate management if shocked

↓

Protect airway and keep NBM
Insert two large-bore cannulae (14–16G)

↓

Draw bloods FBC, U&E, LFT, glucose, clotting screen
Cross-match 6 units

↓

Give high-flow O_2

↓

Rapid IV crystalloid infusion *Up to 1L*

↓

If remains shocked, give blood
Group specific or O Rh-ve until cross-match done

↓

Otherwise slow saline infusion[1]
to keep lines open

↓

Transfuse as dictated by haemodynamics

↓

Correct clotting abnormalities
Vitamin K, FFP, platelet concentrate

↓

Set up CVP line to guide fluid replacement
Aim for >5cm H_2O
CVP may mislead if there is ascites or CCF
A Swan-Ganz catheter may help

↓

Catheterize and monitor urine output *Aim for >30mL/h*

↓

Monitor vital signs every 15min until stable, then hourly

↓

Notify surgeons of all severe bleeds

↓

Urgent endoscopy for diagnosis ± control of bleeding

Rockall scoring system for prognosis in acute GI bleeding

	Score			
Variable	**0**	**1**	**2**	**3**
Age	<60	60–80	>80	
Shocked?	No	SBP >100 Pulse >100	SBP <100 Pulse >100	
Comorbidity?	None		Any major	Renal/liver failure, or malignancy
Diagnosis	Mallory-Weiss or normal	All other diagnoses	Malignancy	
Bleeding visible?	None/spot		Visible blood/clot spurting vessel	

Score <3 means an excellent prognosis; >8 means a high risk of death

1 Avoid saline in patients with decompensated liver disease (ascites, peripheral oedema) as it worsens ascites and, despite a low serum sodium, patients have a high body sodium. Use whole blood or salt-poor albumin for resuscitation, and 5% dextrose for maintenance.

▸**When to act now** Headache, T°↑, neck stiffness, altered mental state: if any 2 co-exist, give benzylpenicillin, 1.2g IM/IV, before admitting, if the patient is not yet in hospital.[37]

Organisms Meningococcus or pneumococcus. Less commonly *Haemophilus influenzae; Listeria monocytogenes.* CMV, cryptococcus (p411), or TB (p399) if HIV +ve.

Differential Malaria, encephalitis, septicaemia, subarachnoid, dengue, tetanus.

Features[39]

Early: Headache, leg pains, cold hands and feet, abnormal skin colour.

Later:

- Meningism: neck stiffness, photophobia, Kernig's sign (pain + resistance on passive knee extension with hip fully flexed).
- Conscious level ↓, coma.
- Seizures (~20%) ± focal CNS signs (~20%) ± opisthotonus (p425, **fig 1**).
- Petechial rash (non-blanching—**fig 1**; may only be 1 or 2 spots, or none).

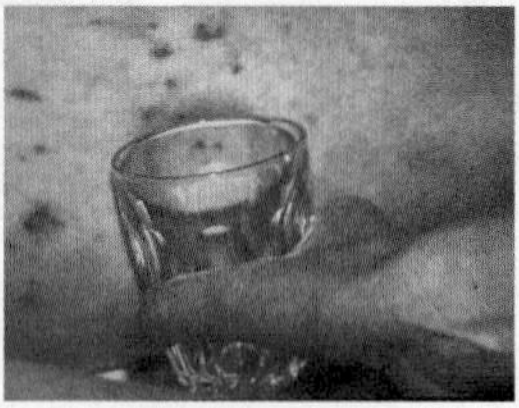

Fig 1. Glass test for petechiae.[38]
Courtesy of Meningitis Research Foundation

Signs of galloping sepsis: slow capillary refill; DIC; BP↓. T° and pulse: ↑ or normal.

Management[40 41]

▸Start antibiotics (below) immediately; see FLOWCHART for acute management

- *Signs of disease causing meningitis:* zoster; cold sore/genital vesicles (HSV); HIV signs (lymphadenopathy, dermatitis, candidiasis, uveitis); bleeding ± red eye (leptospirosis); parotid swelling (mumps); sore throat ± jaundice ± nodes (glandular fever, p401); splenectomy scar (∴ immunodeficient).
- *If ICP raised*, summon help immediately and inform neurosurgeons.
- *Prophylaxis:* (discuss with public health/ID) • Household contacts in droplet range. • Those who have kissed the patient's mouth. Give **rifampicin** (600mg/12h PO for 2d; children >1yr 10mg/kg/12h; <1yr 5mg/kg/12h) or **ciprofloxacin** (500mg PO, 1 dose child 5-12yrs: 250mg stat): neither is guaranteed in pregnancy, but are recommended.

Antibiotic therapy for meningitis

▸Local policies vary. If in doubt, ask. The following are suggestions only, where the organism is unknown:

- <55yrs: **cefotaxime** 2mg/6h slow IV.
- >55yrs: **cefotaxime** as above + **ampicillin** 2g IV/4h (for *Listeria*).
- **Aciclovir** (p834) if viral encephalitis suspected.
- Once organism isolated, seek urgent microbiological advice.

Investigations

- U&E, FBC (WBC↓≈immunocompromise: get help), LFT, glucose, coagulation screen.
- Blood culture, throat swabs (1 for bacteria, 1 for virology), rectal swab for viruses. Serology, eg EBV (p401); HIV (serial IgG for seroconversion, p412; contact lab).[42]
- Lumbar puncture (p782) is usually done after CT but safe without if no mass lesion or raised ICP suspected (eg ↓conscious) or CI: suspected intracranial mass lesion, focal signs, papilloedema, trauma, middle ear pathology, major coagulopathy. Measure opening pressure (7-18cm CSF is normal; in meningitis may be >40; typically 14-30). Send samples for MC&S, Gram stain, protein, glucose, virology/PCR, and lactate (see FLOWCHART for interpretation and normal values).
- In aseptic meningitis (usually self-limiting) do CSF PCR: 46% are from enteroviruses (eg Coxsackie A & B; echoviruses); 31% herpes simplex type 2 (HSV2); 4% HSV1). HSV meningitis is self-limiting if immunocompetent, unlike HSV encephalitis (a different entity).[43] For mumps etc, see *OHCS* p142.
- CXR (signs of TB? If so, consider TB meningitis, p399).

ABCs: high-flow O_2; IVI + fluid resus. Ask a nurse to draw up cefotaxime 2g. If immunocompromised, get help; add **ampicillin** 2g/6h IV for *Listeria*, also if >55yrs old.

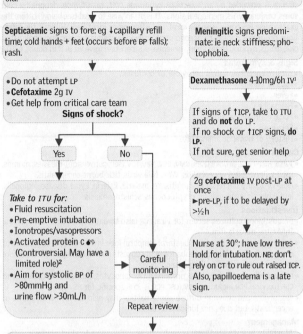

Septicaemic signs to fore: eg ↓capillary refill time; cold hands + feet (occurs before BP falls); rash.

- Do not attempt LP
- **Cefotaxime** 2g IV
- Get help from critical care team

Signs of shock?

Yes →

Take to ITU for:
- Fluid resuscitation
- Pre-emptive intubation
- Ionotropes/vasopressors
- Activated protein C (Controversial. May have a limited role)[2]
- Aim for systolic BP of >80mmHg and urine flow >30mL/h

No →

Careful monitoring

Repeat review

Meningitic signs predominate: ie neck stiffness; photophobia.

Dexamethasone 4–10mg/6h IV[1]

If signs of ↑ICP, take to ITU and do **not** do LP.
If no shock or ↑ICP signs, **do LP.**
If not sure, get senior help

2g **cefotaxime** IV post-LP at once
►pre-LP, if to be delayed by >½h

Nurse at 30°; have low threshold for intubation. NB: don't rely on CT to rule out raised ICP. Also, papilloedema is a late sign.

Subsequent therapy: Cefotaxime 2–4g/8h IVI (eg for 10d); ↓dose in renal failure; see p379 and *datasheet* (SPC). **Maintenance fluids:** avoid over- and under-hydration (despite ICP↑). **Isolate** for 1st 24h. If response to the above is poor consider pre-emptive **intubation & ventilation** ± **inotropic/vasopressor** support (p804). Inform CCDC, p373.

Lumbar puncture in meningitis

CSF in meningitis	*Pyogenic*	*Tuberculous* (p399)	*Viral ('aseptic')*
Appearance	Often turbid	Often fibrin web	Usually clear
Predominant cell[1,2]	Polymorphs	Mononuclear	Mononuclear*
Cell count/mm³	Eg 90–1000 or more	10–1000	50–1000
Glucose	<½ plasma	<½ plasma	>½ plasma
Protein (g/L)	>1.5	1–5	<1
Bacteria	In smear & culture	Often none in smear	None seen or cultured

▶There are no certain rules

Normal values: ≤5 lymphocytes/mm³ may be normal, so long as there are no neutrophils. protein: 0.15–0.45g/L. CSF glucose: 2.8–4.2mmol/L: *Causes of ↓CSF glucose*: sepsis; parasitic meningitis eg from eating snails (do CSF eosinophil count); also herpes encephalitis, hypoglycaemia, sarcoid, CNS vasculitis). A CSF lactate level of ≥3.5mmol/L (31.5mg/dL) predicts bacterial meningitis quite well.[44]

* Predominant cell type may also be lymphocytes in TB, listerial, and cryptococcal meningitis.

1 **Dexamethasone** 0.15mg/kg/6h IV eg from just *before* 1st antibiotic dose; evidence is good, esp. for pneumococcal meningitis and in children. *Avoid in:* septic shock, known meningococcal disease, immunocompromised, TB, post-op meningitis. 2 **Drotrecogin alfa** *(activated)* is approved by NICE for very limited indications. It has anti-thrombotic and anti-inflammatory actions.

►Suspect encephalitis whenever odd behaviour, ↓consciousness, focal neurology or seizure is preceded by an infectious prodrome (T°↑, rash, lymphadenopathy, cold sores, conjunctivitis, meningeal signs). It is often wise to treat (see below) before the exact cause is known—usually viral, and often never identified. Without the infectious prodrome consider *encephalopathy:* hypoglycaemia, hepatic encephalopathy, DKA, drugs, hypoxic brain injury, uraemia, SLE, beri-beri (give vit B_1 if in doubt, p707).

Signs & symptoms

- Bizarre encephalopathic behaviour or confusion
- ↓GCS or coma
- Fever
- Headache
- Focal neurological signs
- Seizures
- History of travel or animal bite.

Causes

- *Viral:* HSV-1 & 2, arboviruses, CMV, EBV, VZV, HIV (seroconversion), measles, mumps, rabies, Japanese B encephalitis, West Nile virus, tick-borne encephalitis.
- *Non-viral:* any bacterial meningitis, TB, malaria, listeria, Lyme disease, legionella, leptospirosis, aspergillosis, cryptococcus, schistosomiasis.

Investigations

- *Bloods:* blood cultures; serum for viral PCR (also throat swab & MSU); toxoplasma IgM titre; malaria film.
- *Contrast-enhanced CT:* focal bilateral temporal lobe involvement is suggestive of HSV encephalitis. Meningeal enhancement suggests meningoencephalitis. Do before LP. MRI is alternative if allergic to contrast.
- *LP:* typically moderately ↑ CSF protein and lymphocytes, and ↓glucose (p833). Send CSF for viral PCR including HSV (CSF PCR is 95% specific for HSV-1).
- *EEG:* urgent EEG showing diffuse abnormalities may help confirm a diagnosis of encephalitis, but does not indicate a cause.

Management

►Mortality in untreated viral encephalitis is ~70%. ►►Aim to start **aciclovir** within 30min[45] of the patient arriving (10mg/kg/8h IV over 1h) for 14 days as empirical treatment for HSV (21 days if immunosuppressed). Adjust aciclovir dose according to eGFR: use every 12h if eGFR 25-50; every 24h if eGFR 10-25. Consult product literature if eGFR <10. Specific therapies also exist for CMV and toxoplasmosis (p404).

- Supportive therapy, in high-dependency unit or ITU environment if necessary.
- Symptomatic treatment: eg **phenytoin** for seizures (p836).

Cerebral abscess

Suspect this in any patient with ↑ICP, especially if there is fever or ↑WCC. It may follow ear, sinus, dental, or periodontal infection; skull fracture; congenital heart disease; endocarditis; bronchiectasis. It may also occur in the absence of systemic signs of inflammation.

Signs: Seizures, fever, localizing signs, or signs of ↑ICP. Coma. Signs of sepsis elsewhere (eg teeth, ears, lungs, endocarditis).

Investigations: CT/MRI (eg 'ring-enhancing' lesion); ↑WBC, ↑ESR; biopsy.

Treatment: Urgent neurosurgical referral; treat ↑ICP (p840). If frontal sinuses or teeth are the source, the likely organism will be *Strep. milleri* (microaerophilic), or oropharyngeal anaerobes. In ear abscesses, *B. fragilis* or other anaerobes are most common. Bacterial abscesses are often peripheral; toxoplasma lesions (p404) are deeper (eg basal ganglia). **NB:** ask yourself: is there underlying immunosuppression?

This means seizures lasting for >30min, or repeated seizures without intervening consciousness. Mortality and the risk of permanent brain damage increase with the length of attack. Aim to terminate seizures lasting more than a few minutes as soon as possible (<20min).

Status usually occurs in known epileptics. If it is the 1st presentation of epilepsy, the chance of a structural brain lesion is high (>50%). Diagnosis of tonic-clonic status is usually clear. Non-convulsive status (eg absence status or continuous partial seizures with preservation of consciousness) may be more difficult: look for subtle eye or lid movement. For other signs, see p489. An EEG can be very helpful. ►*Could the patient be pregnant* (any pelvic mass)? If so, eclampsia (*OHCS* p48) is the likely diagnosis, check the urine and BP: call a senior obstetrician—immediate delivery may be needed.

Investigations

- Bedside glucose, the following tests can be done once ℞ has started: glucose, blood gases, U&E, Ca^{2+}, FBC, ECG.
- Consider anticonvulsant levels, toxicology screen, LP, culture blood and urine, EEG, CT, carbon monoxide level.
- Pulse oximetry, cardiac monitor.

Treatment See FLOWCHART. Basic life support—and these agents:

1. ***Lorazepam:*** 2-4mg as a slow bolus over ~30s into a large vein. If no response within 10min give a second dose. Beware respiratory arrest during the last part of the injection. Have full resuscitation facilities to hand for all IV benzodiazepine use. (Alternative: ***diazepam*** as Diazemuls® but it is less long-lasting—give 10mg IV over 2min; if needed, repeat at 5mg/min, until seizures stop or 20mg given—or significant respiratory depression occurs.) The rectal route is an alternative for diazepam if IV access is difficult.[1] ***Buccal midazolam*** (Epistatus®) is an easier to use oral alternative; dose for those 10yrs old and older: 10mg (1mL); if 1-4yrs old, 0.5mL; if 6-12 months old, 0.25mL; squirt half the volume between the lower gum and the cheek on each side. While waiting for this to work, prepare other drugs. If fits continue...
2. ***Phenytoin infusion:*** 18mg/kg IVI (roughly 1g if 60kg, and 1.5g if 80kg), at a rate of ≤50mg/min (don't put diazepam in same line: they don't mix). Beware BP↓ and do not use if bradycardic or heart block. Requires BP and ECG monitoring. 100mg/6-8h is a maintenance dose (check levels). If fits continue ...
3. ***Diazepam infusion:*** 100mg in 500mL of 5% dextrose; infuse at about 40mL/h (3mg/kg/24h). Close monitoring, especially respiratory function, is vital. It is most unusual for seizures to remain unresponsive following this. If they do, allow the idea to pass through your mind that they could be pseudoseizures (p720), particularly if there are odd features (pelvic thrusts; resisting attempts to open lids and your attempts to do passive movements; arms and legs flailing around).
4. ***Dexamethasone:*** 10mg IV if vasculitis/cerebral oedema (tumour) possible.
5. ***General anaesthesia:*** This requires expert guidance on ITU.

As soon as seizures are controlled, start oral drugs (p496). Ask what the cause was, eg hypoglycaemia, pregnancy, alcohol, drugs, CNS lesion or infection, hypertensive encephalopathy, inadequate anticonvulsant dose (p494).

1 Diazepam Rectubes®: give 0.5mg/kg stat dose—eg ~3 10mg tubes PR (respiratory problems at this dose are *very* rare: all survived). If your back is still against the wall with no response after 10min, try 1 last 10mg tube. Halve dose if elderly. *For children's Stesolid® regimen* (it is different), see *OHCS* p206.

Management of status epilepticus

Open and maintain the airway, lay in recovery position
Remove false teeth if poorly fitting, insert oral/nasal airway, intubate if necessary

↓

Oxygen, 100% + suction (as required)

↓

IV access and take blood:
- U&E, LFT, FBC, glucose (eg BM test®), Ca^{2+}
- Toxicology screen if indicated
- Anticonvulsant levels

↓

Thiamine 250mg IV over 10min if alcoholism or malnourishment suspected.
Glucose 50mL 50% IV, unless glucose known to be normal

↓

Correct hypotension with fluids

↓

Slow IV bolus phase—to stop seizures: eg lorazepam 2-4mg.
Give 2nd dose of lorazepam if no response within 2min.

↓

IV infusion phase: If seizures continue, start phenytoin, 18mg/kg IVI, at a rate of ≤50mg/min. Monitor ECG and BP.
100mg/6-8h is a maintenance dose (check levels).
Alternative: diazepam infusion: 100mg in 500mL of 5% dextrose; infuse at ~40mL/h as opposite

↓

General anaesthesia phase: Continuing seizures require expert help with paralysis and ventilation with continuous EEG monitoring in ITU

NB: ►**never** spend longer than 20min on someone with status epilepticus without having help at the bedside from an anaesthetist.

►If the pupils are unequal, diagnose rising intracranial pressure (ICP), eg from extradural haemorrhage, and summon urgent neurosurgical help (p486). Retinal vein pulsation at fundoscopy helps exclude ↑ICP.

Initial management (See FLOWCHART) Write full notes. Record times.

- Involve neurosurgeons at an early stage, especially with comatose patients, or if raised ICP suspected.
- Examine the CNS. Chart pulse, BP, T°, respirations + pupils every 15min.
- Assess anterograde amnesia (loss from the time of injury, ie post-traumatic) and retrograde amnesia—its extent correlates with the severity of the injury, and it never occurs without anterograde amnesia.
- Nurse semi-prone if no spinal injury; meticulous care to bladder & airway.

Who needs a CT head?

If any of the following are present, a CT is required immediately:

- GCS <13 at any time, or GCS 13 or 14 at 2h following injury
- Focal neurological deficit
- Suspected open or depressed skull fracture, or signs of basal skull fracture
- Post-traumatic seizure
- Vomiting >once
- Loss of consciousness AND any of the following:
  - Age ≥65
  - Coagulopathy
  - 'Dangerous mechanism of injury' eg RTA, fall from great height
  - Antegrade amnesia of >30min

When to ventilate immediately:

- Coma ≤8 on Glasgow coma scale (GCS; p802)
- P_aO_2 <9kPa in air (<13kPa in O_2) or P_aCO_2 >6kPa
- Spontaneous hyperventilation (P_aCO_2 <3.5kPa)
- Respiratory irregularity

Ventilate before neurosurgical transfer if:

- Deteriorating level of consciousness
- Bilateral fractured mandible
- Bleeding into mouth, eg skull base fracture
- Seizures

Risk of intracranial haematoma in adults

- Fully conscious, no skull fracture = <1:1000
- Confused, no skull fracture = 1:100
- Fully conscious, skull fracture = 1:30
- Confused, skull fracture = 1:4

Criteria for admission

- Difficult to assess (child; post-ictal; alcohol intoxication)
- CNS signs; severe headache or vomiting; fracture
- Loss of consciousness does **not** require admission if well, and a responsible adult is in attendance

Drowsy trauma patients (GCS <15 to >8) smelling of alcohol: Alcohol is an unlikely cause of coma if plasma alcohol <44mmol/L. If unavailable, estimate blood alcohol level from the osmolar gap, p682. If blood alcohol ≈ 40mmol/L, osmolar gap ≈ 40mmol/L. Never assume signs are just alcohol.

Complications *Early:* Extradural/subdural haemorrhage, seizures. *Late:* Subdural, p486, seizures, diabetes insipidus, parkinsonism, dementia.

Indicators of a bad prognosis Old age, decerebrate rigidity, extensor spasms, prolonged coma, ↑BP, P_aO_2↓ (on blood gases), T° >39°C. 60% of those with loss of consciousness of >1 month will survive 3–25yrs, but may need daily nursing care.

For *Spinal cord injury & Persistent vegetative states*, see *OHCS* (p766–p774 & p776).

Immediate management plan for head injury

ABC

↓

Oxygen, 100%
Intubate and hyperventilate if necessary
Immobilise neck until injury to cervical spine excluded.

↓

Stop blood loss and support circulation
Treat for shock if required (p804)

↓

Treat seizures with lorazepam ± phenytoin (p836)

↓

Assess level of consciousness (GCS)
Antegrade and retrograde amnesia

↓

Rapid examination survey

↓

Investigations:
U&Es, glucose, FBC, blood alcohol,
toxicology screen, ABG & clotting

↓

Neurological examination

↓

Brief history
When? Where? How? Had a fit? Lucid interval? Alcohol?

↓

Evaluate lacerations of face or scalp
Palpate deep wounds with sterile glove to check for
step deformity. Note obvious skull/facial fractures[1]

↓

Check for CSF leak, from nose (rhinorrhoea) or ear
Any blood behind the ear drum?
If either is present, suspect basilar skull fracture: do CT
Give tetanus toxoid, and refer at once to neurosurgeons

↓

Palpate the neck posteriorly for tenderness and deformity
If detected, or if the patient has obvious head injury,
or injury above the clavicle with loss of consciousness,
immobilize the neck and get cervical spine radiographs

↓

Radiology
As indicated: cervical spine, chest X-rays; CT of head

1 Periorbital (raccoon sign) or postauricular (Battle sign) ecchymoses.

There are 3 types of cerebral oedema:
- Vasogenic: ↑ capillary permeability—tumour, trauma, ischaemia, infection.
- Cytotoxic: cell death, eg from hypoxia.
- Interstitial: eg obstructive hydrocephalus.

Because the cranium defines a fixed volume, brain swelling quickly results in ↑ICP, which may produce a sudden clinical deterioration. Normal ICP is 0–10mmHg. The oedema from severe brain injury is probably both cytotoxic and vasogenic.

Causes
- Primary or metastatic tumours.
- Head injury.
- Haemorrhage (subdural, extradural, subarachnoid, intracerebral, intraventricular).
- Infection: meningitis, encephalitis, brain abscess.
- Hydrocephalus
- Cerebral oedema
- Status epilepticus

Signs & symptoms
- Headache; drowsiness; vomiting; seizures.
- History of trauma.
- Listlessness; irritability; drowsiness; falling pulse and rising BP (Cushing's response); coma; Cheyne–Stokes respiration
- Pupil changes (constriction at first, later dilatation—do not mask these signs by using agents, such as tropicamide, to dilate the pupil to aid fundoscopy).
- ↓visual acuity; peripheral visual field loss.
- Papilloedema is an unreliable sign, but venous pulsation at the disc may be absent (absent in ~50% of normal people, but *loss* of it is a useful sign).

Investigations
- U&E, FBC, LFT, glucose, serum osmolality, clotting, blood culture, CXR.
- CT head.
- Then consider lumbar puncture if safe. Measure the opening pressure!

Treatment

The goal is to ↓ICP and avert secondary injury. Urgent neurosurgery is required for the definitive treatment of ↑ICP from focal causes (eg haematomas). This is achieved via a craniotomy or burr hole. Also, an ICP monitor (or bolt) may be placed to monitor pressure. Surgery is generally *not* helpful following ischaemic or anoxic injury. ***Holding measures*** are listed in the FLOWCHART.

Herniation syndromes

Uncal herniation is caused by a lateral supratentorial mass, which pushes the ipsilateral inferomedial temporal lobe (uncus) through the temporal incisura and against the midbrain. The IIIrd nerve, travelling in this space, gets compressed causing a dilated ipsilateral pupil, then ophthalmoplegia (a fixed pupil localizes a lesion poorly but is 'ipsi-lateralizing'). This may be followed (quickly) by contralateral hemiparesis (pressure on the cerebral peduncle) and coma from pressure on the ascending reticular activating system (ARAS) in the midbrain.

Cerebellar tonsil herniation is caused by ↑pressure in the posterior fossa forcing the cerebellar tonsils through the foramen magnum. Ataxia, VIth nerve palsies, and +ve Babinskis (upgoing plantars) occur first, then loss of consciousness, irregular breathing, and apnoea. This syndrome may proceed very rapidly given the small size of, and poor compliance in, the posterior fossa.

Subfalcian (cingulate) herniation is caused by a frontal mass. The cingulate gyrus (medial frontal lobe) is forced under the rigid falx cerebri. It may be silent unless the anterior cerebral artery is compressed and causes a stroke—eg contralateral leg weakness ± abulia (lack of decision-making).

Immediate management plan for raised intracranial pressure

ABC

↓

Correct hypotension and treat seizures

↓

Brief examination; history if available
Any clues, eg meningococcal rash, previous carcinoma

↓

Elevate the head of the bed to 30°–40°

↓

If intubated, hyperventilate to ↓P_aCO_2 (eg to 3.5kPa)
This causes cerebral vasoconstriction and reduces ICP almost immediately

↓

Osmotic agents (eg mannitol) can be useful *pro tem* but may lead to rebound ↑ICP after prolonged use (~12–24h)
Give 20% solution 1–2g/kg IV over 10–20min (eg 5mL/kg). Clinical effect is seen after ~20min and lasts for 2–6h. Follow serum osmolality—aim for about 300mosmol/kg but don't exceed 310

↓

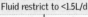

Corticosteroids are *not* effective in reducing ICP except for oedema surrounding tumours
eg dexamethasone 10mg IV and follow with 4mg/6h IV/PO

↓

Fluid restrict to <1.5L/d

↓

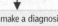

Monitor the patient closely; consider monitoring ICP

↓

Aim to make a diagnosis

↓

Treat cause or exacerbating factors
eg hyperglycaemia, hyponatraemia

↓

Definitive treatment if possible

Diabetic ketoacidosis (DKA)

Mechanism Lack of insulin results in ↓ cellular uptake of glucose. Hence ↓ production of pyruvate by glycolysis. AcetylCoA is thus generated by fat breakdown to make up deficit, but acetylCoA does not fix carbon in the cycle as all lost as CO_2. Fixed carbon normally comes from carboxylation of pyruvate (this is impaired for reason above). Some fixed carbon comes from breakdown of gluconeogenic fatty acids (hence early protein catabolism) but this does not adequately compensate. There is an excess of 2C acetyl CoA relative to the C4 acid in the TCA cycle, so excess converted to ketone bodies (also ↑acetone, hence fruity-smelling breath).[46]

Typical picture Gradual drowsiness, vomiting & dehydration in type 1 diabetic (very rarely type 2) ►Do glucose in *all* those with unexplained vomiting, abdominal pain, polyuria, polydipsia, lethargy, anorexia, ketotic breath, dehydration, coma, or deep breathing (sighing 'Kussmaul' hperventilation). ***Triggers:*** Infection, eg UTI; surgery; MI; pancreatitis; chemotherapy; antipsychotics;[47] wrong insulin dose/non-compliance.

Diagnosis Requires *acidosis* (*p*H<7.3) + *hyperglycaemia* + *ketosis.* Tests: ***Urine:*** Ketones+ MSU. ***Blood:*** Lab glucose, U&E, HCO_3^-, amylase, osmolality, ABG, FBC, blood culture. Plasma osmolarity = 2[Na⁺]+[urea]+[glucose] mmol/L. Anion gap: p684. *CXR.*

Pitfalls in diabetic ketoacidosis

- *Plasma glucose* is usually high, but not always, especially if insulin continued.
- *High WCC* may be seen in the absence of infection.
- *Infection:* often there is no fever. Do MSU, blood cultures, and CXR. Start broad-spectrum antibiotics (eg co-amoxiclav, p378) early if infection is suspected.
- *Creatinine:* some assays for creatinine cross-react with ketone bodies, so plasma creatinine may not reflect true renal function.
- *Hyponatraemia* is common, due to osmolar compensation for the hyperglycaemia. ↑ or ↔ [Na^+] indicates severe water loss. As treatment commences Na^+ rises as water enters cells. Na^+ is also low due to an artefact; corrected plasma [Na^+] = Na^+ + 2.4[(glucose –5.5)/5.5].
- *Ketonuria* does not equate with ketoacidosis. Anyone may have up to ++ketonuria after an overnight fast. Not all ketones are due to diabetes—consider alcohol if glucose normal. Test plasma with Ketostix® or Acetest® to show ketonaemia.
- *Recurrent ketoacidosis:* blood glucose may return to normal long before ketones are removed from the blood, and a rapid reduction in the amount of insulin administered may lead to lack of clearance and return to DKA. This may be avoided by maintaining a constant rate of insulin, eg 4-5U/h IVI, and co-infusing dextrose 10-20% to keep plasma glucose at 6-10mmol/L—the extended insulin regimen.
- *Acidosis* but without gross elevation of glucose may occur, but consider overdose (eg aspirin) and lactic acidosis (in elderly diabetics).
- *Serum amylase* is often raised (up to ×10) and non-specific abdominal pain is common, even in the absence of pancreatitis.

Management (p843). ►Set up IVI: dehydration is more lethal than hyperglycaemia.

- Monitor potassium, glucose, creatinine, HCO_3^-, hourly initially. Aim for a fall in glucose of 5mmol/h, and correction of the acidosis. The use of venous HCO_3^- as a guide to progress may prevent the need for repeated arterial blood gas sampling.
- Flow chart of vital signs, coma score, urine output/ketones; catheterize if no urine passed for 3-4h or comatose/shocked; monitoring CVP may guide fluid replacement.
- Find and treat infection (lung, skin, perineum, urine after cultures).
- Give LMW heparin SC until mobile (↑plasma osmolarity, ↑risk of DVT & PE).
- Change to SC insulin when ketones are ≤1+ and eating (p201).

NB: if acidosis is severe (*p*H<6.9), some give IV bicarbonate (eg 3mL/kg of 2.74% over 1h, and recheck arterial *p*H);[48] others never give it because of effects on the Hb-dissociation curve and cerebral circulation—discuss with your senior.

Complications Cerebral oedema (get help if sudden CNS decline), aspiration pneumonia, hypokalaemia, hypomagnesaemia, hypophosphataemia, thromboembolism. ►Talk with the patient: ensure there are no further preventable episodes.

Management plan for diabetic ketoacidosis

Check plasma glucose: usually >20mmol/L;if so give 4-8U soluble insulin IV

↓

Tests: Blood: Lab glucose, U&E, HCO_3^-, osmolality, blood gases, FBC, blood culture. *Urine:* Ketones, MSU. CXR.

↓

NG tube only if nauseated/vomiting/unconscious

↓

Insulin Give via a pump dilute to 1 unit/mL (care in mixing), start at ~6U/h for an average adult. Expect blood glucose to drop by ~5mmol/L per hour; if poor response, double or quadruple the rate. When blood glucose <10mmol/L, ↓rate to 3U/h and continue until food by mouth is possible. Don't stop the pump before routine subcutaneous insulin has been started. If no pump, load with 20U IM, then give 4–6U/h IM while glucose is >10mmol/L (then ↓ to 2-hrly).

↓

Check GCS, glucose, U&E, and HCO_3^- regularly (hourly initially)

↓

Continue fluid replacement, K^+ replacement

↓

What precipitated the DKA? Prevent the next one!

Fluid replacement

- Give 1 L of 0.9% saline stat. Then, typically, 1L over the next hour, 1L over 2h, 1L over 4h, then 1L over 6h—adjusted according to urine output.
- Use 5% dextrose when blood glucose is <10mmol/L
- Those >65yrs or with CCF need less saline more cautiously

Potassium replacement

- Total body potassium is invariably low, and plasma K^+ falls as K^+ enters cells with treatment.
- Don't add K^+ to the 1st bag. Monitor urine output hourly; start adding K^+ when urine flows at >30mL/h.
- Check U&E hourly initially, and replace as required:

Serum K^+ (mmol/L)	Amount of KCl to add per litre of IV fluid:
<3.0	40mmol
3–4	30mmol
4–5	20mmol

Less will be needed in renal failure or oliguria.

Other emergencies: Hyperosmolar non-ketotic coma & hypoglycaemia: p844.

Hypoglycaemic coma Usually *rapid* onset; may be preceded by odd behaviour (eg aggression), sweating, pulse↑, seizures. ***Management:*** ➡Give 20–30g dextrose IV, eg 200–300ml of 10% dextrose. This is preferable to 50–100mL 50% dextrose which harms veins. Expect prompt recovery. Glucagon 1mg IV/IM is nearly as rapid as dextrose but will not work in drunk patients. Dextrose IVI may be needed for severe prolonged hypoglycaemia. Once conscious, give sugary drinks and a meal.

Hyperglycaemic hyperosmolar non-ketotic (HONK) coma Typically those with type 2 DM are at risk of this.[49,50] The history is longer (eg 1wk), with marked dehydration and glucose >35mmol/L. Acidosis is absent as there has been no switch to ketone metabolism—the patient is often old, and presenting for the 1st time. Osmolality (p842) is >340mosmol/kg. ►*Occlusive events are a danger* (focal CNS signs, chorea, DIC, leg ischaemia/rhabdomyolysis[51]), DVT—so *fully* heparinize, p344.[52,53]

Rehydrate with ~9L of 0.9% saline IVI over 48h, eg at ½ the rate used in ketoacidosis. Replace K^+ (p842) when urine starts to flow. Wait 1h before using insulin (it may not be needed, and avoid rapid changes to avoid pontine myelinolysis).[54] If it is needed, 1u/h might be enough. Look for the cause, eg MI, drugs, or bowel infarct.

Hyperlactataemia is a rare but serious complication of DM with metformin use or septicaemia. Blood lactate: >5mmol/L. Seek expert help. Give O_2. Treat sepsis vigorously; optimise tissue perfusion.

Thyroid emergencies

Myxoedema coma The ultimate hypothyroid state before death. *Signs & symptoms:* Looks hypothyroid (p212); often >65yrs; hypothermia; hyporeflexia; glucose↓; bradycardia; coma; seizures. May have had radioiodine, thyroidectomy, or pituitary surgery (so signs of hypopituitarism, p224). He may have been psychotic (myxoedema madness)[55] just before the coma (eg precipitated by infection, MI, stroke, or trauma).

Examination: Goitre; cyanosis; BP↓ (cardiogenic); heart failure; signs of precipitants.

Treatment: Preferably on intensive care.

- Take venous blood for: T3, T4, TSH, FBC, U&E (Na^+ often↓), cultures, cortisol, glucose.
- Take arterial blood for P_aO_2.
- High-flow O_2 if cyanosed. Ventilation may be needed. Correct any hypoglycaemia.
- Give T3 (liothyronine) 5–20µg/12h IV slowly. Be cautious: you may precipitate manifestations of ischaemic heart disease. Alternative regimens involve levothyroxine.[56]
- Give hydrocortisone 100mg/8h IV—vital if pituitary hypothyroidism is suspected (ie no goitre, no previous radioiodine, no thyroid surgery).
- IVI 0.9% saline. Be sure to avoid precipitating LVF.
- If infection suspected, give antibiotic, eg cefuroxime 1.5g/8h IVI.
- Treat heart failure as appropriate (p130). Get help. Ask if pressors are needed.[57]
- Treat *hypothermia* with warm blankets in a warm room (+warm drinks if possible). Beware complications (hypoglycaemia, pancreatitis, arrhythmias). See p860.

Further ℞: T3 5–20µg/4–12h IV until sustained improvement (~2–3d) then levothyroxine 50µg/24h PO. Hydrocortisone + IV fluids as needed (hyponatraemia is dilutional).

Hyperthyroid crisis (thyrotoxic storm) *Sign & symptoms:* ♀:♂ ≈4:1. Severe hyperthyroidism: T°↑, agitation, confusion, coma, tachycardia, AF, D&V, goitre, thyroid bruit, acute abdomen (exclude surgical causes), heart failure, cardiovascular collapse.[58]

Precipitants: Recent thyroid surgery or radioiodine; infection; MI; trauma.

Diagnosis: Do not wait for test results if urgent treatment is needed. Do TSH, free T4 & free T3. Confirm with technetium uptake if possible.

Treatment: Ask an endocrinologist. **Grand strategy: 1** Counteract peripheral effects of thyroid hormones. **2** Inhibit thyroid hormone synthesis. **3** Treat systemic complications. See FLOWCHART for how to put this into effect[59]. If you are not making headway in 24h, consider thyroidectomy if you can find a good anaesthetist and surgeon.[60,61]

Management plan for thyrotoxic storm

IVI 0.9% saline, 500mL/4h. NG tube if vomiting.

↓

Take blood for: T3, T4, TSH, cultures (if infection suspected).

↓

Sedate if necessary (eg chlorpromazine 50mg PO/IM). Monitor BP.

↓

If no contraindication, and cardiac output OK, give propranolol 40mg/8h PO; max IV dose: 1mg over 1min; may need repeating, eg 5 times at ≥2min intervals. In asthma and if cardiac output is poor, use of propranolol has caused cardiac arrest in thyroid storm, so ultra-short-acting β-blockers have a role, eg IV esmolol (p819). Get help.

↓

High-dose digoxin may be needed to slow the heart, eg 1mg over 2h IVI.

↓

Antithyroid drugs: carbimazole 15–25mg/6h PO (or via NGT, if needed); after 4h give Lugol's solution 0.3mL/8h PO well-diluted in water for 1wk to block thyroid.

↓

Hydrocortisone sodium succinate 100mg/6h IV or dexamethasone 4mg/6h PO.

↓

Treat suspected infection, eg with eg cefuroxime 1.5g/8h IVI.

↓

Adjust IV fluids as necessary; cool with tepid sponging ± paracetamol.

↓

Continuing treatment: After 5d reduce carbimazole to 15mg/8h PO.

Addisonian crisis

Signs & symptoms: Patients may present in shock (pulse↑; vasoconstriction; postural hypotension; oliguria; weak; confused; comatose)—often (but not always!) in a patient with known Addison's (eg when oral steroid has not been increased to cover stress such as pneumonia), or someone on long-term steroids who has forgotten their tablets. Remember bilateral adrenal haemorrhage (eg meningococcaemia) as a cause. An alternative presentation is with hypoglycaemia.

Precipitating factors: Infection, trauma, surgery.

Management: If suspected, treat before biochemical results.
- Take blood for cortisol (10mL heparin or clotted) and ACTH if possible (10mL heparin bottle, to go straight to laboratory).
- Hydrocortisone sodium succinate 100mg IV stat.
- IV fluids: eg 0.9% saline.
- Monitor blood glucose: the danger is hypoglycaemia.
- Blood, urine, sputum for culture, then antibiotics (eg cefuroxime 1.5g/8h IVI).

Continuing treatment
- Glucose IV may be needed if hypoglycaemic.
- Continue IV fluids, more slowly as guided by clinical state. Correct U&E imbalance.
- Continue hydrocortisone sodium succinate, eg 100mg/6h IV or IM.
- Change to oral steroids after 72h if patient's condition good. The tetracosactrin (=tetracosactide) test is impossible while on hydrocortisone.
- Fludrocortisone may well be needed if the cause is adrenal disease: ask an expert.
- Search for (and vigorously treat) the underlying cause. Get endocrinological help.

Hypopituitary coma

Think of decompensated chronic hypophyseal failure whenever hypothermia, refractory hypotension ± septic signs *without* fever occur with short stature or loss of axillary/public hair ± gonadal atrophy.[62] ►Waiting for lab confirmation may be fatal. It *usually* develops gradually in a person with known hypopituitarism. If rapid onset due to pituitary infarction (eg postpartum Sheehan's, p224) subarachnoid haemorrhage is often misdiagnosed as symptoms include headache and meningism.

Presentation: Headache; ophthalmoplegia; consciousness↓; hypotension; hypothermia; hypoglycaemia; signs of hypopituitarism (p224).

Tests: Cortisol; T4; TSH; ACTH; glucose. Pituitary fossa CT/MRI.

Treatment: ►Hydrocortisone sodium succinate, eg 100mg IV/6h.
- Only after hydrocortisone begun: liothyronine (L-tri-iodothyronine sodium), eg 10µg/12h PO or by slow IV: 5–20µg/12h (4-hrly may be needed).
- Prompt surgery is needed if the cause is pituitary apoplexy (p226).

Phaeochromocytoma emergencies

Stress, abdominal palpation, parturition, general anaesthetic, or contrast media used in imaging may cause dangerous *hypertensive crises* (pallor, pulsating headache, hypertension, feels 'about to die', T°↑, LVF, ↑ST segment, VT and cardiogenic shock).[63] NB: low-osmolarity IV contrast may be OK.[64] *Treatment:* ►Get help. Take to ITU.
- **Phentolamine** 2–5mg IV.[65] Repeat to maintain safe BP (alternative: labetalol, p134).
- When BP controlled, give **phenoxybenzamine** 10mg/24h PO (increase by 10mg/d as needed, up to 30mg bd PO); SE: postural hypotension; dizziness; tachycardia; nasal congestion; miosis; idiosyncratic marked BP drop after 1st dose. The idea is to ↑the dose until BP is controlled and there is no significant postural hypotension. A β_1-blocker may also be given at this stage to control any tachycardia or myocardial ischaemia/dysrhythmias (p108).
- **Surgery** is usually done electively after 4–6wks to allow full α-blockade and volume expansion. When admitted for surgery the phenoxybenzamine dose is increased until significant postural hypotension.

• Seek expert help promptly, [illegible] protein 2 [illegible] and [illegible] should [illegible] be rapidly [illegible] have [illegible]. See p[illegible].

Definition [illegible] loss of [illegible] function characterized by a rise in [illegible] creatinine and [illegible] with [illegible] of urine.

Causes

• Hypovolaemia, or low cardiac output

• Glomerulonephritis

• Sepsis

• Drugs

• Urinary obstruction

• Hepatorenal syndrome [illegible]

Investigations

• U&E, Ca²⁺, PO₄, [illegible], [illegible], ESR, LFT, [illegible] protein, [illegible] hepatitis, [illegible] antibodies (ANA, ANCA, complement [illegible]), Blood cultures.

• Urgent urine microscopy and cultures. White cell casts suggest infection, but are seen in interstitial nephritis, and red cell casts suggest an inflammatory glomerulonephritis.

• USS of the renal tract.

• ECG, CXR.

Management See [illegible] for acute measures. Underlying causes are:

1. *Treat precipitating causes*: Treat acute blood loss with blood transfusion, and sepsis with antibiotics. [illegible] ARF is often associated with severe disease that needs monitoring and treatment. For example, a breathless patient with renal failure may need to be managed on ITU, not a ward [illegible] management of the respiratory failure.

2. *Treat life-threatening hyperkalaemia*: See [illegible].

3. *Treat pulmonary oedema, pericarditis, and [illegible]*: [illegible] dialysis may be needed. [illegible] [illegible] below [illegible] consider [illegible] of blood before [illegible] complications.

4. *Treat volume depletion*: [illegible] urine output. Use a large-bore line in a large vein [illegible] can be [illegible] of [illegible] volume depletion [illegible].

5. *Treat sepsis*.

6. *Further care*:

• [illegible]

• [illegible] of [illegible]

• If [illegible] but dialysis [illegible] consider renal biopsy.

• [illegible] with [illegible] daily, [illegible].

Prognosis Depends on cause; [illegible] mortality [illegible] [illegible], [illegible] [illegible] [illegible] [illegible] is worse [illegible] [illegible] higher mortality.

Urgent dialysis if

• K⁺ persistently high (>6.5mmol/L)

• Acidosis (pH <7.2)

• Pulmonary oedema and [illegible] substantial diuresis

• Pericarditis (by [illegible]) early dialyse [illegible] on the heart is [illegible].

• High catabolic state with rapidly progressive renal failure.

Acute renal failure (ARF)

►Seek expert help promptly: BP, urinary protein & sediment, serum K^+, creatinine, and ultrasound *must* be rapidly known. Have them to hand. See p298.

Definition Acute (over hours or days) deterioration in renal function, characterized by a rise in serum creatinine and urea, often with oliguria or anuria.

Causes[66]
- Hypovolaemia, or low cardiac output
- Glomerulonephritis
- Sepsis
- Drugs
- Obstruction (p642)
- Other, eg hepatorenal syndrome (p259), vasculitis (p558)

Investigations
- U&E, Ca^{2+}, PO_4^{3-}, FBC, ESR, CRP, INR, LFT, CK, LDH, protein electrophoresis, hepatitis serology, auto-antibodies (ANA, ANCA, complement, anti-GBM, ASOT; see p555), blood cultures.
- Urgent urine microscopy and cultures. White cell casts suggest infection, but are seen in interstitial nephritis, and red cell casts suggest an inflammatory glomerular condition (p294).
- USS of the renal tract.
- ECG, CXR.

Management See FLOWCHART for acute measures. Underlying principles are:

1 ***Treat precipitating cause:*** Treat acute blood loss with blood transfusion, and sepsis with antibiotics (p382). ARF is often associated with other diseases that need more urgent treatment. For example, someone in respiratory failure *and* renal failure may need to be managed on ITU, not a renal unit, to ensure optimal management of the respiratory failure.

2 ***Treat life-threatening hyperkalaemia:*** See FLOWCHART.

3 ***Treat pulmonary oedema, pericarditis, and tamponade:*** (p814) Urgent dialysis may be needed. If in pulmonary oedema, and no diuresis, consider removing a unit of blood, before dialysis commences.

4 ***Treat volume depletion:*** if necessary. Resuscitate quickly; then match input to output. Use a large-bore line in a large vein (central vein access can be risky in obvious volume depletion).

5 ***Treat sepsis.***

6 ***Further care:***
- Has obstruction been excluded? Examine for masses PR and *per vaginam*. Is the bladder palpable? ►If remains anuric despite fluid challenge an ultrasound is mandatory to exclude obstruction. Bilateral nephrostomies relieve obstruction, provide urine for culture, and allow anterograde pyelography to determine the site of obstruction.
- If worsening renal function but dialysis independent, consider renal biopsy.
- Diet: high in calories (2000–4000kcal/d) with adequate high-quality protein. Consider nasogastric feeding or parenteral route if too ill.

Prognosis Depends on cause (ATN mortality: surgery or trauma—60%, medical illness—30%, pregnancy—10%). Oliguric ARF is worse than non-oliguric—more GI bleeds, sepsis, acidosis, and higher mortality.

Urgent dialysis if:
- K^+ persistently high (>6.0mmol/L).
- Acidosis (pH <7.2).
- Pulmonary oedema and no substantial diuresis.
- Pericarditis. (In tamponade (p814), only dialyse *after* pressure on the heart is relieved.)
- High catabolic state with rapidly progressive renal failure.

Management of ARF

Catheterize to assess hourly urine output, and establish fluid charts

↓

Assess intravascular volume BP, JVP, skin turgor, fluid balance sheet, weight, CVP, attach to cardiac monitor. Consider inserting a central venous cannula.

↓

Investigations *(see p848)*

↓

Identify and treat hyperkalaemia—see below
Use a cardiac monitor

↓

If dehydrated, give fluid challenge.
250-500mL of colloid or saline over 30min

↓

Reassess
Repeat fluid challenge if still dehydrated. Aim for a CVP of 5-10cm

↓

Once fluid replete, continue fluids at 20mL + previous hour's urine output per hour

↓

If volume overloaded, consider urgent dialysis. A nitrate infusion, furosemide or 'renal dose' dopamine may help in the short term, especially to make space for blood transfusion etc. but does not alter outcome

↓

Correct acidosis with sodium bicarbonate, eg 50mL of 8.4% IV

↓

If clinical suspicion of sepsis, take cultures, then treat vigorously. Do not leave possible sources of sepsis (eg IV lines) in situ if not needed

↓

Avoid nephrotoxic drugs, eg NSAIDs, care with gentamicin. Check *Data Sheet* for all drugs given.

Hyperkalaemia

The danger is ventricular fibrillation. K^+ >7.0mmol/L will usually require urgent treatment, as will lower values with ECG changes:
- Tall 'tented' T waves ± flat P waves ± increased PR interval (see p689).
- Widening of the QRS complex—leading eventually, and dangerously, to a sinusoidal pattern and VF/VT.

Treatment:
- Monitor ECG.
- 10mL calcium gluconate (10%) IV over 2min, repeated as necessary if severe ECG changes (may cause skin necrosis if extravasation: avoid injecting into small peripheral cannulae). This provides cardio-protection (raises threshold potential); it does not change serum potassium levels.
- Insulin+glucose, eg 50mL of 50% glucose with 10U of rapidly acting insulin given into a large vein (unless hyperglycaemic) over ~30mins. Monitor for hypoglycaemia. This regimen may need repeating. NB: insulin moves K^+ into cells.
- Nebulized salbutamol (2.5mg) also makes K^+ enter cells.
- Polystyrene sulfonate resin (eg Calcium Resonium®, 15g/6-8h in water) orally or, if vomiting makes the PO route problematic, as a 30g enema (followed by colonic irrigation, after 9h, to remove K^+ from the colon).
- Dialysis (see *urgent dialysis if:*, p848).

Diagnosis Mainly from the history. The patient may not tell the truth about what has been taken. Use *MIMS Colour Index*, *eMIMS* images, *BNF* descriptions, or the computerized system 'TICTAC' (ask pharmacy) to identify tablets and plan specific treatment. Clues may become apparent:

- *Fast or irregular pulse:* Salbutamol, antimuscarinics, tricyclics, quinine, or phenothiazine poisoning.
- *Respiratory depression:* Opiate or benzodiazepine toxicity.
- *Hypothermia:* Phenothiazines, barbiturates.
- *Hyperthermia:* Amphetamines, MAOIs, cocaine, or ecstasy (p855).
- *Coma:* Benzodiazepines, alcohol, opiates, tricyclics, or barbiturates.
- *Seizures:* Recreational drugs, hypoglycaemic agents, tricyclics, phenothiazines, or theophyllines.
- *Constricted pupils:* Opiates or insecticides (organophosphates, p855).
- *Dilated pupils:* Amphetamines, cocaine, quinine, or tricyclics.
- *Hyperglycaemia:* Organophosphates, theophyllines, or MAOIs.
- *Hypoglycaemia:* Insulin, oral hypoglycaemics, alcohol, or salicylates.
- *Renal failure:* Salicylate, paracetamol, or ethylene glycol.
- *Metabolic acidosis:* Alcohol, ethylene glycol, methanol, paracetamol, or carbon monoxide poisoning—p854.
- ↑*Osmolality:* Alcohols (ethyl or methyl); ethylene glycol. See p682.

Management See FLOWCHART for a general guide to management.

- *Take blood* as appropriate (p852). Always check paracetamol and salicylate levels.
- *Empty stomach* if appropriate (p852).
- *Consider specific antidote* (p854) or oral activated charcoal (p852).
- *If you are not familiar with the poison* get more information. The *Medicines Compendium* is useful (**medicines.org.uk**). If in doubt how to act, phone the Poisons Information Service: in the UK phone 0844 892 0111.

Continuing care Measure temperature, pulse, BP, and blood glucose regularly. Use a continuous ECG monitor. If unconscious, nurse semi-prone, turn regularly, keep eyelids closed. A urinary catheter will be needed if the bladder is distended, or renal failure is suspected, or forced diuresis undertaken. Take to ITU, eg if respiration↓.

Psychiatric assessment Be sympathetic despite the hour! Interview relatives and friends if possible. Aim to establish:

- *Intentions at time:* Was the act planned? What precautions against being found? Did the patient seek help afterwards? Does the patient think the method was dangerous? Was there a final act (eg suicide note)?
- *Present intentions.* Do they still feel suicidal? Do they wish it had worked?
- *What problems* led to the act: do they still exist?
- *Was the act* aimed at someone?
- Is there a *psychiatric disorder* (depression, alcoholism, personality disorder, schizophrenia, dementia)?
- What are his *resources* (friends, family, work, personality)?

The assessment of suicide risk: The following increase the chance of future suicide: original intention was to die; present intention is to die; presence of psychiatric disorder; poor resources; previous suicide attempts; socially isolated; unemployed; male; >50yrs old. See *OHCS* p338. There is an increased risk of death in the first year following initial presentation.

Referral to psychiatrist: This depends partly on local resources. Ask advice if presence of psychiatric disorder or high suicide risk.

Mental Capacity Act or the Mental Health Act: (in England and Wales) may provide for the detention of the patient against his or her will: see *OHCS* p400.

Emergency care in acute poisoning

ABC, clear airway

↓

Consider ventilation (if the respiratory rate is <8/min, or P_aCO_2 <8kPa, when breathing 60% O_2, or the airway is at risk, eg GCS <8)

↓

Treat shock (p804)

↓

If unconscious, nurse semi-prone

Further management

Assess the patient

↓

History from patient, friends, or family is vital

↓

Features from the examination may help (see p850)

↓

Investigations

- Glucose, U&E, FBC, LFT, INR, ABG, ECG, paracetamol, and salicylate levels
- Urine/serum toxicology, specific assays as appropriate

↓

Monitor

- T°, pulse & respiratory rate, BP, O_2 saturations, urine output ± ECG

↓

Treatment

- Supportive measures: may need catheterization
- ↓Absorption: consider gastric lavage ± activated charcoal, see p852

↓

Specific measures, see p852; for antidotes, see p854

Consider naloxone if ↓conscious level and pin-point pupils

Plasma toxicology For all unconscious patients, paracetamol and aspirin levels and blood glucose are required. The necessity of other assays depends on the drug taken and the index of suspicion. Be guided by the poisons information service. More common assays include: digoxin; methanol; lithium; iron; theophylline. Toxicological screening of urine, especially for recreational drugs, may be of use in some cases.

Gastric lavage Rarely used. Lavage after 30–60 min may make matters worse. ►*Do not empty stomach* if petroleum products or corrosives such as acids, alkalis, bleach, descalers have been ingested (*exception:* paraquat), or if the patient is unconscious or unable to protect their airway (unless intubated). ►Never induce vomiting.

Gastric emptying and lavage If comatose, or no gag reflex, ask for an anaesthetist to protect airway with cuffed endotracheal tube. If conscious, get verbal consent.

- Monitor O_2 by pulse oximetry. See p156.
- Have suction apparatus to hand and working.
- Position the patient in left lateral position.
- Raise the foot of the bed by 20cm.
- Pass a lubricated tube (14mm external diameter) via the mouth, asking the patient to swallow.
- Confirm position in stomach—blow air down, and auscultate over the stomach.
- Siphon the gastric contents. Check pH with litmus paper.
- Perform gastric lavage using 300–600mL tepid water at a time. Massage the left hypochondrium.
- Repeat until no tablets in siphoned fluid.
- Leave activated charcoal (50g in 200mL water) in the stomach unless alcohol, iron, Li^+, or ethylene glycol ingested.
- When pulling out tube, occlude its end (prevents aspiration of fluid remaining in the tube).

Activated charcoal reduces the absorption of many drugs from the gut when given as a single dose of 50g with water, eg salicylates, paracetamol. It is given in repeated doses (50g/4h) to increase elimination of some drugs from the blood, eg carbamazepine, dapsone, theophyllines, quinine, phenobarbital, and paraquat. Lower doses are used in children. Do not use with petroleum products, corrosives, alcohols, clofenotane, malathion or metal salts (eg iron, lithium).

⚠ **Help on the web:** UK GPs and other NHS workers and departments may register with *toxbase* at www.spib.axl.co.uk for free up-to-date toxicological advice.

Benzodiazepines Flumazenil (for respiratory arrest) 200μg over 15s; then 100μg at 60s intervals if needed. Usual dose range: 300–600μg IV over 3–6min (up to 1mg; 2mg if on ITU). May provoke fits. Use only after expert advice.

β-blockers Severe bradycardia or hypotension. Try atropine up to 3mg IV. Give glucagon 2–10mg IV bolus + 5% dextrose if atropine fails then infusion of 50μg/kg/h. If unresponsive, consider pacing or an aortic balloon pump.

Cyanide This fast-killing poison has affinity for Fe^{3+}, and inhibits the cytochrome system, ↓aerobic respiration. ***3 phases:*** • Anxiety ± confusion • Pulse↑ or ↓ • Fits ± shock ± coma. ***Treatment:*** ▸▸100% O_2, GI decontamination; if consciousness↓ either sodium nitrite + sodium thiosulfate, or dicobalt edetate 300mg IV over 1–5min, then 50mL 50% dextrose IV (repeat once if needed); or hydroxocobalamin 5g over 30 min (70mg/kg) repeated once is required. *Get expert help*. See p859.

Carbon monoxide Despite hypoxaemia skin is pink (or pale), not blue as carboxyhaemoglobin (COHb) displaces O_2 from Hb binding sites. ***Symptoms:*** Headache, vomiting, pulse↑, tachypnoea, and, if COHb >50%, fits, coma, & cardiac arrest. ▸▸Remove the source. Give 100% O_2. Metabolic acidosis usually responds to correction of hypoxia. If severe, anticipate cerebral oedema. Give mannitol IVI (p841). Confirm diagnosis with a heparinized blood sample (COHb >10%) quickly as levels may soon return to normal. Monitor ECG. *Hyperbaric O_2 may help: discuss with the poisons service if is or has been unconscious, pregnant, COHb >20%, or failing to respond.*

Digoxin ***Symptoms:*** Cognition↓, yellow-green visual halos, arrhythmias, nausea, & anorexia. If serious arrhythmias are present, correct hypokalaemia, and inactivate with digoxin-specific antibody fragments (Digibind®). If load or level is unknown, give 20 vials (800mg)—adult or child >20kg. Consult Compendium/SPC (p850). Dilute in water for injections (4mL/38mg vial) and 0.9% saline (to make a convenient volume); give IVI over ½h, via a 0.22μm-pore filter. If the amount of digoxin ingested is known, the SPC will tell you how many vials of Digibind® to give, eg if 25 tabs of 0.25mg ingested, give 10 vials; if 50 tabs, give 20 vials; if 100 tabs, give 40 vials.

Heavy metals Enlist expert help.

Iron Desferrioxamine 15mg/kg/h IVI; max 80mg/kg/d. **NB:** gastric lavage if iron ingestion in last hour; consider whole bowel irrigation.

Oral anticoagulants If major bleed, treat with vitamin K, 5mg slow IV; give prothrombin complex concentrate 50U/kg IV (or if unavailable, fresh frozen plasma 15mL/kg IVI). For abnormal INR with no (or minimal) bleeding, see BNF. If it is vital that anticoagulation continues, enlist expert help. Warfarin can normally be restarted within 2–3d. **NB:** coagulation defects may be delayed for 2–3d following ingestion.

Opiates (Many analgesics contain opiates.) Give naloxone eg 0.4–2mg IV; repeat every 2min until breathing is adequate (it has a short $t_{½}$, so it may need to be given often or IM; max. 10mg). Naloxone may precipitate features of opiate withdrawal—diarrhoea and cramps, which will normally respond to diphenoxylate and atropine (Lomotil®—eg 2 tablets/6h PO). Sedate as needed (see p11). High-dose opiate misusers may need methadone (eg 10–30mg/12h PO) to combat withdrawal. Register opiate addiction (*OHCS* p362), and refer for help.

Phenothiazine poisoning (eg chlorpromazine) No specific antidote. *Dystonia (torticollis, retrocollis, glossopharyngeal dystonia, opisthotonus):* try procyclidine, eg 5-10mg IM or IV. Treat *shock* by raising the legs (± plasma expander IVI, or dopamine IVI if desperate). Restore body temperature. *Monitor ECG.* Avoid lidocaine in dysrhythmias. Use lorazepam IV for prolonged fits in the usual way (p836). *Neuroleptic malignant syndrome* consists of: hyperthermia, rigidity, extrapyramidal signs, autonomic dysfunction (labile BP, pulse↑, sweating, urinary incontinence), mutism, confusion, coma, WCC↑, CPK↑; it may be treated with cooling. Dantrolene has been tried (p574).

Carbon tetrachloride poisoning This solvent, used in many industrial processes, causes vomiting, abdominal pain, diarrhoea, seizures, coma, renal failure, and tender hepatomegaly with jaundice and liver failure. IV N-acetylcysteine may improve prognosis. Seek expert help.

Organophosphate insecticides inactivate cholinesterase—the resulting increase in acetylcholine causes the SLUD response: salivation, lacrimation, urination, and diarrhoea. Also look for sweating, small pupils, muscle fasciculation, coma, respiratory distress, and bradycardia. *Treatment:* Wear gloves; remove soiled clothes. Wash skin. Take blood (FBC & serum cholinesterase activity). Give atropine IV 2mg every 10min till full atropinization (skin dry, pulse >70, pupils dilated). Up to 3 days' treatment may be needed. Also give pralidoxime 30mg/kg slowly IV (in the UK, the Poisons Information Service will tell you how to get it; it is diluted with ≥10mL water for injections). Repeat as needed every 30min; max 12g in 24h. Even if fits are not occurring, diazepam 5-10mg IV seems to help.

Paraquat poisoning (Found in weed-killers.) This causes D&V, painful oral ulcers, alveolitis, and renal failure. Diagnose by urine test. Give activated charcoal *at once* (100g followed by a laxative, then 50g/3-4h). ►*Get expert help.* Avoid O_2 early on (promotes lung damage).

Ecstasy poisoning Ecstasy is a semi-synthetic, hallucinogenic substance (MDMA, 3,4-methylenedioxymethamphetamine). Its effects range from nausea, muscle pain, blurred vision, amnesia, fever, confusion, and ataxia to tachyarrhythmias, hyperthermia, hyper/hypotension, water intoxication, DIC, K^+↑, acute renal failure, hepatocellular and muscle necrosis, cardiovascular collapse, and ARDS. There is no antidote and treatment is supportive. Management depends on clinical and lab findings, but may include:

- Administration of activated charcoal and monitoring of BP, ECG, and temperature for at least 12h (rapid cooling may be needed).
- Monitor urine output and U&E (renal failure p299), LFT, CK, FBC, and coagulation (DIC p346). Metabolic acidosis may benefit from treatment with bicarbonate.
- Anxiety: diazepam 0.1-0.3mg/kg PO. IV dose: p836.
- Narrow complex tachycardias in adults: consider metoprolol 5-10mg IV.
- Hypertension can be treated with nifedipine 5-10mg PO or phentolamine 2-5mg IV. Treat hypotension conventionally (p804).
- Hyperthermia: attempt to cool, if rectal T° > 39°C. Consider dantrolene 1mg/kg IV (may need repeating: discuss with your senior and a poisons unit, p850). Hyperthermia with ecstasy is akin to serotonin syndrome, and propranolol, muscle relaxation and ventilation may be needed.[67]

Snakes (adders) *Anaphylaxis* p806. *Signs of envenoming:* BP↓ (vasodilatation, viper cardiotoxicity) D&V; swelling spreading proximally within 4h of bite; bleeding gums or venepuncture sites; anaphylaxis; ptosis; trismus; rhabdomyolysis; pulmonary oedema. *Tests:* WCC↑; clotting↓; platelets↓; U&E; urine RBC↑; CK↑; P_aO_2↓, ECG. *Management:* Avoid active movement of affected limb (so use splints/slings). *Avoid incisions and tourniquets.* ►Get help.[68] Is antivenom indicated (IgG from venom-immunized sheep)?—eg 10mL IV over 15min (adults *and* children) of *European Viper Antiserum* (from Monviato) for adder bites; have adrenaline to hand—p806. Monitor ECG. For foreign snakes, see *BNF*.

Salicylate poisoning

Aspirin is a weak acid with poor water solubility. It is present in many over-the-counter preparations. Anaerobic metabolism and the production of lactate and heat are stimulated by the uncoupling of oxidative phosphorylation. Effects are dose-related, and potentially fatal: • 150mg/kg: mild toxicity • 250mg/kg: moderate • >500mg/kg: severe toxicity. Levels over 700mg/L are potentially fatal.

Signs & symptoms Unlike paracetamol, many early features. Vomiting, dehydration, hyperventilation, tinnitus, vertigo, sweating. Rarely; lethargy or coma, seizures, vomiting, ↓BP and heart block, pulmonary oedema, hyperthermia. Patients present initially with respiratory alkalosis due to a direct stimulation of the central respiratory centres and then develop a metabolic acidosis. Hyper- or hypoglycaemia may occur.

Management *General:* p850. Correct dehydration. Gastric lavage if within 1h, activated charcoal (may be repeated, but is of unproven value).

- Paracetamol and salicylate level, glucose, U&E, LFT, INR, ABG, HCO_3^-, FBC. Salicylate level may need to be repeated after 2h, due to continuing absorption if a potentially toxic dose has been taken.
- Monitor urine output, and blood glucose. If severe poisoning: salicylate levels, serum pH, and U&E. Consider urinary catheter and monitoring urine pH. Beware hypoglycaemia.
- Correct any metabolic acidosis with 1.26% HCO_3^- (sodium bicarbonate).
- If plasma salicylate level >500mg/L (3.6mmol/L), consider alkalinization of the urine, eg 1.5L 1.26% HCO_3^- with 40mmol KCl IV over 3h. Aim to make the **urine** pH 7.5–8.5. **NB:** monitor serum K^+ as hypokalaemia may occur.
- Dialysis may well be needed if salicylate level >700mg/L, and if renal or heart failure, seizures, severe acidosis, or persistently ↑plasma salicylate. ECG monitor.
- Discuss any serious cases with the local toxicological service or national poisons information service.

Paracetamol poisoning

150mg/kg, or 12g in adults may be fatal (75mg/kg if malnourished). However, prompt treatment can prevent liver failure and death. ►1 tablet of paracetamol = 500mg.

Signs & symptoms None initially, or vomiting ± RUQ pain. Later: jaundice and encephalopathy from liver damage (the main danger) ± renal failure.

Management *General measures* p850, lavage if >12g (or >150mg/kg) taken within 1h. Give activated charcoal if ≤1h since ingestion. Specific measures:

- Glucose, U&E, LFT, INR, ABG, FBC, HCO_3^-; blood paracetamol level at 4h post-ingestion.
- If <8h since overdose and plasma paracetamol is above the line on the graph (see **fig 1**), start N-acetylcysteine.
- If >8h and suspicion of large overdose (>7.5g) err on the side of caution and start N-acetylcysteine, stopping it if level below treatment line and INR/ALT normal.
- N-acetylcysteine is given by IVI: 150mg/kg in 200mL of 5% dextrose over 15min. Then 50mg/kg in 500mL of 5% dextrose over 4h. Then 100mg per kg/16h in 1L of 5% dextrose. Rash is a common SE: treat with chlorphenamine, and observe; do not stop unless anaphylatoid reaction with shock, vomiting, and wheeze (≤10%). An alternative (if acetylcysteine unavailable) is methionine 2.5g/4h PO for 16h (total: 10g), but absorption is unreliable if vomiting. Benefit is lessened by concurrent charcoal.
- If ingestion time is unknown, or it is staggered, or presentation is >15h from ingestion, treatment *may* help. ►Get advice.
- The graph may mislead if HIV+ve (hepatic glutathione↓), or if long-acting paracetamol has been taken, or if pre-existing liver disease or induction of liver enzymes has occurred. ►Beware ↓glucose—do BM hourly; INR/12h.
- Next day do INR, U&E, LFT. If INR rising, continue N-acetylcysteine until <1.4.
- If continued deterioration, discuss with the liver team. Don't hesitate to get help.

Criteria for transfer to a specialist unit:

- *Encephalopathy* or ICP↑. Signs of CNS oedema: BP >160/90 (sustained) or brief rises (systolic >200mmHg), bradycardia, decerebrate posture, extensor spasms, poor pupil responses. ICP monitoring can help, p840.
- *INR* >2.0 at <48h—or >3.5 at <72h (so measure INR every 12h). Peak elevation: 72-96h. LFTs are *not* good markers of hepatocyte death. If INR is *normal* at 48h, the patient may go home.
- *Renal impairment* (creatinine >200μmol/L). Monitor urine flow. Daily U&E and serum creatinine (use haemodialysis if >400μmol/L).
- *Blood pH <7.3* (lactic acidosis → tissue hypoxia). • *Systolic BP* <80mmHg.

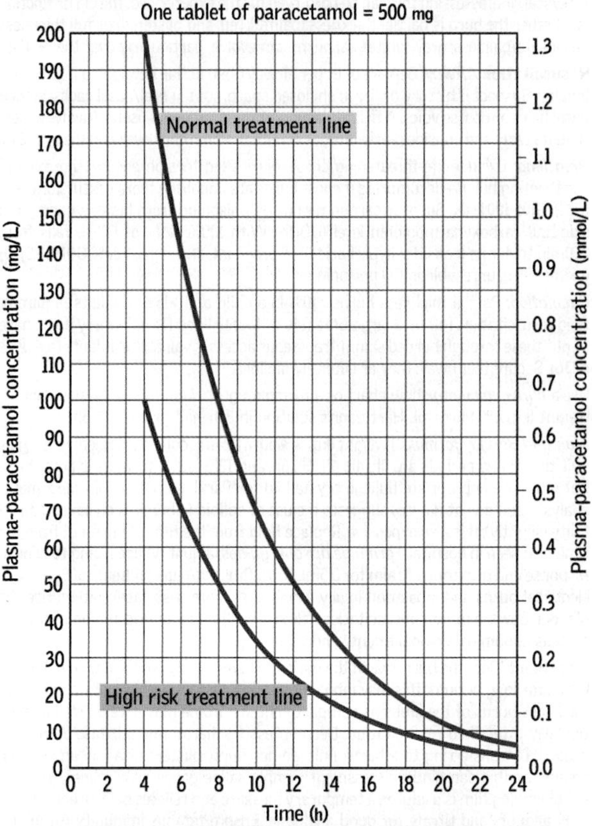

Fig 1. Plasma concentration of paracetamol *vs* time. Patients whose plasma-paracetamol concentrations are above the **normal treatment line** should be treated with N-acetylcysteine by intravenous infusion (or, provided the overdose has been taken **within 10–12h**, with methionine by mouth, see *Paracetamol poisoning*, p856). Patients on enyzme-including drugs (eg carbamazepine, phenobarbital, phenytoin, rifampicin, and alcohol) or who are malnourished (eg in anorexia, in alcoholism, or those who are HIV-positive) should be treated if their plasma-paracetamol concentrations are above the **high-risk treatment line**.

We thank Dr Alun Hutchings for permission to reproduce this graph.

Resuscitate and arrange transfer for all major burns (>25% partial thickness in adult and >20% in children). Assess site, size, and depth of burn (BOX 2, to help calculate fluid requirements). Referral is still warranted in cases of full thickness burns >5%, partial thickness burns >10% in adults or >5% in children or the elderly, burns of special sites, chemical and electrical burns and burns with inhalational injury.

Assessment *Burn size* is important to assess (see BOX) as it influences the size of the inflammatory response (vasodilatation, increased vascular permeability) and thus fluid shift from the intravascular volume. Ignore erythema. *Burn depth* determines healing time/scarring; assessing this can be hard, even for the experienced. The big distinction is whether the burn is partial thickness (painful, red, and blistered) or full thickness (insensate/painless; grey-white). **NB:** burns can evolve, particularly over the 1st 48h.

Resuscitation ***Airway:*** Beware of upper airway obstruction developing if hot gases inhaled. Suspect if history of fire in enclosed space, soot in oral/nasal cavity, singed nasal hairs or hoarse voice. A flexible laryngo/bronchoscopy is useful. Involve anaesthetists early and consider early intubation. Obstruction can develop in the first 24h.

Breathing: Exclude life-threatening chest injuries (eg tension pneumothorax) and constricting burns—decompress if chest burns are impairing thorax excursion (*OHCS* p731). Give 100% O_2. Suspect carbon monoxide poisoning from history, cherry-red skin and carboxyhaemoglobin level (COHb). With 100% O_2 $t_{1/2}$ of COHb falls from 250min to 40min (consider hyperbaric O_2 if: pregnant; CNS signs; >20% COHb). SpO_2 (oximetry) is unreliable in CO poisoning.

Circulation: Partial thickness burns >10% in a child and >15% in adults require IV fluid resuscitation. Put up 2 large-bore (14G or 16G) IV lines. Do not worry if you have to put these through burned skin, intraosseous access is valuable in infants (see *OHCS* p236). Secure them well: they are literally lifelines.

Use a ***burns calculator*** flow chart or a formula, eg: ***Parkland formula*** (popular): 4 x weight (kg) x % burn=mL Hartmann's solution in 24h, half given in 1st 8h.

Muir and Barclay formula: [weight (kg) × %burn]/2=mL colloid (eg Haemaccel®) per unit time. Time periods are 4h, 4h, 4h, 6h, 6h, and 12h. Either formula is acceptable but must use appropriate fluid, ie crystalloid for Parkland not colloid. **NB:** a meta-analysis (somewhat flawed) suggests the use of colloid (albumin) can cause ↑ mortality (slightly); it is also expensive. Replace fluid from the time of burn, not from the time first seen in hospital. *Formulae are only guides:* adjust IVI according to clinical response and urine output; aim for 0.5mL/kg/h (1mL/kg/h in children), ~50% more in electrical burns and inhalation injury. Monitor T° (core & surface); catheterize the bladder. Beware of over-resuscitation ('fluid creep') that can lead to complications such as abdominal compartment syndrome.

Treatment 'Cool the burn, warm the patient'. Do *not* apply cold water to extensive burns for long periods: this may intensify shock. Take care with circumferential full thickness burns of the limbs as compartment syndrome may develop rapidly particularly after fluid resuscitation. Decompress (escharotomy and fasciotomy) as needed. If transferring to a burns unit, do not burst blisters or apply any special creams as this can hinder assessment. Simple saline gauze or Vaseline® gauze is suitable; cling film is useful as a temporary measure and relieves pain. Use morphine in IV aliquots and titrate for good analgesia. Ensure tetanus immunity. Antibiotic prophylaxis is not routinely used.

Definitive dressings There are many dressings for partial thickness burns, eg biological (pigskin, cadaveric skin), synthetic (Mepitel®, Duoderm®) and silver sulfadiazine cream alone (Flamazine®) or with cerium nitrate as Flammacerium® (on a named-patient basis[UK]); it forms a leathery eschar which resists infection.[69] Major full thickness burns benefit from early tangential excision and split-skin grafts as the burn is a major source of inflammatory cytokines causing SIRS (systemic inflammatory response syndrome) and forms a rich medium for bacterial growth.

Smoke inhalation

Initially there is laryngospasm that leads to hypoxia and straining (leading to petechiae), then hypoxic cord relaxation leads to true inhalation injury. Free radicals, cyanide compounds, and carbon monoxide accompany thermal injury. Cyanide compounds (generated eg from burning plastics) bind reversibly with ferric ions in enzymes, so stopping oxidative phosphorylation, causing dizziness, headaches, and seizures. Tachycardia and dyspnoea soon give way to bradycardia and apnoea. Carbon monoxide is generated later in the fire as oxygen is depleted. NB: COHb levels do not correlate well with the severity of poisoning and partly reflect smoking status and urban life. Use nomograms to extrapolate peak levels.

- ▸▸100% O_2 is given to elute both cyanide and CO.
- ▸▸Involve ICU/anaesthetists early: early ventilation may be useful, consider repeated bronchoscopic lavage.
- ▸▸Enlist expert help in cyanide poisoning: there is no one regimen suitable for all situations. Clinically mild poisoning may be treated by rest, O_2,. IV antidotes may be used for moderate poisoning: eg sodium thiosulfate is a common 1st choice. More severe poisoning may require eg hydroxocobalamin and sodium nitrite.

Lund & Browder charts[1]

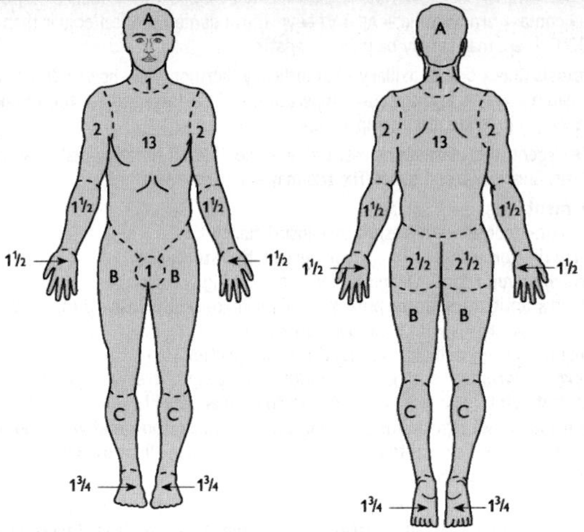

Relative percentage of body surface area affected by growth

Area	Age 0	1	5	10	15	Adult
A: half of head	9½	8½	6½	5½	4½	3½
B: half of thigh	2¾	3¼	4	4¼	4½	4¾
C: half of leg	2½	2½	2¾	3	3¼	3½

1 Accurate but time-consuming compared with the '**Rule of nines**': arm: 9%; front of trunk 18%; head & neck 9%; leg 18%; back of trunk 18%; perineum 1%. The rule of nines generally overestimates burn area (better than underestimating). **A modified rule of nines for children:** from birth up to 1yr, surface area of head and neck is 18% and each leg is 14%. For each year after, the head loses 1% and each leg gains 0.5%—so adult proportions are reached by age 10yrs.

We thank Professor Tor Chiu for help in preparing this topic.

Hypothermia

►***Have a high index of suspicion and a low-reading thermometer.*** Most patients are elderly and do not complain, or feel, cold—so they have not tried to warm up. In the young, hypothermia is usually from cold exposure (eg near-drowning), or is secondary to impaired consciousness (eg following excess alcohol or drug overdose).

Definition Hypothermia implies a core (rectal) temperature <35°C.

Causes In the elderly, hypothermia is often caused by a combination of:
- Impaired homeostatic mechanisms: usually age-related
- Low room temperature: poverty, poor housing
- Impaired thermoregulation: pneumonia, MI, heart failure
- Reduced metabolism: immobility, hypothyroidism, diabetes mellitus
- Autonomic neuropathy (p509); eg diabetes mellitus, Parkinson's
- Excess heat loss: psoriasis
- Cold awareness↓: dementia, confusion
- Increased exposure to cold: falls, especially at night when cold
- Drugs: major tranquillizers, antidepressants, diuretics, alcohol

The patient *How frozen I then became: I did not die, yet nothing of life remained.*[1] So don't assume that if vital signs seem to be absent, the patient must be dead: rewarm (see below) and re-examine. If T° <32°C, this sequence may occur: ↓BP → coma → bradycardia → AF → VT → VF. The abdomen can feel 'colder than clay'. If >32°C, there may simply be pallor ± apathy.

Diagnosis Check oral or axillary T°. If ordinary thermometer shows <36.5°C, use a low-reading one PR. Is the rectal temperature <35°C? Infra-red ear thermometers can accurately reflect core temperature.

Tests Urgent U&E, plasma glucose, and amylase. Thyroid function tests; FBC; blood cultures. Consider blood gases. The ECG may show J-waves (**fig 1**).

Treatment
- Ventilate if comatose or respiratory insufficiency.
- Warm IVI (for access or to correct electrolyte disturbance).
- Cardiac monitor (both VF and AF can occur during warming).
- Consider antibiotics for the prevention of pneumonia (p162). Give these routinely in patients over 65yrs with a temperature <32°C.
- Consider urinary catheter (to monitor renal function).
- *Slowly rewarm.* Do not reheat too quickly, causing peripheral vasodilatation, shock, and death. Aim for a rise of ½°C/h. Old, conscious patients should sit in a warm room taking hot drinks. Thermal blankets may cause too rapid warming in old patients. The first sign of too rapid warming is falling BP. Treat by allowing patient to cool down slightly.
- Rectal temperature, BP, pulse, and respiratory rate every ½ hour.

NB: advice is different for sudden hypothermia from immersion; here, if there has been a cardiac arrest, and T° <30°C, mediastinal warm lavage, peritoneal or haemodialysis, and cardiopulmonary bypass (no heparin if trauma) may be needed (*OHCS* p724).

Complications Arrhythmias (if there is a cardiac arrest continue resuscitating until T° >33°C, as cold brains are less damaged by hypoxia); pneumonia; pancreatitis; acute renal failure; intravascular coagulation. ***Prognosis:*** Depends on age and degree of hypothermia. If age >70yrs and T° <32°C then mortality >50%.

Before hospital discharge Anticipate problems. Will it happen again? What is her network of support? Review medication (could you stop tranquillizers)? How is progress to be monitored? Liaise with GP/social worker.

1 In the last round of the 9th circle of *Hell*, Dante tells how those betraying their benefactors are encased in ice (*canto XXXIV*) 'Com'io divenni allor gelato e fioco...Io non mori e non rimasi vivo.' **Human records:** • Mitsuaka Uchikoshi appears to have 'hibernated' for 24 days on Mount Rokko (core T°≈22°C). • Erica Nordy came to life in 2 hours after her heart stopped (core T°: 16°). NB: being encased in ice is a hazard that goes with paragliding: here the cause is not so much neglect of benefactors, as being treated within violent storm clouds as an item of hail.

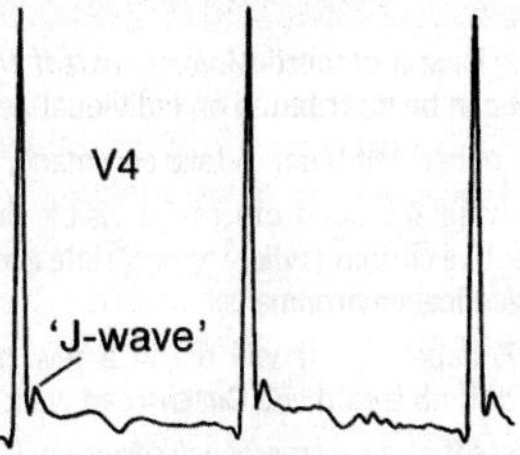

Fig 1. J-wave in hypothermia.

Courtesy of Dr R Luke & Dr E McLachlan

Planning All hospitals have a detailed *Major Accident Plan*, but additionally the tasks of key personnel can be distributed on individual *Action Cards*.

At the scene Call the police; tell them to take command.

Safety is paramount—your own and others. Be visible (luminous monogrammed jacket) and wear protective clothing where appropriate (safety helmet; waterproofs; boots; respirator in chemical environment).

Triage: See OHCS p797. Label **RED** if will die in a few minutes if no treatment. YELLOW = will die in ~2h if no treatment; **GREEN** = can wait. (**BLUE** = dead).

Communications are essential; each emergency service will dispatch a control vehicle and will have a designated incident officer for liaison. Support medical staff from hospital report to the medical incident officer—he is usually the first doctor on the scene: his job is to assess then communicate to the receiving hospital the number and severity of casualties, to organize resupply of equipment and to replace fatigued staff. He must resist temptation to treat casualties as this compromises his role.

Equipment: Must be portable and include: intubation and cricothyrotomy set; intravenous fluids (colloid); bandages and dressings; chest drain (+flutter valve); amputation kit (when used, ideally 2 doctors should concur); drugs—*analgesic:* morphine; *anaesthetic:* ketamine 2mg/kg IV over >60s (0.5mg/kg is a powerful analgesic without respiratory depression); limb splints (may be inflatable); defibrillator/monitor ± pulse oximeter.

Evacuation: Remember that with immediate treatment on scene, the priority for evacuation may be reduced (eg a tension pneumothorax - **RED** - once relieved can wait for evacuation and becomes YELLOW), but those who may suffer by delay at the scene must go first. Send any severed limbs to the same hospital as the patient, ideally chilled—but not frozen.

At the hospital a 'major incident' is declared. The *first receiving* hospital will take most of the casualties; the *support* hospital(s) will cope with overflow and may provide mobile teams so that staff are not depleted from the first hospital. A control room is established and the medical coordinator ensures staff have been summoned, nominates a triage officer, and supervises the best use of inpatient beds and ITU/theatre resources.

Blast injury may be caused by domestic (eg gas explosion) or industrial (eg mining) accidents, or by terrorist bombs. Death may occur without any obvious external injury (air emboli). Injury occurs in 6 ways:

1 *Blast wave:* A transient (milliseconds) wave of overpressure expands rapidly producing cellular disruption, shearing forces along tissue planes (submucosal/subserosal haemorrhage) and re-expansion of compressed trapped gas—bowel perforation, fatal air embolism.
2 *Blast wind:* This can totally disrupt a body or cause avulsive amputations. Bodies can be thrown and sustain injuries on landing.
3 *Missiles:* Penetration or laceration from missiles are by far the commonest injuries. Missiles arise from the bomb or are secondary, eg glass.
4 *Flash burns:* These are usually superficial and occur on exposed skin.
5 *Crush injuries*: beware sudden death or renal failure after release.
6 *Psychological injury:* Eg post-traumatic stress disorder (OHCS p347).

Treatment Approach the same as any major trauma OHCS p724. Rest and observe any suspected of exposure to significant blast but without other injury. Gun-shot injury: see OHCS p722.

Sources: I Greaves 1999 *Pre-hospital Medicine*, Arnold; S Mellor *Recent Advances in Surgery* 14, Churchill Livingstone, London 1991 53-68.

Index

►For drugs, consult the disease you want to treat, not the drug

Abbreviations: **F** indexes a notable figure or image; dis = disease; syn = syndrome.

D

F

G

H

O

Q

R

S

V

W

XYZ

All indexes can be improved: let us know how at ohcm8.index@oup.com

Key references

Chapter 1 Thinking about medicine

★38 Editorial: Welcome clinical leadership at NICE. *Lancet*. 2008. 372: 601. p10

Chapter 2 History and examination

★80 Developed from: Evaluation of a mental test score for assessment of mental impairment in the elderly. Hodkinson HM. *Age Ageing*. 1972. 1:233–8. p70

★81 The Mini-Mental State Examination is now subject to copyright owned by PAR. See: www.minimental.com/ p70

★123 Download TYM test and notes for marking from: www.elderguru.com p85

Chapter 3 Cardiovascular medicine

★5 S Capewell. *BMJ*. 2000. 320: 951–2. p89

★20 HC Bucher. *BMJ*. 2000. 321: 73–7. p110

★21 Fox KA. *Lancet*. 2002. 360:743–51 p110

★28 *J Am Coll Cardiol*. 2007. 50:2173–95 p112

★29 *J Am Coll Cardiol*. 2001. 38:478–85. p112

★31 C Junghans. *BMJ*. 2006. 333: 1080. p112

★34 *Eur Heart J*. 2002. 23: 1809–1840 p114

★38 (p114) and ★125 (p152). Driver and Vehicle Licensing Agency: At a glance guide to the current medical standards of fitness to drive. www.dvla.gov.uk p114

★39 NICE: Implantable cardioverter defibrillators (ICDs) for arrhythmias www.nice.org.uk p116

★46 NICE CG36: The management of atrial fibrillation www.nice.org.uk p124

★51 Cain M. *N Engl J Med* .2008. 358: 2725 p124

★53 Reynolds MW. *Chest*. 2004. 126:1938–45 p125

★58 Gage BF. *Circulation*. 2004. 110:2287–92. p125

★61 NICE Chronic Heart Failure Guidance www.nice.org.uk p128

★67 NICE: CG5 Chronic heart failure: full guideline www.nice.org.uk p128

★72 NICE: Chronic Heart Failure 2003; Guideline 5 www.nice.org.uk p130

★74 Lechat P. *Circulation*. 1998. 98:1184–91. p130

★77 Pitt B. *N Engl J Med*. 1999. 341:709–717. p130

★78 Packer M et al. for the RADIANCE Study. *N Engl J Med*. 1993. 329:1–7 p130

★88 Maisel A. *N Engl J Med*. 2002. 347: 161. p131

★89 Fuat A. *Brit J Gen Pract*. 2006. 56: 3272. p131

★90 Lemos J. *Lancet*. 2003. 362: 316. p131

★94 Beckett NS. *N Engl J Med*. 2008. 358:1887–98. p132

★95 Latest British Hypertension Society guidelines. www.bhsoc.org p133

★98 ALLHAT Officers and Coordinators for the ALLHAT Collaborative Research Group. *JAMA*. 2002. 288:2981–97. p134

Chapter 4 Chest medicine

★8 (p160) & ★12 (p161) British Thoracic Society Guidelines for the Management of Community Acquired Pneumonia in Adults 2001. *Thorax*. 2001. 56:(suppl IV)

★9 BTS Update on the management of community acquired pneumonia in adults 2004. www.brit-thoracic.org.uk p160

★11 An update of the BTS guidelines for the management of community acquired pneumonia in adults. www.brit-thoracic.org.uk p161

★13 BTS Draft guidance on pneumonia 2009 update www.brit-thoracic.org.uk p161

★30 NICE Guidance on The Diagnosis and Treatment of Lung Cancer www.nice.org.uk p170

★33 (p172) & ★37 (p174). 2008 British Guideline on the Management of Asthma. *Thorax*. 2008. 63 Suppl:iv1-121.

★43 Steiner M. Thorax. 2003 58:739. p176

★48 National clinical guideline on management of chronic obstructive pulmonary disease in adults in primary and secondary care. *Thorax*. 2004. 59 Suppl 1: i1-i232. **and** O'Driscoll. *Thorax*. 2008. 63: vi1-vi68. p181

★54 BTS Guidelines for the Management of Suspected Acute Pulmonary Embolism. Thorax. 2003. 48:470–484. p182

★55 BTS Guidelines for the Management of Spontaneous Pneumothorax. Thorax. 2003. 58 Suppl: ii39 -ii52. p182

★57 Iannuzzi MC. *N Engl J Med*. 2007. 357:2153–65 p186

★58 Interstitial lung disease guideline (BTS, TSANZ and ITS). *Thorax* 2008. 63: v1-v58 p188

★64 Management of Obstructive Sleep Apnoea/Hypnopnoea Syndrome in Adults. www.sign.ac.uk p194

★65 TA139 Sleep apnoea - CPAP: guidance www.nice.org.uk p194

Chapter 5 Endocrinology

★37 W Duckworth. *N Engl J Med*. 360: 129. p200

★40 Gutschall MD. *Public Health Nutr*. 2009. 12:1846–54. p200

★41 ADA and EASD consensus statement on management of hyperglycaemia in type 2 DM. Nathan DM. *Diabetes Care*. 2008. 31:173–5. p200

★43 & ★46. American Diabetes Association and the European Association for the study of diabetes. *Diabetes care*. 2006 29 1963–72 p200

★47 Singh. *Am J Ther*. 2008. 15: 506–11. p200

★48 Derosa G. *J Clin Pharm Ther*. 2009. 34:13–23. p200

★ 53 Westman EC. *Nutr Metab (Lond)*. 2008. 5:36. p201

★64 Belch J. *BMJ* 2008; 337:a1840 p202

★67 NICE 2008 recommendation: Chronic kidney disease. www.nice.org.uk p202

★99 Hypoglycemic Disorders: Endocrine Society Clinical Practice Guideline. *J Clin Endocrinol Metab*. 2008. 94:709-28. p207
★124 G Brent. *N Engl J Med*. 2008. 358: 2594 p211
★200 Consensus statement on hirsutism. Martin KA. *J Clin Endocrinol Metab*. 2008. 93:1105-20. p222
★217 Malkin C. *Eur Heart J*. 2006. 27: 57-64 p223

Chapter 6 Gastroenterology

★18 Anderson JW. *Nutr Rev*. 2009. 67:188-205. p237
★19 Lim CC. *Mol Nutr Food Res*. 2005. 49:609-19. p237
★38 Moayyedi P. *Cochrane Database Syst Rev*. 2005. (1):CD002096. p242
★43 Kahrilas PJ. *N Engl J Med*. 2008. 359:1700-7. p244
★50 Kuipers, E. *Lancet*. 2008. 371:1486 p247
★64 Cooper GS. *Gastrointest Endosc*. 2009. 70: 229-35. p252
★70 Gralnek IM. *N Engl J Med*. 2008. 359: 928-37. p253
★79 Villanueva C. *Drugs*. 2008. 68:2303-24 p254
★118 Giannini EG. *CMAJ*. 2005.172: 367-79. p265
★122 Giboney PT. *Am Fam Physician*. 2005. 71:1105-10. p265
★150 Mpofu C. *Cochrane Database Syst Rev*. 2004. (2):CD000279. p272
★162 Pearson DC. *Cochrane Database Syst Rev*. 2000 . (2):CD000067. p275
★178 NICE 2008. Irritable bowel syndrome in Adults. www.nice.org p277
★179 Brenner DM. *Am J Gastroenterol*. 2009. 104: 1033-49. p277

Chapter 7 Renal medicine

★3 Grossfeld GD. *Am Fam Physician*. 2001. 63:1145-54. p286
★5 Isbel NM. *Aust Fam Physician*. 2005. 34:907-13. p286
★6 McDonald MM. *Am Fam Physician*. 2006. 73: 1748-54. p286
★8 Carroll MF. *Am Fam Physician*. 2000. 62:1333-40. p286
★9 NICE clinical guideline 73. Chronic Kidney Disease. www.nice.org.uk p286
★18 Scottish Intercollegiate Guidelines Network. Management of suspected urinary tract infection in adults. A national clinical guideline. 2006. www.sign.ac.uk p293
★19 Hull RP. *BMJ*. 2008. 336: 1185-9. p294
★22 Isbel NM. *Aust Fam Physician*. 2005. 34: 898-992. p294
★46 Meyer TW. *N Engl J Med*. 2007. 357:1316-25. p304
★60 George JN. *N Engl J Med*. 2006. 354: 1927-35. p308
★66 Braun WE. *Cleve Clin J Med*. 2009. 76: 97-104. p312

Chapter 8 Haematology

★68 Guidelines for the management of the acute painful crisis in sickle cell disease. British Committee for Standards in Haematology, Sickle Cell Working Party. *Br J Haematol*. 2003. 120: 744-52. p335
★103 Ranmal R. *Cochrane Database Syst Rev*. 2008. (4):CD002969. p348
★109 Duffy MJ. *Clin Chem*. 54: 1770-9 p348
★123 Dighiero G. *Lancet*. 371: 1017-1029. p352

Chapter 9 Infectious diseases

★41 Glasmacher A. *Clin Microbiol Infect*. 2005. 11 Suppl 5:17-23. p379
★92 WHO malaria factsheet. www.who.int p394
★115 Guidelines For Malaria Prevention In Travelers From The United Kingdom. www.hpa.org.uk p396
★120 Clinical Guideline 33. Tuberculosis. 2006. www.nice.org.uk p398
★134 CDC Sexually Transmitted Diseases Treatment Guidelines. *MMWR*. 2006. 55(No. RR-11). p400
★140 Sampathkumar P. *Mayo Clin Proc*. 2009. 84: 274-80. p400
★165 Review of NICE technology appraisal, guidance 58. 2009. www.nice.org.uk p402
★213 Tobian AA. *N Engl J Med*. 2009. 360:1298-309. p408
★242 Best Practice Guidance HIV post-exposure prophylaxis: Guidance from the UK Chief Medical Officers' Expert Advisory Group on AIDS. 19 September 2008 www.dh.gov.uk p412
★253 Guidelines for the Use of Antiretroviral Agents in HIV-1-Infected Adults and Adolescents. November 3, 2008. aidsinfo.nih.gov p413
★262 Correll T. *Pharmacotherapy*. 2008. 28: 90-101. p414
★264 De Clercq E. *Verh K Acad Geneeskd Belg*. 2007. 69:81-104 p414
★325 Background document: The diagnosis, treatment and prevention of typhoid fever www.who.int p426
★326 E Mintz. *N Engl J Med*. 2009. 360: 1060. p426
★348 Giraudon I. *Euro Surveill*. 2009. 14:8-12. p431
★369 & 370. Q fever. www.cdc.gov p434
★399 & 400 Chappuis F. *Nat Rev Microbiol*. 2007. 5: 873-82. p439

Chapter 10 Neurology

★23 Dib et al. *Neurology*. 2002. 58: 1660-5. p462
★37 Bushnell et al. *BMJ*. 2009. 338:b664 p463
★56 Klein C. *J Inherit Metab Dis*. 2005. 28: 425-39. p472
★57 E Louis. *Lancet Neurol*. 2005. 4:100-110. p472
★58 Jankovic J. *J Neurol Neurosurg Psychiatry*. 1999. 67:646-50. p472
★61 Skidmore F. *Curr Treat Options Neurol*. 2005. 7: 231-236. p472

★85 Sandercock et al. *Cochrane Database Syst Rev*. 2008. (3): CD000029.pub2 p476
★86 Halkes et al. *Lancet*. 2006. 367: 1665–73. p476
★87 Bhatt et al. *N Engl J Med*. 2006. 354:1706–17. p476
★88 Sacco et al. *N Engl J Med*. 2008. 359: 1238–51. p476
★89 Brown & Humphrey (for Assoc British Neurologists). *BMJ*. 1992. 305: 1071–4. p476
★102 Rothwell PM, et al. *Lancet*. 2007. 370: 1432–42. p480
★104 Rothwell et al. *BMJ*. 1997. 315: 1571–7. p480
★152 Frank, RM. *Int J Geriatr Psychiatry*. 2000. 15: 317–24. p490
★153 Royall et al. *J Neurol Neurosurg Psychiatry*. 1998. 64: 588-594. p490
★167 McGuiness et al. *JNNP*. 2008. 79: 4–5. p492
★174 Birks J. *Cochrane Database Syst Rev*. 2006 (1): CD005593. p493
★182 The 1981 Classification of the International League Against Epilepsy p495
★183 Luders H, et al. *Epilepsia*. 1998. 39: 1006–13. p495
★194 Marson et al. *Lancet*. 2007. 369: 1000–1015. p496
★205 Wade D. *J Neurol Neurosurg Psychiatry*. 2003. 74:158–62. p498
★210 LeWitt PA. *Ann Neurol*. 2008. 63: 295–302. p499
★219 Brex et al. *N Engl J Med*. 2002. 346: 158–64. p500
★223 Polman et al. *N Engl J Med*. 2006. 354: 899–910. p500
★228 McDonald et al. *Ann Neurol*. 2001. 50: 121–7 p501
★253 Engström M, et al. *Lancet Neurol*. 2008. 7: 993–1000. p504
★254 Sullivan FM, et al. *N Engl J Med*. 2007. 357: 1598–607. p504
★283 B Halliwell. *Lancet*. 2000. 355: 1179–80. p511
★336 Freeman W. *Neural Netw*. 1997. 10:1175–1183 p521

Chapter 11 Oncology and palliative care

★2 Meyer TJ, Mark M. *J Health Psychol*. 1995. 14: 101–108. p523
★30 Verdecchia et al. *Lancet Oncol*. 2007. 8: 784–96 p531
★38 Remy C. *Br J Anaesth*. 2005. 94: 505–13. p534
★47 A Lindblom. *BMJ*. 2000. 320: 424–427. p538

Chapter 12 Rheumatology

★2 M Doherty et al. *Ann Rheum Dis*. 1992. 51: 1165–9. p542
★4 Speed C. *BMJ*. 2004. 328: 1119–21. p544
★12 Management of Septic Arthritis. *Drug Ther Bull*. 2003. 41: 65–68. p546
★17 Caldwell B, et al. *J R Soc Med*. 2006. 99: 132–40. p547
★21 The American Rheumatism Association 1987 revised criteria for the classification of rheumatoid arthritis. *Arthritis Rheum*. 1998. 31: 315–24. p548
★22 & ★23 O'Dell JR. Therapeutic strategies for rheumatoid arthritis. *N Engl J Med* 2004;350:2591–602 p549
★26 Brennan A, et al. *Rheumatology (Oxford)*. 2007. 46: 1345–54. p549
★38 Hoffman RW, Maldonado ME. *Clin Immunol*. 2008. 128: 8–17. p554
★40 & ★44 Rahman A. *N Engl J Med*. 2008. 358: 929–39. p556
★45 Tan EM et al. *Arthritis Rheum*. 1982. 25: 1271. p557
★46 1997 Update of 1982 American College of Rheumatology Revised Criteria for Classification of Systemic Lupus Erythematosus. www.rheumatology.org p557
★57 American College of Rheumatology 1990 Criteria for the Classifcation of Fibromyalgia. *Arthritis Rheum*. 1990. 3: 160–172 p560

Chapter 13 Surgery

★2 Practice guidelines for preoperative fasting and the use of pharmacologic agents to reduce the risk of pulmonary aspiration. American Society of Anesthesiologists. Task F. *Anesthesiology*. 1999. 901155–6. p568
★16 Guenaga KF et al. *Cochrane Database Syst Rev*. 2005. (1):CD001544. p572
★17 Bucher P et al. *Arch Surg*. 2004. 139: 1359–64; discussion 1365 p572
★27 Janssen MC et al. *Neth J Med*. 2005. 63: 81–90 p580
★57 ACC/AHA guideline update on perioperative cardiovascular evaluation for non-cardiac surgery. www.americanheart.org p590
★62 Wahbah AM et al. *Hepatogastroenterology*. 2000. 47: 1691–4. p592
★63 Parks RW et al. *Br J Surg*. 1994. 81: 437–9. p592
★83 Early Breast Cancer Trialists' Collaborative Group. *Lancet*. 2000. 355: 1757–70. p604
★84 Early Breast Cancer Trialists' Collaborative Group. *N Engl J Med*. 1995. 333: 1444–55. p604
★85 Early Breast Cancer Trialists' Collaborative Group. *Lancet*. 351: 1451–67. p604
★88 Veronesi U et al. *N Engl J Med*. 2003. 349: 546–53. p605
★101 Burger JW et al. *Ann Surg*. 2004. 240: 578–83; discussion 583–5. p614
★108 Flossman E, Rothwell PM, British Doctors Aspirin Trial and the UK-TIA Aspirin Trial. *Lancet*. 2007. 369: 1603–13. p618
★113 McLoughlin and Byrne. *World J Gastroenterol*. 2008. 14: 3798-3803. p618
★121 NHS Bowel Cancer Screening Programme, cancerscreening.org.uk p619

★128 For an exposition on the proposed development of cancer services in the UK see: The NHS Cancer Plan: www.dh.gov.uk p621
★148 Tice JA et al. *Am J Med*. 2008. 121: 885-93. p628
★178 Johansson M et al. *Br J Surg*. 2005. 92: 44-9. p637
★244 The UK Small Aneurysm Trial Participants. *Lancet*. 1998. 352: 1649-55. p656

Chapter 14 Epidemiology

There are no key references in Chapter 14.

Chapter 15 Clinical chemistry

★2 Modification of Diet in Renal Disease Study Group, Levey A et al. *Ann Intern Med*. 1999. 130: 461-70. p683
★29 Kanis JA, et al. *Osteoporos Int*. 2008. 19: 385-97. p696
★40 Ridker PM et al. *N Engl J Med*. 2008. 359: 2195-2207. p700
★48 JBS2 Joint British Societies guidelines on prevention of cardiovascular disease in clinical practice. *Heart*. 2005. 91(suppl): v1-52. p704

Chapter 16 Eponymous syndromes

There are no key references in Chapter 16.

Chapter 17 Radiology

There are no key references in Chapter 17.

Chapter 18 Reference intervals

★3 Ahmed A. *J Gerontol A Biol Sci Med Sci*. 2007. 62: 323-9. p766
★4 Nicolau et al. *J Antimicrob Chemother*. 1995. 39: 650-5. p766

Chapter 19 Practical procedures

There are no key references in Chapter 19.

Chapter 20 Emergencies

★5 Rivers et al. *N Engl J Med*. 2001. 345: 1368-1377. p804
★6 Dellinger RP et al. *Crit Care Med*. 2008. 36: 296-327. p804
★9 Resuscitation Council UK: Emergency treatment of anaphylactic reactions. www.resus.org.uk p806
★10 BNF 56 (September 2008), page 174 (adrenaline in anaphylaxis) p807
★12 ESC Guidelines for the management of acute myocardial infarction with ST-segment elevation. *Eur Heart J*. 2008. 29: 2909-2945. p808
★15 Guidelines for the diagnosis and treament of non-st segment elevation. *Eur Heart J*. 2007. 28: 1598-1660 p810
★16 Antman EM. *N Engl J Med*. 1996. 335: 1342-9. p810
★22 (p816) & ★23 (p818) Resuscitation Council (UK) Adult tachycardia algorithm. www.resus.org.uk
★25 (p820) & ★27 (p821) 2008 British Guideline on the Management of Asthma. British Thoracic Society Scottish Intercollegiate Guidelines Network. *Thorax*. 2008. 63 (Suppl): iv1-iv121
★28 Management of exacerbations of COPD Thorax. 2004. 59(Suppl): i131-i156. p822
★29 BTS Update on the management of community acquired pneumonia in adults 2004. www.brit-thoracic.org.uk p826
★30 BTS Guidelines for the Management of Suspected Acute Pulmonary Embolism, 2003. *Thorax*. 2003. 48: 470-484. p828
★33 BSG Non-variceal upper GI haemorrhage: guidelines. *Gut*. 2002. 51 (suppl): iv1-iv6 p830
★34 Scottish Intercollegiate Guidelines Network. Management of acute upper and lower gastrointestinal bleeding. A national clinical guideline. 2008. www.sign.ac.uk p830
★37 SIGN advice [Scottish intercollegiate guidelines network] p832
★39 Thompson MJ. Lancet. 2006. 367: 397-403 p832
★40 & ★41 Heyderman RS; British Infection Society. *J Infect*. 2005. 50: 373-4. p832

Useful doses for the new doctor

►These pages outline typical adult doses, and the commoner side-effects, of medications that a new house officer will be called upon to prescribe. If in any doubt, consult a drug fomulary (eg British National Fomulary, BNF, www.bnf.org).

Drug	Dose and frequency	Notes
Analgesics	(see p454 for more details on analgesia)	
Aspirin	300-900mg/4-6h PO, max. 4g/24h	SE of NSAIDs: gastritis; bronchospasm; hypersensitivity. CI: GI ulcer/bleeding; NSAID-induced asthma; coagulopathy. Avoid aspirin in children (risks Reye's syndrome).
Diclofenac	50mg/8h PO/PR	
Ibuprofen	400mg/6h PO, max. 2.4g/24h	
Paracetamol	0.5-1g/4-6h PO, max 4g/24h	Avoid if hepatic impairment.
Codeine phosphate	30-60mg/4h PO/IM max. 240mg/24h	Patients with chronic pain (eg malignancy) may require higher doses. SE of opioids: nausea and vomiting; constipation; drowsiness; hypotension; respiratory depression, dependence. CI: Acute respiratory depression, acute alcoholism. Use carefully in head injury, as may hinder neurological assessment.
Dihydrocodeine tartrate	30mg/4-6h PO, OR 50mg/4-6h IM/SC	
Meptazinol	200mg/3-6h PO, OR 50-100mg/2-4h IM/IV	
Oxycodone	5mg/6h PO	
Pethidine	50-100mg/4h PO/IM/SC	
Tramadol	50-100mg/4h PO/IM/IV	
Morphine	5-10mg/4h PO/IM/SC	
Antibiotics	(see p366-374)	
Antiemetics		
Cyclizine	50mg/8h PO/IM/IV	
Metaclopramide	10mg/8h PO/IM/IV	May cause extrapyramidal SE, especially in young adults.
Ondansetron	8mg/8h PO, or 4mg IM/IV	
Antihistamines		
Chlorphenamine	10-20mg IM/IV, maximum 40mg/24h OR 4mg/6h PO	SE of antihistamines: Drowsiness; urinary retention; dry mouth; blurred vision; GI disturbance; arrhythmias. Drowsiness is less commoner with newer drugs, eg cetirizine, fexofenadine.
Cetirizine	5-10mg/24h PO	
Levocetirizine	5mg/24h PO	
Fexofenadine	120-180mg/24h PO	
Loratadine	10mg/24h PO	
Desloratadine	5mg/24h PO	
Gastric acid reducing drugs		
Cimetidine	400mg/6-12h PO	SE of H_2-blockers: GI disturbance; ↑LFT.
Ranitidine	150mg/12h PO	
Omeprazole	20-40mg/24h PO	SE of PPIs: GI disturbance; hypersensitivity. ►Acid-reducing drugs may mask symptoms of gastric cancer; use with care in middle-aged patients.
Esomperazole	20-40mg/24h PO	
Lansoprazole	15-30mg/24h PO	
Pantoprazole	20-40mg/24h PO	

Drug	Dose and frequency	Notes
Heparins	(see p334 for more details on anticoagulation)	
Unfractionated heparin	DVT prophylaxis: 5000u/12h sc	SE of heparins: bleeding; thrombocytopenia; hypersensitivity; hyperkalaemia; osteoporosis after prolonged use. CI: coagulopathy; peptic ulcer; recent cerebral bleed; recent trauma or surgery; active bleeding.
Enoxaparin	DVT prophylaxis: 20–40mg/24h SC. DVT/PE treatment: 1.5mg/kg/24h SC until warfarinized. Unstable angina: 1mg/kg/12h sc for 2–8d	
Tinzaparin	*DVT prophylaxis:* 3500U/24h SC (eg starting 2h pre-op). *DVT/PE treatment:* 175U/kg per 24h SC till warfarinized.	
Dalteparin	*DVT prophylaxis:* 2500–5000U/24h SC. *DVT/PE treatment:* 200U/kg/d SC (18,000U/24h maximum). *Unstable angina:* 120U/kg/12h SC (up to 10,000U/12h maximum) for 5–8d.	
Hypnotics		
Temazepam	10–20mg PO at night	SE: Drowsiness; dependence. Zopicolone also causes bitter taste and GI disturbances. CI: Respiratory depression; myasthenia.
Zopiclone	3.75–7.5mg PO at night	
Tranquilizers		
Haloperidol	2–5mg IM/IV initially, then every 4–8h till response, maximum 18mg in total.	SE: Extrapyramidal effects, sedation, hypotension, antimuscarinic effects, neuro-leptic malignant syndrome.
Others		
Naloxone	*In opiate overdose:* 0.8–2mg IV repeated every 2–3min to a maximum of 10mg if respiratory function does not improve. *To reverse opiate-induced respiratory depression:* 100–200µg IV every 2min.	SE: tachycardia; fibrillation. Can precipitate opiate withdrawl.
Flumazenil	*To reverse benzodiazepines:* 200µg IV over 15s, then 100µg every 60s if required, up to 1mg maximum.	SE: convulsions (esp. in epileptics); nausea and vomiting; flushing. Avoid if patient has a life-threatening illness controlled by benzodiazepines (eg status epilepticus).

See also: laxatives (p248), inhalers (p175), digoxin (p116) insulin sliding scales (p591), fluids (p680), oxygen prescribing (p181).

▸▸Cardiorespiratory arrest

Ensure safety of patient and yourself. Confirm diagnosis (unconscious, apnoeic, absent carotid pulse).

Causes MI; PE; trauma; tension pneumothorax, electrocution; shock; hypoxia; hypercapnia; hypothermia; U&E imbalance; drugs, eg digoxin.

Basic life support Shout for help. Ask someone to call the arrest team and bring the defibrillator. Note the time. Begin CPR as follows (**ABC**):

Airway: Head tilt (if no spine injury) + chin lift/jaw thrust. Clear the mouth.

Breathing: Check breathing then give 2 breaths after 1st set of compressions, each inflation ~1s long. Use specialized bag and mask system (eg Ambu® system) if available and 2 resuscitators present. Otherwise, mouth-to-mouth breathing.

Chest compressions: Give 30 compressions to 2 breaths (30 : 2). CPR should not be interrupted except to give shocks or to intubate. Use the heel of hand with straight elbows. Centre over the lower ⅓ of the sternum; aim for 4cm compression at 100/min.

Advanced life support For algorithm and details, see over. Notes:
Place defibrillator paddles on chest as soon as possible and set monitor to read through the paddles if delay in attaching leads. Assess rhythm: is this VF/pulseless VT? The following assumes monophasic defibrillator.

- In **VF/VT**, defibrillation must occur without delay: 360J (150-360J biphasic).
- **Asystole and electromechanical dissociation** (synonymous with pulseless electrical activity) are rhythms with a poorer prognosis than VF/VT, but potentially remediable (see box next page). Treatment may be life-saving.
- Obtain IV access and intubation if possible.
- Look for reversible causes of cardiac arrest, and treat accordingly.
- Check for pulse if ECG rhythm compatible with a cardiac output.
- **Reassess ECG rhythm.** Repeat defibrillation if still VF/VT. All shocks are 360J.
- Send someone to find the patient's notes and the patient's usual doctor. These may give clues as to the cause of the arrest.
- If IV access fails, adrenaline, atropine, and lidocaine may be given down the tracheal tube but absorption is unpredictable. Give 2-3 times the IV dose diluted in ≥10mL 0.9% saline followed by 5 ventilations to assist absorption. Intracardiac injection is not recommended.

When to stop resuscitation No general rule, as survival is influenced by the rhythm and the cause of the arrest. In patients without myocardial disease, do not stop until core temperature is >33°C and pH and potassium are normal. Consider stopping resuscitation after 20min if there is refractory asystole or electromechanical dissociation.

After successful resuscitation:

- 12-lead ECG; CXR, U&ES, glucose, blood gases, FBC, CK/troponin.
- Transfer to coronary care unit/ITU.
- Monitor vital signs.
- Whatever the outcome, explain to relatives what has happened.

When '*do not resuscitate*' may be a valid decision (UK DoH guidelines)

- If a patient's condition is such that resuscitation is unlikely to succeed.
- If a mentally competent patient has consistently stated or recorded the fact that he or she does not want to be resuscitated.
- If the patient has signed an advanced directive forbidding resuscitation.
- If resuscitation is not in a patient's interest as it would lead to a poor quality of life (often a great imponderable!). ►*Ideally, involve patients and relatives in the decision **before** the emergency.* When in doubt, resuscitate.

UK Adult Basic Life-Support Algorithm 2005[1]

The algorithm assumes that only one rescuer is present, with no equipment. (If a defibrillator is to hand, get a rhythm readout, and defibrillate, as opposite, as soon as possible.)

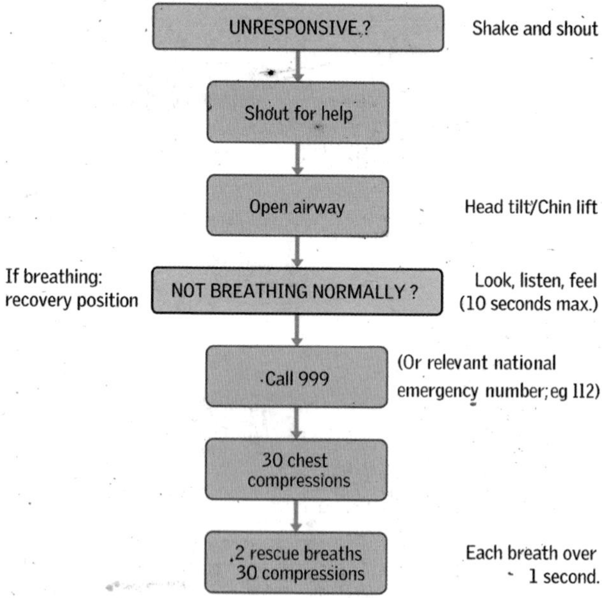
UNRESPONSIVE ?
Shake and shout
Shout for help
Open airway
Head tilt/Chin lift
If breathing:
recovery position
NOT BREATHING NORMALLY ?
Look, listen, feel
(10 seconds max.)
Call 999
(Or relevant national emergency number; eg 112)
30 chest compressions
2 rescue breaths
30 compressions
Each breath over 1 second.

Send or go for help as soon as possible, according to guidelines

Managing the airway

You open the airway by tilting the head and lifting the chin—but only do this if there is no question of spinal trauma.

Use a close-fitting mask if available, held in place by thumbs pressing downwards either side of the mouth-piece, palms against cheeks.

Chest compressions

Cardiopulmonary resuscitation (CPR) involves compressive force over the lower sternum, with the heels of the hands placed one on top of the other, directing the weight of your body through your vertical, straight, arms.

Depth of compression: 4cm.

Rate of compressions: 100/min.

Remember that these are guidelines only, and that the exact circumstances of the cardiorespiratory arrest will partly determine best practice. The guidelines are also more consensus-based than evidence based (p644), and are likely to be adapted from time to time, for example, as consensus develops about the best recovery position—eg semi-lateral position, with under-most arm either straight at the side, in dorsal position, or in the ventral position cradling the head with the upper-most arm crossing it (more stable, but possible risk to arm blood flow).[2]

1 Keep abreast of new guidelines (due 2010); see www.resus.org.uk/pages.blsalgo.pdf 2 A Handley 1993 *Resuscitation* **26** 93–95